Research Administration and Management

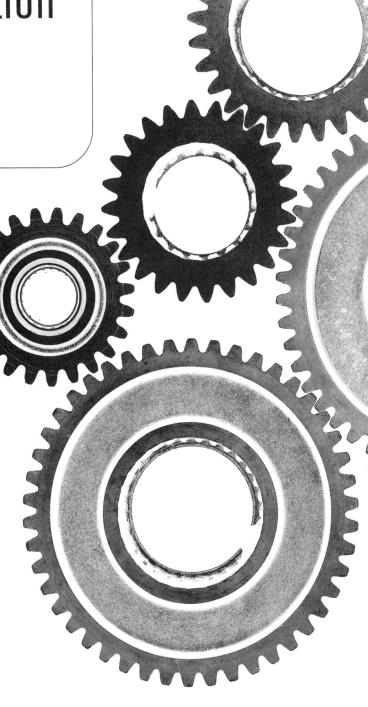

Elliott C. Kulakowski, PhD, FAHA

Director, Office of Sponsored Projects and
Adjunct Professor of Pharmacology and Toxicology
University of Utah

Lynne U. Chronister, MPA

Associate Vice Chancellor for Research Administration
University of California, Davis

JONES AND BARTLETT PUBLISHERS

Sudbury, Massachusetts

BOSTON   TORONTO   LONDON   SINGAPORE

World Headquarters
Jones and Bartlett Publishers
40 Tall Pine Drive
Sudbury, MA 01776
978-443-5000
info@jbpub.com
www.jbpub.com

Jones and Bartlett Publishers Canada
6339 Ormindale Way
Mississauga, Ontario L5V 1J2
CANADA

Jones and Bartlett Publishers International
Barb House, Barb Mews
London W6 7PA
UK

Jones and Bartlett's books and products are available through most bookstores and online booksellers. To contact Jones and Bartlett Publishers directly, call 800-832-0034, fax 978-443-8000, or visit our website, www.jbpub.com.

Substantial discounts on bulk quantities of Jones and Bartlett's publications are available to corporations, professional associations, and other qualified organizations. For details and specific discount information, contact the special sales department at Jones and Bartlett via the above contact information or send an email to specialsales@jbpub.com.

ISBN: 978-1-4496-3440-7

Library of Congress Cataloging-in-Publication Data
Research administration and management / [edited by] Elliott C. Kulakowski and Lynne U. Chronister.
    p. ; cm.
  Includes bibliographical references.
  ISBN 0-7637-3277-X (casebound)
  1. Research—United States—Management. 2. Science and state—United States. 3. Technology and state—United States.
  [DNLM: 1. Research—organization & administration—United States. 2. Guideline Adherence—organization & administration—United States. 3. Technology Transfer—United States. Q 180.A1 R432 2006] I. Kulakowski, Elliott C. II. Chronister, Lynne U. III. Research Enterprise.
  Q180.U5R3816 2006
  001.4′068—dc22
                                        2005012147
6048

Production Credits
Acquisitions Editor: Kevin Sullivan
Production Director: Amy Rose
Associate Editor: Amy Sibley
Production Assistant: Alison Meier
Marketing Manager: Emily Ekle
Manufacturing Buyer: Amy Bacus
Composition: Auburn Associates, Inc.
Cover Design: Kristin E. Ohlin
Cover Image: ©Ablestock
Printing and Binding: Malloy, Inc.
Cover Printing: Malloy, Inc.

Printed in the United States of America
15 14 13 12 11   10 9 8 7 6 5 4 3 2

Contents

Part III   Pre-Award Administration

Part IV   Post-Award and Financial Requirements

Part V   Responsible Conduct of Research

Chapter 60   **How to Organize a Technology Transfer Office   641**
Patricia Harsche Weeks, MS

Chapter 61   **Elements of an Intellectual Property Policy   653**
Elliott C. Kulakowski, PhD, FAHA

Chapter 62   **Industrial Research Collaborations before a Product Is Developed   663**
Colin Cooper

Chapter 63   **Identifying and Triaging Technologies   693**
Joseph Fondacaro, PhD

Contributors

Melissa S. Anderson, PhD
Associate Professor of Higher Education
University of Minnesota

Rebecca Barnett
Summer Intern
Slocum & Boddie, P.C.

Concetta Bartosh, JD
Consultant

Kathryn A. Bayne, MS, PhD, DVM
Associate Director
Association for Assessment and Accreditation of
   Laboratory Animal Care International

Kenneth L. Beasley, MAT, PhD, CRA
Retired Research Administrator

Bryan Benham, PhD
Assistant Professor of Philosophy
University of Utah

Vincent Bogdanski, MBA
Senior Research Administrator
Colorado State University

Jeffrey R. Botkin, MD, MPH
Associate Vice President
Research Integrity Professor, Pediatrics and
   Medical Ethics
University of Utah

Howard W. Bremer, JD
Consultant and Emeritus Patent Counsel
Wisconsin Alumni Research Foundation

Joe R. Brown, MHS
Research Privacy Specialist
University of Kentucky

Jayne Carney, MS, PhD, MBA
Consultant to Technology Commercialization Office
University of Utah

William H. Caskey, MS, PhD
Director, Research and Grants Administration
The Children's Mercy Hospital

John S. Child Jr., JD, B.Litt.
Patent and Trademark Attorney
Dann, Dorfman, Herrell and Skillman, P.C.

John Chinn, MBA
Compliance Director
Carnegie Mellon University

Katherine Chou, MS, MBA
Director, Office of Technology Transfer
Thomas Jefferson University

Lynne U. Chronister, MPA
Associate Vice Chancellor for Research
   Administration
University of California, Davis

Dale Clark
Graduate Assistant
University of Utah

Cheryl Coffin, MD
Department of Pathology
Primary Children's Medical Center

Colin Cooper
Assistant Director of Research
University of Liverpool

Gail De Vun
Special Projects Manager
Division of Public Health Sciences
Fred Hutchinson Cancer Research Center

Michael R. Dingerson, PhD
Retired Professor, Department of Education
   Leadership and Counseling
Higher Education Program
Old Dominion University

Matthew D. Finucane, MS, CIH

Director, Environmental Health and Radiation
Safety
University of Pennsylvania

Jerry Fife

Assistant Vice Chancellor for Research Finance
Vanderbilt University

Joseph Fondacaro, PhD

Director, Intellectual Property and Venture
Development and
Research Professor of Pediatrics
Cincinnati Children's Hospital Medical Center

Leslie P. Francis, PhD, JD

Dean, College of Humanities and Professor of Law
University of Utah

Edward F. Gabriele, MDiv, DMin

Director, Office of Research Integrity
MedStar Research Institute

Jo Anne Goodnight

SBIR/STTR Program Coordinator
National Institutes of Health

Jim Hanlon

Manager Human Resources & Administration
TRIUMF, Vancouver BC

John E. Harkness, DVM, MS, MEd

Retired University Laboratory Animal Veterinarian
College of Veterinary Medicine

Patricia Harsche Weeks, MS

Vice President, Planning and Business Development
Fox Chase Cancer Center

Steve Highlander, PhD, JD

Partner
Fulbright and Jaworski, LLP

Janet M. Holdsworth

Midwest Higher Education Compact

David Huizenga, JD, PhD

Intellectual Property Attorney
Needle and Rosenburg, PC

Ellen Hyman-Browne, JD, LLM, MPH

Director of Research Compliance
New York University School of Medicine

Michael Kalichman, PhD

Adjunct Professor of Pathology and Director of the
UCSD Research Ethics Program
University of California, San Diego

Karen S. Karp, MS, DEd

Professor, Mathematic Education
University of Louisville

Rosemarie Keenan

Administrative Manager, Division of Public
Health Sciences
Fred Hutchinson Cancer Research Center

Cindy Kiel, JD, CRA

Director of Sponsored Projects
University of Nevada, Reno

Robert Killoren, MA, CRA

Associate Vice President for Research
The Pennsylvania State University

William S. Kirby, MA

Independent Consultant

Richard Kordal, PhD

Director, Intellectual Property Office and
University Patent Office
University of Cincinnati

Greg Koski, PhD, MD, CPI, DSc (Honorary)

Associate Professor of Anesthesia, Harvard
Medical School
Senior Scientist, Institute for Health Policy
Massachusetts General Hospital

Elliott C. Kulakowski, PhD, FAHA

Director, Office of Sponsored Projects and Adjunct
Professor of Pharmacology and Toxicology
University of Utah

Helene Lake-Bullock, PhD, JD

Research Compliance Officer
University of Kentucky

Marcia Landen, MS

Executive Director, Sponsored Research Services
Indiana University Bloomington

Lisa A. Lapin

Assistant Vice Chancellor of Media Relations
University of California, Davis

Robert S. MacWright, PhD

Executive Director and CEO, Patent Foundation
University of Virginia

Michael McCallister, PhD

Director of Research and Sponsored Programs
University of Arkansas Little Rock

Judy McCormick

Associate Director for Contracts, College of
    Agricultural Sciences
The Pennsylvania State University

David R. McGee, PhD

Director of Technology Transfer
University of California, Davis

Christopher McKinney, MBA, DA

Director, Office of Technology Transfer and Enter-
    prise Development, and Lecturer, Department of
    Electrical Engineering and Computer Science
Vanderbilt University

Pamela F. Miller, PhD

Director of the Office of Sponsored Projects
University of San Francisco

Geraldine P. Mineau, PhD

Research Professor, Huntsman Cancer Institute
University of Utah

Victoria J. Molfese, PhD

Ashland/Nystrand Chair in Early Childhood
    Development and Professor
University of Louisville

Mark A. Munger, Pharm D

Professor, Pharmacotherapy
University of Utah

Paul Nacon

Director
Maximus Higher Education Practice

Roberta A. Nixon

Director of Internships and Corporate Outreach
Department of Biomedical Engineering
University of Virginia

Sandra Nordahl, CRA

Manager, Sponsored Research Administration
San Diego State University

Michael Owen, PhD

Associate Vice-President Research
Brock University

Chris B. Pascal, JD

Director, Office of Research Integrity
Department of Health and Human Services

Tim Quigg, PhD

Associate Chairman, Computer of Administration
    and Finance
University of North Carolina Chapel Hill

Fred Reinhart, MBA

Assistant Vice President for Research and
    Technology Commercialization
Wayne State University

Kathleen D. Rigaut, PhD, JD

Partner
Dann, Dorfman, Herrell and Skillman

Lawrie Robertson

Division Administrator, Division of Public Health
    Sciences
Fred Hutchinson Cancer Research Center

John A. Rodman, MBA

President and CEO
Research and Management System, Inc.

Janet E. Scholz

Senior Licensing Manager
The University of Manitoba

William Schweri, MS

Director, Federal Relations
University of Kentucky

Ada Sue Selwitz, MA

Director, Office of Research Integrity
University of Kentucky

Patrick A. Shea, JD, PC

Private Detective

Rick Shindell

President
Zyn Systems

Joseph B. Shultz, PhD

Administrative Fellow
University of Minnesota

Amy J. Sikalis, MPA

Administrative Director, Office of Research, and
The Institute for Health Delivery Research
Intermountain Health Care

Bev Silver

Administrative Manager
Division of Public Health Sciences
Fred Hutchinson Cancer Research Center

John D. Sites Jr., CRA

Senior Contract Administrator
Utah State University

J. Michael Slocum, JD

President
Slocum and Boddie, P.C.

Hope Slonim, JD

Senior Staff Attorney
United States Patent and Trademark Office

Brad Stanford

Project Manager
Office of Naval Research

Bruce Steinert, PhD

Research and Grants Administrator
Children's Mercy Hospital

Kathleen Sybert, PhD, JD

Chief, Technology Transfer Branch
National Cancer Institute

James Taylor, JD

Grants and Contracts Officer
University of Utah

Cary E. Thomas MBA, CMA

Senior Associate Dean, Finance and Administration
Keck School of Medicine
University of Southern California

Louis G. Tornatzky, PhD

Vice President for Business Planning and
    Development
Select University Technologies, Inc.

Daniel Vasgird, PhD, CIP

Director, Office of Research Integrity and
    Compliance
University of Nebraska, Lincoln

Paul G. Waugaman, MPA, MA

Principal
Technology Commercialization Group LLC

Dorothy Yates

Interim Assistant Vice Chancellor
University of Colorado, Denver and Health
    Science Center

Abby Zubov

Director, Audit Services
University of California San Francisco

Preface

This book on the leadership and management of the research enterprise was written for any individual who is involved in the leadership, development, management, or support of research. This text is designed for all of us who are students throughout our lives and look for creativity in problem solving and lifelong experiences. Individuals who are senior research administrators, well-versed in the intricacies of leading a complicated and sometimes immense research program will hopefully find some creative solutions to challenges faced by their peers. For those less senior research administrators, we hope that this is a reference text that will enable them to grow in the profession and continue to be the cornerstone of the infrastructure for forging a strong research program.

Each year, hundreds of men and women enter the profession of research administration. Many of them do not even realize that they are joining a profession! This book will give them the direction, information, and motivation to learn and develop the skills to become the next generation of leaders in administration of research. For the thousands of scientists, scholars, and leaders who rely on the research administrator, this text will provide a resource for them. Furthermore, the glossary and list of acronyms located in Appendix A and Appendix B will help establish a common language.

This book is the second comprehensive text ever written about the management of the research enterprise. The first text, authored by Kenneth L. Beasley, Michael R. Dingerson, Oliver D. Hensley, Larry G. Hess, and John A. Rodman, was published in 1982. Ken Beasley, Mike Dingerson, and John Rodman are contributing authors of this text and have fostered the advancement of the profession into the 21st Century. The profession, the responsibilities, and depth of required knowledge has grown exponentially since the publication of the first definitive text. This book was written in the hope that the profession will continue to grow and prosper, and that we can continue to contribute to the growth of knowledge and the quality of life globally.

Those of us for whom research administration is a career hope that in the very near future students will enter undergraduate or graduate school planning a career in research administration. Cleveland State University is developing graduate programs in the field of research administration. We hope that the cycle has begun and that this text can provide the foundation for an advanced certification or a degree program in research administration at many institutions across the country.

Acknowledgments

Few books that are ever written are the result of a single author's knowledge. This book is no exception. It represents the collective thoughts of hundreds of individuals from higher education, government, and the private sector. Over eighty-five individuals, most of whom label themselves as research administrators, contributed their knowledge and experience through the text that they provided. This sharing, this collaborative spirit, is one of the keystones of the profession of research administration. It is a core value to share information and to support others who have chosen research administration as their vocation and the multitude of constituents with whom we collaborate and lead. We thank the many authors who are the heart of this book.

The publisher, Jones and Bartlett, and the editors and staff have been patient and encouraging and always willing to hold the hand of two neophyte authors. We are grateful.

Thanks must be given to three professional associations who have, for almost forty years, been the motivating and codifying force behind the development of research administration as a profession. Both of us have been presidents of the Society of Research Administrators International and members of the National Council of University Research Administrators, and we represented our institutions at the Council on Government Relations. Without these three organizations guiding and supporting us over many years, this book could not exist. We received from them more than we gave.

A special and heartfelt thanks must go to those who supported us on a daily basis, the research administrators at the University of Utah and the University of California, Davis. Many people both contributed to the text and encouraged us even during hectic weeks and months.

Two people actually had to put up with us days, nights, and weekends: Roxanne Kulakowski and Robert Adams. Thank you both for your enduring love, support, and encouragement.

Elliott C. Kulakowski and
Lynne U. Chronister

Introduction to the Administration of the Research Enterprise

CHAPTER

1

Introduction: Leadership and Management of the Research Enterprise in the 21st Century

Lynne U. Chronister, MPA, and Elliott C. Kulakowski, PhD, FAHA

According to a US Census Bureau report, as of October 3, 2004 there were 6,391,856,082 people living across the globe—294,430,115 living in the United States alone.[1] In many ways, the research carried out in universities, in industry, in government laboratories, and in independent research organizations touches the lives of almost every one of the world's billions of people. The definition of *research*, according to Webster's dictionary, is of French origin and means *to investigate thoroughly* and the *investigation and experimentation aimed at the discovery and interpretation of facts, revision of accepted theories or laws in the light of new facts or practical application of such new or revised theories or laws*.[2]

The investment in the research enterprise is enormous. In 1999, the collective R&D expenditure of the major industrialized "group of seven" countries (Canada, France, Germany, Italy, Japan, United Kingdom, and United States) was $461 billion.[3] The National Science Foundation further reported that in 2000 $265 billion was spent on R&D in the United States with private industry supporting over 68% or $181 billion of overall funding.[4] Within the Federal Fiscal Year 2005 budget, a record-breaking $132.2 billion was slated for federally funded R&D.[5]

While we can quantify funding, the magnitude of the impact of research is immeasurable. Research is a major driving force behind the fact that, in little more than a century, many societies have and are advancing from primarily agrarian to highly technologically sophisticated societies.

Research has both a direct and indirect impact on society. Medical research has directly led to cures for diseases and reductions in morbidity and mortality. The indirect impact is less tangible with medical advances having economic impact, such as workers losing fewer days from work because of illness. Research in agri-genetics has led to disease and drought resistant crops that have increased crop yields, allowing developing countries to feed their own populations and allowing more people to move into technological positions, thus raising the economies of these countries. Telecommunication and information technology industries also are a direct result of research advances. The resulting impact is greater internationalization of education, commerce, and economic development. This transformation of need and ideas to public benefit and knowledge represents the power of research.

While research and development are critical to the advancement of understanding of our universe and the quality of our lives, the administration of the research enterprise is essential for channeling research into areas of greatest benefit to society. As our dependency on research and development has expanded, the need for competent leaders and managers of the enterprise has grown concomitantly. Most institutions have centralized the leadership and management of research in a central office of research led by a chief research officer, vice president or vice chancellor for research. In addition, research institutions including academic institutions, nonprofit research institutes, federal laboratories, and industries have developed an entire network of individuals devoted wholly or in part to supporting and promoting the research function.

For purposes of this book, the term *research* will be used interchangeably with *sponsored programs* or *projects* to reflect a broader range of creative processes seen in academia. These disciplines include scientific and technical disciplines, social and behavioral sciences, and the arts and humanities.

The research enterprise at institutions grows in response to both strong leadership and steady management, each of which has a multitude of overlapping functions. Leadership involves setting a vision. Whether at the central or unit level, no research institution or program will reach its highest level of achievement without a commonality of vision and shared goals. National, regional, and local policy-setting is a critical component of a strong research program as is involvement in the economic growth and health of the nation and region. The research leader fosters innovation and a culture and environment that allow the research and researcher to flourish. Concomitantly, the leadership must instill the highest level of integrity in the conduct of research. It can be a delicate balance that can be achieved with a solid infrastructure guided by strategic planning and metrics for achievement.

Management of the enterprise involves the implementation of the vision that is set collectively by institutional leaders and the scientists and scholars who create and innovate. Managers include the individuals at the central and departmental level who handle the process of project or proposal development, submission, and oversight of the business end of research and scholarship. The research manager implements regulatory and fiscal policy set by government, sponsors, and institutions. The breadth of responsibility includes, but is certainly not limited to, dissemination of funding information, communication of policy and processes, proposal preparation, award negotiation and management, financial management, regulatory research compliance oversight and implementation, facilities management, and intellectual property protection and technology transfer.

Innovation in Research Administration

In his book, *How Breakthroughs Happen*, Andrew Hargadon discusses the nature of innovation.[6] He describes innovation, in part, as the "recombination of old people, objects, and ideas in new ways." One such example cited by Hargadon is Thomas Edison's success at his Menlo Park laboratory, where Edison's laboratory spawned dozens of inventions

and he and his colleagues were as much *technology brokers* as they were inventors. Hargadon writes that technology brokering is a "strategy for exploiting the networked nature of the innovation process. . . involves combining existing objects, ideas. . . and people in ways that, nevertheless, spark technological revolutions." In much the same way, research administrators are the brokers of innovation. One role that the research administrator assumes is as facilitator of the translation of innovation into a benefit to the public. In part, this is accomplished through devising a solid management and administrative process that allow scientists and scholars to devote their energy to the creative process. However, the administration of research involves devising pathways to enhance building technological and scholastic revolutions into creative solutions and cultural insights.

The vast expansion of our capacity to do research has fostered this relatively new profession of research administration. Research administration has evolved to become a synergistic, highly complex, sometimes highly bureaucratic and legalistic profession that requires a breadth of knowledge and skill unequaled in most business and management professions. Research administrators have a multitude of titles with the common goal to support and to provide leadership for research and development. With some large not-for-profit research institutions, including universities, expending about one billion dollars on research and development, the management of the institution's enterprise parallels the breadth and responsibility for leading a large corporation.[7] The individuals involved in the administration of the enterprise must be well-trained, engaged, and knowledgeable. This book is designed to enhance the knowledge and skills of those engaged in the administration of research as leaders and managers and the scientists and scholars who are the creative energy behind innovation.

This book has been organized to reflect the major categories of information and knowledge that encompass the administration of the research enterprise. The content of the book will assist the administrator from small, developing research programs to large, multifaceted and complex research organizations. The chief research officer (CRO) or vice president or vice chancellor for research and the newly initiated research administrator will find information useful to developing professionally and gaining the knowledge, skills, and abilities to grow a research program. The profession is somewhat defined by the environment since institutions do not necessarily assign responsibilities uniformly. Not all research offices will have responsibility for every facet of research administration discussed in the text. However, the major cradle-to-grave responsibilities are represented. The book is organized by major functionalities: infrastructure, pre-award activities, post-award activities, technology transfer, and research compliance.

This is the first book on research administration and management in nearly a quarter of a century. The scope and depth of knowledge needed by research managers at all levels have grown dramatically over this period of time with new fields of research and increased fiscal and regulatory compliance requirements directed to manage the changing research enterprise. While the book focuses primarily on the administration and management of research in the United States, it is no way intended to be the definitive guide for how research should be managed throughout the world. However, the general concepts presented in the book have universal application, and international colleagues have contributed to the writing of the book.

Organization and Content of the Text

Part I: *Introduction to the Administration of the Research Enterprise*   In Chapter 2, the history and fundamental structures, responsibilities and roles of research administration are detailed. Kenneth Beasley describes the history of the growth of the research enterprise and the development of the need for a system, as well as policy and procedure for managing the enterprise. In Chapter 4, Robert Killoren and Lynne Chronister provide a framework for understanding the structure and function of research administration units or programs. Michael Dingerson follows with a treatise on what a vice president or vice chancellor for research needs to know and understand in order to lead the enterprise.

Part II: *The Infrastructure for Research Administration*   This section describes many of the services, programs, and auxiliary units necessary to create and maintain a vibrant and supportive unit that has the capacity to facilitate critical research and scholarship. With the expansion of the breadth of research programs, ever-increasing responsibilities have fallen under the purview of a research administration unit, and many of these are described in Part II. Development, training, and support systems for administrators of research are outlined by Michael McCallister and Marcia Landen. Some of these infrastructure functions include the management of change written by Lawrie Robertson and associates. In an ever-changing environment, this is a critical

component of management. Lynne Chronister and Lisa Lapin discuss the area of public relations, marketing, and communication in an environment that is designed to foster client service.

As an outgrowth of client service, the foundation of research productivity continues to locate and disseminate information on funding opportunities and sources of support including internal grant programs. Lynne Chronister discusses some modes of support for interdisciplinary and institutional research. William Schweri discusses the promotion of research through the lobbying and advocacy processes. Jim Hanlon outlines human resource issues in the research environment and Cary Thomas discusses working with boards of advisors and trustees. Paul Waugaman, William Kirby, and Louis Tornatzky provide information on benchmarking research productivity and administrative support and the development of the entrepreneurial culture.

Bruce Steinert and Elliott Kulakowski discuss the critical components of developing a clinical trials office, and J. Michael Slocum discusses the legal issues involved in clinical trials. One area that requires particular attention is use of human body parts in research and developing a tracking and processes unit. Lynne Chronister and David McGee have provided a description of this central research function. With expanding research endeavors, especially those involving human subjects, greater risk is engendered by the institution. J. Michael Slocum outlines the process of working with counsel and the management of risk.

Part III: *Pre-Award Administration*   The most basic and, probably, the first unit developed as an institution begins to seek and accept external funding is a sponsored programs unit. A pre-award sponsored programs function generally refers to the activities that take place prior to accepting an award. Pre-award administration emphasizes the proposal development and submission process and the award acceptance and negotiation phase. This section outlines some of the basic knowledge needed to understand the pre-award function and provides details of some of the technical considerations that must be addressed by a pre-award office. Part III begins with a discussion by Dorothy Yates on the fundamentals of sponsored programs offices. These offices are generally responsible for facilitation of the proposal development and submission and award acceptance and negotiation. William Caskey has provided a section on the basics of budgeting for research. Tim Quigg has outlined the role of the research administrator at the departmental level.

The growth of research has spawned the need for well-trained managers within colleges, departments and large research programs. Victoria Molfese and Pamela Miller provide insight into developing successful proposals, and Pamela Miller discusses understanding the review process.

John Rodman and Brad Stanford describe some of the principles and processes involved with the advent of large-scale computing and electronic business processes, Electronic Research Administration (ERA) as a primary business process. Cindy Kiel and J. Michael Slocum provide much of the background for the legal issues involved in sponsored projects administration including clinical trial administration, federal contracting, contract negations, and working with industry. Sandra Nordahl and J. Michael Slocum discuss the terms and conditions common to grant or contract documents. Since research is rapidly becoming a global process, John Sites discusses the issue of international collaborations.

Part IV: *Post-Award and Financial Requirements* This section delineates the post-award and financial requirement of acceptance of external funding. The post-award process is carried out both centrally and at the unit and program level and includes the management of the budget and expenditures, cost sharing among sponsors, reporting of effort on projects. Jerry Fife describes the post-award processes and various responsibilities generally assigned to individuals knowledgeable with accounting and financial management. Much of the post-award financial activity is driven by federal circulars, as discussed by Sandra Nordahl in Part III and compliance standards, which are described by Amy Sikalis. Paul Nacon lays the foundation for budgeting and finance by detailing the development and negotiation of facilities and administrative rates also defined as overhead or indirect cost. Cary Thomas has provided text on financial reporting by institutions. Even with the most rigorous post-award process, the grant or contract may be audited. Abby Zubov has outlined the auditing process as it relates to externally funded programs.

Part V: *Responsible Conduct of Research* Institutions and individuals who accept the responsibility of conducting research also must accept the responsibility of following laws, regulations, and commonly accepted practices relating to the conduct of the research. Integrity in designing, conducting and reporting of research is one of the most critical elements of a research program. In his chapter on edu-

cation in the responsible conduct of research, Chris Pascal frames many of these issues and broadens the concept of misconduct beyond the federal definition. Elliott Kulakowski describes the process of dealing with instances where integrity has diminished and investigations into misconduct must be implemented. Edward Gabriele discusses the role of leadership in developing a spirit of integrity. Dan Vasgird and Ellen Hyman-Browne describe how an institution can develop a proactive research compliance and integrity program.

The many elements of responsible research include cultivating mentorship, which is discussed by Melissa Anderson, Janet Holdsworth and Joseph Shultz. Michael Kalichman provides guidance on data management and Bryan Benham, Dale Clark, and Leslie Francis discuss responsible authorship. Increasingly, *conflict of interest* has become a concern as research programs have become more collaborative and involve industry and other private sector entities in research, and this is addressed by Elliott Kulakowski and John Chinn. Greg Koski discusses the challenges of building a program to foster research while ensuring protection of our research subjects. Michael Owen addresses the special issues and concerns associated with protection of volunteers in social and behavioral research settings. The advent of the Health Insurance Portability and Accountability Act (HIPAA), which has brought new dimensions to human subject research, is profiled by Ada Sue Selwitz, Helene Lake-Bullock, and Joe Brown. Jeffrey Botkin is the lead author on the section discussing the questions of use and protection of human tissue.

Another issue related to proper research conduct includes the welfare of animal subjects in research. Kathryn Bayne and John Harkness have described the policy and practices that must be put in place in order to conduct research with animals. Matthew Finucane has outlined the various health, safety and environmental regulations, policies and programs that support research programs. Bryan Benham discusses the impact of bio-terrorism on the research endeavor.

Part VI: *Technology Transfer* The product of research may take a variety of forms, few of them mutually exclusive. The process of transferring this product is generally defined as *technology transfer*. The product may be tangible, for example, a new medical devise, or intangible in the form of a new process for developing transgenic plant varieties. The management of the process is complex, involving numerous best practices, regulations, and national and international laws. Colin Cooper discusses a framework for collaboration with industry in the development of a product. The basis for patenting inventions and the components of the Bayh-Dole Act are described by Steve Highlander and Howard Bremer. Elliott Kulakowski and Patricia Harsche Weeks provide guidelines for developing intellectual property policy and establishing a technology transfer office. The intricacies and requirements of the material transfer agreement are defined by Fred Reinhart. Copyright, trademarks, and trade secrets are elements of the intellectual property and technology transfer processes for a research institution are described by David Huizenga and Hope Slonim. Concetta Bartosh and Kathleen Sybert both describe other issues integral to intellectual property management including non-disclosure agreements and Cooperative Research and Development Agreements (CRADAs). James Taylor describes relevant to research and intellectual property management issues related to the Patriot Act, Export Control, and the International Treaty on Arms Regulations (ITAR).

Joseph Fondacaro defines the process of patenting and licensing as beginning with determining the potential value of a technology. John Child and Kathleen Rigaut discuss the process of applying for US patent protection and Robert Macwright describes the licensing process. Katherine Chou outlines the complex elements of a license. Richard Kordal and Christopher McKinney provide information on negotiation and marketing of technology.

Jayne Carney and Janet Scholz give guidance to the spin-off process of new companies from university-developed technology. Elliott Kulakowski elaborates on the importance of these companies to economic development. Roberta Nixon, Jo Anne Goodnight, and Rick Shindell discuss the SBIR/STTR process as it supports the development of new technologies by both established and new small businesses.

Summary

It is recognized that research today is so specialized that researchers must collaborate across many disciplines, seeking researchers from multiple institutions and multiple nationalities, and from public, not-for-profit and industrial sectors if the world is to be understood, if problems are to be solved, and if quality of life universally is to be improved. Multidisciplinary international research is not uncommon and communications among investigators has never been easier. Fiscal, regulatory, intellectual property and other governmental requirements are different in nearly every country in the world. There is a need to understand each other's culture and requirements. Future editions of the book will look to incorporating differences.

The administration of research is broad in scope and complexity. In this edition, the authors have attempted to ensure that the major functions and responsibilities that encompass or relate to the leadership and management of research are addressed.

• • • References

1. US Census Bureau, "World Population Clock Projection," www.census.gov/ipc/popclockworld (accessed October 4, 2005).

2. *The Merriam-Webster Dictionary*. 10th ed., s.v. "Research."

3. National Science Foundation, "National Patterns of R&D Resources: 2002 Data Update," http://www.nsf.gov/sbe/srs/nsf03313/start.htm (accessed January 3, 2005).

4. National Science Foundation, "U.S. and International Research and Development: Funds and Alliances," *Science and Engineering Indicators 2002,* http://www.nsf.gov/sbe/srs/seind02/c4/c4s1.htm#fn1 (accessed January 3, 2005).

5. American Association for the Advancement of Science, "Defense and Homeland Security *R&D Hit New Highs in 2005; Growth Slows for Other Agencies*," http://www.aaas.org/spp/rd/upd1104.htm (accessed August 25, 2005).

6. Hargadon, A. *How Breakthroughs Happen: The Surprising Truth About How Companies Innovate*. Boston: Harvard Business School Press, 2003.

7. National Science Foundation, "U.S. Academic R&D Continues to Grow as More Universities and Colleges Expand Their R&D Activities," *InfoBrief,* May 2004, http://www.nsf.gov/srs/infbrief/nsf04319/start.htm (accessed January 3, 2005).

2

The History of Research Administration

Kenneth L. Beasley, MAT, PhD, CRA

Research administration is the support required for success in research programs. Research administration is practiced in organizations that conduct research: institutions of higher education, industrial research laboratories, independent profit and not-for-profit research companies, medical research institutions, and government research laboratories and centers. There are many research administrative positions within a single organization or agency. These positions have diversified responsibilities that have evolved from the following management areas: 1) the conduct of research and its impact on the entire organization, and 2) the oversight and compliance of the sponsor's management and fiscal requirements as stated in the grant or contract. The administration of these two responsibilities is often divided within the organizational structure between a person with a research or organizational management background and a person with a business management background. Sometimes, organizational responsibility for research administration is vested in a single executive, usually a vice president for research, laboratory director or provost. Research administration is not the direction of an individual research project; that duty is the responsibility of the principal investigator. The scientific direction of an individual project is usually referred to as project management.

Before World War II, research administration was vested with and was the responsibility of scientists and their research staff members. A senior administrator, such as a president, vice president, director or dean provided for the general management of research in an organization. In the years immediately after 1945, a new type of research administrator emerged to create a new professional position and launch the rapid growth of research administration.

Federal support of research is a function of the federal government's science policies. Thus, the history of research administration requires knowledge of national science policies that support research and create the opportunities for success. While most of the material in this chapter refers to the sciences, where most of the federal money goes, the term *research* is used in a broad connotation to also include applied research and research in nonscience fields.

Prelude: Federal Science Policy and Practice, 1787 to 1940

Among the delegates to the 1787 Constitutional Convention were proponents of federal policies to support science development, a national university and public works. During the debates on the powers of Congress, Charles Pinckney of South Carolina submitted a proposal entitled, "The power to 'establish seminaries for the promotion of literature and the arts and sciences,' to 'grant charters of incorporation,' to 'grant patents for useful inventions.' and to 'establish public institutions rewards and universities for the promotion of agriculture, commerce trades and manufactures.' "[1] James Madison of Virginia offered a similar proposal for discussion as an addition to the Constitution when he succinctly called "for the power to establish a university and to 'encourage by premiums and provisions, the advancement of useful knowledge and discoveries.'"[2] The most famous scientist among the delegates was Benjamin Franklin, who proposed that the Constitutional powers of Congress include "cutting canals where deemed necessary."[3] Franklin's argument was that a good transportation system developed better commerce as well as training for scientists and engineers.

These proposals were caught up in the debate over limited government and the big state versus the little state controversy. With one exception, the proposals were all defeated. The exception, which concerns research administrators, was the approval of Congress (Article I, Section 9) "to promote the Progress of Science and the useful Arts, by securing for limited times to Authors and Inventors the exclusive Right to their Writings and Discoveries."[4] This power established the patent and copyright systems.

From the start, it was not the United States federal policy to support science or research; the only time the word *science* appears in the Constitution is within the patent clause. This vague reference stood as US science policy for almost 150 years. However, the general policy was breached often during that period through actions that supported science in specific projects, usually for an applied purpose or for programs to build a science base.

> The Federal Government had been a continuous patron of science since the Constitutional Convention of 1787. This support of science came largely through the individual programs of the many Federal Bureaus and departments created during the nineteenth and early twentieth centuries.[5]

Important Congressional actions related to scientific research during this period include:

- The Smithsonian Institution
  The Smithsonian Institution was established in 1846 by a grant from James Smithson. The purposes of the Smithsonian Institution as stated in the original charter called for the "increase and diffusion of knowledge. Headed by eminent science administrators, the Smithsonian Institution played a leading role during the nineteenth century in various aspects of scientific research, including anthropology, biology, geology, and astronomy."[6] The Smithsonian Institution was financed from the original 1846 grant, but also received additional federal money for research.

- The Morrill Act
  The Morrill Act in 1862 provided each state with land to build a college with emphasis on developing the agricultural and mechanical arts. The land could be used by the new institution or sold to obtain funds to create the college. These public institutions, known as the land grant colleges, focused on applied education for the workplace instead of the classical education offered at most other institutions of higher education. The second Morrill Act of 1890 provided a yearly operating grant to the land grant colleges. While the original act did not specifically emphasize research, these institutions soon developed research programs and experiment stations in the sciences, agriculture, and engineering. The land grant universities built a base as strong research universities in the twentieth century.

- The National Academy of Sciences (NAS)
  The National Academy of Sciences was founded in 1863. The enabling act stated the academy was "to assist any department of the government with science related questions when requested. Such assistance was to take the form of investigations, examinations, experiments and reports."[7] In effect, NAS became a quasi-government agency at the government's expense to conduct research for the federal government.

- The Hatch Act
  The 1887 Hatch Act was the culmination of the extramural research activities of the Department of Agriculture. The Act established state-owned agricultural research stations in each state with the stations receiving support from the Department of Agriculture. The system permitted the Department of Agriculture to conduct research in all states and, with the addition of county agents, gave the Department grass roots political contacts.

- Allison Commission
  In 1884, when Congress became concerned about the haphazard manner in which the federal government was conducting science, the Allison Commission was formed to investigate the practices and recommend a national science policy. The Commission asked the NAS to conduct the investigation. "The Academy report, submitted in 1884, favored the creation of a Department of Science to conduct research not undertaken in university research laboratories or within private enterprise."[8] The report was adopted and Congress finally had a recommendation that would both coordinate and support federal research. "Nevertheless, after extensive hearings and debate, the Allison Commission

shelved the proposal on the grounds that centralized agencies ultimately did not serve the general welfare of the nation."[9] Congress had officially recognized the amount of federal research support in an uncoordinated system, but it rejected the recommendation and stayed with the status quo of no centralized program of control and support of research.

- World War I

A strong interest in research developed during the onset of the war as a means to help win the war and two organizations were established to enlist scientists to apply research in the development of military capability. In 1915 the Naval Consulting Board (NCB) was appointed with Thomas A. Edison serving as chair. The Naval Consulting Board was "charged with soliciting and screening proposals for improved weapons technology."[10] Concerned about research in other areas, the National Academy of Sciences recommended the creation of the National Research Council (NRC) to utilize scientists to assist the war effort. President Woodrow Wilson appointed members to the NRC in 1916. The contributions of these two groups were minimal in World War I. "Neither the Naval Consulting Board or the National Research Council achieved great success in either weapons development or overall policy coordination during the war."[11] The experience of both organizations did demonstrate, however, that a team approach to science research and a working relationship with the federal government were essential to achieving results. After the war, the Naval Consulting Board was reorganized and continued as the Naval Research Laboratory and NRC was continued under an Executive Order.

The prior examples represent only some of the federal research support activities from the start of our nation until 1940, during which time the official policy of not supporting research was observed more in the breach than in practice. Prior to the 1940s, however, the federal government had yet to establish a program of national grants to scientists to pursue basic research.

On the eve of World War II, science support in the United States primarily came from:

1. The federal government through mission oriented research by various agencies.
2. Universities through internal support of their basic research mission. The development of basic research in American universities developed in the research institutions in the early years of the twentieth century. "By the 1930s, universities were the undisputed leaders in the conduct of basic research. As an indication of this, government, industry and private foundation support of science often took the form of funding basic research done within the universities."[12] The universities were also recognized for their applied research in areas that received federal funding such as agriculture and engineering.
3. Industrial research laboratories for support of their research and the development of products. Industry realized that a team approach to research and development was the best road to product development and invested in bringing scientists together in the laboratory to focus on an area of promise. The best-known industrial laboratories included American Telephone and Telegraph (Bell Laboratories), Eastman Kodak, Dupont, General Electric, Corning Glass, and Westinghouse.
4. Private foundations through grants to institutions and individuals. The Rockefeller Foundation, the Carnegie Institution, and the Guggenheim Foundation were among the most noted of the private foundations. Since the private foundations made grants to individuals, they were an important source of support for university faculty, especially faculty with expensive facility and equipment needs.

There were few research administrators with an overall responsibility for multiple projects before World War II. Research administrators at that time were the scientists themselves, managing a specific project or the head of a team focused within an area of investigation. They had to seek and secure the support they needed to conduct research.

An example of research administration before 1940 is the work of Ernest Orlando Lawrence, an eminent physicist and Nobel Prize laureate for his work in inventing the cyclotron. A professor at the University of California, Berkeley, Lawrence was indefatigable in his research to develop the cyclotron and constantly in need of money to build a more powerful machine. He continually and successfully asked the University of California for resources. Lawrence received large grants from major foundations and he obtained a used magnet for an early cyclotron from a San Francisco power company warehouse. Lead was needed to shield the cyclotrons, especially as each version grew larger.

> He solved the lead problem with his usual inspiration and boldness; through the president's office, he asked for the loan of lead from

American Smelting and Refining Company in San Francisco, pointing out the merits of his work and the fact that it would cost them very little in time and expense to allow its use. The request was granted and 350 tons of quarter inch sheeting arrived in time to shield the improved model.[13]

With the help of project scientists and graduate students, he managed the details of the research and the administrative requirements of the sponsors. He received practically no support from the federal government. Lawrence's work in funding research was typical of the major research scientists of his time.

In summary, research was respected by the framers of our Constitution, but except for the patent and copyright provisions, was not supported in the Constitution. In the period from 1789 to 1945, US scientists conducted research by contracts for applied research requested by federal agencies. There was no federal office to coordinate and control research supported by government money. There were no federal grants to individuals to support basic research. The higher education system in the United States was considerably smaller in the 1930s than it is today. According to the United States Census Bureau's *Statistical Abstract (1997)*, there were only 1,690 colleges and universities in 1938; by 1995 that number more than doubled to 3,706. After World War II, the sheer number of students also increased significantly. Many of the institutions of higher education in 1938 were small liberal arts colleges and teacher preparation schools that focused on undergraduate education and training. The number of universities with a strong emphasis on research and doctoral programs was small before World War II. Again, according to the Census Bureau's *Statistical Abstract (1997)*, the number of Ph.D. degrees awarded in physics alone in 1936 was 138, compared to 1,655 in 1995. The relatively low amount of financial support of research by outside sources had not yet created a need for research administration as an administrative function to support researchers.

A Model System of National Research Coordination and Support, 1940 to 1945

In September of 1939, Germany invaded Poland and World War II started in Europe. Although the United States remained neutral at the time, national leaders were preparing for the defense of the country should war come. Within the US science community attitudes about the war in Europe were mixed. Overall, the federal government, led by President Franklin D. Roosevelt, decided to organize for war and, as part of preparation, two leaders of the scientific community came to the fore as advisors to President Roosevelt on how to mobilize scientific research for war. One of these men was Vannevar Bush, President of the Carnegie Institute in Washington, D.C. and former Vice President and Dean of Engineering at the Massachusetts Institute of Technology. A noted researcher, he held several patents and was a founder of the Raytheon Corporation. Bush had also conducted research on anti-submarine detection devices at a naval laboratory in New London, Connecticut during World War I. Bush became the president of the Carnegie Institution in 1939 and, in that role, made connections with the leading research programs throughout the nation and provided Carnegie funds to enhance existing research programs and to start new programs. More than anyone else in the nation, Bush was aware of the state of scientific research and the individual scientists at the forefront of discovery. Another important science leader of the time was James B. Conant, a soft-spoken organic chemist of note who had been President of Harvard University since 1933. During World War I, Conant had worked for the US Chemical Warfare Service. Later, as President of Harvard during the onset of World War II, he had taken a strong position on intervention in the war for fear that the totalitarian states would squash democracy in Western Europe.

In May 1940, Bush submitted a paper to President Roosevelt calling for an organization to enlist and direct the scientific community in the defense of the country. Bush insisted that the organization report directly to the President of the United States. President Roosevelt agreed with Bush's recommendations and on June 27, 1940, he created the National Defense Research Council (NDRC), appointing Bush as the NDRC Chair. The purposes of the organization were to centralize scientific research to defend the country and engage scientists in targeted research projects. The research projects would be conducted primarily through contracts with universities, industrial laboratories, private research companies and federal research activities. As NDRC Chair, Bush had access to support funds for personnel, laboratories, equipment, and supplies for mission research programs deemed promising to national defense. In June 1941, the structure was reorganized as the Office of Science Research and Development (OSRD). The final structure was a tripartite organization consisting of the National Defense Research Council, the Committee on Medical Services and the Office of the Executive Director. NDRC, then headed by Conant, supervised all research in the sciences. There were nineteen research divisions within the NDRC, each named for a mission area (radar, electrical communications, fire control, new missiles and chemical engineering, etc.). The Committee on Medical Research conducted all medical research in six divisions: general medical, surgery, physiology, aviation medicine, chemistry and malaria. Bush became the Executive Director of the OSRD and the Office of the Executive Director, and as such was the administrative arm in charge of procurement, contracting and managing the business aspects of the program. The office also served as liaison with research and development in the armed services. In OSRD Bush had created a central structure to coordinate and support a national scientific research program. He had also, knowingly or unknowingly, built a model for the new federal research policy for the nation after the war.

The successes of OSRD during World War II were unparalleled and included advances in radar, penicillin, proximity fuses, communications, and improved ordnance. The OSRD's most notable achievement was its Manhattan Project, the creation of the atomic bomb. In 1943, when the project promised a significant role in the war and required a larger amount of money and people, the project was turned over to the US Army.

In addition to its research and development accomplishments, OSRD also developed the system for procuring and managing research awards. Through contracts, the government established the rules for project goals, financial management and reporting. The basic management agreements between the sponsoring agencies and the research laboratories were developed as part of the OSRD management system. This system was continued after the war as part of government grants and contracts.

As World War II portended ultimate victory for the Allies, both the scientific community and the Washington political establishment looked to the future and the continuation of federal support of science. On September 17, 1944, President Roosevelt sent a letter to Vannevar Bush commenting on the success of OSRD, stating that he saw, "no reason why the lessons to be found in this experiment cannot be profitably employed in times of peace for the improvement of national health, the creation of new enterprises bringing new jobs, and the betterment of the national standard of living."[14] The President asked Bush how to extend the use of science and improve science education in the post

war world. Bush immediately formed four committees, each working on a different question posed by the President. Following his own experience and beliefs and the reports of the four committees, Bush completed his recommendations and submitted them to President Harry S. Truman in a June 1945 report, *Science: The Endless Frontier.*

> The central theme of the summary was that the nation's health, economy and military security constantly required the deployment of new scientific knowledge; that the federal government was obligated to ensure basic scientific progress and the production of trained scientific manpower; and that a new federal agency—he called it the National Research Foundation—should be established with funds and authority to promote these purposes.[15]

Bush pointed out that the National Research Foundation's main goal was to coordinate all federal research, and he placed medical research under the foundation and placed military research in a Division of National Defense associated with the National Research Foundation. Bush's recommendations became the blueprint for a science policy in which all federal research was coordinated under one agency and support was provided for individual research, team research, and programs to increase scientific training.

The OSRD programs were the training grounds for many of the first wave of research administrators after the war. In addition to the scientific personnel, OSRD needed people to manage nonresearch requirements, including contracting, personnel management, purchasing, accounting, and reporting. As part of OSRD, many of the research scientists had learned management skills that prepared them for the new research administration of the future.

In summary, the OSRD was the nation's first central government agency that coordinated, controlled, and supported scientific research. The OSRD's success created a demand to continue federal supported research for peacetime improvements.

A Pluralistic National Research System and the Start of Research Administration, 1945 to 1950

During the period from 1945 to 1950 a proposed central agency to control all federal research programs was being considered by the research community, Congress and the President. There were different views on the responsibilities and control of the new agency, and it took five years to establish a new federal research policy and supporting system.

The different viewpoints on a new science policy revolved around several issues, but the foremost issue was whether to have a central agency to control all federal research or to delegate different research areas to different federal agencies.

During the five-year delay, several important decisions were made that changed Bush's proposed central coordinating research agency into the pluralistic system we still have today. New research support came soon after World War II and the infusion of research awards created a need for federal award recipients in the public and private sectors. Existing funding agencies, such as the National Institutes of Health and the Office of Naval Research, were ready to make awards at the beginning of this period. A look at the developments during these five critical years explains the creation of a pluralistic national research policy and the emergence of research administration to support it.

Creating the National Science Foundation: Differences and Delays

When *Science: The Endless Frontier* was released in 1945, there was broad acceptance of the proposed program of support with recommendations for a new national science policy and a new coordinating agency. However, there was political opposition to certain details in the report and some reservations among scientists. In July 1945 Senator Warren G. Magnuson of Washington had submitted a bill to establish the National Science Foundation (NSF) much along the lines of Bush's recommendations. Senator Harley M. Kilgore of West Virginia, however, soon introduced a separate bill differing from the Magnuson bill in: "1) the governing structure of the proposed National Science foundation, 2) patent policy associated with publicly financed research, 3) federal support of the social sciences, 4) geographical distribution of Federal research grants."[16]

Regarding control and accountability, Bush had recommended an independent civilian/science agency as proposed in Magnuson's bill, while Kilgore proposed a government organization that reported to the President. The second issue concerned public funding of research projects that were patented and profited for private firms. The basic question was whether the discoverer or the government would own patent rights for research that had been funded by the government. The third issue concerned the

belief that the social sciences, in general, contributed to national good and, thereby, should be supported by the government (for example, during the Depression, many government-funded projects had been awarded to social scientists). A final issue of concern between the Magnuson and Kilgore proposals regarded pressure from both scientists and legislators to distribute the federal research awards to a broader number of recipients, including institutions that had not already participated in OSRD programs. It was pointed out that "OSRD had spent 90 percent of its funds at only eight institutions, about 35 percent at the MIT Radiation Laboratory alone."[17]

Senator Kilgore's bill prescribed a National Science Foundation that reported to the President, called for federal ownership of patents, the inclusion of the social sciences in grant awards and distribution of grants geographically.

Congress passed a compromised bill in 1947, but President Truman vetoed the bill fearing that "the proposed legislation would place NSF in the hands of private citizens unaccountable to the Federal Government, thus producing an absence of administrative accountability."[18]

After the veto, President Truman appointed a Scientific Research Board that studied the issues, citing recommendations in the Steelman Report. The five-volume report detailed the state of science in the United States. While the report agreed with Bush's earlier recommendations about the need for federal coordination and support of science, the Steelman Report favored some positions in line with Senator Kilgore's proposal. A compromise bill was finally accepted by both sides and signed into law by President Truman on May 10, 1950.

The NSF's mandate was to fund basic research in the physical, mathematical, engineering biological, medical and other sciences, mostly following Bush's original recommendations with some compromises in two of the disputed areas. The disagreement over control and accountability was resolved by assigning control of NSF to a director and members of a National Science Board, as appointed by the President and confirmed with the advice and consent of the Senate. In 1958 support was extended to specifically include the social sciences. Regarding the distribution of awards, the legislation rejected a formal program or formula for dispersing funds and accepted Bush's position that awards should be made on merit. Lastly, the legislators took the position that patent policy would not be addressed in the bill. The resulting "no change" decision meant that patents could continue to be awarded to individuals and corporations.

The five-year delay and lower than expected appropriations in its early years resulted in a slow start for NSF. "Although Bush had called for a budget of $33.5 million for NSF in the first year, its initial budget was $3.5 million. By its fifth year, NSF had a $16 million budget, rather than Bush's target of $122.5 million."[19] The following table presents the NSF expenditures for basic research in the 1960s.

TABLE 2-1	NSF Expenditures to Support Basic Research.[20] (In millions)
1962	$88.7
1963	$107.2
1964	$112.4
1965	$119.5
1966	$157.8

While not fully the organization that Bush recommended, NSF developed into the primary source of support for basic research and the training of scientists in institutions of higher education. Research administrators with pre-award responsibilities during the past fifty years are all familiar with NSF programs, application forms, and guidelines.

Military Research Expands

In 1945, there were only two military branches, War and Navy, and each occupied a cabinet position. The research divisions of both branches started before World War II and, during the war, carried out research programs in support of the war. They coordinated their research activities with OSRD programs. With the close of the war, the Secretaries of War and Navy established a Joint Research and Development Board with representatives from both services and Vannevar Bush serving as a civilian chair.

The Navy was the first military service to establish a strong program of research funding when it created the Office of Naval Research (ONR) in 1946. The OSRD management system was the model for ONR.

Its research support was carried out largely through contracts with universities—a continuation of the principal method used by OSRD—and its contracts were awarded on the basis of scientific merit. Its support of research was both generous and relatively free of administrative or programmatic restrictions, thus helping to insure academic freedom.[21]

Because ONR programs supported basic research by individual scientists, it became the major source of basic research until NSF was organized and funded. There were many questions about ONR supporting research in areas that did not seem feasible to Navy needs.

Although ONR's main purpose was to support scientific research related to the Navy's defense mission, it was charged with sponsoring a broad array of basic research. Indeed, many of the early research projects had little apparent bearing on defense issues.[22]

ONR became a source of science support for basic research in 1946. ONR began a program of liaison with American universities and faculty. Its practices refined the OSRD system and became the model for NSF when it was established. The first director of NSF, Alan T. Watermen, had been the first chief scientist for ONR.

Following the Navy's lead, the two other military service branches, Army (formerly the War Department) established the Army Research Office (ARO) and the newly established Air Force, initiated the Air Force Office of Science Research (AFOSR). In the early days, only ONR was funding research projects on campuses. The Army Research Office and the Air Force Office of Science Research would catch up to the Navy in the 1950s and 1960s. The amount of university research expenditures by ONR is reflected in Table 2-2.

The actual military expenditures for university basic research began in 1947 and continued until the Mansfield Amendment to the Department of Defense Appropriations Bill in 1969. Section 203 of the bill stated:

None of the funds authorized to be appropriated by the Act may be used to carry out any research project or study unless such a project has a direct or apparent relationship to a specific military function or operation.[23]

TABLE 2-2	ONR Expenditures for University Research Contracts.[24] (In millions at selected intervals. All expenditures including basic research)
1947	−$22.3
1952	−$35.7
1957	−$29.5
1962	−$73.2
1967	−$82.9
1969	−$96.8

National Institutes of Health

As a part of OSRD, The Committee on Medical Services conducted research that was successful in developing new medicines and practices that saved many lives in the war. With strong public and legislative support for continuing medical research after the war, the Public Health Service (PHS) proposed that medical research be placed in one of its divisions, The National Institutes of Health (NIH). NIH conducted medical research in its own laboratories before the war. The proposal was approved in 1945 and NIH took over the responsibility for medical research from OSRD. A Division of Research Grants was created at NIH to administer the extramural research support program. The new program provided support for medical schools, large medical research grants, and individual research grants. NIH became the agency for a national program to improve the nation's health. NIH was independent from Bush's conception of a coordinated national research system under the NSF. The extramural grant award program of NIH was started five years before NSF was established.

NIH research contracts started at a low level in 1945, but they have continued to increase substantially over the years because of their positive impact on health and the backing of members of Congress. The rise in expenditures up to 1995 is presented in Table 2-3.

The Atomic Energy Commission

Immediately after World War II, there was a debate on the future of research in atomic energy. Nuclear research was clearly an important key for the future of the nation's defense, but such research also held the promise of many benefits in the fields of energy and medicine for peaceful uses. Bush felt ongoing research was necessary in all fields and research in atomic energy should be coordinated under his proposed National Research Foundation. The Army, which had performed the later task of developing the atomic bomb, felt it should continue nuclear research for the nation's defense. The Navy shared the same viewpoint. Yet, there were strong concerns by scientists and civilians that atomic energy research and development should be under civilian control. In the end, President Truman signed the Atomic Energy Act in August 1946, which was noted for "its de-emphasis of the military role in regulation and its promotion of civilian application of nuclear power."[25] The new Atomic Energy Commission (AEC) followed the OSRD model and conducted research through contracts with universities,

TABLE 2-3	NIH Obligations for Grants, 1945 to 1995.[26] (In thousand of dollars. Amounts are presented in five-year intervals and include research grants, fellowships, training, facilities and centers)
1945	$142
1950	$43,823
1955	$54,214
1960	$292,910
1965	$774,520
1970	$771,259
1975	$1,306,475
1980	$2,343,220
1985	$4,018,137
1990	$6,140,937
1995	$8,085,349
2000	$13,218,410
2005 Appropriation	$20,529,913

industries, profit and not-for-profit research organizations, and medical research institutions. The AEC also established a research network of federal laboratories that were government-owned and contractor-operated. The establishment of AFC created an immediate source of federal money to support nuclear research that was independent of any other agency. The primary benefactors of the AEC contracts and grants were the physicists, chemists and engineers.

In summary, during the period from 1945 to 1950, several federal research support programs were initiated or continued as independent agencies not under the control or coordination of a single national research agency. This pattern of establishing independent funding agencies for research arose to fill the vacuum when the start of the NSF was delayed and continued after 1950 with the establishment of extramural support programs in most federal agencies. Bush's concept of federal research support and coordination through a single federal agency was replaced by a pluralistic system with many federal agencies having their own research support programs. This pluralistic system is still in place as the national research policy.

The period from 1945 to 1950 marked sudden availability of federal money marked specifically for research and other programs. Prior to World War II, federal money was granted only for projects the agencies wanted performed, the mission-oriented projects. By enabling authorization and the appropriation of funds to the new funding agencies, contracts and individual grants began to fund research in universities, industrial laboratories, profit and not-for-profit institutes, and medical research institutions. This flow of money also required that recipients of federal awards pay attention to the institutional research policy, the application and procurement process, the financial and reporting requirements of the sponsors, and overall coordination of the research program. Recipient institutions had to create research administrative systems and employ qualified people to manage research programs. Present day research administration was born to fulfill this institutional need.

The Emergence and Growth of Research Administration, 1950 to the 1980s

As OSRD ceased its role in research development at the end of the war, some of its research centers on university campuses were continued as basic research centers devoted to discoveries that would lead to peacetime needs. Likewise, many OSRD projects at industrial and independent laboratories continued research and development to produce new products for the postwar economy. Research universities, not involved in OSRD contracts, sought to increase their research capabilities and projects. In higher education, the race was on to build facilities, attract capable faculty researchers and secure outside contracts and grants. This pursuit of research excellence immediately challenged the prewar administrative structure of the universities. The expanded research program brought new requirements that had not been present before. A new structure was created to manage these requirements and coordinate the research activities. This new function was called research administration.

The infusion of federal dollars had an impact on two of the traditional divisions of a university. These areas were the academic division that promoted and maintained research and the business affairs division that managed contracts. This dual responsibility for research grants and contracts led to two different management areas. The academic leaders were concerned about the research goals of the institution, the relationship of research to the instructional program and the quality of the research performed. The business officers were concerned about the terms of the grant or contract and the management of awards in areas such as contracting, negotiating, award obligations, expenditures, cost control, accounting, financial reports, and audits. In most institutions these two responsibilities did not merge to supervise federal grants and contracts, although cooperative

agreements were usually made. Consequently, research administration came from two parallel areas with different responsibilities and different outlooks on those duties.

The term *research administration* was an early generic title. Recognizing that all external funds are not solely used for research but also for sponsored activities such as training, pilot or development grants, and support for work in the arts and humanities, alternate titles like the Administration of Sponsored Programs or Research and Sponsored Programs Administration are more common today.

The placement of research administration in institutions varied widely according to the university. Many schools used a centralized approach and placed all research administration in an institutional-wide office under a vice president, dean, or director. As the responsibilities grew, offices were established at lower levels in the institutional hierarchy but were the responsibility of the central office.

Another pattern was that of a decentralized function with responsibility of research administration distributed to deans or directors of research centers. The research officers in this model were responsible to the division director, but usually, coordination with a senior official was required. Other combination arrangements were also practiced. When the volume of research in an institution reached a high level, research administrators were placed in departments with a lot of research projects. For example:

- In the 1970s, when the University of Illinois's School of Chemistry had a research volume larger than most state colleges and universities, a business officer with assistants was appointed to manage the School of Chemistry's needs.
- The California Civil Service System has a position title of Laboratory Business Officer (LBO). Most of the LBO's have an academic background in business, in management or accounting. In the early days of the Society of Research Administrators, a large number of the new members were Laboratory Business Officers from the University of California.

The individuals occupying the new positions were called Vice President for Research, Dean for Research, Dean of the Graduate School and Director of Research, Research Director, and Laboratory Director. Responsibility for research administration placed in the Business Affairs Division of universities had titles such as Vice President of Business Affairs for Research, Research Business Manager, Contracts and Grants Manager and Director of Grants Management.

Since the inception of the profession, the three basic functions of the research administrators include:

- Providing needed services for researchers to enhance their success,
- Overall administration of the institution's research mission, and
- Working with sponsors to help achieve their goals and abide by their regulations.

Thus, the research administrator operates in a milieu consisting of the researcher, the institution and the sponsor. I have described the role of the research administrator as the mediator-expeditor for different parties in the research process.[27] This central role is portrayed in the following diagram:

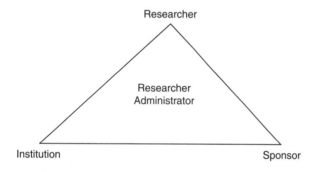

Waves of Growth of Research Administrators

The First Wave

The nation's research organizations that established the new administrative function multiplied rapidly after 1945. As the offices were created, the institutions began to seek qualified individuals to assume the new responsibilities. The first wave of the qualified candidates came from the former scientists and science administrators with OSRD. Many of these new research administrators were scientists, but they were also overall administrators for team projects. They developed skills in leadership, management, fiscal matters, the procurement of contracts, employment, purchasing, patents, and many other areas. Former OSRD members were prepared by experience and many knew the federal personnel who contracted with them for services. Many OSRD graduates were the ideal research administrators for the new positions. A look at three prominent postwar research administrators illustrates the career path of the first wave of research administrators.

Eric Walker   Born in England in 1910, Walker immigrated to Canada in 1921 and moved to the United

States in 1923. He received three degrees from Harvard, culminating in a Doctorate in Electoral Engineering in 1935. His first position was as a professor and head of the Electrical Engineering Department at Tufts. He later held the same position at the University of Connecticut. Just after the United States entered World War II, Walker returned to Harvard as the Associate Director of the Underwater Sound Laboratory developing sonar for underwater detection. After the war, he became head of the Department of Electrical Engineering and director of the Applied Research Laboratory (formerly the Ordinance Research Laboratory) at Pennsylvania State University. His research and administrative skills soon led to appointments as Dean of the School of Engineering (1951), Vice President for Research (1956), and in the same year, President of the University. He was always an advocate for research administration as an important position to further the research goals of a university. Many of his speeches and papers were dedicated to improving research administration. Dr. Walker was the founder of the National Conference on the Administration of Research. The name was later changed to the National Conference on the Advancement of Research. When Walker retired as President at Penn State, he became the Vice President for Research at the Aluminum Company of America (ALCOA). According to the former President and Chairman of the Board at ALCOA, Krome George, "Walker worked diligently to change the research laboratories to enable them to meet corporate needs more effectively. One of his goals was to integrate the research function with the management function so it would be a part of the corporate culture."[28] Walker was clearly a strong early leader in founding and improving research administration in all sectors.

Raymond Woodrow   Woodrow was born in New York City in 1913. His formal education included a degree in physics, Phi Beta Kappa from Williams College in 1934, a Masters Degree in Engineering from MIT in 1937, and advanced engineering study at the University of Pittsburgh while working for General Electric. Woodrow was employed by OSRD in the following administrative roles: Technical Aid in the Liaison Office concerned with liaison with other nations; Deputy Chief of the Transition Office handling the transition of OSRD research knowledge to production devices; and Associate Project Engineer and General Manager of the Radiation Laboratory at MIT. After the war, Woodrow took a new position at Princeton University as Executive Officer and Secretary of the Committee on Project Research and

Invention. While at Princeton his responsibilities in research administration increased over the years. He was a prolific author on research administration topics, both academic and financial management. He served as Associate Treasurer of Princeton and finally as Assistant for Special Studies to the Chair of the University Research Board. Woodrow was a part of many professional associations for research administration. He was an early leader and president of the National Council of University Research Administrators (1959), active in the National Association of College and University Business Officers, the Council on Government Relations, and in the University of Denver Biennial Conference on Research Administration. Perhaps Woodrow's greatest contribution to research administration is the 1978 book, *Management for Research in US Universities*. In the book he points out that research administration exists to serve the research scientists. He discusses the different motives and methods of researchers and those who are research administrators. He emphasizes "for" research as the common denominator to avoid a dilemma of the different motives and methods.

> Among the different things research administrators do, a universal feature is, or should be, to provide support for research. The common denominator is administration for research. There is a vast difference between administration for connoting support and service and administration of connoting direction and control.[29]

Woodrow was a great leader for research administration and certainly deserves accolades for his ideas, writings, and leadership.

Howard Wile   Wile was active in almost every professional development activity for research administration after 1945. His name appears frequently in correspondence, minutes of meetings or historical narratives in the early years. Wile received his BA degree from Dartmouth College and went on for an MBA from the Harvard Business School. During World War II, he worked at the MIT Radiation and Electronics Research Laboratories. When the war was over he was employed as an Administrator of Research at the Brooklyn Polytechnic Institute. Wile was recognized as a skilled research administrator because

> He had lived intimately with the technical problems that worried the academic research community, and he was familiar not only with the principal issues but with the details of regulation

and rule making inherent in the federal relationship. He was, in addition, a quietly skillful communicator, able to explain to the institutions, to the federal agencies, or to education associations the meanings of the problems coming to the Committee attention.[30]

Wile's important influence and role in research administration included:

- Attendance at the first and later meetings of the National Conference on the Advancement of Research;
- Founding of the Council on Governmental Relations, serving as its Executive Director for eleven years;
- Member of the Planning Committee for the first University of Denver Biennial Conference;
- Founding of the National Council of University Research Administrators and serving as its Advisor to the organization for a number of years.

Wile was instrumental on many fronts in the professional development of research administration.

The Second Wave

The number of research administrators expanded rapidly as the amount of federal money for research also expanded. The second wave of research administrators followed close behind the OSRD "graduates." Almost all of the large research universities realized they needed research administrators to manage their research program. The second wave of research administrators came from several sources: scientists with administrative experience, scientists with no administrative experience, retired military officers with contracting and management experience in the service, business managers, and people with industry, government or independent research laboratory backgrounds. The number of federal programs for research and other projects continued to increase in the later part of the twentieth century. The *1995 Catalogue of Federal Domestic Assistance* lists "over 1,300 grant programs by more than 50 Federal agencies"[31] with programs that provide money for a wide variety of projects.

These additional programs continue to reinforce the necessity of adding a research administration office.

The Third Wave

The third wave of research administrators came primarily from the state colleges and universities, many of which had been teachers colleges into the 1950s. While most of these institutions were not considered major research universities, many sought to become more research-oriented. As a result, many training opportunities were developed that would assist them to achieve this goal. Most of the third wave research administrators started in the 1960s and early 1970s.

The Fourth Wave

A fourth wave of research administrators filled positions at small colleges and community colleges. The primarily private undergraduate colleges sought support for projects such as institutional grants for laboratory equipment, curriculum improvement, and research grants for faculty. The community colleges sought funds for vocational training and improvement of facilities and equipment to serve special populations. This fourth wave came primarily in the 1970s and the 1980s. (The dates of these separate waves are approximate, based on the rosters of professional research organizations and observations of the author.)

Since 1945, other research entities in the nation increased administrative staff members to manage federal research projects. Awards to medical institutions, whether connected to a university or not, grew just as fast, if not faster, as other funded areas. Research administrators were hired for medical schools, hospitals and medical research institutions to manage federally supported research. Similarly, research dollars for Veterans Administration Hospitals also increased with the establishment of money for research administration.

During this period, both for-profit and not-for-profit research organizations had new access to contracts from government agencies and, as a result many new research institutes were founded. Several for-profit research companies established main offices in the DC area to be near the funding agencies.

While industry did not receive individual grants for research scientists, the government did need industry's expertise for some large research and development projects. The government recognized that industry had the required team experience to fulfill project scopes and therefore industry increasingly was allowed to bid on federal contracts. The government also began to tap many industrial companies for program management for which new research administrators were employed to manage the projects to specifically meet federal procurement and management regulations.

The Growth of Professional Associations, 1947 to the Present

It did not take long for the practitioners of research administration to create organizations to discuss practices and exchange ideas. The first organizations provided an opportunity for research administrators with similar interests to learn from each other. Five organizations had an early impact on the development of research administration. The story of the founding of these five organizations yields insight into the growth of the profession.

The National Conference on the Advancement of Research (NCAR), 1947

The concept for NCAR was developed in the greater Boston research community by Eric Walker and his colleagues in 1945. Several research administrators were seeking a solution to common problems and issues through friendly open discussion.

> Walker liked to say that NCAR was born in a bar, or at least a restaurant, in Cambridge, Massachusetts in the spring of 1945. Leaders of research activities in the Boston area would meet to discuss problems, and they decided it would be helpful to hold a conference of administrators to discuss issues and pass on experiences.[32]

After World War II, Walker went to Penn State, where he and several research administration associates planned and held the first meeting of NCAR on campus in October 1947. The invitation list consisted of upper level research administrators from higher education, industry and government. (Much later, in the 1970s, not-for-profit research organizations were also invited.) At the first meeting there were 170 attendees and some of the nonuniversity affiliated attendees included Philco Corporation, Navy Electronics Laboratory, Dupont, National Research Council, National Bureau of Standards, Brookhaven National Laboratory, Armour Research Foundation, Ontario Research Foundation, and Eastman Kodak. Several members were also active members of the Industrial Research Institute (IRI). The university attendees comprised 50% at the first gathering, coming from the established research universities, which received the majority of federal awards.

The NCAR administrative structure was minimal, with attention paid primarily to its annual meeting and publishing of the proceedings. At first there was only one continuing officer, the secretary-treasurer, who was later joined by an executive secretary, who maintained the records and was custodian of the funds. There were no dues. There were two NCAR committees: the Conference Committee of twenty-five members with rotating terms that directed NCAR, and the Program Committee that planned and conducted the annual meeting. There was no national office. The conferences were self-supporting: the host representative(s) arranged for the facilities, activities, set the conference fee, and took responsibility for conference costs.

The annual conference consisted of a meeting with a central theme, featuring keynote speakers. The presentations pertained to current science developments and national research policies with time allotted for follow-up discussion. The two-day conferences were informal and usually held at a resort location, at a university or a research setting with time set aside for informal discussions, visits to nearby research facilities or recreation.

One early discussion regarding a national organization for university research administrators occurred among university attendees at the 1959 NCAR conference in Vermont. During this discussion the concept for the National Council of University Research Administrators (NCURA) was born.

In the early 1970s, NCAR participants discussed the purpose and future of the organization: whether NCAR was a forum for research discussions or an action group to promote science research. At this time, NCAR changed its name to the National Conference on the Advancement of Research. The industrial attendees advised the conference attendees that NCAR should not become an action group, noting, "The role of the Conference should be to help identify and clarify issues for the participants, rather than develop a collective position."[33] In summarizing the role of NCAR, Martin Berger of Occidental Research Corporation stated:

> NCAR, to the best of my knowledge, is the only major organization in which the four major sectors for research—government, industry, university and not-for-profit—deal with these issues together... NCAR provides a forum for trying to provide that synergism, for trying to deal with research issues. and trying to find out how each can contribute to solving each others' problems.[34]

For further information, see *NCAR 50th Year*, an NCAR published booklet written by William T. Moye, historian for the US Army Research Laboratory.

Former Secretary-Treasurers and Executive Secretaries of NCAR include:

Merritt Williamson, Penn State University, 1956–1963; Robert Ramsey, Penn State University, 1964–1966; Paul Ebaugh, Penn State University, 1967–1968; Shirley (Sandy) Johnson, Denver Research Institute, 1969–1983; Norman Waks, MITRE Corporation, 1984–1987; Lieutenant General Austin Betts, Southwest Research Institute, 1988–2001.

In summary, the inspiration for NCAR came from research administrators before the close of World War II: NCAR's founders had already gained experience with OSRD during the war. NCAR's annual conferences brought together the foremost science research administrators from the four main sectors of research to discuss issues and problems to improve all aspects of research administration. NCAR and its leading members were the pioneers of research administration.

Council on Government Relations (COGR), 1948

Another organization that developed to meet the growing contract and business needs of higher educational institutions was the Council on Government Relations (COGR). COGR grew through several iterations from regional committees to an independent national council. It has been the preeminent organization to interact with federal agencies to serve the grants and contracts, compliance, accounting, technology transfer needs and reporting needs of colleges and universities accepting federal awards.

As research support at universities increased significantly after World War II, many institutions had problems in the financial and management requirements of the federal contract system that had been used during the war. Known as "The Green Book," the regulations did not specifically address contract issues of universities. The Green Book business policies were originally established in 1942 in a War Department memorandum titled, "Explanation of Principles for Determining Costs Under Government Contracts." At the time, there were many new questions about the contract rules, and the business affairs office of most institutions were responsible understanding such matters. Working with newly formed COGR, Howard Wile observed:

> The leadership of higher education was generally pleased by this new relationship, feeling that the institutions and the nation were benefiting mutually from what was sometimes referred to in

those early days as a 'partnership' between government and the academic community. Yet many institutions discovered immediately that the new relationship brought with it complex new problems of financial management.[35]

The first problem faced by universities involved costing policies for direct and indirect costs that were based on an arbitrary percentage of salaries and wages. The wages were unevenly assigned to institutions. R. B. Stewart, Purdue University, had worked at OSRD during the war and was later employed at the War and Navy Departments in the late 1940s and early 1950s. He had extensive experience with university business management and was a recognized consultant with the government on contract program management. In 1946, Stewart assembled a group of business officers from sixteen universities to address the cost problems with federal contracts. The group completed a memorandum of understanding and a list of recommendations that were later discussed with representatives of the War and Navy Departments. These discussions produced a new set of guidelines, called *The Blue Book for University Research Contracts*. The Blue Book guidelines determined new cost practices between the universities and the government contractors for the next ten years. The book was a welcomed early guide to understanding federal contract policies, but the book did not address all issues and it was realized that a more complete set of guidelines would be needed in the future. The success of the Stewart and his group was the first instance of a partnership between universities and agencies in determining the cost guidelines for awards.

Recognizing that a permanent mechanism was needed to work with the government on research issues, Stewart and his colleagues, working on an ad hoc basis, sought the establishment of an ongoing group under the auspices of an association of business officers. There was no national association for business officers at this time—only five independent regional associations. One of these, the Central Association of College and University Business Officers, passed a motion at its 1948 meeting endorsing "the establishment of a committee representing the five associations of college and university business officers to cooperate with R. B. Stewart in all relationships involving fiscal matters between the several financial agencies of the Federal Government and the institutions of higher education."[36] The

Committee on Government Relations was established that year as a permanent group representing all of the five associations. The original committee was also called the Middlebrook Committee on Federal Relations after W. T. Middlebrook of University of Minnesota, an early delegate to the Central Association. He later chaired COGR for several years. In 1979 the committee changed its name to the Council on Government Relations.

A major task of COGR in the 1950s was the completion of a complete set of guidelines for the management of contracts and grants in educational institutions. The first phase of this task required working with business officers and other higher education organizations that were involved in business practices in relation to government requirements. A coalition agreement was needed in preparation to negotiate with federal officials. In 1950, the independent business officer associations formed a federation, which allowed COGR to work with a single association. COGR played a leading role in building a coalition of higher education interests and with the government produced a guide, *Circular A–21, Cost Principles for Educational Institutions* in 1958. Amended several times since its first issue, Circular A–21 replaced the Blue Book and was considered a major achievement of COGR.

The success of COGR, along with the overall rise in business issues connected with government-supported projects, resulted in the need for a permanent COGR staff in Washington, DC to keep up with issues and to communicate with agencies. In 1960, the Federation of College and University Business Officers voted to establish an office in DC and to employ a full-time executive director. Support for the new office came from COGR membership fees. Before opening its DC office, COGR consulted with the American Council on Education to ensure that its purposes and practices did not conflict with the Council's Commission on Federal Relations and its Committee on Sponsored Research. Through discussion and practice, a separate role for COGR was established.

In 1962, COGR gained a stronger association base when the National Association of College and University Business Officers (NACUBO) replaced the Federation. COGR and NACUBO enjoyed a successful relationship for thirty-one years. In 1993, COGR separated from NACUBO and became an independent organization.

Led by the board, executive director, president and the support of volunteers, COGR played a seminal role in enhancing the business aspects of research administration. COGR continues to be well-regarded for its information and action in support of research supported by federal funds.

For complete information on the founding of COGR see the informational book by Tom Ewing on the occasion of its 50th anniversary in 1998, *COGR 1948–1998: An Association of Research—Intensive Universities.*

The University of Denver Biennial Conference on Research Administration, 1954

While not as well known as other research organizations, this series of biennial conferences sponsored by the University of Denver has influenced the development of research administration in several ways. The first meeting was held out of economic necessity in 1954. The Denver Research Institute (DRI) was established in 1947 to meet the needs in the mountainous West for applied research. In the 1940s, this area of the country had few research facilities, but had much available open land on which to locate new research facilities. Subsequently, "DRI was built mainly on weapons technology, defense contracts."[37] When the flow of contracts to DRI continued to increase during the 1950s, the staff began to have questions about grant management regarding allowable costs, patents and copyrights, ownership of equipment and cost sharing. DRI was still small and with few resources. To find answers to their questions about managing federal contracts, DRI staff first discussed visits to the top twenty research universities and institutes in the country, but decided it would be far less expensive to bring the most knowledgeable research administrators to Denver instead. They decided the best way to attract the expertise to Denver was to hold a conference in the summer vacation period in the mountains.

The first organizer of the meeting was George Cannetta, DRI's business manager. The first meeting was held on the campus of the University of Denver, June 1954; there were thirty-five attendees. Subsequent meetings were held at resort facilities in the mountains. The second meeting was held in 1956 at the Brinwood Ranch near Estes Park, Colorado, with fifty-five people in attendance. The background of the mountains and the pristine environment created a congenial and relaxing setting for the attendees. The meeting was informal and the business program was augmented with local entertainment such as ranch activities and participant events, including a contest in writing limericks about the meeting. There was also ample time to get to know each other and discuss the issues of research admin-

istration. Except for the first meeting when the participants had scattered lodging around Denver, the resort locations provided opportunities for greater communication and friendship. An important conference rule was stated in the Program and General Information Brochure at the first conference, "All sessions will be closed and no notes of the proceedings will be kept or published. Panel discussions will be at round tables to facilitate general participation by all present."[38] The "keep it within the walls" requirement encouraged open discussion of the issues. The attendees praised the conferences for providing the opportunity to talk to each other about common problems in a pleasant and pristine atmosphere.

The biennial conferences emphasized the business practices for research grants and contracts between higher education and the contracting agencies. The individuals attending the conferences were mostly business officers and academic research administrators from the foremost research universities. The participants were the most knowledgeable people in the field. The University of Denver had brought the leading experts in research administration together to discuss issues and explore solutions. While not an action organization, each conference was a powerful forum. To point out the power base for influencing federal policy and agency programs Sandy Johnson said that "one year he looked around the meeting room and realized that the administrators of 80 percent of the country's higher education research were sitting there with him."[39] The topics at the early conferences, like those of COGR meetings, were concerned with the business office and the management of federal contracts. Troublesome issues at the second DRI conference included discussion about:

> The fact that different government agencies made their own interpretations and regulations; that the government wanted time and effort reports from professors; that the universities felt that research and teaching could not be separated completely; that professors do not and should not be required to work by the clock, that the government wanted segregated the space used for research from that used by instruction; that the universities wanted the inclusion of departmental and Dean's overhead; the need to clarify consultants time and procedures: and that the universities did not have a profit to use in order to help defer additional costs and work load incurred with government contracts.[40]

These were typical questions asked by universities across the nation. The early conferences occurred at the time when contract management regulations were guided by the Blue Book, then replaced by Circular A21.

The Denver Biennial Conference was the site for the first discussion of a national organization for college and university research administrators. The participants at the third conference in 1958 spoke about the need for an organization just for research administrators from academic institutions, which led to the formation of the National Council of University Research Administrators.

National Council of University Research Administrators (NCURA), 1959

NCURA was created by a group of academic leaders who pointed out the need for an organization to serve the special needs of institutions of higher education in managing research contracts with the government. The founders of NCURA were research administrators from established research institutions who knew each other from previous OSRD positions or through attendance at the existing professional association for research administrators. Through a progressive series of meetings at different locations, the founders developed the basic purposes and structure of NCURA. The idea for the NCURA first arose at the June 1958 Biennial Conference of the University of Denver. The discussion pointed out the need for information related specifically to higher education research administration. The discussion resulted in a plan for a clearinghouse of information for practitioners in colleges and universities. Following up on these plans, a small group of research administrators met in November 1958 at the Cornell Aeronautical Laboratory in Buffalo, New York, and "agreed that there was need for some kind of group or organization that would look beyond business and fiscal matters into the broader aspects of research administration."[41] Following this meeting, Ray Ewell of the State University of New York at Buffalo, and William Wheadon of Syracuse University made plans for a group of research administrators in the east to meet and discuss common problems. The opportunity for this meeting arose at the annual meeting of the National Conference on the Administration of Research in Vermont in October 1959 where it was agreed to establish a national organization for all higher education research administrators. A month later in New York City, five research administrators met to formulate a set of recommendations to present at an organization meeting to be held in Chicago. These individuals were: Ray Ewell, State University of New York; William Wheadon, Syracuse University; Donald Murray, University of Pennsylvania; Sidney Roth, New York University, and John Hastie, Cornell University.

The first meeting of the NCURA was held on January 1960 in Chicago, where the purposes and administrative structure of the new organization were adopted at the meeting. Ray Ewell was elected as the first national chairman. Ewell was Vice President for Research at the State University of New York at Buffalo. Before becoming Vice President for Research at SUNY-Buffalo, Ewell had been a chemist directing the Incendiaries and Flame Throwers research unit of the OSRD Fire Warfare Division. As Howard Wile notes in his early history of NCURA, there were forty-five people representing forty universities in seventeen states at the meeting. The name of the new organization, National Council of University Research Administrators, was approved. According to the "Twenty-Five Year History of NCURA, ROOTS," the minutes of the Chicago meeting reflect passage of the following objective, "The discussion and exchange of ideas on research policies in universities through national and regional meetings, workshops and seminars."[42] The original purposes of NCURA included promoting the development of research administration; providing a forum to improve research administration practices; dissemination of information and exchange of ideas; and improving research administration as a professional field. Membership in NCURA was open to individuals practicing research administration in institutions of higher education or affiliate entities. Most of the original members of NCURA were the leaders of research administration in their respective institutions. The responsibilities of the original members were split between overall research administration in the academic area or business and financial management of research grants and contracts in the business area.

NCURA did not prepare a formal charter or bylaws until they were developed at the fifth meeting and unanimously approved by mail. The early meetings were held at various locations in tandem with other organizations. The seventh meeting, held at the Mayflower Hotel in Washington, DC was the first meeting planned and directed for NCURA members only (subsequently the meetings have all been held in DC). NCURA has always maintained a close relationship with federal funding agencies and their support programs. Federal directors of funding programs frequently speak at NCURA annual meetings to inform the NCURA members of program opportunities and application requirements.

The annual meeting fulfilled the NCURA purposes in the early years. Topics on a broad range of areas in research administration were covered by speakers at plenary sessions or in separate sessions. As the council increased its membership, the annual meeting expanded to include featured national speakers, workshops before the meeting, roundtable discussion sessions, presentations of awards and social activities. NCURA has seven regional organizations with each area holding a spring meeting. A variety of conferences, workshops, seminars and videoconferences are part of the education and professional development goals of the council. NCURA has a publication program that includes a professional journal, a newsletter, books, manuals, workbooks, and monographs. It extends services to its members through electronic means such as teleconferencing.

In summation, NCURA was created by a need for an organization that addressed concerns and proposed solutions just for higher education research administrators. Its founders were all leaders in other organizations for research administration and many of them were graduates of the OSRD research programs during World War II. These individuals were veterans who volunteered their experiences to found an important organization for higher education research administrators. The successors to the NCURA founders have built that base into a large, effective organization that has developed the profession of research administration for its college and university members.

The Society of Research Administrators International (SRA), 1967

The four research administrator organizations discussed in the earlier sections were all founded by individuals employed at the higher levels of administration in their respective places of employment. As the number of research dollars increased in higher education, industry, profit and not-for-profit organizations, and medical research centers, the volume of work at all levels also increased. By the middle 1960s, many of the larger research institutions extended research administrative positions to the departmental and laboratory levels. The individuals in these positions had concerns about their roles in the broad scope of research administration. They also wanted programs to develop their skills and opportunities for advancement. The Society of Research Administrators International (SRA) was founded under this environment.

An organization of laboratory and academic business managers was formed at Yale University in 1966. The organization was named the Management Issues Forum (MIF). The purpose of MIF was to provide information and a forum for the discussion of university programs for its members. The group of about twenty-five people met monthly and discussed topics, usually with appropriate Yale administrators. The first chair of MIF was Ken Hartford, the University's Laboratory Business Manager in Biology. The MIF program was well received from the start. Based on this success, Ken Hartford published an article in *Laboratory Management* (1966) describing this interactive forum. In response to the article, many laboratory business managers wrote to Hartford requesting information on MIF and how they could start a similar organization. Hartford was amazed at the response and wondered if a national organization could serve many more laboratory business managers the way MIF served those at Yale. He placed a notice in *Science* in 1966 requesting anyone interested in a new organization for research administrators meet with him at the December 1966 meeting of the American Association for the Advancement of Science. The following three people showed up to meet with Hartford: T. Jack Stacy, Manager of Plans, Programs and Resources at the Midwest Research Institute, Kansas City, MO; David Meyer, Laboratory Business Manager in Biology at the University of Massachusetts; Richard Nicholson, Research Center Business Manager, Archer, Daniels, Midland Company. These four research administrators from varied research entities were harbingers for a broad base of membership for a new organization. As former SRA president Ken Beasley stated

> It is significant to note that the four founders were: all business managers for scientific research; 2) represented higher education, industry and a nonprofit research laboratory; and 3) felt the need for an organization to provide the exchange of mutual concerns between these sectors.[43]

The meeting resulted in a plan to test the interests in a new organization for research administrators by holding an organizational conference on June 1967 at the University of Massachusetts at Amherst.

One hundred people attended the Amherst meeting, including four women participants. The meeting sessions were in a lecture hall with Hartford presiding. The attendees came from the three sectors: university, industry and not-for-profit, with the universities having the highest representation.

For the conference, Nicholsen had prepared a preliminary constitution and bylaws for discussion, amendment and acceptance. The meeting consisted of going through both of these proposed documents, line by line, until there was an acceptable organization and the attendees were willing to commit to its creation. Discussions were lively, but in the end, the constitution and bylaws were approved for referral to the attendees at the next meeting in 1968, when they were later adopted. At the end of the meeting the following enacting resolution was passed. "We, the research administrators, present, hereby constitute ourselves into an organization."[44]

According to its constitution, the original purposes of SRA were to promote the exchange of information, encouraging research on research administration; develop professional standards; and improve the relationship between research administration and the general administration of the university, industry, profit and not-for-profit companies, medical research institutions, and federal agencies. The founding members stressed the need for education, recognition, and advancement. Attaining greater skills in research administration was an important goal of SRA. The emphasis was more on improving practices than on learning about what was going to happen in the granting agencies.

Another principal goal of SRA was to open the membership up to all research administrators regardless of the type of research organization or the administrative level of the applicant. The concept was that all research administrators could learn from each other and the open door membership policy recruited everyone to participate and learn. The Society formed five sections as regional parts of SRA. Canadian members joined SRA in the first years and, through the efforts of Justin Crawford, a Canadian group was formed and started regular meetings. In 1975, a Canadian section was chartered and led the way to broader international activities and membership.

Early Society programs focused on the goals of education and professional development. The annual meeting in the fall rotates by sections to different cities in the United States and Canada. The sections all have spring meetings. The meetings have keynote speakers, breakdown sessions, workshops, and social programs. Like other organizations, SRA has special workshops, seminars, teleconferences, and other means of electronic communications.

In the late 1980s and early 1990s, SRA pursued establishment of a certification program as a means of establishing levels of knowledge and professional qualifications for research administrators.

After a vigorous debate on the certification program, the SRA declined to pursue certification as a Society activity. The proponents of certification for research administrators continued, though, with their efforts through an independent organization, the Research Administrators Certification Council (RACC). International research administration has continued to be an active area for SRA. Many research administrators from other nations have attended SRA programs and Society members have attended conferences and presented programs in Europe and Asia. The publications of SRA include a professional journal, a member newsletter, books, pamphlets, and manuals. As part of the electronic age, SRA also uses teleconferences and other electronic means of communications.

In the 1990s, SRA began to add "International" to its name to represent its increasing international membership and its programs in Europe and the Far East (the name was officially changed to the International Society of Research Administrators with the adoption of new bylaws at the 2000 annual meeting).

In summary, the Society of Research Administrators International was founded to provide education and advancement for its members and became an open door organization for all research administrators, regardless of rank, employer, or location. Its policies and programs reflect the desire to serve this broad constituency through traditional and innovative activities. The original goals of SRA members were the improvement of practices in their everyday responsibilities and advancement in their profession. While keeping those early goals, SRA has developed into a large organization with many constituencies.

Organizations for Specific Areas

The five early organizations discussed earlier have been the leaders in building the profession of research administration. Later organizations were created to serve specific areas (e.g., the use of humans in research, patents and copyrights, animal care and use, conflict of interests, and the use of recombinant DNA). These specialized organizations attracted members with responsibilities in each specific area. Like the other organizations, the goals of these specialized groups were to educate and provide a forum for discussion. These special organizations will both increase and become more important as research administration becomes more specialized.

The five organizations described in this section have been successful in meeting the needs of their members. A major reason for their success is the enthusiasm and contributions of member volunteers. The size of the staff at each of the organizations is not large enough to achieve all that each has accomplished. The willingness of members to contribute their knowledge, talent, and time has extended the work of the staff members in all five organizations. The volunteers and staff have played a major role in building the profession of research administration.

Research Administration in Our Society

Research administration, in the 1980s and as it is generally known today, was conducted primarily in higher education, industry, for-profit and not-for-profit institutes, medical research institutions, government research agencies and laboratories. Recognition of research administration as a profession was not universally accepted in the 1950s and 1960s, but the profession has grown over time with the demonstration of competency. Changes in the practice of research administration have come, but the basic purposes and responsibilities of research administration continue.

Some of the significant changes in recent years have been:

1. Federal compliance regulations have increased. The first wave of research administrators in the 1940s did not have the plethora of regulations that are required today. The federal regulations of the time exclusively addressed grant and contract business areas. Today, the compliance regulations have increased the workload of research administration in many areas and often require additional staff and expertise.

2. The increased workload in research administration has led to differentiation of staff. Most of the early research administrators had general responsibilities in either the academic or business affairs divisions. Today, the requirements of the sponsors and the internal policies of the grantee organization require specialized duties with advanced training. The age of a few generalists has passed. Research administrative duties have evolved into an overall responsible administrator leading a group of specialists in required areas. The need for cross-training is evident.

3. The number of female research administrators has increased many times since 1945. The first research administrators were almost entirely male. Margery Hoppin of University of Iowa became the first female NCURA president in 1978. Lorraine Lasker of News York Medical College was appointed the first female president of the International Society of Research Administrators in 1975. Today, the membership of NCURA and SRA are more than 50 per cent female.

4. The last change has had a tremendous impact on the practice of research administration. Electronic research administration has changed the way business is done in the office and in communication with sponsors. The cyber world has brought grant information, application guidelines and forms, electronic submission of proposals, tracking of grant applications, making awards, instant reports of expenditures, schedules of reports due, federal regulation information, record keeping, and inventories of faculty research interests. This is only a partial list of the use of computers in research administration. Research administrators have to be competent with a computer in today's work environment. A computer specialist is also required to install and maintain new systems of electronic research administration in the office.

A summary of the history of research administration must start with a reminder of its role as a handmaiden to the research community and its success in enhancing research results. The definition of research administration is the administrative support required for success in research programs. Research administration is not an entity unto itself, rather it provides a service function for investigators. Raymond Woodrow emphasized this basic necessity in his book, *Management for Research in US Universities*, by stressing the word "for" in his title. Thus, success in research administration is the measurement of success in the research programs being served.

The American research enterprise expanded rapidly after World War II. The experiences of OSRD during the war, coupled with the ideas and initiatives of Vannevar Bush after the war, changed federal science policy from a haphazard approach of unrelated applied research projects to comprehensive funding for basic and applied research. The first result of the new national research policy was a major increase in support for research. The second result was a simultaneous increase in successful research that changed the lives of people around the world. The rise and leadership of US research since 1945 is a worldwide success story. Since 1945, US colleges and universities have become the preferred educational choice for international students, especially at the graduate and professional levels. The investment in research has and will continue to pay off for our society. Research will continue to unravel the unknown and change the future. For example three research areas that will have a tremendous impact on the future are: high energy physics with the promise of efficient, inexpensive, and non-polluting sources of energy; DNA research with the promise of eliminating diseases and sickness; and nanotechnology with the promise of incredibly small control systems.

As handmaidens to research, research administrators have played a major role in these accomplishments. The rise of research support dollars and the rise of research administration parallel each other. The scientist at the bench, the sociologist studying rural communities, and the educator determining effective learning styles do not have to spend their time with the administrative details of the grant or contract. Achieving the research goals of the institution is the goal of research administrators. Fiscal accountability and regulatory compliance with the sponsors are managed by the research administrators. Assistance in many ways helps the principal investigator make discoveries. Research administrators mediate differences and expedite programs. This new profession arose from a need to manage the rapid growth of research awards. It expanded and increased efficiency with experience and sharing information through professional associations. The number of research administrators will continue to increase and the research administration roles will continue to develop to and there will be continued need to adapt to changes in research policies. As research administration continues to mature, it is important to remember that it does not exist for itself: the fundamental purpose of research administration is to enhance the ability to carry out successful research.

• • • References

1. Dupree, A.H. *Science in the Federal Government: A History of Policies and Activities to 1940.* Cambridge, MA: The Belknap Press of Harvard University, 1957, 4.

2. Ibid, 4.

3. Ibid, 4.

4. U.S. Constitution, art. I, sec. 8.

5. U.S. Congress. House. Task Force on Science Policy, Committee on Science and Technology. "A History of Science Policy in the United States, 1940–1985." *Science Policy Background Report No. 1.* 99th Cong., 2d sess. Washington, DC: U.S. Government Printing Office, 1986, 5.

6. Ibid, 6.

7. Ibid, 7.

8. Ibid, 7.

9. Ibid, 7.

10. Ibid, 8.

11. Ibid, 8.

12. Ibid, 9

13. Childs, H. *An American Genius: The Life of Ernest Orlando Lawrence.* New York: E.P. Dutton & Company, Inc., 1968, 191.

14. Bush, V. *Science: The Endless Frontier; A Report to the President on a Program of Post War Scientific Research.* Reprint. Washington, DC: National Science Foundation, 1990, ix.

15. Ibid, ix.

16. U.S. Congress. House. Task Force on Science Policy, Committee on Science and Technology. "A History of Science Policy in the United States, 1940–1985." *Science Policy Background Report No. 1.* 99th Cong., 2d sess. Washington, DC: U.S. Government Printing Office, 1986, 17.

17. Bush, V. *Science: The Endless Frontier; A Report to the President on a Program of Post War Scientific Research.* Reprint. Washington, DC: National Science Foundation, 1990, xii.

18. U.S. Congress. House. Task Force on Science Policy, Committee on Science and Technology. "A History of Science Policy in the United States, 1940–1985." *Science Policy Background Report No. 1.* 99th Cong., 2d sess. Washington, DC: U.S. Government Printing Office, 1986, 30.

19. Ibid, 37.

20. Schaffter, D. *The National Science Foundation.* New York and London: Frederick A. Praeger Publishers, 1969, 59.

21. U.S. Congress. House. Task Force on Science Policy, Committee on Science and Technology. "A History of Science Policy in the United States, 1940–1985." *Science Policy Background Report No. 1.* 99th Cong., 2d sess. Washington, DC: U.S. Government Printing Office, 1986, 33.

22. Ibid, 33.

23. U.S. Congress. House. Task Force on Science Policy, Committee on Science and Technology. "A History of Science Policy in the United States, 1940–1985." *Science Policy Background Report No. 1.* 99th Cong., 2d sess. Washington, DC: U.S. Government Printing Office, 1986, 62.

24. Schaffter, D. *The National Science Foundation.* New York and London: Frederick A. Praeger Publishers, 1969, 132.

25. U.S. Congress. House. Task Force on Science Policy, Committee on Science and Technology.

"A History of Science Policy in the United States, 1940–1985." *Science Policy Background Report No. 1.* 99th Cong., 2d sess. Washington, DC: U.S. Government Printing Office, 1986, 28.

26. *NIH Almanac.* Washington, DC: NIH Publication 97-5, September 1997: 115.

27. Beasley, K. "The Research Administrator as Mediator-Expediter." *Journal of the Society of Research Administrators* 2, no. 1 (1970): 4.

28. George, K. Interview by Kenneth Beasley in Del Ray Beach, FL, March 2003.

29. "Woodrow R. Woodrow's acceptance speech as recipient of the Society of Research Administrators Distinguished Contributions to Research Administration Award." *SRA Newsletter* 10, no. 2 (1977): 1.

30. The Council on Government Relations. *A Historical Review.* Washington, DC: 1997, 25.

31. Office of Management and Budget. *Catalogue of Federal Domestic Assistance.* 1995 ed. Washington, DC: Government Printing Office, 1995, xi.

32. Moye, W.T. *NCAR 50th Year: National Conference on the Advancement of Research*, 1997, 2.

33. Ibid, 2.

34. Ibid, 3.

35. Wile, H. *The Committee on Government Relations: A Historical View.* Washington, DC: National Association of College and University Business Officers, September 19, 1975, 1.

36. Ibid, 4.

37. Seckinger, S. S. *We Gather Together: An Account of the Biennial Conferences on Research Administration.* Denver: University of Denver, 1982, 1.

38. Ibid, 15.

39. Ibid, 30.

40. Ibid, 20.

41. Murray, D. S. *Memorandum to the Ad Hoc Committee for Establishing NCURA: Summary of the Meeting at the Cornell Aeronautical Laboratory.* Ithaca, NY, November 12, 1958.

42. Wile, H. "The Twenty-Five Year History of NCURA: ROOTS." *NCURA Newsletter* (June 1980): 5.

43. Beasley, K. "The Premise and the Promise of the Founding Years of SRA." *SRA Journal* 20, no. 1 (1988): 5–9.

44. Nicholsen, R. "History of the Society of Research Administrators." *SRA Journal* 1, no. 1 (1969): 70.

The Future of Research Administration in the 21st Century: Looking into the Crystal Ball

Elliott C. Kulakowski, PhD, FAHA, and Lynne U. Chronister, MPA

Introduction

> Providing effective support to the extraordinary research enterprise that has grown up since the Second World War will be a challenge.
>
> *(Source: Erich Bloch, 1990)*[1]

Research administration and management as a profession is growing and evolving. The future will be filled with new challenges, but it will create many opportunities for researchers and its managers and leaders. The statement that "if you are doing things the same way five years from now as you are today, you will be far behind" applies to the future of research administration. Research managers need to be prepared to take advantage of what the future holds.

Research administration has a basic core of knowledge that remains relatively constant. However, research administrators in the future will need to be more knowledgeable, better trained and have different skills in a totally different high technology environment. This book attempts to present the state of knowledge of research management. Research and its management are conducted within the context of the politics of the times. The political realities of post-September 11th on the United States continue to alter the types of research that are supported by the federal government. Research support is shifting away from basic and applied research to a more developmental focus. The National Science Foundation definitions of basic, applied, and developmental research are as follows:

"**Basic Research:** The objective of basic research is to gain more comprehensive knowledge or understanding of the subject under study without specific applications in mind. In industry, basic research is defined as research that advances scientific knowledge but does not have specific immediate commercial objectives, although it may be in fields of present or potential commercial interest.

Applied Research: Applied research is aimed at gaining the knowledge or understanding to meet a specific, recognized need. In industry, applied research includes investigations oriented to discovering new scientific knowledge that has specific commercial objectives with respect to products, processes, or services.

Development: Development is the systematic use of the knowledge or understanding gained from research directed toward the production of useful materials, devices, systems, or methods, including the design and development of prototypes and processes."[2]

Collectively, basic and applied research is referred to as *fundamental research*. Much focus today is upon the problem-based or functional research that is specifically directed toward solving societal problems.

In this chapter we will discuss that in the future there will be less of an emphasis on fundamental research and more emphasis on developmental research. With the change in research priorities, the growth of research supported by traditional funding agencies will show little growth except for those areas that support the mission of the Department of Homeland Security and the Department of Defense. Export control regulations will be more strictly enforced and foreign trainees and researchers will have less access to US technologies and development research opportunities. At the same time the federal government will streamline proposal submissions and certain research management procedures while other regulations, such as those related to the responsible conduct of research, will be of decreasing federal importance unless there is a major public tragedy.

From the institutional perspective, the research manager will have a new set of skills. Electronic research administration will lead to a near paperless office. While the office will be more streamlined, it should not be interpreted as a cost-saving measure. Staff will be expected to do more with their new skills and the cost of ever-improving technology is high. The increased emphasis on multidisciplinary research will become more worldwide and research managers will need to be more versed in issues related to international research. With an increased emphasis on cost of research and ever-expanding budgets, it is critical to review the fiscal environment wherein research is supported and enhanced. These realities are explored in the following section of the text.

The National Fiscal and Policy Context for the Administration of the Research Enterprise

The United States has over 3,300 public and private, not-for-profit and for-profit colleges and universities. Since World War II, research has been a cornerstone of the tripartite mission of many of those institutions. Research and development (R&D) operate in an environment that is dictated in large part by the political and socio-cultural environment within which we live. What political party is dominant and the level of fiscal and social conservatism or liberalism heavily influences research policy, priorities, and the requisite funding for research foci.[3] The correlation is not exact, with embryonic stem cell research a prime example. The debate over stem cell research is a prime example of the influence of politics on research. In 2002, the federal government policy restricted research using embryonic stem to a few lines. Federal support for research was limited and, as a result, many researchers immigrated to the United Kingdom and European countries that did not have the restrictions imposed by the US government. However, in 2004 and 2005, selected states, led for example by Proposition 71 in

California, set in motion the policies and funding necessary to broaden stem cell research with state and private funding. California set aside up to $3 billion as investment into stem cell research and other states followed with smaller but critical investments. Some of the critical social and fiscal environmental factors are described in order to put into context the leadership and management of the research enterprise.

Fiscal Environment Supporting the Research Enterprise

While recognizing that funding for research and development is a means to an end and that the returns on investment include enhancement of quality of life, not just monetary gain, the fiscal environment is still a critical driving force. In recent years, universities internationally have focused extensive resources on enhancing their research capacity. In 2002, the expenditures for research at US universities were estimated at $36.3 billion. With over $283 billion dollars in all sectors invested in research, including academics, government, and the private sector, external support for research has become a major source of revenue for institutions and a large percentage of a research institution's total expenditures. Over $54 billion is expended on basic research, which is a main emphasis at US academic institutions.[a]

Sources of Support

With competition increasing for research funding, researchers and administrators are seeking nontraditional, as well as established sources of grant and contract mechanisms of support. Historically, government, industry, and, more recently, nonprofit foundations have been the primary supporters of research. The portfolio of sponsors has expanded to include a much broader support base. State and local governments are seeking university research support especially in the areas of health, transportation, agriculture, public service, and utilities and the environment. In 2002, state and local support at colleges and universities reached a high of $2.5 billion.[b] Some of the funds are competitive or block grants

---

[a]www.nsf.gov/sbe/srs

[b]www.nsf.gov

from federal sources and a smaller percentage are allocated from the state revenues. In addition, states frequently look to colleges or universities to carry out surveys, planning, and training activities. Figures for non-R&D support are not nationally available, but in some states they are a critical source of research and service funding.

Agricultural research is supported jointly by the US Department of Agriculture and state and county allocations for experiment stations and agriculture extension services. Commodity boards, such as those for dairy and rice, and associations, such as the cattlemen's association, provide targeted support for research. These boards generally require flexible policies on the part of the recipient because of somewhat stringent funding requirements. Other types of trade associations, like the building and construction trades, may also provide limited funding for research. Foundations such as American Heart Association and March of Dimes, that are disease-specific, and similar foundations that target specific diseases, account for a considerable amount of financial support for colleges and universities. In 2002, these sources other than government and industry accounted for $2.7 billion of the R&D support.[c]

In 2003, industry spent $193.7 billion on R&D with a modest amount contracted out to research institutions.[d] Industrial outsourcing of research and development has fluctuated but has shown strong increases over the past 50 years. In 1953, industry support for R&D at colleges and universities was recorded by the Office of Management and Budget (OMB) at $19 million. By 2002, this number increased to $2,188 billion.[e] This figure is down from 2001, a year when industry felt the lowering of the economy in many sectors and federal support for industry decreased. With constant dollars there still have been increases in the support from industry over the last five decades. Generally the research dollars are noncompetitive with most of the support targeted to very specific industry-relevant research.

The federal government established itself in the early 1950s as the largest source of R&D funding to colleges and universities. In 1953 the federal government funding for research totaled $255 million, increasing to $2,283.8 billion in 2003 with the majority of the nondefense funds targeted to health-related research. Understanding the sources of sup-

port assists in long-range planning for institutions seeking external support and information regarding how to invest institutional dollars. Since 1953, institutional R&D support has increased from $35 million to $7.2 billion in 2002.[f] With the advance of support for large and collaborative science, it is critical to leverage various private and public sources of support in order to achieve successful research programs.

Mechanisms of Support of Research and Development

The mechanisms for the award or transfer of research and support for other scholarly activities to recipients are competitive, noncompetitive, or quasicompetitive. They include grants, contracts, cooperative agreements, gifts, purchase orders, and many others. While government entities do not provide gifts or donations, industry, foundations, private individuals, associations, and other private sources do make gifts and donations to support basic research and other scholarly programs. The most common form of providing support both for large programs and centers, as well as for individual projects, is through the granting process. The majority of federal support and much of foundation support use the grant or cooperative agreement mechanism for making awards. Grants come with fewer constraints on the deliverables expected from the award. Cooperative agreements anticipate more oversight and collaboration with the sponsor.

Industry and some programs sponsored by federal agencies make awards through contracts that are much more restrictive in both the implementation of the award and the expected outcomes. Increasingly federal sponsors are using the "Other Agreement," an award mechanism that is most closely aligned to a contract, and which gives even more latitude and flexibility to the sponsor to attach terms and conditions to the award. Federal flow-through funds are subawards from a prime recipient and the subrecipient could receive a subgrant or subcontract depending on the type of prime agreement.

Earmarked or directed funding has had a fluctuating history. Some administrations and some congresses have favored the earmarking process while others have not been as aggressive in targeting funds to causes or constituents. Regardless,

[c]www.nsf.gov/sbe/srs

[d]www.nsf.gov/sbe/srs

[e]www.whitehouse.gov/omb/reports

[f]www.nsf.gov/sbe/srs

billions of dollars have flowed to institutions for support of a wide variety of programs and projects. Generally these funds are authorized and funds appropriated to a federal agency that in turn will make a grant or contract award to the named recipient. In some instances, earmarked funds will require a quasicompetition for funds. Some institutions are supportive of the process of earmarking. Other institutions, including the University of California, have policies that do not support earmarking if competitive programs are available.

Investment in Research and Development

Knowledge of the national and international trends in funding for research is necessary to project strategic investments in research at institutions. One measure that is used internationally to reflect the health of the research and development investments is the R&D expenditures as a percent of the Gross Domestic Product (GDP), the measure of a nation's total economic activity. In 2003, the United States ranked fifth in overall R&D support as a percent of GDP behind Sweden, Finland, Japan, and China. Government funding was ranked fifth, while industry funding in 2003 for R&D as a percent of GDP ranked sixth. The United States ranked first in total dollars invested in R&D with Japan and China as second and third respectively. That same year, the United States expended 38% of all R&D invested worldwide, down from 40% the prior year. This percentage includes government and private sources. As impressive as these percentages are, they represent less than a 2% increase in R&D as a percent of GDP growth since 2000. The United States ranked 7th in rate of growth for R&D funds in 2002.[g]

Despite declining economic growth, industry historically has expended the largest actual dollar amount on R&D. In 1999 industry provided $169.3 billion or 68% of total US R&D. By 2003 the percentage has declined to 63%; however, industry actually performed 68% of all R&D in that year. In contrast, the federal government supported 30% of all R&D and performed 9% of the research. In 2004 the federal government budgeted $127 billion for R&D, and in 2005, $132B was appropriated, the largest amount ever approved by Congress.[4] However, according to the OMB, the amount of dollars available for R&D are declining

in constant dollars.[h] The actual dollars available for discretionary programs is decreasing rapidly because of the growing number of entitlements.

Federal Support for Research

Change in budgets from 1998 and 1999 during the Clinton administration and the budget passed by Congress for 2005 under the Bush administration exemplify the effect that administrative priorities have appropriations. In 1998 and 1999, a high priority was placed upon balancing the federal budget and reducing the debt. Energy conservation, health-related research and wellness and the environment were high priorities. The R&D budget for 1998 was $76.3 billion. In 1998 the defense R&D was budgeted at $41 billion while the 2005 defense appropriation was $70.3 billion, plus $1.2B for the Department of Homeland Security (DHS), almost equal to the entire R&D budget for 1998. Nondefense in 1998 was budgeted at $35.5 billion however by 2005, the nondefense appropriation of $60 billion represented severe decreases from the previous four years. Of the 24 federal agencies sponsoring R&D, only the DHS, the Department of Defense (DOD), and NASA saw reasonable budget increases for 2005. Some budgets were drastically cut in the 2005 budget. DOD Medical Research was cut 86% and the Department of Energy's Clean Coal Research Program was eliminated. NASA received large increases in Exploratory Science, part of the Moon to Mars program.[5]

Total Cost Research

Knowledge of federal policies, priorities, and appropriations, along with national and international fiscal and programmatic trends, are critical components for developing or sustaining a strong and vibrant research program at any institution. Information regarding new policy directions aids in identifying future federal and industrial support for research. An additional component necessary for the research administrator is to have a full understanding of the total cost of research. The funds provided by external sponsors of research represent only a fraction of the total cost of research, even when overhead costs are factored in through the addition of indirect cost (IDC) or facilities and administrative (F&A) rate. The institutional cost of R&D

---

[g]NSF, Science and Engineering Indicators, 2000, www.compete.org.

[h]www.whitehouse.gov/omb.

through cost-sharing or matching funds, indirect cost-recovery and direct institutional support do not constitute total project costs. The NSF estimated that in 2002 universities invested $7.2 billion in research but that did not include the cost of compliance. With the increased number of unfunded mandates, the cost of administering research has grown tremendously. The Health Insurance Portability and Accountability Act (HIPAA), implemented in 2003, is a prime example of a compliance mandate the cost of which is borne solely by the institutions and providers. The Council on Government Relations (COGR) reported in a 2003 study on the cost of compliance that a sample of 25 institutions "average incremental expenditures range from approximately $1.8 million per institution in 2000 to approximately $4.1 million of projected expenditures per institution in 2003."[6] Only one of the twenty-five institutions reported that their administrative costs did not exceed the 26% cap that OMB incorporated into the allowable administrative costs of the facilities and administrative (indirect cost) calculations in 1991.

As institutions work through the long-term strategic planning process, one objective should be to do projections on both the total anticipated revenue as well as the total cost of the research enterprise. While the F&A rate is designed to cover those costs not directly budgeted, the administrative portion of the formula as of 2005 is still capped at 26%. This means that the full cost of administration, including escalating compliance costs, are not fully accounted for in the F&A. Another factor is that the institution does not recover the fully allowable F&A and may not recover more than 50% of potential F&A revenue.

Shift in Emphasis of US Federally Funded Research

The future of US federally funded research is changing. In the 1990s there was a resurgence of efforts to support basic science research. There was the Human Genome Project, the doubling of the NIH budget, and support for the doubling of the NSF budget. There was an increased focus on multidisciplinary research, transnational research, clinical research, and the development of the next generation of instrumentation for scientific and clinical diagnostic purposes. The federal deficit looked bright and there a surplus of funds in the government's coffers to a support these efforts.

However the events surrounding September 11, 2001 changed the emphasis on research and research administration for the immediate future. There is a growing shift toward less fundamental research and more toward developmental research with defense applications.[i]

There is an ongoing major expansion of the DOD research budget that will last for at least the next five to ten years. The DHS was created and was responsible for coordinating the homeland security efforts of several funding agencies. New and expanded funding opportunities related to chemical, biological, radiation and nuclear (CBRN) defense both nationally and militarily have become available. While the overall National Institutes of Health budget has been relatively flat, the role of the National Institute of Allergy and Infectious Diseases related to homeland security has grown tremendously, as has its budget to more application-based research. With the first attack on the shores of the continental United States in nearly 200 years, the potential threats to our freedom and safety are real. The shift continued shift to an increase in funding to support CBRN defense programs will continue in the foreseeable future. Research institutions are examining the shift in funding priorities. Investigators are reengineering themselves and their skills or research focus to take advantage of the new funding opportunities.

Export Control

The Export Administration Regulations (EAR) and International Traffic in Arms Regulations (ITAA) are discussed in detail in Part V. The regulations limit the export of certain developmental research information, prohibit the foreign export of certain tangible items or require license from the federal government, and the regulations can be interpreted to restrict technological access by nonpermanent residents of the United States. This can be viewed as technological isolationism or economic nationalism and also may result in immigration restrictions. Regardless of how it is categorized, it has the potential to hamper academic research in the United States.

Current export regulations restrict activities related to developmental research and technology export. Since the advent of the export control

[i]www.aaas.org/spp/rd

regulations, the Department of Commerce, the agency cognizant of implementing EAR, has focused nearly all of its intentions on industry. However, it has come to the attention of federal funding agencies that academic institutions are engaged in a variety of international activities. They are shipping tangible items and restricted data outside of the United States to other academic institutions and commercial entities. While the federal government is shifting its funding priorities toward research development and while academic institutions also are being asked to play a greater role in economic development in the United States, they are collaborating internationally on research development. In addition, academic institutions conduct much of this developmental research with nonpermanent resident foreign nationals and provide training to them, which is controlled by export control laws. The result is that the application of export control regulations as they pertain to academic institutions is receiving a great deal of scrutiny.

The export control regulations do provide for a "fundamental research" exclusion. However, recent reports from various federal agencies suggest that the fundamental research exclusion should be abolished. Currently the definition of basic research is under question as well. The long-standing exclusion is being diluted with a recent clarifying statement that the determination of whether or not research is fundamental can be determined after the conclusion of the research. The fate of the fundamental exclusion is to be determined. The future impact on academia is tremendous. The very cornerstone of academic freedom—the free exchange of ideas—is threatened if the regulations change.

It must be recognized that nonpermanent resident graduate students and postdoctoral trainees conduct much of the research efforts in the United States. The recent trend has been that foreign graduate students make up a growing proportion of students pursuing graduate degrees in the United States. The Chronicle of Higher Education on November 19, 2004 reported that for the first time since 1971 the number of foreign students in the United States has decreased.[7] Yet, American students have not been pursing graduate degrees at nearly the levels necessary to meet the needs of research institutions. Institutions have been forced to recruit foreign trainees to meet their needs. If foreign trainees are restricted from developmental research activities or what they can learn, they will be less inclined to come to the United States to train.[8]

If such policy continues, it will result in technological isolationism that will surely backfire on the United States and the terrorists who attacked the United States will have gained another victory. Even with American and foreign science trainees, there remains a need for more trainees to conduct research. Compounded by a shortage of foreign trainees who are restricted from participation in research in the United States, we will have a major crisis in academia. Additional American trainees cannot overcome the deficit, because they are not pursuing advanced scientific degrees at increasing levels. With appropriate incentives in place, it would still take several years to prime the academic pipeline to produce a sufficient number of trainees and the research enterprise and future technology advances will suffer in the meantime. If the export restrictions are strictly enforced or expanded to include fundamental research, the future of academic research enterprise in university settings will be threatened. The result will be a technological void and a decline in economic development in the United States that could lead to a recession.

Streamlined Federal Research Management Procedures

The Federal Demonstration Partnership (FDP) began in 1980 as the Federal Demonstration Project to identify areas of opportunity where federal processes related to the external funding of projects and educational programs at institutions could be streamlined and to develop and implement such procedures. It was hoped that such procedural changes, whether through guidances or changes in regulations, could reduce the administrative burden for administrators and faculty at the various institutions.[9]

Individuals serving as institutional representatives on the FDP include members from the federal funding agencies, recipients of the funding, and affiliate members. The federal funding agencies include the Air Force Office of Scientific Research (AFOSR), Army Medical Research Command (AMRMC), Army Research Office (ARO), Department of Energy (DOE), Environmental Protection Agency (EPA), National Aeronautics and Space Administration (NASA), National Institutes of Health (NIH), National Science Foundation (NSF), Office of Naval Research (ONR), and Department of Agriculture (USDA). The institutional recipients for federal awards include academic institutions, research institutes, and research hospitals. The affiliate members are comprised of the major research administration organizations in the United States, including the

Council on Government Relations, the National Council of University Research Administrators, and the Society of Research Administrators International. Participants also include the National Academy of Science's Government University Industry Research Roundtable. While originally conceived to be a meeting ground for discussions among administrators, faculty participation was added in 2003 and the FDP continues to evolve.[10]

The FDP has been growing in importance in recent years and its future is bright. Current FDP initiatives and issues can be found at the FDP Web site.[11,12] These include a number of OMB notices, federal agency notices, research business models, e-government initiatives, and other issues. The progress in 2003 and 2004 has been tremendous and the outlook for the future is even greater.

There is a growing perception that, based on its recent successes, the opportunity for the FDP to play an expanded role in management of the federal research enterprise is great. Issues that will be discussed and acted upon by the FDP in the coming months and years include the process of streamlining federal financial management; time and effort reporting; award terms and conditions; research business models; space allocation; contracting; and electronic research administration.

Responsible Conduct of Research

In 2000, the US Public Health Service (PHS) was moving toward requiring institutions receiving PHS support to implement an educational program, Responsible Conduct of Research (RCR).[13] The PHS policy was promulgated as the minimum standards that an institution should strive to achieve in education. However, the standards have subsequently been suspended. While some institutions felt that they were being overburdened by federal regulations, more progressive institutions thought the guidelines were important. Other institutions implemented the policy thinking it was a matter of time before the guidelines would resurface as regulations. The latter two types of institutions established offices for responsible conduct of research and implemented the minimum standards. The structure of these offices differed among institutions. Many of them brought together the human subjects protections program, the animal care and use program, and a conflict of interest committee under a single office. In response, institutions hired associate vice presidents or directors of research

integrity. They also hired or recruited from within their faculty ethicists, philosophers, and lawyers to develop and provide comprehensive training programs for faculty and trainees to discuss and teach the concepts of responsible conducts of research.

The importance of RCR was never more evident than in 2001 when the Office of Human Research Protections and the Office of Research Integrity brought together leaders in the area for what would become the Responsible Conduct of Research Education Consortium.[14] Subsequently, a Responsible Conduct of Research Interest Group was established within the Society for Research Administrators (SRA). Both SRA and the National Council of University Research Administrators (NCURA) also provide a variety of workshops, meeting sessions, and video-conferences on responsible conduct of research topics. Textbooks also have been written to provide the basis for educational programs.

For the most part, institutions, to varying degrees, have attempted to establish appropriate policies, to enforce them and to train their faculty and staff about responsible conduct of research. Time has come for institutions to go beyond the regulations and to begin to examine the underlying ethos behind the regulations. There is a need to take a more Socratic look at the purpose of engaging in responsible conduct of research. There is an apparent sentiment in the current federal administration that implementing such a policy would increase regulatory burden on the institutions. Therefore, it is not being pursued at this time. The future for a more philosophical dialogue and understanding of the underlying reasons for conducting research responsibly may continue at some level, however, it will not be a major endeavor among research institutions in the near future.

The reluctance to initiate new regulation by the Office of Research Integrity has not gone unnoticed. Institutions have observed what they perceive as a change in philosophy within the upper levels of the federal government, and they are beginning to respond accordingly. Programs related to responsible conduct of research cost money. They are unrecoverable costs that either erode an institution's facilities and administrative (F&A) revenues or require the institution to look to other sources of support for these programs when an institution's administrative costs exceed the 26% F&A cap. Institutions are beginning to take some cost saving measures by scaling back such programs or decentralizing them to a college or department level where programs may not be uniformly developed, presented, or emphasized. Columbia University, which once had a strong centralized responsible conduct of research program, appears to be shifting toward a less centralized model whereby training in responsible conduct of research may be at the college level. It is uncertain whether the commitment at a college or department level would be the same as through a centralized office.

In research administration, we have all heard that "the future is electronic" and truly it is. Virtually every nonprofit funder has a Web site today that lists their funding opportunities and criteria. The basic requirements for responsible conduct of research will remain. Strong voices in the federal government, including that of Chris Pascal, the Director of the Office of Research Integrity for the Department of Health and Human Services, will continue to advocate for expanded efforts related to responsible conduct of research.[11] Despite his and others' efforts, the regulatory climate within the federal government appears to signal that this is less of a priority than in the past on regulatory issues. It is unfortunate, but unless a major incident occurs at an institution to raise public and congressional awareness, it is unlikely that in the next four to five years there will be an increased emphasis on responsible conduct of research.

Electronic Research Administration

Whether you are seeking to identify funding sources for an externally sponsored activity, or to find application forms, methods of tracking applications, awards, expenditures, and reporting, the most comprehensive sources are electronic. The future is here today. The increasing availability and sheer number of resources available electronically continue to extend the management challenges of research administration.

While some funding opportunities are still distributed by mail, they are less frequent, and today the sponsor's mailings often refer a potential applicant to their Web site. As fewer funding opportunities are found and initiated in hard copy, applicants are most often directed to Web site resources to identify funding sources. The success of such databases is that they can be available at relatively no mailing cost, can be updated daily, if necessary, and can be available instantly to potential applicants. All the federal agencies post funding opportunities on specific Web sites for example the NIH has the electronic NIH Guide for Grants and Contracts, and the

NSF releases the E-Bulletin. Federal contracting opportunities, whether research related or not, can be found in the Federal Register (www.gpo.gov). In the future electronic funding opportunities for the US federal government will use Grants.gov, where all federal funding announcements related to grants and contracts will be posted. The Community of Science, a for-profit organization, claims to be the world's largest source for identifying funding opportunities and includes federal, as well as industry and nonprofit funding opportunities. Research administration offices within the past ten years have begun to switch from collecting hardcopy of sponsor guidelines and application forms in file cabinets to collecting Web addresses, which saves the time taken to updating paper forms and guidelines, and reduces the space needed for such forms and applications. Through a bookmarker Web search, the latest information can be quickly identified and transmitted to potential applicants in a matter of seconds.

The process of submission of proposals also is changing. While forms are found on Web pages and downloaded, they are nearly always printed off, completed, signed by the principal investigator, walked to the department chair, and dean for approval on internal clearance forms and hand carried to sponsored projects office for signature. Copies are then made and mailed to the sponsor. A new paradigm for proposal development and submission is emerging, but will take several years before it is universally acceptable. The NSF has been a leader in this endeavor within the federal government with the development and implementation of FastLane. However, because of the ease of use and academic support for FastLane that it will be replaced with Grants.gov, which is still in its infancy. The NIH is using Grants.gov on a trial basis for certain programs and is looking at third party companies to manage the submission of grants, but, as of 2005, some flaws in the process remain, for example, for investigators who cannot submit proposals with Macintosh computers.

In addition to the inconsistent functionality of electronic proposal submissions, there is the issue of institutional routing of proposals for approval and final sign-off by the authorized institutional official. Individual institutions and companies are developing such routing systems. In the future the principal investigator will be able to complete the proposal electronically and append it electronically to the online internal clearance form, along with any needed regulatory compliance assurances or approvals. The investigator will then forward the proposal electronically for appropriate approvals by a department chair, who can then forward the proposal to a dean. Following a dean's approval, the entire information package will then be directed electronically to the research office for final review and approval or the package will be redirected back to the principal investigator for submission. There would be no paper copies of any information. The paper file will be replaced with a re-writable CD or the latest state-of-the-art storage media that contains all the information on a particular proposal. Current limitations for implementing this broadly are the ability of the sponsors to capture the large number of proposals, appropriate programs for internal document transmission, and adequate e-authentication acceptable to sponsors.

On the post-award side, many sponsors already provide electronic awards through e-mails. This will be extended in the future to all sponsors. The award information will be captured on the proposal CD or in the research office, transmitted to the principal investigator and the finance office. There are a number of grant-tracking databases available depending on the size of the institution. A number of smaller institutions have developed their own grant-tracking mechanisms that may be Excel- or Access-based. Other more sophisticated systems are available. InfoEd, PeopleSoft, RAMS, Banner, COEUS and other commercially developed software are being adapted by a number of large universities across the country.

International Research Management

The research enterprise in the United States has undergone a tremendous change since World War II. Research investment by the federal government and industry in research at academic institutions, research institutes, and hospitals is at an all-time high. The outgrowth of research has been the development of new inventions. As more and more research is being conducted, the accepted norms for conducting research are also evolving from few regulations, to more, and now to a focus on the ethics of the research.

In the broadest sense this has led to the creation of research administration and management as a career. There are now those who specialize in identifying research opportunities, pre-award, contracting, post-award, grant and contract accountants. In addition, research administrators can specialize in various aspects of technology transfer

including patenting, marketing, and licensing as specialties. There has been a growing focus on regulatory compliance with research administrators specializing in human subjects' protection, animal welfare, conflict of interest, environmental health, and safety, just to name a few. The breadth of research administration can be seen in the various chapters in this book.

As research has grown in the United States, so too has the concept of those engaged in research administration. Research administration, which was once perceived as a clerical position or managed by a part-time faculty member, has grown into a profession as it has become more complex. To keep abreast of the fiscal and regulatory changes, organizations developed to aid institutions. Among them are the Council on Government Relations (COGR), National Council of University Research Administrators (NCURA) and the Society of Research Administrators International (SRA) that deal with the spectrum of research administration issues. Others such as the Association of University Technology Managers (AUTM) and the Licensing Executives Society deal exclusively with technology transfer, and for regulatory issues there are organizations such as the Public Responsibility in Research and Medicine and the recently created Responsible Conduct of Research Education Consortium. New research administration organizations will continue to develop to meet the needs of the profession.

Growth of research administration is not unique to the United States. Different countries have progressed at different paces. Canada developed in much the same time frame as the United States. In Canada there is Canadian Association of University Research Administrators (CAURA) and SRA has a chapter in Canada. Today in the United Kingdom and Australia research administration and management is recognized as a profession and both countries have professional societies. Within the last decade we saw the formation of the Economic Union and the development of the European Association of Research Managers and Administrators (EARMA). We see countries in Africa such as South Africa, Nigeria, and Kenya, where the academic institutions are beginning to see the need for research administration and are seeking appropriate training both at their institutions and at international meetings. Since the end of the cold war there has been a shift in Russia toward a greater focus on economic advancement through research, technologies coming from their institutions and the need to manage it properly. They are exploring means to bring representatives from the United States to

Russia to train them in research administration and are planning to visit American universities for internships. As research becomes more complex and specialized there will be a growth of international research collaborations and a need for a greater understanding of the issues of research administration. To this end, an International Network of Research Management Societies (INORMS) was established in 2001 in Vancouver, British Columbia. This organization of the various international societies of research administration is growing in international societies, and in the next few years it has the potential to serve as the hub for international collaboration of research administrative activities.

Summary

Research leadership and management, collectively labeled research administration, has come a long way as a profession since World War II. However, its roles are still expanding and it will continue to adapt to the changing political environment in which research and other sponsored activities are conducted.

• • • References

1. Bush, V. *Science–The Endless Frontier, (40th Anniversary Edition).* Foreword by Erich Bloch. Washington, DC: National Science Foundation, 1990.
2. National Science Foundation, "Definitions of Research and Development in Science and Engineering Indicators 2002," http://www.nsf.gov/sbe/srs/seind02/c4/c4s1.htm#definitions (accessed December 31, 2004).
3. Smith, B. L. R. *American Science Policy Since World War II.* Washington, DC: The Brookings Institution Press, 1990.
4. Koizume, K. "Analysis of 2005 US Spending Measures Finds Mixed News for R&S," Association for the Advancement of Science (AAAS), www.aaas.org/news (accessed December 2004).
5. Association for the Advancement of Science (AAAS), "Defense and Homeland Security R&D Gain, Other R&D Programs Face Looming Cuts in Slow Moving 2005 Budget," *Analysis of Out Year Projections for R&D*, August 2004, www.aaas (accessed October 18, 2004).
6. Council on Governmental Relations, *Report of the Working Group on the Cost of Doing Business,* June 2, 2003, Washington, DC: CDGR.
7. Bollag, B. "Enrollment of Foreign Students Drops in the U.S.," *The Chronicle of Higher Education.* November 19, 2004, A1.
8. Bollag, 2004.
9. Federal Demonstration Partnership, "About FDP," http://thefdp.org/About_FDP.html (accessed December 31, 2004).
10. Federal Demonstration Partnership "FDP Members," http://thefdp.org/FDP_Members.html (accessed December 31, 2004).
11. Federal Demonstration Partnership. "Current Initiatives," http://thefdp.org/Current_Initiatives.html (accessed December 31, 2004).
12. Federal Demonstration Partnership, "Issues," http://thefdp.org/issues.html (accessed December 31, 2004).
13. U.S. Department of Health and Human Services, Office of Research Integrity, "PHS Policy on Instruction in the Responsible Conduct of Research (RCR)," http://www.ori.hhs.gov/policies/RCR_Policy.shtml (accessed December 31, 2004).
14. Responsible Conduct of Research Education Consortium. Web site, http://rcrec.org (accessed December 31, 2004).

4

The Organization of the Research Enterprise

Lynne U. Chronister, MPA, and Robert Killoren, MA, CRA

In the biological world, form seems to follow function, which helps to explain a few of the more unusual creatures on earth like the giraffe and pelican—but what about the hippopotamus? That must be a case of form gone awry. In the organizational world, function also generally dictates form or structure, though we do occasionally find anomalies. The research enterprise is no different. There are typical organizational structures, but many other forms that are equally appropriate. In this section information will be provided for determining or reviewing:

- functional and service units;
- the structure of the research organization;
- roles and responsibilities, authorities; and
- the costs associated with administration of research.

None of the elements are independent but impact each other and are tightly interrelated. The organization must have common goals and objectives and must communicate regardless of structure, individual and group roles, responsibilities, and authorities. This chapter will capture the essence of both the critical functions and the structures associated with the management and leadership of the research enterprise. Each of the topics discussed is further elucidated in subsequent chapters and sections.

Functional and Service Units within Research Administration

Before embarking on a description of research administration functional and service units, it will

be helpful to get an understanding of the scope—the breadth and depth—of the enterprise we will be examining in this chapter. The research enterprise encompasses all organizations that advocate, fund, manage, practice or report on research. When an institution is significantly engaged in the research enterprise, research administration is woven into the very fabric of the organization: nearly every operation within the institution is impacted in some way or other by the conduct and support of research. For instance, at Penn State, the judicial affairs office, which oversees the student court, called the Office of Sponsored Programs to ask about "NISPOM," the National Industrial Security Program Operating Manual, because of the increasing numbers of background checks being conducted by federal special agents, including investigations into former students' disciplinary records. NISPOM applies to universities such as Penn State that have secure research facilities for conducting classified research. A requirement of NISPOM is that subject organizations "cooperate with Federal agencies during . . . conduct of personnel security investigations of present or former employees and others."[1] "Others" may also include former students. With so many students going into security-sensitive jobs or being called up to active duty overseas, the volume of these background checks is escalating. At Penn State, even though background checks had nothing to do with research, the conditions under which the checks were conducted were there because of the research program being conducted at Penn State's secure facility, the Applied Research Laboratory. New regulations may be extremely pervasive and to some extent invasive as demonstrated by the work student affairs, the graduate school, and other university offices have had to undertake in order to comply with regulations regarding visas for graduate research assistants from foreign countries. The mandate of background checks at all universities where research is conducted has placed a great burden on research administrators at schools throughout the US.

Indeed the spectrum of research administration also reflects the breadth of the research enterprise. Research, although considered one of the three main activities of a comprehensive institution of higher education (teaching, research, and service), actually supports and interacts with the other missions—supporting and enhancing them. Research is integral to the instruction of undergraduate and graduate students. A faculty member engaged in active research makes a better teacher. Student research experiences help prepare students for the "real world" of business and industry. Research is also one of the key driving forces in economic development. Many universities see interactions with business and industry as a clear part of their service mission to the community, state, and nation. There are many other indicators of how closely aligned the research mission is with instruction and service, but the "take home" lesson is that research administration is indeed visible throughout the institutional garment, even if the garment isn't always seamless!

Another indicator of the breadth of this enterprise is that the spectrum of research administration activities spans the entire life cycle of a research project and all its sponsored support: from building faculty expertise and a culture for research and sponsored support, through the identification of funding opportunities; to proposal writing and submission, award acceptance, project management, the handling of research results (including inventions and creative works), project closeout and auditing, and all the physical and administrative infrastructure that supports the whole operation.

A final element to consider by way of introduction is that what a research administration operation does, its very functions and activities, is highly dependent on what that "organization" perceives are its core values. Historically, research administration has been recognized as a service organization. Raymond Woodrow, an early research administrator at Princeton University, said more than 25 years ago that a primary function of research administra-

tion is to create a nourishing climate for research.[2] While that job has grown in scope and complexity over the years, the mission is the same. This means serving the faculty who perform the research, serving the institution by protecting the institution's reputation and finances, serving the sponsor by ensuring proper stewardship of funds and proper dissemination of results, serving the federal government by complying with research regulations, and serving the people by facilitating the creation and dissemination of new knowledge and technologies to their benefit.

All this cannot be accomplished within a single office—even at an institution that has little sponsored activity. How all these functions and activities are organized depends a great deal on how much research and other sponsored projects activity there is, how the institution is organized, and the cultural history of institution—whether it has evolved as a centralized or decentralized organization, whether it has strong departments or strong colleges, and whether it has a good or a poor electronic business system.

In this chapter, we will survey the range of functions and activities involved in research administration. One can consider them organizationally, as units; but what is discussed is not necessarily related to organizational placement, but is related, rather, to the functions and services themselves. In this discussion we will rely on the components of the *Topical Outline of the Essential Elements of Research Administration,* a document produced jointly by the National Council of University Research Administrators (NCURA) and the Society of Research Administrators (SRA) in 1998. Even though the document has aged somewhat, it still provides a strong foundation on which to build. We will look at some options available for organizing these functions within a corporate structure.

The Pre- and Post-Award Research Enterprise

Research administration has been historically divided into two principal functions: pre-award and post-award. Many institutions still divide their operational offices in this manner. While these two categories still exist, the proportion of items falling into the two categories has radically shifted in the last decade or so, so that the number of post-award activities has greatly increased. Instead of using the two categories, we are going to examine nine principal functions of research administration: capacity building and marketing; proposal development and submission; award negotiation and acceptance; research protections and regulatory compliance; project management; financial management; intellectual property and technology transfer; research administration support; and institutional research administration infrastructure management. One could write an entire book covering these functions; in fact most of this book will be devoted to covering some of these functions individually and in more depth. In this chapter we provide a survey to give the student of research administration an introduction to the functions of research administration.

Capacity Building and Marketing

Institutions realize that in order to thrive as research organizations, they must first create cultures which stimulate, promote, assist, and reward those faculty who take on the extra burdens of seeking and operating sponsored projects. In addition, the success of individual faculty members depends heavily on the reputation of the institution. Promoting the successes of the institution in research and sponsored projects is also a task that research administrators need to consider.

Identification of Faculty Expertise and Institutional Research Facilities

Research administration offices should maintain a database of faculty research interests and expertise and a listing of institutional research facilities.

- *Faculty Research Interests.* There are some faculty profile systems available on the World Wide Web, such as the Community of Science (www.cos.com). Through this kind of service, institutions can maintain research expertise databases for use within the institution in matching investigators with funding opportunities, in building multi-investigator or interdisciplinary research projects, but a service like COS also allows other institutions or companies to find research experts at your institution to partner with or obtain services from. Some institutions build their own research expertise databases or have them as a part of their electronic research administration (ERA) systems, either of the homegrown or the vendor variety. The advantage of having the faculty profile database in the overall ERA system is that faculty expertise can be linked electronically to the faculty's grant and contract activity; faculty can keep their profile information current and "port" their information into proposals; and faculty "track records" in proposals and awards is another indicator of expertise and interest that can be employed within the institution. Faculty profiles should

contain such key information about the faculty member as: college, department, contact information; academic degrees and certifications; and research keywords. Additional information might include a list of publications, funded research projects, and an "abstract" of primary research. The obvious problem with all such systems, however, is keeping them updated. The more the profile system is integrated into an overall ERA system for the institution, the more likely it is that the information will be kept current by the faculty.

- *Institutional Research Facilities.* Maintaining a current listing of major research instruments and laboratories that are available for faculty use is a great way of informing faculty who need resources for their research of where they might find them on campus, but it is also a great way of advertising an institution's strengths. If a little "boilerplate" information is also available on the Web site containing the list, faculty can use the descriptive material for proposals. A listing of research centers is also helpful to internal and external "customers or clients."

Identification and Dissemination of Funding Opportunities

One of the principal functions of a research administration office is keeping faculty and institutional officials aware of funding opportunities and deadlines. This means keeping current with information coming out of a host of sponsoring entities including the federal government, state governments, foundations, and corporations. This can be done by monitoring the Web sites of these entities and getting on their mailing lists (either e-mail or "snail mail"). For federal opportunities Grants.gov's FIND Web site posts government-wide grant opportunities. There are a number of vendors who compile funding information for subscribers. Institutions large and small can benefit greatly from this kind of service. The research administration office also needs to find the best way(s) for disseminating the information. Maynard Kohler of Penn State University and one of the first research administrators to envision electronic dissemination of opportunities announcements, once described the process as trying to take a drink from a fire hose. There's just too much information. The principal method is providing a search tool for faculty to pull out matching opportunities from a funding database. But constantly checking databases for new opportunities is time-consuming and usually wasteful. Alert systems (like the National Science Foundation's Custom News Service) that allow faculty to enter keywords describing their interests, which are then used to send matching opportunities out by e-mail, is an improvement on that system. The second way is to proactively transmit opportunities to faculty. The two principal dangers that exist in this latter process are sending too little or sending too much information, either of which can undermine the goal of getting the right information into the right hands or catching the attention of the faculty recipients before they hit the delete key. An ideal system combines faculty research interest profiles with a human being who has a general idea of who is doing what. Funding newsletters, deadline lists, and Web sites are some of the favorite tools for disseminating funding information.

Identification of Research Administration Infrastructure Elements Keeping faculty aware of the services and resources that an institution has available to assist them in research and sponsored programs is a difficult but absolutely essential activity for a research administration operation. A functional and easy-to-navigate, content-rich home page and an accompanying hard copy version is the best way for letting your faculty customers know about what is out there to help them. A complete survey of services and tools available can also let you benchmark against other institutions or against recommended best practices. The list needs to include guidance for faculty on whom they need to see to get help finding funding, building budgets, submitting proposals, monitoring their budgets, appointing personnel and making purchases, etc.

Coordination of large multidisciplinary research is becoming more and more complex. Often single scientists, single disciplines, or even single institutions cannot provide solutions. Thus, multidisciplinary approaches to certain research problems are becoming standard. The National Institutes of Health's Roadmap Initiatives, as an example, stress an interdisciplinary approach to research to cope with the complexity of studying human biology and behavior, recognizing that the "traditional divisions within biomedical research may in some instances impede the pace of scientific discovery."[a] Research administration needs to provide coordination within the institution and among institutions in order to bring together scientists from the various

disciplines, facilitate their working together, and provide the unique management requirements that are required for grants that overlap departments, colleges, and institutions.

Industrial Research Development and Management Both industrial support of research and industry-university research collaborations have been on the rise since the 1980s. While some technical and land grant universities trace their close workings with industry back 80 to 100 years, industry interactions are a more recent phenomenon for most institutions. The Reagan administration was instrumental in fomenting this change. First Reagan stated the principle that it is not up to the federal government to provide for all the costs of fundamental research at US institutions of higher education and science. Industry, he insisted, benefits greatly from the new knowledge generated by universities and therefore should be responsible for supporting to some degree the costs associated with that enterprise. Second, during the Reagan administration, the Bayh-Dole Act was passed, which opened new doors to collaboration between universities and industries, since US research institutions could then own intellectual property developed with federal funding. This change in federal research policy and the recognition of both the industry and university communities led to the creation of the Government-University-Industry Research Roundtable (GUIRR) in 1984 under the National Academies. In addition, government grant programs were specifically developed to encourage and enhance this collaboration. Government, industry, and universities all began to see the importance of industry-university collaborations for enhancing technology transfer from university science to commercial products, promoting regional economic development, and putting university and industry scientists together to meet national needs. Companies received new ideas and solutions to their problems; universities received new sources for much-needed research funding. Unfortunately, this interface is particularly difficult because there is such a cultural divide between nonprofit institutions and profit-driven corporations. Some universities, in responding to resulting pressures, have established research administration operations that promote and facilitate interactions between faculty and companies. Research administrators need to be sensitive to the needs of industry, but also the risks that working with companies can present. The service operations typically "market" university research capabilities to industry, mainly

---

[a]National Institute of Health, "Interdisciplinary Research Overview," http://nihroadmap.nih.gov/interdisciplinary/index.asp.

through personal interactions, but also through specialized brochures and Web sites. For large institutions, one promotional technique is to showcase a particular strength of the university to a particular industrial segment. One institution recently held a "Hydrogen Day" which brought together university faculty and companies that shared an interest and expertise in hydrogen production, storage, sensors and monitors, fuel cells, transports, and national policy. An office that functions directly with companies apart from those associated with negotiating contracts or managing industry financial matters can often act as a liaison between the university and a company if problems or disagreements arise.

International Research Development and Management
Universities have long recognized the benefits of developing an international dimension to the advancement and dissemination of knowledge. Research administration offices need to be able to assist in this activity. First of all, universities have long been committed to the principles of social justice that call for sharing educational, agricultural and technological advances that promote human development especially in the poorest of countries. "In a world moving rapidly toward the knowledge-based economies of the 21st century, capacity building in science and technology (S&T) is necessary everywhere. But the need is greatest for the developing countries."[3] In addition, university faculty collaborate with peers in their fields worldwide; sometimes these collaborations are enhanced by joint research projects that require external funding. Research administrators need to know how to work with foreign governments, US government organizations such as the Agency for International Development, joint research programs sponsored by the National Science Foundation, and others, so that they can facilitate these exchanges. Since the September 11, 2001 terrorist attacks on the United States, international research exchanges have become many times more complicated. Export control and national security issues, visa problems, travel restrictions, and a host of other complications now have to be on the research administrator's radar when working on international projects. In addition, in some respects international research entities are becoming a tough competitor for industrial research funding. Recent congressional testimony from industry says that many companies are so frustrated fighting with US universities over intellectual property clauses in

research agreements that they are finding new partners internationally. It is important that research administrators in the United States gain a better understanding of how their neighbors are working and create better lines of communication. The importance of the international dimension has been reflected in associations of research administrators: The SRA formally changed its name to the International Society of Research Administrators and the National Council of University Research Administrators announced in 2003 the creation of a task force to study the international dimensions of research administration, both developments intended to better prepare their memberships to work in the international arena.

Marketing Research Capacity One of the most difficult and frustrating aspects about university research programs is how little our clients know about what we do for them day in and day out to help promote the welfare of our citizens and the world. All too often, the only university activities that make the news (aside from sports news) are stories of scandals and blunders. Universities in general and university research in particular suffer from poorly managed public relations. Research administration needs to address this problem in some way. Some of the basics that are essential include sending out press releases covering the receipt of major grants and contracts, new discoveries and technologies from which our constituencies will benefit, and the ways that university research creates new jobs and improves local economies. Another essential for many institutions is the publishing of an annual report of research that highlights research projects that are under way and gives some of the institution's statistics in regards to proposals and awards. These kinds of publications can enhance the institution's reputation and promote the research capacity of the institution. But marketing research capacity is not only an external activity; part of creating a culture of sponsored research on campus is to market research capacity internally. University-based newsletters that recognize faculty accomplishments in research and that highlight current research projects and research facilities at the university can inform faculty of the research capacity of their own institution.

Proposal Development and Submission
Preparation and submission of proposals are two primary functions of any research administration

operation. Whether these functions are performed centrally or in a distributive fashion, whether done electronically or on paper, proposal development is the heart of the research administration process. There has always been a direct proportional relationship between the number of proposals submitted and the number of awards received. The way proposals are prepared affects not only success in grant competitions but the whole course of the research project, from how much money is available, to how it is spent, and how much can be accomplished. A truly bad proposal may not be the one that is rejected, but the ill-conceived one that is awarded. Bad proposals that become funded can lead to financial liabilities, contractual defaults, lawsuits, conflicts of interest, ruined partnerships, bad science, and your institution's name on the cover of the Chronicle of Higher Education in a none-too-flattering way.

Budget Building   The budget of a proposal is the financial expression of the project. Every research administration service unit needs to be fluent in the language of budgets, in their construction, the rules and regulations that set up boundaries on allowable and unallowable costs, and in their institution's various rates for fringe benefits, student stipends and tuition remission, facilities and administrative costs, etc. In the preparation of budgets an indispensable tool for any research administration office is some form of electronic budget building capacity. While it is still possible to crunch out a proposal budget with a calculator, a pencil, and a pad of columnar paper, the complexity of today's research, the short turnaround times expected by faculty, and the sheer potential for errors make the use of electronic spreadsheets, budget templates, or proposal development software an absolute essential. These budget building tools range from highly sophisticated software packages to simple spreadsheets that do nothing more than add numbers automatically. The highly dynamic packages lead faculty or research administrators through the budget process like Turbo Tax leads one through the preparation of tax returns. These tools frequently have business rules built right into the software, so that rates are always applied correctly and unallowable costs avoided. Regardless of the tools used, budget building almost always should involve an experienced research administrator working closely with a faculty member. In this manner, the tasks of the project can be converted into the finances needed to accomplish them—with the faculty member providing the description of the science, and the research

administrator translating that into dollar impacts. Since budget building works best with interaction between faculty and administrator, organizationally, the budget building operation ought to be situated as close to the faculty as practicable. Spending time with faculty members during the budget building process can help them understand better what is going to be expected later from them as they manage their project. It also gives research administrators an opportunity to explain some of the logic and purposes for the rules that are established regarding budgets.

Proposal Writing, Editing, and Assembly   The narrative of the proposal is what really sells it to the sponsor. Well-written proposals coherently and cogently make the case to reviewers that this is the project they should select for funding. Some truly great scientists might get away with sloppy language and incomplete sentences in their proposals and still get funded, but this is certainly not the case for everyone else. Dr. Don H. Blount, formerly a program officer of the National Heart, Lung and Blood Institute and now retired from the University of Missouri–Columbia Medical School, used to talk of the phenomenon he called the "cascade of negativity." One typographical error is not likely to affect a priority score, but each additional grammatical error, incomplete sentence, poorly reproduced chart or photograph works almost geometrically in convincing the reviewer that the science is probably just as sloppy as the proposal. On the other hand, poor science, no matter how well expressed, is unlikely to be funded. So research administration operations need to recognize that while they may be able to enhance a well-conceived proposal, they really can not write the proposal for the faculty member. What can research administrators do for faculty who are writing proposals? Here are some helpful services, tools, and activities they typically provide:

- Offer proposal writing classes for new faculty that cover the basics of proposal writing
- Have a prewritten boilerplate describing institutional capacity and facilities
- Provide editorial assistance to faculty who request it (remembering that the really great editor does not rewrite the text but elicits the best writing possible out of the writer)
- Provide faculty mentoring and internal reviewers to help young faculty
- Provide proposal templates for faculty to help them make sure they cover all the necessary sections
- Remind them constantly about the proposal guidelines—emphasizing the importance of

complete compliance with page limits and type-size restrictions

- Coordinate the final packaging of the proposal, ensuring that all the sections are completed
- Have access to proposal and funding information to help prepare statements of current and pending support

Proposal Compliance Reviews and Representations, Certifications, and Assurances Institutional responsibility for ensuring that proposals comply with federal regulations must be taken with the utmost seriousness. This responsibility falls squarely within the realm of research administration. Other offices may be responsible for ensuring compliance with the regulations themselves: for example, purchasing department keeping track of procurements from small, minority, or disadvantaged businesses or the affirmative action office being responsible for monitoring compliance with civil rights laws. Research administration, however, must maintain contacts with all the offices that oversee compliance to be able to make the proper representations, certifications, and assurances. The first hurdle in accomplishing this, of course, is knowing all of the requirements. The National Council of University Research Administrators has a compendium of all the various federal compliance issues. This is a great resource, but one can also glean a great deal of compliance information by a careful reading of the proposal guidelines, like the PHS 398 packet. At the proposal stage the primary responsibility of the research administrator is to make sure that key compliance reviews are completed as necessary. Checklist forms are a good aid for this. Most internal review forms or electronic processes have a compliance checklist that is completed by investigators, identifying when human research participants will be involved, animal experimentation undertaken, the use of biohazardous materials is proposed, or when the financial holdings of a researcher might present the potential for a conflict of interest. With "just-in-time" processes in effect at some agencies, actually having all the reviews completed at the time of proposal submission is not always required, but having a record of what compliance issues are raised in the proposal makes it easier to track completion and approval at a later date.

Coordination of Multi-Institutional Proposals Federal agencies have stressed the necessity of a team approach to many research problems. It is no wonder then that the number of collaborative arrangements between institutions is increasing. At the proposal stage research administrators are called on to assist faculty in the integration of the various work scopes. Research administrators at the various institutions can work as a team in this particular effort, sharing information with one another as the proposal is being built, keeping each other notified of target dates and deadlines for wrapping up the various parts of the proposal. When a single proposal is to be submitted, one institution's research administration office is called on to do the final assembly of the proposal. From each collaborating institution the prime recipient needs to make sure it has a statement of work, a budget, and an institutional endorsement, at a minimum. Ensuring that all the pieces are there at the proposal stage makes issuing a sub-award at a later date a much easier task. The coordination of multi-institutional proposals can sometimes be helped by electronic communications, but frequently agency electronic proposal submission processes make it more difficult to submit proposals. Part of the research administrator's job is to make sure that coordination is begun early enough to head off problems.

Proposal Review, Approval, and Submission This is most likely the area that witnessed the genesis of the research administration profession. For early generations of research administrators it was the most important responsibility they had. It represents the first official point of intersection with outside sponsors. What is transmitted by the institution to the sponsor must be accurate, responsive, cohesive, and an excellent representation of the quality and reputation of the submitting institution. The proposal is the first document establishing the legal history of a contractual relationship and what is contained therein is of utmost importance. Regardless of how an institution delegates the responsibility and authority for review, approval, and submission, the task itself requires a high level of technical skill, a great attention to detail, and the endurance and mental toughness of a marathon runner to get through major deadline periods! As mentioned before, most institutions have some type of internal approval form or electronic process that is completed during the proposal review process. It is the final check for the accuracy of the budget, application of the correct rates, identification of investigators and their levels of effort, space commitments, regulatory compliance reviews, type size and space limitations, adherence to proposal guidelines, cost sharing commitments, appropriate commitments from subrecipients and collaborators identified in the proposal, the terms and conditions of award if the proposal is successful, concurrence of department heads and deans, and the overall appearance of the proposal. Usually all this must be done within a very short period of time in order to meet the deadline. The approval given to the proposal by an authorized official represents the commitment of the institution to dedicate the resources and best efforts of university personnel to accomplish the scope of work within the budget proposed. Even when the proposal is for a grant (assistance and not procurement) it becomes, in a sense, a contractual offer. Sometimes, in the case of a response to an request for proposal (RFP), the proposal is in fact a binding contract that can be executed and awarded by the agency without further negotiation. The authorized official is a specifically assigned representative of the corporation submitting the proposal. There needs to be a clear line of delegation indicating the signer's legal capacity to execute legal documents, in this case the proposal. The research administration organization is responsible for ensuring the timely submission of the proposal. This means being aware of impending deadlines, tracking proposals through the review process, and using the appropriate method of transmission. While research administrators have tried for years to get faculty to submit proposals early enough before the deadline for thorough review, inevitably some proposals always come in at the last moment. New electronic submission techniques press the deadline crunch even more. In these situations, research offices should have a conditional submission process that allows the proposal to be submitted but makes the faculty member aware that if problems surface with the proposal, the faculty member would be responsible for revising the proposal or withdrawing it.

Award Stage

Award Review and Approval   The award process may actually begin at any point after the proposal is submitted when the agency begins to work with the institution in arranging for a grant. Thus, this function includes providing "just-in-time" submissions of compliance information, working up and submitting revised budgets or statements of work, or providing other clarifications to the sponsor prior to the official award notice. Unfortunately, the "award" activity actually also includes receiving and processing "rejections" or, as many sponsors word rejections, proposals that have been "approved but not funded." The research administration office needs to appropriately

log the status into the proposal database and ensure that the principal investigator (PI) and the appropriate academic office are informed. Rejected proposals have to be "pulled" and processed according to the office protocol. The research administrator may also work with the PI in getting the agency's documentation on the review process, which may contain suggestions helpful to revising and resubmitting the proposal for reconsideration. Upon receipt of the award notice, the details of the award need to be reviewed against the proposal, with any discrepancies noted for follow-up. The award terms and conditions also need to be examined. With federal awards, this is normally a transparent process, since the terms are usually known before submission occurs. However, with certain foundations and other not-for-profit organizations, the institution may not have seen the award terms and conditions. Negotiations may even be called for in some instances with grants [see next section]. Normally grants are issued unilaterally, formal approval is therefore not usually required, but where it is, then obtaining the sign off of the authorized official is required. In some instances, formal acceptance is not required, but the sponsor asks for an acknowledgement that the award has been received. Such acknowledgement does not legally require an authorized official's signature (although some institutions may require it in their procedures). With unilateral awards, formal acceptance "contractually" takes place by the setting up of an account and spending money on the project.

Contract Negotiations   Contract awards are quite different and require a great deal more work of the research administration office. Negotiations are to be conducted by authorized representatives of the institution only. This is a situation in which the old adage, "too many cooks spoil the broth," is really true. PIs, their staff assistants, and department heads need to be told politely that, while their input is important, it needs to be channeled through official university negotiators. The negotiation process needs to be adjusted to the particular situation at hand. "Negotiations" with federal contracts is more a process of arguing for the application of proper FAR clauses. To assist research administrators with this activity the research administration office should have a list of FAR clauses that are acceptable to the institution, those that are not (with the reasons stated), and the appropriate alternate clauses. Sometimes, however, "real" negotiations do occur with federal contracts, over such issues as the applicability of publication restriction clauses. The federal process also basically applies to federal "flow-through" contracts from industry or from another nonprofit institution. However, straight industrial contracting is usually a very real negotiation. This function may be the most challenging among all the others undertaken in the research administration enterprise. Research administration negotiators need to balance the needs and desires of the faculty member, the best interests of the institution in avoiding excessive risks and liabilities, and compliance with university policies with the concerns and needs of the company, all in the interest of arriving at a win-win solution. All through the negotiation process it is critical to keep the PI informed and to consult with the PI from time to time on issues that might be impacted by the scope of work proposed and the potential for the creation of new technologies and knowledge. Research administration offices should have a "library" of contract clauses that work with the various groups of sponsors. These should include not only the language but the rationale for employing each particular clause or alternate. For a research project to be successful a well-reasoned and fair contract is essential. If the parties cannot agree on the nature and terms of their relationship, it is hard to imagine that their scientific collaborations will be any more successful. Using national norms in negotiations is very important, such as the NIH statement on developing sponsored research agreements with industry published in the NIH Guide in July of 1994 or the series of reports from the National Academies on model industry-university agreements, or the more recent report from the Business-Higher Education Forum, *Working Together: Creating Knowledge.*

Award and Account Establishment Upon the acceptance of the award, the emphasis shifts to concern about getting the research project underway. The research administration operation is responsible for coordinating the smooth transfer of documentation and data from the pre-award function to the post-award. A summary of the award terms and conditions should be transmitted to the various offices that will be responsible for the conduct of the project and the financial reporting and invoicing. Some institutions find it extremely helpful, particularly with new faculty, to establish orientation meetings with the PI and the lab staff to ensure that all understand both the financial and scientific responsibilities that the grant entails. The next activity is creating the proper account in the institution's accounting system that will allow project funds to be spent. Clear procedures for setting up the

account and informing the PI and department of the account need to be in place.

Compliance

Protection of Human Research Participants The fundamental healing axiom, "first do no harm," is paramount in research as well. Research administration is responsible for ensuring that sufficient infrastructure is in place within the institutional environment to support the operation of federally mandated Institutional Review Boards (IRB), including the selection of members, providing adequate training and preparation to members, keeping detailed minutes, and the preparation and maintenance of IRB documentation. The administration needs to ensure that IRB membership is adequately diversified, has community members to reflect community standards, and possesses adequate expertise appropriate to the types of research supported. The supporting research office also oversees the submission and processing of protocol applications, maintenance of records, reporting of adverse events, and the development and enforcement of institutional policies and guidelines for conducting research involving human research participants. Special attention needs to be paid to the potential for conflicts of interest among investigators and the institution itself that might arise in conjunction with research involving humans. The institutional systems and procedures should be built upon the Belmont Report's basic ethical principles of respect for persons, beneficence, and justice. Research administrators need to ensure that the system provides for informed consent of and an assessment of the risks and benefits to all human research participants, and appropriate training for all those engaged in the conduct of human research. Research administrators also need to ensure that institutional policies are kept current with policy changes and the introduction of new federal regulations, for example, the effects of the Health Insurance Portability and Accountability Act (HIPAA) of 2002 on the conduct of human research.

Humane Care and Use of Animals Research administration generally oversees the operations of the Institutional Animal Care and Use Committee (IACUC) that is federally mandated for research that is conducted utilizing animals. This includes selection of members that reflect the diversity of the research community engaged in animal research, veterinary experts, community members, researchers, and research administrators. The IACUC, with the assistance of research administration, has the responsibility of ensuring that animals used in research, testing, or education within the institution are treated humanely and within the regulations and standards established by federal, state, and local governments. Research administration needs to develop appropriate policies and procedures on animal research and offer adequate training programs for those engaged in animal research. The office overseeing animal research often takes the lead in the accreditation process under the Association for Assessment and Accreditation of Laboratory Animal Care (AAALAC).

Conflict of Interest   An institution's ability to perform research in an objective and unbiased manner is key to its continued success and to fulfilling its role to society to advance new knowledge, to protect society from false claims, and to warn society of dangers. It is also an important service to the academic community and the nation. The institution needs to ensure that this reputation for unbiased research is not threatened when the financial holdings of individual researchers or the institution itself might call into question the objectivity and honesty of research conducted. At many institutions this responsibility is within the domain of research administration. Oversight would include: the development of policies and procedures compliant with federal and state regulations and standards; the operation of a conflict of interest committee (including establishing membership); administrative support to the committee (including preparing the agenda for meeting and maintenance of minutes and other documentation); development of disclosure mechanisms and review principles; disseminating findings and enforcing decisions, including the enactment of sanctions; and reporting as appropriate to federal sponsors.

Security and Export Controls   Some institutions, by the nature of the research they perform, may fall under regulations governing the levels of security provided to certain kinds of research and the control of access to and dissemination of information and materials covered by the Export Administration Regulations (EAR) or the International Traffic in Arms Regulations (ITAR). A select group of US institutions perform government classified research in secure facilities. Research administrators at these operations must oversee strict requirements regarding facility security, clearance of persons entering the premises, storage of classified information, and the enforcement of appropriate federal regulations and institutional policies. Other institutions may

fall under these requirements because of contractual restrictions placed on the publication or other dissemination of certain security sensitive research. But research administrators at all institutions need to be aware of applicable US regulations that affect the actual export or the "deemed" export of restricted materials or information to foreign persons. This area is under a great deal of flux at the time of the writing of this chapter. Recent interpretations made by the inspectors general of a number of federal agencies and confirmed by the Department of Commerce present significant challenges to the open conduct of research at all US universities and nonprofit research institutions. In addition to concerns over the security of information, research administration needs to address the security of biological and other extremely dangerous substances that have come to be known as "select agents." The Centers for Disease Control and Prevention (CDC) is currently charged with regulating the possession of biological agents and toxins that can pose a serious threat to health and safety. Possessing or using select agents requires an institutional registration, which is reviewed and approved by the CDC. Research administrators need to keep current on new and changing requirements affecting security and export controls.

Research Integrity   One of the most prized possessions of a university is its reputation. This reputation is built from the ground up in the way that research is proposed, reviewed by peers, conducted in the laboratory, and reported at conferences and in the literature. It is research administration's role to promote sound practices that lead to research being conducted with the highest level of integrity, to ensure that those engaged in research are properly trained in the responsible and ethical conduct of research, and, whenever failings or abuses are found, to investigate them, appropriately report findings to sponsors and the community, and to sanction those who have been determined to have committed scientific misconduct. A research administration office needs a thorough grounding in the requirements of the federal government promoting research integrity, which needs constant updating. Complete policies and procedures must be established to govern how the institution deals with suspected cases of scientific misconduct.

Ombudsman–Whistleblower Hotline   A research administration office needs to have its eyes and ears open to effectively monitor the conduct of research. While we may not enjoy the policing role, one can remember the motto of many police departments, "to serve and protect," and be comforted with the notion that in our vigilance, we as research administrators arc both serving and protecting our institution and the reputation of the research enterprise. As research is conducted at the ground level, so, too, our knowledge of what is occurring in the research program has to come from the ground level. Therefore, it is essential for an institution to provide a way for suspected abuses to be reported, without fear of reprisal, by those who work in the laboratories or departmental administrative offices. Research administration should establish appropriate policies and procedures to encourage faculty, staff, and students with questions, suspicions, or allegations to report these to the proper authority.

Health and Safety   The faculty, staff, and students of a research institution need to be provided a safe and secure environment in which to work and study. Research administration's role in this is to ensure that the institution has properly addressed health and safety concerns and has strong policies and procedures in place to effect that and that training is provided to those working in, maintaining, and cleaning scientific laboratories. For schools with agriculture and animal research programs, this means providing a sound health monitoring program for those engaged with working with animals. For schools working with radioactive material, it means having the appropriate individuals complete the approved training and certification. As stated in a section above, research administration needs also to be aware of what, if any, "select agents" may be present on campus, to provide adequate safeguards for them, and to ensure that the proper registrations have been made with the federal government. The research administration office needs to keep thoroughly up-to-date with federal requirements and restrictions.

Project Management

Assisting the Principal Investigator   A basic tenet of research administration is that researchers research and administrators administer. Most institutions do actually put the primary responsibility for the conduct of a research project, both the scholarly/scientific aspects of a project and the fiscal management, on the principal investigator. And this responsibility is appropriate. But researchers need to devote most of their time and energies on advancing the academic goals of the project; they need to rely on their research administrators to see to the details of the fiscal management of the research project. How

research administration supports the principal investigator (PI) in project management depends in large measure on the size and cultural history of institutions. A small institution can run a highly centralized project management system to support PIs, but a large multicollege institution must rely on a more decentralized support system. In any case, the research administration infrastructure supporting project management needs to be "as close" to the PI as possible to really facilitate the management of the project. In most institutions, this means having project management and financial research administrators assigned to large program projects, to large centers, and to individual departments. Assisting the PI means serving the needs of the project, but it also means knowing when and how to say, "No." Research administrators are also responsible to the institution and must ensure compliance with institutional and sponsor regulations and requirements.

Human Resource Management   At the initiation of a project the research administrator needs to coordinate with the PI the hiring of new project personnel and the assignment of current staff to the project. Salary distribution must be in conformance with OMB Circular A-21 and within the scope of the project and the budget. As the project continues, changes in personnel and effort must be monitored and effected in a timely manner; required approvals must be obtained in advance. The effort of all personnel must be reported in accordance with institutional procedures to comply with federal regulations.

Purchase Requisitions   The research administrator is the front-line "purchasing agent" and "property manager." This begins with fulfilling due diligence in purchasing the right items, in a fair and competitive manner, and processing them within institutional procedures. Purchases must be in compliance with the project budget and within institutional or sponsor requirements, including prior approval if necessary. Procurement regulations for federal grants are covered by the Office of Management and Budget (OMB)'s Circular A-110. According to this circular, the institution is the responsible authority for the settlement of all contractual and administrative issues associated with procurement, without recourse to the federal agency. This includes handling disputes, claims, protests of award, source evaluation, and all other contractual matters. All university personnel involved in directly handling purchases, including research administrators, must comply with the institution's standards of conduct governing the award and administration of procurements and contracts. These standards as well as all policies and procedures governing procurements must be in writing and a part of the institution's official regulations. An institution's procurement system is subject to periodic review by the federal government.

Subawards and Subcontracts Administration Closely related to procurement activities is the management of subawards and subcontracts. When an institution provides project funding to outside entities to accomplish a portion of the scope of work, it takes on the role and responsibility of the sponsoring agency in terms of oversight given to the subrecipient. Under federal sponsorship these duties are identified under OMB Circulars A-110 and A-133 or, in the case of contracts, under the Federal Acquisition Regulations. The research administration office is generally the preferred unit to serve as the subcontracts administration operation. The institution needs to have in place written policies and procedures governing subawards and subcontracts. These need to cover the full range of activities. Subawardees and subcontractors are usually identified at the proposal stage by the PI. They generally are considered collaborators on the project. Proposals from potential subrecipients need to include a scope of work, a budget, required representations, certifications, and assurances, and be signed by an authorized official of the subrecipient. When subrecipients are not identified in the proposal, agencies frequently require prior approval before subcontracting out a portion of the work. In these cases, too, it is important to make sure that competitive procurement practices are employed. In making an award to a subrecipient, it is absolutely essential to flow down to the subrecipient the appropriate terms and conditions of the prime award. With federal grants this can be done with the model subaward agreement form developed by the Federal Demonstration Partnership (FDP). This form can even be adopted for use with nonfederal sponsors who have given your institution grant assistance, as opposed to a contract. Subcontracts require individual attention to flow down terms and may require negotiation. Once subawards or subcontracts are issued, research administration attention turns to subrecipient monitoring. Even at the award stage it is important to verify that a potential subrecipient has the proper infrastructure to carry out the project and provide sound financial management of funds. The research administrator needs to confirm that the subrecipient has a "clean bill of health" by checking the status of its A-133 audit. Once the project is under way, the principal investigator and financial research administrators working with the project need to be clearly charged with the responsibility to review invoices against budgets and progress reports against the scope of work and certify to the institution prior to making payment that the subrecipient is performing well. Anomalies and discrepancies must be tracked down (even if such investigation requires a site visit) and resolved. The research administrator must also be involved in the closeout of the project.

Payroll The research administrator, usually at the department or college level, needs to ensure that all project personnel are correctly entered into the payroll and paid from the proper accounts to match their efforts. This function is usually coordinated through the payroll office. However, the research administrator is the responsible party for ensuring compliance with A-21, Section J.8, which deals with compensation for personal services. The research administrator needs thorough knowledge about regulations governing academic year and summer appointments, distribution of effort and what constitutes 100% effort, and limitations on supplemental compensation.

Project Monitoring (Deliverables) The effective research administration operation has procedures in place to track performance of project goals and deliverables. This is usually done using electronic research administration tools, but can also be done separately on electronic spreadsheets or even on paper ones. While contracts containing milestone payments and deliverables are less frequently seen at universities, they are far from rare, especially as universities engage more in contract support of federal, state, and industry sponsors. Since the university investigators may be unaccustomed to working towards the accomplishment of milestones and production of contract deliverables (such as prototypes, manuals, brochures, samples processed, etc.), it is very important to provide them assistance and to keep them focused on output requirements. Contracts with deliverables, unlike grants, do not allow investigators the flexibility to follow their own course. Many a faculty member has been burned because of a lack of understanding of the contract model.

Technical and Administrative Reporting Related to the above section, even when working with grants, it is important to monitor the progress of the project and keep up with reporting requirements. Research administrators provide an important service to researchers by frequently reminding them of responsibilities under their research agreement for submitting reports. The simplest way to do this is through an electronic research administration (ERA) system. As the award comes in, reporting requirements are entered into the system (either on the award or accounting side) and the system takes care of sending out notices reminding project staff of deadlines. If no system exists, then maintaining a separate spreadsheet of requirements and manually sending out notices is sufficient. More attention is being paid by agencies to the delivery of required reports. The inspectors general of the various federal agencies have emphasized the importance of agency grants managers verifying receipt of required reports before closing projects. Institutions that are chronically delinquent in meeting reporting requirements can face sanctions that include withholding of awards all the way to disbarment from receiving any awards. One important detail is to ensure that all required copies are transmitted. Another reason for ensuring that all reports are submitted is that reports provide the measurement of real success in the research project. It is crucial to this nation's universities and research institutes to maintain the confidence of the people, whose tax dollars support the research.

Clinical Trial Management   A growing area of project management and financial research administration is administering clinical trials. Whether funded by the federal government or by companies, clinical trials present unique challenges to the research administrator. At some institutions, clinical trials are a major component of a medical school's or hospital's research program. Some research administrators have become clinical trial specialists, whose full-time job is preparing proposals, negotiating awards, and managing clinical trials. Some major medical research institutions have whole departments that do nothing but manage clinical trials. Much of what is done to support clinical trials parallels all the services being covered by this survey of research administration functions. The difference is chiefly the focus on clinical trials research. Some additional areas of expertise are required of research administrators in clinical trials, for instance, the recruitment of human research participants. The list of services of Rush University Medical Center's Clinical Trials Office demonstrates the breadth of activity:

- Identification of investigators
- Completion of regulatory documents
- Budgeting and contract negotiation
- IRB application submission
- Study initiation, patient recruitment and follow-up
- Study coordinator support
- Ongoing quality control monitoring[b]

Another example from the University of Iowa's Clinical Trials Office:

- Negotiate acceptable terms and conditions of clinical trials contracts
- Develop and implement marketing programs to increase clinical trials at the University
- Serve as a resource for faculty and staff concerning the clinical trials process
- Inform faculty of clinical trials opportunities
- Coordinate activities with the Human Subjects Office for expedient review of protocols and agreements
- Set up meetings between corporate visitors and our investigators[c]

The management of clinical trials, like research administration itself, requires the research administrator to wear many hats.

Financial Management

A growing area of research administration is financial research administration. Once solely the domain of many central offices, financial management of grants and contracts has undergone some changes across the country. Many institutions have experienced tremendous growth in sponsored research, which has required new organizational models designed to try to keep up with the burgeoning workload. These distributed models have pushed much of the responsibility and authority for fiscal management out to individual colleges, institutes and centers, and even large research-intensive departments. This section will attempt to cover the central and distributed aspects of financial research administration.

---

[b]Source: Rush University Medical Center Web site, http://www.rush.edu/research/clinical-trials-office. html.

[c]Source: The University of Iowa Clinical Trials Office Web site, http://research.uiowa.edu/cto/.

Expenditure Monitoring

The research administration support function should provide faculty with support in tracking and approving expenditures on grants and contracts. This service is needed not only to keep the PI on track with expenditure "burn rates," but also to protect the institution from unallowable expenses being charged on projects. In addition, support is provided to prevent running an account into deficit, or from running too big of a surplus of funds (which can be a problem on fixed price agreements causing pricing questions. On Department of Defense projects—big surpluses can be de-obligated by the agency and pulled back to support more pressing military needs). To accomplish this takes an accurate and timely account reporting system. Research administrators, who find that the central accounting system cannot support this kind of monitoring, often become experts in spreadsheet management, creating "shadow systems" to track and reconcile expenditures.

Accounting and Financial Reporting

Typically this research administration function is managed centrally by a research accounting office or equivalent. OMB Circular A-110 identifies the range of responsibilities for accounting and financial reporting:

- Operating financial management systems
- Managing payments
- Accounting for cost sharing and matching requirements
- Accounting for program income
- Making budget revision approvals
- Undertaking audits
- Determining allowability of cost
- Establishing fund availability

Accounting and financial management requires a robust central, auditable accounting system that provides an accurate, current and complete disclosure of each individual sponsored project's financial activity. It must be able to identify the source and application of each sponsored project expenditure. A-110 requires that these records shall contain information pertaining to Federal awards, authorizations, obligations, unobligated balances, assets, outlays, income, and interest.

Financial Compliance: Expenditure Review, Cost Sharing, Allowable Costs, Program Income, and Effort Certification

Financial compliance is usually a shared responsibility among the central research administration unit, the college or department research administrators, and the investigators. As mentioned earlier, except for smaller institutions, few central offices are engaged in reviewing individual expenditures simply because of the workload volume. This activity is one generally carried out by research administrators at the unit level. Expenditure review requires checking each expenditure against what is allowable, reasonable, and allocable to the grant under the approved budget. Allowable costs are determined first by OMB Circular A-21, Section J, then by the award document, and finally by the budget that has been approved. Most budget modifications on research grants can be approved by the institution under the expanded authorities, but research administrators need to check the terms of each grant to ensure compliant budget revisions. Institutional written policies need to cover both cost sharing and program effort, as directed by OMB Circular A-110, Sections 23 and 24. Research administrators need to be particularly sensitive to these targeted audit categories and constantly watch for any clarifications that may be issued by OMB regarding cost sharing and program income. Financial research administrators need to ensure that local procedures capture both cost sharing and program income in accounts or cost centers where it is easy to identify the link to the grant and to monitor dollar levels. Effort certification is also a target for auditors. Institutional research administration operations need to ensure that the institution has a workable and auditable effort verification system in place and unit research administrators need to ensure that all personnel charged to grants or included in the institutional facilities and administrative cost pools certify their effort in a timely manner.

Closeout Closeout activities are normally the responsibility of both central research administration operations and their counterparts in a central research accounting operation. Closeout requires a final reconciliation of the budget and expenses, carried out by the central fiscal people, usually in collaboration with unit financial research administrators; submission of all required technical reports; final invention statement; and additional documentation necessary for closing out contracts. Institutions have 90 days after the ending date of the project to liquidate all financial obligations.

Audit Research administrators across the university usually participate in audits because it takes both central research administrators (both financial and academic) and unit research administrators to handle most audit questions. Audits can be a breeze if an institution has good systems and everyone is following institutional policies and procedures. They can become very rough, however, if appropriate expense monitoring and close scrutiny of details are not a part of the research administration process. Audits come in many varieties, from the A-133 single audit, usually performed by an institution's certified public accounting firm, to programmatic audits by federal agencies, to internal audits. In addition, the institution is subject to certain other periodic reviews of property systems and procurement systems.

Intellectual Property

Invention Disclosures   Since the early 1980s and predominantly due to the passage of the Bayh-Dole Act, research administration operations at universities have taken on the management of institutional intellectual property. The Bayh-Dole Act, codified in CFR Title 37, Part 401, sets forth the requirement for researchers working at universities and nonprofit institutions to file disclosures on all inventions funded in part by federal funds. A part of this activity is also ensuring that all employees of the university who are engaged in research have signed an intellectual property agreement and have it on file with the intellectual property office.

Licensing   Bayh-Dole also sets forth requirements for patenting and licensing technologies. Most universities and other research institutions have a separate office that manages patents and licensing. Negotiations for intellectual property licenses parallel in many ways what research administrators do in research contracts, taking the process one step further. Whereas the research agreement may simply grant an option for a license, the license agreement itself spells out all the details of the license, including royalties, due diligence required of the licensee to bring the product to market, and sublicensing rights. One of the Bayh-Dole stipulations is that US companies be given preference for receiving licenses on federally funded research and among this pool of companies preference is to be given to small businesses.

Technology Transfer   Technology transfer is a vital and growing part of university research administration. It is one way in which universities and nonprofit research institutions give a return on the country's investment in research. The goal of technology transfer is to turn research results into practical benefits for society. Research administration is a key to the success of transferring technology and includes the review of researcher invention disclosures; the identification of potentially marketable technologies and the companies that may have an interest in the technology; and by marketing the technology to these potential licensees.

Copyrights   Another frequent product of research is copyrightable works. Many institutions give back to faculty rights to scholarly works and textbooks that are not commissioned specifically by the institution, but products that come from grants or contracts usually are considered the property of the institution, since ownership and licensing may be determined by the sponsored agreement. Copyrightable works from sponsored programs might include software that is developed by researchers. Frequently the Intellectual Property Office also manages copyrights.

Research Administration Support

Institutional Policy and Procedure Development and Maintenance   As one can readily see from all the above research administration functions, a master set of research administration policies and procedures is absolutely essential in complying with federal regulations and giving good stewardship to all sponsored funds. Usually this task falls to a senior research administrator at the institution, frequently at the assistant or associate vice president level. The research administrator charged with this obligation needs to keep current on all federal regulatory changes affecting research. This can be done by participation in any number of research administration organizations, but primarily the Association of American Universities, Council on Governmental Relations, Federal Demonstration Partnership, National Council of University Research Administrators, Society of Research Administrators, Association of University Technology Managers, Applied Research Ethics National Association/Public Responsibility in Medicine & Research, American Association of Medical Colleges, and others. Policy development is generally best done in a collegial manner, vetting policy drafts through faculty and fiscal and academic administrative channels. Education is also an important factor in promulgating and disseminating research policies. Finally, policies must be strictly enforced and sanctions levied against violators in an appropriate degree.

Electronic Research Administration   Electronic research administration (ERA), once a subject unto itself, has now been nearly fully subsumed into the standard operating procedures of research administration itself. Hardly a day goes by for any research administrator in the country that does not involve a number of ERA transactions. ERA computer applications, many of which are fully integrated into ERA systems, cover the full spectrum of research administration functions. We use ERA to find funding opportunities, to market our institutions, to prepare proposals and budgets, to submit proposals, to review and approve animal and human research protocols, to negotiate awards, to receive and set up awards, to issue subawards, to rebudget accounts, to request prior approvals, to process and monitor expenditures, to file invention disclosures, to report on results, and to close projects. On the horizon for ERA are further integration of systems and (hopefully) the standardization of federal ERA systems under the Grants.gov initiative.

Research Administration and Research Integrity Training

As stated above, training is an integral part of any promulgation and dissemination of research administration policies and procedures. Certain training programs are mandated by the federal government, for example, the training that is required on the subject of human research participants before anyone can work on a project involving human subjects. In addition, certain federal regulations, like the US Sentencing Guidelines, place responsibility for certain illegal acts of employees on the employer, if adequate policies are not in place and training programs have not been initiated to communicate institutional policies and procedures to employees. The Office of Research Integrity has recommended training in the following areas of research integrity:

1. Data acquisition, management, sharing, and ownership
2. Mentor/trainee responsibilities
3. Publication practices and responsible authorship
4. Peer review
5. Collaborative science
6. Human subjects
7. Research involving animals
8. Research misconduct
9. Conflict of interest and commitment

In addition, auditors look for what educational programming the institution provides to the financial management of research projects to ensure that not only does the institution have policies, but employees are aware of the policies and know how to comply with them.

Institutional Research Administration Management

Property and Facility Management (Space Management)

OMB Circular A-110, Section 30, covers the requirements of the institution in regards to property management. These minimum regulations must be incorporated into the institution's policies and procedures. Research administrators are frequently involved with the institution's property management office, which should have the primary responsibility for managing property purchased on grant or contract funds. When dealing with research equipment acquired in association with a grant or contract, research administrators need to pay special attention to whether the equipment is considered government furnished equipment (GFE) or exempt equipment. GFE requires labeling the equipment as federally owned property and reporting on all federally owned equipment on an annual basis. Basically, nothing can be done with GFE without the written concurrence of the institution's federal administrative contracting officer. GFE cannot be modified, upgraded, traded in, assigned to another project, moved to another PI or institution, scavenged for parts, scrapped, or declared salvage, without federal approval. Ownership to exempt property vests immediately in the institution, but still has a number of restrictions on its use, especially for nonproject related purposes. The research administrator's role in all this is primarily ensuring that the investigators on the project know what they can and cannot do with what equipment. As everyone knows, space issues on campus are the most hotly contested of all academic matters. Research administrators need to make sure that space requirements for sponsored research are identified and addressed at the proposal stage. There is nothing like a PI showing up with a multimillion dollar grant saying, "Now, where's my space to do this project?" Many institutions are incorporating space allocations into their ERA system and relating that data to research activities (both sponsored and nonsponsored) to ensure that those investigators who need the space the most are given it in preference to those who are not producing. Having solid space data helps keep the issue focused on space requirements and less on personalities.

F&A Rate Development

The development of institutional facilities and administrative cost rates is a specialized field of financial research administration. OMB Circular A-21 governs how indirect cost rates are developed. Basically one divides what it costs to administer and support research by the modified total direct costs of research (both sponsored and organized research) at the institution. This yields a percentage that reflects the costs for which institutions should be reimbursed when conducting research. F&A costs are a much-misunderstood aspect of financing the full costs of research. Research administrators at every level in the institution need to be thoroughly conversant with F&A costs so they can adequately reflect their nature to inquiring faculty and staff. The more everyone knows about F&A the better the full costs of research can be recouped and the research infrastructure of the institution maintained.

Cash Management   This is generally a function performed by the central office for financial research management. A primary tool for proper cash management is a strong cost receivables and billing system. Many federal agencies are using electronic financial reporting and payment systems. These greatly improve an institution's cash position. But still there are many agencies and other sponsors for whom paper invoicing is required. Usually, the investment of research administrators who focus on cash management on research grants and contracts pays for itself out of improved cash management.

Records Management and Retention   OMB Circular A-110, Section 53, sets forth the requirements for maintaining appropriate project related documentation on grants. This is a research administration function that affects all layers and the entire breadth of the institution's research program and infrastructure. Records are to be kept on proposals and awards, protocols and compliance approvals, financial actions, inventions and patents, personnel actions and effort reporting, requisitions and expenditures, and technical reports. This takes the coordinated actions of many research administrators. Records need to be maintained for a minimum of three years from the date of the submission of the final financial report or, for grants requiring quarterly or annual reports, from the time of the submission of these periodic reports, unless an audit is started during that period. This task, too, requires the cooperation of research administrators across the university. A special aspect of records management and retention is now the storage and destruction of electronically stored documents. Many ERA systems are incorporating electronic records. Institutions need to obtain permission from their cognizant federal agency prior to relying solely on electronic records, but whether these records are the official records or just back-up records, the ease

of access and the minimal storage space required of electronic records is something that really can benefit research administrators.

This ends the survey on the functions of research administration in the university and nonprofit research institution environments. One can readily see the scope and depth of expertise that research administrators must have and the breadth of coverage that research administration requires at a major research institution.

Organizational Structure for Administration of Research

The focus of this portion of the chapter is on structure of the research unit and is primarily relevant to universities, foundations, and not-for-profit and independent research institutes. Industry and for-profit research organizations are beyond the scope of this chapter but will have many of the same functions and responsibilities. In mission, scope, and responsibility an independent research institute will mirror closely a large research unit within a university. In middle to large universities, based upon level of extramural support, there is generally an office of record for research named Office of Research or a similar title. At the middle to large institution there is a chief research officer (CRO) at the vice president or vice chancellor level. Some universities, primarily public, administer the research program through a separate foundation. Still a vice president will be the CRO or chair of the foundation. Some foundations, such as Fred Hutchinson Cancer Institute, have a structure similar to a university and are frequently linked to an institution of higher education.

Central versus Decentralized Structure

The issue of whether the research functions should be centralized or decentralized to some degree has paralleled the general shifts in institutional policy regarding central control and responsibility. Since the late 1990s there has been a noticeable shift toward consolidation of traditional pre-award and post-award financial responsibilities into an office of research. The rationale for this stems from greater need for accountability and coordination of all research related administrative activities. Consolidation of the two functions can occur when administrative structures are either central or diffuse, but policy and oversight generally remains at the central level. The smaller research institutions have greater need for centralization from a management or administrative responsibility. The centralized structure can avoid redundancy and promote consistency.

In her 1995 book, *Moo*, Jane Smiley wrote about an unnamed midwestern, land grant university, perhaps fictional, perhaps not. In her treatise, the research function resided with an unfriendly development officer. Thankfully, this model does not find itself too often in nonfictional research universities in the United States. However, at institutions with small research programs and little extramural support, the responsibilities and authorities may be distributed. No central office will coordinate the various functions of research administration. In some of these schools, a dean or faculty member may assume the role of CRO and the signatory for grant proposals may be the president. When an institution assumes research as one arm of its mission, a sponsored programs office is usually established to manage the administrative responsibilities. As the volume of extramural funding and commitment to expanding the research mission increase, additional central structures, including a chief research officer, are added.

A large institution will have a central research office but may decentralize some of the various functions. For instance, Stanford University has decentralized part of the function of the sponsored programs office. Each department in Stanford's School of Medicine has its own sponsored programs officer with signatory authority. The individuals in this position must go through extensive training and testing. Large medical schools, such as those at Johns Hopkins and Ohio State, have sponsored programs personnel in departments or colleges. With decentralized functions, the office of research assumes an even greater coordinating and policy and oversight role. With the advent of the Sarbanes-Oxley Act (PL 107-204), the government is requiring even greater accountability on the part of the chief research officers and research managers. This may demand or encourage even greater central control. There is no *right* structure; the structure must fit the culture of the institution.

Sponsored Programs Offices

In 1999, Bill Kirby and Paul Waugaman looked at the reporting channels for sponsored programs offices at universities. The survey looked at universities with varying levels of extramural support. The outcome was that the largest percentage of the sample had a vice president for research and the sponsored programs office reported to that office. Next, the second largest reporting structure was with a sponsored programs office reporting to the vice president for administration but this occurred primarily in very small offices. Based on this survey and the functions that accrue to a large research office, a unit might be organized as is the University of California, Davis. Figure 4-1 shows the main functions and the reporting structure used to support the major areas of responsibility.

The Role of Research Administration in Universities

During and after World War II, Vannevar Bush began promoting the responsibility and benefits of federal support science and the role of universities in forging a national research agenda. Out of his efforts and those of other prominent scientists emerged the Office of Naval Research and the National Science Foundation. Regulators and the laws and regulations that they pass and protect grew in number and scope, generating the need for newly created positions at organizations that were in receipt of federal support for research. An organization that receives federal and other external funding for research, education, or other sponsored projects must commit to assuring the sponsor that they will adhere to generally accepted accounting principles and will comply with the laws, regulations, and program-specific requirements. Who or where in the organization this responsibility is vested is determined by the organization. There is no externally required or prescribed requirement that an office of research is established at the senior leadership level. However, if form and responsibility are to follow function, the creation of a central research administration is logical.

Roles and Responsibilities of the Research Administrator

Over the past 50 years universities began assigning responsibility for some oversight and coordination of research activities to an individual, generally a faculty member, who handled the administrative activities part-time. As the regulations, requirements and competition for funds expanded, so did the roles and numbers of responsible individuals. Gradually an entire body of knowledge and requisite skills emerged and the administration of research became a recognized unit within research-intensive organizations. Whereas in the 1970s a large university may have had only a few research administrators, it now requires literally hundreds of faculty, staff and high level administrators to manage the research enterprise. The research itself may encompass thousands of faculty, undergraduate, graduate, and post-doctoral students, and technical and staff support.

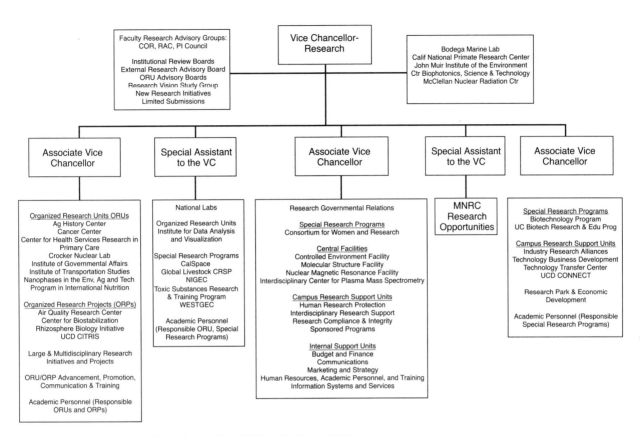

FIGURE 4-1 Organization Chart, University of California, Davis, 2004

The Research Administrator

The label *research administrator* is relatively new and describes generally someone who leads, manages or supports the research enterprise. The research administrator may provide service centrally or at the department or program level. Over the past 40 to 50 years, administration evolved from the responsibility assumed as part of another job to very specialized positions and leaders and managers with an enormous breadth of knowledge. In some large institutions, the research enterprise, because of its scope and complexity, parallels the management of a large business, and the scope of the research administrator has expanded to encompass this scope. Identified below are generic descriptions of typical members of the positions that form the leadership and administrative team in a central research program.

Chief Research Officer (CRO) In the university structure, the CRO is generally a researcher who has risen up the administrative ladder to the title of "vice president" or "vice chancellor for research." With the advent of large independent research organizations, the CRO may also serve as the chief

executive officer (CEO). While the organization is the legal receiver of all grant and contract funds, the authority to commit the institution, the authorizing official usually is delegated to the CRO. The CRO may assume a national leadership role in policy development and help set research priorities. At the home institution the CRO is responsible for fostering a research culture and environment and potentially leading the university in regional economic development. It is also this position that must instill, along with the president or chancellor, the highest level of research integrity. The CRO is generally the authorizing signatory for external proposals and awards and ultimately has responsibility of the management of the research enterprise at the institution.

Associate Vice President or Vice Chancellor Larger institutions may have multiple associate positions. Traditionally, these individuals are research faculty who have assumed administrative roles. Responsibilities may be directed to specific discipline areas, colleges, or research units or programs. Increasingly, large institutions are also promoting individuals to this role who have skill and experience managing research units such as sponsored programs, research compliance, and technology transfer but who may not have had a faculty position. Sponsored programs offices, technology transfer, and research compliance may report to associate vice president. Development and oversight of training programs may rest with the associate.

Assistant Vice President or Chancellor The position of assistant vice president or chancellor is generally an administrative position and may have responsibility for the administration of the budget and human resources and other central management functions. Additionally this may be the title for the head of the sponsored programs function.

Special Assistant to the Vice President With the expansion of research programs and the increasing complexity of research, special assistants to the CRO assume responsibility for specialized programs. For example, a special assistant may be appointed to oversee expansion of an institution's nanotechnology related programs. These are generally faculty who assume part-time or temporary administrative positions.

Director of Sponsored Programs The director of sponsored programs has responsibility over all aspects of the process of proposal submission and contract negotiation. In smaller offices, this individual may also have the management of grant accounting and research compliance. The director frequently has signature authority for proposals and awards and may further delegate that authority to senior research officers. Efficient processes of awards, negotiations of grant and contract awards, training, and management of the budget and human resources of the office are the director's responsibility. Some universities have a separate research development office or the director of sponsored programs may be responsible for this function.

Director of Technology Transfer Institutions with separate technology transfer offices will have a director who will oversee staff experienced in the legal and technical aspects of protection of intellectual property (IP), licensing of patents and other IP, and, potentially, development of spin-off companies and regional economic development. Responsibility for material transfer agreements (MTAs) and nondisclosure agreements (NDOs) and industrial collaborations may fall under the director of technology transfer.

Director of Research Development Research development may be the responsibility of the vice president or vice chancellor or may rest with a director, who takes responsibility for maintaining data and information on grant or contract opportunities, disseminating the information to researchers and scholars, and offering assistance to individuals seeking specific research opportunities. The director may also be responsible for training and assistance in proposal development.

Director of Interdisciplinary Research With the emphasis at the federal level for large-scale, multidisciplinary or interdisciplinary research, the director may assume responsibility for development teams of researchers and preparation of complex or institutional proposals.

Director of Extramural Accounting The director must have extensive knowledge of financial compliance and federal, state and institutional regulations and policies regarding the expenditure and accounting for externally supported research and scholarship. This individual oversees the process of establishing extramural accounts, tracking and approving expenditures, and requesting draw-downs or reimbursements for sponsored projects. Institutional reporting to sponsors may rest with this office.

Director of Research Compliance Research compliance positions in medical schools and hospitals generally oversee billing compliance and clinical investigations. Compliance officers and directors who are part of a research office team ensure that a campus has all the requisite research related policies and procedures to carry out compliance. In addition, the office may be responsible for scientific misconduct investigations and conflict of interest reviews and management teams.

Director of the Human Subjects Office The human subject office/IRB director manages the office that provides support for the institution's institutional review board (IRB) committees. The human subjects or IRB offices oversee process, policy delineation, training, and coordination of the members and committees charged to protect human subjects in research. As part of this role, the director oversees policy development, ensures policy compliance, sets training programs, establishes efficient review processes and maintains records and committee minutes, and tracks and audits compliance with IRB decisions.

Director of Animal Care and Use   The director of the institutional animal care program supports the institutional animal care and use committee (IACUC). The director ensures compliance with federal, state, and institutional policy and promotes the humane treatment of animals in research. The animal care office supports the IACUC by setting processes that are efficient and appropriate, develops and delivers training programs for investigators who use animals in research, assists investigators in designed appropriate protocols, and oversees the procurement and care of animals used in research.

Authorities Delegated to the Research Leadership

Generally, signature authority for the multitude of documents signed daily in research offices is legally vested in the highest authority at the institution. The high authority may be the chair of the board of trustees, the regents, the president or CEO, or other governing body. At a public institution, signature authority may be a matter of state law. In order for the institution to function, signature authority is delegated to the responsible operational unit, for example, the vice president or chancellor for research. The CRO may then re-delegate signature authority to directors and possibly senior research officials assuming there is not an institutional or state prohibition against lower tier delegation. All delegations should be in writing to protect both parties and the institution. Faculty and administrators may sign documents without clear understanding of the implications of what has been signed and without delegated signature authority.

Summary

This chapter began with a discussion of the forms and functions commonly associated with the leadership and management of the research enterprise at a university or independent research institution. The functions described are extensive and range from research initiation and proposal development to the dreaded audit from an internal or external entity. Likewise, the model for the structures and positions needed to be created to handle the expanding multitude of required functions has been outlined. The model developed in this chapter placed most of the functions within one central unit. This may or may not be effective in all institutions. For example, the post-award accounting function traditionally has been situated within a business unit. Currently there is a trend toward incorporating all research functions, including research accounting, within a central research office. There are good arguments for keeping an arms-length relationship between a research office and the accounting function as well as equally good arguments for the efficiency of having a "one-stop shop." As an institution reviews its organizational structure and its strategic plan, it might review whether or not it has established a structure that optimally accommodates all of its clients and accomplishes all critical functions. Sometimes, for historical reasons or to accommodate individual skills or personalities, we end up with the hippopotamus. But like the hippo, the form and function meld into a workable creature. In conclusion, each research institution must define for itself the most workable, effective, and efficient form and function.

• • • References

1. Department of Defense, Department of Energy, Nuclear Regulatory Commission, and Central Intelligence Agency. *National Industrial Security Program Operating Manual.* Washington, DC: US Government Printing Office, 1995, sec. 1-204.

2. *Management for Research in U.S. Universities.* Washington, DC: National Association of College and University Business Officers, 1978, 1.

3. InterAcademy Council, *Inventing a Better Future: A Strategy for Building Worldwide Capacities in Science and Technology,* 2003, http://www.interacademycouncil.net/report.asp?id=6258 (accessed August 26, 2005).

5

University Research Development and the Role of the Chief Research Officer

Michael R. Dingerson, PhD

Have you ever pondered why one university makes substantial, even striking progress in advancing its research program, while a similar institution struggles to stay even or makes only modest progress? What is it that distinguishes an institution that doubles and redoubles research funding in a short period of time? What are the understandings and ingredients that go into a successful formula for developing the university research enterprise? Why is it that so many institutions declare their intent to grow their research programs, yet few accomplish their goals? Why is the rapid growth of university-sponsored programs such a rare phenomenon? These and other related issues are addressed in this chapter. Unfortunately, there is not enough space in this text to go into the complete details of these issues, but the major and critical details that are key to the successful endeavor of research enterprise are addressed. This chapter is intended to provide a generic philosophy and model of institutional research development, one adaptable to individual institutional circumstances.

The chief research officer (CRO) is the individual with primary responsibility for research development and administration on a campus or in other research-performing organizations. In a university, he or she usually holds the title of vice president for research, associate vice president for research or a similar title, sometimes combined with a graduate studies administration title such as dean of graduate studies. Depending on the nature and history of the institution's sponsored research program, he or she spends little time on the development aspects of his or her responsibilities compared with the always-pressing administrative responsibilities. This may not be a problem at the top-ranked universities where the research mission is ingrained into the fabric of the institution, but it can be a major concern within those institutions that are ranked in the second 50 and in those outside the top 100 in funding, and particularly in institutions with aspirations for changing their research cultures and to greatly increase sponsored project funding. It is to the latter type of institution, the mid-level research university, which this chapter is primarily addressed.

Among those in research, the term "research administration" is generally understood as involving all functions necessary to support and manage sponsored project activities within an organization. These functions are generally divided into pre- and post-award activities. The term "research development"—not to be confused with "research and development"—is less understood, and is a term rarely, if ever, used within most universities. It is, in essence, a pre-award type function that focuses on the nature and capacity of the overall institutional research program rather than on services provided to faculty such as those available in preparing and submitting proposals, for instance. It is the institution that is to be "developed" in this context. It is an institutional change, even institutional transformation activity that involves leadership from the CRO in developing and following a comprehensive plan of what the institution aspires to be and how it intends to accomplish its aspirations.

A journey into the literature of most topics within research administration will produce a plethora of articles and other manuscripts. Conduct a literature search on the topic of "research development" and little or nothing will surface. Why is this? Because the issue of research development has been below the radar screen for research administrators. These individuals have seen their role as primarily support and management, not as institutional planning and change. I was one of five co-authors who produced a 1982 book entitled, *The Administration of Sponsored Programs*.[1] I argued vociferously with my colleagues without success to include the term "development" in the title. Not only was I voted down four to one then, but there is little evidence in the literature that this issue is getting any more attention now. The book did include a chapter, which I authored, entitled "Developing the Capacity for Project Support" that only scratches the surface on some of the issues.

If the issue is not prominent in the literature, then why should we consider it important? It is of critical importance because understanding the philosophy, policies, activities, and implementation of a comprehensive institutional development undertaking is the primary, if not the only, way an institution can have a successful, major transformation in its research enterprise. This transformation is not just doing more of the same in terms of sponsored research; few if any institutions can double and redouble their sponsored project activity by doing more of the same. It is a "different" institution that does so. This less practiced route to development is explored in this chapter.

Even if we understand more about the process of institutional transformation, are there reasons we should care about research development beyond the obvious added resources and possible increased prestige? Is the institutional disruption, the turmoil that is created by asking faculty to be more research focused and to undertake more, to do different kinds of things, to hire different kinds of colleagues worth the possible gain? Each institution will want to answer this question for itself, but looking to the future, institutions may only be able to answer in the affirmative. Why?

There may be a "perfect storm" coming in the research funding arena within higher education in the near future. For those midlevel institutions struggling with advancing their research missions, achieving distinction may be harder than in any time in our current memories. At a time when more and more institutions are competing for funding opportunities, there is at least a peaking if not an actual decline in available funds. For instance, recently the US Congress committed to doubling

the budget of the NSF but in actuality that agency's budget was reduced $110 million in FY 2005 over the previous year (NSF Annual Reports, 2005). Many believe this is only the beginning of an ominous trend that will be unavoidable as tax revenues decline, the deficit grows, and competition for available funds from areas like health care become more extreme. In addition, those research funding agencies that rely on endowments are not experiencing the returns on their investments they were used to in the 1990s and that trend is expected to continue into the future as far out as most have been willing to predict. Overall then, there very likely may be substantially fewer dollars being pursued by a greater number of more capable research institutions. In general, the midlevel university may find itself in jeopardy regarding whether it is able to support its research missions. It is quite possible that there will be a "shaking out" of institutions that today consider themselves research universities. Institutional research programs do not grow and prosper by natural forces; they require strong, focused leadership. Those institutions attempting to make substantial changes in their research profile requiring strong, effective leadership are more likely to succeed.

While success in this regard requires the concerted and genuine commitment and engagement of faculty and administration—particularly that of central administration and of the deans—it is the job of the CRO to develop, communicate, convince, represent, implement, evaluate, celebrate, and do whatever else is necessary to make it happen. This chapter addresses the issues and activities of significance, describes the role of the CRO and its importance, and delineates the roles of others in transforming the institutional research profile.

Why Is Rapid Growth of Research a Rare Occurrence?

Why is it that CROs have generally thought about their sponsored projects programs in a piecemeal fashion rather than recognizing their programs as part of an institutional system? I believe there are several reasons. A first reason is noted previously: there has been little or no literature to inform CROs about the philosophy and issues. This results in the research development role being poorly understood or not understood at all.

A second reason is that CROs generally end up in their positions because they have been successful funded researchers and they see the world of sponsored projects through those experiences. To them, the most important issues are developing and implementing better policies and providing better services. They basically think about ways to do better what is currently being done; they don't think of their function as an institutional change/transformation function. Their typical answer to research growth is for the faculty to improve the quality of proposals they write and submit more proposals to a broader selection of funding agencies. These are important activities, indeed, but they limit what growth the institution can expect. They are necessary activities in making an institution a more research-oriented place and they improve the possibilities of increased funding, but they will not by themselves result in major advances.

A third reason is that the CRO position (and other research administration positions held by faculty) have been seen as a stop-out in a career, not as a career. Today's CRO may stay in his position for a longer time than in the past but by the time an individual gets in this position (and it may be their first research administration position) they are likely to be a senior administrator fixed in their ways and seeing the problems of the institution in a limited context. They have not had the experiences that would provide them with a mental model of what is possible.

Another reason is that the CRO is almost always under pressure to respond to immediate problems and issues happening as a result of lack of planning and systems thinking. In general, I believe that research administration offices are almost always understaffed, at least understaffed to the degree that the CRO does not have time to spend on the important larger and longer-term issues of planning, representing, and advancing the overall institutional research effort. This problem is further exacerbated by the fact that institutions do not have the fiscal will and/or flexibility to address adequate staffing for the research office often because presidents do not understand the nature and magnitude of the problems. Mundane administrative responsibilities, whether institutionally assigned or self-assigned, are the bane of the CRO. How many institutions require the CRO to affix his signature to all proposals leaving the institution, and how many CROs pride themselves on reading every proposal that leaves the campus? These kinds of activities are not only a waste of a senior administrator's time but take away from the very activities that could help the institution distinguish itself in terms of research growth.

Finally, it takes a very aggressive, confident, and accomplished individual to undertake a role that is very visible, possibly controversial, and in many ways antithetical to the stereotypical faculty personality and role. Few have been knowledgeable, able, or willing to undertake the kind of role that is being described here. This is a very important aspect of a research development undertaking that may go unrecognized by many because it is inconsistent with most people's expectations and there have been few role models of this type in these positions. My experience is that there is no single issue more important than this: it is at the heart of a successful research development effort.

The word "system," as discussed in the earlier section, is a useful term to describe the philosophy that is being advanced in this chapter. The success of developing a university research program growing at a rapid pace and with the capacity to continue along such a growth path into the future, is based on understanding the ingredients that go into creating a comprehensive plan and implementing it within and outside the institution. The plan will be only as strong as its weakest elements. There are many critical players but none more critical than the CRO because it is his or her role to create and communicate the vision and to work tirelessly on its implementation. Before we go into more depth about the CRO role, it will be important to delve into the other key roles needed to make the research development plan a success.

The President

The president is obviously very important to successful institutional change efforts and is responsible for resource allocation and policy directions that are critical to any effort to increase sponsored project activity. It is often the president who calls for action on the research agenda. It may be to move from one classification, such as in years back from Carnegie Doctoral I to Carnegie Research II, a very important distinction in the world of institutional competition for dollars and prestige. Make no doubt about why the president is interested in improving the research profile of his institution—his or her reputation and the reputation of the institution are riding on it.

A common goal of midlevel institutions is to move into the top 100 in sponsored research, a distinction that brings enormous bragging rights, possible increases in state funds for the public institutions, enhanced prestige, and all the rewards that come with the acknowledgment of the latter including the ability to recruit a higher quality student and faculty. The ability to attract higher quality individuals to the institution (or to a department) is one of the hallmarks of success in a growing research environment and one that provides its own momentum into the future. A university that can attract a top-level researcher faculty member is able to attract other similar talent, allowing the institution over time to hire from a pool of candidates that it may not have been able to touch earlier. This is one of the major long-term keys to changing the nature of the institution and improving its research prospects.

For the president to play a successful role in this activity, he or she must believe in what the institution will accomplish in research. The president must be willing to mention the term "research" in each and every public presentation and internal meeting in which the institutional mission and future is relevant. He or she must fully support the institutional development plan, be willing to get actively engaged in its implementation, be willing to support policies that make it possible for the plan to succeed and be willing to allocate resources that help make it all happen. He or she must be consistent, create realistic expectations followed by responsive financial commitments, be willing to create and evaluate institutional expectations, and be able to lead in highly visible institutional celebrations. He or she must walk the walk and talk the talk to make it work. Faculty will know immediately or shortly if the president is not a genuine believer and supporter.

Unfortunately, too many presidents do not understand the issues sufficiently and have the impression or belief that increasing the institution's research profile is just a matter of existing faculty doing more, that there is not an institutional cost to this activity and that grant funds are out there for the easy picking if faculty will just write more proposals. Faculty know better but it seems that some individuals who end up in presidencies think all of this happens in sort of a magical way with little or no investment—just declare it and it will happen. Not so! And, while the "road work" will be done by the CRO, deans, department chairs, faculty, and others, the president must be seriously on board for any of this to succeed. The president must be able to convincingly articulate what is to be accomplished and why it is important for the institution and good for the faculty. The president must set clear goals and, again, be consistent and frequent with the research message.

Vice President for Academic Affairs/Provost

The academic vice president must be as overtly supportive as the president and must address the impor-

tance of the evolving research mission nearly as often as the president. This is the individual with direct responsibility for the functions and personnel of the institution who will lead in the transformation of the research program. The vice president must be on board and be able to articulate the vision for the future as effectively as the president. The person in this position is particularly important in the areas of faculty evaluation, promotion and tenure, merit salary rewards, and new hires. This person is also responsible for other incentives and investments and possibly in funding the expansion or initiation of promising research programs. These issues and others under this position's jurisdiction will be discussed later. The importance of this position in the success of a research development is critical.

Deans and Chairs/Department Heads

It is in the colleges where "the rubber meets the road," particularly within departments. The deans and chairs must buy into the new mission with the same level of zeal as the president, vice president, and CRO. If not, they must be replaced. They have multiple roles, targets of activity to meet, investments to be made, evaluations of performance to conduct, and active leadership to be provided in the development of their departments and individual faculty. More of what this includes will become apparent in later sections. What is important at the outset is that the deans and chairs are supportive of the new research mission and are active supporters of its accomplishment. It is easy for one or more deans and chairs to "hide" from this mission but it is important to the institution that these individuals are truly on-board and aggressive in their developmental and support roles.

In those institutions in which the chairs have had a coordination-type role, there is a need to transition to a head-type role in which the chair plays an instrumental part in the policy and decision matters of the department, in the development of the research activities of the department, and in the individual and collective careers of the faculty. This sort of change can be very shocking for some individuals and institutions but is necessary to focus the institution's resources most effectively in the direction of developing the overall research program. The chair must also face the issue of the allocation of faculty time to particular responsibilities. This means that if faculty are not or have not been active in research they will be assigned other activities, including teaching more and conducting more service activities. It is not wise to make the responsibilities issue a confrontation that creates anxiety in tenured faculty who know they will neither be willing nor able to go along with the new priorities of the institution. It should be made clear that they will not prosper in terms of the reward structure for the future but that their services to the institution are valuable and respected. At the same time, the institution should do everything possible to find ways to use these people effectively and to ease them to retirement as soon as possible. Overt buy-out programs and other incentives for senior faculty to retire are often very good institutional investments that will accelerate the transition to a new institutional research profile.

Research Administration Infrastructure

Universities are notorious for understaffing research administration offices. There are two sources of workload pressure on these operations that are frequently not well recognized and/or respected by those allocating funds for new staff positions. The first is the stealth-like growth of regulatory requirements emanating from federal and state sources. These are often costly issues that are a hard-sell to campus administrators until the institution is in some sort of compliance bind which, of course, is the research administrator's greatest fear. The second source of workload pressure for these offices is the growing number of proposal submissions along with expectations of increased support from faculty sensing the pressure from the administration to increase research funding.

These are pressures that cannot be ignored but they also cause difficulties in other ways as well. The first is that these offices frequently have stressed-out staff members who spend the vast majority of their time in administrative duties—getting the proposals out the door, etc., rather than in proposal development activities. This often means that there is no qualified assistance for new faculty and others who need help in such activities as identifying possible funding sources, drafting a proposal, or finding a colleague from another department who may strengthen the pending research. A modest amount of these kinds of services is important in any institution seeking sponsored projects. It is critical in the institution seeking to transform its research program. These activities can be centralized up to a point in the development of the institution's program but they must either be transferred to the colleges or initiated there anew as growth in activity proceeds. Having a single individual in each college, with a title of associate dean or something similar which faculty will respect, responsible for research, is a proven functional way to support research development and administration in the colleges while allowing for a coordinated

overall institutional effort out of the CRO's office. A university council of research deans is an excellent mechanism to foster important communications and to develop plans, projects, and policy.

Policy Development Important for Research Growth

The most important policies that must be considered in a growing research environment are those related to assignment of time, salary administration, and promotion and tenure. Some discussion of faculty responsibilities was included in the previous section. What is important here is to recognize that faculty teaching assignments for research-active faculty must be driven down over time to allow these faculty to expand the base of sponsored project activity. Assuming that a normal faculty load is four courses or the equivalent per semester, teaching assignments should decline to two, one or even no courses (for short periods) depending on other responsibilities. It is not possible for faculty to maintain substantial teaching assignments and be expected to be successful in attracting major external resources. On the other hand, it is not advisable to keep research-unproductive faculty on light teaching assignments. Accountability in this matter is very important. Faculty should be expected to produce what is considered reasonable in their assignment or the assignment should be expected to change. This is a delicate balancing act for the chair and an important issue of integrity for the department and institution. Fair treatment is critical both to faculty morale as well as to the productivity of an individual or a unit.

It is equally as critical that salary administration be conducted with integrity. While this is a difficult issue under any circumstances, it is even more so when the institution is changing its mission and the reward structure has changed to reflect that. Merit salary increases must be awarded for accomplishments that are in keeping with the pronounced expectations of the institution and department. Across-the-board increases in salary should be avoided and any new allocation of salary funds should be preceded by extensive discussions of what is coming in terms of the priorities with the authorities that will make the evaluations of faculty performance. The administration of salary increase funds in any way that is inconsistent with the new expectations for the institution as communicated will diminish the commitment of the faculty and retard the outcomes for the institution.

The most difficult policy issues are related to promotion and tenure. These policies will most likely require review and revision in the context of the enhanced mission for research. At the least, the interpretation of these policies will need to become more strict. The importance of communicating these issues cannot be overstated. If the changes are substantial, there will be the possibility for campus-wide turmoil. It is the responsibility of the provost, president, CRO, deans, chairs and others to explain with a consistent dialog why these policies must change and why this is important for the institution and the individual faculty in the institution. Of particular concern are those who were hired with one set of expectations who will now be judged on another. These people need to be advised to prepare themselves for the new future of the institution or seek more compatible employment elsewhere. Opportunities for professional development need to be provided and every effort should be made to incorporate these individuals into ongoing research activities to which they might contribute. The reality is that not many of these people will be "saved," though some will, and the humane thing to do with them as a group is to assist them in any possible way to continue to have productive careers.

Incentive Policies and Activities

As the institution communicates the new vision of its research mission and begins to change its expectations for performance and for promotion, tenure and merit salary issues, it is very important that new and/or expanded, well-funded programs be made widely available to faculty to assist in their developing research and sponsored projects activities and for disseminating the results of their research.

An initial and critical aspect of this is the faculty start-up package for new hires. This can include support for equipment, reduced teaching loads in the first two years, summer salary for the first and second summers, small-project research support, and travel to professional meetings.

In most circumstances, these are very substantial expenses to the institution, upwards of one-half million dollars in cases where the equipment issues are a major cost. This is a difficult issue for universities to deal with effectively because of the usual lack of flexible resources for these kinds of expenses during any fiscal period. This requires planning and an ongoing commitment by the institution to provide an annual amount that will address the new faculty start-up issue each year. This is also a major credibility issue with the faculty. The concern of having a new faculty member come on-board without the capability to energize a competitive research program is unthinkable. The institution would be

better off to postpone or deny the hire if funds are not available to provide a competitive start-up package. The institution must show its genuine commitment to the new mission by not falling down on this kind of expectation. Sometimes it is possible to work out equipment rental or sharing arrangements with another institution as an interim condition for a new faculty member. While these are possibly inconvenient, they are often workable and not only show the seriousness of the institution to meet its commitments but provide the new faculty member an opportunity to meet individuals in his research area that could be important in future collaborations.

Funds must be made available for faculty to attend professional meetings for the purpose of networking and to disseminate the results of their research. It is important to be almost lavish with this kind of support to demonstrate to the faculty the measure of the institution's new commitment to research and sponsored projects and to its understanding of the importance of the networking and dissemination processes to the development of the faculty and to the future research growth of the institution. It is better to "waste" resources supporting this important activity than to provide too few resources for the challenges facing the faculty. While it is important to adequately fund this activity, it is equally important to communicate clearly that institutional funds will be used primarily for developmental efforts and on a short-term basis and that faculty will be expected to generate funds for these kinds of activities in the future from their grants and contracts. It is important to be aware of the possibility (actually probability) of faculty getting used to having institutional resources available for this kind of activity and that with each allocation should come the notice that these kinds of expenses are being covered for developmental purposes and that faculty are expected to generate these funds themselves in the future. If this is done properly, the institution will get its message across and the faculty will understand that it is a temporary activity to help them wean themselves off internal resources onto external resources. Faculty do understand that the institution does not have the resources required to support this kind of activity as an ongoing expense but communicating this effectively to avoid hard feelings is very important.

It is critical that the institution have a small-grants program in place for supporting new faculty and those developing new areas of research or who are between grants. There may be other reasons to have such a program and it is very important to be explicit about the program's purposes and priorities. Supported projects should be significant. The review of proposals must have a peer-review process to be conducted with integrity, and those awarded funds must be held accountable for dissemination of results and the preparation of external submissions based on the work. An important function of the research office is to follow up internal awards with assistance in identifying possible funding sources and in offering to assist in the proposal preparation process.

Faculty need to know that if the institution makes a commitment to their research they will be expected to keep their end of the bargain by being accountable. Every legitimate effort to assist faculty to interact with an external funding agency must be pursued. The purpose here is to generate familiarity with the process and to help a developing faculty member gain one step in the ladder of success to larger externally funded projects. There is no doubt that success breeds success in this activity as does removing the mystery that some feel it holds. A small-grants program properly managed by the CRO allows all of these issues to be productively addressed.

In institutions with commitments for major changes in research, it is important that new incentives be considered. Much of what is occurring in these institutions will require more of a business approach to growth activities. This could mean that new forms of rewards need to be considered and developed—forms that have been generally considered an anathema in higher education. Overload salary policies and opportunities need to be explored as do bonuses for exemplary accomplishments in scholarship, research, and external funding. The institution may also need to consider a separate not-for-profit corporation to undertake activities like the aforementioned that are difficult or impossible to undertake within the organization framework of the institution. Award programs also need to be developed for research-related activities which include appropriate professional and financial recognition for exemplary performance in selected areas.

New and or strengthened incentives and rewards are critical in generating the appropriate and responsive environment in which research and sponsored project growth can occur. It is very important that these efforts be conducted with integrity to avoid any perceptions of unequal or unfair treatment. This is sometimes difficult to do but is very important to the intended outcomes. It is

also important that the institution not try to "low ball" the funding for these efforts. Again, it is better to spend too much rather than too little on these programs, particularly in the early years when the integrity of the programs and the overall aspirations of the institution are subject to most questions. It is penny-wise and pound-foolish, to repeat an overused phrase, to skimp in any way on efforts such as these which are at the heart of the institution's efforts to provide incentives and rewards and to assure the integrity of the institution's intentions.

Role and Importance of the Chief Research Officer

It is at the desk of the CRO that all the issues of research development find their nexus. The CRO is the person who is the visible embodiment of all the research and sponsored projects aspirations held by the institution and energized by the president and provost. It is the leadership of the CRO that will make the difference in the overall success of the institution in meeting its goals. Just as the faculty must be held accountable, the president must hold the CRO accountable for the institution's goals in research.

As was noted earlier, the overall research development effort is only as strong as its weakest element. The elements have been discussed in the previous pages and must be the categories of concern for the CRO as he or she drafts and develops an institutional research development plan. The plan is very important to bring clarity to exactly what the institution is seeking with its research development efforts. The CRO is likely to start with a mandate from the president that is ill-defined, yet clear in its orientation; the purpose of the CRO's plan is to clarify the details. The ability to communicate consistently and effectively is based on a realistic and well understood plan that will result in the buy-in of the faculty. The president may start with a statement something like the following: "we must increase our institutional research profile; our future success in attracting better students and faculty and becoming a better institution is contingent on being in the top 100 universities in federal funding in five years." That may be a lofty and worthy goal yet there will only be fuzzy understandings at best across campus of how to achieve this goal. It is the job of the CRO to create a vision (the plan) for the institution that will remove the fuzziness and bring clarity to the issues that will be unmistakably understood by those who are to play a role in how this is going to be achieved. Of course the CRO cannot do this in a vacuum nor can he or she do it in an arbitrary fashion. In a sense, the CRO is required to develop this plan while seeking the voluntary commitment of the faculty. There is a good chance of arriving at a mutually shared plan that will achieve the institution's goals with the right conditions, realistic goals, serious commitments from the institution for programs and rewards, and the active involvement of the faculty. All of these components must be in place within a context of high integrity—of the faculty toward the administration and vice versa. A project cannot proceed when the goal is unrealistic or when there is administrative cynicism toward the faculty and from the faculty to the administration in return.

It is the president's responsibility to set the tone and to clearly establish the institutional goals. Institutional aspirations will need to be repeated by the president and provost as often as possible. Making the goals a part of the campus culture is important from the outset. It will be important for the president to meet with the deans to be sure the goals are clear and to make it known that any dean not on board should step down or will be replaced by the provost. This can be done professionally and effectively without hurting any individuals, if done with care. Deans who step down from their positions should be treated with the utmost of respect and should be afforded positions of significance if possible. This may sound harsh but at this point institutional accountability is critical from top to bottom and the institution that is serious about these undertakings must have all key staff consistent in their thinking and actions. This does not mean that there are not differences of opinion about how to accomplish the goals, for there surely will be, but there must not be differences in the goals that are eventually arrived at for the institution.

The CRO must be the primary communicator in keeping the dialog going between the administration and faculty. He or she must be able to deliver resources for new programs and incentives, be able to effectively address the teaching load issue, and must have a sympathetic ear for real faculty issues when they arise. The CRO is the focal point from the administration to move the institutional agenda forward and the focal point for the faculty, deans, and chairs in turning the institution's aspirations into goals, programs, and activities. The CRO may want to identify a key group of senior faculty to serve as a sounding board for the many issues. The involvement and endorsement of a group like this can be very important in the eventual acceptance and success of the plan.

The university with a fast growing research program will be successful because it will concentrate on developing larger, group activities around institutional research strengths. There will be more group activities and fewer individual-investigator activities in the future institutional research profile. A university cannot double its external research funding by doing more single-investigator projects; there is simply not enough manpower within the institution to accomplish this. This issue is one of the major fallacies put forward by those who do not understand these issues or who view research development through a limited lens of experience. It will be accomplished by getting successful researchers involved in larger efforts, helping them become research leaders in a sense, while they provide new opportunities for those who have been minimally active. The CRO must take the responsibility of forming groups of faculty within the institution who have similar or intersecting interests. It is his or her responsibility to provide leadership to the development of these groups as he or she searches for a natural leader to take over each group. The CRO may want to take such actions as to provide resources for a seminar series, send research office staff to consult about possible sources of external resources, and provide other support to keep the group intact in ways that might make sense for future proposal submissions.

Another responsibility of the CRO is to initiate and establish interfaces with other universities and other possible collaborators such as national labs and private research groups. It is important to have standing groups of individuals and organizations that are ready to respond to a proposal opportunity on short notice. This is usually not possible if a group has to be established for this purpose from scratch. Standing research groups, like multiuniversity consortia, are critical to these kinds of efforts. They are effective and important ways for an institution to extend its capabilities and to generate resources that an institution would not be competitive for without a partner. It takes a particularly mature institution and CRO to establish and work through these kinds of arrangements because compromise and the sharing of dollars and credit are at the core of successful partnerships of this kind. Presidents are sometimes difficult to convince that activities of this type are good for the institution. It is the CRO who is responsible for convincing the president of the importance of these activities and for identifying those opportunities, with the assistance of the faculty, and to provide the leadership to bring them to fruition. The CRO must always be looking for permanent leadership for these activities, possibly leaving behind a staff member from the research office to support the activity as he or she moves to other agenda. However, the CRO must continue to provide material and moral support to these groups and must not lose contact with their efforts. The CRO must also be a participant or a leader in celebrating their successes.

The CRO must also provide leadership in the institution's efforts to secure funding directly from the state legislature and from the US Congress. Commonly known as "pork barrel funding," these initiatives can be very important in supporting important projects and in building institutional capacity for future research activities. While these kinds of activities may be distasteful to some, there is over $2 billion being spent at the federal level in this way on university campuses annually. As long as this process is going on, the CRO must lead his or her institution in this activity either as a single institutional entity or as part of a multicampus effort to secure funds for specified activities. This source of funds has been particularly important to some campuses in establishing or expanding research centers and in acquiring new facilities. Multicampus activities within a state are particularly important possibilities for federal pork barrel funding. It is the role of the CRO to initiate, communicate, and direct this effort from beginning to end. The CRO's staff must prepare the materials used to communicate an initiative and he must take the lead in personally presenting the institution's priorities to elected officials and their staff. The president may want to get involved in some of this but it is up to the CRO to assemble the plan, the materials, and the strategy for pursuing these opportunities. It is sometimes advisable to seek professional assistance in this kind of activity. The CRO must select someone with whom he or she can work effectively. It is also advisable for the CRO to know if this kind of decision is a good one for the institution as well, since some elected officials would rather work with people from the institution than with a professional lobbyist. This can be a very delicate issue that must be managed very carefully by the president and CRO.

The CRO must have resources to make all of these programs and activities available. He or she must have flexible funds to respond to any problem or opportunity as it arises. He or she must not be handicapped in the progress of the institution's growth because resources are not available. The investment dollars available to make all of this happen are just that—investments. If an institution does not have or is not willing to make resources available for these purposes, it should not be embarking on an effort to generate substantial growth in research and sponsored projects. Not only will it not be successful but faculty will become cynical and withdrawn and everything will be more difficult to achieve in the future. While universities are frequently undercapitalized in their ventures, this should not be the reason for failure at research development. If capitalization is an issue, some well-funded activities should be initiated while others are postponed rather than mount a comprehensive effort for which adequate funds are unavailable.

The CRO must lead in the celebration of the institution's successes. The CRO must recognize individual accomplishments, arrange activities in which individuals can be recognized for their work, and create forums where the future of the institution in terms of sponsored research can be celebrated and discussed. A major outside speaker is sometimes a good idea when doing this as well; it builds pride amongst the faculty in addition to spreading the message that this university is serious about its research mission. An annual dinner, inviting all faculty who have submitted proposals is a positive motivator as is a research fair where faculty and students set up posters to communicate their undertakings and results. Any productive activities that bring attention to the research agenda should be considered. It is up to the CRO to know what is appropriate and to what magnitude these activities should occur.

The CRO must be an optimist about the future of the university's research program and its ability to grow to meet its aspirations. He or she must be a source of exuberance and confidence in the research plan and communicate its importance within the institution to faculty and to individuals and groups outside the institution. However, the CRO must not be perceived as being out of touch with reality; enthusiasm must always be within a context of realism. The institution's demonstrated success is a powerful influence in convincing faculty to get involved in research endeavors. Less effective is proof-of-concept evidence for the research development plan and how these successes are benefiting faculty and the institution.

Over the course of this process, there comes a tipping point when all the commitments of time and other resources bring a cascade of successes. This will be an obvious occurrence to the CRO; faculty will voluntarily bring external funding opportunities, large projects will receive funding due to the hard work of a productive group of faculty which the research office has been staffing, and the research development effort will seem to run on its own steam in a sense. This means that the faculty will take charge of the development effort themselves; and where the CRO was originally needed as a catalyst to get the program started, involvement will become infrequent or cease. Activities will evolve under "local leadership" and grow with sometimes boundless energy. A true litmus test for when an institution has "arrived" in this context is that there is no discussion of the research mission when a new individual comes on board—it is all a given, and the new person will correctly assume that he or she is there to continue what has been established by those who preceded. It is clear that *the* mission is research. At this point, the CRO may take a brief vacation.

The Bottom Line

An institutional research development undertaking is a complex and difficult task that has specific ele-

ments that must be considered. The single most important issue, however, is the leadership provided by the chief research officer. There is no substitute for informed, able, and persistent leadership, in a context of total accountability, in rapidly achieving the institution's aspirations in research. This chapter has explored the issues and activities, from an overview perspective, that each institution must consider in arriving at a comprehensive research development plan. Of course like most issues in higher education and life in general, the devil is in the details. The purpose of this chapter has been to present and discuss the issues while leaving the final crafting of a specific plan to those who know their institution best.

• • • Reference

1. Beasley, K.L., Dingersen, M.R., Hensley, O.D., Hess, L.G., and Rodman, J.A., *The Administration of Sponsored Programs.* San Francisco, CA: Jossey-Bass, 1982.

II

The Infrastructure for Research Administration

6

The Research Administrator as a Professional: Training and Development

Marcia Landen, MS, and Michael McCallister, PhD

Introduction

Research administrators work in an intricate world at the interface between the research project and the research institution where they help to balance the motives for research with the institution's ability to conduct it. Motives are the human elements: a researcher's search for knowledge, the desire for individual tenure or institutional prestige, or anything else that motivates the people involved. The institution's ability to conduct research is more practical, including physical facilities, financial capabilities, and the large administrative infrastructure required to support the research function. Each research project brings the potential for institutional and personal rewards, as well as institutional and personal jeopardy.

Complementary factors govern both the work and the types of people who can effectively do the jumble of work we call research administration. Talents, abilities, aptitudes, interests, and education all play a role. We seek and nurture people who can see and understand life in the borderlands, who can keep those borders open and commerce flowing. What kinds of people are effective at the borders? Those who understand the cultures, speak the languages, and understand the systems of commerce. Research encompasses many cultures, not only national and ethnic cultures but also disciplinary cultures and styles of and approaches to research itself.

All of this requires special people who possess global and systemic understanding along with the ability to communicate with and appreciate the multiplicity of people who constitute the research enterprise. Successful research administrators must have an affinity for the creative process in a variety of disciplines, an acceptance for the mixture of ways research and its administration is done, and an appreciation for what constitutes a contribution to the field. Research administrators are brokers, translators, intermediaries, and helpers who value the long-term process. But mostly, research administrators are believers in the vital importance of research.

Traditionally a research administrator's role involves some or all of these tasks:

- Understanding the nature of the principal investigator (PI)'s research
- Assisting the PI with pending funding opportunity information
- Promoting positive relationships between the PI and research sponsors
- Helping the PI apply for a grant or contract, especially through assistance with budgets, forms, deadlines, approvals, and signatures
- Recording and reporting on related institutional information
- Ensuring that the PI's proposal complies with institutional policies and sponsor requirements
- Assisting the PI with the financial and managerial aspects of awards
- Ensuring the integrity of the institution's financial and nonfinancial processes related to the research function.

The traditional view of research administration has subpopulations (e.g., pre-award, compliance, technology transfer) and responsibility levels (e.g., vice president, contract negotiator, department secretary) in discrete functional units, usually separated by physical location and reporting line. Central pre-award and post-award offices, for example, have seen themselves as two distinct components bound only at the point of award. However, the need for professional development cuts across these lines. The need for training research administrators in a more global mode of problem solving, rather than training for a specific task, is new.

A look at the contemporary state of research administration shows a trend toward decentralization, meaning that people not traditionally part of the central research administration function have become a recognized part of the research administration team. This is evidenced by the growth in training specifically for departmental administrators by professional organizations as well as by an increase in institutional programming for this group. Change brings resistance. The institution's leaders and change agents are more likely to foster success if issues are made clear. All research administrators should feel confident that because of what they do, problems get solved. While research administrators are not "teachers" in the traditional pedagogical sense, they are nonetheless educators, facilitators, skill builders, change agents.[1]

Research Administration as a Profession

We tend to think of our membership in the research administration community as belonging to a particular profession. But discussion and definition of the concept "profession" is wide-ranging. A Google search on "definition of profession" yields 1.7 million hits. One appealing definition comes from the Australian Council of Professions: "A profession is a disciplined group of individuals who adhere to ethical standards and uphold themselves to, and are accepted by the public as possessing special knowledge and skills in a widely recognized body of learning derived from research, education and training at a high level, and who are prepared to exercise this knowledge and these skills in the interest of others."[2] This definition implies, and most definitions explicitly state, that a profession includes a code of ethics for its members with recognized professional standards of behavior, along with recognized professional education and training.

The idea of "profession" is also a topic of academic study by business faculty, sociologists, communication researchers, historians, and others.

Evetts,[3] in a meta-analysis of some of the research done in sociology, notes that the meaning of professionalism is not fixed. She states, "The ideology of professionalism that is so appealing to occupational groups and their practitioners includes aspects such as exclusive ownership of an area of expertise and knowledge and the power to define the nature of problems in that area as well as the control of access to potential solutions." Research administrators function as an occupational group with ownership of expertise and knowledge, and in this aspect with the markings of a profession.

Therefore, we must have or must develop specialized training toward a recognized level of professional proficiency. In the absence of a generally accepted education and certification program, we have thus far tended to our own. Initial efforts include the Certified Research Administrator examination and designation[a] and certificates of completion for various administrative specialties available through conference sessions or specialized workshops of the professional organizations. In working toward a discernable and generally accepted body of knowledge, The Society of Research Administrators (SRA) and the National Council of University Research Administrators (NCURA) cooperated to put together a topical outline of competencies for research[b] development. The intent was to clarify the breadth and depth of research administration across subspecialties.

As research administration grows as a profession, this culture of professional development will lead to a better understanding and definition of the profession itself and, ultimately, to clearer professional standards. We value these things as insiders, however the majority of research administrators rely primarily on on-the-job-training and their network of colleagues to gain proficiency in their areas of responsibility. Attempts at formal education programs have been largely elusive.

Developing Successful Research Administrators

Research administrators play many different roles: compliance officer, cheerleader, consoler, advocate, and, perhaps the least appreciated role, crisis coun-

[a]http://www.cra-cert.org

[b]http://www.srainternational.org/newweb/Publications/topicaloutline/index.cfm

selor.[4] What qualities and skills does a successful research administrator possess? First, every research administrator generates and/or interprets information, and therefore, the administrator's ability to interpret and find meaning in textual or numeric data is crucial. In describing the successful administrator, Fish states that he or she must possess "the ability to sift through mounds of data while at the same time continually relating what the data reveal to the general principles and aspirations of the enterprise."[5] Fish talks about college and university administrators in general, but the discussion appropriately applies to issues of research administration, within or outside of academia, as well.

Secondly, successful research administrators are communicators at many levels. McCallister and Miller state, "Clear communication between researchers and research administrators fosters a partnership between the two groups that can help minimize problems in the proposal process and post-award process."[6] Communication among and between research administrators is also vital to the problem-solving and problem-prevention roles we play. Likewise, open communication between the research institution and the sponsor is vital to the success of a research project, and research administrators have key roles to play in fostering that interaction. Communication to a larger audience (e.g., the press and public) is sometimes a requirement of senior-level administrators, but all research administrators could (and should) engage in this at some level as advocates for research.

Third, successful research administrators are problem solvers who demonstrate high levels of honesty, integrity, and ethics. Solving problems frequently means fixing what someone else broke, answering ambiguous questions, weighing risk vs. reward, and finding innovative solutions to a new problem. From this, research administrators derive gratification from other people's successes as they support and facilitate the success of researchers. You will never hear a successful research administrator say, "If it weren't for the researchers it would be a great job."

Formal, professional preparation for a job in research administration is currently nonexistent. Research administrators represent all academic fields, and this diversity of expertise is a strength when working with a breadth of research disciplines. Research administrators have disparate, assorted, and diverse backgrounds: They may or may not have any training in any type of research methods, or they may be highly trained scientists embarking on a second career in administration. In all cases, it is impossible to learn how to be excellent by taking a course, reading a text, or passing a test. Learning excellence comes from learning from others, modeling behaviors, practicing creativity, and sharing one's own strengths and knowledge.

Given that formal education in research administration is nascent and that skills training is available only periodically, how does a professional learn and grow? A visit to any research office with multiple staff will show a definite line and staff arrangement—some people are managers and others are managed. What is the yardstick? An examination of positions announcements from the November/December 2003 NCURA newsletter[7] and a week's listing on SRA's Web site[8] show that mid- to senior-level positions are advertised in these national forums.

Vice Chancellor/Vice President/ General Counsel:	3
Assistant/Associate VC/VP:	3
Director:	18
Assistant/Associate Director:	4
Administrator/Coordinator/Manager/ Specialist:	17

Entry-level jobs seem to almost always be filled from the local applicant pool. And this makes sense, given the lack of preparation available for a career in research administration. Recruiting on college campuses, at job fairs, and even at professional conferences in any formal way is nonexistent. Moving up usually means moving out, with reliance on personal and professional networks and a bevy of skills collected along the way.

There are no "preprofessional" training programs for research administrators, and ongoing, organized training of any kind is relatively rare. The professional organizations provide some training, but access is limited to those with travel budgets and/or registration fees. Quality is generally good, but because the audience of research administrators attending is almost always generic, training is not always directly transferable to one's own institutional problems or processes. Training at the institution itself may be more specific, but it is generally not based on the bigger picture. So, it is apparent that most research administrators take responsibility for training themselves, using knowledge gained both inside and outside of the institution. On-the-job, experiential learning is the standard for this learn-by-doing field. Those who manage staff can provide mentoring, staff development, job shadowing, and cross-training, but the predominant form of training is still to be thrown into the deep end of the pool with the instruction, "Swim!"

This is a simplistic description, of course, but it does point out one strength of research administration professionals: *they take the initiative* to learn and grow, to stay current within the world of sponsors, regulations, technology, legislation, and other influencers of the research agenda. In the absence of a career ladder, the excellent people take the responsibility to prepare themselves for migration to other opportunities.

Research institutions must ensure that there is sufficient and adequately trained staff so that their institutional integrity is promoted. Each institution is unique in its administrative structure, management information systems, financial tools, and research-related practices and policies. Even more, they are all different in their missions, cultures, and values. Institutions are responsible for training their research administrators to master their work tools, processes, and values.

- Work tools are the things one needs to function productively. Examples are access to technology and training in its efficient use, knowledge of and the ability to apply rules and regulations appropriately, and proficiency with the institution's management and financial database(s) and software.
- Institutional processes are the things that create and distribute information, such as electronic and paper paths for seeking and moving data. Examples are institutional processes for proposal routing, financial transactions, and obtaining various approvals. Research administrators must know who is responsible for what, how information flows, and, less tangibly, the formal and informal power structure for decision making.
- Institutional values evolve based on the needs of the institution and could be called the general discourse of business. This encompasses the institution's common vocabulary and practices. Examples include the types of research allowable—e.g., is classified research conducted?—contracting language and its (in)flexibility, and recognition of universal issues as a basis for making and defending institutional decisions (e.g., institutional conflict of interest policies).

Training staff to successfully use their work tools and to master institutional processes is generally accomplished through on-the-job training supplemented by "how to" workshops or seminars through external providers. Some examples include specialized training in the Federal Acquisition Regulations, training from the vendors of any of the funding opportunity websites, use of Adobe Acrobat, public speaking seminars, etc. These are important, but not enough.

Research administrators also need access to universally accepted training programs, as well as access to peers through professional research administration organizations in order to learn about and keep abreast of the greater research administration community. There are few unique or "new" problems in research administration, other administrators have solved the same issues and we can learn from them. Just as research is more and more a collaborative venture, so is research administration, which is increasingly complex, sophisticated, evolving, and not place-bound.

In order to apply knowledge of skills and processes and values, research administrators must also learn about the institution. This cannot be accomplished by remaining safely cloistered in an administrative office. Successful research administrators serve on committees, visit research labs and facilities, go to art openings, visit the libraries, volunteer as a human subject for a study, and take research methods classes. In short, successful research administrators demonstrate that they are part of the research community not only through the job they do, but through their active participation in the institution's community.

Responsibilities of the Supervisor

Eavesdrop on a conversation among research administrators. It will quickly become evident that these people are conversant with an outlandish amount of minutia; their conversations are largely unintelligible to the ordinary observer. Yet, the role of the research administrator is that of problem solver for researchers, sponsors, and others within and outside of their institution, most of whom are not research administrators. Their knowledge store becomes the basis for answering questions or facilitating a process. In order to be successful in this problem-solving role, research administrators must possess qualities of self-assurance, personal initiative, and communication skills developed through support of their supervisors. Adequate training and development must be provided so that workers are confident in their ability to make independent decisions appropriate to their roles. Micro-managing kills the individual problem solver, and smart people cease to be independent because they no longer own their jobs. The result is that an otherwise skilled research administrator has been reduced to a clerk with routinized responsibilities.

Nurturing the problem solving abilities of research administrators requires a healthy working environment, the institutionalization of professional development, provision of appropriate tools, and the encouragement of work styles within norms of the institution.

- *Environment.* Offices of research administration are environments of people working together for a common goal. Diversity in its truest sense (gender, race, religion, ethnicity, political affiliation, age, disciplinary training) provides the most opportunity for varying viewpoints and, in turn, for problem solving for disparate researchers and sponsors. Hiring people of similar backgrounds with similar expectations and similar skills deprives the group of a richness of knowledge. Instead, cultural understanding, curiosity, and even appreciation for eccentricity should be encouraged.
- *Institutionalization of professional development.* Professional development should be an ongoing expectation, not the occasional opportunity. Supervisors and staff should routinely set mutual goals for ongoing professional development in the areas of knowledge attainment, skills enhancement, and/or personal growth.
- *Tools and job flexibility.* Some of these will be imposed by institutional policy and practice, some should be self-chosen by the employee. An employee can't very well choose the institution's accounting system, but there are other choices an employee can make, such as having a choice between a laptop and desktop workstation. Other examples are large and small, such as flexibility in working hours, participation in workgroup decision making, and freedom to question status quo or suggest change.

When hiring entry and mid-level staff, general aptitude and values are more important than specific experience in the area. Kutger notes that supervisors must find ways to identify and hire people who can learn the skills, perform the duties of the job, and fit into the new environment.[9] She cautions supervisors to be careful not to limit the applicant pool by being too specific about education and experience requirements, since there is a risk of eliminating some of the "unlikely" applicants who, with training, would be a success. Instead, she suggests that supervisors look for demonstrated competencies such as planning and organization, communication skills, flexibility, cooperation, and responsibility. Skill sets can be learned.

Developing the Individual

Because there is no academic preparation for a career in research administration, people happen into the field, then many "find themselves" in research administration, since the work enables the use of a range of interests, skills, and talents. Once hired, the professional may see his or her career as a curriculum, or a desire for ongoing learning.[10] The field is so broad and no one research administrator can know everything, so training can be both complicated and never ending. Learning the skill needed for effective research administration is a lifelong learning process. Perhaps the larger training goal is not the improvement of skills as much as it is the improvement of learner attitudes and behaviors that include competence, commitment, and confidence, as suggested by Merriam and Caffarella.[11]

The starting point for every learning experience is the problem or concern of the adult learner.[12] Once the problem or concern is identified, there are four aspects of adult education that are particularly pertinent to the research administrator:

1. implementing the learner-centered instructional strategy,
2. valuing the learner's experiences,
3. teaching skills, and
4. recognizing the role of the educator as a change agent.[13]

Therefore, the most successful programs address identified needs of the research administrator. What problems need to be solved? What processes need to be facilitated? What does the research administrator want to accomplish? How can the researcher be better served?

But organized training programs are not generally learner-centered. The well-regarded National Council of University Research Administrators (NCURA) Fundamentals workshop, for example, serves as an overview of research administration at colleges and universities. It is an excellent introduction to the vocabulary of research administration, and provides the new research administrator with a sense of community and a fundamental knowledge of the role. However, large training programs may be more about teaching than learning. It is an efficient way to be exposed to a lot of ideas, but it is not an ideal way to train people to actually *do* anything. Research administrators should take advantage of these types of programs for exposure to broad topics, for the community it provides, and to meet people who later will become a resource. But real learning takes place colleague to colleague.

The professional organizations are excellent resources for information, for networking opportunities, and for developing one's own leadership experience through volunteer activities. Training inside and outside of the institution are two sides of the same coin—both are important. Colleague-to-colleague learning generally takes place at the institution itself. Examples of institutionally based training programs include:

- One-on-one, on-the-job training
- Issue-centered impromptu group discussions
- Planned programs for specific audiences, or about a specific topic, or both
- A series of required programs or experiences that lead to a certification or other formal recognition for completion
- Programs provided outside of the research administration area, such as a seminar on institutional human resources policies

Most of these types of training opportunities happen without an inordinate amount of planning. On-the-job training takes place for all new employees, and for all employees when something about their job changes. Impromptu discussions among staff should be encouraged for optimal group problem solving and learning. Planned programs take a bit of preparation, but are generally short with only one or a few issues discussed. The series of programs leading to a formal certificate or completion is by far the most complex of these. Some institutions have invested heavily in this kind of training for their research administrators. An excellent example of this is the Research Administrator Instructional Network (RAIN) at the University of Michigan.[14] RAIN trains departmental and other research administrators according to a well-established curriculum based on particular policies and practices of the university, using the work tools that will be needed on the job. Participants meet one full day a week for four weeks. [See the RAIN Web site at http://www.research. umich.edu/rain/rain.html for course details.]

The needs of the individual for professional development will change throughout the course of a career. The new hire needs more specifics, more "how to" training, more grounding. Senior people need a broader approach, less canned programming and more discussion of policy and universal issues. For them, the mass market conference sessions are not nearly as valuable as the exposure to and discussions with other leaders in the field to spot trends, identify common concerns, and engage in collegial problem solving. Senior leaders are less likely to be interested in the changes to the National Science Foundation (NSF) Fastlane electronic administration system, for example, and more likely to care about human resource concerns, strategic planning, forecasting, resource allocation, and policy issues.

Two good examples of professional development for senior research administrators come from the Society of Research Administrators International (SRA). Some years SRA provides a retreat solely for senior members of the research administration community so that they can devote several days to a contemporary theme. Sessions are less structured with very few lectures and a high degree of discussion and individual participation. SRA's western section also taps their senior members during an "old gray heads" roundtable discussion at their spring section meeting to identify needs and solve organizational problems, as well as to recognize these experienced people as a resource for discussion, leadership, and opportunities. Ultimately, responsibility and personal interest will drive the growth and training for senior research administrators.

Identifying Training Needs

There are so many aspects to research administration, from externally imposed regulations to internal processes, that it's hard to know what training is required for any individual staff member. The traditional approach to identifying training topics focuses on finding common group-sized programs and then developing a presentation. This can be effective for certain things that lend themselves to lecture/discussion (Federal regulations are a good example); however, this approach does not satisfy the individual staff member's need for broad knowledge and skills.

One way to determine a more personalized training plan is to reverse engineer the job: what is required at that institution, in that job or related group of jobs?

A job analysis can be conducted using the following steps:

- Understand the overall position requirements. *What is the purpose of the job?*

- Articulate the tasks performed. (*What does the person in this job do?*)
- Group tasks into related categories. *What are the different kinds of activities required?*
- Identify the demands and challenges of the position. *What makes the job difficult, non-routine, or different from other jobs?*
- Identify the skills, education and experience required. *What must a person know to be successful in the job?*

Once the particulars of any job are defined, then it becomes easier to see the breadth and depth of training required, or to answer that final question, "What must a person know to be successful?"

Another approach for determining training is to conduct a needs assessment. This can be a very formal process that includes surveys and interviews, or it can be a more informal approach that consists primarily of asking people what they need to do their job better. A supervisor might use several approaches, such as having individual discussions with staff members about what staff say they need, having observation sessions of the work group to assess strengths and weaknesses, and tracking patterns or clusters of common problems.

Personal interest is also an important consideration. It is natural that an individual will have greater interest in some aspects of the job and less in others. In a large enough shop it might be reasonable for a staff member to be a specialist in a given area, but this is not always possible or desirable. Therefore, it is important to ensure training and development in all job aspects, while encouraging personal interests as well. Remember, too, that a person is never completely finished learning the business of research administration.

Training decisions are usually a combination of what a supervisor identifies as needed, what an individual staff member wants to learn, and what a research institution requires. Supervisors know that certain skills and experiences are needed and they must either hire staff with the requisite knowledge or train existing staff in acquiring new knowledge and skills. A staff member can also contribute to his or her own training agenda by identifying skills or content that will lead to improved job performance. The institution itself can also dictate certain types of training, such as compliance with institution-wide policies and practices.

The SRA/NCURA Topical Outline[c] can also serve as a menu to choose areas for specialized train-

[c]http://www.srainternational.org/newweb/Publications/topicaloutline/index.cfm

ing and identify the components applicable to an individual's responsibilities and the organization's goals and seek external training or plan for in-house or online learning opportunities.

No matter how training is planned, the learner's primary intention is to gain certain definite knowledge or skills.[15]

Evaluation

Evaluating the usefulness of training is a constant, if difficult, responsibility for the research administrator/supervisor because an individual's general development and growth are incremental and continuous. As discussed, much of the training offered by professional organizations is generic, an investment in developing the professional preparation of the research administrator. Informal one-on-one training is easy to assess and the teaching when the learner has conquered the task. But formal evaluation tools are not off-the-shelf items, and most research administrators are not trained in evaluation methodologies. Fortunately, evaluation does not have to be complex or lengthy; we just have to find out if the training made a difference.

One way for supervisors to know if their training expenditures are worthwhile is to combine training evaluations with the annual performance review. Evaluating training is related to evaluating an individual's job performance because the whole purpose of training is to improve an individual's performance. This requires some recordkeeping of the training opportunities that an employee has experienced in the last year combined with a focused interaction during the evaluation to ascertain the employee's self-report. This serves two functions: learners provide feedback on their perceptions of how well the training benefited their growth, and supervisors can decide if they want to continue investing in the type of training they supported or if an alternate training plan should be considered for the next cycle.

Office evaluations of generic "services" are actually evaluations of the staff and their effectiveness and their ability to work in a complex environment. These are also the outcomes of training and professional development, but only in the context of the group. To find out how much each staff person has grown, each evaluation must be personal and focused on the individual and their particular set of responsibilities. Evaluating each worker doesn't have to involve an intimidating call into the boss's office. Those formal kinds of discussions can be supplemented with a short survey or sampling of customer opinions and satisfaction levels. This can be done by telephone or other method, and while it may be time consuming, only the customers truly know if the individual was helpful, efficient, informed, or whatever other attribute is being sought.

Co-workers can also be involved in evaluation of training in support of processes, work flow and related topics. These evaluations will give the supervisor important information into a worker's contribution at each step of the research project's processing. This does not have to be a formal peer evaluation process, although it can be, but some type of tracking or acknowledgment of ideas, improvements, cooperation, and leadership is essential.

In the end, though, it will come down to the supervisor's daily interaction with staff and researchers, keeping track of skirmishes and victories, the little innovations that are often unnoticed, the instances when staff volunteer to help each other, and other times when your research administrators demonstrate that they know what they're doing.

Conclusion

Professional development must be an integral part of the culture of research administration. No one individual can know everything, but all research administrators can increase their knowledge and grow in this profession. This is, indeed, similar to how researchers constantly grow in their work, discovering more about their chosen fields. If smart, creative people are hired, then they must be nurtured and developed so that their brain is fed and their skills are built. We must provide opportunities for people to grow and we must build into that growth a feedback loop (evaluation) to prepare what they need next. There are many methods of training to encourage growth in understanding, knowledge, and skill that training programs provide, although there is no substitute for a manager that pays attention to the performance and needs of staff. It is vital for people to work together with their different talents and jobs in an environment and culture that values innovation, synergy, learning, and service. In this way, research administration can fulfill its goals of serving the researcher, protecting the institution, and ensuring that the sponsor's needs are met.

••• References

1. McCallister, M. "The Adult Education Mind-Set: An Effective Model for Research Administrators as Research Educators." *SRA Journal* XXVI, nos. 3 and 4 (1994/1995):41–43.

2. Australian Council of Professions site. 2004, http://www.professions.com.au/constitution.html (accessed August 12, 2004).

3. Evetts, J. "The Sociological Analysis of Professionalism: Occupational Change in the Modern World." *International Sociology* 18, no. 2 (2003): 395–415.

4. Blankinship, D.A. "Personality Priorities, Stress Management and the Research Administrator." *SRA Journal* XXVI, nos. 3 and 4 (1994/1995): 29–35.

5. Fish, S.A. "First Kill all the Administrators." *Chronicle of Higher Education*, April 4, 2003: B20.

6. McCallister, M., and Miller, C. "Forging Partnerships between Researchers and Research Administrators through Orientation Programs." *SRA Journal* XXV, no. 1 (1993): 17–21.

7. National Council of University Research Administrators. *NCURA Newsletter* XXXV, no. 4 (September/October 2003), http://www.ncura.edu/data/newsroom/newsletters/pdf/septoct03.pdf (accessed September 19, 2005).

8. Society of Research Administrators. "Jobs, 2003," http://www.srainternational.org/NewWeb/Publications/newsletter/index.cfm (accessed December 12, 2003).

9. Kutger, A. "Hiring the Unlikely to Do the Unusual." *The Journal of Research Administration 1*, no. 1 (2000): 9–16.

10. Ibid.

11. Merriam, S., and Caffarella, R. *Learning in Adulthood*. San Francisco: Jossey-Bass, 1991.

12. Knowles, M. *The Modern Practice of Adult Education: From Pedagogy to Andragogy*. New York: Cambridge Book Company, 1980.

13. McCallister, M., 1994/1995.

14. Hawkins, E., Randolph, J., and McCallister, M. "Training the Staff Close to Home: You Don't Have to Wait for a Big Meeting." Presentation at Society of Research Administrators International meeting. Vancouver, British Columbia, Canada, October 2001.

15. Cross, K. *Adults as Learners*. San Francisco: Jossey-Bass, 1987.

7

Planning for Success

Lynne U. Chronister, MPA

This book offers data, information, policies, processes and procedures, suggestions, best practices, and strategies for developing or enhancing the research enterprise. The ultimate goal of a research administration unit is to facilitate the growth of a productive, dynamic, and respected program that is carried out in an environment that promotes integrity and public benefit. Achievement of this goal requires a solid funding base and supportive administrative structure and, most critically, a short- and long-term plan for increasing institutional competitiveness. In *Competitiveness in Academic Research*, Roger L. Geiger states that "Institutional strategies for enhancing research competitiveness cannot be formulated in isolation; they will depend on institutional goals as well as opportunities in the research environment."[1] The plan can be developed through relatively informal processes or by initiating a formal strategic planning process. Whatever process is used, it is critical to involve all of the stakeholders in the process, to communicate broadly the goals and responsibilities, and to develop an achievable roadmap and implementation process. Outlined in the proceeding section are two viable processes that can be used to plan for success. As with any plan, the most critical component is implementation and evaluation to avoid the well-designed plan from collecting both dust and cynicism on the part of stakeholders.

Basic Planning

Ideally, an organization will commit to a formal, on-going strategic planning and implementation process.

However, not all institutions have the resources, inclination, or infrastructure to develop a comprehensive strategic plan and roadmap for increasing the effectiveness and the efficiency of their enterprise. The development of a basic plan is necessary for increasing the effectiveness of an operation and determining the optimal use of scarce human and financial resources. A simplified process that has worked effectively is a one-day session with key individuals that answers basic operational questions and provides a near-term roadmap for the organization. The facilitator should be someone experienced in meeting facilitation, perhaps a member of the research team.

Step One: Prepare a list of key issues to be addressed by the group and ask the participants to review the issues prior to the group meeting.

Step Two: Set a one-day planning session that is structured to respond to the following questions:

- What does the organization want to achieve over the next one or two years?
- What are we currently doing to achieve these results?
- What is working or leading toward success?
- What is not effective or generally criticized?
- What should we be doing that we are not currently doing?

Step Three: Answers to the above questions will lead to determination of the following:

- What can we stop doing—either because it isn't working or we can declare that activity a success?
- What activities should be continued?

- What new activities should be initiated to achieve success?

Step Four: The facilitator should prepare a summary of the answers and disseminate them to the participants for comment and then, based upon comments, prepare an action plan that includes timelines and responsible parties. Follow-up progress reports are a critical part of the process.

Strategic Planning Processes

According to John M. Bryson, strategic planning is "a disciplined effort to produce fundamental decisions and actions that shape and guide what an organization is, what it does, and why it does it."[2] Strategic planning is not a "quick fix" nor can an organization assume that an effective plan can be developed in a matter of days. A timeline for completing the plan and implementing the agreed upon objectives will indicate that it is an ongoing process. The first decision in the process is to determine who should be included in the process. If the implementation of the plan is to be successful, key stakeholders must be involved in the development and planning process. A delicate balance must be met to assure that everyone feels included and to ensure that the group is not too large that it becomes untenable to meet and gain any level of consensus.

Step One: Identify a strategic planning facilitator. To better assure a successful and inclusive process, it is important to bring in a qualified and experienced facilitator. It is extremely difficult to assign strategic planning facilitation to a member of the affected group. They cannot then participate in the process on an equal level with other members and they must "fit it in" to what is very likely an already heavy workload.

Step Two: Get agreement among the individuals involved on the process to be used and the timeline for the planning process. Do so well in advance; at least two days should be set for bringing the planning group together. Prior to that, information regarding expectations, current achievements, perceived barriers, and demographic information should be gathered by surveying the group. The survey may include a larger group of stakeholders than those identified to participate in the group planning session. This information will be made available to participants prior to the planning session.

Step Three: It will take at least two days of formal group strategic planning for a thorough plan to emerge. The outcome of the process will be a plan and a roadmap for achieving the vision of the organization. Included in the plan should be an analysis and roadmap.

Part I. Organizational Analysis

- The Vision: This statement should identify how the organization wants to be viewed in the future. It should be creative, concise, inspirational, and empowering. The visioning process requires letting go of preconceived ideas.
- Mission Statement: The mission statement reflects the organization's identity or why it exists and gives it a purpose for existing. The mission statement should reflect the values and core competencies of the organization.
- Core Values: The values statement identifies how an organization conducts itself and sets the philosophical guidelines under which it operates. The core values will provide the standard against which the strategic issues are assessed.
- Identify Stakeholders: A stakeholder is a person, group, or organization that can lay claim to resources or is affected by or can affect, the product or outcome.
- Identify Existing Mandates: These describe what an organization is required to do. They may originate in law, regulations, by-laws, or board guides and may be formal or informal.
- SWOT Analysis: This process involves identifying the strengths, weaknesses, opportunities and threats (SWOT) or barriers to an organization's success. Strengths and weaknesses are generally internal, while opportunities or threats are external to the organization.

Part II. Organizational Roadmap

- Setting Goals: Goals describe generally what actions need to occur. They translate the mission policy, clarify purpose, and are the basis for assessing priorities.
- Identifying Objectives: Objectives are the essence of an organization's plan for the designated timeframe. Objectives provide a basis for a detailed action plan. They must be realistic, consistent with goals and values, and must be measurable.
- Operational Plan: One outcome of the planning process should be a written action plan that includes: activity, responsible party, timeline, and measure for success. The plan should specifically identify the individual responsible for scheduling progress reports and updates.

Summary

In *Engines of Innovation*, Mark B. Myers and Richard S. Rosenbloom state that "...in today's global competitive arena, renewal and adaptation of the research establishment is an important goal for any firm investing significantly in scientific research."[3] While the reference was to industrial research entities, the statement is equally true for the academic and other not-for-profit research organizations. Successful research programs are effective and efficient and adaptive to the social, political, and economic environment. The cornerstone of an adaptive or competitive research institution is appropriate planning. The brief discussion of planning processes will hopefully encourage development of an operational and strategic plan for the research enterprise.

• • • References

1. Geiger, Roger L. *Making the Grade: Institutional Enhancement of Research Competitiveness. Competitiveness in Academic Research*, edited by Albert H. Teich. Washington, DC: AAAS, 1996.

2. Bryson, John M. *Strategic Planning for Public and Nonprofit Organizations*. San Francisco: Jossey-Bass, 1995.

3. Mowery, David C., and David J. Teece. *Strategic Alliances and Industrial Research, Engines of Innovation*, edited by Richard S. Rosenbloom and William J. Spencer. Boston, MA: Harvard Business School Press, 1996.

8

Change Management Theory Put to Practice as Stakeholders' Advocates: A Case Study

Lawrie Robertson, Bev Silver, Rosemarie Keenan, and Gail De Vun

By exploring process of change at a large private research institution, this case focuses on how to first create a process that considers and accommodates the needs of those directly affected by a changed work environment. This case study details the change resulting from the impact of planning, construction, and relocation of nearly 1,000 faculty and staff into a new research building. In this case, specific change principles were identified prior to initiation and systematically applied to influence the change process for the benefit of those affected. Written from the perspective of research administrators involved in planning and leading a change process, this case underscores the value of applying a systematic series of steps to ease the transition experience from a current to a new work environment. It illustrates how research administrators with a clear vision and the willingness to engage can positively influence the change experience for the scientists and staff they serve. It concludes with specific ways research administrators can influence change processes on their campuses as part of their service role.

Introduction

Change is all around us—from the way we conduct science to ever-developing community landscapes. Change is fundamental to the evolution of the research process: its idea, test, analysis, results, replication, and conclusion. In addressing changes in the work environment, research managers have

the opportunity to view their role as being active advocates for their constituents. In approaching change issues, effective managers will choose to engage early, adapt their approaches to respond to evolving work and research circumstances, and help faculty and staff sustain morale and focus during periods of uncertainty and transition.

Definitions

For purposes of this article, *change* is defined as *a movement from a current state to a new and different state*. Another key term is stakeholder. A *stakeholder* is defined as *anyone whose pattern of work or involvement with a group is influenced by the change*. In the illustrating case, anyone who needed to interact with activities within the building was viewed as a stakeholder.

Change Management Considerations

Reactions to institutional change processes are influenced by such factors as an organization's culture, values, norms, traditions, formal and informal decision structures, leadership style, and previous history of change processes. In shaping any change management plan, these factors should be considered and respected.

If change is a constant or is managed poorly, institutional change fatigue or resistance can reduce a system's ability to respond to new initiatives. If there is no history of stakeholder involvement in the changes influencing their work environment, it will be more challenging for managers to initiate this involvement or to proactively reduce negative responses to the change. On the other hand, when change processes are guided by a set of principles and specific objectives, those engaged have a common compass to chart their way.

Change Management Principles: The Compass

While the literature frequently discusses the importance of applying a series of principles to manage change processes, rarely is any complete listing of these steps offered as a guide. These principles are truths about the components of a systematic approach to influence the change experience. In the following case, principles mentioned in the literature were compiled to serve as the compass for guiding the change. A group of research managers used these steps to guide their involvement in assisting over 1,000 constituents to prepare for their relocation to a new building. This effort included the building's design, space allocations, construction details, and relocation processes. These managers believed that structuring the change plan to follow the principles below offered the best chance to positively influence how their stakeholder constituents would experience the transition from current to future:

1. Define the change, outcome vision, and challenges to achieve this vision.
2. Assess the culture: its norms, values, change history, traditions, and expectations.
3. Identify, enroll, and clarify roles for: stakeholders, decision-makers, sponsors, champions, and idea validators.
4. Determine the schedule and constraints to develop an appropriate change management plan, communications strategy, and support structure.
5. Communicate, coordinate, and celebrate.
6. Monitor, adjust, and evaluate.

Applying the Principles in the Real World: A Case Study

It was four years prior to the Division of Public Health Science's (PHS's) February 2004 relocation to its long-awaited new research building. The move would complete the consolidation of the Fred Hutchinson Cancer Research Center onto a single campus. Three PHS managers had been designated to coordinate the division's part of the building design and move processes.

To discuss the project's schedule and launch, the PHS trio met with representatives from the Center's facilities department and the architectural team. Quickly, it became clear that different mental models (i.e., ways of viewing things) and definitions of project success factors were at play. Each group (facilities planners, architects, division representatives) appeared to have its own definition of a successful project outcome. In simplistic terms, facilities' central goals were to bring the project in on time, remain within budget, and create a building that would be cost-efficient to operate. For the architects, this building would be the centerpiece of a 14-year campus development plan, a building that would represent the best in design and function. PHS managers were focused on the need for the building to be designed to complement and support the division's research and to incorporate input from its faculty and staff at every step. Each group, however, shared a common vision of satisfied occupants following move-in.

Principle 1: Define Change, Outcome Vision, Challenges

Defining the Change

In tackling any change, change leaders first need to formulate a common understanding of what is changing, its components and dynamics, the desired change outcome, and the challenges to this outcome. From the PHS trio's perspective, the essential change was defined as the impacts of transitioning over 1,000 scientists and staff, several hundred support personnel, and thousands of current and future study participants into a new 365,000 square foot population sciences building located at the center of Fred Hutchinson's new campus. After the relocation, specific changes would include new faculty and project adjacencies, more expansive floors, closer proximity to colleagues on the campus, changed office sizes and furnishings, and altered commutes. To guide their actions, plans, and communications, the PHS trio chose to create a four-year transition plan prior to launch that would be attentive to the above change principles and focused on the interests of PHS stakeholders: the division's faculty, staff and study participants.

Outcome Vision

To clarify the transition plan's intent, it was important to articulate both a vision and goals that could be broadly understood as well as supported by PHS' leadership. This overall vision was summarized as: *an inclusive planning process leading to minimum tears at move-in.* This vision focused on the PHS stakeholders' process expectations and the desired outcome result.

Identify Challenges

Three phases typify most change processes: initiation, transition, and transformation. Of these, the most challenging and precarious is the transition phase. Change literature indicates that transition is a period of uncertainty often characterized by low stability, disorientation, misunderstood intentions, decreased productivity, emotional stress, undirected energy, feelings of lack of control, valuing past patterns, and increased conflict. Often this fear and unease manifests as resistance to the change or denial through an unwillingness to engage. Here, all involved in leading or supporting the change must focus on clarity, communications, and sustained will. Avenues must be provided for sharing feelings and reservations while instilling confidence that group interests will be considered.

The length of a change process can stress a system. For PHS stakeholders, four years would represent a prolonged period of transition requiring sustained attention to these issues. Numerous challenges that would need to be shared with and understood by all involved lay in the path ahead. During this planning, design and move period, consideration would need to be given to the diverse interests of over 1,000 scientists and staff, several hundred support personnel, and thousands of current and future study participants. Focused attention would be required at each stage: in anticipation of the change, during transition, and in the transformed work environment following the relocation.

Uncertainties of a changing work environment influenced anticipation of the new setting. As one of four scientific divisions (with Basic Sciences, Clinical Research and Human Biology), the Division of Public Health Sciences would be the last to have a building constructed on the new campus. It had been separated from the rest of the center for over a decade, which led to a sense of autonomy. Consolidation would mean a loss of much of this autonomy.

The PHS building would feature an integration of the division's previously separate office, lab, and clinical facilities. The work environment would be transformed from a high-rise vertical setting into a low-rise horizontal arrangement, with each floor approximately three times the size of current floors. Two of the most critical challenges for the trio were to find ways to make a long complex planning process seem inclusive and responsive to PHS faculty and staff and then assist these stakeholders to transition to the coming environment. Uncertainty about the impacts and loss of group autonomy was also expected to be an issue. It was assumed that new work patterns would begin to emerge as participants prepared for the relocation and associated impacts and these new patterns would prepare faculty and staff for additional postrelocation challenges.

Principle 2: Assess Culture, Norms and Values, Traditions, and Expectations

Culture

Each organization has a unique culture and history; therefore it is important that the change plan responsively address group process expectations and traditions. As representatives of a scientific division with longstanding traditions for openness, consensus decision-making, and responsiveness to its faculty, the PHS trio understood the need for an inclusive process. While motivated to create an innovative science facility, the design process also had to be sensitive to stakeholder expectations for frequent communications and input opportunities.

Norms and Values

Group perspectives are influenced by both stated and unstated norms and values. In planning this process a PHS norm would be that the planning steps be consistent with the division's core values and follow a clear set of project goals monitored by faculty leaders. In concert with the center's central values of scientific excellence, respect, openness, and innovation, the following PHS core values had been established and were discussed with every new employee at quarterly orientations over the prior decade.

1. Science is the primary focus of division activities.
2. World-class scientists require world-class staff.
3. Every person deserves good treatment and respect.
4. Every employee is important to our results.
5. Contributions are what count most.
6. All center staff are partners in achieving PHS' goals.
7. Professional development and innovative thinking are encouraged.

8. Importance is placed on two-way communication, openness, and sharing.
9. Horizontal relationships are often most important.
10. Everyone deserves a safe and secure work environment, assured by individual actions.
11. Everyone is responsible for protecting the confidentiality of protected health information.
12. We are all in the solutions business!

Traditions

Traditions offer groups a sense of history, continuity and common purpose. Because PHS members enjoyed a long tradition of openness and frequent stakeholder communications, active group consultation in major division-wide projects would be an expectation. Success in this project would require the design process to create a building retaining several historic elements perceived to be central to the division's research success. These included: arrangements of related research groups, largely private offices for all, logical office adjacencies, and arranging spaces to support collaborative research methods.

Change History

Individual perceptions and expectations are also influenced by previous change experiences and the potential impact of this change on that stakeholder. Therefore, during the transition period every stakeholder tends to anticipate the process uniquely according to her or his personal change history and outlook. Before being willing to engage in broader issues, each individual needs to first understand how this change affects him or her personally.

In PHS' case, previous change history for most members served to benefit this project. A decade earlier, many of the affected stakeholders had experienced a successful facility planning and relocation process into the current leased high-rise space one mile from the new campus. This process had been inclusive and well-communicated, which had resulted in enhanced space arrangements and most experienced minimal work disruption. Many of those hired after the relocation shared some space related history either as part of their current or previous center jobs. A number of internal hires had some experience with the four previous scientific and administrative building projects on the new campus. Over the past decade, others had lived through one or more of the multiple renovations and floor additions to the current high-rise space. For most, previous center change processes were viewed positively.

Past experiences also provided the PHS trio with insights concerning both stakeholder process expectations and considerations for planning and designing an effective postrelocation work environment. Going last had its advantages. In being the last division building on the new campus, PHS managers learned much from noting the experiences of previous center construction projects.

Expectations

Culture, values, norms, traditions, and history provide the context for stakeholder expectations. For PHS scientific leaders, their active engagement in the design process would present a unique opportunity to create an ideal collaborative research environment while retaining valued traditions. This balance could be achieved through more interactive horizontal adjacencies rather than isolated vertical groupings, integrating new lab and clinic facilities with offices, and taking best advantage of proximity to other center scientists and research facilities to expand PHS' collaborative research approach. Thus, PHS faculty and staff expected to be involved, consulted, and effectively represented. As advocates for the scientists and staff, the PHS management trio understood that they would be expected to take an activist role in the building's planning rather than merely reacting to centrally developed plans. Fortunately, center leaders, the facilities department, and the architects also understood this expectation.

Principle 3: Identify, Enroll, and Clarify Roles

Stakeholders, Sponsors, Champions, and Idea Validators

During the transition period, several different roles can influence how the change takes place. These include those directly affected, those who desire the change, those who sustain the will to change, and those who endorse the process. From day one, PHS's change managers chose to broadly define a stakeholder as *anyone who needed to work in the building or participate in the research conducted within the building.* However, they placed specific attention on the needs of those within the PHS family.

The center had a longstanding tradition of all essential decisions being made by the scientific leadership with major fiscal and policy decisions reviewed by the center director and an engaged board of directors (*sponsors*). As noted, this project would complete the integration of the center within a single campus guided by a campus master plan endorsed by the board. Over the previous decade, PHS space assignments and design decisions were made by the division's scientific executive committee composed of the four scientific program heads plus the division director and associate division director. Despite a change of division directors at the midpoint, both leaders and the executive committee eagerly accepted and consistently acted as change *champions* and key decision makers. At a more subtle level, the trio recognized that certain staff and faculty are perceived by peers to be *idea validators*. While not always formal decision makers, these are the people who others look to for either endorsement or resistance. Identifying and involving these persons would be essential to achieving the project vision and uncovering early signs of potential looming issues.

Clarify Roles

To support a change initiative and ease stakeholders through each of the three phases, all participants must be clear about who advises and who decides. At the initial stage of the planning process, change managers should clarify: the roles of each set of participants; how and when to best engage each group; and methods for monitoring and assessing the impacts on the range of stakeholders as the process unfolds. For the PHS advocates, this effort included understanding who the various PHS stakeholders were (staff, faculty, and study participants) and what stakeholders would need to know to effectively influence the changes for each group. It was then important to determine how to secure feedback on decisions from all of the players—stakeholders, validators, design team members, champions, and sponsors—as they transitioned from launch through outcome. To effectively engage this range of participants, the role, scope, and limits for each group would have to be understood by all involved. Roles were first spelled out in an introductory e-mail sent to everyone at the project's commencement.

Clarify Terminology

Terminology can be a barrier to active participation and an impediment to understanding the context or importance of decisions. Mastering a whole new set of terms and decision approaches would be required if the PHS team wished to be respected partners in the design and construction tasks. For example, within their paradigm, facilities staff and contractors viewed the project in terms of meeting construction deadlines driven by such milestones as

permits, construction drawings, demolition, excavation, and physical construction. From a designer perspective, the architects developed plans, recommended features, and set design milestones. To guide their design tasks, initially the architectural team sought to convince PHS to endorse a set of project design goals developed by the architects. Quickly, it became apparent the PHS team would need to not only master construction and *design speak*, but also continuously assert for process and decision criteria defined by PHS leaders.

Understanding each change participant's terminology, constraints, and decision processes can enable the research representatives to insert their own set of critical process and decision points without delaying the master schedule. While formal authority for final decisions and the overall budget resided with the center director and board, most of the actual decision authorities for design details were given to the division's scientific leadership— the division's executive committee (EC). In response to the architects, at an early stage the PHS EC decided to create its own design goals to assess input and guide its decisions toward its vision for a successful outcome. Like the principles, the EC's statement of goals provided a structure. The EC goals focused on creating a building that could perform the following tasks:

1. Facilitate scientific opportunities;
2. Function effectively (flexibility, integration, technology, convenience to study participants, security);
3. Promote a productive work environment (adjacencies, maximum daylight, private offices, shared space, air quality);
4. Sustain the strengths of the PHS culture and traditions (neighborhoods, promoting collaborations, parity between groups).

Subsequently, PHS would assess all design decisions in terms of their consistency with the EC's goals.

Principle 4: Determine the Change Schedule and Constraints to Develop an Appropriate Change Management Plan, Communications Strategy, and Support Structure

Determine the Schedule and Constraints

Schedules, constraints and critical paths drive construction projects. Within any project schedule are essential completion points. These milestones must be met for the project to be completed on time and within budget. From the architect's perspective, the critical design milestones included: programming (determining how space requirements match building capacity), blocking and stacking (allocating spaces to groups with respect to horizontal and vertical relationships), schematic design (designing the general spaces for the groups), design development (confirming and finalizing interior space details), construction drawings (documents required for bidding and constructing), and interior finishes (colors, flooring, carpeting, doors, relight selections). The facilities group was concerned with construction milestones that included: construction documents, master use permit, street/alley vacation, building permit, demolition, construction, furnishings, commissioning, and move-in. These were brought together into a master schedule spanning the four years from launch through relocation.

Constraint appreciation enables stakeholders to understand what is possible and what is not. In addition to design and construction deadlines, other larger constraints impacting the process included the overall project budget and center standards for research facilities.

Develop Change Plan

To achieve their vision of positively influencing the project on behalf of PHS stakeholder interests would require the PHS management trio to create a process plan addressing the following items:

1. Stakeholder communications. A communications plan recognizing PHS stakeholders' need to be periodically informed, even during periods when there is nothing major to report, and to ensure that these communications are interpreted as communicated.
2. Internal PHS requirements. How to fit the PHS process and decision steps within the master project design and construction schedule, identifying windows of opportunity within each design and construction milestone.
3. Consultations. Mechanisms for stakeholders and idea validators to be consulted and clearly influence the process.
4. Decision processes. Building in division control mechanisms, guided by the division, determined goals and channeled through the division's scientific policy making process.
5. Celebrations. Activities to recognize project milestone achievements to keep the process on everyone's radar screen and to make it real so people would remain engaged.

Communications Strategy

Essential to the plan's success would be its launch, decision processes, early and frequent communications, and the actions required to permit the scientific leadership and other stakeholders to reach closure within each phase of the master design and construction schedule. Periodically, the PHS trio also needed to clarify support from board and center leadership who originally sponsored the change. To have decision leverage, PHS needed to ensure that the right people within the center would be willing to continuously advocate (champion) for PHS's desired change outcome from design decisions through move-in.

Support Structure

Following the creation of an overall vision and basic communications plan, it was decided that two input structures would be required—consultation and decision making. Consultation would be achieved by channeling stakeholder input through a single project/group/lab representative selected by the group members. Selected representatives would comprise the space planning effort committee (SPEC). Meeting periodically, the SPEC representatives would be expected to discuss issues with their group and advise the design team on the group's space requirements in SPEC meetings and one-on-one consultations between SPEC members and the architectural planners. As a whole, the SPEC would serve as a forum for updates between twice yearly all-staff briefings. Between SPEC meetings on larger issues, a small group of seven key administrators—the space coordination team (SCT)—would focus on the details. This smaller group would hold frequent meetings (at times, weekly) with the architects and facilities planners to cover every conceivable detail of the design, features, and relocation planning. In addition, special efforts were planned to consult informally with those viewed as key *idea validators* and those providing support services to the new building to ensure that emerging issues could be dealt with proactively.

Ensuring that the science did come first meant giving special attention to faculty members' input. As part of an intern's project, each faculty member participated in a one-on-one interview. This survey covering fifty-three interviews would be used to place faculty in interest clusters and to arrange support spaces. This survey sought to identify the following:

1. Faculty reactions to the initial planning process and communications;

2. General goals for the building design and challenges expected from the changed space arrangements;

3. Specific goals for their new space and working relationships;

4. Adjacencies to individual faculty, staff, or shared resources they most wanted to be near.

When major policy decisions were required, a meeting of PHS's EC would be called. These meetings needed to be planned several weeks in advance due to travel schedules and required the SCT to anticipate and consolidate all of the looming policy issues for a single review meeting. Examples of these decisions included PHS's design goals, standards for office sizes and group space allocations, placement of groups within the building, provisions for future initiative growth space, provision of private offices for staff, office layouts and window shades, and colors for interior finishes for the cafeteria, break rooms, and clinics. The original project goals guided these decisions. For example, consistent with the goal to bring a maximum of outside light into interior offices, the EC reduced the size of relight window shade so they covered no more than two-thirds of the glass surface. Successful engagement requires an investment of resources. To support the consultation and decision structures, the management trio and division director decided to dedicate PHS staff positions to the project. Their efforts would focus on coordinating input, identifying and bird-dogging project details important to PHS stakeholders, and representing division interests at construction team meetings. To be credible to all parties, these staff needed to have both the expertise and standing as valued participants by the facilities staff, architects, and various other external stakeholders while being viewed as effective advocates by division's stakeholders.

Starting four years out, PHS leaders allocated funds to pay for the time of two experienced PHS staff to be devoted to project planning. The two were selected for their extensive experience in coordinating division space remodels, planning new floor arrangements, purchasing furniture, and detailing space occupancy logistics. Both had already established reputations with facilities planners as value-adding professionals who understood the demands of construction projects. In turn, with access to the construction team, they quickly earned the respect of the design and construction professionals. Subsequently, a young PHS information technology (IT) professional emerged as an equally regarded partner in the IT planning effort. With this expertise in place, PHS was positioned to monitor all elements of the project (including frequent on-site inspections) that could influence the success of the final building.

Principle 5: Communicate, Coordinate, Celebrate

Communicate

Project introduction sets the stage for how the project is perceived and how well the path ahead is understood. It can also announce the vision that will guide the transition journey. Four years prior to occupancy, the project was launched with a presentation at the division's semiannual all-staff meeting and an e-mail was sent to all faculty, staff, and affiliates. Both briefings covered the following topics:

1. About the project: Vision, overview of the activities to date, timetable for major tasks ahead, and what was to have been achieved by each milestone;

2. Communications: Creation of a Web site, periodic e-mail updates;

3. Input Opportunities: How to participate, SPEC role (with a listing of the representatives), description of other roles and responsibilities.

Over the next four years, every subsequent semiannual all-staff meeting and new staff orientation would include a formal update presentation on the project. Thus, early on it was recognized that sustaining clear communication channels involved more than internal audiences (PHS stakeholders and leaders). Additional communication links were needed between various groups across the institution having responsibility for major elements of the building's design, construction, occupancy, and ongoing operations. PHS's change managers asserted that its personnel would need to include access to groups that had not previously viewed the *client* (now PHS) as an active player in the design and construction processes. These groups included the construction management team (facilities, architects, and general contractor), central information technology planners, furniture vendors, and building systems engineers.

A challenge in a large change process involving hundreds of stakeholders is to find ways for the individuals to feel that they have some direct influence over the change that they will be experiencing.

In addition to the faculty interviews, a second "making the project real" opportunity emerged with the furniture selection process. Much of the current furniture had exceeded its useful life. Since the moving of groups from current to new spaces had to be staged over weekends with a minimum disruption to the science, it was decided that new furniture would be purchased for the building. While the EC had already settled on four basic office configurations for each of the standard office sizes, it was left to each full-time faculty and staff person to select the furniture arrangement that best suited their work practices. The SCT concluded that individual interviews would be used to collect this information. This interview process was seen as providing an opportunity for most stakeholders to influence the one part of the building they cared most about, their own offices.

To support the interviews, digital photos were taken of every current office and a three-month period was set aside to conduct fifteen-minute one-on-one interviews with every faculty and staff member assigned to individual offices. In advance, the employee groups were divided into three interviewing phases. At the start of each phase, an orientation was conducted. Participants were encouraged to visit working offices originally designed as mock-ups, and to chat with colleagues about furniture options. A Web site with a Web database was established to facilitate preparation for these interviews. In the end, over 695 faculty and staff chose to participate in the interviews. Several have since indicated that nothing has more reinforced why they believe that the center is a great place to work than the experience of being asked about their personal space and being given a choice.

Remaining steps in the communications and planning process will cover preparations for the move, premove tours, publication of transition orientation brochures for employees, and study participants, a postmove open house (including the construction workers as special guests), and an evaluation of the process from the diverse set of people who were considered stakeholders—PHS employees, study participants, the design team, center support personnel, and center leadership.

Coordinate

Transition period anxieties related to change uncertainty are influenced by how the details are managed. Following the launch, the trio started the task of working with individual groups to define basic space needs and special requirements. These included establishing parameters for space allocations (in most cases the current group space allocation was used), office sizes (a faculty standard and staff standard), support spaces and storage, specialized spaces (assay rooms, lactation room, clinic exam room, exercise testing), lab and shared resource standards, and meeting spaces. Also considered was the need for shared conference rooms and other common spaces (reception, cafeteria, break rooms, and coffee bar).

Using the EC design goals as a guide expected future scientific collaborations and desired faculty adjacencies were the first criteria in assigning group locations within the building. In addition to input by the EC, faculty interview results helped to determine desired faculty and staff adjacencies. Generally, faculty sought to be near colleagues with common research interests and placed a higher priority on proximity to other faculty than the staff who worked on their projects. Once faculty adjacencies and related research group blocks were established, a floor placement pattern began to emerge. Other key considerations included investigator collaborations with lab colleagues and proximity to clinic exam rooms and other specialized research spaces. The EC took this information and placed the various groups by scientific program in horizontal adjacencies on each floor with a *faculty row* facing the scenic lake view. Because one program was too large for a single floor, the EC created a vertical adjacency pattern supported by connecting stairs and the elevators.

Celebrate

Special events offer a means for both celebrating the completion of major milestones and making the change real to less engaged stakeholders. As this project moved through each successive step, the SCT assessed ways to engage PHS stakeholders. The first opportunity was to celebrate the completion of the excavation. Since the Fred Hutchinson Center was named after a Hall of Fame baseball manager, the baseball theme, *If They Build It, PHS Will Come!* was used for a "bottoming out ceremony." To inject an element of fun in promoting the event, four baseball-type cards were designed. Each card highlighted a different building feature on the front and gave interesting facts about the project on the back. Randomly shuffled, one card was sent to each employee with an invitation to the event and a promise that they could get the complete set of four by attending the celebration. Popcorn, crackerjacks, peanuts, hot dogs, and sodas were provided at a ceremony next to the site. The ceremony provided stakeholders with an opportunity to get an update on progress, see the site, and hear champions and sponsors affirm their vision for the project. Additionally, the reports at the semiannual PHS all-staff meetings offered regular opportunities to report on the completion of each milestone (programming, assigning groups to floors, demolitions, completion of excavation, exterior windows/brickwork, commissioning and opening). The goal of the postmove open house celebration was to provide closure.

Principle 6: Monitor, Adjust, Evaluate

Monitor

Throughout any significant change process, the transition between the change announcement and change completion can be a trying time for all involved. Frequently, changes fail during this period due to the lack of ongoing communications with stakeholders, sponsors, champions, idea validators, and others critical to sustaining the process. Other undermining factors are a lack of continued commitment from champions and sponsors, inadequate monitoring systems, or the failure to appreciate the range of persons who should be consulted. A lack of attention to stakeholder interests often results in their initial enthusiasm evolving into change resistance.

The most dangerous phrase during any change process is: *I assumed*. This often reflects an inattention to details or too narrow view of those whose input could enhance the outcome. For example, in selecting conference room chairs, it would be important to seek the input of those responsible for setting up various meeting layouts (block, theater and classroom). For the PHS building, a number of projects assumed that any new equipment or small items (like plates, pots, and pans for the human nutrition lab) for the new expanded spaces would be covered within the construction budget—they were not. By not asking the right questions, a faulty assumption can linger and the opportunity to address the issue can be missed.

Therefore, opportunities to ask questions should to be built into the planning process. Managing change to benefit stakeholders requires a means to uncover and attend to details throughout the transition period. It is a constant process of asking who has been left out, who needs to be consulted, what has been ignored, and what information is needed by the various players to remain informed and sustain their support?

Responsibility for monitoring project progress and adjusting process steps was given to the SCT. This group of senior managers met on a nearly weekly basis to identify and discuss all possible details. Notes were taken to document requests and persons assigned to track recommendations. Along with the design team, the SCT periodically consulted with the SPEC on complex issues affecting multiple groups and then provided feedback for use by the EC to make major policy and design decisions.

Adjust

Change processes are dynamic. It is not possible to predict every issue that will surface. Creating mechanisms to monitor and adjust plans allows the manager to anticipate and respond quickly to emerging issues or points of resistance. Importantly, ideas or new strategies that enhance the likelihood of change acceptance can surface during the transition period. The SCT made several adjustments to the original plan including the decision to conduct individual furniture interviews, allowing time to deal with scientific reorganization impacts resulting from the new division director's recruitment plans, and addressing an evolving lab bench space allocation policy.

Evaluate

Following the relocation, the center planned to celebrate the building with a community open house. After working out all of the bugs inherent in settling into a new facility, the PHS management trio plans a comprehensive evaluation of the process. At the core will be the PHS stakeholders' assessment of their involvement and its impact. The trio will also seek evaluative input from other design/construction team members, sponsors, and champions. The assessment focus will be on lessons learned and opportunities for enhancing future large-scale change processes.

Conclusion: Lessons Learned and Next Steps

This case illustrates how having a clear plan of action supported by awareness of change principles and the issues of importance can lead to a successful change outcome. Research administrators willing to engage can make a difference. Conscientious decisions were made by PHS administrators prior to launch to play an activist role in guiding the project toward the division's vision of a successful project outcome. By continuously asking what needs to be considered, who needs to be consulted and informed, what is being overlooked, and what needs to be changed or adjusted, PHS change managers were able to find ways to positively influence the change in a manner that both honored the division's cultural expectations and kept the project within an externally driven schedule.

Lessons Learned

In retrospect, the following recommendations for research administrators appear to be the critical success factors and lessons learned from this case:

- Take time for essential preplanning, vision creation, role clarification, and launch.
- Understand the diversity of stakeholder interests involved, the potential value of their input, and how to best secure that input.
- Roles need to be clear and constraints understood.
- Invest in staff dedicated to the project who are credible to a range of stakeholders. Create benchmarking goals to assess input and guide decisions.
- Recognize that different mental models influence perceptions, communications, and expectations.
- Communicate in a manner that is heard—recognize the difference between issuing communications and effectively communicating.
- Update stakeholders frequently (even when there is nothing significant to report) and celebrate milestones to keep everyone engaged.
- No process is perfect or without setbacks or surprises, but it is important to keep seeking perfection.

Throughout, the PHS trio kept asking the team these valuable assessment questions:

1. Who or what has been overlooked?
2. What strategies are needed to keep the project on course and to achieve our vision?
3. What needs to be changed or adjusted so we can look back with minimum regrets?

Considerations for Research Administrators and Managers

It is understood that the center had numerous positive characteristics that created a strong foundation for success. However, even in the midst of a less supportive environment, there is much that a research administrator can do to positively influence an outcome for stakeholder constituents. When given the opportunity to lead or participate on a change team:

- Define the change, its characteristics and the guiding change management principles.
- Focus on what can be done, what you can control or influence.
- Understand that the most dangerous phrase is *I assumed*.
- Appreciate your institution's norms, values, and past change history—manage accordingly.
- Evaluate and build upon lessons learned from past experiences in your environment.
- Understand and respect culture, mental models, decision processes, and traditions.
- Define appropriate outcome vision, process steps, mechanisms, and communications.
- Understand the differing mental models, visions, definitions of a successful outcome, and work styles of various interest groups in a change process—adapt your methods for impact.
- Clarify, coordinate, communicate, celebrate.
- Assess, adjust, and evaluate.
- Start early to outline possible input opportunities and the needed components to structure and implement your contributions to the change management process.

Change will happen. In serving their constituents, it is up to research administrators to be prepared to adapt and respond. By actively engaging in the process, research administrators can influence how their stakeholders experience significant changes directly impacting them. However, when engaging change, it is vital for administrators to understand the rules that govern that specific change process. Next, administrators need to identify the steps they can take to systematically guide stakeholders through the transition phase and positively influence the change experience. Those who understand the process of change and have a plan are apt to have a more satisfying transition and change outcome for themselves and their constituents.

• • • Recommended Reading

Barnes, B. Kim. *Exercising Influence*. Berkeley, CA: Barnes & Conti Associates, 2000.

Bridges, William. *The Way of Transition: Embracing Life's Difficult Moments*. Cambridge, MA: Perseus Publishing, 2001.

Driscoll, Dawn-Marie, and Hoffman, W. Michael. *Ethics Matters: How to Implement Values Driven Management*. Waltham, MA: Center for Business Ethics, 1999.

Johnson, Spencer. *Who Moved My Cheese?* New York: G. P. Putnam's Sons, 1999.

Nadler, David A., Gerstein, Marc S., and Shaw, Robert B. *Organizational Architecture: Designs for Changing Organizations*. San Francisco: Jossey-Bass, 1992.

O'Toole, James. *Leading Change: The Argument for Values Based Leadership*. New York: Ballantine Books, 1995.

Robbins, Harvey, and Finley, Michael. *Why Change Doesn't Work: Why Initiatives Go Wrong and How to Try Again and Succeed*. Princeton, NJ: Peterson's/Pacesetter Books, 1996.

Whyte, William Foote, and Whyte, Kathleen King. *Making the Mondragon: The Growth and Dynamics of the Worker Cooperative Complex*. Ithaca, NY: Cornell University Press, 1988.

9

Human Resources in a Research Environment

Jim Hanlon

Introduction

In order to succeed and, indeed, excel as a research administrator, it is important to adapt to the research environment, as it is unlikely that the general environment will change to meet one's expectations. This is particularly true for the human resources manager.

Administration is necessary to support the scientific or research mission of our institutions and human resource (HR) administration should be both supportive and protective of the people behind the research. The author has heard that "…it's not that the scientists think administration is a necessary evil, they just don't think it is necessary at all." While this is somewhat of an overstatement, there is some truth in it. When working in the research environment, an administrator cannot be too bureaucratic and must understand that the research, not its administration, drives the institution. Policies and procedures that follow the best practices in the field of research administration should exist, but one must also be cautious with application.

Sound human resource management is crucial to the effective operation of any institution, whether of a nonprofit or commercial nature. The end product of a nonprofit research institution is the science or education mission that it delivers, while the product of a commercial research facility may be more bottom-line oriented with an emphasis toward applied research. In either case, if the agreed upon program is not delivered as promised, then funding will cease. The converse being that if a strong program is delivered, funding may increase. To make this happen, one must only look at the cal-

iber of the institution's researchers and staff, and the facilities and equipment that exist. While the focus of this chapter is on human resources issues, the importance of facilities and equipment should not be understated because these can attract strong candidates as well as a demanding salary. Indeed, in some cases these can be used as leverage in attracting new personnel.

This chapter makes several references to the institution where the author is employed; for clarification, the following is a brief overview of its governance. Tri-University Meson Facility (TRIUMF) is Canada's national laboratory for particle and nuclear physics. It was originally established as a consortium of three universities. There are now six universities that own and operate the laboratory and all operating funds come via a contribution from the Government of Canada through the National Research Council of Canada (NRCC).

"Human resources are the cornerstone of a scientific laboratory."[1] This statement can be made for any institution conducting research—a university, research institute, academic research hospital, or the research department of a for-profit company. The motto of the Human Resources Department at TRIUMF is, "We believe our most important resource is Human."

This chapter briefly touches on the major areas of human resource management that are most pertinent to the research environment with which the author is most familiar: an independent research institute.

Figure 9-1 gives an overview of the major areas of human resources responsibility. Note that all

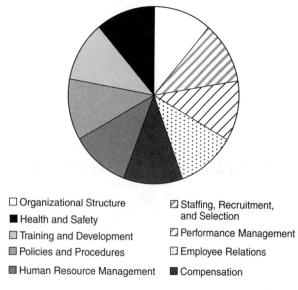

☐ Organizational Structure
■ Health and Safety
☐ Training and Development
■ Policies and Procedures
■ Human Resource Management

☑ Staffing, Recruitment,
   and Selection
☑ Performance Management
⊡ Employee Relations
■ Compensation

FIGURE 9-1 Human Resources Overview

areas are given an equal amount of importance and to operate effectively the human resources department must deal with these issues concurrently.

Organizational Structure

Fundamentally the organization must have clear divisions and lines of responsibility. If one expects people to be accountable for their actions then one must give them the responsibility and authority for which they are accountable or they cannot be held accountable. In many cases organization structures fail because people are held accountable for events over which they really have no control. Secondly, the published organization chart should be factual. This means that in some cases, group leaders or department heads may be only figure heads with another person actually dealing with the responsibilities of directing that specific area of the facility. The organization chart should also clarify the governance of the institution. Figure 9-2 is a sample organization chart taken from TRIUMF.

One might ask, "How does human resources fit into the organization?" Human resources (HR) should and must play a major role: the HR function should be involved in organizational design and work design, as well as in designing and interrelating information systems, budgeting processes, and all other critical functions in the organization. HR should be an integral component of strategic and business planning by the management team.[2]

Using TRIUMF's model as an exemplar structure for any research institution, employees can be sorted into the following categories:

Research Scientists. These employees are primarily research scientists and research engineers who may be considered equivalent to faculty in universities and are eligible to receive grants from funding agencies. The lead investigator on a grant is referred to as the principal investigator (PI).

Research Associates (RAs). These are recently graduated PhDs who are given up to a three-year appointment. This category may also include research scientists whose salary is being paid from a research grant where long-term funding is not assured. There are some RAs at TRIUMF who have had their three-year appointments extended several times. This happens when research grants are extended over a period of several years.

Visiting Scientists. These are scientists who are on sabbatical from another laboratory or university who have chosen to take a term leave from their current position to join the research program at the facility they are visiting. Many institutions have a program in place where a scientist can periodically take a leave with a reduced salary to conduct research at another facility. In TRIUMF's case, if a visiting scientist were to come to TRIUMF for a one-year period for example, TRIUMF would make up the difference in his or her salary from that paid by the home institution.

Post Doctoral Fellows (PDFs). These are newly graduated PhDs within five years of receiving their PhD who are given a one- or two-year appointment. These scientists gain experience, are trying to establish themselves in their field of research, and do not typically have their appointments renewed because they will move on to a continuing appointment at another institution or take up a faculty position at a university.

Administrative, Professional, and Supervisory Staff. This group is made up primarily of senior management, some with engineering or science degrees, and employees who function in office and clerical positions.

Technical Staff. These include trades people and those employees with design, mechanical, and electrical training who fulfill a support role and perform other technical or routine functions. At TRIUMF the ratio of technical support to research scientists and engineers is on the order of two-to-one.

Students. Student employees, either at an undergraduate or graduate level, are hired for a specific term.

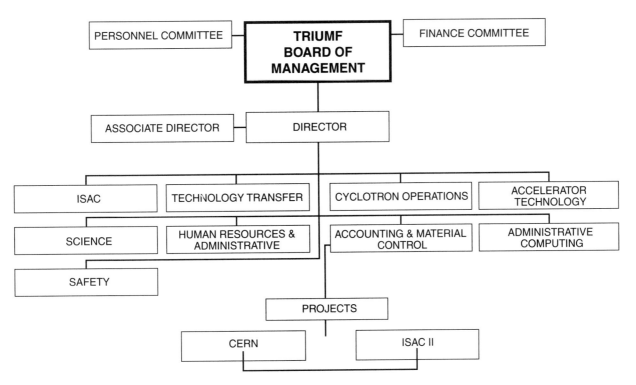

FIGURE 9-2   TRIUMF Organization Chart

For a typical physics project, a research team might include:

PI (lead research scientist) (1)

Research Scientist (1)

Research Associate (2)

Engineer (1)

Technical (3)

Student (3)

Staffing, Recruitment, and Selection

This is one of the most crucial areas of responsibility for the human resources manager. It is very important to recruit the right person for the right job and the job fit is crucial. When a research scientist or research engineer is recruited, one is usually looking for an accomplished individual who either brings knowledge to the institution or has the foundation and skill set to grow intellectually in his or her field of research and ultimately reap rewards for the institution. This fit is not as clear when hiring senior administrative and other support staff. Often when people are hired, they either succeed or fail. There is no in between. Those coming from a fast-paced manufacturing climate or an aggressive business culture may not be able to adapt to the collegial and sometimes competitive nature of a research environment.

When the author first started working in a research environment, his background was in distribution and manufacturing. He did not understand what the "drivers" were in this business. In a research enterprise it is delivering the best science that drives the institution, unlike a business where a strong bottom line is the objective.

The quality control process that exists in a research institution is that of "peer review," the process by which colleagues assess and judge the output of the projects and the research record of the individual scientists.

In the author's experience, scientists are very critical when judging one another and the merit of any proposed research project. In addition, all promotions for research scientists and research engineers are based on peer review. HR can play an important role in this process by ensuring that review criteria are used consistently and fairly to ensure that careers are not negatively impacted by errors with the review process.

Recruitment

When a need for particular research talent has been identified, a search process is launched by a search committee, usually made up of senior scientists and managers who are familiar with the job requirements. The HR department should be involved in the hiring process, as it serves as the source of information interview process, including the institution's policies on the screening of potential candidates, benefits, and hiring policies and guidelines. As a talent search may extend internationally, HR should supply search committees with the immigration regulations. While HR plays a lesser role to that of the search committee when going through a recruitment process, HR research administration plays more of a traditional role in the recruitment of administrative and technical support positions, similar to HR's role in other industries.

At TRIUMF, scientists hired into permanent positions are given two consecutive two-year appointments and, in the fifth year, a decision is made to grant either a one-year termination appointment or tenure, where employment can be terminated under only the most serious of circumstance. The scientist faces, technically, a five-year probation period.

Some institutions use employment contracts but in most cases institutions prefer to rely on the "letter of offer" used when the applicant was hired. At TRIUMF we follow this practice. The letter of offer should outline the terms of employment and should include working conditions, length of employment, status, terms of probation, salary and benefits, lab space, monetary support, moving expenses and any details pertinent to the particular offer. The applicant should sign this letter as a condition of employment. Often a candidate will write a response fine-tuning and sometimes attempting further negotiation. This can be avoided by ensuring that all questions are answered in the letter of offer.

Immigration

In the effort to establish and support best science, institutions strive to recruit the most qualified scientists, oftentimes foreign nationals, whose credentials must be presented to the immigration department for clearance. The laws vary within Canada and the United States but the North American Free Trade Agreement (NAFTA) makes hiring a foreign national from Canada, the United States, or Mexico easier in many instances.[3]

With respect to Canada and the United States, in almost all cases a foreign worker requires a valid work permit. These steps must be followed before applying for a work permit:

1. An employer must first offer a job.
2. The immigration department must normally provide a labor market opinion or "confirmation" of the job offer. Some types of work are exempt, such as those covered under the NAFTA.

3. After receipt of confirmation that a foreign national may fill the job, the successful candidate for the position must apply for a work permit.

Collaboration agreements are sometimes in place with institutions in other countries and are a good tool for bringing visiting scientists into the country.

In both the United States and Canada, human rights laws are in place to protect the rights of the candidate and the rights of the citizens. The HR department must ensure that these rights are not violated.

Termination

In some cases it is necessary to terminate an employee. This should only be done after serious consideration. The employee must be given proper notice and employers are bound to comply with either state or provincial legislation. Cases of "wrong fit" should be discussed with the employee. In these cases, the employee can leave by mutual agreement with an appropriate settlement being made. The HR department must be involved in this process in order that the rights of the employee are not infringed and the institution not charged with wrongful dismissal.

A defined probation period gives the employer the opportunity to seriously assess the employee and when poor performance is noted, the employee may be immediately advised. The probation period at TRIUMF for nonscientists is six months.

The author recalls one case where performance was an issue with an employee, but the supervisor was reluctant to terminate the individual. The supervisor insisted on extending the probation period and then after the decision to terminate was made, waited several months before advising HR. When the employee was finally advised, HR found out that the employee had just purchased a home near our facility one month earlier. Imagine the tone of the exit interview when this information was revealed!

Performance Management

The debate on whether or not an annual performance appraisal is warranted continues and some supervisors and institutions do not think they are worthwhile. At TRIUMF we feel that performance appraisals afford employees an opportunity to focus on their strengths and overcome identified deficiencies, thereby becoming more satisfied and productive.

The following is taken from the TRIUMF HR policy on performance management:

TRIUMF recognizes that the organization's success depends to a large extent on the performance of its employees. TRIUMF's Performance Planning and Review Program is an essential component to ensure our success. The goals of Performance Planning and Review are:

1) To support the accomplishments of TRIUMF's program of work.

2) To plan work assignments, review and evaluate individual employee performance.

3) To identify individual employee training and development needs.

4) To provide an opportunity for individual employees to achieve their maximum potential.

5) To recognize and reward the efforts of employees.

The decision to institute a formal performance management system at TRIUMF was made for two reasons:

1. Salary Administration

With continued pressures on rising salary costs and funding increases barely keeping up with inflation or the cost of living, management felt that a system had to be in place that would reward employees for strong performance. This system had to apply to all employees and those employees with a poor performance record would not be entitled to a salary increase. The salary administration system also had to accommodate younger scientists who were establishing their careers and clearly performing at levels beyond normal expectations. A system that awarded salary increases equally across the board was no longer adequate.

2. Staff Reduction

Around the same time, the laboratory had to reduce staff by 15% as a result of a reduction in funding due to a federal government austerity program. When managers were suddenly required to reduce staff, no clear employee information was available that could identify the strong performers from those who were not performing to TRIUMF's expectations. Decisions to reduce staff when required should be based on concrete information, not perception. Now that a performance system is in place, those employees who have been identified as needing improvement are encouraged to improve their performance, and, if required, are offered courses in those areas where weaknesses have been identified. Those who have demonstrated leadership and strong performance are given opportunities for career growth and advancement.

In any event, the author feels strongly that all employees should have the opportunity to discuss performance issues with their immediate supervisors at least once a year to keep communication clear and to avoid cases when an employee is surprised by his or her supervisor's assessment. It is important for the employee to be in sync with both the job and the supervisor—in other words, that the employee and supervisor's expectations are the same. TRIUMF HR looks at all performance reviews and notes issues or requests for reclassification, and follows up with any of these issues throughout the year. The performance management system has become a successful tool and is generally supported by all staff.

Employee Relations

Fair and ethical treatment of employees creates an environment of mutual respect. When an employee has an opportunity to have regular input into his or her career progress, productivity will improve. Employee issues are important and have a direct impact on employee morale, enthusiasm, and ultimate performance. HR should make every effort to understand each issue when it arises and help the employee resolve them in a timely manner. The HR department, in some institutions, designates an employee relations manager who is responsible for dealing with all issues that may arise between the institution and the employee. However, at many institutions this is a part-time position. The HR professional has a vast number of tasks to complete and when an employee comes into human resources with a problem, it may be perceived as a burden for the human resource person, but a critical issue for the employee. Timeliness really is of the essence in many cases when employee issues are involved.

It is very important for HR to create a climate of open communication within the institution and support a common sense approach to behavior In some cases one may not be motivated to treat others the way one would want to be treated. In these instances, it may be wise to have a definition of the organization's "Golden Rule" for dealing with people.[4] It is best not to take word-of-mouth information at face value and to always have proper documentation to support any recommended actions. In institutions where labor unions exist, a labor relations officer may be designated to handle collective bargaining units.

At TRIUMF, employee concerns may be taken to one of three representative groups that have been established within the organization in addition or as an alternative to contacting the HR department. These representative groups function as employee liaisons to management, and act on behalf of the employees they are representing. The three representative committees are referred to as the board appointed representative committee (BARC), the technician employee liaison committee (TELC), and the professional and supervisory representative committee (PSRC). While these committees operate formally, they have no negotiation rights and, therefore, no collective agreements are required between these organizations and the institution.

Compensation

Compensation is one of the most difficult areas of the HR manager's job. The institution's funding level and changing demographics within the organization will also have an impact on this process. How does one ensure that people are paid a fair salary that is in line with their qualifications and experience and at the same time compete with other institutions for people from the same talent pool?

There are a number of ways salaries can be administered, ranging from annual scale or cost of living increases, graduated career progress or range progression based on years of experience, to pay for performance. In some cases where the total salary budget is allowed to increase by the rise in the cost of living for the previous year, the institution may award salary increases based on this allowed increase but with a bit of a twist. If salaries were budgeted to increase at 3% per year as an example, some employees might receive no increase based on poor performance, while others could receive an increase in the order of 8%. The total payroll budget would increase by a total of 3% but the distribution for each employee would be completely different. With a performance management system in place, management can implement this type of salary administration system and award significant salary increases without having to make arbitrary decisions.

Improvements in the institution's benefits plan may be an alternative to salary increases when funding is low or stagnant. The ability to increase salaries is contingent on funding or revenue levels. If the institution offers a good research product, then funding may increase and the ability to issue salary increases goes along with it.

Some will say that by reducing staff numbers, more money will be available for salary increases for those who are left. This may be true, but it is only possible to reduce staff numbers based on changes in the institution's program. Furthermore, shifting more work on often already overworked employees should be considered very short-sighted.

A further comment should also be made that working in a research environment is not only about wages. Employees make their decisions to work at a certain research institution based on the entire package, including salary, benefits, and working conditions. In addition, some institutions offer employment packages that offer flexible benefits and lifestyle enhancing/balancing benefits and these can be offered to employees with no impact on the institution's salary budget.

Human Resource Management

HR staff should recognize all employees, visitors, and managers in the organization as customers. If the HR staff does the job correctly, then principal investigators (PIs) and departmental managers will know that the HR professionals are an important resource. HR should be a strategic partner in bringing the HR perspective to the general management of the company. The HR manager's role is to develop policies and programs and share responsibilities with department managers.

To ensure that HR can deal with issues that continually arise in a timely manner, it is very important to have an HR Management Information System (HRMIS). This database system should include all information related to the employee and should be able to generate management reports that will assist department managers with staffing, reorganization, succession planning, and general organizational issues.

HR Management (HRM) is moving away from being a transaction-based, paper-pushing, hiring-and-firing support entity, toward becoming an integral part of the management team dealing with responsibilities concerning decision making, profitability, and strategic planning. HRM is the use of HR to achieve organizational objectives.[2]

Policies and Procedures

As discussed earlier, organizations need HR policies and procedures, but these cannot be too bureaucratic both in language and application.

TRIUMF's HR philosophy is stated in the following:

TRIUMF is committed to providing leadership and direction to its employees through the development and support of policies and procedures that contribute to an individual's personal and professional growth, and to overall internal equity. Recognizing the unique cultural framework that exists within TRIUMF, we strive to foster an environment based on respect for individuals, recognizing that this type of atmosphere contributes to overall co-operation and teamwork. TRIUMF further supports this philosophy with the following:

> Employment and all related decisions at TRIUMF are determined by ability and performance. Factors such as age, gender, sexual orientation, religion, race, color or handicap are not considered in these decisions. The working environment will at all times be supportive of the dignity and self-esteem of its employees, and TRIUMF will rely on mutual respect, co-operation and understanding between all of its staff. All employees have the right to be free from harassment of any kind in our workplace. Inappropriate conduct expressed verbally or physically towards another employee, regardless of who initiates it, and to whom it is directed, will not be tolerated.[5]

Some policies have been established as a result of labor legislation and can appear quite autocratic to many within the organization. The application of these policies in a way that can be widely supported can sometimes be a challenge.

At TRIUMF, the director, the board of management personnel committee, and the board of management approve all personnel policies and procedures. This is done only after all employee groups have had an opportunity to comment on any new policies or proposed changes to existing policies.

In a research environment, policies cannot be enforced by decree. When bringing in new policies, it is key to buy in from all parties in order to encourage cooperation, understanding, and adherence to the policy. All employees must be treated consistently with the application of the policy.

Training and Development

Training and development of staff are very important and HR's role in this area is to identify demonstrated staff weaknesses and to point out areas where the development of employee skills would enhance the institution. Employees should always be encouraged to grow and develop their job skills and department managers should also work with their staff to identify training and development needs.

At many institutions, leadership development might be better described as the development of "technically correct leaders"—leaders who improve in managing their tasks. HR should promote leadership development and work with senior managers to identify potential leaders, or provide current leaders with the appropriate training to develop higher visions, self-confidence, and good coaching skills on how to position their staff for success. Developing leadership is about both personal and professional growth. In many cases, there is a "command and control" leadership style with newly promoted leaders that just does not work in the long term.

TRIUMF's training and development policy is shown below:

> Subject to budgetary constraints and operational requirements, TRIUMF will support employees in acquiring, updating or developing the knowledge and skills required for them to meet their present and future work requirements.

> It is the responsibility of the employee to:

> - consult the supervisor on his/her development needs; and
> - complete the relevant application (training request) as per these procedures

> It is the responsibility of the Supervisor to:

> - assist the employee in identifying his/her development needs
> - endorse attendance at a training event as per these procedures
> - review all applications for Training Support
> - make a recommendation to the Division head for approval or denial of Training request[5]

Health and Safety

The employer has a responsibility for the health and safety of its employees for work-related activities. The employer also has a responsibility to the environment and those who may be impacted by the operations of the facility.

Following is TRIUMF's Health and Safety policy:

MISSION

The mission of the TRIUMF Office of Environment, Health and Safety (EH&S) is to provide TRIUMF management and staff with the tools and information to minimize the impact of TRIUMF operations on the environment, to ensure a healthy workforce and a safe workplace, so as to enable TRIUMF to maintain excellence in scientific research.

RESPONSIBILITIES

It is the responsibility of TRIUMF management to demonstrate by example TRIUMF's commitment to safety, and to support, develop, and require the leadership of supervisory staff in occupational health and safety matters.

It is the responsibility of all workers at TRIUMF to abide by all of the policies and procedures adopted by the TRIUMF management and to ensure personal and public safety. All workers shall practice safety in personal work habits and encourage the same among fellow workers. They shall initiate suggestions for new methods of improving safety, report hazardous conditions to their supervisors, group, or senior manager, and cooperate in the solution of safety problems in the workplace.[5]

Most institutions require new employees to attend an orientation that includes standard lab safety procedures as well as policies and procedures unique to their institution. Annual review is required of many procedures and this should be identified in performance reviews.

Conclusion

The author has identified a number of issues that should be considered of prime importance to the HR manager and key areas of responsibility for the HR department. Of these, it is worth emphasizing the following main points.

Communication

Communication is key to the success of any relationship and this is essential to a productive work environment.

Leadership Skills

Scientists or academics usually direct research institutions and while they may be technically expert in their area of competence, they are sometimes lacking in the leadership skills required to run a facility efficiently, and therefore must rely on others within the organization. It is the responsibility of the human resources manager to identify these areas of weakness to senior management and work with them so they can acquire the necessary skills or resources to do their jobs properly.

Institutional Culture

The culture in a research institution is very unique and crucial to the scientific program. This culture involves an organization of "peers," not necessarily bosses and subordinates, and all HR initiatives must take this into consideration. HR must acknowledge the critical importance of the culture at an institution and should also help to define that culture. HR should try to reinforce, reward, and act in a way that is always consistent with the culture. New administration, in trying to improve the efficiency of an organization by exerting pressure to have an overall shift in the culture, will result in inefficiencies and poor morale.

Management by Persuasion

In a research environment, it is not about managing by the power of the position, but by ideas and persuasion. Leadership plays a crucial role in this process. The HR administrator cannot decree what must be done, but must demonstrate that it is worthwhile for the mission of the institution. If senior management or senior scientists cannot be convinced that something is worth doing, then it is not worthwhile or one has failed in the task.

Employee Retention

One can never stress enough the importance of retaining current staff. In a competitive climate, human resources should work with senior managers to develop a strategy for retention. Career development and natural progression through the organization can be a powerful retention strategy, and may be one of the biggest in a nonprofit organization. How many times has a new employee been hired and left disillusioned after several months? Does the institution have a proper orientation process, one that covers a several month period? With all the time and expense taken to bring in a new scientist to an institution, if he or she leaves after earlier deciding that this was the place he or she wanted to be, then the institution has failed with either the recruitment or orientation process. A mistake that many institutions often make is in going outside the organization to recruit senior people or leaders. Succession planning is very important and can be tied into a system for retaining staff.

HR can help move an organization toward excellence and the role of the HR department is shifting from an administrative function to a strategic one. To be truly effective there must be linkage between the organization's objectives and the HR initiatives. HR can offer the strategies, tools, motivation, and support to create this excellence but then must be true a partner with both the senior management of the organization and its management board.

• • • Endnotes

1. Gelès, Claude, Gilles Lindecker, Mel Month, and Christian Roche. *Managing Science: Management for R&D Laboratories*. New York: Wiley, 2000.

2. Downie, Bryan, and Mary Lou Coates. *Managing Human Resources in the 1990s and Beyond*. Queen's University, Kingston, Ontario: IRC Press, 1995.

3. Citizenship and Immigration Canada, "You asked about . . . immigration and citizenship," http://www.cic.gc.ca/english/pub/you-asked/section-18.html (accessed July 15, 2005). U.S. Citizenship and Immigration Services. "Immigration Information," http://uscis.gov/graphics/shared/lawenfor/bmgmt/inspect/nafta2.htm (accessed July 15, 2005).

4. Phin, Donald. "Building Powerful Employment Relationships," Presentation at the HRMA conference, Vancouver, Canada, March 25, 2002.

5. TRIUMF, Canada's National Laboratory for Particle and Nuclear Physics. Human Resources Policies and Procedures and Environmental Health and Safety. Internal documents not available for public access. For public access, see http://www.triumf.info/ (accessed July 15, 2005).

Immigration
Citizenship and Immigration Canada
http://www.cic.gc.ca/english/

Human Resources and Skills Development Canada
http://www.hrsdc.gc.ca/en/home.shtml

US Citizenship and Immigration Services
http://uscis.gov/graphics/exec/whereis/index.asp

Safety-Related Organizations
Canada
Canadian Centre for Occupational Health and Safety
http://www.ccohs.ca/

Canadian Radiation Protection Association
http://www.crpa-acrp.ca/

Canadian Nuclear Safety Commission
http://www.cnsc-ccsn.gc.ca/

Health Canada
http://www.hc-sc.gc.ca/index_e.html

Canadian Environmental Assessment Agency
http://www.acee-ceaa.gc.ca/

International
World Health Organization
http://www.who.int/en/

International Commission on Radiological Protection
http://www.icrp.org/

United States
National Council on Radiation Protection and Measurements (NCRP)
http://www.ncrp.com

National Institute for Occupational Safety and Health
http://www.cdc.gov/niosh/homepage.htm

US Department of Labor Occupational Safety & Health Administration
http://www.osha.gov

• • • Additional Resources

Human Resources
Big Dog's Human Resource Development Page
http://www.nwlink.com/~donclark/hrd.html

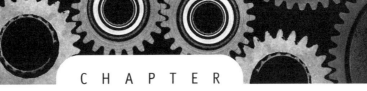

CHAPTER

10

Media Relations

Lisa A. Lapin

Research administrators have been successful in their academic environments largely because they have been good teachers—successful at communicating their expertise to students, granting agencies, and academic peers. Do you know how to take what you would say in a fifty-minute classroom lecture or in a twenty-page grant proposal and teach it to a television journalist in five minutes? Would you be ready to answer your office phone and conduct an interview with a reporter on the other end? Mastering a few simple principles can make research administrators ready to be effective communicators under such circumstances, whether facing a hostile news reporter, speaking to a crowd of two hundred, taking part in a departmental meeting, or simply speaking across the dinner table.

Benefits of Media Relations

There is inherent risk in media relations. Unlike academic publishing, there is no peer review prior to a newspaper article publication and it is unlikely that television news programs can be previewed prior to airing. Internet news sites run only very brief versions of in-depth news stories. Radio audiences are passive listeners, not likely to absorb great detail. Overall, there is little control over the final media outcome, though an astute research administrator knows how to control the media interaction at the outset, even prior to an interview. Media interaction presents risk of poor messaging. Given the risk, what is the benefit of media relations to the

research unit? To the campus? To you as an individual representative?

Research administrators must consider a number of principle issues and conditions when dealing with media:

The news media are very influential. A single newspaper article can prompt a series of legislative hearings. Media coverage is a way to reach audiences that influence public opinion and can influence funding for research. These include elected officials, funding agencies, voters, prospective faculty and students, and potential donors. Numerous research institutions have stories about funding that was obtained because granting agencies or foundations learned about a research project through the mainstream media.

Research institutions rely on public taxpayer funds, and often have a goal of developing research discoveries that can change lives and influence policies. Research units have an obligation to explain their purpose to those upon whose goodwill and financial support we depend.

The public often has misinformation and misperception about the purpose of research. Basic research can often be misunderstood and viewed as frivolous. Other areas of research, including biotechnology and genomics, are sometimes feared and little understood. Thus, the news media present an opportunity to provide a broader education and increased understanding about new areas of science.

Media coverage is free publicity. Most research units do not have extensive marketing or advertising budgets to purchase television airtime or newspaper space. In an average US metropolitan area, a 30-second commercial spot during the local TV newscast costs between $1,000 and $3,000; 30 seconds on national news, such as NBC Nightly News, can run $75,000. Print advertising in a major metropolitan daily newspaper can cost $15,000 for a half-page ad that runs just once.

There can be an advantage to having research covered in the mainstream press. Popular press accounts of articles that appear in science journals can enhance the attention the articles receive in scientific circles.

Forms of News Media

Where do most people get their news today? Most people associated with academic and research environments often assume that most people receive their news from newspapers because newspapers cover stories in more detail and depth. However, the Roper Polling organization in repeated surveys has found that seven out of ten members of the general public receive their news each day from television.[1]

What is deemed the most credible source of news and information? Again, it is not newspapers, but television. When television viewers see the visual image of someone talking on camera, they see the direct source of the information, rather than relying on a journalist to translate information into writing. Therefore, it is particularly important that research units learn how to make the best use of the television medium, despite the fact that the average TV news story is 90 seconds or less.

The Internet is taking on increasing importance as a news source. A 2002 Pew Research Center study of internet usage asked thousands of Americans where they got their news "yesterday."[2] Of the total general public, 54% went online for news, 55% watched television news, and 46% read the newspaper. However, of the cohort of those studied who were under the age of 30, there was a dramatic skew toward the Internet where 74% went to Internet sites for news, 44% watched television, and 29% read a newspaper. This information does not render newspapers obsolete: the printed media remains the primary originator of news that then forms the basis for television and radio reports, and it is often newspaper-operated Internet sites that are frequently visited for news.

It is important to know that information that "makes news" or is deemed "newsworthy" and generates interest from journalists is often that which is about conflict or controversy. Research

administrators can anticipate that when they are approached by news media for interviews, the journalists are also speaking to someone with an opposing perspective. Research discoveries that are out of the ordinary and go against common understanding (for example, that chocolate can be good for your health) are often the discoveries that generate the greatest media attention. For example, one of the most widely reported recent scientific stories was about a University of California, Davis study of a chemical process that infused antibacterial agents into textiles—creating not only sterile hospital clothing and bedding, but smell-proof socks.

Working with Print and Broadcast Media

In many respects, it can be easier to work with a print reporter (those from newspapers and magazines) than a television journalist. Print reporters often conduct interviews with a notebook or, occasionally, with a tape recorder, which ensures that words are accurately recorded. Most often, print journalists conduct interviews by phone, which is a less intimidating circumstance that allows the subject of the interview to look up information in files, reference information on the computer, and refer to prepared notes and talking points.

A television interview can be a daunting experience. Often, there is a two-person crew, the reporter and the camera person. There are bright lights and attached microphones. During a television interview, the subject of the interview needs to think quickly and to communicate simply and concisely: there is no opportunity to look at reference materials. The manner presented on television establishes an impression and intimacy with the television audience; viewers make judgments about the credibility and integrity of someone appearing on television in a matter of seconds. Therefore, body language, facial expressions, gestures and visual appearance take on greater importance. Audiences are often won by the attitudes of interviewees.

When interacting with either a print or broadcast journalist, several key points apply. It is important for the subject of the interview to understand the reporter's time frame. In most cases, journalists are reporting daily news and have stringent deadlines: returning their phone calls at the end of the day or the next day can result in a missed opportunity. When seeking news sources, journalists most often go with the sources who promptly return calls.

It is wise to assume limited knowledge on the part of the journalist. Most television and newspaper reporters are generalists who know little about the subjects they have been assigned to cover, particularly in the fields of scientific research. It is the responsibility of the interviewee to provide background information and to educate the reporter prior to the beginning of the main interview. Give the reporter any papers or fact sheets about the subject in advance to help him or her ask more informed questions and to improve the resulting content of the news story in a more complete context.

In interviews with both newspapers and television media, the interviewee needs to consider visual impact and content of a report. Newspaper stories accompanied by photos almost always receive better placement than those without visuals, and television stories rely almost entirely on visual impact. Television stories have a person on camera giving them information and background verbally. The subject of an interview often has an opportunity to dictate the location of a television interview to make the most appropriate use of background. Demonstrations of equipment, processes, and examples of discoveries are also very valuable for example, a cyclotron in action or a greenhouse full of a new breed of food crop. Visual demonstrations enhance the reporter's ability to tell the story—and your institution's positive coverage.

Primary Media Assumptions

Be safe and assume that everything you say to a reporter—even in a social situation—may appear in print or on the air and that nothing is "off the record." Reporters frequently fail to honor agreements with news sources to use information only as "background" or "not for attribution." Many reporters make promises to not use names, but ultimately, the information can be traced to the source. If the subject of an interview should not be speaking or using his or her name with the news media, he or she should refrain from providing any information altogether.

Negative attention can be attracted when news sources say "no comment" or do not return the calls of journalists requesting information. A comment of "no comment" can immediately convey a tone of dishonesty to the public. Even when nothing can be said on record legally—situations involving, for example, legal cases, personnel matters, or client confidentiality—it is important that an institution presents some message to the reporter. Take

for example a case where a university professor may be under investigation for conflict of interest with respect to a research grant. An appropriate media response would be, "I am not at liberty to discuss this specific case, but let me tell you about our process for conducting investigations into alleged conflict of interest. We convene a committee, we review all documentation, we interview involved parties, etc." This type of response will often satisfy a reporter and certainly will protect the institution's reputation.

A subject of a media interview should expect mistakes to appear in print or on the air and it is important to let reporters know as graciously as possible about errors in stories. Many people fear making an enemy of a journalist, but it is important to let reporters know of any errors so that they are not repeated in the future. In print media, corrections are often buried within the publication, but electronic record is corrected online for anyone who references the story in the future. For televised stories, watch the first newscast and call the assignment desk to report any errors so that errors can be edited for subsequent broadcasts of the story.

With regard to any print media, do not expect to read copy beforehand—most major news organizations have a policy against allowing news sources to preview news stories prior to publication. This is difficult for many in the academic community where peer review is the norm. However, media organizations insist on reporting what their journalists observed without interference from sources. But if information is highly technical or sensitive, ask that the reporter call you back, as a courtesy, and read back to you just your quotes. Another way to ensure that an interview is accurately reported is to ask the journalist, before the end of the interview, to repeat back for you your main points. Ask them at the time of the interview, *What do you think you will quote me saying? What main point that I have made will you be putting in your story or on the air?* This presents an opportunity to clarify any points or facts that the reporter may not have understood.

Successful Interview Preparation

Before the start of an interview, it is important to immediately turn the tables and ask the reporter some questions:

> *What is the subject?*
> *Why have you been asked for the interview?*

Are you the right spokesperson?

Has the reporter contacted the media relations office at your campus or institution (if there is one)?

Who is the reporter? What is his or her usual "beat"?

What does he or she know about the subject he or she has have been assigned to cover? Has the reporter ever written about it or talked about it on the air before?

What is the deadline?

Who else is being interviewed?

What type of background material has the reporter read or seen?

It is highly recommended that the interviewee then take a minimum of 15 minutes to prepare before launching into the interview. Ask the reporter if his or her call can be returned, but by all means, be respectful of deadlines. The reporter's answers to the questions above should indicate the reporter's agenda, who he or she works for, how much he or she knows, and who else he or she is talking to, including anyone who might have something negative to say about the research or subject at hand. All of this information contributes to the substance of what to discuss in an interview and what factual information to include.

The most successful interviews are those in which the interviewee has taken time to prepare and has developed "messages" or "talking points" to deliver during the interview. A strong message is one that answers the questions: *Why should my audience care about this topic?; What is the value of this research to my audience?; What questions are we trying to answer that are relevant to society at large?* The answers to these questions will provide information that should resonate with newspaper readers or television viewers—creating those "a ha" moments where the audience reaches a deeper understanding of the value of research. Write down two or three primary points to make in an interview and practice them out loud prior to meeting with the reporter. Keep in mind that, with the exception of specialized media such as scientific journals, the audience for most news media is the general public.

It is important to speak simply to reporters, keeping in mind that newspapers and television aim their news coverage to the understanding of a high school sophomore. Be brief; the average length of a sound bite today is seven seconds. The best communicators receive more airtime, but it is still crucial to be succinct.

Conclusion

Although the experience can be daunting, it is to the advantage of research administrators to take advantage of opportunities to interact with the news media. Even a few minutes spent in proper preparation will make the time spent with the news media more productive. Used effectively, media relations can be added to the other tools at your disposal to communicate the value and importance of research. Positive coverage of research accomplishments will result in broader awareness among the public, and among the opinion leaders who determine levels of research funding and support.

• • • References

1. Roper Center for Public Opinion Research, University of Connecticut, Roper Public Affairs & Media Poll, 1992 and 1996, US Public Opinion on News Media iPoll database.

   "Which Is Your Main Source of News?" The Washington Post, telephone poll of 1,011 adults, April 19–23, 1996.

   Carroll, Joseph. "Local TV and Newspapers Remain Most Popular News Sources," The Gallup Organization, Dec. 20, 2004 (survey data also being used by Roper).

   Witt, Evans. "Necessary Embrace: The Public and the News Media," Public Perspective, July/August 2002.

2. "Public's News Habits Changed Little by Sept. 11," The Pew Research Center for People and the Press, Washington DC, Biannual News Consumption Survey, June 9, 2002.

11

Working with Boards of Trustees and Advisory Boards

Cary E. Thomas, MBA, CMA

While there are many books and professional guidance readily available for members of nonprofit boards, in direct contrast, little has been written to provide guidance to the research administrator on the supporting roles they should be ready to play in the essential work of governing and advisory boards.

This chapter first explores the roles of a governing board, and then the roles of advisory boards, in each case highlighting the roles and responsibilities of a research administrator in connection with these boards.

Board of Trustees

A board of trustees plays a vital role in the management of a nonprofit organization, especially one engaged in research. The members of the board of trustees can be legally liable for the acts of the nonprofit organization, so they are interested in assuring that the organization is run in a legal and compliant way! Thus the goals of the board are consistent with the goals of a research administrator.

In the classic textbook, *Boards That Make A Difference*, author John Carver describes his view of an "ideal" organization as one that is led by a strong board in partnership with a strong CEO. When such a leadership structure is in place, the primary role of the board is to monitor executive performance.[1]

Carver poses the question, "With Boards operating at policy arm's length from operations and delegating so much authority to the CEO, how can it know that its directives are being followed?"[2]

Carver goes on to answer his own question by pointing out that three types of information are commonly provided to boards: decision information, monitoring information, and incidental information. Decision information supports the choices or new directions that the board is being asked to endorse, and so should provide a complete picture of the decision, all the options, and should explain why the recommended option is the best choice. Monitoring information lets the board know how approved plans are progressing. Incidental information is used neither to make decisions nor to monitor results, thus Carver discounts their value, but believes this is the most common information provided to boards!

The task of the research administrator when providing information to the board is to understand which type of information is being provided and to provide the appropriate detail, content, and context. Table 11-1 shows examples of the three information types commonly found in research organizations.

Carver also outlines the board's responsibility in policy formulation, charting the strategic plan for the organization and evaluation of CEO performance.[3]

While all of these responsibilities are essential to any nonprofit organization, the board of a research enterprise faces some unique challenges. These challenges can be grouped into the following areas: assuring that the board understands the unique business model of a nonprofit research organization; clear and regular board communication; and the role of the board in management of the research organization. As detailed in the following section, the research administrator can play a vital role in each of these areas.

TABLE 11-1	Information Needs of Boards	
Information Type	**Subject Matter**	**Relevant Information**
Decision Information	Construct a new facility or remodel an old facility	Growth in research volume, projections of future research volume, Space as a percentage of research expenditures, space per employee.
	Initiate a new program and/or recruit new faculty	Measurement of the opportunity (field of research is expanding or shrinking), the impact of outcomes of the new program, its costs and the identified sources of funds.
	Capacity planning	Growth rate, both past and projected, of research; changes in the type of research and the kinds of facilities and equipment necessary for quality research, staffing impact.
Monitoring Information	Progress of research programs	Number and quality of publications, invention disclosures, patents issued, licenses granted, absorption of use of CORES, etc.
	Audit findings	Background of findings, management's response, and the expected impact.
	Allocation of resources	Comparison of space allocated to the financial impact of the program, trends in space per indirect cost recovery.
	Funding: actual vs. budget	A comparison of results versus budget, the percentage variance, and the likely impact on year-end performance.
	Implementation of the strategic plan	Metrics of the degree to which programs and milestones are being achieved.
Incidental Information	Grant growth, funding hit rate, indirect cost trends, mixture of funding resources	See sections that follow for concrete examples of typical reports.

The Unique Business Model of Sponsored Research

Most board members come to their positions either from the for-profit world or from the philanthropic world. Each of these environments has a business model that makes perfect sense for most people familiar with a traditional management perspective. A consistent problem for board members of institutions engaged in research is that the business model of research—especially research conducted under federal costing and compliance policies—often does not make sense to those unfamiliar with the workings of research. This is especially true in the case of facilities and administration, or "indirect" expenses. Other chapters of this book describe the nuances of the financial model used for research management, especially funding infrastructure and administrative expenses, so the subject matter will not be repeated here.

Some items the research administrator needs to be sure his or her board members understand include:

- In most cases, revenue is not recognized until funds have been expended. For example, gifts or grants received are first recorded as temporarily restricted assets and are not recognized as revenue earned until the funds are expended for their intended purpose!
- Budget surpluses in one area cannot always be used to cover budget deficits in another.
- If the facilities and administration cost accounts have recoverable income to match them, reducing these "overhead" costs will reduce expenses, but will produce no positive result because there will be a matching reduction of income.
- Not all research expenditures will generate their proportionate share in indirect cost recovery; this especially true for large equipment contracts or multi-institutional agreements.
- When indirect costs are in equilibrium with indirect recovery (income), increases in non-federal expenditures will decrease both the income recovered from federal funds and the indirect cost recovery rate.

Board Communication

A well-informed board contributes to good non-profit management. The major communication issues confronting management of the research enterprise as it interacts with the board are:

- Determining what issues are relevant for board notification;
- Identifying issues that are of such a magnitude that board involvement is required;
- Developing a routine, timely, informative reporting system; and
- Providing a conduit for appropriate management-board interchange.

Board Notification Nothing is more satisfying to management or more rewarding to board members than good news. Since all news is not good, effective communication of bad news is a must.

There are dual dangers in keeping the board informed of relevant information. The first is that the board may become preoccupied with smaller matters that do not merit board attention. The second is that events or circumstances that warrant the board's attention may not be communicated in a timely or clear way. Navigating between these extremes requires skill and judgment. The following points provide criteria regarding situations that should be brought to the attention of the board:

- Any situation that has the potential to cast the institution in a bad light, jeopardize its reputation, or create negative publicity.
- Any existing or potential financial condition that materially impacts the capital or operating budget of the organization.
- Any change in key administrative or scientific personnel that impacts the ability of the organization to continue the orderly conduct of its science or operations.

Board Involvement Under normal circumstances, the board's role is one of oversight rather than direct involvement. However, sooner or later every organization faces issues that are of such importance or magnitude that the board should be promptly notified and should become fully involved. If the organization is well managed, these issues should rarely occur. For organizations involved in research, especially research involving human subjects, there are risks that can lead to such issues. The following list details issues that call for the board's attention:

- *Conflict of interest transactions involving board members.* It is not uncommon for the members of a nonprofit board to come forward with a financial transaction between the board member and the organization. Typically the board member is engaged in a business that provides goods or services and wants to offer a transaction favorable to the nonprofit organi-

zation. For example, a board member may want to offer the nonprofit organization a contract for insurance coverage at rates that are lower than any other provider could offer due to favorable treatment by the board member. In such a case, the board member is called an "interested person."

Many state laws, and most organization's bylaws require such a transaction to be approved by a majority of the board members with the "interested person" (or persons) excluded from participating in either the discussion of the transaction or the vote on its approval. Typically, management of the nonprofit organization would impartially study the transaction, gather timely and independent information regarding the transaction, and make an assessment of the degree to which the transaction is favorable to the organization. The research administrator may be called upon to participate in the impartial collection of facts and their presentation.

- *A charge of impropriety against any board member.* It would be highly unusual for the research administrator to have any role in such an issue, but it is mentioned here for completeness.

- *A charge of impropriety against the CEO or other corporate officer.* Organizational personnel at any level, including the research administrator, should report through appropriate compliance channels any suspicions of wrongdoing, failure to meet regulatory requirements, or a lapse in good practices of operational and financial propriety. Depending on the veracity of alleged wrongdoing and the severity of the allegations, the research administrator may be required to participate in an investigation in an impartial, diplomatic, and tactful manner.

- *Any event that threatens the reputation or integrity of the organization.* Responsible conduct of research, ethical business practices, and the protection of human and animal research subjects lie at the core of quality research management. The research administrator needs to be mindful of these imperatives, must keep abreast of the issues and associated regulations, should be an integral part of a robust compliance program, and a potential source of support to his/her board in these matters.

- *Any significant litigation or threat of litigation.* Sadly, litigation is an all-too-common part of contemporary life even in the world of nonprofit management. The research administrator should be aware of real or threatened litigation, seek and understand attorney-client rules and relationships, and be especially cautious regarding activities, information, and events that have or may have an impact on such cases.

Board Reporting   A quality reporting regimen characterized by frequent, informative, succinct, and useful information is the hallmark of good management. Volunteer board members will be better informed and more fully engaged if they can rely on clear, detailed reports, in a format that is consistent and useful, which is delivered regularly in advance of board meetings.

Clear reports will be those that "paint a picture" for the board member and will be produced in the same format consistently so that board members can adapt to the content and style of the report, thus easily gleaning the message to be conveyed. The value of reports is greatest if, following Edward Tufte's principle, reports "should show...data in a comparative perspective."[4] For example, a report that specifies that the current year research volume is forecasted to be $X million, while an interesting statistic, is much more useful to board members if it is reported as $X million which is a 20 percent increase over the prior year and is the highest level of research in the history of the organization.

Determining how much information to present to board members is more art than science. The author believes that the number of pages is inversely proportional to the value of the report: if you can't tell the story in a few pages (or better yet, within a single page), you are dealing in too much detail! Board members want to know the trend, the likely result, or the bottom line. They are relying on you, the members of management, to know (and manage) all the details. However, while keeping the report concise, be sure not to omit any relevant facts.

The management and staff responsible for preparing reports should consider the essence of the nonprofit organization's mission, the metrics by which it is managed, and the information that most clearly communicates them. For a research enterprise, the following examples should be considered as minimum metrics for reporting:

- Grant and contract *applications*. Both the number of applications and the dollar amount, submitted in the current fiscal year, with a comparison to the same metrics for prior years. Such a report shows if the organization is continuing to pursue with vigor expansion of research. For those organizations with a diversity of funding, the simple report could be expanded to show applications by funding agency or programmatic area.
- Grants and contracts *awarded*. Both the number and the dollar amount, received in the current fiscal year, with a comparison to the same metrics for prior years (ideally, as of the same time period of the prior year). Such a report shows if the research-funding base is continuing to expand or is stagnant or shrinking. Some organizations prefer to contrast these two reports by providing a measure of the ratio of awards to applications (some times referred to as a "hit rate," i.e., Professor Jones is awarded 25 percent of the grants for which she applies). While this can be a meaningful metric, the complexity of resubmittals of grants, and the wide difference in workload associated with competing versus noncompeting awards frequently demands that any conclusions from such numbers be tempered with anecdotal information or analysis.

- A report of indirect cost recovery (income) contrasted to current indirect costs (expense). Such a report shows the degree to which these essential costs are tracking the funds to pay for them. A variation of this report measures each grant's capacity to pay its fair share of indirect costs, giving management a measure of grants that are unable to carry their full load, and for those which cannot, the need to tap other funds to pay for unrecovered costs.
- To the extent that philanthropy is an important component of the nonprofit's financial profile, a report of the gifts received (or released from restrictions) compared to the same period in prior years, and to the budgeted level of giving should be a standard report. In any such reports it is essential to differentiate between restricted and unrestricted funds. Reports that track gift income by source (e.g., annual giving, major gifts, earnings on endowment funds, etc.) and the uses to which these gift funds are to be deployed exhibit a high level of quality reporting.
- Operational reports for long-term projects: implementation of mission-critical information systems; progress on renovation or construction projects; status of major recruitment programs for faculty, scientists, or key management positions; capital, endowment, or other major fundraising campaigns are essential.

The fundamental message for those involved in research management is that every board should expect, and is entitled to receive, reports that show how the research organization is performing. Thus, the collection of reliable information upon which such reports are based must be part of the management information system; staff needs to understand how the metrics are collected and how to report them in consistent, reliable ways.

Interchange between the Board and Management   The role of a board is to define the strategic plan of the organization, supervise the CEO, and assure that the CEO implements the strategic plan. The role of the CEO is to manage the affairs of the nonprofit organization, implement the strategic plan, and keep the board informed of progress. When boards and management are performing their respective roles well, the interchange between them is regular but infrequent, formal but informative, and characterized by candor and trust. Normally most interaction between management and the board is accomplished at regular board meetings. There are two cases in which more detailed or more frequent communication is warranted: standing committees and ad hoc committees. In many cases the research administrator can and should play a supportive role to these board committees.

Standing Committees Standing committees provide an effective tool for board oversight of essential functions at a level of detail not possible during the normal course of board meetings. Standing committees are frequently composed of a mixture of board members, members of the nonprofit organization and in some cases outside experts, volunteers, or members of the community at large. Minutes should be kept of all standing committee meetings, should be approved by the members present, and should be provided to the board at its regular meetings (or in advance). Examples of standing committees include:

- *Finance Committee.* The finance committee meets more frequently than the board as a whole reviewing the financial statements of the organization and monitoring financial performance. Board members with financial expertise are ideal candidates for the finance committee. Frequently professional accountants from the community at large are invited to be members of the finance committee, typically providing valuable advice and independent insight. The chief financial officer of the nonprofit should be a member of the committee, possibly augmented by financial staff members. Of particular importance to a finance committee of a research organization is the ability of the members of the committee to understand and apply the financial principles of research finance. Among these are the concepts of cost-reimbursable research expenditures, the matching of direct research income and expense, the arcane and complicated aspects of indirect cost recovery, provisional, awarded, and experience rates for indirect costs, the nature of restricted versus unrestricted gifts, and more. Support of the finance committee is an essential task of the research administrator. In addition to the financial reports provided to the board (as outlined earlier), the research administrator is commonly asked to provide more detailed reports for the finance committee.

- *Audit Committee.* In the wake of the 2002 Sarbanes-Oxley Act,[5] audit committees are increasingly becoming commonplace in nonprofit organizations. Although their size is small (typically three members, one of whom should be adept at nonprofit accounting) and their scope is limited, this is an essential committee. No members of management should serve on this committee. The typical roles of the audit committee are: to hire the audit firm; to negotiate and approve the audit firm's engagement letter; to receive the audit and transmit it to the board; and to resolve any differences between management and the external auditors. The audit committee will probably also secure tax services for preparation of the federal form 990 and any other required state information returns.

  The research administrator can support the audit committee by providing historical costs of audits and the cost of preparation of the nonprofit's federal form 990 and other information returns.

- *Compensation Committee.* Oversight of top management's performance and associated compensation packages is, by definition, a very personal matter. Most boards prefer to have a compensation committee review performance and recommend salary, bonus, and benefits of the CEO and potentially other top executives. The committee should be guided by a clear policy that details the timing and frequency of performance reviews (typically at least once per year and normally at the conclusion of a fiscal year). The compensation committee should expect to receive a written report containing a statement by the executive(s) of the degree to which prior period goals were attained and a list of accomplishments during the review period.

  The research administrator can and should provide staff support to the compensation committee by providing information such as: salary survey data for comparable institutions to support salary adjustment decisions; reports demonstrating the degree to which critical goals were achieved by top executives; the financial impact of key accomplishments (which might bear on considerations of the awarding of a bonus); and other information, as requested.

- *Executive Committee.* The primary purpose of an executive committee is to be available to handle issues requiring board approval for those rare cases where a decision cannot wait for a regularly scheduled board meeting. The executive committee is typically composed of the officers of the organization. Bylaws typically specify a minimum notice period for the calling of an executive committee meeting, the number of members that constitute a quorum, and the degree to which the executive committee can act on behalf of the board.

The research administrator may be asked to provide information to the executive committee as part of its deliberations.

- *Investment Committee.* The purpose of the investment committee is to implement the investment policy of the board, to hire the investment manager, and to monitor the performance of the investment manager on a regular basis. A good investment policy will provide guidance on the roles of the investment committee members versus the role of the professional investment manager.

The research administrator typically has minimal interaction with the investment committee. However, there are times when research expenditures such as major construction projects or the acquisition of major equipment can have an impact on the investments of the nonprofit organization, and the research administrator may need to provide details on depreciation schedules, timing of cash expenditures and recovery of costs and other financial information.

Ad Hoc Committees   The use of ad hoc board committees provides the board with a tool to assist management with long-range planning, recruitment of a new CEO, reaching wide-ranging decisions, and other nonroutine tasks. The research administrator should be ready to participate in ad hoc committee work as appropriate and to provide information and perspective.

Advisory Boards

Advisory Boards are characterized as having a role of limited but focused scope, their role is advisory only (they have no management of governance authority or responsibility), and their duration is temporary. Common examples of advisory boards in a nonprofit research environment include:

Scientific Advisory Board

The scientific advisory board usually reports to the CEO on the scientific direction and composition of the organization. Such a board would have representatives with specific subject matter expertise in the scientific field(s) of the organization whose own research programs, experience, and academic credentials enrich the ability of the board. The scientific advisory board should meet with the CEO and the scientific staff at least annually. The board may pose specific areas of inquiry or the scientific staff may make presentations concerning recent scientific advances, publications, discoveries, patents, and program growth, but in either case an interactive dialogue between the scientific staff and the board is essential. The scientific advisory board should prepare a written report of its findings, conclusions, and recommendations.

The research administrator may be called upon to participate in the work of the scientific advisory board by providing information on grant applications, success rates, the viability and utility of shared scientific cores, and other areas of inquiry.

Advisory Board on Philanthropy or Major Fund-Raising Campaigns

Significant campaigns to raise funds for a research institute can be critical to expanding programs. Boards commonly rely on an advisory board to plan, orchestrate, and execute such campaigns.

The research administrator can be a helpful resource or even a member of such a committee or board by providing insight on critical needs for funding, worthy programs that are not fundable by normal or routine funding mechanisms, and ideas for programs that will prospectively have great impact.

Conclusion

The research administrator is a vital source for reliable, consistent, and informative materials that can have a direct impact on the work of boards of trustees and advisory boards. Further, a well-informed research administrator is engaged in the institution's compliance program and is fully informed of current regulations and ethical practices so that he or she can be a vital component of the institution's internal control system and the management of a fully compliant research institution.

• • • References

1. Carver, John. *Boards That Make a Difference: A New Design for Leadership in Nonprofit and*

Public Organizations. San Francisco: Jossey-Bass Inc., 1997, 109.

2. Ibid, *109.*
3. Ibid, 112–114.
4. Tufte, Edward R. *The Visual Display of Quantitative Information.* Cheshire, CT: Graphics Press, 2001, 32.

5. To protect investors by improving the accuracy and reliability of corporate disclosures made pursuant to the securities laws, and for other purposes (Satibannes-Oxley) P.L. 107-204, 2002. H. R. 3763

12

Communication and Marketing

Lynne U. Chronister, MPA

Research units have traditionally focused on communications and public relations. This is a critical function of good research administration practice, as it keeps our internal and external constituents abreast on new developments, newsworthy events, new initiatives, and other important information. Our institution—the faculty and staff and our sponsors, partners, and local and regional communities—have a need to be well-informed about services, priorities, research, and scholarly strengths and resources.

Marketing is a newer concept for research units and has long been considered contrary to academic culture because it is associated with commercialism. This unfortunately is a misconception as marketing serves a greater purpose than to sell a product. It is both an art and a science that enables achievement of a unit's strategic objectives. These objectives vary by the function of the unit and should be identified, understood, and prioritized through market research of client segments. Market research helps identify and understand a client base: who they are, what they want, and their preferred choice in media. This understanding drives marketing priorities; selection of message and media; additions and modifications to services and systems; and selection of evaluation metrics. Some areas that marketing addresses are awareness (of products, services, facilities, research strength) misconceptions (perceived delays and difficulties, lack of customer service); and decision making (sponsorship research or event).

Marketing Plan

A well developed marketing plan is critical in order to establish solid and successful relationships with client groups. Many resources for plan development are available online and in print. Another valuable and often overlooked resource is business schools, where graduate and postgraduate students can often assist in planning and development. Top management involvement and support is also key to development and execution. Marketing plans have several main components: audience, format, and media. Integration across media is important to reach all audiences. Consistency in message and design across media is also important to build identification and brand value with a client group.

Measures of Success

It is important to know the return on your marketing effort. Marketing actions alter client behavior or perception and the selection of measures is determined by the objectives of the plan. It is important to limit measurement to aspects that can be directly or indirectly affected by marketing efforts. The metrics need to be well thought through to ensure that the numbers are reliable, relevant, and reasonably accurate. As your marketing efforts progress, these measures help to compare the effectiveness of various programs (direct mail, online advertisements, etc.) and to plan for future marketing activities.

Client Satisfaction

Of all measures, client satisfaction is the most important. There are many areas along the relationship continuum where satisfaction can be lost: beginning with marketing, the communication they receive, to the courtesy received at initial contact. Quality and speed of service, ability to meet their needs, to postservice support and communication are critical components. Depending on the client group, there are some key, often overlooked, areas that directly affect customer satisfaction.

Good market research provides information that can ultimately improve clients' attitudes and beliefs about the research unit. However, marketing is not a substitute for good business practice and it is critical that the unit be able to deliver to the marketing message. Universities are increasingly using electronic information management systems (e.g., grant processing and award management; IRB proposal submission and tracking, and intellectual property management) to improve processes and client satisfaction. In addition, materials provided to clients by research units are forms of indirect marketing communication and include research manuals, policy manuals, principal investigator handbooks, etc. It is critical that these client materials, which tend to be highly detailed, are well written and designed. Easy-to-navigate reference or FAQ sections help clients better utilize products and information, thereby delivering positive marketing effects.

Often customer satisfaction stems from a lack of knowledge about policy, new system functions, or new information materials. Client education and training, including online and in-person tutorials, as components of marketing, can greatly improve customer satisfaction. Some institutions have mandatory training for faculty and staff who receive external funding. In addition to in-person training, interactive Web technology can provide easy, effective means to train and certify researchers on a 24/7 basis.

It is important to always listen to your client groups and open forums provide clients an opportunity to network, air issues of concern, and resolve issues in a group setting. At the University of California, Davis, the Associate Vice Chancellors for Research Administration and for Business and Finance lead a monthly breakfast meeting in an open forum of 75 participants. Such forums provide an opportunity to meet and better understand the needs of a client group; seek them out and get involved.

If such forums don't exist at your institution, research vice presidents can help to facilitate opportunities for client groups by establishing advisory boards. Such boards can help to guide client group concerns by serving specialized functions; advising on policy and direction; helping to set priorities and goals; disseminating information; and carrying out key fact-finding. Committees and boards can serve as strong advocates for research development and compliance. A principal investigator's council, for example, can offer feedback from productive researchers regarding quality of service, resource allocation, and review of internal grant programs; a council of associate deans for research can provide support for campus priorities and promulgate interdisciplinary research. An external advisory board comprised of alumni, industrial, and governmental leaders can provide invaluable external expertise and perspective on organization and direction for the research enterprise in relation to the world outside the university. These board members can also serve as connections to external partnerships.

Media

Most people are familiar with traditional print (annual reports, brochures, newspapers) and other news media, such as television and radio. However, many clients prefer to receive electronic messaging. There are a number of new media and format options available today for communication and marketing that include:

Electronic Newsletters. These communication modes have become common because of ease of development and dissemination and relative low cost. Most university faculty and staff are accustomed to receiving information electronically. Electronic newsletters can provide information on funding opportunities from membership and subscription services (e.g., "Community of Science" or www.cos.com). Electronic newsletters also provide general news: announcements on national and institutional policy and procedure changes; funding opportunities; and grants and contracts awards. Weekly news bulletins sent to central research administration staff and directors are a simple, effective way to communicate regularly, especially within a large research organization.

List Serves. For principal investigators and department administrators this can be a valuable vehicle for sending information internally. Use of the list serve should be conservative and should require active subscription, rather than establishing a list serve and spamming information to entire populations.

Web Sites. These often have information on policies, procedures, funding opportunities, contact information and organization charts, training opportunities, as well as updates on ongoing research and scholarship. Web sites can also serve as great marketing tools to communicate marketing messages to a target audience.

Trade Shows/Conferences. Trade fairs (for example, the Bio 2004 and the Advocacy Day on the Hill sponsored by the Coalition for National Science Funding) are examples of excellent opportunities to showcase both outstanding research supported by the National Science Foundation (NSF) and emerging biotechnology. Development cost, assembly, travel, and fees can be high and discretion should be used in determining the cost benefit of participation.

Promotional Items. These items have great internal and external marketing value. Traditionally these are given to prospective and current clients to improve and maintain brand awareness. Examples include pens, mouse pads, calendars, memory sticks, external boards, or other special, more expensive, customized items.

Staff Development Courses. At many institutions, human resource offices offer classes in research administration and regulatory compliance.

Recognition. Name badges worn by research staff for on- and off-campus events are simple but effective marketing and serve to let the campus community know that leadership does value involvement in campus activities. Campus pins designed for special purposed committees such as an institutional review board (IRB) or other campus groups signify pride in the work of the committee or area of study and the contribution of these individuals to the body of knowledge in research and scholarship.

Print Materials. One-page descriptions of resources and research programs can be included in information packets to distribute to campus visitors or sent in response to requests for information.

Summary

Communication and marketing can be achieved by many methods and use a range of tools. The key to success is a communication and marketing plan that includes outcomes and sets a level of expectation among research staff. For example, because of the nature of a research compliance program such as the IRB or a sponsored programs office, it is easy for the staff and leadership to assume a gatekeeper role. Setting expectations and providing training in communication for research personnel should be built into the overall communications and marketing plan. The results will be research units that are technically competent, but also serve the needs of their clients and the institution.

• • • Suggested Reading

Lindsay, A. W., and R. T. Neumann. *The Challenge for Research in Higher Education.* Hoboken, NJ: ASHE_ERIC Higher Education Reports, 1988.

Ouellette, L. P. *I/S At Your Service: Knowing and Keeping Your Clients.* Dubuque, IA: Kendall/Hunt Publishing Company, 1993.

Overton, G. W., and J. Carmedelle Frey. *Guidebook for Directors of Nonprofit Corporations, Section of Business Law.* Chicago, IL: American Bar Association, 2002.

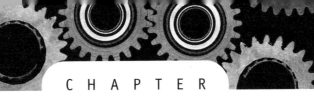

13

Policies and Management of Human Tissue in Research

Lynne U. Chronister, MPA, and David R. McGee, PhD

The use of human tissue and body parts is a critical, emotionally-charged issue in basic and clinical medical and health research and instruction and training. There is little information about how to develop and manage programs which involve use of human tissue nor are there clear regulations or policies on the role of internal review boards in approving use of human tissue in research and instruction. Generally, hospitals and medical schools have policies that govern use of cadavers in medical instruction; those institutions have internal review boards (IRB), which have authority over the establishment of program policies that involve collection and research use of human tissue. What is often lacking at many institutions, however, is a comprehensive policy that covers use of human tissues and human bodies in research for all campus units—a policy that needs to be closely aligned with existing policies and procedures for handling use of human tissue and human bodies and body parts.

Considerations for such area-wide policy development and management include defining what constitutes tissue and body parts and determining whether a single policy can cover all usages or multiple policies are needed. There does not seem to be a universal definition. In the United Kingdom, the House of Parliament is seeking to establish a human tissue authority and defines human tissue broadly to include human bodies, body parts, organs, and tissues. Similarly, the Ministry of Health in New Zealand proposes to define human tissue broadly to include organs, body parts, and bodies. If differentiated, human body parts and organs might be described as discernable or recognizable tissue

mass. Tissue would include any human cell recognizable microscopically and human fluids.

In addition to distinguishing between human tissue, body parts, and organs, an institution may decide to differentiate in the policy and management between: a) banked tissue and b) tissue used discretely for a single project and then disposed. Banked tissue requires maintenance of inventory and tracking that is more rigid than for discrete use. Regardless of the definition, use of tissue has some special considerations: a) there is the potential for transmission of pathogens to anyone who may come in direct contact with that tissue or through contamination left by the tissue; b) documented permission must be obtained from the patient source or someone having proper authorization to make dispensation of that human tissue; and c) appropriate maintenance of confidentiality under the Health Insurance Portability and Accountability Act (HIPAA) is required. Additionally, the very possession and use of human tissues has initiated a number of very complex ongoing ethical issues. Adequate security procedures need to be in place and policy made regarding use of human tissue at the university and public access to records.

Management of the Use of Human Tissue in Research

Institutions must develop and promulgate policies regarding acquisition, handling, storage, and disposal of human tissue, as there is potential for human pathogen carryover and transmission and public concern about the issue of human tissue use itself in general. Therefore, it is critical that policies be in place prior to initiating an inventory. Policies may already exist that can be applied to human tissue handling. A biological safety committee or equivalent should make existing and new policies. Depending on the situation, the university IRB may also have oversight. Some of the issues that must be considered include: inventory, safety, confidentiality of records, record-keeping, acquisition, usage, storage, shipment or sale, disposal, and security. Policy on management of tissue should include a requirement for training, roles and responsibilities, including those of faculty and committees (e.g., the IRB), and the consequences of improper management of tissue. It should be understood that the checklist serves only as a general guideline. It is expected that every institution has unique situations and policies that require additional modifications or practices.

Safety

Safety of personnel is paramount. Some major categories relating to safety include the training of researchers, technicians, and inventory and shipping, and receiving personnel. Some of the safety considerations include: pathogenic and radioactive tissue handling, use of solvents and aerosols, skin protection and wound management, and emergency response cleanup.

Human Tissue Inventory

Inventories are not merely an accounting of material at one point in time. Done properly, an inventory program can provide valuable information regarding research directions, sharing of tissue assets, economical efficiencies, and lab safety. It is an ongoing, dynamic process. Each laboratory will have intralab record keeping of tissues obtained and the dispensation of each tissue as well as any subsamples created in the lab. This can be accomplished through a number of means depending on the size of sample population in any lab. Laboratories that have only a few samples will be able to keep simple, manual accounting ledgers. For those labs in which the sample size becomes very large, bar coding of sample containers can be easily done in order to keep precise track of a sample. An inventory of body parts used across the institution for research is critical, as is knowledge and oversight of all human tissue

banks. Inventory of human tissues must occur in order to:

- Promote safety for all personnel,
- Ensure compliance with government regulations,
- Provide a means of monitoring experiments involving human tissue, and
- Ensure the ethical use of human tissue.

Confidentiality

Strict policies and practices, with concurrent legal counsel review to comply with maintenance of confidentiality are critical. Examples of confidentiality issues include, but are not limited to: compliance with HIPAA, public disclosure under the Freedom of Information Act (FOIA), preventing access of nonauthorized personnel to records, database maintenance and security.

Acquisition and Shipping of Human Tissue

Issues and practices regarding the acquisition and shipping of human tissue include due diligence prior to contracting, source of tissue, release from donor, tissue type, pathogen testing of tissue prior to shipping to the university, radio-labeled tissue, and receipt of tissue. Careful documentation of the shipping information is critically important. Both parties must have authorization to ship or to receive the tissues. Prior to shipment, paperwork must be accurate relating to tissue preparation, pathogen screening, verification of appropriate licensure, trained shipping and receiving staff, monitoring equipment, inventory procedures, and confirmation of available storage facilities.

Disposal

Improper disposal of human tissue can have serious legal repercussions and very negative public reaction. Generally, proper disposal can be readily achieved through knowledge of regulations, acquisition of appropriate disposal equipment, validation of equipment, and contracting with appropriate waste disposal companies

Security

Personnel must understand the security measures that need to be maintained. Proper inventory control is essential. Unless accurate records are kept, it is not possible to accurately account of potential security breaches.

Summary

With the advent of areas such as adult and embryonic stem cell research and the ability to genetically characterize tissue, the use of human tissue in research is critical. Ethics, legal safety, and security dictate that tissue, as well as anatomical specimens, be acquired and handled respectfully and carefully and that its use and storage be well tracked and documented.

13-A

Use of Human Tissue in Research

In a general sense, the procedures for handling human tissues are similar to those used when handling radioactive materials and when handling controlled drug substances in the lab. First, all personnel involved in the use of or in shipping/receiving human tissue must have proper safety and record-keeping training. Knowledge of regulations and compliance with those regulations are essential. An inventory of all radioactive material is maintained for each individually ordered radioactive material starting with the actual purchase order, then receipt, usage (including all subsamples and storage), and disposal. Possession limits by type of isotope, specific activity, experimental protocol, etc., are approved in advance of starting an experiment by a campus radiation safety officer, who, in turn, has been approved by the state radiological health branch. Specific procedures for clean-up, monitoring, storage, and waste disposal are mandated by the state of California. Similarly, the use of controlled drug substances in the lab is through federal DEA permits. Strict inventory, restricted, secured storage, and usage history are required. For human tissues, a biological safety committee should have general oversight and similar procedures for handling and accounting of material should be established.

Inventories are not merely an accounting of material at one point in time. Done properly, an inventory program can provide the university with much more valuable information regarding research directions, sharing of tissue assets, economical efficiencies, and lab safety.

Human Tissue Samples Have Unique Problems

Human tissue samples have special considerations: (1) there is the potential for transmission of pathogens to anyone who may come in direct contact with that tissue or through contamination left by the tissue; (2) documented permission must be obtained from the patient source or someone having proper authorization to make dispensation of that human tissue; and (3) appropriate maintenance of confidentiality under HIPAA is required. Additionally, the possession and use of human tissues has initiated a number of very complex ongoing ethical issues. Adequate security procedures need to be in place and policy made regarding use of human tissue at the university and public access to records.

Establishment of Policies and Practices for Human Tissue Handling

It is essential that the university develops and promulgates policy regarding acquisition, handling, storage, and disposal of human tissue. Because of the potential for human pathogen carryover and transmission and given the public interest, such policies must be in place prior to initiating an inventory. Policies that can be applied to human tissue handling may already exist. A biological safety committee or equivalent should make existing and new policies. Depending on the situation, the university IRB may also have oversight.

Procedures and policies for the following need to be in place:

- **Training programs**—All parties (lab personnel, inventory personnel, and committees) must receive training to ensure compliance with regulations and university policies.
- **Faculty responsibilities**—Faculty must be clearly informed regarding the proper procedures for obtaining and disposal of human tissue samples.
- **Institutional review board (IRB)**—The IRB may have mandated oversight for some human tissue programs. The biological safety committee will work closely with the IRB to ensure appropriate participation of both committees is maintained.
- **Biological safety committee (BSC)**—This committee provides oversight of use of human tissue at the university to ensure compliance with policies and regulations.
  - Formal charter of operations, responsibilities, authority
    - Composition:
      - Scientists
      - Physician(s)
      - Administrative
- **Inventory control staff**—This will be composed of university employees who have received specific training in the inventory of human tissue samples.
- **Safety, usage, shipping/receiving, inventories**—See comments in safety section for more specifics in these areas.
- **Reporting of safety hazards, safety violations, and emergency situations**—The university needs to inform all employees how to report various problems and potential violations.
- **Investigation of lost samples**—All human tissue samples must be accounted for. Lost samples have to be investigated. The university will need to have a policy that describes the conduct of such investigations.

Safety

Safety of personnel is paramount. Some major categories relating to safety are provided herein. These must be in place prior to initiating an inventory.

- **Safety/administrative training of personnel handling tissue samples**—The campus health/safety physicist should be able to design the safety training.
  - Scientists

- Inventory personnel
- Shipping/receiving personnel
- Biological safety committee members
- **Tissue sample handling**
- **Pathogens**—Human tissues received have the potential to have unknown human pathogens. Some experiments will require diseased human tissue.
- **Solvents**—Some human tissue will be in solvents that have their own health/safety hazards including but not limited to carcinogens, teratogens, mutagens, inhalation toxicity, transdermal toxicity, flammable hazards, etc.
- **Radioactively labeled samples**—Human tissue samples may commonly contain radioactive material in which case special, additional safety, usage, personnel monitoring, and disposal precautions must be observed. Inventory personnel may be required to wear radiation safety badges and/or monitoring rings or use other monitoring devices (e.g., GM counters to determine if sample containers are contaminated).
- **Aerosols**—Aerosols can be created whenever there is water present. Human tissue frequently is hydrated and there is a potential for accidental aerosol exposure. This is particularly true when tissue samples are received and divided into multiple samples. Protective clothing and the use of a validated biological safety cabinet are required.
- **Puncture wound hazards (e.g., from bones, scalpels, etc.)**—Human tissue samples may contain sharp objects that can penetrate containers, bags, etc. In addition, scalpel and needle wounds are possible.
- **Protection of skin**—Gloves selected for solvent resistance and allergenicity should be worn by anyone handing any human tissue or a human tissue-containing vial, jar, bag, etc. Those persons handling human tissues, including inventory personnel, should wear protective clothing. Other protective gear may be required. The policy should contain instructions regarding disposal of protective gear.
- **Prevention of inhalation**—Powdered and aerosol preparations should be done in a biological safety cabinet. Inventory personnel should avoid open containers.
- **Appropriate hand washing stations**—Inventory personnel should ensure that prior to starting an inventory and at the conclusion of an inventory, hands are thoroughly washed.
- **Access to eye wash, emergency shower**—Inventory personnel should know where there are emergency eye and shower wash facilities.

- **Access to biological safety cabinet, fume hood**—As described elsewhere, lab personnel should have available appropriate safety cabinets and fume hoods. All equipment should receive annual service and certification that the equipment meets operating specifications.
- **Disinfectants**—selection of appropriate type and use before and after handling. The surface used for observation of samples and recording of inventory data should be disinfected before and after the inventory. The selection of disinfectant should be appropriate to the tissue and equipment.
- **Emergency response cleanup**—The university no doubt has policies, procedures, and contracts already in place for emergency response. This should be verified and personnel conducting an inventory as well as lab personnel should received written or posted information detailing what to do in the event of an emergency.
  - University emergency response team
  - Outside professional emergency response firm

Confidentiality of Records

The university will need to establish strict policies and practices—with concurrent legal counsel review—to comply with maintenance of confidentiality. Examples of confidentiality issues include but are not limited to:

- Compliance with HIPAA
- Public disclosure of information under FOIA
- Preventing access of nonauthorized personnel to records
- Database maintenance/security

Record-keeping

- **Training**—OSHA and local safety compliance agencies require that periodic, documented safety training be conducted. Usually training must be taken and a copy of the course syllabus kept on file.
- **Material transfer agreements (MTAs)**—MTAs contain many contractual terms that relate to usage, reports, confidentiality, ownership of IP, etc. During an inventory, it is important to be able to distinguish between samples owned by the university from those owned by another entity. A separate inventory may need to be maintained for those human sample materials that are owned by another party.

- **HIPAA considerations**—The HIPAA requirements for confidentiality may be very complex depending on where and under what conditions the university obtains human tissue samples. Records, databases, etc. must take into account HIPAA.
- **Hazardous waste Manifests**—Disposal of human tissue will frequently require hazardous waste manifests or other disposal documentation. These records must be maintained in a separate, cross-referenced file that is ready for inspection by government agencies without notice.
- **Inventory records**—Inventory records created by the inventory control personnel will have to be cross-referenced and indexed for tracking all samples. Raw inventory records must be maintained even after transfer to electronic or other record forms.
  - Establish university-wide inventory form.
  - Establish laboratory log form.
  - Establish/modify university MTA form for intra-campus transfer of material.
  - Establish exception report forms (e.g., lost material, inventory gain/losses).
  - Establish university database with limited access/read access only.
  - Establish record room for file maintenance.
  - Training record file.
- **Usage history records**—The use of each human tissue sample must be tracked and records of usage maintained. The use of sample identification numbers and bar coding may be appropriate.
- **Disposal records**—Final disposal (including cross-reference to hazardous waste manifests) must track each sample number and be reflected on current inventory.
- **Conformance to labeling standards**—Uniform, official university labels should be used for all human tissue. There are some specific regulatory agency requirements for labeling to be considered. Labels should not contain information that could violate HIPAA regulations
  - Conformity to NIH and OSHA, and in California, UC standards and CAL-OSHA.

Acquisition of Source of Human Tissue

- **Due diligence prior to contracting**—It is critically important to thoroughly investigate the entity or person providing the human tissue prior to placing an order or receipt of any human tissue.

- Reliability of source's data—The investigator should ensure the data regarding the tissue type, condition of tissue, special preparation of tissue, etc. has been thoroughly confirmed.
- Physical and on-site audit of source's policies and practices—It is appropriate to conduct an on-site inspection of the tissue provider's physical facilities and to review its record keeping and procedures for handling, storage, and processing of human tissues to ensure regulatory compliance and appropriate preparation of the tissue has been made.
- Appropriate, signed patient release form—Many tissue banks, hospitals, etc. have not obtained an appropriate patient release form for tissue. Some forms frequently contain important limitations for use (e.g., research only, no commercial applications), ownership and intellectual property rights. The university should receive copies of the patient release form (that has been redacted to protect patient confidentiality) or a signed form from the tissue provider that clearly provides all limitations of the patient release form used for that sample (some providers use more than one release form type).
- Approval by biological safety committee/IRB—See comments elsewhere in this appendix.
- **Source of tissue**—Every source of tissue will have different issues regarding its own policies and practices. A thorough review of these is mandatory before accepting any tissue.
  - Tissue banks
  - Blood banks
  - Research institutes and universities
  - Hospitals, clinics
  - Volunteers—Great care needs to be taken to ensure that all HIPAA information is kept confidential and that there has been complete release of the tissue to the university.
  - University personnel—In addition to that above for volunteers, it is extremely important that employees have not been pressured to provide any tissue.
- **Contract negotiations**—Inventory staff need to be advised of any outstanding contractual issues for any human tissue samples. For example, if the tissue belongs to the provider (e.g., a corporation), then the inventory of that nonuniversity owned tissue may have to be kept on a separate inventory since such tissue may be returned in the future to the provider. Also, it is possible that the identification of certain tissues may be protected under confidentiality agreements.

- Compliance with contracts regarding IP rights, return of tissues, ownership and confidentiality.
- Appropriate licenses for both parties; acquisition of appropriate patient releases
- **Release from donor**—The IRB will need to provide a university patient release form for tissues received directly from a patient. Tissues received indirectly from a patient must be accompanied with adequate documentation that establishes authority to ship and use such tissue.
- **Tissue type**—Tissue can come as a solid or liquid. Frequently, whole organs or large liquid volumes will be divided into multiple aliquots. Prior to receipt of samples, appropriate equipment and training must be done.
  - Solid, liquid, combination
- **Diseased tissue**—It is common to require diseased human tissue for experiments. All samples must be clearly labeled. Direct handling by inventory personnel should be avoided.
  - Verification of pathogen(s)—The investigator should verify that the tissue does contain the pathogen and that there is proper labeling, storage and safety precautions regarding the diseased tissue to avoid exposure to all staff.
- **Pathogen testing of tissue prior to shipping to university**—It is a common practice to require that the tissue provider test the tissue for the presence of certain identified pathogens not intended to be in the sample. Documentation should be provided with each shipment that the tests were performed and the actual data from those tests (e.g., testing for hepatitis B and C, HIV, others)
- **Radiolabeled tissue**—Some human tissue will contain radioactive isotopes. This will represent additional considerations for receipt of material, usage, storage, and disposal. Tissue containing S35 or P32 may be able to be stored until radioactive decay has occurred such that it is below the specific activity if allowed under the terms negotiated by the university in its radioactive materials license. Other isotopes such as I125 may require periodic urine samples and special biomonitoring of users of this material. It will be up to the BSC and the RSO whether inventory personnel will have to have special monitoring for certain isotopes. Tissue samples that are both radioactive and contain organic solvents may be classified as mixed waste and proper disposal will depend on the amount and type of isotope and the amount and type of solvent. Inventory personnel will need to be trained in working with radioactive material and have appropriate, certified monitoring equipment available during inventory.

- Appropriate radioactive materials licenses for shipping and receiving parties; receipt of a copy of the shipping party's license prior to shipping—maintain on file.
- Adherence to university procedures for monitoring for radioisotopes in packaging, training of personnel for safe handling, transport, inventory, storage, use and disposal of radioactive material.
- Availability of certified equipment for monitoring and verification of specific activity and isotope (e.g., GM counters, LS counters).
- Appropriate storage facilities and labeling of radioactive materials.
- **Receipt of tissue**—The receipt of tissue samples is an important event in that it involves a large number of considerations and activities associated with its arrival. This is the point at which there is the greatest opportunity for error in record keeping and exposure of personnel (shipping/receiving and scientists) to hazardous conditions. Below are listed some examples to consider:
  - Verification of shipping documentation (e.g., sent to intended recipient, receipt of complete shipment).
  - Accompanying patient release form or verification form of compliance.
  - Verification of pathogen-free samples (if required).
  - Visual inspection of all packaging; monitoring of packages and containers.
  - Safety clothing.
  - Safety equipment.
  - Generation of aerosols.
  - Creation of aliquots of samples (if required).
  - Proper use of preservatives for samples.
  - Bag selection (if appropriate) to prevent sample deterioration and leakage.
  - Labels that conform to OSHA requirements for content.
  - Label types that are appropriate to storage conditions (for example, selection of label adhesive for use at -80°C; label ink that has the proper solubility and stability for storage and use conditions).
  - Initial inventory of samples.

Usage of Tissues

- **Approval by biological safety committee/ IRB**—Generally, the acquisition of human tis-

sue samples may be expected to be under the authority of some reviewing body at the university. The establishment of a biological safety committee (if one does not already exist) comprised of scientists, a physician, and administrators concerned with human tissue samples is appropriate. Depending on the specifics of the request and source of tissue, the university IRB may also have to be consulted.

- **Documentation of use by scientist user**—Perhaps the biggest potential problem associated with inventory is going to be determined by how well the principal investigator (PI) keeps track of the use of human tissue between inventories. If the PI does not engage in diligent record keeping, then there will be irreconcilable inventory gains and losses.
- **Effect on inventory**—An inventory is only as accurate as the data. Persons other than the inventory personnel will record most of the data between inventories. **Repeated training and accountability of all concerned personnel is absolutely essential to having an accurate inventory.**

Storage of Human Tissues

Storage conditions will normally be dictated according to the tissue type and the demands of the experiments. However, because of the numerous public relations issues that surround the use of human tissue, additional storage conditions may need to be imposed in order that the tissue be physically secure from outside, unauthorized access. Inventory records will need to accurately reflect locations of all material. Movement of samples between inventories will need to be entered on the laboratory inventory log.

- **Selection of storage conditions**—Generally, tissue will be stored at room temperature, 4°C, –60°C, or –80°C. It may have to be physically isolated from all other tissues if contamination issues are of concern. It may also have to be secured by locks and other security measures depending on the situation.
- **Selection of storage equipment**—Storage equipment ranges from refrigeration equipment (freezers, refrigerators, walk-in rooms, closets, file cabinets, safes, fenced off areas holding storage barrels, etc.)
- **Data/chart recorders**—Data recorders and other monitoring devices are important and inexpensive ways to verify storage conditions,

not only for experimental purposes but for ensuring that deterioration of the sample does not occur so that inventory and disposal can be made more easily.

- **Over/under temperature and flood alarms**—Human tissue will generally be stored either in environmentally controlled conditions as described above or in other places (e.g., open rooms). It is advisable that each device or area be equipped with a temperature and/or water sensors that have audible alarms and that are monitored by an alarm company 24 hours per day so that notification of responsible personnel can be made if the storage conditions are not maintained.
- **Selection of storage rooms**—Storage room selection will vary widely according to the individual situation.

Shipment of Tissues to and from the University

The university will, on occasion, receive or ship human tissue samples. Careful documentation of the shipping information is critically important to ensure that the shipper and the addressee are correct and that each has the proper qualifications to ship or receive the tissues. Prior to shipment, it is important to make sure that paperwork relating to tissue preparation, pathogen screening, appropriate, verified licenses, trained shipping/receiving staff, monitoring equipment (if required), inventory procedures, and storage facilities are available. In addition, attention must be paid to legal authorization to ship certain samples (for example, is the tissue owned by a third party?). Examples of common issues for shipping are:

- **Identification of named receiving party**—Verification that receiving party is authorized to receive/handle/dispose of tissues.
- **Returning shipment to sender**—Need to know the procedures for returning a tissue sample to the shipping entity.
- **Intra-campus shipment**—Need to establish appropriate procedures and record keeping forms to allow shipment from one lab to another.
- **Inter-campus shipment**—Need to establish appropriate procedures and record keeping forms to allow shipment from one campus to another.
- **Record keeping**—Maintain complete records regarding each sample's history.

Disposal

Improper disposal of human tissue can have serious legal repercussions and very negative public reaction. Generally, proper disposal can be readily achieved through the following means:

- **Knowledge of local, state, and federal regulations**—This sounds simple, but the regulations do change at all levels. Compliance with one does not necessarily mean complete compliance with other government agencies. Contracting with regulatory consulting firms can be money well spent.
- **Acquisition of appropriate disposal equipment**—Different tissues and different forms of samples require different disposal methods. Equipment, therefore, varies. Examples include autoclaves, fume hoods, biological safety cabinets, waste storage cabinets, barrels with liners, GM counters, LS counters, air monitoring sensors, etc.
- **Validation of equipment**—Equipment must be maintained in operating order that conforms to design specifications and regulatory specifications. When outside contract validation is required, records must be maintained.
- **Contracting with appropriate waste disposal companies**—It is extremely important to only contract with waste disposal companies whose credentials and operating histories have been thoroughly verified. Such due diligence by the university is essential.

Conducting an Inventory

An inventory program is never a finished task. Because of the dynamic nature of research, the amount of tissues present at the university is continuously changing. Periodic inventories must be made but are immediately out of date. Due to the potentially large number of tissues to be inventoried, an inventory of the entire university may literally be a continuous process.

The inventory team is only one part of those involved in keeping track of material. Each laboratory will have to learn—and reliably practice—intra-lab record keeping of tissues obtained and the dispensation of each tissue as well as any subsamples created in the lab. This can be accomplished through a number of means depending on the size of sample population in any lab. Laboratories that have only a few samples will be able to keep simple, manual accounting ledgers. For those labs in which the sample size becomes very large, bar coding of sample containers can be easily done in order to keep precise track of a sample. This is routinely done in genomic laboratories where many thousands of samples containing gene sequence variants have to be tracked. Given the emphasis at UC Davis in genomics research, the university likely has in place suitable laboratory management software that can be applied to human tissue sample tracking.

It should be expected that the inventory itself would provide information that may lead to new policies. In addition, inventories commonly result in the discovery of unexpected samples that must be included as inventory gains and samples that, for various reasons, need to be disposed of (inventory losses). Samples that are unable to be located will also be an inventory loss but investigations of lost samples will have to be conducted.

Inventory Control

Inventories are almost always conducted for two reasons: (1) as a means of ensuring cost-effective use of raw materials and (2) to ensure that adequate product can be delivered to a customer. Neither of those reasons applies to the human tissue inventory program. Instead, some of the primary reasons for the inventory of human tissue are: (1) to promote safety for all personnel, (2) to ensure compliance with government regulations, and (3) to provide a means of monitoring experiments involving human tissue for ethical reasons.

- **Classification of tissues by usage**—Normally inventory can be grouped according by using a system based on identified characteristics. In the case of human tissue, it may be possible to do so, but only after the initial inventory has been completed.
- **Variation in degree of control of tissues**—Some tissue will require extremely strict control (for example, pathogen containing tissue or radioactively labeled tissue). Other tissue will require lower levels of control (for example, freeze-dried, pathogen-free tissue).
- **Types of inventory records**—Refer to "Record Keeping." In typical industry inventories, there are three types of inventory records, which are listed below. For human tissue inventories, all records will necessarily fall into either of the first two categories. The third does not apply.
  - Very accurate; complete—Records that conform to strict standards for completeness and accuracy must be kept. This type of record is required for that tissue requiring the strictest control. Anything less and the inventory is a

waste of time. Pathogen and radioactive tissues would be examples of tissues requiring this type of record.
  - Normal, good records—Records for those tissues not requiring the strictest control.
  - No records or very simple records—Does not apply to human tissue inventories.
- **Ordering of tissue**—See other comments throughout this appendix regarding ordering parameters.
- **Only ordering the minimum needed (if possible)**—Just as ALARA (as soon as reasonably available) has been used for inventory control and usage of radioactive materials for decades, the same concept applies to human tissues. Sometimes, however, the amount available cannot be preselected and one must take what is available. Accurate inventories may be able to provide available, on-campus tissue sources to faculty that might otherwise have ordered that tissue.
- **Quantity discounts/IP sharing**—When ordering repeated, multiple tissues from a single source, frequently a contract will specify minimum ordering and discount rates. In addition, since human tissues are being used for research, intellectual property ownership, and royalties may play a major role in the future applications of a tissue sample. Inventory personnel must be made aware of special conditions for tissues under contract.
- **Segregation and identification of inventory owned by another entity**—As stated earlier, it may be necessary to segregate tissues because of contractual provisions or to ensure safety (e.g., radioactive or pathogens).
- **Determination of shelf life/when to dispose of tissue inventory**—During the first inventory, the PIs will need to estimate shelf life of samples. This can be monitored by inventory personnel to assist PIs with timely disposal of tissues that have an expired shelf life.
- **Frequency of inventories**—Campus-wide inventories should be conducted once a year.
- **Notification of departments of upcoming inventories**—Advance notice to all affected faculty should be made as early as possible with dates of inventory, names of inventory personnel (if known) or a contact person, the length of time at their lab, the reason for the inventory, and what is needed from the PI.

Security

It is very important that from the start university personnel understand the security measures that need to be maintained. An important, fundamental component of security is proper inventory control. Unless accurate records are kept, it will not be possible to accurately know when and to what degree security breaches may have occurred. The list below contains typical security measures that can be implemented very easily.

- **Storage alarms**—Monitored temperature and flood alarms as described earlier.
- **Burglar alarms**—Monitored door and window alarms.
- **Locks**—All types ranging from padlocks to cipher locks.
- **Limited access**—Only authorize personnel who really need to work with tissues.
- **Selected personnel for public disclosures**—Only allow those personnel who are trained, experienced, and knowledgeable about human tissues to speak for the university.
- **Confidentiality of records**—Do not allow records and other media to contain confidential patient information or unnecessary and extraneous information.
- **Database maintenance/drive access**—Have the information systems department develop and implement limited, tiered access (for example,

access to those who can enter data into the human tissue databases, those who have read-only access, and those who have no access at all).

- **Emergency procedures**—Emergency procedures need to be in place prior to inventory because an emergency can occur at any time, including during an inventory.
  - Automatic notification of named response personnel—Each lab should have posted the names and phone numbers of personnel to be notified in the event of an emergency. This is common in labs and is probably already in place.
  - Notification of emergency response teams—Emergency response teams may be composed of trained lab personnel, campus emergency response teams, and contracted emergency teams. Phone numbers for all teams should be posted near an exit door for each lab.
  - Maintenance of files at those sites—It can be of enormous benefit during an emergency for the responding team to have up-to-date documentation of the potential hazards and their locations. Most fire departments, for example, appreciate periodic tours of facilities by lab supervisors and frequently ask for files containing floor plans that can be kept at the fire station with locations of hazardous materials.

14

Performance Measurement

Paul G. Waugaman, MPA, MA, William S. Kirby, MA, and Louis G. Tornatzky, PhD

Introduction

Historically, research-performing organizations in the public, nonprofit sector (educational institutions and independent research organizations) have had little incentive to measure performance or competitiveness. Internal improvements could be easily measured by the level of sponsored research revenue, and there was little interest in comparative analysis.

This has changed as a number of environmental factors have shifted. First, the rate of growth of federal research support slowed down, which seemed to researchers and research organizations like a cut in support, because funds available for new, competitive awards dropped and stayed low. Second, organizations performing medical research (almost half of the federal funding for research) faced sharp drops in funding from institutional funds and other resources including funding from health services revenues, which dwindled as insurance companies set forth major cost-restructuring and as a result of Medicare and Medicaid reforms. Third, because the value of endowments and the income from endowments dropped as stock values dropped, institutions became even more strapped for revenues to indirectly support research. Finally, the federal cap on reimbursement of administrative costs as part of an institution's facilities and administrative costs began to bind as institutions' internal costs continued to rise. This final factor has had a direct impact on research administration, forcing institutions to plan and implement major control measures to make research administration more efficient and cost effective.

There is a growing concern among institutional leaders to demonstrate to institutional stakeholders (both external and internal) that:

1. The resources dedicated to research are being used wisely and that the institution's performance justifies continued investment in research, and
2. The institution is wisely managing the precious resources supporting research (Holmes et al., 2000).

It is, therefore, important that any research management activity include a component of performance evaluation. These evaluations can work at two levels:

- The competitiveness and health of the institution's research enterprise;
- The effectiveness and efficiency of the institution's research management activity.

At both of these levels, benchmarking is at the heart of performance evaluation. Benchmarking can work well as the vehicle for performance measurement and evaluation and when deciding what practices and activities can be changed in order to improve performance. Benchmarking studies can be carried out at two levels. Internal benchmarking can be used to compare like activities and different departments or units of a single organization.

External benchmarking can compare like activities at separate institutions in order to objectively identify the "best practitioners," or to benchmark an institution's performance in comparison with other institutions that are considered the best "peer" institutions or "role-model" institutions.

This chapter discusses the technique of benchmarking and suggests examples of internal and external benchmarking to be used for performance and practice.

Benchmarking in Research Organizations

Benchmarking has evolved over the past 20 years into a powerful tool for performance analysis and total quality management. Its concept is simple: if you want to know how well your organization is doing at some task or function, you need to know how well others are doing at the same task or function. Benchmarking has been defined as follows: "Benchmarking is the systematic comparison of elements of the performance of an organization against that of other organizations, with the aim of mutual improvement" (McNair and Leibfried, 1992).

In his book, *Thriving on Chaos*, Tom Peters writes, "…the term 'what gets measured gets done' has never been so powerful a truth"(Peters, 1987).[3] Benchmarking has been embraced by many companies and industries. Companies have seen the value of benchmarking in assessing their competitive positions and adopting "best practices," which improve outcomes and bottom lines. Benchmarking (Spendolini, 1992) has developed into an important tool in the for-profit environment for managing and improving quality and productivity. Benchmarking and related methodologies have become accepted practice in program evaluation as well as in the not-for-profit sectors (Fetterman et al., 1996).

By contrast, the educational sector has been slow to adopt the metaphors and methods of benchmarking, especially in the management and administration of research and other externally-sponsored activities. Morris and Hess (1989), Lowry and Walker (1992), and Hansen (1989) have discussed the need to evaluate and measure the effectiveness of research administration activities. What are the organization's results in comparison to what it intended to achieve? Have its improvement interventions resulted in any improvement? How is it doing in comparison to similar activities at other institutions? These are basic questions of organizational effectiveness. However, most managers and employees in research administration have remarkably little information about the effectiveness of their services or operations. Most information they do have is primarily about activities (e.g., proposals prepared) or accounting for resources (e.g., staffing levels), with few details about performance. In an informal survey, Lowry and Walker estimated that only slightly more than half of research support offices have engaged in any form of evaluation. We doubt that this situation has changed significantly in the past ten years as budgets have tightened and research administrators increasingly perceive that they are overworked.

The reasons for the lack of attention to measurement and evaluation are varied and complex. Nevertheless, it appears that sponsored research managers are increasingly being asked to document performance by higher management and to make compelling business cases for new resources where they are overworked and understaffed. Therefore, there is a general need for more knowledge and skills on how to do so.

Developing performance measures addresses an important question of strategic management: How do we know we're on track? An organization may have a picture of what it wants to achieve, and how it plans to get there, it then needs a way to gauge its effectiveness. Managers use a variety of information and data in gauging how an organization is doing. Most, however, rely heavily on informal qualitative data to stay in touch with how things are going operationally with customers and with "competitors."[1] This type of information is indispensable, but in order to have an objective basis for answering these questions, managers also need systematic qualitative and quantitative indicators that are both valid and reliable. Getting such data is at the heart of using benchmarking for quality assessment. Doing this involves a cyclical discipline that includes:

1. Identifying an important domain of organizational activity;

---

[1]It is important for research administrators to know who their customers and competitors are. The paramount class of customers are the institution's research performers, the people who generate the resources and the institution's reputation. A "customer" relationship with research sponsors is incidental. Just as researchers who submit applications and research proposals are in competition with other researchers, institutions are in competition for research dollars, the best reputation, and ultimately, the best researchers.

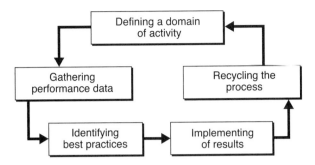

FIGURE 14-1 The Benchmarking Process

2. Gathering performance data therein (preferably quantified)
3. Identifying "best practices" used in exemplary peer organizations to enhance performance in that activity;
4. Adopting or adapting those practices in one's own organization;
5. Recycling the whole process.

Figure 14-1 depicts the process graphically, and one can describe each of those steps in more detail.

Defining a Domain of Organizational Activity

Benchmarking is, at its foundation, a set of applied social science research methods and procedures. The first step derives from core organizational goals and objectives. That is, it derives from identifying which areas or *domains* of organizational activity are inseparable from the core organizational mission. For a research university, this typically involves aspects of research and education; for a manufacturing firm it might involve aspects of the production process. It is important when initiating the benchmarking process to identify a *domain* of activities, rather than single, discrete behaviors. From a benchmarking perspective, a domain subsumes a cluster of interrelated individual and organizational behaviors. However, the domain is typically understandable to organizational participants because of its label and descriptors.

For example, the activity generally known as *sponsored programs administration* was the selected domain for a multiyear benchmarking effort (Kirby and Waugaman, 2000, 2001, 2002, 2003). Although this domain would appear to be synonymous with research administration in universities and research institutions, several important research administration functions were excluded from the domain: technology management, research compliance (human subjects, use of animals, etc.), and managing conflicts in interest, to name a few. Within the defined domain, many

opportunities for performance measurement exist, most of which fall into three subdomains identified by the reasons for managing sponsored projects:

- Fostering and promoting an environment resulting in increased activity and revenue (competitiveness);
- Using available staff and financial resources for sponsored programs administration (efficiency and productivity);
- Providing service to researchers engaged in sponsored programs activities (service).

Some additional examples of organizational activity domains are presented in Table 14-1.

Gathering or Identifying Benchmark Performance Data

A key aspect of benchmarking involves understanding empirically how one is doing relative to peer or similar organizations. It is interesting to note that, in the area of science and technology policy, much of this comparison function is built into public data sources such as the *Science and Engineering Indicators* series produced by the National Science Foundation (National Science Board, 2002). Therein, one may find data on countries, regions, states, industry sectors, disciplines, institutions, and so on, displayed in literally hundreds of comparative tables of indicators of science and engineering activity domains. However, there may be many domains of organizational activity that are of keen interest to one or more groups of organizational stakeholders (internal or external) for which there are no existing performance data suitable for benchmark comparisons. This necessitates gathering primary data in the activity domain. For example, in technology transfer benchmarking research recently conducted by the coinvestigators (Waugaman et al., 1994, 2001; Tornatzky, Waugaman, and Casson, 1995; Tornatzky, Waugaman, and Bauman, 1997), it was found that there was a strong interest among some university-linked stakeholders in examining the geography of technology transfer, that is, to better understand how well universities are doing in terms of licensing deals that might impact state or regional economic development. To this end, metrics were developed (e.g., percent of licenses involving state-based companies) that served as understandable and useful performance benchmarks for this area, and two waves of performance benchmarking were conducted.

In other cases, it may be logistically difficult to gather quantitative measures of performance in a domain, and researchers may have to rely on informal ratings of a more qualitative nature. For

TABLE 14–1	Overview of Benchmarking Methodology			
Activity/ Problem Domain:	**University/Industry Technology Transfer**	**Sponsored Programs Administration**	**Technology Business Incubation[i]**	**Migration of Science and Engineering Students[ii]**
Performance Benchmarking	Primary survey data collected from 50 technology managers at research institutions in the South. Resulted in regional benchmarking summary (Tornatzky, Waugaman and Bauman, 1997), and institutional "report cards," in terms of 7 quantitative performance measures.	Primary survey data were collected from over 90 research organizations (academic and independent) in three rounds. Each survey resulted in institutional reports using quantitative performance measures. A database of longitudinal comparative performance data and general summary reports are available to participants.	From among 600 incubators that exist nationwide, ratings were collected from a panel of industry experts to identify a group of 54 exemplary technology business incubators.	Using states as units of analysis, database from the National Survey of Recent College Graduates (NSRCG) was used to develop performance measures of retention and net migration of recent science and engineering graduates. Incorporated into a national report (Tornatzky et al., 1998).
Practice Benchmarking	One metric (licensing to local startups) was further analyzed to identify "best practitioner" institutions. Qualitative data collected on practices and policies that support working with start-ups, and incorporated into report (Tornatzky, Batts, et al., 1995).	Collection of practice data began with the third round, and is focusing on three areas of SPA activity: incentives for researchers, training in research administration, and coordination of activities and delegation of authority.	Extensive survey and interview data collected from 54 incubators on their organizational practices and procedures. 200-page guidebook produced (Tornatzky, Batts, et al., 1995).	First approximation to practice benchmarking via regression analysis of state policy and economic predictors of retention and net migration.
Implementation of Results	Several approaches used: (1) regional "Keeping it Home" conference held in collaboration with University of Mississippi; (2) 3,300 copies of 1997 performance benchmarking and best reports disseminated; (3) implementation projects conducted with several universities.	Encouraged use of benchmarking data by consultants, self-study groups, etc. at participating institutions. Presentations at professional meetings.	600 copies distributed to stakeholder organizations in the South; and several hundred elsewhere.	3,000 copies of reports distributed to date.

[i]Tornatzky, L. G., Y. Batts, N. E. McCrea, M. S. Lewis, and L. M. Quittman. 1995. *The art and craft of technology business incubation: Best practices, strategies, and tools from 50 programs.* Research Triangle Park, NC: Southern Growth Policies Board.

[ii]Tornatzky, L. G., D. Gray, S. A. Tarant, and J. Howe. 1998. *Where have all the students gone? Interstate migration of recent science and engineering graduates.* Research Triangle Park, NC: Southern Growth Policies Board.

Tornatzky, L. G., D. Gray, S. A. Tarant, and C. Zimmer. 2001. *Who will stay and who will leave? Individual, institutional, and state-level predictors of state retention of recent science and engineering graduates.* Research Triangle Park, NC: Southern Growth Policies Board.

example, in a best practices benchmarking effort (Tornatzky et al., 2002), the study team needed to identify "best practitioner" universities in the domain of promoting regional and community economic development in the so-called new economy. Since no relevant performance database existed, and it would be very expensive and time-consuming to develop one, the study team surveyed a national group of economic development practitioners and scholars, and obtained their nominations of the universities they perceived to be doing a good job in this field. From the resulting responses, a list of 16 universities with the highest numbers of nominations emerged. This group was the source of the 12 universities whose case studies made up the final report.

Various other approaches to gathering performance benchmarking data are provided in Table 14–1.

Identifying Best Practices

Defining and benchmarking organizational "best practices" requires a different analytic strategy. The comparative performance benchmarking described above often creates an institutional impetus for change and self-improvement, as the objects of study (particularly those in the bottom of the rankings) search for ways to do better. This often motivates institutions to better understand the policies and practices that exemplary organizations have adopted, and which they in turn can emulate. Seen from the perspective of classical experimental or quasi-experimental design (Cook and Campbell, 1979), best practices are analogous to clusters of independent or predictor variables that are associated with changes in outcome or dependent variables. Analytically then, the benchmarking challenge becomes to confirm positive relationships between specific practices and policies and performance outcomes.

However, it is here where benchmarking analysis deviates from traditional research methodology. In the latter, it would be sufficient to achieve acceptable levels of statistical significance in terms of an experimental treatment, or achieve a respectable r^2 in multiple regression analyses. However, this is insufficient (albeit an often necessary precursor) from the perspective of *defining and documenting* organizational best practices. Organizational practice involves a much richer mix of behaviors, roles, norms, and incentives. In order to be meaningful for organizational participants, best practices need to be documented via qualitative methods and described in plain language.

For example, as a result of the technology transfer benchmarking studies of the mid-1990s, it was evident that two interrelated factors were important to successful outcomes measured in the numbers of licenses awarded, the numbers of licenses awarded to local businesses, and the license revenue stream. These two factors were success at start-up business creation and faculty culture supportive of technology transfer. For investigating best practices in start-up business development, interviews were conducted with a sample of institutions that were doing well, and a similar sample of institutions that were underperforming. The study resulted in a monograph outlining best institutional practices in a number of areas relevant to success in business start-ups (Tornatzky, Waugaman, et al., 1995):

- Technology match
- Institutional mission and goals
- Faculty personnel policies, practices, and culture
- Business support systems and capital resources
- Technology transfer office operations

For looking at faculty culture, a different approach was taken. Rather than collecting data from a sample of institutions, all recipients of a series of prior benchmarking reports were asked to provide information about good and bad practices and their personal experiences with them. Volunteered information was followed up by loosely structured telephone interviews with the providers. The resulting report identifies good practices in areas of activity including acknowledgement programs, mission statements, and tenure and promotion review criteria (Tornatzky and Bauman, 1997).

As a final example, a national science and technology policy group documented model agreements regarding the disposition of intellectual property in industry-sponsored research (Government-University-Industry Roundtable, 1993). See Table 14-1 for illustrations of various approaches to identifying and documenting best practices.

Implementating Benchmarking Results

Performance and practice benchmarking can enable organizational members to understand how they are doing (e.g., relative to peers) and what they need to do to reach another level of performance. Here again benchmarking differs from more traditional approaches in that the research team typically has a client/partner relationship with the institutions that are the objects of the research (Rossi, 1993; Fetterman et al., 1996). That is, not only do the participating institutions help the research team define domains to study and useful benchmark measures, but they expect that the researchers in turn will be actively involved in disseminating results to individual organizations and to the entire cohort of institutions studied. Benchmarking results may be disseminated either in an institution-specific (e.g., confidential) version, or in more aggregate or generic versions.

Examples of institution-specific reports are available from both the technology transfer and sponsored programs administration studies. The first example is the technology transfer performance studies, in which "report cards" were prepared for all participating institutions after each round of data collection. These report cards provide the institution's ranking on each of 18 measures, as well as information on the median scores of all survey participants and median scores of all participants in the Association of University Technology Managers' annual licensing survey for the same year, if available. The second example is the sponsored programs administration benchmarking study, which provides reports for participants at the study Web site.[2] Not only do participants have access on a secure Web site to a prepared report which reflects up-to-date data, they also have an opportunity to construct individual reports for their internal use using sophisticated computing resources at the Web site. This approach, although expensive, allows participants maximum flexibility preparing and using benchmarking data for a number of institutions for internal studies and evaluations.

As an example of the practice of wider public dissemination is *Innovation U.*, which is a collection of case studies covering the critical organizational practices and policies at identified "best practitioner" institutions. *Innovation U.* has been widely disseminated through partner channels and the case-study institutions. Other examples are provided in Table 14–1. In addition, implementation of results can be conducted in more interactive ways such as via conferences, briefings, and planning sessions.

Recycling the Process

Integral to most longitudinal benchmarking programs is the concept of "continuous improvement" and repetition of performance and practice bench-

marking studies. For example, the Southern Technology Council conducted four waves of performance benchmarking of university-industry technology transfer, at two year intervals. These, in turn, have been punctuated by best practice analyses that derive from the performance studies. The sponsored programs administration program has evolved through three rounds of data collection to focus on the specific questions of interest to the participants as a result of their experiences with previous surveys in the series.

Using Comparative and Internal Performance Data for Performance Measurement

The most common uses of performance benchmarking data are to drive improvement as part of the self-evaluation and improvement cycle that is part of any management role. Typically, such efforts begin with some form of diagnostic review. More often than not, such reviews are initiated because there are qualitative or other indicators (e.g., faculty complaints, audit findings, misconduct, etc.) that point to problems. In other instances, management simply wants to know "how we are doing relative to other like institutions." In both situations, the results of diagnostic reviews are used to identify areas where improvement is needed. Based on an analysis of underlying causes of problem areas, goals or improvement targets are set and management makes policy or administrative changes in order to address the underlying issues and lead to improvement. These steps are known as interventions, or changes in the normal operation. The diagnostic review is then repeated to determine if the interventions have had the desired effect, adjustments are then made, and the process is recycled. In some cases, the measurement cycle becomes institutionalized. In effect, a "report card" is instituted and used for longitudinal tracking on several key indicators.

The following sections discuss some of the factors that should be taken into account in using comparative data and provide selected examples of how some institutions use such data.

> **Internal Measures.** Good comparative data offers an advantage over internal performance data in that it provides an external reference that helps provide an indicator of "where we should be." However, good comparative data is

---

[2]www.higheredbenchmarking.com

often not readily available for some types of performance measures, and developing it requires considerable resources and expertise that are not usually available to most research administration offices. The development of internal performance data for "self comparison" purposes is often necessary. For example, comparative data about processing times for various parts of the grant life-cycle (e.g., proposal processing times, account set up times, etc.) are simply not available and would be extremely difficult to develop. Yet, they are key measures of process efficiency and effectiveness that most offices should track.

Examples of Metrics Used in Research Administration. Some indicators commonly used in performance benchmarking include:

1. *Workload and Staffing Metrics*
   - Proposals submitted per central office of sponsored programs (OSP) full-time equivalent employee (FTE)
   - Active awards per central post-award financial administration (PAFA) FTE
   - Research expenditures per OSP and PAFA FTE
   - OSP cost per proposal submitted
   - PAFA cost per award managed
   - Active PIs per staff FTE (OSP & PAFA)
   - OSP and PAFA costs as a percent of total research expenditures
   - Percent of sponsored programs receivables over 120 days old (effectiveness metric)
   - Median OSP and PAFA staffing

2. *Institutional Research Competitiveness Measures*
   - Percent of faculty that are active PIs
   - Proposals submitted per faculty FTE
   - Sponsored research revenue per faculty FTE
   - Median active award size
   - Research expenditures as percent of total institutional expenditures
   - Success rates (percent of proposals submitted that are funded)

3. *Internal Process Metrics*
   - Timeliness of award set up process
   - Timeliness of proposal routing and approval process
   - Lead time for proposal routing and approval process

- Proposal "defects" delaying routing and approval process
- Number of cost transfers over ninety days
- Percent of late final scientific reports
- Percent of late final financial reports

Limitations of Comparative Data

Comparative data must be used with care. Just as reliance solely on qualitative data to have a picture of "how we are doing" is insufficient, so, too, is overreliance on quantitative data. Both types of data must be used together to see the whole picture. Some of the more obvious concerns follow:

Validity and Reliability. Typically comparative data is not representative of all institutions because the source is generally a self-selecting group of cooperating institutions. While the data can often be controlled for such things as research volume and other demographic variables, the overall sample is not random and survey populations will change from year to year.

Lack of established definitions for such terms as "full-time equivalent," "research faculty," "proposal" etc., and general lack of consistency in reporting such data create difficulties in generating accurate comparative data. Moreover, some survey responses are estimates because some institutions do not keep precise data in all the areas surveyed. All these factors affect the quality of the results.

Institutional Comparability. There is no way to establish truly homogeneous peer groups for institutions. Major factors, such as mission, research strengths, location, organizational structures, salary levels, etc. create unique financial and operating patterns. Peer group comparisons that lead to administrative or financial policy changes require sensitivity to the many factors not readily apparent from the statistics. In our experience, comparisons with groups of institutions with similar research expenditure volumes provide a good, all purpose "peer group" for comparison on most research administration metrics. Another approach is to control the number of variables when selecting a comparison group. For example, a comparison group could include land-grant universities with research expenditures between $50 million and $75 million, regardless of other characteristics.

Myth of the "Typical" Institution. There is no typical institution, and institutions should use comparative data only as one indicator of performance. Most surveys will result in high variations in reported data. It is futile to try to point to some standard of performance such as the "median" that should be met. A more useful and meaningful method is to compare an institution's data to a "normal" range of values, rather than on a nonexistent benchmark.

Use of Median and Quartile Data. The median represents the value that will split the group of institutions in half for a given measure: one-half of the institutions will be above the median, while one-half will be below. For that reason, the median institution will be different for each performance measure in a multimeasure survey.

The first quartile is the value for a statistic that separates the lowest 25% of the institutional values from the top 75% of the institutional values. The third quartile is the value that separates the lowest 75% of the values from the top 25% of the values for each statistic.

The interquartile or median range is the range of values from the first quartile to the third quartile. It represents the range comprising the middle half of all institutions. For comparative analysis it is often more useful to use the median range as a reference rather than the median. The median range indicates the "normal" range for institutions on a particular statistic. If an institution's score on a given measure falls outside the median range, the performance should be examined because the score indicates a value higher or lower than 75% of all institutions.

Example of Institutional Report Cards. The University of Missouri-Columbia developed a report card consisting of seventeen measures taken from the SRA-BearingPoint Sponsored Programs Survey (Kirby and Waugaman, 2000–2003). Measures were normalized by transforming each

measure on the survey into a percentile ranking. These rankings can be displayed in a graphic array showing year-to-year change. Each line on the graph in Figure 14-2 represents a year's scores on each measure, and where the score stood in comparison to the other large institutions in the survey by percentile.

Another example shows how the median range can be used to compare an institutional performance metric with a peer group. Figure 14-3 compares central OSP staffing for a hypothetical "Demonstration U," with a staff of 13, with the median range for all institutions in its peer group (14-24). The comparison shows that Demonstration U's staffing is in the first quartile, below 75 percent of the institutions within the peer group. This result can then be examined together with performance data on workload, productivity, competitiveness, customer satisfaction, or other variables to determine the adequacy of staffing. Low scores on competitiveness and customer satisfaction would indicate that the office needs more manpower.

Looking at Institutional Practices

The challenge for most highly research-intensive institutions is to foster high levels of growth in high quality research in a way that is consistent with the institution's mission, goals, and financial health. At the same time, the institutions need to facilitate institutional and federal accountability, while providing high quality and efficient service to the researchers. Optimizing the achievement of these goals simultaneously requires clarity of purpose and conscious trade-offs in the most stable of environments. However, a confluence of related factors and developments over the past ten years has trans-

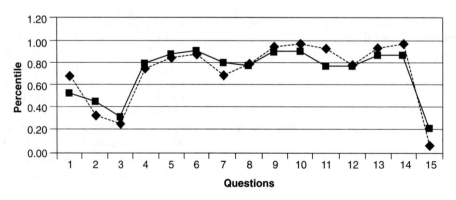

FIGURE 14-2 Percentile Ranks against Peers

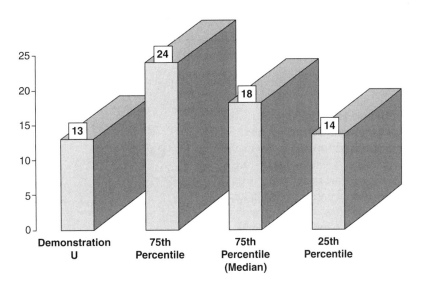

FIGURE 14-3   Central Sponsored Programs Staffing

formed the way institutions have approached research administration and complicated the challenge of reaching these multiple goals. These factors include such things as:

- Unprecedented competition for federal research support due to the entry of new "competitors" (teaching institutions, independent research organizations, small companies, etc.),
- Continued pressure by the federal government for cost containment, especially in indirect costs,
- Increased regulatory oversight by government agencies, and
- A technology explosion that has only been applied piecemeal to the business of research administration.

Thus, the effectiveness of an institution's research administration system needs to be evaluated in four key areas:

- How well does the institution foster an environment that results in increased research activity and revenue *(Competitiveness)*?
- How well does it use and leverage available resources *(Efficiency)*?
- How well does it serve its faculty to support research competitiveness?
- How well does it maintain requisite sponsor accountability?

In order to answer these questions, institutions need a combination of quantitative data that can help identify strengths and weaknesses in perform-

ance when compared to similar or peer institutions and "practice" information that can provide models for effective change.

In addressing the aforementioned performance issues we have documented in previous surveys several trends that are characteristic of highly research intensive institutions.

First, there has been a trend toward decentralization of research administration activities from central administration to academic units. Decentralization may be a key factor in improving service and fostering an environment that promotes faculty involvement in sponsored research, and in return helps faculty recruitment.

A second and related trend has been devolution of certain research administration authorities from central offices to administrators in academic units. This devolution of authority closer to where decisions are made also may be a key factor in both service enhancement and process efficiency.

Finally, survey data appear to show a trend toward a combination of pre- and post-award functions under a single executive. The reasons for doing so usually include:

1. Better integration between financial and nonfinancial aspects of research administration, and
2. Improved service by presenting a single face to the "researcher-customer" and creating a more seamless process.

Thirty-four percent of the institutions reported a structure that combined central pre-award and post-award financial functions in FY 2000. This is up from 25 percent in FY 1998.

While decentralization and combination trends may have contributed to some institutions' improved ability to handle workload and service demands, they are not issue-neutral. Many institutions are not making the necessary investments in the tools and technology infrastructure needed to support research and financial information needs in a timely and accurate manner. Their ability to support grants management functions are often severely constrained by limited integration of key grants management applications with university financial and administrative systems. In a decentralized environment, this makes it problematic for PIs and academic units to effectively manage their awards even though there is an institutional expectation that this has become a delegated responsibility. At some institutions significant investments in research administration support and staff at academic unit levels and the accompanying decentralization and devolution of authorities is resulting in considerable variation in quality due to insufficient training and lack of necessary oversight. This factor may contribute to increasing federal audit and compliance risk. Thus, clarity about roles and responsibilities, effective training mechanisms, and improved communication and information access have become critical success factors.

Two significant questions posed by decentralization, remain:

> *How do institutions effectively leverage departmental administration resources in a decentralized administrative environment while maintaining quality and compliance?*
>
> *Are there working models that effectively address the corollary issues of defining roles and responsibilities, training, information access, compliance assurance, communication, and quality control?*

Summary

As research becomes more competitive, research administration functions must become more businesslike in their approach to using resources and doing business. Adopting an attitude of self-evaluation and continual improvement is necessary. Self-evaluation requires solid data about internal activities and valid comparisons with competitor institutions. This need has been recognized by business and by other kindred activities such as health care and to some degree, educational services. There are methods and resources that can help the research manager benchmark and evaluate the functions for which he or she is responsible. These need to be considered essential tools in the research manager's toolbox.

• • • References

Cook, T. D., and D. T. Campbell. 1979. *Quasi-experimentation: Design and analysis issues for field settings.* Boston: Houghton-Mifflin.

Fetterman, D. M., S. J. Kaftarian, and A. Wandersman, eds. 1996. *Empowerment evaluation: Knowledge and tools for self-assessment and accountability.* Thousand Oaks, CA: Sage.

Government-University-Industry Research Roundtable. 1993. *Intellectual property rights in industry-sponsored university research.* Washington, DC: National Academy Press.

Hansen, S. 1989. Evaluating sponsored programs at predominantly undergraduate institutions. *Journal of the Society of Research Administrators* 21(1): 23–32.

Holmes, E. W., T. F. Burks, V. Dzau, M. A. Hindery, R. F. Jones, C. I. Kaye, D. Korn, et al. 2000. Measuring contributions to the research mission of medical schools. *Academic Medicine* 75(3): 304.

Kirby, W. S., and P. G. Waugaman. 2000. Performance benchmarking in sponsored programs administration: Results from the 1999 nationwide data collection. Contributed paper, SRA international annual meeting, St. Louis, MO, October, 2000.

Kirby, W. S., and P. G. Waugaman. 2001. Performance benchmarking in sponsored programs administration: Using the Web to analyze results from the FY 1998 and FY 2000 nationwide data collection. Contributed paper, SRA international annual meeting, Vancouver, BC, October, 2001. Reprinted in the *Journal of Research Administration* 33(1): 37–40.

Kirby, W. S., and P. G. Waugaman. 2002. Moving to best practices in benchmarking sponsored programs administration. Contributed paper, SRA international annual meeting, Orlando, FL, October, 2002.

Kirby, W. S., and P. G. Waugaman. 2003. Performance benchmarking in sponsored programs administration: Selected preliminary practice data from the 2002 SRA-bearing point nationwide survey. Contributed paper, SRA international annual meeting, Pittsburgh, PA, October, 2003.

Lowry, P. and C. S. Walker. 1992. The need to evaluate research support offices in institutions of higher education. *Journal of the Society of Research Administrators* 23(4): 35–41.

McNair, C. J., and K. H. J. Liebfried. 1992. *Benchmarking*. New York: Harper Business, 3.

Morris, D. E., and L. Hess. 1991. Self-evaluation project for research business office services. *Journal of the Society of Research Administrators* 23(1): 25-34.

National Science Board. 2002. *Science and engineering indicators*. Washington, DC: National Science Foundation.

Peters, T. 1987. *Thriving on chaos: Handbook for a management revolution*. New York: Knopf, 486–488.

Rossi, P., and H. E. Freeman. 1993. *Evaluation: A systematic approach*. Thousand Oaks, CA: Sage.

Spendolini, M. 1992. *The Benchmarking Book*. New York: American Management Association.

Tornatzky, L. G., and J. S. Bauman. 1997. *Outlaws or heroes? Issues of faculty rewards, organizational culture, and university-industry technology transfer*. Research Triangle Park, Southern Technology Council.

Tornatzky, L. G., and P. G. Waugaman. 2002. *Innovation U: New university roles in the knowledge economy*. Research Triangle Park, NC: Southern Growth Policies Board.

Tornatzky, L. G., P. G. Waugaman, and J. S. Bauman. 1997. *Benchmarking university-industry technology transfer in the South. 1995–1996 data*. Research Triangle Park, Southern Technology Council.

Tornatzky, L. G., P. G. Waugaman, and L. Casson. 1995. *Benchmarking university-industry technology transfer in the South: 1993–1994 data*. Research Triangle Park, NC: Southern Growth Policies Board.

Tornatzky, L. G., P. G. Waugaman, L. Casson, S. Crowell, C. Spahr, C., and F. Wong. 1995. *Benchmarking best practices for university-industry technology transfer: Working with start-up companies*. Research Triangle Park, NC: Southern Growth Policies Board.

Waugaman, P. G., and L. G. Tornatzky. 2001. *Benchmarking university-industry technology transfer in the South and the EPSCoR states: 1997–1998 data*. Research Triangle Park, NC: Southern Growth Policies Board.

Waugaman, P. G., L. G. Tornatzky, and B. S. Vickery. 1994. *Best practices for university-industry technology transfer: Working with external patent counsel*. Research Triangle Park, NC: Southern Growth Policies Board.

15

Institutional Enhancement of Research and Scholarship

Lynne U. Chronister, MPA

Universities and other research and educational institutions establish systems and programs to support their education, research, and service missions. Each of these missions may be enhanced by funding from grants and contracts. An institution that makes it a priority to develop their level of research and scholarship by increasing external funding requires additional resources, including funding, be directed toward that goal. Mechanisms and programs to achieve this goal include incentives and awards for faculty who compete for grant and contracts. Also required is the institutional infrastructure and support necessary for faculty to increase their ability to compete for external funding. Discussed in this chapter are:

1. Systems to motivate and reward faculty for developing grantsmanship skills and research competencies
2. Programs to assist in identifying external sponsors
3. Processes for promoting and managing grant programs, when the number of submissions are limited by sponsors,
4. Options for establishing internal grant programs.

Motivating and Rewarding Faculty

Reward structures at universities and independent research institutions are complex and are interwoven with the overall culture and environment of the institutions. A tenure-based system necessarily differs in comparison to a system of motivation and rewards for contract or soft-money researchers. Structures, e.g., internal grants discussed in this section, provide motivation to faculty who are unsure of the degree of their national competitiveness that is needed to succeed in local competition for funds. The development of grant proposals is time-consuming and faculty with large teaching loads find it difficult to devote resources to the process. Releasing faculty from teaching duties to develop proposals or to provide graduate student or clerical or administrative support can motivate faculty to seek external support, especially if it the support offered is a condition of proposal submission.

Monetary rewards for exceptional performance in successful efforts that generate external funding for research must be handled within the guidelines imposed by federal, state, and institutional policy and regulation. For instance, an institution may want to reward a researcher who brings in significant federal funding by increasing salary or by providing a time-limited stipend. However, a stipend is not generally an allowable cost under OMB A110 and it is not acceptable to increase salary and charge the federal sponsor only for the duration of, and as an outcome of, the federal funding. Any salary increase should be permanent. For institutions whose researchers are part of clinical practice plans, this becomes a balancing act with many sources of support.

Other rewards may include increased travel funds, equipment, or additional staff and graduate student support. Standard reward programs include dinners and recognition of faculty as outstanding researchers or entrepreneurs. In addition, appointments as a distinguished faculty or endowed chair are two of the highest forms of institutional recognition that an institution can bestow as performance rewards.

Identifying External Sponsors

There are literally thousands of different sources of external support and over $100 billion dollars distributed annually for research, development, scholarship, education and training, and procurement. Sources range from federal, state, and local government, private and public foundations, to business and industry. Identification of such sources can be incomprehensible for less experienced faculty and sometimes even experienced faculty. One means of providing assistance to faculty and enhancing the institution's mission is to set up an office or designate an individual to untangle the maze of funding opportunities, assist in locating appropriate opportunities, and to facilitate the building of networks and contacts with potential sponsors.

At a minimum, institutions may assist in locating funding by subscribing to print and electronic newsletters and searchable databases. In support of the services offered by the research development staff, library resources that offer electronic and print funding opportunities, funding priorities, and announcements of new policies and directions are necessary. Federal government and large, private foundations generally provide information on standard grant programs, as well as information about special grant opportunities. Much information about grant opportunities can be found on the Web, for example www.nsf.gov. All federal Web sites end with ".gov." Contract opportunities with government entities are posted in the Federal Register or through subscription services. Search engines such as Community of Science, SPINPlus and IRIS provide searchable databases for current grant and contract opportunities with key word or phrase indexes and list deadline information, links to program announcement sites, as well as tools for developing and sharing bio-sketches and faculty expertise. Other online assistance can be attained through organizations such as the American Association of State Colleges and Universities Grant Resource Center. Some institutional libraries also subscribe to many print and online services.

Establishing a Research Development Office

The number of individuals who staff an office determines its level of service, but some basic principles and processes can be followed to build a successful service regardless of staff size.

The most common structure is to implement the development function within the sponsored programs office. The development office may also be established as a separate unit reporting to a director or chief research officer. In some institutions this function may reside solely within a university relations or university development office. The quality and experience of the staff is critical to the success of a development service, for example, its familiarity with the interests, expertise, and needs of the faculty. This enables the staff to review and analyze the plethora of relevant information available and to notify specific faculty. Too often a shotgun approach is taken in the dissemination of funding information (e.g., a nuclear physicist receives proposal information about marine biology). However, it is important to identify interdisciplinary opportunities as well.

When several hundred researchers and scholars seek information on funding opportunities and advice on approaching a potential sponsor, the research administration must know or learn about, at least in general terms, the funding portfolio and priorities of all major government and private sponsors. Providing instruction to faculty and staff on use of the searchable databases and effective electronic search is important. Research offices might consider teaming with the library or human resource offices to offer training.

Making contact with potential sponsors prior to proposal can present an opportunity to succeed in the bid for funding. Depending on the program and the nature of the opportunity, telephone calls, e-mails, meeting at professional conferences, and in-person visits to program officers can be both appropriate and beneficial (conversely, a negative impression can be given if such contact efforts are poorly conducted). Less senior or less successful researchers and scholars may disclose to potential sponsors that their institutions lack funding support or that they need funding to advance their careers in particular areas of expertise. Faculty who have succeeded in funding can mentor junior faculty and offer invaluable advice on how to develop relationships with sponsors. The staff of the development office should encourage and coordinate these efforts by initiating workshops where senior faculty can share their insights. The expertise of senior faculty who have worked at an agency or industry is also of great value.

Promoting and Managing Limited Submissions

With the thousands of funding opportunities, a select number require that the institution predetermine which faculty within the institution is eligible for proposal submission or who will be nominated for a particular award or fellowship. Over one hundred of these sponsors restrict the number of applications or proposals that an institution is allowed to submit. Some programs limit only one submission per institution within a submission cycle, while others may merely allow several. An institution should determine the process that works best for its culture, but also must select the official who makes the final determination of eligibility. The ease of electronic collection and transmittal of information allows an institution to easily maintain a list of limited submissions on a Web page and to send announcements of impending competitions. The institution may set up a formal or informal process of review. Final decisions should be made centrally in order to avoid confusion or speculation. A vice president for research may ask that all nominations come to his or her office for review, and the decision-making process or final decision may be a collaborative one among campus units.

Establishing Proposal Review and Decision Making

Two processes are described which differ in level of review and level of decision making. Both have advantages and disadvantages and can be expanded or modified to respond to campus culture.

A formal process for announcing and reviewing limited submissions better assures success in competing for these funding opportunities. The steps involved might include:

1. *Maintenance of a Web-based list of limited submission opportunities and updating of the list at least monthly.* Review the list weekly or create an electronic tickler system to remind the limited submission coordinator of an upcoming deadline. Ideally, this reminder should be sent out three to four months in advance. If an-

nouncements are sent out prior to formal announcements by the sponsor, either confirm the process and priorities with the sponsor or indicate that this has not yet been confirmed. When a limited submission program is published or identified, an announcement is drafted by a limited submission liaison. This announcement is then broadcast to the campus community via the e-mail list of deans, department chairs, and other communications point people.

2. *Applicants submit preproposals by the campus deadline stated in the announcement.* Preproposals should be three pages and should include an abstract and a description of the project. The preproposal should be sent to the school or college and a copy sent to the limited submission coordinator in the office of research.

3. *Review of preproposals should occur within one week of receipt, using the sponsor's guidelines to rank the most competitive candidates and proposals.* The top three proposals and rankings for all proposals should be sent to the limited submission coordinator in the office of research.

4. *The office of research may consult with the involved schools or colleges if necessary to assist in final ranking or to suggest collaborations.* The office of research should review preproposals and inform selected principal investigators within one week of receipt of the rankings from the school, college, or division.

A less formal process may be more appropriate for some institutions and may involve sending requests to the vice president for research or other designated individual. The investigator would be informed within a short period of time whether or not he or she has approval to move forward with a submission. The process is simple and decisions can be made quickly. The downside is lack of broad campus involvement.

Internal Grant Programs

Extramural grants and contracts are the primary sources of support for research and other projects within most not-for-profit institutions. However, institutions may determine that an effective method to further their missions and support faculty research and scholarship is to establish an internal grant program. These funds generally are made available on a competitive basis to enhance an institution's ability to attract extramural support, provide support for high-risk early stage research, as start-up or seed funds for researchers and other scholars, or as an additional means of distributing funding across campus units. In addition, comparatively small amounts of funding enhance the ability of arts and humanities faculty to carry out scholarly research and artistic expression and to publish and exhibit their work.

Available resources are a factor in determining the level of support an institution can provide. Public institutions may have additional state funds from which to draw but are very likely limited in the availability of that revenue for support for research and program enhancement. Private institutions may have more flexibility in uses of their fund sources and may be better positioned to provide internal support for academic and research development. Options for sources of internal support vary by institution; however, the most common sources include:

- Base funding from state or region
- Facilities and administrative funds
- Unrestricted gift funds
- Endowment
- Bond funds
- Interest on investments

Rationale and Uses of Internal Support for Research and Scholarship

Increasingly scarce resources have dictated that even well-endowed institutions must carefully review funds allocated for new academic initiatives, including those for research and scholarship. This environment has led to scrutiny of existing support and increased concern that investments are being made strategically. Institutions must determine the anticipated outcome of internal investments prior to allocating resources or at a point where a strategic review is appropriate. Long-standing internal support programs may no longer be relevant to the current goals and vision of the institution. Programs that exist merely to support vested interests of campus groups or support declining programs may not be effective use of state or private funds. A strategic review of existing programs or strategic plan will assist in leveraging internal funds to achieve long-term goals. Examples of uses of internal funds include:

- Support innovation and discovery
- Equitable allocation of scarce resources

- Expansion of innovative academic programs
- Graduate student support
- Support for external advisory boards
- New laboratory build-out
- Faculty start-up packages
- Support artistic and scholarly growth
- Promote extramural support
- Enhance economic development
- Support for research outreach
- Sabbatical support
- Visiting scholars and researchers
- International collaborations

Institutions may use a variety of mechanisms to manage and distribute funds, including providing cost-sharing, matching funds, graduate student stipends, research support programs for undergraduates, base administrative support for research programs, centers and institutes, administrative support for proposal development, and internal grant programs. Funds may be accessed through either a competitive or noncompetitive process, depending on such factors as a central versus decentralized administrative structure, the degree of shared governance, use of funds, and established priorities. If not maintained centrally in an academic or research office, noncompetitive funds may be distributed to schools or colleges, other units such as an academic senate or faculty research committee, graduate schools, undergraduate research offices, or outreach and international offices.

Internal grant programs reflect institutional culture and priorities: some are used for a single purpose, e.g., matching funds. In contrast, funds may be distributed to a variety of grant programs administered centrally or by designated units. Some options for targeting funds include:

- Seed funds and pilot projects
- Bridge funds
- Scholarship and arts
- Innovative education and training
- Matching grants
- Junior faculty enhancement programs
- Travel grants
- Technology enhancement and development
- Equipment grants

A short description of a variety of programs help to identify new options for internal grant programs, for example:

Equipment Match. This program provides cost sharing or matching funds for equipment when required by an external sponsor. The percentage of equipment cost-sharing or matching funds is usually defined by the funding agency. Requests may be limited to a specific dollar amount requiring cost sharing by the college or school. Matching funds are committed only for capital equipment (equipment of at least $5,000).

Cost Sharing. Matching funds are provided for proposals to government and not-for-profit organizations when required by the sponsor. Nonrequired cost sharing may be considered; however, all required matching requests would take precedence over nonrequired cost sharing

Multidisciplinary Proposal Support. This support encourages faculty to develop large interdisciplinary proposals (e.g., multimillion dollar projects related to the sciences) that usually cross department or college boundaries. The institution may provide project development support (e.g., clerical, travel, supplies and expendables, or grant writing assistance). It is required that a major grant proposal be submitted to an external sponsor within 18 months of the date of the internal award.

Basic Research Grants Program. This program supports the development of new research centers and institutes. Base support is provided for clerical and administrative salaries and basic operating costs. Funds may be time limited or renewable upon an internal or external review.

Principal Investigator Bridge Program. A principal investigator bridge program may provide one-time funding to principal investigators (PIs) who have lost or stand to lose their primary extramural funding. Funds ensure continuation of a research project for an interim period until extramural support can be reestablished.

Intellectual Property Grant Program. This program encourages faculty who have promising ideas that could lead to the capture of significant and valuable intellectual property to complete the research or data gathering and analysis that will likely lead to a patent with major potential for benefiting society.

The Publication Assistance Fund. This fund assists ladder faculty, particularly those early in their careers, with the publication of books or monographs and exhibitions or performances of works of art. The intent of the fund is to defray certain costs that would not normally be covered by the publisher, thus enhancing the possibility of the work to be published.

Research Buyouts Program. Funding for faculty is reassigned for time-limited or special administrative appointments or to aid in recruitment.

Junior Faculty Research Fellowships. Nontenured faculty may apply for funds to develop new scientific processes or for developing or learning new research methodology. The fellowships may be used as summer salary compensation for the candidate with the expectation of devoting full time to research or study in the summer of the awarded year. No additional salary compensation may be received during the awarded fellowship.

Research Travel Grant Program. Reimbursable expenses are funded for participation in research meetings. These grants support presentation of original work of one's own scholarship, including fine arts, or for the one time special circumstances of familiarizing oneself with a new field of scholarship in a highly visible forum. Support may be available to undergraduate and graduate students and postdoctoral fellows for travel to collaborating research laboratories.

New Faculty Research Grant Program. This program is available to faculty during the first three years of a tenure track position. Proposals are evaluated on the basis of the significance of the project and need.

Managing Internal Grant Programs

Regardless of what unit manages an internal grant program, certain management principles and objectives should be observed to avoid the criticisms that are frequently levied against external competitions, including concerns over subjectivity in the review and awarding process. When initiating a grant program or reviewing an existing program some questions to consider include:

- *Has the program been broadly communicated to the institutional community? Is the program described on the research Web site or other appropriate site?*
- *Has a standard process for submission that includes timelines and forms been developed?*
- *Is the submission process clear, concise, and easily understood? Is contact information listed? Is there information about where the proposal is to be submitted?*
- *Are consistent deadlines set for submission and do the deadlines compete with any critical external funding?*
- *Have consistent review criteria been established and published?*
- *Has the review team been oriented to the review criteria and the scoring or ranking process? Is the team aware of the need for confidentiality? Does any member of the team have any conflict of interest regarding any of the proposals?*

- *Is there a standard letter prepared that is sent to those not funded? Is there a letter that is sent to the investigators who are funded? If so, does the letter give information about the fund account and grants management process?*
- *Is feedback provided to the principal investigators of projects that are and are not approved?*
- *Is there a feedback system in place to provide feedback from the submitters regarding the submission and review process?*

Evaluating Internal Program Support

Program evaluation is especially critical when resources are scarce and when significant funding has been put into a program. Thorough program evaluation is a matter of the chief research officer's credibility, as steward of institutional funds. If institutional funds are put into a program on a continuing basis, it is necessary to continue review of the program to assure the community that the program is accomplishing its research and scholarly mission. In the event that reviews indicate need for revision of the program or process, the changes should be made and subsequently monitored to provide the institution documentation to substantiate continued support or elimination of the program. As part of the evaluation process, it is important to question whether the evaluation process in place routinely and effectively reviews the efficacy of the grant program and whether the evaluation ties into the strategic purpose of the program. For example, if the purpose of the internal grant program is to increase success in external funding, how successful have the investigators been in receiving external funding? Or does a program aimed at scholarship or artistic expression have a sufficient baseline of publications, books, or exhibitions showings? Whatever the program's purpose, the tracking and evaluation process should be simple and straightforward or the likelihood of abandoning the evaluation increases.

Summary

Institutions with a set goal to develop or expand their extramural awards have varying levels and types of internal support, which may include how to locate funding opportunities, a coordinated process for limited submissions, and institutional grant programs. To attract and maintain external program funding, institutions must have solid evaluative structures in place demonstrating effective program management in order to ensure continued research program development.

16

Support for Institutional and Interdisciplinary Projects

Lynne U. Chronister, MPA

Opinions on whether we should or should not provide support for preparing grant proposals vary widely. Two trends have fostered the need for institutional support for proposal development: the increased emphasis on large multidisciplinary programs and regional centers of excellence and, second, the increased competition for limited dollars. Much of funding previously directed toward single-investigator research has been redirected toward big science, for example NSF Centers, the NIH Roadmap Initiative, and Department of Homeland Security (DHS) Centers of Excellence. Individuals with specific expertise and skill in coordinating and writing proposals are increasingly critical members of proposal writing teams. The increase in site visits to potential awardees has grown with the trend toward large and multidisciplinary proposals. Institutions can offer assistance for a full range of proposal development activities and coordination of site visits. The type and level of support depends on institutional goals, priorities, resources, and culture.

Small and nonresearch intensive universities often require heavier teaching loads than larger institutions or research-intensive universities. Smaller institutions often set the goal to expand levels of nondonation external support. To support this effort, an experienced proposal writer can provide general assistance to faculty who wish to seek grant or contract funds or are charged by the administration to focus on certain areas of strength. The proposal development function may reside in the development office or a sponsored programs office. Frequently a proposal writer may be asked by administration to identify sources of funding in addition to assisting in the proposal writing.

With public and private funds becoming more aligned with problem-solving and multidisciplinary programs larger and more research-oriented, institutions often establish support units to assist in coordinating and assembling large proposals. Increased competitiveness also has motivated departments and colleges to create proposal development teams in addition to centrally supported teams.

Structuring a Proposal Development Function

The administrative support provided to the content experts is a key component of the proposal development function. A proposal development office or function, in turn, ideally includes at least five areas of administrative support: director of research development, experienced scientific writer, budget developer, proposal editor and assembler, and computer support. Responsibilities of four of these positions are provided to demonstrate the type of support that can be offered by a professional research development group.

Faculty support (stipend, summer salary, reassignment of teaching or clinical workload) may be necessary to allow a principal investigator to devote sufficient time to lead the proposal effort. For most research proposals, faculty leadership is critical to assure "buy-in" and collaboration among researchers across departmental and college units as well as across institutions. It may be necessary to provide a buy-out or stipend because of the effort that must be devoted to developing a large competitive proposal. Few professional proposal writers are able to design and prepare a competitive proposal without the assistance of a subject expert, regardless of the subject. A team effort is required.

Director of Research Development:

- Coordinates the activities of teams of faculty and staff in the preparation of major grant proposals for large-scale, interdisciplinary research or training programs.
- Assumes lead responsibility for grant proposal preparation, including assemblage of faculty written contributions, editing, obtaining supporting documents and forms, and producing and establishing grant application project schedule.
- Coordinates the written contributions of participating faculty and staff, edits technical writing or writes about specialized subjects to make the contributions consistent in style and content.
- Participates with lead faculty and staff on project development and grant proposal teams involving collaborations with other institutions or agencies.

Proposal Writer:

- Develops a database of background materials for use in future grant applications and develops internal grant application protocols to facilitate preparation of these applications.
- Develops a broad range of standard boilerplate descriptions of university resources and programs for inclusion in proposal applications.
- Assists in identifying new grant initiatives and other funding mechanisms for large interdisciplinary research programs.
- Assists in preparation of select portions of proposals.
- Assists in editing and reviewing scientific and technical proposal sections.
- Assumes responsibility for designing and preparing the administrative structure and evaluation and dissemination of sections of proposals.

Budget Developer:

- Works with faculty researchers to develop budgets that adhere to proposal guidelines and follow costing principles and university requirements.
- Identifies financial data needed from partner

schools and colleges (internal and external) and other institutions and coordinates receipt and analysis of data.
- Works with faculty to identify all expenditure categories of the budget including consultants, equipment, lease costs, travel, and subcontracts for proposed research activity.
- Applies expert level knowledge of federal cost allowance practices to ensure sensitive costs are adequately identified and justified in proposals.
- Advises faculty of policies governing the expenditures of their research funds.
- Prepares subcontracts and consortia agreements with partner institutions.
- Identifies and applies indirect cost rates for participating institutions.
- Completes all budget-related forms for complex grant applications. Delegates authority to approve grant budgets on behalf of the research development unit.
- Trains school, college, and departmental staff on budget preparation for large contracts and grants.

Finally, the budget developer must understand, interpret, and apply federal, state, and university rules, regulations, and policies and have the skill to interpret and apply OMB Circulars A-21, A-110, and A-133.

Proposal Editor and Assembler:

- Coordinates and compiles sections of grant applications and ensures consistent technical dimensions (e.g., typeface, spacing, margins, templates for tables, charts, diagrams, sequence, pagination):
  - Integrates graphics into narrative.
  - Recommends appropriate format and presentation of grant application manuscripts.
  - Examines page proofs for accuracy.
  - Assembles proposal package and forwards to the appropriate office.
- Conducts research to create and update "boilerplate" sections of grant applications; identifies and incorporates appropriate "boilerplate" sections into grant applications; edits "boilerplate" language to make it compatible with specific grant application.
- Edits copy for stylistic consistency according to sponsor style guidelines, logical content and rational development of content. Coordinates editorial changes of multiple writers and reviewers of parts of grant applications.
- Maintains "critical path" calendar for grant application tasks. Generates and updates grant application production schedules. Communi-

cates regularly with faculty and key staff about assignments and schedules. Alerts director to potential barriers to meeting schedules.

Functional Issues in Proposal Development

The successful support team receives multiple and overlapping requests for assistance, which necessitates that the team establish a process for requesting assistance, priority setting, time management, and communication. The request process should fit within the existing structure of the institution and kept as simple as possible both for the requester and review team. A sample process that can be easily modified to fit institutional need and structure is provided.

- A packet requesting support to be submitted to the director should consist of:
  - *Project summary and submission deadline*
  - *List of investigators with short bio-sketch for each*
  - *Cost sharing and resource requirements*
  - *Copy of the program announcement*
  - *List of external collaborators and partners*
- The director should review the packet and forward it with recommendations to the chief research officer and to the review committee. The director's recommendations should include conflicting commitments and available resources in the proposal support unit.
- The review committee should respond within one week in order to allow sufficient time to develop a competitive proposal.

Reviewing and Setting Priorities

An advisory group should be established or the expertise of an existing group used to review requests (for example, an associate dean for the research advisory council might review and prioritize requests for support for responding to a request for proposals from units across campus). It is important that qualifications of individuals involved in the review process and selection criteria of proposals be considered including the experience of the principal investigator; depth and breadth of expertise available to collaborate on the project; cost-sharing options and other institutional

resources; timelines and deadlines; and level(s) of collaboration across disciplines. When a project generates controversy, a determining selection factor might include assessment of support across units, as well as of the level of support from the surrounding community.

While flexibility is crucial in any collaborative project, it is important for the proposal support unit to communicate to the content team what services they are able to provide, what is required from the team, and the timeline for completing the proposal. The support unit should prepare a materials packet for the investigators, which includes a proposal development checklist, sample timeline, and list of available boilerplate information.

Organizing for a Sponsor Site Visit

Awards can be won or lost depending upon the success of the site visit. The research development team is responsible for the coordination of the site visit: this requires the team's ability to coordinate planning for such visits well in advance of a visit. As part of preparation for the site visit, the research development officer staff assures that all the members of the research team, as a team of participants, have a clear, consistent understanding of the proposal, its design, and preparation to share with site visitors. Evidence that some of the participants have not met prior to the visit suggests that the program is poorly coordinated and indicates a lack of preplanning. A timetable within a checklist can assist in the previsit planning and, while the orientation and focus of any visit is determined most often by the potential sponsor, a checklist can assist in the smooth conduct and organization of the visit.

Summary

Establishment of a proposal development service within a unit or the central research function helps the institution to facilitate timely requests for large institutional and interdisciplinary proposals. The cost of such service ranges depending on the level of support provided. Most faculty or departments do not have the time or resources to devote to the large roadmap-type initiatives and the institution may be unable to respond without a level of proposal development support.

Since most institutions are able to devote only a limited amount of resources to a proposal development office, it is important that they set up a process and time period (three to four years) in which to measure the success of the office's efforts. Success of a program should be based on the number of proposals submitted and subsequently awarded to the institution, as well as overall satisfaction with the office's performance and services as part of the institution. If, over a period of time, the proposal development office shows little return on investment, the office should be realigned or the level of resources and staffing reevaluated.

••• Suggested Reading

Scafidi, Gia, and Diane Krieger. How Many Academics Does It Take? *USC Trojan Family Magazine,* Autumn 2004.

17

Institutional Development Offices and Research Offices: Gifts and Grants

Lynne U. Chronister, MPA

Relationship between Development Offices and Research Offices

Institutional development or advancement offices and research offices have very similar missions and numerous common goals. The offices primarily function for the purpose of facilitating the generation of external support for research, scholarship and education, including the requisite infrastructure and capital improvement that supports the institution. Despite sharing mission-critical goals and objectives, or possibly because of it, often there is some rivalry between the two offices. When offices do collaborate, the relationship is often found to be mutually rewarding. Identifying the environmental and technical disparities and misperceptions between the two offices can help build a foundation for collegiality and cooperation. Making these distinctions can also assist the institution on the whole to differentiate between a gift, grant, or contract, which are known in the development sphere as *exchange transactions*, which, if not clearly understood, can lead to the serious legal and accounting repercussions detrimental to the institution's research missions.

Working Together

The benefits of advancement and research collaboration can result in greater support for the institution, faculty, and students. The leadership of the two functional areas should meet regularly to collaborate in the development of relationships with sponsors and donors. Joint training of research and development officers, including workshops, can help to clarify common goals. Workshops might include discussions, led by research officers or by external speakers, on the characteristics of donations and contracts or exchange transactions.

The importance of research and development officers working together is also enhanced when their institution fosters increased collaboration with business and industry. When both research administration and advancement offices are seeking support from the same industry, it can appear that the institution is disorganized if the effort is not collaborative.

As universities are encouraged to become partners in regional economic development and to be responsive to the needs of industry, more faculty are developing close associations with industry. They may have consulting and research relationships with industry as founders, officers, or scientific advisors of companies. A faculty member who starts a new company based upon technology that they developed at the institution while retaining appointment must be especially careful. For example, making a donation back to a campus laboratory may be inappropriate and could pose legal issues. These close associations, even when encouraged, can present challenges for research administration, development officers, and faculty alike.

Points of Concern between the Development and Research Offices

The issues between development and research offices that can become contentious are generally those related to credit and accountability, but differences, such as basic definitions, also cause confusion and concern. The terminology and interpretation of language used by development officers is different from that of the research officer. To facilitate communication, it is important to understand the variations in language. For example, the term "grant" is used by a development office to mean a type of gift but a research unit would consider a grant a contractual arrangement. The Council on the Advancement and Support of Education (CASE) is the international association that services the development community. Located in Washington, DC and London, CASE has over 3,000 institutional members from elementary through university levels.[1] The CASE Management Standards provide guidance for university and other education institutions. CASE defines grants or contracts as *Exchange Transactions* that signify the reciprocity attributed to revenue from sponsors as opposed to donors. Grants or donations may be labeled a contribution by CASE definition.

Definitions

CASE discusses gifts, grants, and contracts from the development perspective.

> A Gift is an unconditional, voluntary, non-reciprocal transfer of assets (including unconditional promises) to a not-for-profit organization. The donor may have certain expectations but there cannot be any actual control over expenditure of funds or any quid pro quo. The donor may not benefit from the execution of the gift. (Case, 76)

CASE also discusses the intent of the donor or awarding agency and the legal obligation of the awarding agency as two discriminating factors.

> A grant may be donative in nature, bestowed voluntarily and without expectation of tangible results. A contract always carries explicit quid pro quo between the source and the institution. (Case, 76)

Other definitions, including a legal definition, can assist in understanding the difference. According to CASE, one legal definition of a gift states:

> A gift is a voluntary transfer of property to another made gratuitously and without consideration. A contract is a promise or promises constituting agreement between the parties that gives each a legal duty to the other and also the right to seek remedy for breach. A grant shares the attribute of both a gift and a contract. (Case, 76)

Accountants look to the definitions provided in the Federal Accounting Standards (FASB) or Government Accounting Standards (GASB). FAS 116 states:

> A contribution is an unconditional transfer of cash or other assets... in a voluntary nonreciprocal transfer. (Case, 76)

A gift may be either restricted or unrestricted. An unrestricted gift is donated to the organization with no strings attached. The funds can be used at the discretion of the institution. A restricted gift is targeted toward a particular use, for instance, a scholarship fund or a specific research program. Generally, confusion arises when trying to determine whether a transfer of funds should be categorized as restricted or fall into a restricted account under OMB A-21 principles.

Who Gets Credit?

A point of concern is who receives credit for the gift or an award. The relationship between a donor and the institution, faculty member, or development officer plays a major role in solicitation and receipt of a gift. The condition of a contract or grant is somewhat less subjective, although the reputation of the institution and the faculty (in addition to the quality of the work proposed) are major factors in the review of a grant or contract proposal. A development officer may be more engaged and directly involved in soliciting a gift than a research administrator would be for most awards. The development officer has greater personal investment in the decision about whether or not the funds are posted as a gift or grant or contract. A research administrator may not be judged specifically by the dollars generated by grants and contracts but also has a vested interest in where the credit is placed. Institutions' national rankings are determined in large part by the dollars that they are awarded and expend. The greater number of

---

[1] www.case.org

awards posted, the higher the rankings or reputation. One of the first questions asked by one research administrator to another is, "What is your research volume?" A second motivating factor for the research administrator is allocation of internal resources. The greater the volume of proposals and awards, the more likely funds will be budgeted for additional staff and staff support. So, the question of who gets credit can be difficult because of the accounting for the funds and personal vested interests.

The standards for how gift funds are accounted for and reported are provided by the Federal Accounting Standard Board (FASB) for private institutions and the Government Accounting Standards Board (GASB) generally used by public institutions. In addition, the research administrator will look to Circular OMB, A-21 for additional assistance in understanding Organized Research and to the Cost Accounting Standards Board (CASB) and FASB and GASB to set criteria for reporting of gifts. Under these standards, restricted grants that are accounted for in the research reports can be reported. However, the institution must make it clear that the restricted funds are identified as restricted funds. This allows an institution to credit a grant, not a contract, as both a sponsored-programs award and as a gift. The reverse is not true—a gift should not be reported in the grant and contract awards. The Internal Revenue Service and the Department of Justice also look at issues such as unrelated business income tax (UBIT) and recording of gifts and other transactions that result in defrauding the government. The Federal Drug Administration has a requirement in 21 CFR 54 for reporting of gifts by individual researchers.

Gifts in Support of Research

Restricted gifts can fund research but only if they are truly donative in nature. They do not require the establishment of a restricted grant account. It is generally unacceptable for preclinical or clinical trials to be supported by a gift from a pharmaceutical manufacturer, but an unrestricted gift donated to the university from a private citizen could be used to fund an internally sponsored clinical trial. Care should be taken to ascertain that there is no conflict of interest nor connection between the donor and institution nor research team. Funds provided to

support research are not contributions if their potential public benefits are secondary to the potential proprietary benefits to the sponsor. If intellectual property developed either directly or indirectly from gift funds is transferred to the donor, the transfer of funds should have been under a contractual arrangement that describes the disposition of potential intellectual property.

One motivation for characterizing funds as gifts as opposed to a grant or contracts is avoidance of an institution's facility and administrative rate (F&A). Routine labeling of awards as gifts in order to channel all funds, minus any gift tax, to the project may be interpreted by the federal government as financial misconduct and perhaps even fraud. If the amount becomes material and affects the calculation of the F&A negotiated rate, the outcome may be a higher F&A rate. For accounting purposes, research is classified as organized or instructional research under OMB A-21. Any research support affects either the organized or instructional research base and can have an impact on the outcome of the negotiated F&A rate. A higher rate assessed to government grants and contracts results in overpayment by the government and a possible interpretation that an institution is defrauding the government sponsor. This outcome can be alleviated if the F&A is waived on the gift and counted as cost sharing. However, the optimal solution is appropriate classification of the funding as organized research.

In clinical research, gifts and bonuses are frequently informal and may be part of the formal acceptance of support for clinical trials. Institutions are beginning to develop policies dealing with the efficacy of this practice. A clinician may receive gifts of travel, cash, or other tangible gifts from a pharmaceutical company, perhaps to encourage use of a particular therapeutic line. If at the same time, that clinician is researching the effect of the same company's new drug, a conflict of interest will exist. The question is whether or not the practice should be allowed or the conflict managed by oversight from the institution. Similarly, the same researcher or the clinical coordinator may agree to accept bonus payments in the form of a donation for early enrollment of subjects. Again, there is a potential or real conflict of interest. One solution for cash donations is for the institution to accept the gift or bonus payment and establish the policy that the researcher or research team has no control over the funds and do not directly benefit from the gift or bonus payment.

Equipment and Patent Donations

Equipment donations can be valued assets to a research and instructional program and can be accepted by the institution as a gift if certain conditions are met. The institution cannot accept equipment as a gift and agree to any requirement to perform specific research using the donation. No strings can be attached to the donation regarding specific research functions that the institution will be required to perform. For instance, a company might donate an MRI machine to a laboratory on the condition that research on the use of a new therapeutic for hyperactive children must be the primary use of the instrument. Especially if that company would benefit from the outcome of the research, it should be considered an exchange transaction, not a donation. Additionally, if equipment title does not accompany the donation, it cannot be considered a gift because the full benefit has not accrued to the institution.

Patent donations have been somewhat controversial since corporations expanded the process of donating patents to universities and other nonprofit entities. The IRS is concerned that corporations are using the patent donation process as a mechanism to defer or avoid corporate taxes. Corporations donate patents at the potential market value. If only 2% to 3% of all patents have value, the IRS contends that the patents may not actually be considered business assets. Universities accept the patent and book them as charitable donations, generally at much less than the valuation determined by an accounting firm.

Universities also should set criteria for accepting donations of patents in part because of the cost of maintenance. The research office and technology transfer offices should coordinate the donation with the advancement and finance offices to determine appropriate process and valuation for institutional purposes. Some the considerations include:

> Does the technology match a research area at the institution?
>
> Is there a researcher interested in furthering the patented technology?
>
> Are funds available to further develop the technology?

The institution must be willing to work within specific timelines for acceptance and be willing to devote significant staff time to the process. Cost for accepting and maintaining the patent and the cost of any regulatory requirements must be factored into the decision about whether or not to accept patent donations (Martin, 2003).

Legal and Regulatory Considerations

Institutional requirements for compliance with legal, statutory, and regulatory requirements do not lessen when funds are accounted for as gifts. Compliance with federal and state laws and institutional policies are irrespective of source of funds. The requirements for compliance with human subject rules and regulations must adhere to institutional policy. Most, if not all institutions of higher learning, extend the requirement for review and oversight of all human subjects research regardless of funding source. The consequences of bypassing the institutional review board (IRB) generally extend to all human subjects research. Protection of animals is equally critical and no research should be conducted without appropriate institutional animal care and use committee (IACUC) review. All of the Environmental Health and Safety requirements are imposed, as are the safety and security laws including research that could be impacted by immigration laws, the Patriot Act, and other bioterrorism regulations.

Conflict of interest policies should cover projects that are supported by gifts, as well as by contractual arrangements. The opportunities, both real and perceived, can be equal to conflict of interest on any contractual arrangement. A faculty member who has a consulting arrangement with a donor or who owns stock or equity with a donor is subject to the same opportunities for the relationship to influence outcomes or conflicts of interest. Management or oversight of gifts should be equivalent for gifts and grants and contracts. Similarly, falsification, fabrication, and plagiarism, while infrequent, are as great a concern when gift funds support research as when the research is contractual. Misconduct in scientific endeavors is blind to source of funding.

The legal liabilities that an institution accepts may be equivalent or even greater with acceptance of gift funds. Whereas contractual and restricted grants must comply with mutually accepted terms and conditions, contributions come without the legal protections contractually defined. Despite this, the institution is accountable for compliance and liable for legal and regulatory infractions. A gift transaction provides no opportunity to obtain indemnification from the donor for liability that the recipient might incur in the performance of the research. Thus, the entire liability rests with the researcher and the institution. For example, a gift made to the institution of a particular biological material could be found to be toxic or otherwise hazardous. If this material was not transferred under a material transfer agreement (MTA), all liability for damages caused could fall back to the receiving institution.

Acceptance of a donation with a verbal agreement to provide access to any invention or other intellectual property (IP) can be a serious problem. Intellectual property generally belongs to the institution and may be licensed out exclusively or nonexclusively. An informal agreement or arrangement that the donor would have rights or access to the IP is contrary to university and possibly federal policies and could result in negating any effort to patent or license the technology. In a worst-case scenario, the institution may patent and license the invention, only to find out that the IP had earlier been disclosed to the donor. Informal agreements of any nature increase the risk to the institution.

Making Determinations: Important Questions to Consider

Questions that should be asked frequently when determining the nature of funds and whether they are to be handled as a gift or contractual arrangement include:

- *Who will be the primary beneficiary?* If it is the donor or sponsor, the award should be handled under a contractual arrangement.
- *Does the donor derive a tangible benefit other than a potential tax credit?* If so, the funds awarded are not gifts.
- *Is there a quid pro quo? Is the institution or principal investigator required to provide the donor with any deliverable?* Assurance to the donor that the funds were used for the purpose for which they were donated does not constitute a quid pro quo.
- *Can the sponsor require the institution to return the gift if the donor is unsatisfied with the outcome of a project which it supported?* If the funds were provided with no expectation of outcome or deliverable, then they can be properly considered a contribution. For example, a donor contributing to a scholarship fund rightfully expects that the funds would be used for that purpose. However, if the sponsor was unsatisfied with the outcome of a research project and requested a refund, the funds were not contributed. Gifts are considered irrevocable while restricted grants and contracts can be terminated for poor or nonperformance or unavailability of funds as well as a variety of other reasons.
- *Can a project that is funded on a cost reimbursement basis be considered a gift?* There may be exceptional circumstances where it would be appropriate, but generally the receipt of funds as reimbursement would not be counted as a gift.

- *Can funds be provided partially as a gift and partially as a contractual arrangement?* Funds can be transferred as both a gift and contract. However, intent and use of the funds should be reviewcd, as well as any relationship between the sponsor and recipient. It is difficult to separate a portion of a project supported by a gift and the portion that is contractual. For instance, an institution may agree to a contractual arrangement to develop a new nano-particle. The sponsor also provides funds to support a graduate student. If the student works on the same project it may be construed as circumventing the contractual process. A gift must have charitable intent and the expectation and distinction between the gift and contract must be clear.
- *Can an individual donate funds to the institution and take a tax credit?* This is best answered by a tax specialist on a case-by-case basis, but one option is to ensure that the donor does not derive direct benefit from the donation and has no control over use of the funds. For example, the employee may donate the funds to a scholarship program administered by the alumni office, which would not be under the control of or benefit the individual.
- *Can gift funds be used as matching or cost sharing for federal grants and contracts?* Gifts are a viable and desirable source of matching funds and cost sharing. However, if the funds are used to cost share federal dollars, the funds become restricted and are subject to OMB Circular A 21 and any specific sponsor restrictions. The funds should be handled using whatever cost-sharing methodology is consistently used by the institution.
- *Can government funds be counted as gift funds?* It is not likely that either state or federal funds would be transferred as gift funds. Generally public funds come with restrictions that exceed minimal requirements to be counted as a contribution and as a general rule, governments are not legally authorized to make gifts to not-for-profit organizations.

Summary

The collaborative efforts between the offices of research and development can benefit the individual interests, goals, and missions of each. Tension that arises from the offices may be generated from lack of communication and differing requirements and need for reporting and accounting for donations and grants and contracts. The fact that numerous laws and requirements determine how and to whom reporting is made increases the importance of good communication.

• • • References

CASE. *Management and Reporting Standards for Annual Giving and Campaigns in Educational Fund Raising*, 3rd ed. Washington, DC: Council for the Advancement and Support of Education (CASE), 2004.

Martin, David. Patent Donations—The Tale of Intangibles. Special Report Prepared for Department of Treasury, Internal Revenue Service, 2003.

18

Federal Relations, Advocacy, and Lobbying in the Research Environment

William Schweri, MS

Why should research administrators concern themselves with, and engage in, federal relations? We are already busy in our careers—sending new program information to the right researchers; helping researchers develop competitive proposals; assisting them to get their proposals out the door to meet the next, fast approaching deadline; reviewing another subcontract; analyzing data for the report that is already late; and juggling a dozen projects at one time. Research administrators do seek to stay current on events in the executive branch of the federal government. There is a high priority placed on staying informed about the latest changes in regulation, interpretations of cost principals, implementation of new funding programs, or changes in proposal submission deadlines. Often, research administrators lack knowledge about happenings in Congress. On Capital Hill, policy decisions are made which set the annual R&D funding levels, provide direction for new programs, and initiate changes in current funding programs. Put simply, Congress enacts new laws that directly impact the programs in the executive branch which fund research. While research administrators have traditionally focused on events in federal funding agencies, they have neglected to note events in Congress that drive funding levels, regulations, and policies. Research administrators need to know the basics about congressional funding and relations to be efficient and effective. This chapter provides a basic outline for research administrators on how to successfully manage federal relations.

The Changing National Priority for Research

After Sputnik was launched in 1957, science became a top priority in the United States. Science also became the focus for national defense. The support for and understanding of the federal-university-private partnership had never been greater. Since the end of the Cold War, however, there has been a lower priority placed on R&D funding by Congress. The members of Congress understand that the development of new knowledge and technology is critical to the new economy (based on early innovation) in the United States. However, the need for science as an economic driver has never reached the same level of importance as science as a driver for national defense, nor will it in the near term.

Congress reacts to public opinion and sets priorities based on greatest need. The management of the largest budget deficit in US history, funding of critical social programs such as Medicare and Social Security, and the costs of national and homeland defense are all issues that weigh heavily on decisions made in Congress. Research is but one issue, and from a budget standpoint, a small piece of the larger picture (the administration proposed a $2 trillion budget for FY 2005). The American Association for the Advancement of Science (AAAS) reported in its analysis of the FY 2004 Federal budget, "a $127 billion federal research and development (R&D) investment in FY 2004, a $9.5 billion or 8.1 percent increase" over FY 2003 (AAAS, *Highlights*, 2004). This increase was concentrated in defense, health, and homeland security. The administration's proposed budget request for total federal R&D in FY 2005 is $132.0 billion, $5.5 billion or 4.3 percent more than FY 2004. The AAAS's *Highlights, 2004* reports "the entire increase would go to Department of Defense (DOD) development of weapons systems and R&D in the new Department of Homeland Security (DHS), leaving all other federal R&D programs collectively with declining funding. Total research (basic and applied) would stay flat (up 0.2 percent) at $55.7 billion, even including DHS' expanding research efforts" (AAAS, 2004).

In addition to flat R&D budgets, the research enterprise has been damaged by the numerous allegations of ethical misconduct ranging from conflicts of interest to inadequate protections for research subjects. It is obvious to anyone who reads the newspaper that there have been numerous, well-publicized instances of scientific misconduct in recent years. In his book, *Science, Money and Politics*, Daniel Greenberg outlines a series of events beginning with the endorsement of commercial products by professional associations and ending with the death of a subject attributed to gene therapy (Greenberg, 2001). Greenberg describes in Chapter 22, "The Ethical Erosion of American Science," how the interplay of greed, the lack of institutional ethical surveillance and enforcement, and the pressure to be first with a discovery have eroded the ethical foundation of the enterprise (Greenberg). This has caused a loss of trust in the mind of the American public and where public opinion goes, Congress is soon to follow.

In the current environment, research is not an entitlement and frankly, it never has been. It certainly has had a higher priority in the budget process than it enjoys now, but there has never been a set percentage or a specific budget number that is set for research. In a tightening discretionary budget picture, research has some tough competition with higher priorities winning. While the National Institutes of Health (NIH) budget was doubled by Congress over a five-year period, other R&D budgets have not increased. The basic research funding at National Aeronautics and Space Administration (NASA), Department of Energy (DOE), Department of Defense (DOD) and National Science Foundation (NSF) has remained rather static, not enjoying the same largess bestowed on NIH (AAAS, 2005).

Advocacy

Never has there been more need for those who are supporters of science to take a leadership role and become vocal advocates for research. An advocate should be differentiated from a lobbyist. A lobbyist conducts activities with the objective of influencing public officials and public policy; he/she seeks to secure passage of legislation by his/her influence. An advocate is an individual who pleads the cause of another. While both might use similar methods, the advocate makes the case for his or her issue at various levels including personal, community, state, and federal. The advocate often becomes an opinion leader in the community or institution. The lobbyist usually focuses on the members of a legislative body in an attempt to influence policy outcomes. Personal advocacy for research may be no more than an individual engaging a friend or acquaintance in a conversation detailing an important discovery by a local scientist and why it will make a difference in people's lives. The same activity can be applied to community leaders, state legislators, and congressional staff. Articles about new discoveries and their potential impact in local, statewide, and national newspapers and magazines serve to highlight the importance of research. Advocacy tends to be informative in nature and education is the intended outcome. With considerable knowledge of new discoveries and ongoing research projects, research administrators can be excellent individual advocates for research. They can also be very helpful to their institution's federal relations effort.

Research administrators can provide aggregate institutional data about the amount of activity (numbers of people, numbers of sponsored projects, and amount of funding) in a specified area of research. They can identify senior experts in their unit or institution who can be engaged in a variety of ways, providing expert advice or testimony to Congress. Research administrators can give specific examples of problems created by federal policies and how much it actually costs to comply with federal regulations. They can also identify problems in new policies before they are enacted into law and offer solutions that will work at a practical level.

An example of this is the response that Senate Bill § 2031 received when introduced by Senator Leahy (D-Vermont) in the Senate Judiciary Committee. The proposed legislation would have presented many problems for state universities. § 2031 was written to "restore Federal Remedies for infringements of intellectual property by States" (Intellectual Property Protection Restoration Act of 2002).

The proposed legislation would do that by "limiting ownership of intellectual property" by states that did not waive sovereign immunity relating to that property infringed upon (Leahy, 2002). In short, the legislation would have made it impossible for a state university to prosecute an infringement of its intellectual property if the state did not waive sovereign immunity to allow for suits concerning state infringement. The ploy was to hold the universities' ability to protect intellectual property (rendering the IP useless to the university) in order to get states to allow software manufacturers the ability to seek relief from illegal use of their software by state agencies through a partial waiver of sovereign immunity. This would have been devastating to state universities trying to develop new technology for commercialization. Clearly, states would not provide even a partial waiver of sovereign immunity. The cost of a partial waiver in comparison to the amount gained through university royalties would have been astronomical and the anticipated increase in litigation made the suggestion of a partial waiver a ridiculous proposition from the standpoint of the state.

Mr. Rich Harpel, formally with the National Association of State Universities and Land-Grant Colleges (NASULGC), organized an effective campaign to amend the legislation. He sought the cooperation of a number of major state universities, a number of university associations including the American Association of Universities, and the National Governors Association. Research administrators in intellectual property offices at numerous universities provided information about the potential impact of the legislation. This information was used to make the case for the losses that would be incurred through royalty income, numbers of new start-up companies lost, and the overall loss of new economic development that this legislation would cause. In the end, § 2031 did not make it out of the Judiciary Committee because a majority of the members realized that the negative impact outweighed the benefits. In addition, many members of the committee thought it inappropriate to hold the universities hostage in an attempt to stop states from illegally using software.

University Government Relations

Universities engage in government relations for a variety of reasons at the state and federal level. Federal relations and state relations efforts usually seek to preserve institutional interests and advance new

interests. This is usually done in a systematic way coordinated by an office of state relations and an office of federal relations. Sometimes these activities are found in the same unit (often reporting to a VP for external affairs or community relations) and sometimes they are separate offices reporting to two different upper level administrators. Frequently, the office of federal relations reports to the chief research officer but this is not always the case. Regardless of where they reside within the institution, the offices are systematically engaged in facilitating new opportunities, advancing the institutions interests and responding to faculty concerns. Frequently, researchers will be notified through their contacts within a federal agency or by their professional society that there is a change being contemplated which will have a positive or negative impact on their area of science on the funding that supports their work. Responding to these proposed changes and seeking to diminish the potential for a negative impact while supporting the potentially useful outcomes is important to the individual researchers and to the institution.

The primary areas of impact for federal relations include research policy, authorization, appropriations, and regulatory development. There are various stages of the budget process and the reauthorization process that might provide an opportunity to have a positive impact for research issues. The administration sends a budget request to Congress in early February. This request is the culmination of months of work to develop a budget proposal and budget justification by each of the agencies in the executive branch. The Office of Management and Budget, acting for the President, compiles the budget proposal. After the budget request is received by Congress, the House and Senate pass a budget resolution that initiates the budget process.

It is in the appropriations process that considerable effort is expended to secure funding for individual projects and for supporting recurring budget increases in programs that benefit an institution. For example, if an institution relies heavily on a particular program in the Centers for Disease Control, it is in the institution's best interest to support a budget increase in that program. There are numerous disease-related groups (most are nonprofit associations) that work to increase funding for the specific disease important to the associations' members. Every year, there are attempts to increase funding for diseases such as diabetes, various cancers, neurological degenerative diseases (e.g., Parkinson's), and heart disease. It is also during the appropriations process that various constituent groups request direct appropriations for specific projects (also known as "earmarks"). As each of the appropriations bills is passed independently in the House and Senate, a conference committee is formed of members from both houses to work out the differences in the two bills. The conference report is then taken back to the floor of the Senate and House for a floor vote. Once passed, each appropriations bill is sent to the President for signature or veto. There are opportunities to increase funding for research in the appropriations process until the conference process is completed.

University Strategy

Effective federal relations efforts at the university level are normally organized and systematic. The most effective federal relations efforts are based upon a well-developed strategy, are highly organized and, most important, institutionalized. The internal organization for advocacy usually is centered in the president's office with support from an office of federal or governmental relations. These offices may report to various upper level administrators but to be effective they must coordinate the overall effort of the university. It is critical that everyone in the institution understand the federal relations policy and how it is translated into practice. Communication is the key factor in maintaining a systematic approach to federal relations. Communication must be clear from the unit level up and from the president down within the organization. In addition to vertical communication, there has to be clear horizontal communication so that units, colleges, and upper level administrators are engaged as necessary. Above all, information must flow through the office of federal relations.

The decision-making process to set institutional priorities should be transparent (although the outcomes may not be). All concerned parties should know how institutional priorities are set and, generally, what they are. This is important to ensure that the message from the university to the delegation is the same, regardless of the messenger, and that the possibility of miscommunication that might be confusing to the members and their staff is reduced as much as possible. Congressional staffers appreciate a uniform message and a set of priorities that are not constantly in a state of flux. This makes their job easier, and with precious little time, they can concentrate their efforts on those items that are most important. Administrators and faculty are

often asked by their professional society or a group representing their area of research to contact their congressional representatives in support of an issue or to voice concern over problematic language. It is important to consider where these requests rank on the priority list and whether it is in the institution's best interest to support the request. By all means, an individual—as an individual—should contact his/her elected representative when he/she wishes. Individuals do not, however, have the right to act on behalf of the institution unless that authority is delegated to them. Contacts by researchers and administrators who have not communicated with the federal relations office first are likely to cause some confusion among the delegation. Frequently, in cases where there is excellent rapport with the delegation staff, there will likely be a follow-up phone call from staff to the federal relations office to determine the institutional priority, if any, placed on a request that has come from anyone suggesting that they are speaking for the institution.

When faculty members are asked to respond to a grassroots request to contact their congressional representatives there are a number of issues that need to be considered. Most important is whether this issue affects them directly. A few years ago, the American Physical Society sent out a message to all of their members asking that they contact their congressional representatives to ask them to support funding for a new accelerator facility. A number of researchers sent letters and made phone calls. One staff member became curious about the sudden influx of calls and letters and returned the calls of a few of the faculty. When he asked faculty how the new accelerator would impact their research, he was told that it would not impact their research and that they would not use the facility. They were simply trying to be good members of their professional society and respond to the call for assistance. Needless to say, this diminished the staff member's interest in working on the issue. These contacts would have been much more effective if they had come from researchers who intended to use the facility and could explain, in lay terms, how the new facility would benefit their work and even better, how it would benefit the district or the state.

Do Your Homework

When working with members of the delegation and their staff, it is critical that information that fully characterizes the issue being discussed be gathered.

It is not enough to know only one side of an issue—indeed, this will frequently lead to failure. All aspects of an issue must be explored and counter arguments to the opposition's position must be developed. A complete understanding of who is interested in an issue must also be considered. Frequently, there are numerous groups focusing on an issue from their own unique perspective. Knowing who is supportive of your position and who is not supportive is very important. This is often critical information to provide to the delegation staff and it is important for the institution. Sometimes, the friends of an institution may be on the opposing side. This can be a sensitive situation for the university and should be dealt with in a forthright manner. In other situations, friends outside the institution might make very effective advocates if they agree with the institution's position and have a strong relationship with the member of Congress. Gathering information is the first logical step in preparing to contact a member of the delegation.

Before making contact with the delegation, it is also important to determine where an issue falls on the university's priority list. This usually determines the degree to which an issue is pursued or how hard it will be worked and that, in turn, will determine how the delegation will be notified. Everyone engaged in an effort to advocate a position must understand where the issue resides on the priority list. If different individuals approach the delegation with differing degrees of intensity, there will be unnecessary confusion. External priorities must also be taken into account. It is too easy to create confusion by focusing on an issue that is not consistent with the external priorities that an institution has as a part of its mission or message.

In developing a case for or against an issue, having the facts is an absolute necessity. More importantly, facts should be carefully formatted into a clear, concise picture that makes the case for or against an issue. Factual information about the impact of a policy or funding for a new program is very useful to staff. Research administrators are particularly good at organizing summary information that can be used in an effective manner. For example, when requesting an increase in funding for a research program, it is critical to know how much work in the specific area is being conducted by your institution. Determining the number of sponsored projects in a specific area such as energy, cancer, or education is very important in that it makes a clear case for the expertise found in an institution. The total funding from a specific program, number of researchers supported, new dol-

lars leveraged with federal dollars and specific outcome measures (adoption of a process, a new company formed based on new intellectual property, numbers of people served, or extension activity) are useful in making the case for increasing a program budget. Increasingly, delegation members are asking for assessment measures to demonstrate that the funded project was worthwhile and produced the anticipated results.

Who Should Be Involved?

From an institutional standpoint, it is necessary to involve those individuals who either have something to contribute to the process or those who can support a request. The upper level administration must be involved in the setting of priorities and faculty must work with their unit heads and deans to ensure institutional support for a project. If they are to succeed, new programs must fit within the priorities of the unit and college. Without the backing of the college and unit, it is unlikely that upper level administrators will place a high priority on a project and that needed resources will be made available. The sponsored projects staff can provide substantive information about the current volume of work in an area and demonstrate that the critical skills necessary for a new project are extant. They can also provide trend data indicating growth or decline in an area of funding. This information can be invaluable in making the case for support.

The alumni association and public affairs office can also play a role. For projects that will impact a specific part of a state, it is very useful to have individuals from that area contact their congressional representative. This is frequently done using business owners who have a vested interest in the research or who will likely benefit from the research. This allows an institution to reach out to a congressional representative from another part of the state for assistance on projects important to their district. The public relations office is also very useful in assessing the potential public reaction to a new project. Controversial projects are usually avoided because the institution, the member, and the community are seeking win-win situations. That is usually not the case when there is opposition to a controversial project at the local or state level. The public relations office can also play an effective role in developing a strategy to thank a delegation member for his/her hard work on behalf of the institution.

For large projects, it may be necessary to involve entities outside the institution. Frequently, consortia are developed between two or more institutions where there is complementary expertise and common interest in a project. Consortia are made up of universities, other nonprofit agencies, state agencies, or private companies. Frequently a consortium is formed with institutions from different states. This is useful politically. In this case, the members from more than one state can lend support to the project and enhance the probability of securing funding. Each of the consortia members must bring research strengths to the effort and they need to be complementary. A well-integrated effort from a number of institutions is more likely to secure support than a loose amalgam of noncomplementary partners. In addition, larger consortia can often focus on a larger project that will benefit a number of states.

It is important to include federal agency staff in early conversations to ensure that the focus of the proposed project fits within the agency's mission and objectives. It is critical that the proposed project fit with in an agency's funding authority. The key is to find the right agency and program, and then target the project to that program. Often, an agency will have considerable interest in a project but does not have the budget to support the activity. When this occurs, it is necessary for the institution to try to raise the level of funding in the agency budget sufficient to fund the proposed project. Another reason to involve the agency is that if it expresses interest in the project, that information can be communicated to the congressional staff to help support the development of the project. Of course, some agency staff never see projects they do not like if it means an increase in their budget and Congressional staffers are well aware of that.

Working with Congress

All institutions must develop and maintain an excellent working relationship with the delegation. This includes the members, the staff in Washington, and the staff at the state and local (district) level. Frequent communication and interaction is the key to developing this relationship. Hosting visits to an institution by members and staff is an excellent way to educate them about areas of strength and areas of emergent interest. Field trips to the state, hosted by a number of partners, are also very useful because they tie other activities in the state to programs at the institution. The best time to plan a visit

or field trip is during a recess for holidays or during the summer recess in August. Visits to campus should be scheduled to expose the members and staff to the top researchers in an area of emphasis or to a facility that supports a broad range of researchers with similar interests. It is important to expose them to the areas of research that are being promoted for new or additional funding. A schedule with the names of the researchers, their titles and addresses should be provided in advance of the visit. Social and athletic events also provide an excellent opportunity to get to know the staff and members better. Every opportunity should be used to maintain a close working relationship. An example of a field trip that focused on biotechnology was recently conducted by the University of Kentucky. A senior staff member who worked on agricultural issues in Senator McConnell's office took the lead in organizing the delegation staff for the field trip. Over a three-day period, the visiting staff received a primer on biotechnology in lay language from an internationally known researcher, they learned about current and planned research activities, and they saw how biotechnology is being commercialized. They met new entrepreneurs starting new companies and visited companies that are well established to see how biotechnology is driving new products and services. They learned about the challenges that these companies face to remain viable in the competitive market. The field trip was accomplished with the cooperation of a number of companies working with the university. During the field trip, the visiting staff had dinner with representatives of the leading biotech firms in Kentucky and were the guests of the university at an athletic event. Events like this can impart a lot of information very quickly to the visitors. This is useful information for staff because they can and do use it in their jobs. It is always better to have a knowledgeable advocate working to support your activities.

Making Contact

There are a number of different ways to contact the delegation when working an issue or promoting a project. Letters are the most common way of communicating. These come from individuals, groups, and institutions. Since the events of September 11, 2001, and the subsequent anthrax attack, heightened security has slowed the mail service to Capitol Hill offices. Most letters are now faxed to the office of a congressional representative or senator and the original may or may not be sent in the post. Meetings with staff to brief them on an issue of concern or to describe a new project can also be effective. However, congressional staffers have more than enough work and limited time; therefore, meetings should be used only when necessary. Meetings should be kept short and on point. A breakfast or luncheon briefing for a group of staff on a new project held at the institution or on Capitol Hill can be an efficient use of time. This is especially true if a project will impact all of the state and support is being sought from the entire delegation. A breakfast briefing can provide all of the information necessary in a short time, allow the staff to consider how they can work together, and provide a uniform message to everyone.

Preparation

Meetings, briefings, and even phone calls must be carefully prepared for in advance. The central issue has to be clearly and concisely defined. If a bill is to be discussed, the bill number and the part of the bill to be addressed must be cited. For example, in title VII of the L/HHS bill last year, a number of primary care physicians asked for increased funding for primary care resident fellowships. Most were well prepared with a briefing document that noted the specific legislation, last year's funding level, the administration request, and the amount needed to continue the program. Most institutions had hard facts about the number of residents funded by the program in primary care departments, the amount of funding received, and why this is important to the medical school and the state. This is the appropriate way to seek support. Staff should not have to look up basic information. We should provide it to save the staff time and to focus their efforts quickly. A few of the primary care physicians seeking support were not so well prepared and they were much less effective in their attempt to seek support. In his 1996 book, *Working with Congress: A Practical guide for Scientists and Engineers*, William G. Wells describes a comment from a senator who says, "they were with me for twenty minutes, and when they left, I still had no idea why they had come to see me" (Wells, 1996, p. 68). It is wise to make a clear request early in the conversation and end with the request as well. It may well be that a member cannot help with your particular issue, but if the member does not know what you are asking him or her to do, he or she certainly will not be able to help. Every contact should begin with a clear statement of what you want followed by facts that make your case.

Timing

In his book, Wells notes that timing is important; in fact, it is everything. Recently a group went to Washington to request support from their senators for a project in their community in the FY 2004 budget cycle (Wells, 1996, p. 67). They went to visit in August 2003. The timing was bad. First, they were told that the appropriations process, which began in February 2003 for FY 2004, was far along in the process and it was too late to make an addition. The second problem they encountered was that the Congress was in summer recess and the members and many staffers were either back in their respective states or on vacation. To be effective in federal relations, one must become knowledgeable about the congressional process and stay up to date on the congressional calendar. It is also helpful to know a bit about your delegation and the staff. Where are they from? What are their interests? Do they have ties to your institution (alumni, friend, or a family member connection)? These are all good things to know and can provide clues as to how well they might know an issue and whether they may have more than passing interest in a topic. This also allows you to avoid ignorant gaffes during conversation.

Briefing Document

One of the most effective ways to work with Congress is to develop a one-page briefing document. This is something that can be handed to members and staff at a visit, faxed to the office, or included in a thank-you letter (or e-mail) after you have contacted them initially by telephone or in person. A briefing document should be clear and concise. It should have a descriptive title, identify the institution, make a specific request, and clearly describe the issue (bill number and section), name any partners, explain any anticipated impact on the institution and state, and include factual information (for example: amount of funding, number of people served or affected, effectiveness to date, etc.). It is usually much more important to explain the local and state impact to members of the House. While they might be interested in the national significance of a project, they are more interested in how it will impact their district. A well-written briefing document can be very helpful to staff. It focuses their attention quickly on the specific legislation in question, provides a justification for the project or position, and makes clear what you are requesting. It is also important to indicate how a project, if that is the nature of the request, will be sustained after federal funding ends. It is not always easy to reduce a complex issue into one page but it is necessary. A well-written briefing page saves a lot of time, which is always appreciated.

Networking and Leveraging

Building a competitive project that will be received well by the federal government often involves more than one institution and sometimes a number of partners. Building a winning team is critical to the success of any project, but for congressional projects, there is more to it than having the best science. Building a project with a team that may include a variety of partners (for-profit, nonprofit, unaffiliated medical institutes, service providers, as well as state and federal agencies) does revolve around good science. It is almost impossible to hide a weak team member. But there is more that has to be considered. First, it is important that the scientists can work together. There may be reasons why they cannot or will not work together, and if this is the case, the project is probably doomed to failure. The compatibility of the researchers is the first concern, if they want to work together on the project, they will find a way to do it. They may also find areas where they need additional expertise. They will need to consider what expertise they need and who should be included to fill those needs. Before a decision is made to include a new team member, it is necessary to consider which of the potential team members will bring the most to the effort. Assuming that there exists ample scientific expertise, the political potential of the new team member must be considered. Frequently, joint projects are developed by institutions in states that have congressional members on key committees (e.g., appropriations committees). Recently, a team joint project was developed among a group of engineers who had very similar interests and worked together well. They did not consider the political ramifications of the team. As a result, they had two member institutions in states that brought nothing to the table politically. One state did not have any appropriators on important committees, and the other had an appropriator but he was a junior member of the minority party. The project was not funded because there was not enough political muscle to support the project.

It is also important to assess the relationship that an institution has with its delegation before an invitation to join a team is extended. If an institution is in a state with a powerful congressman or senator but has a poor relationship with that member, it is unlikely to attract support from that member for the project. Networking and developing clear lines of communication are critical to the team development process. Again, it is important to seek the advice and council of various people within the institution to ensure that the strongest team is built. Once the team is built, communication remains important. Without the ability to communicate at various levels among consortia members, there is a diminished likelihood of success. It is important that administrators communicate with their counterparts and that the scientists likewise communicate with theirs. Obviously, within the institution it is also critical that there be clear and frequent communication among researchers and administrators.

It is often the case that a project can attract both state and federal support. In addition, if there are business partners, there may be an opportunity for them to invest in the project as well. Leveraging a commitment from the state and/or an industry partner or an industry association can be beneficial. Congressional members usually like to see support from the state or industry because it demonstrates the need for the project, reduces federal costs, and implies a lower level of risk for all of the funding sources. Frequently, leveraging agreements are built like a house of cards. Funding is available if, and only if, the state, federal and industry funding is secured. It becomes an all-or-nothing proposition. If one funding source is lost, all of the funding is lost. Some leveraging agreements involve two sources of funding and are quite simple. Others can be quite complex as in the case of a multipartner consortia. Large consortia may include multistate support, multiagency support, and industry support. Generally, the larger the leveraged deal, the bigger the payoff, if funded. The risk is often worth the expenditure of time, effort, and other resources.

Working on the Big Issues

There are many major issues that impact all of a particular sector. Often these issues are the focus of large professional associations. This is certainly the case with higher education. In her 1998 book, *Lobbying for Higher Education*, Constance Cook provides an excellent insider's view of how the higher education community is organized to push forward its agenda. She describes the coordinated efforts of what she calls the big six higher education associations including the American Council on Education and its five largest members, the Association of American Universities (AAU), National Association of Independent Colleges and Universities (NAICU), National Association of State Universities and Land-Grant Colleges (NASULGC), American Association of State Colleges and Universities (AASCU), and American Association of Community Colleges (AACC) (Cook, 1998). These associations work in concert on the large legislative activities such as the reauthorization of the Higher Education Act. They also work independently (or two or three together) on issues such as increases in the level of funding for science and engineering. They provide an invaluable service working on the major issues that are important to the higher education community; these are issues upon which there is consensus. These associations often focus on the macro level, while the member institutions work on the same issues at the micro level. This can be a very effective strategy.

There are many issues upon which there is no consensus and others which are important to an individual institution. Many institutions have found it both necessary and productive to hire firms to represent them (Heinz 1993, p. 30). Usually an outside firm is hired to represent the institution as a whole, to represent the interests of a unit, or to work on a specific project or initiative. Outside firms typically have only one or two specific points of contact to keep communications clear and priorities in order. The firm must know the university's strengths and research capabilities to be effective. A firm can open doors not previously available to the institution and expand the network of the institution. An outside firm can also do some things that the institution cannot do or does not wish to do, and, most importantly, a firm can make indirect approaches to potential supporters or partners.

Summary

In summary, success in federal relations requires clear communication, careful planning, an organized approach, and institutional support. Control of the facts and data to support a position or a project is critical. Research administrators can bring an effective set of skills and experience to any federal relations initiative that involves research. Their command of institutional data on the quantity and quality of an institution's research activity can be very useful in making the case for support. With a basic understanding of the federal relations process, research administrators can be productive members of the team working to develop support for a project.

References

AAAS. Congressional Action on Research and Development in the FY 2004 Budget. *AAAS R&D Budget and Policy Program* in cooperation with the Intersociety Working Group. Washington, DC: American Association for the Advancement of Science, 2004.

AAAS. Congressional Action on Research and Development in the FY 2004 Budget. *Highlights.* http://www.aaas.org/spp/rd/ca04high.htm (accessed June 5, 2004).

AAAS. R&D Programs Face Another Rough Year in 2006; Cuts for Many, Gains for Space and Homeland Security. 2006. http://www.aaas.org/spp/rd/prel06pr.htm (accessed May 15, 2005).

Cook, Constance Ewing. *Lobbying for Higher Education: How Colleges and Universities Influence Federal Policy.* Nashville, TN: Vanderbilt University Press, 1998.

Greenberg, Daniel S. *Science, Money, and Politics: Political Triumph and Ethical Erosion.* Chicago: The University of Chicago Press, 2001.

Heinz, John P., Edward O. Laumann, Robert H. Salisbury, and Robert L. Nelson. *The Hollow Core: Private Interests in National Policy Making.* Cambridge, MA: Harvard University Press, 1993.

Intellectual Property Protection Restoration Act of 2002, § 2031, 107 Congress, 2nd Session, 2002.

Wells, William G. Jr., *Working with Congress: A Practical Guide for Scientists and Engineers.* 2nd ed. Washington, DC: American Association for the Advancement of Science, 1996.

19

Establishing a Clinical Trial Research Program

Bruce Steinert, PhD, and Elliott C. Kulakowski, PhD, FAHA

Introduction

The body of scientific knowledge advances at an ever-increasing rate and the resulting medical therapies save countless lives each day. The translation of discoveries from the laboratory to practice depends on clinical research. Advancing technology, changing social attitudes, and some notorious ethical misdeeds have combined to shape the development process for new medical products: lengthy, expensive, and highly regulated. A recent survey of the pharmaceutical industry found that bringing a new drug to market costs more than $800 million dollars.[1] Much of this expense includes the cost of research at academic medical centers, hospitals, and research institutes to support the approval process required to bring a new product to market.

Clinical research is funded by a variety of sources including pharmaceutical, biotechnology, diagnostic procedure and medical device manufacturers, federal and state agencies, foundations, and individual hospitals and universities. The underlying concepts for administering studies supported by this diverse collection are similar, although each has unique requirements. In the interest of brevity, this discussion focuses on industry-sponsored pharmaceutical studies. This chapter explores clinical research administration and the establishment of a clinical trials research program.

Drug Approval Process

The entire drug approval process from discovery to approval by the Food and Drug Administration (FDA) for marketing can take as long as 15 years. The drug development process begins with "preclinical" research. Preclinical research includes the initial discovery and analysis of the new compound, screening for metabolic activity, and testing in research animals. By the time the new compound is ready for testing in humans, much is already known about its chemical properties, processes for manufacture, purification, and delivery. Its pharmacokinetics and pharmacodynamics (absorption, distribution, metabolism, excretion, and toxicity) have been measured in a number of animal species. The clinical (human) investigation of the compound starts with the filing of an investigational new drug application (IND) with the appropriate regulatory agency [e.g., Food and Drug Administration (US), European Federation of Pharmaceutical Industries and Associations (European Union); Ministry of Health, Labor and Welfare (Japan)]. The IND incorporates the results of preclinical research and describes the manufacturer's overall plan to continue the testing in humans.

Clinical trials are categorized according to how much is known about the compound or device being tested.[2] The studies supporting a marketing approval application are comprised within three phases. In Phase I studies, the first testing of the new article in humans is based solely on the preclinical results. These studies are of short duration and limit the research population to a few dozen "healthy" research participants who do not have the disease for which the drug is intended. Similar to animal studies, the drug is examined for its pharmacokinetic and pharmacodynamic properties and the potential side effects of the new compound are examined. Phase I studies often involve lodging the research subjects within the research facility, precisely scheduled sample collections, and complex chemical and statistical analyses. These studies tend to be conducted by experienced investigators at well-equipped study sites.

Phase II and III studies are more complex and build on the knowledge gained in the Phase I studies and involve progressively larger study populations for longer time periods. The goal of the Phase II and III studies not only includes additional safety data, but also an investigation of the efficacy of the therapeutic agent in a population with the condition intended to be treated. Phase II studies generally have more restrictive inclusion criteria for study participants, while Phase III participants may have other co-morbidity illnesses.

In some cases, the FDA may require a manufacturer to collect additional data on effectiveness and safety of an approved drug.[3] In addition, the sponsor of the study or a research institution may propose other studies to gain more insight into the agent in a more diverse population. Such studies are called Phase IV or "postmarket studies" and can involve tens of thousands of patients. Because the drug in Phase IV studies has already been approved by the FDA for marketing, these studies tend to be simpler in design and can be accomplished by less experienced staff and institutional support. These are excellent studies for a novice investigator to gain research experience before tackling the more complex investigations.

Reasons to Conduct Clinical Trials

Institutions conduct clinical trials for several reasons, and there are direct and indirect reasons for conducting clinical trials. William Tester, MD, a Philadelphia oncologist, describes the direct reasons for conducting clinical trials simply as consisting of "smiley faces, microscopes, and dollar signs."* The

*Tester, William, personal communication, 2000.

studies are done simply for the benefit of the patient, "the smiley faces." Physician researchers also conduct clinical trials for the knowledge that can be gained, which Dr. Tester represented as microscopes. These can be Phase II, III, or IV. A particular study may or may not benefit a particular study participant, but adds new knowledge that can possibly aid future patients with the same illness. It also is anticipated that every study will result in new knowledge about the investigation's drug or device, whether positive or negative from Phase I through Phase IV. Finally, studies are conducted because they generate revenue for the physicians or their institution. Every study conducted involves all three study phases. The difference is that, for example, some studies may provide more knowledge about a particular drug, while having little direct benefit to a particular patient. This often occurs in early studies of new therapeutic agents, but as a particular agent is shown to be beneficial to patients, the focus of the studies changes to the benefits that are provided to a patient.

There also are indirect benefits for physicians being involved in clinical trials. They can mean an increased reputation to the investigator. The investigator is able to publish the results of the studies in which he/she participated and it can increase his/her reputation. This can lead to other sponsors wanting the investigator to do more studies and as the investigator's reputation becomes well-known and received, more patients are attracted. Similarly, the reputation of the physician's affiliated institution is enhanced. People want to be treated at academic medical centers that are performing cutting edge research because they want access to the latest treatments for their diseases.

Reasons to Establish a Clinical Trial Research Program

There is much work to be done prior to initiating any clinical trial regardless of phase or complexity, however. Clinical trials can be managed by individual physicians, by sections within departments such as the pulmonary section within a department of medicine, at the departmental level, or at the level of the hospital, medical school, or at the institutional level. A coordinated clinical trial research program (CTRP) may be most effective. The CTRP can be administered through a single clinical trials office within the institution, within a major department such as a department of medicine, or it can be established as a virtual program that is highly integrated and distributed throughout the institution's various departments, but draws upon the most efficient use of expertise and facilities. The more localized the program, the fewer services it generally provides.

The program infrastructure needed for a given clinical trial will vary greatly depending on the investigator and institution, so this discussion centers on the needed expertise, rather than making assessments about staffing levels or position descriptions. Institutions with a few Phase III or IV studies conducted by experienced investigators may well provide adequate support at the department or clinic level using incumbent medical and administrative staff in conjunction with their nonresearch responsibilities. However, as the research program gains experience with more and increasing complexity of studies, the need for central administrative support and facilities becomes rapidly apparent. A CTRP can provide services at a level of standardization and efficiency not possible at department or clinic level.

Academic Medical Centers (AMC) were once the leaders in conducting clinical trials research, but because of their long and cumbersome processes, the pharmaceutical industry began to conduct more studies at sites not associated with academic medical centers. In response to the loss of clinical trial activities that AMCs were experiencing, many institutions implemented processes to streamline their clinical trial activities and to become more competitive for industry studies.

CTRPs were established to provide a variety of services. The services might include training; standard operating procedures; establishment of a centralized pool of clinical research coordinators; identification of potential studies; protocol review; materials preparation for review by the institutional review board (IRB); patient research participant recruitment; case report form review; business development; budget development; contract negotiation; and invoicing. It should be noted that each and every CTRP does not include all of these topic areas and other sites may offer other services.

Training

The success of any clinical trial program depends on the training and education provided to participants, including physicians, clinical research coordinators (usually nurses or physician assistants),

other support personnel, and patients who eventually agree to participate in the clinical research studies. A list of organizations that provide training and a list of training resources is in Table 19-1.

Physician Researchers

The ultimate responsibility for any clinical trial research rests with the physician investigator.[4] However, the study sponsor has the responsibility to select investigators who are "qualified by training and experience" in the conduct of clinical trials through Phase IV. This requires the investigator to be more than the health-care provider for subjects enrolled in the trial. The same is true of the other medical and administrative staff.

Medical school curricula do not generally place much emphasis on clinical research, so it is left to the institution and investigator to establish appropriate staff development goals. Being a physician investigator is a challenge. The new physician investigator must become familiar with clinical trials in general, the procedures of the IRB, contract negotiations, and the role of the institution's research office. At the same time, the academic physician has the increasing pressures of clinical service, teaching, and administrative duties.

To be able to balance all of these activities and to conduct clinical research takes a trained team and the ability to increase efficiency. Data Edge (now a subsidiary of Fast Track Systems, Inc.) once reported that for the period of 1988 through 1995, over half of physicians conducting clinical research completed

TABLE 19-1	Research Associations and Resources

- Association of Clinical Research Professionals (ACRP; http://www.acrpnet.org)
- Association of University Technology Managers (AUTM; http://www.autm.net/index_ie.html)
- Code of Federal Regulations and Federal Register (http://www.firstgov.gov/)
- Drug Information Association (DIA; http://www.diahome.org)
- Institutional Review Board Forum (http://www.irbforum.org/forum/3)
- Public Responsibility in Medicine and Research/Applied Research Ethics National Association (PRIM&R/ARENA; http://www.primr.org/membership/overview.html)
- National Council of University Research Administrators (NCURA; http://www.ncura.edu/)
- Society of Clinical Research Associates (SoCRA; http://www.socra.org/)
- Society of Research Administrators International (http://www.srainternational.org/newweb/default.cfm)

only one clinical trial. In these cases, it can be speculated that the physician investigator was not fully trained to be a successful clinical investigator.

Training to physicians is important. The old medical school model still applies. Physicians learn to conduct clinical trials from more senior experienced physicians. However, this model suffers from the fact that bad habits or outmoded procedures can be taught to the new physician investigator. There are books that are written on how to be a clinical investigator and a physician can attend sessions at their professional associations or participate in clinical investigator training, such as that provided by the Drug Information Association. Finally, institutions that conduct significant numbers of clinical trials have established their own internal training programs for physicians.

Clinical Research Coordinators

While the principal investigator (PI) has ultimate responsibility for all clinical and administrative aspects of the study, this does not require the PI to be personally involved in all phases of a study. The regulations permit the PI to delegate, in writing, specific duties to other trained and experienced associates, although the PI maintains supervisory responsibility for all persons working on the study at that site. Appropriate delegation can provide an investigative site with considerable staffing flexibility and cost savings.

The backbone of any clinical research program has become the role of the clinical research coordinator. Clinical research coordinators are generally registered nurses or physician assistants, but there is no requirement for that level of certification. A coordinator, who is also a licensed RN, is be able to take on more clinical research responsibilities than one with lesser qualification, although the reduced labor cost of non-RNs may be advantageous for certain types of studies. In general, study coordinators with clinical responsibility should undergo much the same clinical research training as the investigators.

Coordinators with nonclinical duties should be trained on regulatory and administrative issues. So important is the role of the clinical research coordinator that professional associations have been established for them that offer certification programs, such as the Association of Clinical Research Professionals (ACRP) and the Society of Clinical Research Associates (SoCRA).

Certification is not yet required by study sponsors, but is looked on favorably as a demonstration of achievement and commitment to quality. Research-related training should not be limited to the investigators and coordinators as the impact of conducting clinical research can reach any level of the institution.

Other Clinical Research Support Staff

Physicians or their medical departments or clinical sections cannot be involved in clinical research unless they have the support of the ancillary services provided at the academic medical center. A comprehensive academically-based clinical research program requires that not only the physician investigator and the clinical research coordinators be trained in clinical research, but those involved in any aspect of the clinical research process need to have appropriate knowledge of their role and procedures that need to be followed: this can include, for example, pharmacy, radiology, medical records, and offices that deal with issues of the Health Insurance Portability and Accountability Act (HIPAA).[5] Each of these units does not need to know the level of detail as the physician investigator or clinical research coordinator. The impact of HIPAA on research is discussed in Chapter 53.

However, ancillary personnel need to know their roles and the expectations of them and must have appropriate standard operating procedures for managing clinical research protocols. For example, the vast majority of studies are conducted in collaboration with the involvement of the pharmacy department. If pharmacy is unable to add a study to their workload or is unwilling to participate in a study, it is difficult for it to be involved in clinical research. Pharmacy staff must be trained not only in the importance of why clinical research should be conducted, but also trained in their roles as participants and have the capability to handle, store, track, dispense, report, and dispose of the experimental pharmaceutical agent. In addition to general training, the staff also should be included in any initial physician and coordinator discussions about potential new therapeutic agents that are being planned so that they can ensure the pharmacy can meet any particular study requirements.

The CTRP can be instrumental in implementing a comprehensive training program. The training needed, again, depends primarily on the type research to be conducted and whether the study is supported by federal or nonfederal funds. When the investigators, clinical staff and administrators at all levels understand the regulations, responsibilities, and ethical implications of clinical research, management of the research becomes much easier. Table 19-2 lists some of the important regulatory and nonregulatory topics that should form the core of a comprehensive training program. This list is not intended as a course syllabus, but should suggest the level of information to include. Fortunately, there has been a recent emphasis on investigator and research administrator education. Several professional associations have developed training materials and conduct periodic meetings and training sessions (see Table 19-1). Additionally, many consulting companies will provide onsite training for many aspects of clinical trial management.

Standard Operating Procedures

To be an effective site for conducting clinical trials, there should be standard operating procedures (SOP). The SOP should cover every aspect of con-

ducting a clinical trial, including: training, identification of potential studies, protocol review, IRB support, research participant recruitment, collecting and reporting of data, case report form preparation and review, business development, budget development, billing and invoicing, and contract negotiation. They should describe how an activity is to be conducted and who is responsible for conducting the activity. Such procedures demonstrate professionalism and good business practice, and sponsors very often want to see them before they allow you to conduct a study.

Centralized Clinical Research Coordinators

For some institutions it can be very efficient to have a centralized pool of clinical research coordinators. Large departments that conduct multiple studies may have their own clinical research coor-

TABLE 19-2	Clinical Research Training

Research Overview
- Drug and device development processes
- Ethical background—Belmont Report, Declaration of Helsinki, responsible conduct of research
- Study design—Protocol, randomization, blinding
- Regulations
- FDA—Title 21
- HHS—Title 45
- Department of Transportation—Hazardous materials regulations
- International—International Conference on Harmonization, European directives
- State and local regulations, institution policies governing research

Investigator and Sponsor Responsibilities
- Important study documents and disclosures
- Meetings—Investigator, initiation, monitoring, close-out, audit
- Working with a contract research organization (CRO)
- Grants vs. contracts
- Budget development

Protecting Study Subjects
- IRB requirements—Approval process, continuing review
- Informed consent process—Consent form, vulnerable subjects
- Adverse event reporting, safety monitoring
- Recruitment and retention of study subjects
- Study documentation and record keeping
- Source documents
- Case report forms, queries, corrections, electronic recordkeeping
- Drug storage and accountability
- Record retention requirements

Site Management
- Standard operating procedures
- Staff utilization
- Budget management—Billing

dinators. However, clinical departments may not want highly trained clinical research coordinators on their staff because they do not conduct a significant number of studies to warrant paying the added cost of these higher priced professionals when they are doing studies. In this instance an institution may elect to have a pool of clinical research coordinators.

It has been estimated that a clinical research coordinator may be able to manage about four to six clinical studies at one time, depending on their complexity. These studies would be at various stages in the life cycle of the study. They may consist of studies just beginning, some at the stage of patient recruitment, and some that are in follow-up stage. Staffing should be sufficient to allow coverage of the studies and should allow for contingencies, for example, if one (or more) coordinator is attending a study orientation meeting or is on vacation.

In this case, the clinical research coordinator could be involved in a pulmonary study, a neurology study, and a psychiatry study. Depending on the institution's configuration, it may be advisable for study participants to have offices and examination rooms in a central location for the clinical studies.

Study Identification

The identification of clinical studies for an institution can be a reactive or proactive process. In the reactive model, a pharmaceutical company contacts the institution about a study that is already in progress. In this model, a company learns about a physician investigator at your institution, and then contacts the investigator to determine interest in a study. This is very unproductive for an active clinical research program, because many opportunities may be lost.

In a proactive model, someone within the institution seeks out prospective studies. This may occur at a CTRP, at the department level, or at the institutional level. The individual reviews pharmaceutical-related publications and identifies prospective studies planned to begin within six months to a year or identifies current studies that are recruiting research participants. The individual then prepares a list of such studies, shares the list with appropriate physician researchers to determine their interest, and examines records to identify if there might a sufficient patient population to enroll in the study. If there is an interested physician investigator and an appropriate study population, the pharmaceutical company is contacted. While the institution may or may not be chosen by the company, contact that may result in future opportunities for the institute has been made.

Protocol Review

The study sponsor provides the institution with a copy of the study protocol after a confidential disclosure agreement has been signed (see p. 185). The review of the protocol can be accomplished by the physician investigator, a clinical research coordinator in the physician's office or department, or by a coordinator who is part of the CTRP. Regardless of who reviews the protocol, it is the physician investigator's responsibility to know what is being asked for in the protocol.

The protocol review examines in detail the requirements that the investigative site must meet in conducting the study. One of the most important requirement considerations involves a thorough understanding of the inclusion and exclusion criteria. The review should determine if the study population exists for the study. In addition, the review must identify the number of participant visits and procedures to be performed, in addition to creating a flow chart for the study. The protocol review is also important to identify those procedures that are routine standard of care and those that are solely for research or data collection purposes. This review is also useful in building the budget and in preparation of materials for IRB submission.

IRB Support

Every clinical research study must be reviewed and approved by an institutional review board (IRB) prior to the study being initiated. The IRB is responsible for ensuring that the study is conducted in conformance with the Belmont report;[6] to confirm that there has been a risk benefit assessment; that the risks to the subject have been minimized; and that there is an appropriate informed consent process and document. The IRB can be associated with the institution, a local or a national IRB.

As part of every protocol, the pharmaceutical sponsor includes what it has determined to be an appropriate informed consent document. If the institution has its own IRB, it generally has its own informed consent form template format and certain clauses or language that the institution requires.

Institutions that have a centralized clinical trials office often provide IRB support. These individuals may be research nurses or administrative personnel with appropriate knowledge about IRB regulations and the institutional requirements. This support includes putting the sponsor's informed consent document in the format of the institution, completing the necessary transmittal documentation forms and questionnaire, and submitting the completed package to the IRB. Depending on the practices of the IRB, the clinical trial program staff person who provided IRB support also may attend the IRB meeting along with the physician investigator to discuss the protocol and answer questions. This person also is responsible for responding to any questions identified during the review and making any appropriate modifications to the informed consent document.

The role of IRB support personnel is much less if a centralized IRB is used. In this instance, IRB support may be limited to ensuring that the sponsor obtains the approval from the central IRB and that the appropriate approvals have been obtained by the institution. Where an institution has its own IRB and allows the use of a central IRB, the IRB support staff's role consists of coordination of information between the sponsor and central and institutional IRB.

In an institution that does not have a centralized clinical trial office, there is a need for these activities in every clinical department or clinical section that is engaged in research. These activities often are conducted by the clinical research coordinator. Depending on the size of the research program in a department, such duplication of effort can be costly to the institution. A centralized process appears to make more sense. However, centralized IRB support personnel need the active participation of the investigator and clinical research coordinator as questions and issues arise.

Patient Recruitment

Some clinical trial programs offer integrated patient recruitment. One of the first things an institution must accomplish is to educate potential patient research participants about the need to conduct clinical trials. Once that has been accomplished subjects can be actively recruited into clinical studies.

There are so many bad headlines in the media that talk about all the problems of clinical research. Prospective patient research participants must be educated about the value of clinical trials if they are to be involved in clinical research program. One of the best ways is to have materials about the value of clinical research and have these readily available in the waiting rooms. Information can also be made available on the institutional Web site. Staff with whom participants interact must be able to answer questions about being a clinical research participant or be able to refer patients to someone who can answer their questions. A CTRP can work with the institution's marketing department to develop appropriate handouts and in development of information for the Web site.

Once patients have been educated, they are ready for study recruitment. Patients can be recruited through a centralized clinical trials research program Web site that includes information about specific studies and provides information about whom to contact. Radio, television, and newspapers are also sources for patient recruitment.

Beyond the activities already discussed, some institutions with active clinical trial programs have an individual or a bank of operators available to answer calls from patients or family or friends of a prospective patient about a particular study. Individuals are able to call into a call center, a local number, or toll free number, with general or specific questions about a study that can be answered by friendly and informed operators. Answers about specific studies are often limited, scripted, and approved in advance by the IRB. Call centers allow the recruiter to collect data about a particular subject with consent of potential research participants and use the data for later study follow up. The recruiter can also schedule appointments with physicians for research coordinator if the subject is interested in learning more about a particular study. The patient recruitment database can also be used to collect information about patients who want to become informed about a future study for a specific disease. These types of activities are best conducted through a centralized clinical trial office.

Case Report Form Review

A centralized CTRP can be a useful resource in reviewing case report forms (CRF). A CRF is a document developed by the pharmaceutical company sponsor that is used by the site to summarize information collected about a research participant. The document may be paper or electronic. As data (history, physical, laboratory results, and information for research participant visits) is collected, it is entered into the patient's medical record and abstracted as required on the CRF. When a research participant completes the study, the CRF is submitted to the sponsor of the study. This research participant information allows a pharmaceutical company representative (called a monitor) to verify data as the study progresses.

If there is a sufficiently staffed CTRP at a department level or at a central office, the research coordinator or health information specialist can review the CRF and compare it to the medical record before submission to the sponsor. The completeness and accuracy of the CRF is very important to the sponsor, as it can reduce the amount of time their study coordinator needs to spend at the institution. Reliable data is the most important thing to a sponsor: if the data are complete and accurate, sponsors are more likely to use the study site and/or the investigator for future studies.

Business Development

The purpose of business development (also known as marketing) is to make an institution known. An institution may include the greatest team of clinical researchers in the world, but the institution will not get clinical studies if the pharmaceutical industry does not know about such resources. Business development is best conducted through a centralized CTRP that works closely with a public relations department.

The pharmaceutical industry seeks out researchers who are experts in the medical discipline that relates to the therapeutic agent that they are studying. These individuals are often identified through publications in scientific journals and from presentations that they make at national and international meetings. Being an author or a presenter is one form of marketing. Well-organized clinical trials programs are also effective, active forms of marketing.

Institutions should have a developed, actively advertised marketing message that clearly represents the institution's qualifications and unique qualities. The design must be professional and consistently, widely, and professionally presented.

Advertising can take the form of brochures, Web sites, mailings to pharmaceutical companies and clinical research organizations (CROs), booths at national and international meetings, and included in presentations at professional association meetings.

An institution's brand identity should be easily recognized and associated with the institution's strongest attributes. The message should be simple and catchy and should include a brand identity (logo or phrase); historical background of the institution; a description of the institution's unique qualities and list of services, size and uniqueness of patient population, areas of expertise, contact information; and any other information about pertinent information that "sells" the institution's qualifications.

One institution created as its brand identity, "Advancing Medicine Through Collaboration with Industry," to present itself as a partner in the development of new therapeutic agents' medical devices or biotechnology. The brand logo was used throughout its media campaign.

Exhibiting at Meetings

The largest meetings for the pharmaceutical industry are the Drug Information Association (DIA), and the Association of Clinical Research Professions. Between 1993 and 1997, the number of sites that exhibited at DIA increased from 2 to 17.[7] While more recent figures are not readily available, attendance at these meetings seems to show a growing number of investigator sites exhibiting. The brand identity and message should be consistent with, for example, the brochure. In addition, many of the sites also attempt to attract attendees to their booths by providing small tokens of remembrance (a pen or calculator with the brand logo and contact information, often a Web address). Others hold raffles for gifts (e.g., digital cameras) where business cards of pharmaceutical representatives are collected and drawn and the cards later used as contact information (mailings, e-mails, or calls).

Utilizing the Internet

In 2001, CenterWatch reported on the number of clinical research sites that were utilizing the Internet as a means of marketing, citing that sixty-five percent of all academic medical centers advertised on the Internet and targeted the pharmaceutical industry and prospective patients.[7]

The Web site should contain the institution's brand identity and be consistent with the overall message of the institution. A Web site can be readily updated and expanded and its content can include:

1. An introductory description of the institution;
2. The administrative leaders of the clinical trials research program;
3. An area for potential sponsors that can list the description of what makes the institution unique, departments and subspecialties with biographies and expertise of individual physi-

cian investigators, a list of ancillary services that could be provided such as radiology, pathology, bio-statistical services, and a description of the size and uniqueness of patient population,

4. A link for patients that includes a description of why patients should consider being involved in clinical trials; a list of active studies that are recruiting patients; a brief nonconfidential description of the study and eligibility requirements; and a contact name and number, and;

5. Links to other sites related to clinical trials such as the FDA and clinical research organizations such as ACRP and DIA and general clinical research news items.

It should be noted that any announcements about a particular study should be approved in advance by the IRB and, in some cases, the sponsor to avoid violating any confidentiality agreements that may have been signed with the sponsor.

External Publications and Web Sites

There are a number of Web sites and hardcopy publications that list clinical research sites and their levels of expertise. Again, the brand logo and message should be consistent with the program's mission. These sites publish general information about a site for a fee and may also include a breakdown by specialty. They also may serve as a marketing extension for your program by providing links to your site.

Local Media

Marketing also includes use of local and regional radio, television, and newsprint. General articles or short segments about the institution's clinical trials research and about those conducting state-of-the-art research at the institution attract interest in both the physicians and the institution. For these segments, the institution's public relations department should be engaged to publicize the public benefits about the institution's clinical research. Other types of public education include the direct advertisement of the need to recruit subjects for particular studies. These are targeted types of marketing activities for specific studies and are generally paid for by the sponsoring pharmaceutical company. The benefit of such activity is two-fold: it attracts potential study participants and it gets the name of the institution out in front of the public.

Clinical Trial Budget Development

Developing a budget that meets the needs of the institution and the sponsor is among the more challenging aspects of clinical research administration. The

costs of conducting the study should be an important consideration when evaluating project feasibility. Industry sponsors continually seek ways to accomplish more research at lower cost, which results in a "Catch-22." Charging too little to conduct clinical studies may jeopardize the institution's research program, while high costs will drive sponsors to other study sites. Additionally, there are compliance considerations for health care providers when federal assistance or medical insurers are to be billed for routine medical costs of research subjects. A high level of consistency, accuracy, and regulatory compliance is more readily accomplished by a centralized budgeting process within an organized CTRP than by individual investigators or departments.

Many sponsors prepare study budget projections using benchmarking reports from databases such as CROCAS (Contract Research Organization Capability Assessment Service)* and TrialSpace™ Resource & Cost Estimator.** These compile the costs and capabilities of CROs, contract central laboratory facilities and investigative sites, and provide analyses on cost ranges for various geographical regions.

Budgeting Concepts and Best Practices

This section presents an overview of budgeting concepts and best practice recommendations. Research budgets generally involve three cost categories: direct costs, contingent costs, and indirect costs.

Direct costs are actual costs to the institution for physician and clinical coordinator, time and effort, research related tests, procedures, labor, and facilities required to conduct the study. These are generally negotiated with the sponsor as a per subject cost. However, many institutions build their budgets on a cost per procedure budget and then determine the cost per subject charge. For the purpose of prorating payment for subjects who do not complete all study visits or procedures, negotiating a cost breakdown by study visit is good business practice.

Any professional or other ancillary services should be identified in advance and included in the budget negotiations. Some studies may require professional interpretation of tests (e.g., electrocardiogram or computed tomography scan), while others may request only the machine-interpreted tracings

---

*Information on CROCAS is available at http://fast-track. inverseparadox.com/pdfs/TrialSpace_CROCAS_PBT.pdf.

**Information on TrialSpace is available at http://www. fast-track.com/.

or film images for interpretation elsewhere. These costs need to be established appropriately.

For in-hospital studies, the cost of a bed-day needs to be determined. Will the sponsor be charged the full bed rate, full bed rate plus, the insurance rate, the Medicare rate, or other rate? At minimum, the Medicare rate must be charged.

Additionally, start-up and close-out costs allocable to a particular study should also be considered direct costs. Start-up costs may include such items as protocol review; preparatory chart reviews; administrative fees for contract and budget preparation; establishing study records for pharmacy, laboratory, or ancillary departments; preparation and presentation of the IRB application; IRB review fee; and any equipment or upgrades (e.g., software) needed to conduct the study.

Close-out costs will depend on the type of study. Pharmacy, laboratory, and department records may be closed and may require internal or external audit (e.g., disposition of the investigational product). Study records, case report forms, and source documents should be organized and stored. The length of time needed to archive records depends on the sponsor's marketing application schedule and regulatory requirements of the country to which the sponsor submits licensing application. Data for a Phase I or early Phase II study may need to be stored for a decade or longer. Advances in storage technology can pose a significant challenge to archiving study data. If the data are recorded on media other than paper, a means of retrieving the records (e.g., laptop computer, digital tape reader) should be archived as well. However the data are stored, it is generally a good idea to contact the study sponsor prior to destroying any study-related records. Start-up and close-out costs should be independent of subject enrollment (or IRB approval) and should be non-cancelable.

Sponsors of clinical trials are required to monitor the progress of the trial. This monitoring process is not usually budgeted as a direct cost. However, the number and frequency of these routine monitoring visits should be established in advance as they can be disruptive to clinical staff schedules.

The direct costs of study-related tests, procedures, and services can be difficult to determine. This is not because the calculations are overly complex, but rather that many hospital and medical center accounting systems are designed to track billing and reimbursements using negotiated rates based on treatment codes such as diagnosis-related groups (DRG), current procedure terminology (CPT), or healthcare common procedure coding system (HCPCS) rather than by individual line item. Determining the actual cost of a test or fair market value of a service may require some assistance from the accounting department. Maintaining a current database of research costs by the CTRP can significantly reduce the time needed for budget development.

Some expenses, although directly allocable to the study, do not have predetermined costs. Such items may include investigator or coordinator time for obtaining informed consent. The duration of the consent process varies according to the complexity of the study or study procedures, expected ease of communication with the study subject, or need to use an interpreter. A few such cases will not likely disrupt the conduct of the trial, but if unusual circumstances are anticipated in recruiting subjects, any arrangements should be negotiated with the sponsor in advance. Similarly, not every subject who signs a consent form will meet the requirements for participation for the duration of the study resulting in "screening failures" and early withdrawals. These subjects will be excluded from further study activities and an allowance should be negotiated to cover the costs of study-related procedures conducted prior to the withdrawal.

Additional study costs relate to anticipated, but unscheduled events. These "contingent" costs are only relevant if the triggering event occurs (see Table 19-3) and provision for these events should be negotiated with the sponsor prior to initiating the study.

Indirect costs or facility and administrative (F&A) costs are rare in the for-profit business world. They are generally built into the total budget and are not costed out separately. As a result, the inclusion of indirect costs in clinical trial budgets is tolerated, but not well understood by industry sponsors. In research supported by nonprofit sponsors

TABLE 19-3	Contingent Budget Costs

- Protocol amendments requiring IRB review
- Consent form revision including costs of language translation and certification
- Documentation and reporting of serious or unexpected adverse events
- Monitoring visits in excess of the agreed frequency or duration
- Unscheduled monitoring in preparation to a regulatory agency audit
- Advertising
- Reimbursement of care to treat adverse effects

(e.g., federal or state governments and foundations), indirect costs are intended to cover the costs of non-allocable expenses supporting the research, which are borne by the investigating institution. Their purpose in industry-sponsored studies is the same, although the method of calculation may differ.

The F&A rate for government is determined through a detailed negotiation governed by the type of research institution (e.g., OMB Circulars A-21 or A-122) and an audit of institutional research facilities and expenses (e.g., clinical and nonclinical research facilities, maintenance, equipment, utilities, administration.)[8,9] Research conducted for industry sponsors utilizes these facilities and services and their support is appropriate and necessary. The indirect cost rate applied to industry-sponsored clinical trials should be determined through careful analysis of expenses even though there are no regulations to guide the process.

In the end, however, budget negotiations are just that—negotiations. Within the legal, policy, and ethical boundaries of the parties, there is a wide spectrum of possibilities to meet everyone's needs. Cooperation, communication, and timeliness in budget negotiation set a positive stage for a long-lasting business relationship.

While on the topic of research finances, a trend that is gaining popularity in industry-sponsored clinical trials is the use of incentives to improve performance at investigative sites. Incentives can be categorized into performance-based or enrollment-based incentives. Performance-based incentives generally depend on the investigator achieving specified performance standards such as increasing data entry accuracy or decreasing the number of data queries, timely submission of case report forms (CRF), or addressing data queries within a specified period. The additional payment would ostensibly reimburse the institution for additional labor costs to involve, for example, additional personnel entering or abstracting data, or for performing internal CRF audits prior to submission. Enrollment-based incentives provide additional payments, offer future research contracts, or provide other tangible gains to the institution contingent on a defined enrollment milestone by a certain date or within a specified time period. Such payments are disturbing as they may introduce financial or ethical conflicts of interest for the investigator and institution. Each institution should establish policies to address and procedures to monitor these forms of incentive payments.

It is also critical to determine actual charges that are attributable to standards of care versus what is part of the research study. Standards of care are normal and customary procedures that are part of care for the patient whether or not the patient is part of a clinical research study. The charges associated with the treatment or procedures are billable to the patient or their third-party insurer. The research charges are those directly related to conduct of the clinical study, are in addition to standard of care, and are not subject to third party coverage. For example, if the standards of care included a single echo cardiogram, this would be covered by the patient or their third party payer. However, if a second or third echo cardiogram were required as part of the study, the cost should be borne by the sponsor of the study. The institution must have procedures in place for ensuring that third party payers are not billed inappropriately for charges that are above standards of care, and even more importantly that may result in double-dipping where, for instance, the pharmaceutical sponsor and Medicare are both billed for the same activity.

Clinical Trial Contracting

Generally there are two agreements that must be signed for each clinical trial: the initial confidentiality agreement and the clinical trial agreement. During the course of the study there may be several amendments made, if the protocols change, the study is extended, or when there is additional enrollment of subjects.

Confidential Disclosure Agreement

A confidential disclosure agreement (CDA) is an agreement between the pharmaceutical company and the institution or the investigator, depending on institutional policies. The sponsor will want the signed CDA as assurance that proprietary and confidential information disclosed to the institution and/or investigator is kept confidential. The CDA presents the first opportunity for the institution to manage its risk exposure. It is unlikely that a physician investigator has time, expertise, or institutional authority to negotiate the CDA or subsequent clinical trial agreement.

CDAs should be reviewed, negotiated, and approved by an institutional official with expertise in handling such agreements and signed according to the institutions policies and procedures. The agreement specialist may be an attorney in the institution's legal office or a nonlawyer who is sufficiently familiar with clinical research processes and institutional policies (e.g., indemnification, publishing results, intellectual property ownership, liability, reports to the National Practitioner Data Bank[10]) to make informed judgments. Nonlawyers may include grants and contracts administrators in the sponsored projects office or negotiators in the technology transfer office.

Clinical Trial Agreement

The clinical trial agreement is the major agreement between the institution and the sponsor of the clinical trial. It spells out the terms for the mutual responsibilities of conducting the study. For an academic institution there are four major areas of a clinical trial agreement. They can be considered the four "Ps": protection, publication, property, and payment. Protection includes indemnification, insurance, and subject injury clauses. An academic institution as part of its mission also must maintain its ability to freely publish the results of its research activities. Therefore, publication rights are of utmost importance to academic institutions. Property rights refer to intellectual property. Every clinical trial agreement needs to identify who owns the intellectual property of a study and what are the limits of ownership. This includes what is owned by the sponsor and who would own any intellectual property not related to the clinical trial. Finally, the payment schedule is of importance to the institution to be sure that it receives appropriate and timely payment based on the budget developed.

It is not the intent of this chapter to discuss in detail clinical trial contracts. Those are described in Chapter 20 in this book.[11] It is the intent to make the reader aware that to negotiate clinical trial agreements takes skills that are available through the institution's general council office or the sponsored projects office. Some institutions have separated clinical trial agreement negotiators from their office of sponsored projects and located them in their clinical trials offices. However, others have found this to be cost ineffective and the contract negotiators remain in the sponsored projects office, but are considered part of the virtual clinical trials research program.

While some institutions conduct their contracting through the CTRP, others continue to do it through their sponsored projects office. Recently, we have heard that some institutions that did their clinical trial contracting through a centralized CTRP have reverted to having their sponsored projects office do the contracting because it was found to be more cost effective.

Invoicing for Clinical Trials Activities

One of the biggest issues regarding clinical trials is the appropriate allocation of charges between actual study costs and those considered routine medical costs. There must be appropriate measures in place to appropriately allocate these charges. This may be done at the time that costs are charged or at the end of a research participant's visit or at the end of their enrollment in the study. Staff within a centralized or virtual CTRP must be appropriately trained to review and appropriately allocate the charges. These charges may be for physician and coordinator time, laboratory services, and inpatient hospital charges.

Once charges have been appropriately allocated, invoicing must be done to ensure appropriate payments. This can be done through the department or from staff in a CTRP. There must be an appropriate tracking method for receipt of payment from the sponsor and distribution of funds to the department and for ancillary services.

Summary

Clinical research is vital to continuing improvements in health care. There is no one specific model that works for every institution. An effective and efficient program can be accomplished in many ways: through a decentralized process where departments and physicians manage their own clinical trials, through a centralized CTRP for all related activities, or through a virtual CTRP. Most institutions have a virtual CTRP where some activities are centralized and others are decentralized. The services that are centralized vary greatly among institutions and depend on institutional culture.

• • • References

1. Grabowski, H., J. Vernon, and J. DiMasi. "Returns on Research and Development for 1990s New Drug Introductions." *Pharmacoeconomics* 20, no. 3 (2002):11–29.
2. "Phases of an Investigation," Title 21 Code of Federal Regulations Part 312.21, revised as of April 1, 2004.
3. "Phase 4 Studies," Title 21 Code of Federal Regulations Part 312.85, revised as of April 1, 2004.

4. "Selecting Investigators and Monitors," Title 21 Code of Federal Regulations Part 312.53, revised as of April 1, 2004.

5. Selwitz, A. S., H. Lake-Bullock, and J. R. Brown. "The Impact of Health Insurance Portability and Accountability Act (HIPAA) on Research." In *Research Administration and Management,* edited by Elliott C. Kulakowski and Lynne U. Chronister, 557–565. Sudbury, MA: Jones and Bartlett Publishers, 2006.

6. Department of Health and Human Services. "The Belmont Report," 1979, http://www.hhs.gov/ohrp/humansubjects/guidance/belmont.htm (accessed July 11, 2005).

7. "AMCs Finding and Fueling Growth." *Center-Watch Newsletter* 8, No. 8 (2001).

8. Office of Management and Budget Circular A-21. Cost Principles for Educational Institutions, revised May 5, 2004, http://www.whitehouse.gov/omb/circulars/a021/a21_2004.html (accessed August 28, 2005).

9. Office of Management and Budget Circular A-122. Cost Principles for Non-Profit Organizations, revised May 10, 2004, http://www.whitehouse.gov/omb/circulars/a122/a122_2004.html (accessed August 28, 2005).

10. "National Practitioner Data Bank for Adverse Information on Physicians," Title 45 Code of Federal Regulations Part 60, 1989.

11. Slocum, J. M., "Legal Issues in Clinical Trials." In *Research Administration and Management,* edited by Elliott C. Kulakowski and Lynne U. Chronister, 189–206. Sudbury, MA: Jones and Bartlett Publishers, 2006.

20

Legal Issues in Clinical Trials

J. Michael Slocum, JD

Introduction

The regulation and control of new drugs in the United States has been based on the New Drug Application (NDA) process since 1938. The NDA application is the vehicle through which drug sponsors formally propose that the Food and Drug Administration approve a new pharmaceutical for sale and marketing in the United States (Figure 20-1). The data gathered during the animal studies and human clinical trials of an investigational new drug (IND) become part of the NDA.

The NDA process permits the FDA to decide:

- Whether the drug is safe and effective, and whether the benefits of the drug outweigh the risks.
- Whether the drug's labeling is appropriate and what the package insert and other labeling should contain.
- Whether the manufacturing methods and the quality control are adequate to preserve the drug's identity, strength, quality, and purity.

The documentation required in an NDA is comprehensive, including details on the drug's composition; the results of the animal studies; the specifics of how the drug behaves in the body; and manufacturing, processing, and packaging. However, the core of the NDA is information obtained during clinical tests or trials. The research that develops this information is central to the drug development process and much of this activity is at many major research institutions (Figure 20-2).

Definition of a Clinical Trial

The National Institutes of Health (NIH) define a *clinical trial* as:

A clinical trial (also clinical research) is a research study in human volunteers to answer specific health questions. Carefully conducted clinical trials are the fastest and safest way to find treatments that work in people and ways to improve health. Interventional trials determine whether experimental treatments or new ways of using known therapies are safe and effective under controlled environments. Observational trials address health issues in large groups of people or populations in natural settings.[1]

The NIH identifies several types of clinical trials.[2] These are:

Treatment Trials. Test new treatments, new combinations of drugs, or new approaches to surgery or radiation therapy.

Prevention Trials. Look for better ways to prevent disease in people who have never had the disease or to prevent a disease from returning. These approaches may include medicines, vitamins, vaccines, minerals, or lifestyle changes.

Diagnostic Trials. Are conducted to find better tests or procedures for diagnosing a particular disease or condition.

Screening Trials. Test the best way to detect certain diseases or health conditions.

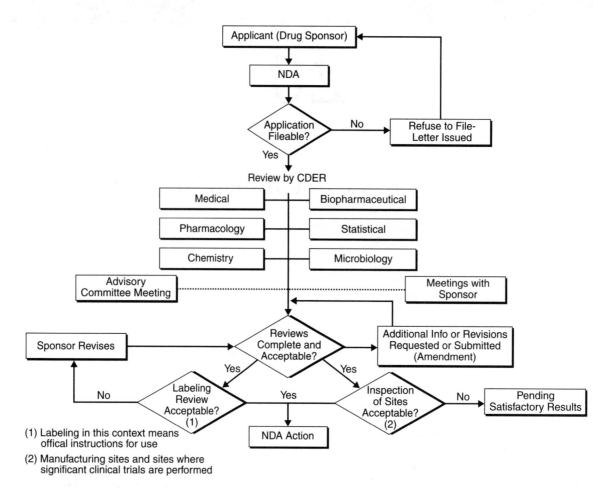

FIGURE 20–1 New Drug Application Process.[3] U.S. Food and Drug Administration Center for Drug Evaluation and Research. NDA review process. Available at: http://www.fda.gov/cder/handbook/nda.htm (accessed July 29, 2005).

<u>Quality of Life Trials (or Supportive Care Trials).</u> Explore ways to improve comfort and the quality of life for individuals with a chronic illness.

The US Food and Drug Administration (FDA) regulates most clinical trials conducted in the United States. Under the applicable federal law, controlled clinical trials are the only legal basis for the FDA to conclude that a new drug or device has shown "substantial evidence of effectiveness, as well as confirmation of relative safety in terms of the risk-to-benefit ratio for the disease that is to be treated."[4]

Clinical Trial Phases

Clinical trials are conducted in phases (Table 20-1). The trials at each phase have a different purpose:

Phase I. The new drug or treatment is tested in a small group of people (20 to 80) for the first time to evaluate its safety, determine a safe dosage range, and identify side effects.

Phase II. The study drug or treatment is given to a larger group of people (100 to 300) to see if it is effective and to further evaluate its safety.

Phase III. A large group is given the study drug or treatment (1,000 to 3,000) to confirm its effectiveness, monitor side effects, compare it to commonly used treatments, and collect information that will allow the drug or treatment to be used safely.

Phase IV. Postmarketing studies delineate additional information including the drug's risks, benefits, and optimal use.

New Drug Development Overview

The clinical trial process starts with a sponsor,[5] (most often, a pharmaceutical company) working to develop a new drug or device. By the time clinical

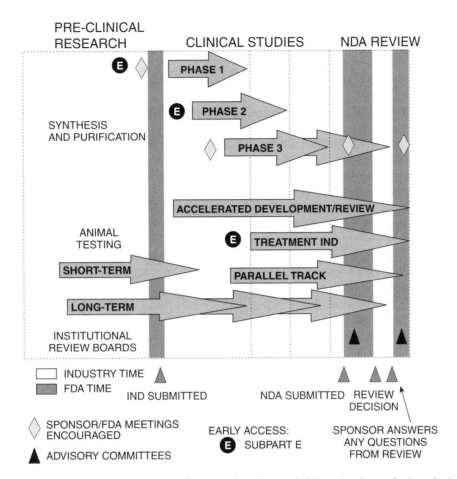

FIGURE 20–2   Drug Development Process in the U.S.[6] U.S. Food and Drug Administration Center for Drug Evaluation and Research. The new drug development process: Steps from test tube to new drug application review. Available at: http://www.fda.gov/cder/handbook/develop.htm (accessed July 29, 2005).

trials commence, the sponsor's own researchers will have analyzed the drug's main physical and chemical properties in the laboratory and studied its pharmacologic and toxic effects in laboratory animals. If the laboratory and animal study results are positive, an application can be filed with the FDA to begin testing in people. This application is called an Investigational New Drug Application. For med-

TABLE 20–1	Phases of Pre-NDA Human Clinical Trials			
	Testing in Humans*			
	Number of Patients	**Length**	**Purpose**	**Percent of Drugs Successfully Tested****
Phase I	20–100	Several months	Mainly safety	70 percent
Phase II	Up to several hundred	Several months to 2 years	Some short-term safety but mainly effectiveness	33 percent
Phase III	Several hundred to several thousand	1–4 years	Safety, dosage, effectiveness	25–30 percent

*Source: U.S. Food and Drug Administration. Testing in humans. Available at: http://www.fda.gov/fdac/special/newdrug/testtabl.html (accessed July 29, 2005).

**For example, of 100 drugs for which investigational new drug applications are submitted to FDA, about 70 will successfully complete phase I trials and go on to phase II; about 33 of the original 100 will complete phase II and go to phase III; and 25 to 30 of the original 100 will clear phase III (and, on average, about 20 of the original 100 will ultimately be approved for marketing).

ical devices, the path to approval is more complicated, but is similar. That application process is briefly covered below.

Investigational New Drug Application

An Investigational New Drug Application (IND) is a request for FDA authorization to administer an investigational drug to humans. Such authorization must be secured prior to interstate shipment and administration of any new drug that is not the subject of an approved new drug application. IND regulations are contained in Title 21, Code of Federal Regulations, Part 312. Copies of the regulations, further guidance regarding IND procedures, and additional forms are available from the FDA Center for Drug Evaluation and Research. In addition, forms, regulations, guidances, and a wide variety of additional information are available online.

Devices

Medical devices are subject to the general controls of the Federal Food, Drug and Cosmetic (FD&C) Act and the regulations in Title 21 Code of Federal Regulations Part 800-1200 (21 CFR Parts 800 to 1299). These controls are the baseline requirements that apply to all medical devices necessary for marketing, proper labeling, and monitoring its performance once the device is on the market. However, it is important to confirm that the product to be approved meets the definition of a medical device in section 201(h) of the FD&C Act. The product might actually be a drug or biological product, or it might be a medical device and also an electronic radiation emitting product with additional requirements.

FDA may assign the device in one of the three classes: medical device, biological product, or radiation-emitting product. Classification identifies the level of regulatory control that is necessary to assure the safety and effectiveness of a medical device and will identify, unless exempt, the marketing process the manufacturer must complete in order to obtain FDA clearance or approval for marketing. Once the device is classified, the sponsor (again, usually the manufacturer) must develop the data and/or information necessary to submit a marketing application and to obtain FDA clearance to market. For many devices, clinical performance data is required to obtain clearance to market. In these cases, conduct of the trial must be done in accordance with FDA's Investigational Device Exemption (IDE) regulation, in addition to marketing clearance.

Clinical Laboratory Improvement Act (CLIA) of 1988

In addition to FDA regulation under the FD&C Act, some diagnostic devices are also subject to the Clinical Laboratory Improvement Amendments (CLIA) of 1988. This law established quality standards for laboratory testing and an accreditation program for clinical laboratories. Some regulation of certain diagnostic tests was transferred from the Centers for Disease Control (CDC) to FDA. However, the CDC still has a role in approval of these devices.

Types of Applications

There are three types of INDs:

1. Investigator IND. Submitted by the physician who initiates and conducts an investigation. The submitting physician is the one who directs the administration or dispensing of the investigational drug. A physician might submit a research IND to propose studying an unapproved drug or an approved product for a new indication or in a new patient population.

2. Emergency use IND. The FDA may authorize use of an experimental drug in an emergency situation that does not allow time for submission of an IND. It is also used for patients who do not meet the criteria of an existing study protocol or if an approved study protocol does not exist.

3. Treatment IND. Submitted for experimental drugs showing promise in clinical testing for serious or immediately life-threatening conditions while the final clinical work is conducted and the FDA review takes place.

For example, a treatment IND was granted for the use of AZT in the treatment of AIDS. The FDA requires any IND application to contain information as follows:[7]

Animal Pharmacology and Toxicology Studies. Preclinical data to permit FDA to assess whether the product is reasonably safe for initial testing in humans. Any previous experience with the drug in humans (often foreign use) is also included.

Manufacturing Information. Information pertaining to the composition, manufacturer, stability, and controls used for manufacturing the drug substance and the drug product. This information is assessed by FDA to ensure that the company can adequately produce and supply consistent batches of the drug.

Clinical Protocols and Investigator Information. Detailed protocols for proposed clinical studies for the FDA to assess whether the initial-phase trials will expose subjects to unnecessary risks. Also, information on the qualifications of clinical investigators—professionals (generally physicians) who oversee the administration of the experimental compound—to assess whether they are qualified to fulfill their clinical trial duties. Finally, commitments to obtain informed consent from the research subjects, to obtain review of the study by an institutional review board (IRB), and to adhere to the investigational new drug regulations.

Once the IND is submitted, the sponsor must wait 30 calendar days before initiating any clinical trials. During this time, the FDA has an opportunity to review the IND for safety to assure that research subjects will not be subjected to unreasonable risk.

Detailed Guidance

The Center for Drug Evaluation and Research (CDER) provides an abundance of information for the investigator, the sponsor, the manufacturer, and the consumer. Most, if not all, of this information is available online.[8] The guidance includes summary information and all of the specific instructions, forms, and regulatory information needed to conduct clinical trials and to undertake the new drug application process (Figure 20-3). Every research manager and administrator should be completely familiar with the material on the site and should regularly review the site for new developments.

The Center for Devices and Radiological Health (CDRH) is responsible for devices. An overview of that organization's process and links to more detailed guidance is available from its Web site.[9] Not all devices require clinical trials as a prerequisite to approval. Those that do are those requiring pre-market approval (PMA). PMA is the process to evaluate the safety and effectiveness of medical devices that support or sustain human life, are of substantial importance in preventing impairment of human health, or that present a potential, unreasonable risk of illness or injury. The detailed requirements for this process are found on the CDRH site.[10]

Sponsor–Investigator Interrelationship

The interrelationship and interaction between the research sponsor (e.g., drug, biologic, and device manufacturers) and the clinical investigator varies from that of close collaborators to strictly arms-length service provider. This is complicated by the fact that the investigator may be a health care provider in private practice, an employee of an institution (either for-profit or nonprofit), a faculty member of an academic institution, a government employee, or perhaps a combination of all of these. In many cases, the investigator may have co-investigators, or subinvestigators with whom the work is shared or split. Therefore, the following discussion must be tempered with the knowledge that there are many more "flavors" to the relationship than can be comprehensively discussed in this text.

Sponsor Obligations

The relationship between the sponsor and the investigator/institution and/or any other parties involved with the clinical trial should be established by a written agreement, executed or acknowledged by the sponsor, the individual investigator(s) and the institution(s). FDA regulations [21 CFR 312.23(a)(1)(iv)] place the responsibility for assuring that a study will be conducted in compliance with the informed consent and IRB regulations [21 CFR parts 50 and 56] on the sponsor. However, sponsors normally rely on the institution and the clinical investigator to have the study reviewed by an IRB. Because clinical investigators work directly with IRBs, they normally assure the sponsor (in the contract or agreement covering the trial) that the IRB is functioning in compliance with the regulations.

The sponsor is responsible for implementing and maintaining quality assurance and quality control systems to ensure that trials are conducted in compliance with the protocol, good clinical practices, and the applicable regulatory requirement(s). A sponsor may transfer any or all of the sponsor's trial-related duties and functions to a contract research organization (CRO), but the ultimate responsibility for the quality and integrity of the

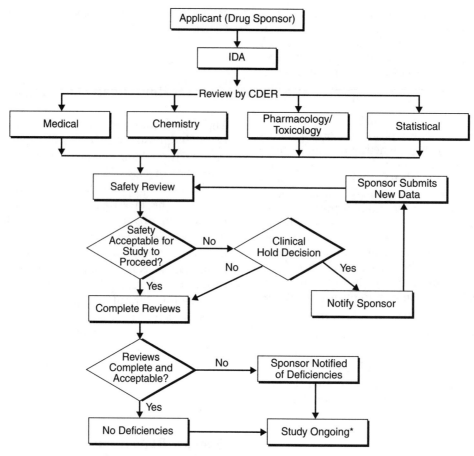

FIGURE 20-3 New Drug Application (NDA) Review Process[11] U.S. Food and Drug Administration Center for Drug Evaluation and Research. NDA review process. Available at: http://www.fda.gov/cder/handbook/nda.htm (accessed July 29, 2005).

trial data always resides with the sponsor. Any trial-related duty and function that is transferred to and assumed by a CRO should be specified in writing

While the investigator is expected to provide and is selected for his or her medical/clinical expertise, the sponsor should designate appropriately qualified personnel who will be readily available to advise on trial-related questions or problems. If necessary, outside consultant(s) may be appointed for this purpose. All of these persons' relationships should be subject to written agreements.

Access to Medical Records

FDA requires the sponsors (or research monitors hired by them) to monitor the accuracy of the data submitted to the FDA in accordance with regulatory requirements. However, the data are normally under the control of the health care institution, or perhaps

the clinical investigator. Most states in the United States have begun to require that the medical records themselves remain the property of the health care institution/provider. These statutes and the Health Insurance Portability and Accountability Act (HIPAA) of 1996 govern the disclosure of such patient medical records to the sponsor and other entities. The agreement between the investigator and provider will need to define the rights to and procedures for access to records identifying the subject.

Confidentiality in Relationship

Most investigators undertake clinical research with an objective of publicizing the results. However, most sponsors pay for such research in order to advance the drug approval process and to obtain commercial advantage. Therefore the relationship between the parties must balance the investigator's need to publish with the sponsor's need to maintain confidentiality of certain information about products under development. Routinely, sponsor information may be confidential, trade-secret, and of commercial interest. However, if the investigator does not have publication rights, then the research is not generally acceptable to the FDA. The level of confidentiality is one that must be individually negotiated in each relationship with care.

Disagreements

The sponsor may normally choose not to conduct, to terminate, or to discontinue studies that do not conform to the sponsor's wishes. For example, the sponsor, clinical investigator, and IRB may reach an impasse about study procedures or specific wording in an informed consent document. It is important to establish just how much independence the investigator will have to continue a study in the face of inconclusive or adverse results. Additionally, the parties will need to set the procedures for termination and for dispute resolution in advance, whenever possible. (Due to the multijurisdictional nature of most clinical trials, it is often not practical to set dispute resolution procedures in advance.)

Additional Guidance

A comprehensive discussion of the relationship between the parties, and the division of responsibility for trials is provided in the International Conference on Harmonization document, ICH E6, *Good Clinical Practice: Consolidated Guidance. Good Clinical Practice* (GCP) is an international ethical and scientific quality standard for designing, conducting, recording, and reporting trials that involve human subjects. This document has been published in the United States *Federal Register*, Vol. 62, No. 90, May 9, 1997, pp. 25691–25709.

Planning and Execution of a Clinical Trial

Clinical trials are usually first conceived by individual researchers, although many trials today are conducted at multiple institutions after the sponsor first designs the trial following initial preclinical research shows a compound or device to be promising. After

these laboratory and animal studies, the treatments with the most promising laboratory results are moved into clinical trials, based on a clinical trial protocol. A protocol is the study plan/procedural blueprint on which the clinical trial is based. The plan is carefully designed to safeguard the health of the participants as well as answer specific research questions. A protocol describes what types of people may participate in the trial; the schedule of tests, procedures, medications, and dosages; and the length of the study. While in a clinical trial, participants following a protocol are seen regularly by the research staff to monitor their health and to determine the safety and effectiveness of their treatment. The following are important issues to address in connection with the development of the protocol:

- Who or what entity will be providing the protocol (i.e., drug company, investigator, government agency, or multi-institutional group)
- Will the protocol specify:
  - The principal investigator
  - The study design
  - Information desired
  - Estimated duration of the study
  - Estimated charges
  - Institution(s) involved
  - Additional protocol requirements
  - Required language for informed consent
  - Adverse experiences which must be reported
  - Grounds for stopping the study or participation in the study
  - Release of patient/subject information to the company, the FDA, and other governmental agencies
  - Medical records and patient privacy issues

The contents of a trial protocol should generally include the topics set out in Table 20-2. However, site-specific information may be provided in a separate agreement, and some of the information listed in the table may be contained in other protocol-referenced documents, such as an investigator's brochure.

The protocol is accompanied by an investigator's brochure (IB). The IB is a compilation of the data relevant to the trial. Its purpose is to provide the information on the rationale for and the procedures to be followed during the trial. These might include the dose, dose frequency/interval, methods of administration, and safety monitoring procedures.

In addition to the protocol and the IB, there are many other documents that must be prepared for the

TABLE 20–2	Clinical Trial Protocol Outline
1	General information
2	Background information
3	Trial objectives and purpose
	A detailed description of the objectives and the purpose of the trial.
4	Trial Design: The scientific integrity of the trial and the credibility of the data from the trial depend substantially on the trial design.
5	Selection and withdrawal of subjects, including subject inclusion and exclusion criteria and discussion of withdrawal issues.
6	Treatment of subjects: The treatment(s) to be administered, including the name(s) of all the product(s), the dose(s), the dosing schedule(s), the route/mode(s) of administration, and the treatment period(s), including the follow-up period(s) for subjects for each investigational product treatment/trial treatment group/arm of the trial.
7	Assessment of efficacy, including the efficacy parameters and the methods and timing for assessing, recording, and analyzing efficacy parameters.
8	Assessment of safety, including safety parameters and the methods and timing for assessing, recording, and analyzing safety parameters.
9	Statistics: A description of the statistical methods to be employed, including timing of any planned interim analysis(es).
10	Access to source data/documents: It is specified in the protocol or other written agreement that the investigator(s)/institution(s) will permit trial-related monitoring, audits, IRB/IEC review, and regulatory inspection(s) by providing direct access to source data/documents.
11	Quality control and quality assurance
12	Ethics: Description of ethical considerations relating to the trial.
13	Data handling and recordkeeping
14	Financing and insurance: Financing and insurance are usually addressed in a separate agreement.
15	Publication policy: Publication policy, if not addressed in a separate agreement.

Source: U.S. Department of Health and Human Services, Food and Drug Administration, Center for Drug Evaluation and Research (CDER), Center for Biologics Evaluation and Research (CBER). Guidance for industry; E6 *Good Clinical Practice: Consolidated Guidance*. April 1996 ICH. Available at: http://www.fda.gov/cder/guidance/959fnl.pdf (accessed July 29, 2005).

clinical trial. These are detailed in the *Guidance for Industry E6 Good Clinical Practice: Consolidated Guidance*.[12] Table 20-3 is from that document.

Multi-Institutional Trials

Documenting Cooperative Arrangements

Many trials are conducted at more than one institution. Such trials may be independently conducted by separate investigators and institutions, conducted cooperatively by several institutions working together, or conducted by one main institution/investigator working with subinvestigators. Examples include research coordinated by cooperative practice groups and participation by investigators and subjects in a clinical study primarily conducted at or administered by another institution. Sometimes, one of the actual research institutions has the

primary responsibility for the conduct of the study and the responsibility for administrative or coordinating functions. At other times, multicenter trials may be coordinated by an office or organization (such as the drug company) that does not actually conduct the clinical study or have an IRB. In each case the research managers and administrators should be aware of the issues that can arise.

The FDA and HHS regulations concerning institutional review boards permit institutions involved in multi-institutional studies to use reasonable methods of joint or cooperative review (21 CFR 56.114 and 45 CFR 46.114, respectively). The cooperative research arrangements between institutions may apply to the review of one study, to certain specific categories of studies, or to all studies. A single cooperative IRB may provide review for several participating institutions, but the respective responsibilities of the IRB and each institution should be agreed to in writing. The agreement for cooperative research

TABLE 20–3	Documents to be Generated and on File Before the Trial Starts
Title of Document	**Purpose**
Investigator's brochure	To document that relevant and current scientific information about the investigational product has been provided to the investigator.
Signed protocol and amendments, if any, and sample case report form (CRF)	To document investigator and sponsor agreement to the protocol/amendment(s) and CRF.
Information given to trial subject—Informed consent form (including all applicable translations)—Any other written information—Advertisement for subject recruitment (if used)	To document the informed consent. To document that forms subjects will be given are not coercive and are appropriate written information (content and wording) to support their ability to give fully informed consent. To document recruitment measures.
Financial aspects of the trial	To document the financial agreement between the investigator/institution and the sponsor for the trial.
Insurance statement (where required)	To document that compensation to subject(s) for trial-related injury will be available.
Signed agreement between involved parties, e.g.:—Investigator/institution and sponsor—Investigator/institution and CRO—Sponsor and CRO—Investigator/institution and authority(ies) (where required)	To document agreements.
Dated, documented approval/favorable opinion of IRB/IEC of the following:—Protocol and any amendments—CRF (if applicable)—Informed consent form(s)—Any other written information to be provided to the subject(s)—Advertisement for subject recruitment (if used)—Subject compensation (if any)—Any other documents given approval/favorable opinion	To document that the trial has been subject to IRB/IEC review and gives the version number and date of the approval/favorable opinion. To identify document(s).
Institutional review board/independent ethics committee composition	To document that the IRB/IEC is constituted in agreement with GCP.
Regulatory authority(ies) authorization/approval/notification of protocol (where required)	To document appropriate authorization/approval/notification by the regulatory authority(ies) has been obtained prior to initiation of the trial in compliance with the applicable regulatory requirement(s).
Curriculum vitae and/or other relevant documents evidencing qualifications of investigator(s) and subinvestigators	To document qualifications and eligibility to conduct trial and/or provide medical supervision of subjects.
Normal value(s)/range(s) for medical/laboratory/technical procedure(s) and/or test(s) included in the protocol	To document normal values and/or ranges of the tests.
Medical/laboratory/technical procedures/tests—Certification or—Accreditation or—Established quality control and/or external quality assessment or—Other validation (where required)	To document competence of facility to perform required test(s), and support reliability of results.
Sample of label(s) attached to investigational product container(s)	To document compliance with applicable labeling regulations and appropriateness of instructions provided to the subjects.
Instructions for handling of investigational product(s) and trial-related materials (if not included in protocol or investigator's brochure)	To document instructions needed to ensure proper storage, packaging, dispensing, and disposition of investigational products and trial-related materials.

(continued)

TABLE 20–3	Documents to be Generated and on File Before the Trial Starts (continued)
Title of Document	**Purpose**
Shipping records for investigational product(s) and trial-related materials	To document shipment dates, batch numbers, and method of shipment of investigational product(s) and trial-related materials. Allows tracking of product batch, review of shipping conditions, and accountability.
Certificate(s) of analysis of investigational product(s) shipped	To document identity, purity, and strength of investigational products to be used in the trial.
Decoding procedures for blinded trials	To document how, in case of an emergency, identity of blinded investigational product can be revealed without breaking the blind for the remaining subjects' treatment.
Pretrial monitoring report	To document that the site is suitable for the trial.
Trial initiation monitoring report	To document that trial procedures were reviewed with the investigator and investigator's trial staff.

Source: U.S. Department of Health and Human Services, Food and Drug Administration, Center for Drug Evaluation and Research (CDER), Center for Biologics Evaluation and Research (CBER). Guidance for industry; E6 *Good Clinical Practice: Consolidated Guidance*. April 1996 ICH. Available at: http://www.fda.gov/cder/guidance/959fnl.pdf (accessed July 29, 2005).

should be documented. Depending upon the scope of the agreement, documentation may be simple, in the form of a letter, or more complex, such as a formal memorandum of understanding. In the case of studies supported or conducted by HHS, arrangements or agreements may be subject to approval by HHS through the Office of Human Research Protection (OHRP) and should be executed in accordance with OHRP's instructions. Whatever form of documentation is used, copies should be furnished to all parties to the agreement, and to those responsible for ensuring compliance with the regulations and the IRB determinations.

Subjects Involved with More Than One Institution

Several issues are raised when a subject who is participating in a research study at one institution is admitted to another facility. Perhaps the most common issues arise when a subject's treatment or hospitalization is not related to the research. In this case, the second facility is providing incidental medical care and is not participating as a research site.

The research managers at the research institution should assure that procedures are in place for rapidly identifying test drugs and devices (e.g., an emergency contact number and unbinding procedure). Any clinical research contract will need to address the possibility that confidential information may need to be provided to the admitting facility for emergency treatment. The investigator at the

research institution remains responsible for test drug administration and follow-up and therefore, should be aware of the hospitalization. The investigator may need to report the event as an unexpected adverse incident if it is possibly related to use of the test article.

When involvement of outside medical facilities or providers is reasonably foreseen and is an anticipated part of the study protocol, the research managers should be aware that other institutions and/or providers will be providing medical care and/or follow-up and should ensure that adequate reporting and safety systems are agreed to and documented before the study begins. These arrangements may be covered by subagreements or by "service contracts." In most cases, the agreements should at least cover treatment procedures, adverse reaction response and documentation, and emergency procedures. The second institution or provider should be given a copy of the signed informed consent document, which is a research summary as well as documentation of consent.

Finally, the second institution or investigator may be treated as an extension of the research activity. In this instance, the second institution is actually responsible for a portion of the research protocol. For instance, a physician at a community hospital may be identified in the protocol as a subinvestigator for subjects residing in that locality. That physician is responsible for conducting examinations of subjects to monitor status and measure effects of the test drug (data collection). These research data are systematically reported to the lead investigator. Because the community hospital is conducting research, it is responsible for complying with the applicable research regulations. The community hospital's IRB must either: a) review; b) approve and be responsible for monitoring the portion of the research conducted at MH just as it would for any other research in the facility; or c) the community hospital may agree to accept the RMC-IRB as the responsible IRB. The research managers must determine and document the respective duties of the lead and subinvestigator(s) and determine the "contractual" relationships between and among the various parties (including the drug company or other sponsor).

Informed Consent Issues

Generally, having a subject sign a second research consent document for the secondary facility should be avoided. Of course, when no research is involved at the second institution, no research-related consent is needed. When the second institution is actually involved in the research, that involvement should normally be included in the initial consent document. It is important that the subject not receive conflicting information and the two institutions and their IRBs should work together to conduct the necessary consent process.

Other Multi-Center Issues

When a company sponsors a multi-center trial it must assure that all investigators conduct the trial in strict compliance with the protocol. While the trial contracts may sometimes vary to accommodate the specific needs of the various institutions, the trial itself must be conducted uniformly. All investigators should be given instructions on following the protocol, on complying with a uniform set of standards for the assessment of clinical and laboratory findings, and on completing the "Case Report Forms" (CRFs). The CRFs should be designed to capture the same data at all multi-center trial sites. For those investigators who are collecting additional data, supplemental CRFs designed to capture the additional data should also be provided.

The responsibilities of the coordinating investigator(s) and the other participating investigators should be documented prior to the start of the trial. Normally, a publication committee should be estab-

lished at the inception of the trial, with a clear mandate for publication review and with guidelines for determining authorship. Drug company sponsors should generally not be on the publication committee, but should have the normal review rights that are generally accorded to sponsors under the Uniform Requirements for Manuscripts prepared by the International Committee of Medical Journal Editors.[13]

Institutional Review Boards

The United States government has adopted a common federal policy for the protection of human research subjects. The federal policy applies to research involving human subjects conducted, supported, or otherwise subject to regulation by most of the federal departments and agencies. The federal policy implements a recommendation of the President's Commission for the Study of Ethical Problems in Medicine and Biomedical and Behavioral Research. The Office of Human Research Protection (OHRP) is the entity within the United States Department of Health and Human Services (DHHS) in charge of implementing the regulation for that department (which is the largest clinical research activity in the federal government). It is a part of the Office of the Director, Office of Extramural Research, National Institutes of Health (NIH). The FDA has concurred in the Federal Policy, but did not adopt the policy in its entirety. Instead, the FDA made selected changes to its own IRB and informed consent regulations that correspond to the federal policy. Under DHHS rules, a department or agency head may determine that procedures prescribed by a foreign institution afford protections at least equivalent to those in the regulations, and on that basis approve the substitution of foreign procedures in lieu of the procedural requirements in the common policy. However, this exception is not available under FDA rules.

Under both the common policy and the FDA regulation, the institutional review board is the group that has the official duty to review and monitor research involving human subjects. Under United States government regulations, the IRB has the authority to approve, require modifications in, or disapprove research. Other governments require the use of equivalent organizations for research conducted in their countries.

The purpose of IRB review is to assure, both in advance and by periodic review, that the rights and welfare of human subjects in the research are protected. To accomplish this purpose, IRBs review the research protocols and related materials (e.g., informed consent documents and investigator brochures) and, where appropriate, require changes to the protocols; or sometimes prohibit the research as proposed. Each research institution may establish its own IRB or use an IRB established by another institution or established as a service provider. Regardless of the specific arrangement, the IRB is subject to the IRB regulations of the applicable federal agencies (e.g., FDA or NIH) when studies of regulated products or treatments are conducted under their jurisdiction. When research studies involving products regulated by the FDA are funded or supported by DHHS, the research institution must comply with both the DHHS and FDA regulations.

Currently, there is no general requirement for IRB registration or licensing in the United States. The form FDA-1572 "Statement of Investigator" for a study conducted under an IND requires the name and address of the IRB that will be responsible for review of the study. IRBs that approve studies of FDA regulated products must be established and operated in compliance with 21 CFR part 56. For US DHHS-supported studies, there is a requirement that the institution provide an assurance called a federal wide assurance (FWA) concerning the use of the IRB. An assurance is an agreement (or a portion of an agreement) negotiated between a research institution and the DHHS. For research involving human subjects, the DHHS regulations require a written assurance that the institution will comply with the DHHS protection of human subjects regulations (45 CFR part 46). Once an institution's assurance has been approved by DHHS, a number is assigned to the assurance. OHRP is responsible for drafting and implementing the DHHS regulations.

Purpose of the IRB Review

The basic purpose of IRB review is protection of the rights and welfare of subjects. A signed informed consent document is evidence that the document has been provided (and explained, as necessary) to a prospective subject and that the subject has agreed to participate in the research. Many institutions also task the IRB with additional responsibilities concerning review of the research for substance, objectivity, etc., but these functions are often better performed by other organizations or managers.

IRB Membership

Common policy and FDA IRB regulations both require an IRB to have a diverse membership. Those regulations also prohibit any member of an IRB from participating in the IRB's initial or continuing review of any study in which the member has a conflicting interest, except to provide information requested by the IRB. Some of the members should be otherwise unaffiliated with the institution and have a primary concern in a nonscientific area. Others must have a scientific (including medical) background (one individual could satisfy two of the membership requirements of the regulations). IRB members may not use proxies. Alternates who are formally appointed and listed in the membership roster may substitute, but ad hoc substitutes are not permissible as members of an IRB.

IRB Procedures

IRBs are required to function under written procedures. Neither the DHHS nor the FDA has developed a model written IRB procedures document for institutions to adopt. The organizations are prevented from doing so due to variations in institution size, the type of research activities, institutional administrative practices, number of IRBs, and local and state laws and regulations. However, both the DHHS and the FDA have outlined the areas in which procedures must be developed. For each required element, the written IRB procedures should provide sufficient step-by-step operational details so that an independent observer can understand how an IRB operates and conducts its major functions. The US FDA regulations do not require (but do not prohibit) public or sponsor access to IRB records. The IRB and the institution should establish a policy on whether minutes or a pertinent portion of the minutes are provided to sponsors. Because they vary greatly, each IRB also needs to be aware of state and local laws regarding access to IRB records. Each IRB should also be completely familiar with the privacy rule under HIPAA.

The IRB system is meant to promote open discussion and debate. Therefore, each member must be provided with sufficient information to be able to fully participate. Each member must receive, at a minimum, a copy of consent documents and a summary of the protocol in sufficient detail to determine the appropriateness of the study-specific statements in the consent documents. In addition, the complete documentation should be available to all members for their review, both before and at the meeting. Some IRBs are using electronic submissions and computer access for IRB members. Whatever system the IRB develops and uses, it must ensure that each study receives an adequate review and that the rights and welfare of the subjects are protected.

Certain kinds of research may be reviewed and approved without convening a meeting of the IRB. This "expedited review" is a procedure through which an IRB may review certain categories of research if the research involves no more than minimal risk. The IRB may also use the expedited review procedure to review minor changes in previously approved research during the period covered by the original approval. After approval many IRBs do not routinely observe consent interviews, observe the conduct of the study, or review study records. However, the IRB has the authority to observe, or have a third party observe, the consent process and the research. When and if the IRB is concerned about the conduct of the study or the process for obtaining consent, the IRB may consider whether, as part of providing adequate oversight of the study, an active audit is warranted. It is good practice to include an auditor or quality assurance officer on the IRB staff to maintain vigilance over controversial studies.

When an IRB disapproves a study, it must provide a written statement of the reasons for its decision to the investigator and the institution. If the study is submitted to a second IRB, a copy of this written statement should be included with the study documentation so that it can make an informed decision about the study. FDA regulations do not prohibit submission of a study to another IRB following disapproval. However, all pertinent information about the study should be provided to the second IRB. Protocol amendments must receive IRB review and approval before they are implemented, unless an immediate change is necessary to eliminate an apparent hazard to the subjects.

IRB Records

The IRB records for each study's initial and continuing review should note the frequency (not to exceed one year) for the next continuing review in either months or other conditions, such as after a particular number of subjects are enrolled. The IRB must maintain copies of research proposals reviewed. The documents to be maintained should include the complete documents received from the clinical investigator, such as the protocol, the investigator's brochure, a sample consent document and any advertising intended to be seen or heard by prospective study subjects. Some IRBs also require the investigator to submit an institutionally developed protocol summary form. All documentation reviewed is to be maintained for at least three years after completion of the research.

Additional Guidance

There is a plethora of guidance available to the IRB from both the FDA and the HHS. This material is quite fluid, and IRB members and research managers should check frequently with the agency Web sites to assure that they are current.

Informed Consent

Twenty-five years ago, problems with the informed consent process were the subject of academic study.

> Probably no aspect of the ethics of human research has received closer review by institutional review boards (IRBs) than that of informed consent. In a recent nationwide survey of IRB practices, modification of consent forms was found to be the most frequent substantive change requested of investigators. However, this survey also found that IRBs were largely ineffective in improving the quality of consent procedures. IRB proposals for modification were largely limited to the content of consent forms.[14]

The problem of obtaining truly informed consent is still a matter of constant struggle. Informed consent is a process, not just the completion of a form. It is both a mechanism to ensure that persons who are the subject of research are voluntarily participating and a protection to the institution and the investigator to reduce the risk of litigation for improperly designed or conducted research. The procedures used in obtaining informed consent should educate the subjects in terms that they can understand. They also should be provided with the documentation of that education and of the careful consideration of the risks and rewards to be obtained by human experimentation.

It is imperative that informed consent language and its documentation (especially containing explanation of the study's purpose, duration, experimental procedures, alternatives, risks, and benefits) be understandable to the people being asked to participate. The consent document must avoid the use of forms or formats that could be interpreted as suggestive or constitute coercive influence over a subject. While the consent is legally important, it is primarily an educational tool, and if it does not serve that purpose, it will not be considered legally sufficient. In recent years, there have been increasingly stringent requirements that the subjects be told the extent to which their personally identifiable private information will be held in confidence. These requirements are covered elsewhere in this text.

If there is more than minimal risk of research-related injury (i.e., physical, psychological, social, financial, or otherwise), then the informed consent must provide an explanation of whatever voluntary compensation and treatment will be provided. Both FDA and the common policy regulations prohibit waiving or appearing to waive any legal rights of subjects. However, if a subject is injured due to negligence or other actionable harm by the institution, the investigator, or the sponsor, he or she may not be required to waive any legal rights. Therefore, subjects should not be given the impression that they have agreed to and are without recourse to seek satisfaction beyond any voluntarily compensation or treatment available.

The consent must identify knowledgeable contact persons to answer questions of subjects about the research, rights as a research subject, and research-related injuries. All three of these issues must be addressed and usually at least two different contacts must be provided. Subjects must be told that their participation is voluntary and that they have a right to withdraw at any time. The consent must point out that no penalty or loss of benefits will occur as a result of not participating or withdrawing at any time. The subjects must also be alerted to any foreseeable consequences to them should they unilaterally withdraw while dependent on some intervention to maintain normal function. There are many additional requirements that involve consent. Some of these requirements can be found in the applicable agency's regulations and additional guidance. Many IRBs impose additional requirements that are not specifically listed in the regulations to ensure that adequate information is presented in accordance with institutional policy and local law.

There are many situations that will call for special handling. For example, when minors are included as research subjects, parental permission must be obtained. Certain populations (including, but not limited to, nonliterate or politically vulnerable populations, such as those who speak English as a second language or not at all or those of certain foreign nationalities) call for special informed consent procedures. Additionally, there are special rules concerning the conduct of research on incarcerated individuals.

The Clinical Trial Agreement

Most clinical trials are sponsored by either a pharmaceutical firm or by the government. In either case, there is an agreement (a contract, grant, or some other type of agreement) that governs the relationship between the parties and the course of the trial itself. These agreements are surprisingly uniform in what they cover, but the particular language used by each sponsoring company is a matter of zealous individual drafting. There have been several efforts to standardize the privately sponsored clinical trial agreement, but for the most part each company continues to adopt uniform language only in response to FDA or other government fiat. Federally funded trials are much more uniform in the language, but there are significant differences that arise among the various departments and agencies.

Important Issues in Negotiating the Clinical Trial Agreement

Almost every clinical trial agreement will require attention to the same seven issues. These are:

1. Publication rights
2. Confidential information
3. Patent rights
4. Subject injury
5. Payment
6. Indemnification*
7. State law[15]

In addition, the clinical research agreement should reference the protocol and other study documents. The agreement may include a more substantive "scope of work" or may only "incorporate by reference" the applicable documents ("incorporation by reference" means including only language

---

*Indemnification is the part of an agreement that provides for one party to bear the monetary costs, either directly or by reimbursement, for losses incurred by a second party. The clauses often also call for one party to defend against third-party claims made against the other party.

that states that the document is considered, or deemed to be included, even though the whole document is not actually copied into the agreement). When drafting the agreement the following issues should be addressed:

- Is the work to be done on a "best efforts" or "completion" basis? That is, will the study organization use its best efforts to complete the study, or will it commit to complete the study unless there is a termination of the agreement?
- What, if any, phases of the work are included (single phase, multiple, or options)? That is, will the work proceed under this contract throughout the entire study as contemplated in the protocol, or does this contract only cover the initial stages of research? If the entire study is not covered, how are the additional phases of the work addressed? Are there options to continue the work? If so, at whose discretion will the work continue?

The clinical trial agreement must also deal with the many issues that surround simply getting the study completed. These issues range from quite practical to highly esoteric. For instance:

- Who is investigator? (Is there more than one, and if so, is only one the primary investigator, with the others subinvestigators?)
- Who provides the IRB and other review/management reviews, etc.?
- Who provides what reports, data, and document management?
- Who/what entity has treatment responsibilities?
- How is the clinical research agreement term calculated? Is the contract "completion" or does the agreement run for a definite period of time?
- What, if any agreement is there concerning extensions or delays?
- What is the effect of a disaster or emergency on the contract? (These clauses are often called "force majeure" clauses).
- There is always a need for provisions in the clinical research agreement to address payment.
- The drafter should consider if the agreement needs to specify the method(s) of payment (e.g., per procedure, per patient, cost reimbursement).
- What needs to be specified concerning time of payment(s)?
- What needs to be said concerning amount?
- Does there need to be specific coverage of the type of contract (i.e., whether the contract is fixed-price or cost-reimbursable)? Note: Many agreements place the details of payment in attachments that the contract drafter may not normally see.

- What needs to be said, if anything, about exclusivity of payor (i.e., are multiple sponsors allowed)?
- An issue that is associated both with costs and with the respective liability of the parties is the coverage of the costs of injury or harm to the subject.
- What should be included concerning costs incurred and associated with the diagnosis and treatment of an adverse reaction involving the study drug or device?
- What language is needed to deal with other compensation if any injury occurs?
- Is it necessary to address routine medical care costs? This is particularly important for devices, the costs of which may be reimbursable under insurance or Medicare/Medicaid.

Another cost issue that may need to be covered is that of referral fees. Many referral fees that might benefit the health care provider are illegal and other fees (to patients for example) may be unethical. However, not all fees are prohibited. Patients are often provided with a small amount for travel, for instance. The agreement may need to address any of these payments (or prohibitions on payments.)

There are many issues concerning the principal investigator that may need to be addressed:

- Can the sponsor approve the principal investigator (PI)? The issue of whether the individual person to be assigned to the contract is under the control of the sponsor or the research institution is often of importance, particularly when there are changes in personnel over time.
- If the PI becomes unable to complete the study, must the sponsor consent to a new PI?
- Can the sponsor follow PI?
- Are there to be multiple PIs?
- What, if any, time commitments must be made by the PI or PIs?

As with any research study, there are records issues to be addressed in the clinical trial agreement. These include:

- Which entity will be charged with records retention?
- What is the minimum and maximum amount of time for retention of records?
- What language is needed to address transfer(s) of study records?
- What language is necessary to address ownership of documents (e.g., patient records vs. study records)?
- What is the applicability of 1996 HIPAA and state laws on patient records?

- What format and specification of the content of the records is needed?

Confidentiality is always an issue and is usually addressed in several parts of the agreement. The agreement needs to deal with information that is disclosed by the sponsor to the institution; information that is disclosed by institution to sponsor; third-party information; and patient/subject information. The drafter may need to specifically address the obligations of investigator, staff, students, and third parties such as subinvestigators, consultants, and nongovernmental auditors.

Agreements should cover the possible promotional activities of the parties. For instance, the use of name of sponsor and institution, the use of PI's name, any trademarks, or other trade name should be covered. Any publicity, press releases, and responses to inquiries from media and financial analysts should be addressed. Advertisements for patients should be covered in the protocol, but additional language may be needed in the agreement. Publications and scientific communications are at the center of the agreement. The drafter will need to specify the institution's/investigator's right to publish the results of the study in accordance with the guidelines established by the "Uniform Requirements for Manuscripts Submitted to Biomedical Journals" cited earlier. Other rights to discuss include nonpublication disclosures (e.g., conferences—where and when?); notification to the sponsor prior to submission; notice if publication contains patent information; the sponsor's right to delay; and publication in nonscientific journals, newspapers, radio, or television.

Just as the institution's primary concern is normally advancing science, the sponsor's primary concern is the accumulation and retention of "intellectual property rights," including patents and trade secrets. It is the ownership of these rights that makes the clinical research costs worthwhile to the corporate sponsor, and most sponsors will not negotiate a great deal over the language required to protect their interests in this area, unless the research is investigator initiated, and unless the research does not involve a drug or device whose intellectual property rights are already owned by the sponsor. In sponsor initiated research, the ownership of all inventions will be demanded by the sponsor, with no licensing of any right for any purpose. Sometimes, the sponsor may accept pure research rights in the institution, and in a few cases, the sponsor may accept institutional ownership with exclusive commercial rights to be transferred

to the sponsor. Rarely, a drafter may see another arrangement offered.

Another issue that may need to be decided includes arrangements for joint inventions. This is particularly important where an investigator has subinvestigators, or where the sponsor is actually collaborating in the research. There are provisions in the patent laws to cover situations in which there is not a specific agreement concerning joint rights, but it is obviously better to deal with the issues that may arise with custom-crafted language.

Data-related issues are arising more and more, as research resulting in vast databases of information becomes more common. Some of these kinds of research include "genomics" and "proteomics." In these cases, the drafter will need to handle the copyright, and "trade secret" ownership of the databases that result. The drafter may also need to deal with administration of intellectual property rights (e.g., with the payment of the filing fees and with preparation of the filings), with transfers of "biological materials" (such as cell lines, DNA and other chemicals resulting from biological or medical activity), and with third party rights (such as background patents and derivative copyrighted works).

For many institutions, indemnification is a major problem area. Indemnification is the part of an agreement that provides for one party to bear the monetary costs, either directly or by reimbursement, for losses incurred by a second party. Corporate sponsors almost always agree to indemnify clinical research organizations and investigators for sponsor-initiated work. This is appropriate as the sponsor stands to benefit from the research. In every case, the indemnification should clearly cover:

- Who indemnifies and who is indemnified?
- From what injuries are the indemnities protected?
- To what extent is there coverage of expenses of claims and suits?
- To what extent is the indemnification limited as to specific injuries?
- To what extent is the indemnification limited to injuries caused by specific acts or omissions?
- Is there any limitation on the scope of causation, i.e., is the indemnification for injuries caused in whole or in part? That is, does the sponsor cover injuries for which it is only partly at fault?
- Is the indemnification limited to covering the substance studied or the procedure performed?
- Is the indemnification limited to covering injuries arising when the study is done in accordance with the provisions of the protocol?

- Does it cover product liability?
- Is there indemnification without prior payment by the institution?
- What are the exclusions from obligation to indemnify?
- What happens if there is a failure of the institution to comply with any applicable governmental requirements or to adhere to the terms of the protocol?

Negligence of the institution, officers, agent or employee, and subcontractors is normally not subject to indemnification. Most states will not allow indemnification of negligence or failure to comply with law. However, the institution and investigator may be indemnified for third-party negligence and the clause should be structured so that only the narrowest exclusion is allowed. Most indemnification offered by sponsors will include conditions to indemnification. Common conditions include notice of any claim or lawsuit, the sponsor's right to defend the lawsuit (often subject to the institution's right to retain the counsel of its choice, if it pays the costs), the sponsor's right to settle the claim (again often subject to restrictions), and the sponsor's right to require the indemnified party to cooperate fully in the investigation and with defense of any such claim or lawsuit.

Additional indemnification issues may include the costs of extra unanticipated tests, treatments and hospitalizations of patients required as a result of adverse events, costs covered by the subject's or patient's medical or hospital insurance or by governmental programs providing such coverage, and nonmedical indemnification (e.g., worker's compensation, third-party injuries, public health costs). All of these other issues are often the subject of other clauses that may deal with them satisfactorily. For instance, the agreement may deal with insurance (malpractice or errors and omissions, automobile and other general liability, etc.). Many institutions are particularly careful to check the status of insurance when a third-party clinical research organization is the sponsor's agent and the only signatory to the contract.

Many clauses in a clinical agreement may deal with compliance with various laws. These include debarment certification (FDA certification), conflict of interest, integrity or objectivity requirements, scientific misconduct, tax issues (including unrelated business income tax [UBIT]), state laws, and the applicability of laws in foreign countries. An additional topic that is often covered includes the institution or investigator status as an independent contractor. This clause concerns whether the spon-

sor must be responsible under workers compensation laws, and the like.

It is common for the agreement to deal with *notices* (to whom, where, and for what). Similarly the agreement usually covers modifications and amendments: Who has the right to require, when and what if required by government, medical situation, or science? The agreement must specify the rights and responsibilities concerning inspections and access to patients, records, and facilities. Questions to address include:

- May the sponsor inspect the institution's procedures, facilities, and study records?
- May information obtained from such inspections be shared?
- With whom may inspection information be shared, and for what purposes?
- What are the detailed procedures to be addressed to allow and document access to patients, records, data, faculty, treatment facility, etc.

The agreement needs to cover the permissible uses of and controls on the study drug/device:

- May drugs furnished for study (study drugs) be used for other studies or for routine treatment?
- When and how is the study drug provided?
- What provisions are required for storage and accounting for the drug or device.
- Who is responsible for lost or broken drugs or devices?
- Are there requirements for Drug Enforcement Agency registration?
- Is there a need to specify what can be done or what cannot be done with derivative compounds or by-products?
- Is there a need to deal with special waste disposal?

Some agreements try to provide details concerning dispute resolution. Because many institutions are government-supported or part of a governmental unit and therefore covered more or less by sovereign immunity, such provisions often must be scrapped. However, if practicable, language in the agreement can be useful in streamlining the means, methods, and place for resolution of disputes. Such provisions might include:

- Method(s) of dispute resolution (e.g., arbitration or mediation in place of litigation).
- Costs and attorney's fees (e.g., if the prevailing party be entitled to these).
- Jurisdiction and venue. (Such clauses are almost always not accepted unless all parties can agree to the institution's jurisdiction as the place for

settlement of disputes and the appropriate choice of law to be applied.)

- Right to jury (many commercial disputes provide for waiver of jury trial).
- Subcontractor disputes, for example, when there are no subinvestigators or when the institution and investigator are coprincipals, it is wise to at least consider how to deal with disputes between the researching parties.

Termination should always be covered in a clinical research agreement and should deal with:

- Reasons for termination.
- Payment on termination (at a minimum, the institution should be paid for its costs to the date of termination and its uncancellable expenses).
- Responsibility for patients/subjects on termination.
- Students and other personnel (academic institutions must deal with students who may have been relying on the research for their academic progress).
- Close-out (the mechanics of closing down the job should be discussed).

• • • References

1. NIAID glossary of funding and policy terms and acronyms. Available at: http://www.niaid.nih.gov/ncn/glossary/default2.htm#clintrial (accessed July 29, 2005).
2. National Cancer Institute. What is a clinical trial? Available at: http://www.cancer.gov/clinicaltrials/learning/what-is-a-clinical-trial (accessed July 29, 2005).
3. U.S. Food and Drug Administration Center for Drug Evaluation and Research. NDA review process. Available at: http://www.fda.gov/cder/handbook/nda.htm (accessed July 29, 2005).
4. Federal Food, Drug, and Cosmetic Act, as amended; United States Code, Title 21, Chapter 9.
5. The sponsor is the person who takes responsibility for and initiates a clinical investigation. The sponsor may be a pharmaceutical company, a governmental unit, a private or academic organization, or an individual. A sponsor-investigator is an individual who both initiates and conducts a clinical investigation and under whose immediate direction the investigational drug is being administered or dispensed. For administrative reasons, only one individual should be designated as sponsor. If a pharmaceutical company will be supplying the drug, but will not itself be submitting the IND, the company is not the sponsor.
6. U.S. Food and Drug Administration Center for Drug Evaluation and Research. The new drug development process: Steps from test tube to new drug application review. Available at: http://www.fda.gov/cder/handbook/develop.htm (accessed July 29, 2005).
7. U.S. Food and Drug Administration Center for Drug Evaluation and Research. Application process. Available at: http://www.fda.gov/cder/regulatory/applications/ind_page_1.htm (accessed July 29, 2005).
8. U.S. Food and Drug Administration Center for Drug Evaluation and Research. Application process: Introduction. Available at: http://www.fda.gov/cder/regulatory/applications/default.htm#Introduction (accessed July 29, 2005).
9. U.S. Food and Drug Administration Center for Devices and Radiological Health. Overview of regulations. Available at: http://www.fda.gov/cdrh/devadvice/overview.html (accessed July 29, 2005).
10. U.S. Food and Drug Administration Center for Devices and Radiological Health Premarket approval overview. Available at: http://www.fda.gov/cdrh/devadvice/pma/ (accessed July 29, 2005).
11. U.S. Food and Drug Administration Center for Drug Evaluation and Research. NDA review process. Available at: http://www.fda.gov/cder/handbook/nda.htm (accessed July 29, 2005).
12. U.S. Food and Drug Administration Center for Drug Evaluation and Research. Guidance for industry; E6 good clinical practice: Consolidated guidance. Available at: http://www.fda.gov/cder/guidance/959fnl.pdf (accessed July 29, 2005).
13. The official version of the Uniform Requirements for Manuscripts Submitted to Biomedical Journals is located at www.ICMJE.org (accessed July 29, 2005).
14. Faden, Ruth R., Lewis Carol, and Barbara Rimer. 1980. "Monitoring informed consent procedures: An exploratory record review," *IRB: A Review of Human Subjects Research* 2(8):9–10.
15. Costic, Phil. 1998. Presentation at the Clinical Trials and Tribulations workshop, Los Angeles, March 25, 1998.

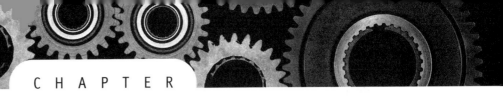

21

Dealing with Legal Counsel and the Management of Risk

J. Michael Slocum, JD, and Rebecca Barnett

Counsel in Research Activities

The multitude of legal issues and documents associated with research mandate that legal counsel be involved throughout the entire process. The role of counsel shifts during the process, depending upon the progression of the research. Counsel's main goals in representing research institutions include:

- Protecting the institution from loss, both financial and to reputation.
- Ensuring that the needs and objectives of the institution are met.

While most research institutions are primarily concerned with beneficial advancements made in the scientific and medical fields, research sponsors are more concerned with reaping the benefits of the research in which they invest.

The Role of Counsel

Counsel's role in the research process varies among different institutions and different types of research foundations. In addition, counsel's role changes throughout the research process from that of adviser, to enforcer, to risk manager, and even to educator. Because of the variety of tasks and responsibilities associated with representing research facilities, institutions, and sponsors, each institution often needs several specialized attorneys. Most institutions have a general counsel department that delegates the tasks required to protect the institution's objectives.

Common Tasks

Although counsel's role in the research process varies among different institutions and research foundations, there are a number of important general tasks assigned to counsel representing research institutions:

1. Counsel is first responsible for a preliminary investigation of the needs and goals of the research institution.
2. It is counsel's role to design a relationship with the research sponsor or third party that suits the needs of the institution. Designing the appropriate relationship for the institution involves drafting and negotiating various agreements. Counsel also advises and assists the institution in several review processes, including regulatory reviews, audits, and internal investigations.
3. One of counsel's most important roles in the research process is compliance assistance. Compliance assistance involves advising the institution on complying with federal, state, sponsor, and institution regulations.
4. Counsel may also help set up programs and actions that help the institution enforce compliance with all clinical trial rules and regulations.
5. Counsel is also involved in ensuring the institution's goals are met in the research process. In this role, counsel may act as a corporate support system, helping the institution design beneficial business relationships with sponsors and partners. Meeting the needs and goals of the institution also involves assistance and management of intellectual property ownership and rights.

Preliminary Investigation and Due Diligence

In order to be effective in meeting the needs of a research institution, counsel must conduct a preliminary investigation. The preliminary investigation should involve meeting with the institution's administrative offices, principal investigators, and possibly the institution's institutional review board (IRB). The preliminary investigation process should be designed to educate counsel on the goals and needs of the institution. Counsel should determine what types of research are being conducted and the appropriate relationships that should be established to effectively conduct the research. The preliminary investigation must also give counsel an accurate depiction of current regulation compliance, so that counsel may advise the institution of necessary changes and improvements. In representing research institutions, counsel has the responsibility of due diligence. The Food and Drug Administration (FDA) defines due diligence as:

> A measure of activity expected from a reasonable and prudent person under a particular circumstance (21 Code of Federal Regulations 60.30)

Practicing due diligence is necessary because of the severe consequences associated with possible compliance and breach of contract issues. See Figure 21-1.

Designing Relationships

In tailoring research agreements and business relationships, the role of counsel can shift dramatically depending upon the client. If counsel represents a study sponsor, the focus of counsel in designing contractual relationships is maximizing the benefit for the client. However, if counsel represents the research facility, often the role is more of a protective nature. Counsel ensures the facility is adequately protected from associated liability and risk, and secures the appropriate publishing and intellectual property rights. Counsel is not responsible for evaluating the merits of the research or business arrangement or for ensuring that the research is ethical or necessary, only that the agreement is legally sound.

Due to a wide range of goals and interests, many types of research agreements exist. Counsel must understand the client's role in the research as well as its financial and intellectual property interests. Possible agreements include research contracts, partnerships, joint ventures, contracts, licensing agreements, and consulting agreements.

Drafting Agreements and Negotiating

Counsel often serves as a mode of communication between the study sponsor and the investigator. Counsel must communicate and address the goals of each party during the drafting of the research agreement. Research agreements usually go through many drafts prior to final review. When specific clauses in a drafted agreement do not meet the needs or goals of a particular party, counsel must give advice on a legally sound way to solve the issue. Counsel often suggests negotiations in the process of drafting agreements to aid in the agreement of parties. Counsel must advise the represented institution or sponsor of the negotiation options that would provide the most protection for the client while assuring the client's goals are met.

Regulatory Review: Compliance Assistance

In the research setting, counsel is not only responsible for ensuring that research agreements meet federal and state regulations, but also meet those established by the institution's human investigation committee (HIC). HICs are set up by research institutions to ensure that research performed on human subjects is ethical, safe, and effective. HIC regulations are based upon the FDA's Good Clinical Practice document, Department of Health and Human Services regulations, Health Insurance Portability & Accountability Act (HIPAA) laws, and state regulations. While the HIC at each institution is more concerned with ensuring that research performed at the institution meets all appropriate regulations, counsel is more concerned with verifying that all contracts and business arrangements are legally sound and that the risk associated with each agreement is minimal.

Because of the multitude of research grants and contracts associated with each institution, most do not require that counsel approve each one. These institutions generally make checklists for the researchers to follow when writing contracts, which set forth the general format and language deemed appropriate by counsel. Reducing counsel involvement in research speeds the initial process and lowers research costs. The following is a model checklist, generated by the general counsel at the University of California, for the review of research grants and contracts:

1. Is the name and status of each contracting party correctly set forth? e.g., 'The Regents of the University of California,' which is described as 'a California corporation.' (Note: Setting forth the "University of California" or some instru-

---

Legal Details

- Full name of the organization/firm (many times the entity conducting the research is a subsidiary, affiliate, or division of the primary organization
- "Ownership" of the organization/firm [501(c) non-profit, for-profit owned by individuals, for-profit subsidiary of non-profit, etc.]
- State registration documents
- Copies of all applicable minutes, resolutions, etc. of the board of directors (and the shareholders, if appropriate.)
- Signatory rights backed by the appropriate decisions
- The charter of the organization/firm and other incorporation documents
- Copies of licenses, franchises, etc. granted to the organization/firm
- A list of relevant lawsuits that were filed against the organization/firm and that the organization/firm filed against third parties (litigation) plus a list of disputes which are likely to reach the courts
- Legal opinions concerning any relevant aspects of duties

Financial Due Diligence

- Balance sheets and income statements, if appropriate
- Information concerning cost principles, cost accounting issues, and accounts payable and receivable policies
- Audit reports, if any
- Internal controls
- Accounting systems used
- Methods to price products and services (particularly important where medical research is undertaken in a clinical (i.e., hospital) environment, since there are many complex rules concerning pricing for medical care and services)
- Sales and customer information (particularly important when government or foreign entities are primary customers)
- Records, filing, archives
- Budgeting and budget monitoring and controls
- Internal audits (frequency and procedures)
- External audits (frequency and procedures)

Technical and Other Issues

- Operating processes (hardware, software, communications, other)
- Need for know-how, technological transfer and licensing required
- Suppliers of equipment, software, services (including offers)
- Manpower (skilled and unskilled) (union issues, security clearance issues, etc.)
- Infrastructure (plant and equipment, government-owned, etc.)
- Transport and communications (issues relating to movement of materials, IP issues, safety and hazardous waste issues, security issues, etc.)
- Import and export restrictions or licensing (where applicable)
- Sites of performance issues (registrations, licenses, visas, application of foreign laws, etc.)
- Technical specification issues (ownership, licenses, publication, export control, etc.
- Environmental issues and how they are addressed
- Leases and real property issues, special arrangements, tax-free bond issues

FIGURE 21-1   Due Diligence Checklist for Counsel

mentality thereof as the contracting party is not correct, as the university and all its instrumentalities do business in the official name of 'The Regents of the University of California.')

2. Is the consideration for the contract sufficiently stated? That is, are the services and/or materials to be rendered and/or furnished by the contractor (The Regents of the University of California) set forth, and are the amount, time and manner of payment to The Regents set forth?

3. Is the effective date of the contract set forth or ascertainable from the provisions of the contract?

4. Is the period of performance and/or duration of the contract set forth?

5. If authorization has been obtained to incur costs prior to execution of a federal contract, does the contract contain a special clause providing for reimbursement of such costs or otherwise ensure reimbursement of such cost?

6. Are there any ambiguous words or phrases included in the contract?

7. Are there any words or phrases inconsistent with words or phrases in other parts of the contract?

8. Is the subject matter of the contract so described that it may be identified with certainty?

9. Is there any document that is attached to the contract which is meant to be a part thereof? If so, has it been correctly identified and made a part of the contract by the following phrase or another phrase to the same effect: '_____, attached hereto, is incorporated herein by this reference.'

10. Is there any recital in the contract that an attached document is made a part of the contract? If so, has that document been attached as recited?

11. If a state of California contract on the standard agreement form 2 is involved, is there a printed clause on the reverse side thereof which reads as follows: 'Contractor shall not be allowed or paid travel or per diem expenses unless set forth in this agreement'? If so, and if travel or per diem expenses are to be allowed or paid to contractor under the contract, is a typewritten statement to this effect set forth in the contract?[1]

As illustrated by the model checklist from the University of California, general counsel addresses federal and state regulations as well as those regulations imposed by the HIC of the particular institution. State laws regarding research often are more stringent than federal laws, so counsel must be very familiar with the laws of the state in which the institution is located.

Compliance with audit and review processes is discussed later in this chapter. The major issue in complying with all review processes is proper record-keeping. Counsel must advise the institution of the appropriate recordkeeping procedures and the appropriate uses and disclosures of the research records kept at the investigator and administrative levels.

Corporate Support

Counsel's role in corporate support varies depending upon the objectives and business goals of the institution. Most likely, counsel's major role in corporate support is to advise the institution on how to appropriately form and maintain beneficial relationships with business partners. Counsel also must ensure that the objectives of the institution are not sacrificed in forming business relationships with corporations and sponsors. Research institutions often do not have financial influence in the corporate world, so negotiations between sponsors and research facilities become difficult. Counsel must appropriately represent the objectives of the institution to corporate sponsors and must also protect the institution from entering into any agreements that may sacrifice its main objectives.

Another important role of counsel in corporate support is protecting the institution's equipment and resources from improper use. The employees of research institutions often are hired by corporations to complete or assist in privately funded research not linked to the institution. Counsel must advise the institution on how to protect itself from inappropriate use of equipment and resources by research staff. Most institutions require that all research staff members sign an agreement protecting it from misuse of resources.

Intellectual Property Assistance and Management

Depending upon the nature of the research, business relationship, or research contract, many possibilities exist in determining intellectual property (IP) rights and ownership. The fundamentals of intellectual property rights in the realm of research were discussed earlier in this text. Counsel must evaluate the needs of the client, design suitable IP agreements, and advise the institution of the necessary procedures and practices for compliance with the IP agreement.

Generally, the sponsor of the research insists on the retention of the IP associated with the research as the benefit for taking the risk of investing in the research. Most sponsors refuse to negotiate this issue. While the sponsor is almost always awarded ownership of the IP, the research institution is normally awarded the publishing rights associated with it. In fact, most IRBs do not approve research unless it is specifically stated that the institution will maintain publication rights.

Counsel not only ensures that the institution obtains the appropriate IP rights and ownership, but must also help the institution manage the IP associated with research. One of the more important aspects of IP management is the confidentiality of information. All employees or students involved in research at an institution must be appropriately informed of the risks associated with the use and disclosure of research results or data. All disclosures of data must specifically follow the confidentiality guidelines set forth in the research contract. If research data is leaked, the institution may be held liable for any damages or costs associated with the breach of confidentiality. Employees and students must also be aware that all research contracts are not identical in the regulations regarding IP ownership, so they must be familiar with the contract specific to the research in which they participate. Counsel must adequately inform the institution of how to protect itself from the risks associated with the ownership and management of IP.

Internal Investigation Activities

Several investigation processes occur during research. The IRB must review the research being conducted at the institution in accordance with the Good Clinical Practice document published by the FDA.[2] Also, the IRB itself is reviewed by the FDA under the bioresearch monitoring program. The FDA can also inspect clinical investigators/investigations at any time during a study. All investigation processes, whether conducted by the IRB or FDA, require the review of study documents and data. In order to comply with FDA regulations, a large number of documents must be generated and kept on file for every clinical trial performed at an institution. Due to the complex nature of many of the documents required for compliance, counsel often drafts and edits many of the documents, or provides a standard template or checklist for use by the clinical investigators in document preparation and maintenance. Table 21-1 details the documents that must be producible for review of most clinical investigations.

The aforementioned documents are produced and recorded prior to and during the clinical trial. Table 21-2 details documents that are produced and recorded after the trial.

With the exception of research approval, the IRB's primary responsibility is to regularly review the research being performed at the institution. The IRB is concerned with safety, informed consent, and regulation compliance issues. It must conduct a review of continuing research no less than once per year. If the IRB finds that an investigator is not following the guidelines agreed upon for the research, the IRB will end the research until appropriate modifications, if possible, are made. The IRB has

the right to all study documents and data and may conduct interviews with those related to the study.[3]

Inspection of an IRB by the FDA is a common occurrence in order to determine if the IRB is operating in accordance with its own regulations as well as those of the FDA. IRB inspections are on-site procedures conducted by an appointed field investigator. The investigator interviews the appropriate persons to obtain adequate information regarding the IRB's policies and procedures. The investigators will then track several studies, either ongoing or completed, that were reviewed by the IRB to ensure that the IRB followed all appropriate policies and procedures. The investigator has complete access to all IRB records and may copy and release the records to the FDA, if necessary. Before writing the review report to send to the FDA, the investigator meets with the IRB chairperson and a responsible institutional representative, often counsel, to review the findings of the investigation. At this time, any misunderstandings can be clarified and suggested or required corrections or reforms can be provided to the institution so mistakes are not repeated. The investigator submits his written report to the FDA. The FDA then sends a letter to the institution outlining any noncompliance issues and suggesting the appropriate corrective measures. Often it is counsel's responsibility to respond to the letter with a statement of intended reform.[4]

The FDA conducts several different types of investigator reviews. Clinical investigator inspections can be classified as study-oriented inspections, investigator-oriented inspections, or bioequivalence study inspections. All classifications of investigator inspections are conducted by the FDA, but the FDA may have different motives for each type. In all FDA investigator reviews, the FDA's representative has unlimited access to all study or investigator records. Confidential information, such as protected health information, may remain confidential unless it is crucial to the investigation.

Study-oriented inspections are almost always related to either new drug applications or product license applications. The investigation consists of two parts: the first part determines the basic facts surrounding the study, and the second involves auditing the study data for validity. Investigator-oriented inspections are normally warranted when an investigator plays a pivotal role in a study related to a product's approval or its effect in the medical field. Investigator-oriented inspections may also occur when a sponsor complains about

TABLE 21-1	Documents for Clinical Investigations[2]			
			Located in Files of	
	Title of Document	**Purpose**	**Institution**	**Investigator/ Sponsor**
8.3.1	Investigator's Brochure updates	To document that investigator is informed in a timely manner of relevant information as it becomes available	X	X
8.3.2	Any revisions to:—Protocol/ amendment(s) and CRF—Informed consent form—Any other written information provided to subjects— Advertisement for subject recruitment (if used)	To document revisions of these trial-trial related documents that take effect during	X	X
8.3.3	Dated, documented approval/favorable opinion of institutional review board (IRB)/independent ethics committee (IEC) of the following: —Protocol amendment(s)— Revision(s) of: —Informed consent form—Any other written information to be provided to the subject—Adver-tisement for subject recruitment (if used)—Any other documents given approval/favorable opinion—Continu-ing review of trial	To document that the amendment(s) and/or revision(s) have been subject to IRB/IEC review and were given approval/favorable opinion. To identify the version number and date of the document(s)	X	X
8.3.4	Regulatory authority(ies) authoriza-tions/ approvals/notifications where required for: —Protocol amendment(s) and other documents	To document compliance with applica-ble regulatory requirements	X (where required)	X
8.3.5	Curriculum vitae for new investigator(s) and/or subinvesti-gators		X	X
8.3.6	Updates to normal value(s)/range(s) for medical laboratory/technical procedure(s)/test(s) included in the protocol	To document normal values and ranges that are revised during the trial	X	X
8.3.7	Updates of medical/ laboratory/tech-nical procedures/tests—Certification or—Accreditation or—Established quality control and/or external quality assessment or—Other validation (where required)	To document that tests remain ade-quate throughout the trial period	X (where required)	X
8.3.8	Documentation of investigational product(s) and trial-related materials shipment		X	X
8.3.9	Certificate(s) of analysis for new batches of investigational products			X
8.3.10	Monitoring visit reports	To document site visits by, and find-ings of, the monitor		X

TABLE 21-1	Documents for Clinical Investigations (continued)			
			Located in Files of	
	Title of Document	**Purpose**	**Institution**	**Investigator/ Sponsor**
8.3.11	Relevant communications other than site visits—Letters—Meeting notes—Notes of telephone calls	To document any agreements or significant discussions regarding trial conduct, adverse event (AE) reporting administration, protocol violations, trial	X	X
8.3.12	Signed informed consent forms	To document that consent is obtained in accordance with GCP and protocol and dated prior to participation of each subject in trial. Also to document direct access permission	X	
8.3.13	Source documents	To document the existence of the subject and substantiate integrity of trial data collected. To include original documents related to the trial, to medical treatment, and history of subject	X	
8.3.14	Signed, dated, and completed case report forms (CRFs)	To document that the investigator or authorized member of the investigator's staff confirms the observations recorded	X (copy)	X (original)
8.3.15	Documentation of CRF corrections	To document all changes/ additions or corrections made to CRF after initial data were recorded	X (copy)	X (original)
8.3.16	Notification by originating investigator to sponsor of serious adverse events and related reports	Notification by originating investigator to sponsor of serious adverse events and related reports	X	X
8.3.17	Notification by sponsor and/or investigator, where applicable, to regulatory authority(ies) and IRB(s)/IEC(s) of unexpected serious adverse drug reactions and of other safety information	Notification by sponsor and/or investigator, where applicable, to regulatory authorities and IRB(s)/IEC(s) of unexpected serious adverse drug reactions and of other safety information	X (where required)	X
8.3.18	Notification by sponsor to investigators of safety information	Notification by sponsor to investigators of safety information	X	X
8.3.19	Interim or annual reports to IRB/IEC and authority(ies)	Interim or annual reports provided to IRB/IEC and to authority(ies)	X	X (where required)
8.3.20	Subject screening log	To document identification of subjects who entered pretrial screening	X	X (where required)
8.3.21	Subject identification code list	To document that investigator/institution keeps a confidential list of names of all subjects allocated to trial numbers on enrolling in the trial. Allows investigator/ institution to reveal identity of any subject.	X	

continues

TABLE 21-1	Documents for Clinical Investigations (continued)			
			**Located in Files of**	
	Title of Document	**Purpose**	**Institution**	**Investigator/ Sponsor**
8.3.22	Subject enrollment log	To document chronological enrollment of subjects by trial number	X	
8.3.23	Investigational product(s) accountability at the site	To document that investigational products(s) have been used according to the protocol	X	X
8.3.24	Signature sheet	To document signatures and initials of all persons authorized to make entries and/or corrections on CRFs	X	X
8.3.25	Record of retained body fluids/tissue samples (if any)	To document location and identification of retained samples if assays need to be repeated	X	X

TABLE 21-2	Documents Preceding and Proceeding during Trial			
			**Located in Files of**	
	Title of Document	**Purpose**	**Institution**	**Investigator/ Sponsor**
8.4.1	Investigational product(s) accountability at site	To document that the investigational product(s) have been used according to the protocol. To document the final accounting of investigational product(s) received at the site, dispensed to subjects, returned by the subjects, and returned to sponsor	X	X
8.4.2	Documentation of investigational product(s) destruction	To document destruction of unused investigational product(s) by sponsor or at site	X (if destroyed at site)	X
8.4.3	Completed subject identification code list	To permit identification of all subjects enrolled in the trial in case follow-up is required. List should be kept in a confidential manner and for agreed-upon time	X	
8.4.4	Audit certificate (if required)	To document that audit was performed (if required)		X
8.4.5	Final trial close-out monitoring report	To document that all activities required for trial close-out are completed and copies of essential documents are held in the appropriate files		X
8.4.6	Treatment allocation and decoding documentation	Returned to sponsor to document any decoding that may have occurred		X
8.4.7	Final report by investigator/institution to IRB/IEC where required, and where applicable, to the regulatory authority(ies)	To document completion of the trial	X	
8.4.8	Clinical study report	To document results and interpretation of trial	X (if applicable)	X

an investigator's performance or when a study participant complains of a rights violation. The inspection processes are normally the same for an investigator-oriented inspection and a study-oriented inspection. At the end of the inspection, the FDA investigator will conduct an interview with the clinical investigator similar to the one conducted in the IRB review process, where the investigator or institution may request counsel's presence.[4]

Audit Assistance

Research institutions performing medical research involving human subjects are subject to many audits. Audits may be imposed on research institutions by the federal or state government or by the institution's IRB. Government audits include audits initiated by the FDA, audits permissible under the Single Audit Act of 1984 and the Single Audit Act Amendments of 1996, and tax audits. The IRB at each research institution has a responsibility under FDA guidelines to regularly review the research performed at the institution. In the realm of research, audits are almost always concerned with the institution's finances or with the ethics and legal compliance of the research. The audits permissible under the Single Audit Act of 1984 and the Single Audit Act Amendments of 1996 and tax audits are more concerned with the financial situation of the research institution. Audits initiated by the FDA and the institution's IRB are more concerned with research safety and compliance with federal and state regulations.

The Single Audit Act of 1984 and the Single Audit Act Amendments of 1996 set standards for obtaining consistency and uniformity among federal agencies for the audit of states, local governments, and nonprofit organizations expending federal awards. Because many research institutions are classified as nonprofit organizations and expend federal awards for research, the institutions are subject to audits by the appropriate federal agencies. OMB Circular No. A-133 specifically identifies the nonprofit organizations that must conduct annual audits. The circular also details the audit procedures and the requirements of the institution during an audit.[5] OMB Circular No. A-133 Subpart B—Audits §___.200 Audit requirements.

Audit Required

Nonfederal entities that expend $500,000 for fiscal years ending after December 31, 2003 or more in a year in federal awards shall have a single or program-specific audit conducted for that year in accordance with the provisions of this part. Guidance on determining federal awards expended is provided in §___.205.

Counsel must be familiar with the requirements set forth in OMB Circular A-133 and must advise the research institution of the procedures necessary for audit preparation. These include:

- Proper financial procedures.
- Proper recordkeeping.
- Appropriate information to submit for audit.
- Records and information legally accessible to the auditors.
- Documents that are not required for the audit.

It is the responsibility of counsel to ensure that the procedures associated with the audit are executed properly and fairly on behalf of the institution. Counsel's responsibilities regarding tax audits are similar in nature to those associated with the audits detailed in OMB Circular A-133. Counsel must advise the institution on appropriate financial procedures and recordkeeping. A key element in audit assistance is giving advice on audit preparation as there are limits on how much time an institution has to submit requested information to auditors.[5]

Litigation

Another major role of counsel representing research institutions is the prediction and prevention of lawsuits, often referred to as risk management. Counsel evaluates the risks associated with research and day-to-day routines and gives advice on how to eliminate or minimize the assumed risks. Two major types of lawsuits are filed against research institutions: litigation between the institution and the research sponsor or litigation between the institution and a third party. While disagreements may arise between the institution and sponsor, actual legal proceedings between the two parties are rare. Disagreements are normally resolved through negotiations made by or under the guidance of counsel. Disagreements between research institutions and study sponsors normally arise from breach of contract issues. If one of the parties does not uphold its contractual obligations, the other party may seek financial retribution for the losses incurred. Breach of contract issues may include, but are not limited to, reimbursement or payment for services, intellectual property use and ownership, confidentiality of study information, and time delay issues.

One of the few court cases involving a university-sponsor breach of contract issue dealt with unexpected and unacceptable time delays on the part of the university. In *Virginia Polytechnic Institute and State University, et al. v. Interactive Return Service, Inc.*,[6] Virginia Polytechnic Institute and State University ("Virginia Tech") was found liable for damages to the Interactive Return Service, Inc. ("Interactive") due to a breach of contract. Interactive concluded a sponsored research agreement with Virginia Tech in January 1995, and agreed to reimburse Virginia Tech for the costs incurred to conduct research and development. However, Interactive stopped making payments in December 1995. Six months later, the two entities entered into an industry project agreement (IPA) with an intellectual property company that addressed funding for the research and intellectual property rights. In December 1996, Virginia Tech stopped working on the project and assigned its rights to the intellectual property company, which, in turn, licensed those rights to a third party. The state Supreme Court held that:

1. There was sufficient evidence from which the jury could have concluded that Virginia Tech waived its right to receive prompt payment from Interactive, and the trial court did not err when it instructed the jury on the issue of waiver;
2. There was no evidence that Interactive was the first party to breach the IPA, and;
3. The evidence was sufficient to support the jury's verdict that Interactive was entitled to damages for breach of contract.[6]

Adhering to the rules and regulations set up by the federal and state government and the institution's IRB normally prevents third-party litigation. Making the best possible effort to conduct research in an ethical manner is another important safeguard against third-party litigation. Third-party lawsuits in the medical research setting are almost always filed by research participants who are unhappy with the way they are treated during a study. Third-party litigation by study participants can result from a variety of safety and privacy issues including improper informed consent process, breach of confidentiality, breach of contract, and liability issues.

Normally, all confidentiality, contract, and liability issues also fall into the category of informed consent issues. Since confidentiality and injury clauses are part of most informed consent documents, and because the informed consent document is considered a contract between the investigator and participant, these issues often overlap one another. Lawsuits filed claiming improper informed consent procedures normally involve the expected risks and benefits associated with a study. If a participant is injured or harmed because he or she was exposed to risks during the study that were not explicitly stated during the informed consent process, the participant has a right to sue for damages. All possible risks and benefits of research studies must be explicitly stated during the informed consent process to adequately protect institutions from liability. Several landmark cases have dealt with informed consent issues in research studies. One of the more famous is *Grimes v. Kennedy Institute, Inc.*, which involved the vulnerable subject population of children. Several families with healthy children were recruited to live in housing with varying amounts of lead poisoning. The families were not made aware of the lead poisoning present in the houses, nor were they informed of the risks associated with exposing children to lead poisoning. Many of the children suffered learning disabilities and cognitive disorders as a result of the exposure. The Kennedy Krieger Institute was found liable for the damages imposed on the study participants.[7]

Confidentiality of study information is an important aspect in the prevention of third-party litigation. Third parties may seek damages if confidential information is used or disclosed inappropriately and without the proper consent. Specific confidentiality issues associated with third-party litigation will be discussed later in the chapter on risk management.

• • • References

1. University of California Office of the President. "Contract and Grant Manual: Legal Authorities and Principles," http://www.ucop.edu/raohome/cgmanual/chap13.html (accessed August 3, 2005).
2. "ICH E6: Good Clinical Practice: Consolidated Guideline," *Federal Register* 62, no. 90 (May 9, 1997): 25691–25709.

3. US Food and Drug Administration. "FDA Institutional Review Board Inspections," http://www.fda.gov/oc/ohrt/irbs/operations.html#board (accessed August 3, 2005).

4. US Food and Drug Administration. "FDA Inspections of Clinical Investigators," http://www.fda.gov/oc/ohrt/irbs/operations.html#inspections (accessed August 3, 2005).

5. The White House, Office of Management and Budget. "OMB Circular A-133 Compliance Supplement," March 2004, http://www.whitehouse.gov/omb/circulars/a133_compliance/04/04toc.html (accessed August 3, 2005).

6. *Virginia Polytechnic Institute and State University, et al. v. Interactive Return Service, Inc.* 267 Va. 642 (Supreme Court of Virginia, April 23, 2004). 267 Va. 642; 595 S.E.2d 1; 2004 Va. LEXIS 67, April 23, 2004.

7. *Grimes v. Kennedy Krieger Institute Inc.*, et al. 366 Md. 29 (Court of Appeals of Maryland, 2001). 66 Md. 29; 782 A.2d 807; 2001 Md. LEXIS 496, August 16, 2001.

22

Special Issues for Land-Grant Institutions

Robert Killoren, MA, CRA, and Judy McCormick

Administration of research at a land-grant college or university presents some unique challenges to the research administrator. Issues concerning cost-sharing, intellectual property rights, assessment of facilities and administrative costs, allocability of costs, project accountability, and the undertaking of research in the national interest all take on a new spin when examined in the context of the land-grant mission.

In this chapter, we examine the background to land-grant institutions. How did they come about? Historically, what distinguishes them from other institutions? What special rules or expectations affect their missions and the way they do business? And finally, how does all this impact research administration?

A Short History of Land-Grant Institutions

Even before there was such a thing as a land-grant institution, Penn State's first president, Evan Pugh, foresaw the unique role that such an institution could play in our country—a role that creates to this day special issues for research administrators working in these institutions. In 1859 he established the Penn State legacy "to seek to make use of [academic] intelligence in developing the agricultural and industrial resources of the country, and protecting its interests."[1] This view of the purpose of an educational institution, while more commonplace today, was a radical departure from the traditional model of education in the 19th century,

which consisted primarily of the teaching of mathematics, rhetoric, and the classical languages.[2]

President Pugh envisioned an educational program that combined a classical education with practical applications. This was a new vision, but it was not his alone; it was shared by a group of a relatively few, but influential educators from across the states who wanted to make higher learning accessible to the ordinary individual in a very practical way. These visionaries pushed for and eventually won support for federal legislation from Representative Justin Smith Morrill of Vermont who authored the Land-Grant College Act of 1862 (now known as the Morrill Act).[3]

The Morrill Act enabled states to sell federal land (thus the term "land grant"), invest the proceeds, and use the income to support colleges "where the leading object shall be, without excluding scientific and classical studies . . . to teach agriculture and the mechanic (sic) arts [engineering] . . . in order to promote the liberal and practical education of the industrial classes in all the pursuits and professions of life."[4]

While much of the later legislation concerning land grants deals specifically with agriculture, the original Act was much broader applying not only to agriculture, but to engineering as well.[5] However, while it was broad in mission, it did target this "liberal and practical education" to the "industrial classes." In many ways, the land-grant institutions initially were started as "blue-collar" colleges. This practical approach to education and the special mission to offer a higher education to the great middle class of workers and farmers in many ways continues today in the student body, the kinds of research projects undertaken at land-grant institutions, and the willingness of land-grant institutions to work closely with industry. While much has changed, much has stayed the same.

One of the first innovations that this new order of schooling required was the integration of research and teaching. In order to teach the practical arts of agriculture and engineering, schools had to do more than just teach a course on agricultural chemistry or applied physics. Farmers, particularly, questioned the value of "book farming" and wanted tangible proof that colleges were committed to their well-being, so professors began searching for practical ways of instruction. Thus, many land-grant schools started demonstration and model farms that became rudimentary research facilities that grew eventually into full-fledged research centers called "agricultural experiment stations," the first of which was established in 1875.[6]

In 1887, the Hatch Act, named after the act's champion, Missouri's Congressman William H. Hatch, was passed establishing agricultural experiment stations to be housed at institutions founded under the original Morrill Act. Institutions were given $15,000 annually "to conduct original researches or verify experiments ... [on subjects] bearing directly upon the agricultural industry of the United States."[7] The framers of the Hatch Act intended to "connect research with teaching in a unified program to advance the land-grant mission of placing practical knowledge in the hands of the public."[8] Penn State President George W. Atherton articulated this when he said, "Let the college investigate that it may teach well, and the station teach that it may investigate."[9]

While the federal government initiated support for agricultural research through the Hatch Act, it would not lend financial support to the land grant mission in the mechanical arts, embodied in engineering. Congress felt that while agriculture benefited an entire cross section of the American population involved in farming and its related industries, advances that arose out of engineering research only benefited a small subset of the populace and only benefited the general public indirectly.[10] Over the next 25 years land-grant colleges struggled to find support for engineering research. Finally, in 1903 the University of Illinois and in 1904 Iowa State University were able to establish engineering experiment stations with the support of state legislatures and private donors. Some universities, like Penn State, while failing to find financial support, still felt that the concept of the engineering experiment station was still valid, especially as a

help to small companies that could not conduct research on their own.[11] The first bulletin of the Penn State Engineering Experiment Station, which was established in 1909, stated its goals as follows:

> ... to carry on scientific investigations concerning the problems of engineering and the mechanic arts; to study and report on engineering methods, materials, and processes relating to manufacturing, transportation, sanitation and water supply, structures, and the various other industrial interests of Pennsylvania; to furnish specific instructions which may prove of use to the masses of the people.[12]

Back on the agricultural side, within the first decade after the passage of the Hatch Act, three major and interrelated developments occurred that helped shape the administration of research in agricultural experiment stations. This first was the establishment in 1888 of the Office of Experiment Stations under the US Department of Agriculture. This office went about establishing standards by which stations would operate and then, in 1895, the office developed a system for reviewing the accounting procedures, management, a station's working arrangements with its college, and the entire research portfolio of each station.

Next, the office implemented the restriction that Hatch Funds could only be used to support the research programs of the stations, and they were not to be used for educational programs. While this helped focus the available limited resources, it created a continuing problem of how to transfer what was learned in the stations to those most needing that information.

This imbalance between research and education led to the establishment of the Smith-Lever Agricultural Extension Act of 1914 that provided funds to create a national system for vocational education for adults located in rural areas and a network of county extension agents who could take the knowledge gained in the experiment stations and transfer that intelligence into the operational arena.

Of special note for research administrators, for the first time the concept of "matching funds" was used. Under Smith-Lever, each state was required to match every dollar over an initial $10,000 of the annual federal grant, perhaps the first recorded instance of a cost-sharing requirement.[13] Likewise, during this early period of development saw the establishment of system of administration, oversight, and accountability that would play out a half-century later in the establishment of such federal

TABLE 22-1	History of Significant Land-Grant Legislation	
Federal Legislation	**Date**	**Purpose**
Morrill Act	1862	Established the original land grant colleges. States could sell federal land and establish a trust to support the college.
Hatch Act	1887	Established agricultural research stations in the land grant colleges; funding set at $15,000 per year.
Second Morrill Act	1890	Provided for annual appropriation for land grant colleges, starting at $15,000. Forbade racial discrimination or required states establish separate institutions with funds divided in a "just and equitable" manner.
Adams Act	1906	Doubled public funding for agricultural research, committed national support to locally directed experimentation, and created annual performance evaluation standards.
Smith-Lever Act	1914	Established agricultural extension programs at each land grant college; funding dependent proportion of rural residence.
Purnell Act	1925	Tripled funds for the Hatch Act.
Bankhead-Jones Act	1935	Increased annual Hatch Act increments, but made appropriations formula based with matching funds from states, also established the discretionary "Special Research Fund."
McIntire-Stennis Act	1962	Encouraged forestry research at land grant colleges.
Research Facilities Act	1963	Provided federal funds for facilities, provided on a matching basis (never well funded).
Rural Development Act	1974	Provided funds for rural sociological research (meager funding).
Equity in Educational Land-Grant Status Act	1994	Conferred land-grant status to 29 tribal colleges.

funding agencies as the National Science Foundation (NSF).

Table 22-1 provides a selective history of significant land grant legislation.

The Land-Grant Milieu

The whole milieu established by the concept of the land-grant institution dictated in great measure the course of these colleges. They tended to focus on applied education and research. Penn State's history exemplifies this concept; its story parallels that of other land-grant institutions. A quick trip around the campus at Pennsylvania's land-grant institution shows a number of historical markers that tell of its land-grant history. There are markers that commemorate:

- The first Penn State Ag Experiment Station building and the fact that agricultural research has helped make American agriculture the most productive in the world.
- The establishment in 1892 of the Penn State Creamery, which offered America's first collegiate instruction in ice cream manufacture

and helped make the university one of the premier international centers for ice cream research.

- The construction of the first engineering building in 1892, "fitted with labs, lecture halls, shops, forges and a foundry," in other words, the tools necessary for a strong practical education.
- The founding of architectural engineering in 1910 to provide "liberal training in both the aesthetic and construction sides of architecture."
- The calorimeter facility built in 1902 to study a large animal's metabolism, citing the international significance of the research performed there that helped lead to feeds of higher nutritive value.
- How the atom was first "seen" at Penn State using a field ion microscope, invented by a faculty member, that had a magnification of more than 2 million times.
- The construction of the first Penn State electronic digital computer in 1953, among the first on any college campus and built with parts donated by industry.[14]

The Penn State archives also reflect how the land-grant concept pervaded the activities of the university. The first meeting of the Penn State College

(Penn State was not designated a university until the 1950s) Council on Research was held on February 6, 1928. The focus of the first meeting was on how to respond to the constant stream of requests from commercial concerns (from "oil producers, anthracite coal interests, millers' and bakers' associations, and other similar groups") that wanted to support research at Penn State.[15] The following questions and concerns were addressed at the meeting:

1. To what extent should the college enter into agreements with commercial concerns and under what conditions?
2. What should be the institutional policy in reference to patents and patent rights?
3. To what extent can the research work of the graduate school best fit into the whole research problem?
4. What studies should be made to avoid duplication of research in the various departments of the college?
5. What is the proper cost accounting in order to determine the conditions under which the college can undertake research problems?
6. How should the name of the college be used in connection with research work for commercial concerns?

No doubt these issues seem very familiar to today's research administrator; the very same issues remain. The fact that these issues were of concern 75 years ago at a land-grant institution demonstrates the long-standing special orientation of land-grant universities toward the practical aspects of higher learning.

In 1934 Penn State published its first edition of "Policy and Procedure in Research." That same year witnessed the chartering of The Pennsylvania Research Corporation to manage Penn State's intellectual property. It also saw the first recorded discussion at Penn State about filing a patent application. The discussion was over the Frear-Haley Photoelectric Colorimeter, a novel faculty invention that gave a rapid determination of lead residues on apples. It was pointed out that while the invention had "rather limited application, and hence is not likely to be a considerable source of revenue to the holder of the patent, if one is granted," that nonetheless, "it is desirable to make application for a patent, since no manufacturer of scientific instruments will consider the manufacture of the apparatus unless assured of exclusive rights."[16]

These historical points demonstrate the rather unique role that the land-grant mission had in defining the purpose and functions of land-grant colleges. This uniqueness has led to some rather special issues for research administrators.

Industry–University Relations

As was previously stated, the land-grant institution in Pennsylvania had a special role to play in working with industry. Figure 22-1 shows industry funding as a percentage of all research funding at Penn State for various years during the period of 1930 through 1955.[17] The chart shows that from 1945 through 1955 Penn State's average level of industry-sponsored research was 15.5%. Even today, more than twenty years after the passage of the Bayh-Dole Act, which served as the major stimulus to the dramatic growth in industry-sponsored research at US institutions of higher education in recent times, Penn State recorded 14.8% level of industry funding, while the national average for the percentage of industry funding at colleges and universities was less than 7%.[18] The extent of Penn State's active involvement is not true for every land-grant institution, but even so, land grants ranked among the top 100 institutions on average performing more industry research than their counterparts.[19]

This connection with industry presents some unique situations for research administrators at land-grant institutions. The first and predominant question that arises is to what extent should a university engage in industry-sponsored research, even one pledged to a land-grant philosophy? Universities, even land grants, must balance what is done with and for industry with its role as an institution

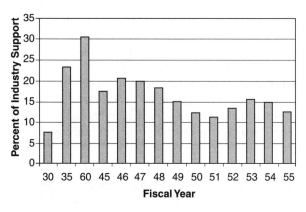

FIGURE 22-1 Penn State Industrial Research Funding
Source: Research at the Pennsylvania State University, A Report to the Committee on Research of the Board of Trustees, May 10, 1957 (Penn State Archives)

of higher education to serve the general public. As one can tell from the Penn State chart of industry-supported research during the 1930s, a significant percentage of total research funding came from industry.[20] What one cannot tell from this particular chart was what was happening specifically in the School of Engineering. There, in some years during this period, more than half of all external support for research was coming from private firms and industrial groups. This level of involvement prompted University President Ralph Hetzel in March 1933 to share his concerns with the Penn State Research Council:

> There is a danger that applied research in cooperation with industries may overshadow and stifle institutional research of a more fundamental nature . . . The question is not whether such investigations should be eliminated, but how far can we go in this line of work without prejudicing the instructional and research programs of an institution that is supported by public funds and unrestricted by contract.[21]

One can note in this communiqué grave concern about a public institution's mission. In response, the research council adopted a general policy that "no school [within Penn State] was to undertake any privately funded research that did not contribute to the overall institutional research program and that did not promise to yield results of public value, as contrasted with value primarily to the donor."[22] This concept was further developed by the School of Engineering, which supported a publicly oriented policy that "no work was done unless the donor clearly stipulated that the School might make public any and all results and could . . . have the right of patent."[23] This internal policy, developed more than 70 years ago, brings up two issues that still dominate research administration concerns, especially at land-grant institutions: those regarding publication and intellectual property rights. The culture of the university is one that is for free and open dissemination and exchange of research results. The culture of industry consists of maintenance of the competitive advantage that secrecy and confidentiality can provide. Operating in this dichotomous environment is difficult for a university research administrator. One approach to use with industry in negotiating from a land-grant perspective is to be up-front with the company in terms of the needs of both parties. The university has a public responsibility to disseminate new knowledge. This derives in great measure from the fact that among the top 100 research institutions in the United States, nearly 60% of total research funding comes from the federal government.[24] Since so much of the total base of research performed by universities and colleges in this country comes from public funds, there is an implied mandate that universities share the findings of all its research with the public.

However, while it is important that research findings of scientific and societal import be made publicly available, this does not mean that universities are required to divulge aspects of a research project that are proprietary to the company. In many cases, universities can acknowledge that specifics regarding the nature of proprietary materials or data, which a company provides a university researcher during the course of the research and identifies as confidential, need not be published in order to publish the scientific results of the research. A compromise is therefore sometimes available to institutions. This might be in the form of a contract clause that states something like the following:

> It is the purpose of this clause to balance Sponsor's need to protect commercially feasible technologies, products, or processes with university's public responsibility to freely disseminate scientific findings for the advancement of knowledge. University recognizes that the public dissemination of information based upon Research performed under this Agreement cannot contain proprietary information [which needs to be carefully defined elsewhere in the agreement] nor should it jeopardize Sponsor's ability to commercialize intellectual property developed hereunder. Further, University acknowledges that commercially sensitive information related to the design or composition of specified products or processes is not of general interest, while its confidentiality may be critical to the commercialization of said products or processes. Similarly, Sponsor recognizes that the scientific results of Project must be publishable and, subject to the confidentiality provisions of the Agreement, may be presented in forums such as symposia or international, national or regional professional meetings, or published in vehicles such as books, journals, websites, theses, or dissertations.[25]

The concepts expressed in this clause give the research administrator a start at balancing the needs of both the university and the company in the spirit of a land-grant mission. [However, in certain contexts such as for research identified on the munitions control list under the International Traffic in Arms Regulations (ITAR), dealing with company proprietary information or materials on a research project can lead to export control issues that affect publication rights and the use of graduate students on projects. Consultation with your attorneys is important.]

Research projects with industry present the same kind of dilemma for intellectual property (IP) issues as for publications. Land-grant universities, as publicly supported entities that have built their research expertise on decades of federal and state support, have a mandate to ensure that inventions are utilized for the public good. This necessarily means that they should exert a significant level of control over patents and copyrights. This usually means that the university must own all IP developed under a research project, a stance that industry often finds puzzling and arbitrary. Their natural reaction is normally, "We paid for the research; we own it."

Once again a balanced approach needs to be taken. A land-grant university recognizes that, unless a company is simply helping a researcher with his or her own research (usually done in the form of a gift or unrestricted grant), the company is sponsoring the research in hopes of solving some specific problems they are having or developing new or improved products for sale. Once again, the research administrator needs to balance the public responsibilities of the university with the competitive advantage the company is seeking through the sponsorship. An introductory clause to an IP section of a research agreement, something like the following, can help bridge that gap:

> The purpose of this clause is to balance Sponsor's ability to reasonably exploit, with due competitive advantage, the commercial viability of technologies, products, or processes with University's responsibility to ensure the broadest public benefit from the results of University research. University recognizes that one of the prime reasons Sponsor has entered this Agreement is an effort to secure, through the creation or enhancement of technologies, a market position with regard to its products or processes. At the same time, Sponsor recognizes that University has an obligation to utilize the knowledge and technology generated by University research in a manner which maximizes societal benefit and economic develop-

ment and which provides for the education of graduate and undergraduate students.

The IP section can then go on to address prompt disclosure of inventions to the sponsor, the university's ownership of IP, and the granting of an option to the sponsor to negotiate a license to the technology. The introductory clause serves to temper the subsequent stance the university takes in regard to IP ownership and sets up the logic behind the offer to license IP to the company.

A unique wrinkle in this area, however, arises for land-grant colleges of agriculture. Because all research under an agricultural experiment station is related to an AES research project regardless of funding source (except for state projects), each project receives some share of federally appropriated funding. This funding may be in the form of partial support for the base salary for faculty, graduate students, or technicians, or for other miscellaneous costs. A provision of federally appropriated funding is that the AES must comply with the Bayh-Dole Act (37 CRF 401.14). Thus, there is a potential link established between every industry-supported research project in an agricultural school and the federal requirement for a nonexclusive license being given to the federal government under the Bayh-Dole Act. At the time of writing this chapter, the USDA is preparing a clarification on how an institution's Bayh-Dole responsibilities interact with a company's rights in the setting of an agriculture research station project. Fundamentally, it is believed that as long as the company is paying all the direct expenses of the research project, then Bayh-Dole requirements are not applicable. However, if any USDA funds are used in direct support of an industry-funded project (for example to pay for the faculty member's time) then the government should be given a nonexclusive, royalty-free license to use any inventions generated under the project for government purposes.

Research Administration Issues Regarding Operating an Agricultural Experiment Station

Establishment of an Agricultural Experiment Station (AES) Research Project in the College

This section discusses the processing requirements for establishing and operating an agricultural experiment station (AES). The procedures discussed in this section represent Penn State's approach to the various requirements established by the USDA, but are representative of procedures that land-grant institutions follow. The history of the USDA's administrative requirements for operating a land-grant institution goes back to the institution of the Office of Experiment Stations that started in 1888. It was the office's third director, Dr. Alfred Charles True, who "initiated a series of policies and procedures which shaped state-federal relations in the public agricultural research partnership to the present day."[26]

The implementation of the Adams Act of 1906 gave Dr. True the necessary federal backing to provide for a real level of coordination and accountability with the agricultural experiment stations. He created the "Project System" for agricultural experiment stations—all research was to be related to a specific project at each station. True's system gave the USDA's Office of Experiment Stations a mechanism to ensure that stations across the country were utilizing federal funds in appropriate ways. Each project proposal was to identify a general area of concern, the specific problem to be addressed, and the experimental methodology to be employed in the research. By combining these three elements, the policy gave reviewers, as well as station personnel, an effective model of solution development for specific agricultural problems. Each project required an itemized budget that gave local station directors and the Office of Experiment Stations the ability to provide a much more sound system of accountability—one that allowed problems to be caught and fixed before serious trouble resulted in disqualifications.[27]

An example of how this plays out today: At Penn's State's College of Agricultural Sciences, all faculty who have a research appointment must have an USDA-approved AES research project or be part of one. Likewise, all research in the college must be conducted under a specific USDA-approved project. This includes all research projects, whether the funding comes from extramural grants and contracts from federal and state government, industry, foundations, and gifts, or from federal and state appropriated funding. Approved projects are assigned a project number that is used on any research expenditure and enables complete financial and scientific reporting of all research under a specific project. Presently, there are approximately 270 approved projects in the Penn State College of Agricultural Sciences.

The procedures for developing a research project at Penn State are as follows:[28]

1. "Review of Past and Current Research to Include a Current Research Information System Search: All projects should begin with a request for information retrieval from the USDA's Current Research Information System (CRIS). This will help to identify ongoing projects in the area of the proposed research and to avoid unnecessary duplication.

2. Prospectus: The prospectus should include the title, personnel, objectives, approach, duration, and advisory committee members. An advisory committee is optional. A prospectus is prepared when a new project and/or new direction of research is initiated.

3. Prospectus Review: The prospectus should be submitted to the lead unit leader who will identify two or three people to review the proposed research. A review form that includes nine criteria must be completed by each reviewer. This form must be signed by the reviewer, the lead unit leader, and the appropriate Associate Dean.

4. Project Development Meeting: To assist in the research planning process, a project development meeting will be scheduled by the Associate Dean with the appropriate scientist(s), unit leader(s), Associate Dean(s), and member(s) of the advisory committee. Project reviewers may also be included. The purpose of the meeting is to clarify the objectives and approach, to identify or discuss other relevant research and scientist(s) for the project, and to explore funding sources for the project. If a prospectus is required, it should be completed and reviewed prior to this meeting. If not, a reviewed draft of the project outline should be available for discussion.

5. Project Outline: The project outline should include in order:
   - a brief, clear, and specific title
   - a statement of justification
   - previous work and present outlook
   - a concise, logically arranged, and numbered series of objectives
   - a number of procedure statements to correspond with each numbered objective
   - literature cited
   - probable duration
   - financial support
   - personnel
   - advisory committee (optional)
   - institutional units involved
   - cooperation

6. Project Outline Review: The project outline should be completed and submitted to the lead unit leader who will distribute it to two or three reviewers for their critique and recommendation. If a prospectus was prepared, the project outline should be sent to the same reviewers.

7. Assurance Statement: The USDA's assurance statement must be completed by the investigator, initialed by the unit leader, and signed by the appropriate Associate Dean. The research project must be reviewed by a standing institutional committee if the work involves: a. the use of recombinant DNA or RNA, b. the use of animals, or c. the use of human subjects. If the project needs to be reviewed and approved by any of the three committees, a copy of the committee's approval letter should accompany the completed assurance form.

8. Signature Sheet: All project leaders, their unit leaders, and members of the advisory committee must be knowledgeable of the proposed project. Their signatures are evidence of their approval of the project.

9. Project Worksheet (HTML Form Submittal): This form is used to provide project information to the USDA's Current Research Information System (CRIS). It should accurately reflect the objectives, the approach, and keywords that other scientists may use to identify and locate the project.

10. Check List for Submission of a Research Project Outline: This checklist, when completed, will ensure that the principal investigator(s) have completed the necessary steps. When all appropriate items on this checklist have been completed, the project outline should be submitted to the Office of the Dean. The Office of the Dean will review the final project proposal and all supporting materials and will submit the proposal to the USDA for approval. The project will officially commence on the date indicated in the approval letter from the Office of the Dean to the unit leader(s).

11. Annual Progress/Termination Reports: At the end of each calendar year a project progress report, or final report, is required to be submitted to the USDA. This report includes a list of publications issued during the current progress report period and will be made available to fellow research scientists and administrators on a worldwide basis. The list of publications for each unit is discussed with the appropriate unit leader during the annual program/budget meetings and is the College's official record of scientific publications."[29]

One of the first steps in establishing a research project is to conduct a review of past and current research in the USDA Current Research Information System (CRIS), a unit of the Cooperative State Research, Education, and Extension Service (CSREES). All research sponsored or conducted by the USDA is required to be documented in CRIS, a documentation and reporting system for ongoing agricultural, food and nutrition, and forestry research. CRIS contains over 30,000 descriptions of current, publicly supported research projects of the USDA agencies, the state agricultural experiment stations, the state land-grant colleges and universities, state schools of forestry, cooperating schools of veterinary medicine, and USDA grant recipients. Project summaries including all progress reports and lists of publications coming out of the research are currently in the CRIS system.[30]

Next, the project prospectus is prepared and submitted to the department head. It is then reviewed by two to three peer reviewers and submitted to the AES Director (who, in Penn State's case, is also the associate dean for research for the college). A project development meeting is held with the appropriate scientist(s), department head(s), research dean, and reviewers. Next, the project outline is prepared and submitted to the department head who will then submit it for review by the same peer reviewers who reviewed the project prospectus. Also, the USDA Assurance Statement must be completed. If the project involves the use of recombinant DNA or RNA, the use of animals, or the use of human subjects, it must be reviewed and approved by the University Office of Research Protections. After the project outline is finalized and all approvals have been obtained, the project worksheet is submitted electronically to USDA for their review and approval.

USDA is required to review project proposals for compliance with the provisions of the appropriate act, such as the Hatch Act. USDA reviews classification coding of projects as they are approved to ensure accurate identification and recording of those that address national research priorities. USDA notifies the director of approval or disapproval of each proposed project and identifies any deficiencies that precluded approval. After the project is approved, notification is sent to the university. This process takes approximately six months.

There are various types of projects, such as Hatch, McIntire-Stennis, Animal Health, State, Regional (multistate, involving two or more state agricultural experiment stations), or USDA grant-specific. The various sources of federal appropriated funding such as Hatch, McIntire-Stennis, or Animal Health can only be expended on projects approved for that source of funding. However, the projects can also be funded by other federal agencies, such as NSF, NIH, or EPA, as well as state, industry, and gifts. Generally, projects are approved for periods not exceeding five years. The institution may extend for not more than one year beyond the approved estimated completion date. Extensions beyond that require USDA approval.

Annual/final progress reports are submitted to the USDA at the end of the calendar year on each project. The reports are submitted electronically. Financial reports on each project are submitted annually to the USDA at the end of the federal fiscal year.

Operation of Agricultural Experiment Station (AES) Research Projects in the College

At Penn State every research expenditure in the college must be associated with an AES research project. Depending on the type of AES research project, it can be funded by numerous sources, such as federal grants and contracts, state, industry, foundations, and gifts. Therefore, except for grant-specific projects or as otherwise restricted, funding from numerous sources are comingled at the project level under an AES research project. A USDA–CSREES-funded grant requires a grant-specific project number and this project number cannot be used in association with any other source of funding.

Facilities and Administrative Costs

One area of concern for research administrators everywhere is indirect costs, or as they are now commonly called in the federal lexicon, "Facilities and Administrative Costs" or simply, "F&A." Since the US Department of Agriculture is the principal funding source related specifically to the land-grant mission, they are important to review.

Are F&A costs allowable under USDA funding? That is a good question, and one that is difficult to answer. It seems that quite frequently F&A policies vary by divisions within the USDA and even within programs within divisions. In some cases, information on whether or not F&A is allowed is conveyed by word of mouth and not by written policy. Even when looking at the written policies, the answer is sometimes ambiguous because the policies are so confusing and in some instances even contradictory.

The basic rule for F&A funding for agricultural research, extension, and teaching is found in Part 7 of the United States Code (U.S.C.), Chapter 64, governing the USDA:[31]

> Sec. 3310. - Limitation on indirect costs for agricultural research, education, and extension programs.
>
> Except as otherwise provided in law, indirect costs charged against a competitive agricultural research, education, or extension grant awarded under this Act or any other Act pursuant to authority delegated to the Under Secretary of Agriculture for Research, Education, and Economics shall not exceed 19 percent of the total Federal funds provided under the grant award, as determined by the Secretary.

In addition, state cooperative institutions (which include institutions under the first Morrill Act, the Second Morrill Act /1890 Land Grant College Funding, the Hatch Act, Smith-Lever Act, McIntire-Stennis Act, as well as those covered under animal health and disease research, aquaculture, and rangeland research provisions) have additional restrictions on F&A recovery:

> No indirect costs or tuition remission shall be charged against funds in connection with cooperative agreements between the Department of Agriculture and State cooperative institutions if the cooperative program or project involved is of mutual interest to all the parties and if all the parties contribute to the cooperative agreement involved.[32]

There are a couple exceptions, however, to this regulation. The above restriction does not apply to international agriculture projects. It also does not apply to some cost reimbursable cooperative agreements that are subject to the following restriction instead:

> Notwithstanding any other provision of law, the Secretary of Agriculture may enter into cost-reimbursable agreements with State cooperative institutions or other colleges and universities without regard to any requirement for competition, for the acquisition of goods or services, including personal services, to carry out agricultural research, extension, or teaching activities of mutual interest. Reimbursable costs under such agreements shall include the actual direct costs of performance, as mutually agreed on by the

parties, and the indirect costs of performance, not exceeding 10 percent of the direct cost.[33]

Typically, in order to figure out what to charge for F&A, one must turn to the program announcement for a specific solicitation. For instance, the National Research Initiative Competitive Grants Program (NRICGP) is a competitive research program. The authority for this program is contained in 7 U.S.C. 450i(b).[34] Under the NRICGP, in accordance with 7 U.S.C. 3310 identified previously, the F&A is restricted to 19% of total federal funds. On the other hand, noncompetitive special research grants are usually line items in the federal budget. Pursuant to Section 1473 of the National Agricultural Research, Extension, and Teaching Policy Act of 1977, as amended by 7 U.S.C. 3319, indirect costs and tuition are not allowable. Finally, the program announcement for Invited Federal Administration Projects for FY 2003 indicates that, for this noncompetitive program, indirect costs are allowable at the institution's federally negotiated rate.

Because the limitation on F&A is legislated in many cases, some USDA academic research services projects that require cost sharing will not even allow the uncollected F&A to count toward cost sharing. So there can be a doubling effect on the lack of full recovery of F&A costs.

Why did all this happen? According to Dr. Daryl Lund of the University of Wisconsin, who has served as executive director of the North Central Regional Association of Agricultural Experiment Station Directors, the caps on indirect costs date back to the early 1990s. Readers will recall that this was the era of the indirect cost scandals that began with questioned costs at Stanford University and ended up with congressional hearings held by Representative John Dingell of Michigan. According to Dr. Lund's account, the rate was quite arbitrarily lowered in the House Appropriations Bill for FY 90 to 25% of total direct costs (TDC). Hearings the next year found that no university turned down grants as a result of the cap and that there were few complaints from universities. Armed with the assurance that they must be on the right track, the FY 91 bill capped the rate at 14% TDC. Again, there was little complaining from the university community, and the USDA reported that millions in funding were available for direct research support. From then on the USDA has stuck with the F&A caps. The rate was eventually raised to 20% of total federal funds (which recalculates to 25% TDC).[35]

Gifts and Grants

Since the agricultural experiment stations have within their purview the research of new products and the dissemination of research results to the agriculture community, many agriculture schools conduct research in collaboration with agriculture companies. Issues of gifts and grants at land-grant institutions through these collaborations, therefore, raise F&A and other concerns as well. What has developed at many agriculture schools is a system of research support that is sometimes colloquially called... "a bag of seed and a check" funding. Basically, agriculture companies provide researchers with new products for testing: seeds, fertilizers, pesticides, herbicides, etc., and along with the product comes a check. Usually the amount of the check is small, frequently just enough to cover some of the costs associated with planting an experimental plot or applying the product.

The rationale behind this system of testing is rather simple: the AES needs to let growers know about what grows best and what products work best in their areas; this is part of their land-grant mission. Either AES researchers can purchase the seeds and products and pay for the full cost of their research out of their station project funds, or they can obtain the seeds and products for free, as well as get a little money to help them. This arrangement has worked well in the past.

Recently, however, a number of circumstances have changed this dynamic. First, there is a heightened interest in intellectual property within both universities and among the agriculture companies. Agriculture companies are much more concerned about their products that are being tested. They have always been concerned to some extent in how the produce of the plants were handled, e.g., protection of "seed varieties." However, now that genetic manipulations and other biotechnical processes can apply to agricultural products, companies are beginning to send out material transfer agreements (MTAs) that place strict legal limits on what can be done with the material subject to the research and any derivative IP. It seems unlikely that universities will continue to accept "gifts" that have such legal ties to them. Certainly university lawyers and tax managers would look askance at the qualifications of these funds as pure gifts.

In addition, the operation of university farms is becoming increasingly costly. Whereas in times past the hidden costs of research may have been buried in the accounts of federal appropriations for agriculture research, now, with shrinking Hatch funding for agricultural experiment stations and reduced state budgets, universities are scrambling to cover some of those basic costs such as replacing tractors, hiring students to help with planting, and tending the field plots.

Can universities afford to accept funding at levels that were applicable ten years ago but not today, and to accept funding that does not recoup any of the institution's facilities and administrative costs? These are questions that many land-grant universities are faced with today.

Select Agents and the Land-Grant University

The Public Health Security and Bioterrorism Preparedness Response Act of 2002 requires the registration of entities that possess or transfer biological agents or toxins deemed a threat to animal or plant health or products derived from them. The regulations most applicable to land grants are listed in 9 CFR 121 and 7 CFR 331 for the USDA, but these regulations are complementary to those issued by the Department of Health and Human Services (HHS), which appear in 42 CFR 73. The USDA has developed a list of livestock pathogens and toxins and a list of plant pathogens that are available through the Animal and Plant Health Inspection Service (APHIS).[36] Likewise HHS has issued lists of viruses, bacteria, rickettsiae, fungi, and toxins that pose harm to human health. Any facility that receives or transfers any agent or toxin that is on these lists is required to register with the Centers for Disease Control and Prevention, Select Agent Program.[37]

Each institution that handles select agents must designate a responsible official (RO) who will have oversight on all matters involving select agents. The RO must implement safety procedures, security measures, and emergency response plans, as well as train appropriate faculty and staff in these areas. The RO must also control all access to and transfer of select agents, report loss or theft of select agents, and provide a complete accounting for all activities related to select agents of toxins. In addition, if in the course of a university's testing of animals, plants, or soils, select agents are identified, these too must be reported by the RO.[38]

Another critical area of responsibility for the institution is the provision of adequate security for laboratories or storage areas containing select agents. This includes limiting and monitoring access to these facilities, e.g., nonlaboratory personnel, such as maintenance staff, may only be allowed on the premises when accompanied and monitored by an approved individual. The university must keep a record of all individuals having authorized access to select agents and toxins and a list of all personnel who have actually accessed a select agent, or those who have accessed an area in which these materials are used or stored.[39]

Some research activities are actually prohibited without the approval of the HHS Secretary. This limit applies to research that proposes to utilize DNA to "deliberately transfer drug resistance traits to select agents that are not known to acquire the trait naturally, if such acquisition could compromise the use of drug to control disease agents in humans, veterinary medicine, or agriculture."[40] The same applies to work involving "the deliberate formation of recombinant DNA containing genes for the synthesis of select agent toxins lethal for vertebrates at $LD_{50} < 100$ ng/kg body weight."[41]

Summary

While many aspects of research administration for land grant institutions are identical to those for other institutions, land grants do have a unique background and a unique mission among American institutions that does present different challenges for the research administrator. The long history of service to the community, the state, and the nation has defined much of the character of land grants and made colleges and universities in the land grant tradition more proactive in working with industry. The challenges facing research administrators in this tradition today are similar to those that existed 100, 75, and 50 years ago—a big mission, not enough money to do everything that is required, and a set of administrative and accounting expectations that place a burden on the institution. But the land grants have survived challenges before, and with the help of research administrators, they will survive the current challenges as well.

• • • Endnotes

1. Penn State Department of Publication, U Ed. "Industry/University Research," Archives of The Pennsylvania State University. RGC 90-0002, 1990, p. 2.

2. Office of University Relations, Penn State University. "A Short Penn State History," 2002, available at http://www.psu.edu/ur/about/history/historyshort.html (accessed June 16, 2005).

3. Kerr, Norwood Allen. *The Legacy: A Centennial History of the State Agricultural Experiment Stations 1887–1987.* Columbia, MO: Missouri Agricultural Experiment Station, University of Missouri, March 1987, pp. 7–8.

4. National Association of State Universities and Land Grant Colleges (NASULGC). "Text of Federal Legislation Relating to Land-Grant Colleges and Universities," 1999, available at http://www.nasulgc.org/publications/Land_Grant/LGTrad_FirstMorrillAct.htm (accessed June 16, 2005).

5. While I will cover a bit the history of the agricultural experiment stations, readers should be aware that similar arrangements (although not federally funded) for engineering experiment stations were also established at many land-grant institutions. Some of the engineering experiment stations still operate today. Examples include the Texas Engineering Experiment Station at Texas A&M and the Engineering Experiment Station at Kansas State University. Their missions are clearly in the land-grant tradition, as the following quote regarding the 1910 establishment of the Kansas State EES suggests:

> The Engineering Experiment Station was established for the purpose of carrying on tests and research work of engineering and manufacturing value to the state of Kansas, and of collecting, preparing, and presenting technical information in a form readily available for the use of the various industries within the state. It is the intention to have all the work of this experiment station of direct importance to Kansas.

McNair, Grayson B. *Illumination for Farm and Town Homes*, Bulletin No. 1, Engineering Experiment Station, Kansas State Agricultural College, December 1914, as cited at: http://www.engg.ksu.edu/more_ees.php (accessed October 5, 2005).

6. Kerr, pp. 11–12.

7. Kerr, p. 20.

8. Kerr, p. 36.

9. Kerr, p. 36.

10. Bazilla, Michael. *Engineering Education at Penn State: A Century in the Land-Grant Tradition.* University Park, PA and London, UK: The Pennsylvania State University Press, 1981, p. 64.

11. Bazilla, p. 65.

12. Bazilla, p. 66.

13. Kerr, pp. 38–58.

14. "Penn State Historical Markers," available at http://www.psu.edu/ur/about/markersalpha.html (accessed on June 16, 2005).

15. Hibshman, E. K., Secretary, *Minutes of the Penn State Council on Research*, February 6, 1928, p. 1, available in the Penn State Archives.

16. Penn State Council on Research, Minutes of October 1, 1934 (University Park, PA: Penn State Archives).

17. "Research at The Pennsylvania State University," report to the Committee on Research of the Board of Trustees, University Park, PA, May 10, 1957.

18. National Science Foundation, Division of Science Resources Statistics, *Academic Research and Development Expenditures: Fiscal Year 2001, NSF 03-316*, Arlington, VA, 2003, Table B-35, R&D Expenditures at Universities and Colleges by Source of Funds: Fiscal Year 2001.

19. Based on the NSF data cited earlier in this section, the national average for nonland-grant institutions ranked in the top 100 is 6.20% and for land grants ranked in the top 100 it is 7.58%.

20. The total numbers for research expenditures are quite small in comparison to today's external support even when adjusted for inflation—e.g., 1935–36 total research expenditures of $430,000 only recalculate to about $5.5 million in today's dollars.

21. Bazilla, p. 119.

22. Ibid, p. 119–120.

23. Ibid, p. 120.

24. National Science Foundation, Table B-35.

25. Penn State University. "Sponsored Research Agreement," http://grants.psu.edu/PSU/Res/SRA-2004.pdf (accessed on June 16, 2005).

26. Kerr, p. 41

27. Kerr, pp. 52–53.

28. The authors would like to acknowledge the assistance of Mary F. Puffer, Manager, Financial and Administrative Services, Penn State College of Agricultural Sciences, for her help in compiling information for this section.

29. Penn State University, College of Agricultural Sciences. "Procedures for Developing a Research Project in the College," available at http://research.cas.psu.edu/FacultyStaffInfo/procedure.htm (accessed June 16, 2005).

30. USDA. "Current Research Information System," available at http://cris.csrees.usda.gov/Welcome.html (accessed June 16, 2005).

31. U.S. Code 64 (2002, as amended) Part 7, § 3310. U.S. Code available on the Web at http://law2.house.gov/ (accessed June 16, 2005).

32. U.S. Code 64 (1985, as amended) Part 7 § 3319.

33. U.S. Code 64 (1998, as amended) Part 7 § 3319a.

34. U.S. Code 64 (1985, as amended) Part 7 § 450i(b).

35. Lund, Daryl. "History of the Indirect Cost Rate Cap on USDA Competitive Grants," May 22, 2003 (updated April 13 2004), available at http://www.wisc.edu/ncra/IDChistory.htm (accessed June 16, 2005). For current rates see http://www.csrees.usda.gov/business/awards/indirect_cost.html (accessed on October 31, 2005).

36. See "Agricultural Bioterrorism Protection Act of 2002," available at http://www.aphis.usda.gov/programs/ag_selectagent_bioterr_toxinslist.htms (accessed 2005).

37. See "Select Agent Program," available at http://www.cdc.gov/od/sap/salist.pdf (accessed October 13, 2005).

38. Federal Register, Friday March 18, 2005, Part II, USDA 74 CFR 331 and 9 CFR Part 121; Part III DHHS 42 CFR Parts 72 and 73.

39. Ibid.

40. Federal Register, Friday March 18, 2005, Part III DHHS 42 CFR Part 73.13(b)(1).

41. Federal Register, Friday March 18, 2005, Part III DHHS 42 CFR Part 73.13(b)(2).

The Academic Entrepreneur: Enabling and Nurturing a Scarce Resource

Louis G. Tornatzky, PhD, and Paul G. Waugaman, MPA, MA

Introduction: The Academic Entrepreneur

Aside from all the details, specific responsibilities, and nuances of the research administration function, there are really only two main objectives:

1. To increase the *scope* of research activity
2. To increase the *quality* of research activity

Both objectives are, of course, instrumental to the larger goal of maintaining (or enhancing) the prominence and reputation of the institution as a whole, and its being considered as among the elite research organizations in the country or world.

To accomplish these objectives, the most important ally in an institution is "the academic entrepreneur," the professor, at any level of rank, who comes up with a seemingly endless array of good research ideas; who writes competitive proposals that are funded at a higher rate than those of peers; and who roams the terrain of his or her discipline, department, or college with a focused intensity looking for the novel opportunity to advance a career.

The academic entrepreneur is relatively rare. Merely 10% to 20% of faculty can be considered as such, and, yet, these faculty carry the majority of research activity for their institutions.

Nearly eighty years ago, a scholar named Alfred Lotka conducted some very insightful research on research which led to the formulation of what came to be known as Lotka's Law about the frequency of publication in a field. He found that of authors contributing to the literature in a field, about 60% have one publication, another 15% have two publications, 7% have three publications, while only 6% of authors produce more than 10 articles.[1] In effect, a relatively small percentage of scholars account for a large fraction of published work. The basic relationship is quite startling, and remains largely true today. One analyst has concluded the following:

> The skew in the frequency distribution of scientists by number of papers published is sufficiently pronounced that one may say that the 10% to 15% of scientists who constitute the productivity (and prestige) elite are responsible for about half of all the science produced.[2]

These dynamics present the research administrator some fairly clear objectives in order to encourage entrepreneurship by enabling the existing high productivity, entrepreneurial members of the faculty and *nurturing* the ambitions of *wanna-be* or *could-be* academic entrepreneurs.

This may be easier to accomplish in non-academic settings where there is a single organizational mission and purpose, and where organizations are strictly adapted to the needs of research. In academic settings competing goals and roles make the research manager's job to enable and nurture more challenging and complex. This chapter discusses ways in which these challenges can be met.

Basic Strategies

There are several strategies that research administrators can employ in order to foster academic entrepreneurs at their institutions:

Providing tools, primarily informational.

Maximizing extrinsic motivation, in terms of career and financial outcomes.

Brokering action, focusing mostly on enabling connections and relationships outside of the nominal structure of the institution.

Influencing personnel policies and practices, to insure that hires of faculty and administrators take into account academic entrepreneurship and research productivity.

Building cultural supports, symbolic gestures and "soft" tactics.

Qualifications to Consider

There are two important qualifications that these strategies must take into account, discussed in the following sections.

The Rise in Research Competition

Academic entrepreneurship and productivity is being played out in somewhat different venues now than it was a generation ago. We note three important changes:

1. *Increasing research activity at universities:* Since 1985, the expenditures for research (in current dollars) conducted by the top 100 institutions in the United States have risen from $9.94 billion to $26.39 billion. In addition, a growing number of other institutions have aspirations to become first-rank research universities. Several universities have publicly stated goals of increasing their research activity and becoming a "top 10" or "top 20" public institution.

2. *More universities are doing well:* Over the period from 1987 to 2001, the share of total academic research expenditures accounted for by the top twenty schools has declined from 34.8% to 31.1%, while the share accounted for by the top 100 schools has only declined from 81.8% to 80.6%. It would appear that institutions in the bottom three quartiles of the top 100 are becoming more robust research performers. This is an indication of the increasing competition among research institutions in the United States.[3]

3. *Federal government share of support is not expanding:* At the same time that overall academic research expenditures have increased, the federal share of research funding has leveled off and started down. The federal share of academic research expenditures peaked at 73.4% in 1965. By 1985, that share had declined to 62%, and further declined to 58.7% in 2001.[4]

One expression of these trends has been a dramatically increased degree of competition among universities for research excellence and associated research funding. In this kind of environment, universities need to hire, nurture, and maintain highly productive research faculty and keep the faculty productive and competitive.

Economic Uncertainties and the Plight of the Publics

From the late 1970s to the early 1990s, America's long romance with its great publicly supported universities began to sour for several reasons. First was the series of economic dislocations, beginning with the massive inflation (exacerbated by a world-wide oil crisis) during the late 1970s, followed by the mid-1980s demise of the durable good manufacturing sector (led by autos) in the midwestern heartland. The onset of massive structural changes in the US economy, emerging realities of globalization, new communication technologies, and declining trade barriers in the early 1990s further contributed to an era of economic uncertainty. Overall, the period from 1975 to 1990 also produced significant challenges for public universities.

Weak state tax revenues during this period also marked a decline in state appropriations to universities, while state support also failed to keep pace with the rising costs of university operations. The declining appropriations support forced institutions to raise tuition and fees for students, and forced institutions to seek alternative sources of revenues, to sustain research support. During this period, when some states experienced record-high 15% to 20% unemployment rates in their major cities, there were reports that many tenured faculty members were giving short shrift to their teaching duties and were under increasing pressure to devote most of their attentions to financial matters, namely the pursuit of federal research grants.

At a time when state universities were being pilloried in the press as havens for idle and politically outrageous tenured faculty, those same universities were being championed in economic development policy circles with the vision that universities' leading edge research activities would feed new-economy business, thus, boosting state economies. From the mid-1980s through the present, states have launched university-affiliated, technology-based economic initiatives, many of these funded with significant amounts of public investment (a list of these programs and activities is maintained by the State Science and Technology Institute).[5]

These developments have placed new sets of external expectations on the university. Not only are institutions expected to serve as excellent instructional resources, but they are also expected to be direct support systems regarding state and regional economic matters.

Rethinking Philosophy and Mission

As a result of these changes, there have been many large-scale efforts over the past decade to rethink the mission and goals of the university and to establish (or reestablish) key priorities, including those related to the purpose and function of university research resources.

Sets of publications and foci of discussions have been dedicated to redefining the nature of "scholarship" in the contemporary university. This school of thought has been led by students of higher education, most notably the 1990 publication of *Scholarship Reconsidered*.[6] The basic argument in *Scholarship Reconsidered* is that faculty life is not entirely defined by research and scholarly publication and teaching duties (which, the book notes, should share comparable stature), but that outreach should also define faculty excellence. Other writers and practitioners have since expanded upon these ideas and have led to campus efforts to develop new, more encompassing definitions of scholarship. These have included descriptions of "outreach scholarship" and expansion of tenure portfolios to include activities that had heretofore been beyond the pale for academics (e.g., involvement in community schools).

There have also been efforts to look more broadly at the missions and goals of universities in the context of the larger society. While much of this has been focused on the evolution of US land-grant universities, the impacts have been more widespread. The most notable of these has been the effort supported and spearheaded by the W. K. Kellogg Foundation, which has resulted in creating a set of metaphors and ideas about *The Engaged University*.[7] Several US universities have taken the language and ideas expressed in these reports and have integrated them with organizational goals and tenure criteria. Virginia Tech University's action in these regards serves as a prime example.[8]

The notions of outreach initiatives and overall university engagement have not been widely adopted by US universities, nor have they had major impact on most faculty review criteria and processes. Nonetheless, given changes in factors

and the increasing pressures to make such changes, the influence of these notions' importance is likely to grow.

Consolidation of Research Activity

A large fraction of research on the most prominent campuses is being conducted via "organized research units" (ORUs). These are centers, institutes, and programs typically structured as multi-investigator, multiyear agglomerations of multidisciplinary or interdisciplinary research projects. The National Science Foundation (NSF) currently supports 294 centers, which account for 8.3% percent of its grant expenditures; while the National Institutes of Health (NIH) supports 1,137 centers, which account for 11.1% of its extramural budget (NSF, NIH, 2003).[9] These figures indicate that the successful academic entrepreneur will more likely than not have to be adept at organizational entrepreneurship, and will need to have the capacity to lead, organize, and politic for centers (or their equivalent). Some of this demands certain skills and understandings, and the how-to literature is fairly informative.[10] These efforts also demand inspiration and motivation from the academic entrepreneur, features less easily transmitted. Therefore, while we do not discount the importance of single investigator and/or single project work, the current state of affairs does signify an increase in opportunities (and responsibilities) for research administrators to activate ORUs and research partnerships that cut across academic units and disciplines.

Academic entrepreneurship also demands a second important qualification: the science-to-technology life cycle. At an increasing rate and ever since the 1980 passage of the Bayh-Dole legislation, US universities have become very active in technology transfer in areas of patenting, licensing, and commercialization. The various policies and practices that are specific to this activity are well-documented,[11] but two facts are significant:

1. Institutions that do well in the area of technology transfer are those that are also, more often than not, among the top-tier of universities from the perspective of research prestige[i] and productivity (e.g., Stanford, MIT, UCSD, Purdue, Virginia Tech).[12]

---

[i]One might conclude the larger, more research-intensive institutions have more technology to pick from, and, thus, are naturally successful at patenting and licensing. However, when one factors out size by normalizing technology transfer performance metrics (such as in the cited work of the Southern Technology Council), the more prestigious institutions still rise to the top.

2. Individual faculty members who are more actively involved in the area of technology transfer (and industry partnerships) are most often among the ranks of the Lotka 15%—the best and brightest.[13]

The Strategies

Information Tools

When fostering academic entrepreneurs, there are two general categories of information that research administration units should disseminate. One concerns the *what* or information about "hot" areas of research and agency funding opportunities; the second focuses on the *how-to* of acting on those opportunities.

Every research administration unit that we have encountered disseminates these types of information to campus stakeholders, but they differ widely in the *scope, medium, currency,* and *focus* of that communication process. We believe that the more information that can be provided (in the richest and "grabbiest" form), the sooner the better. Information should particularly highlight attention to the 10% to 15% of faculty that account for the majority of successful proposals.

In terms of scope, we believe that research management offices should wholeheartedly adopt a Web-based approach to getting information to faculty about funding opportunities and new research initiatives. There are examples of good practices everywhere and electronic tools make this method easier and more effective. The best systems push information to faculty members in a customized fashion that "sorts out signal from noise," giving the individual faculty member the information of most interest. This sort of information service, which should be considered a primary function, too often gets a low priority in favor of other "must-do" jobs, such as getting proposals reviewed, submitted, and setting up new projects following the award. Good information does not stop at agency announcements, requests for proposals, etc., but includes notices about national agenda-setting conferences where agencies often organize and announce changes in federal science and technology policies and legislation—key information to landing opportunities. Information services should link to technology transfer functions and should include news about inventions and licenses and success stories at other institutions that can serve as case studies.

Information services also need to be focused on "how-to" knowledge, such as tips on how to de-

velop a center proposal, how to file an invention disclosure, or how to develop a project budget.

Many institutions have developed short workshops on "grantsmanship" to keep faculty members up to speed on proposal processes and techniques. These workshops can get beyond mere proposal writing and can address more challenging issues such as how to form a project team, develop a relationship with a program officer, and process a proposal through the institutional sign-offs. Despite the importance of the training and staff development, a practice benchmarking survey[14] demonstrates that 73% of participating institutions either had no such programs (or their program was considered at the beginning level—only 27% reported that their training programs were at the advanced stage).

Technology transfer is one of the most prominent and critical topics among faculty. Many universities have implemented "by-invitation" workshops (targeting the most research-productive faculty) on the concepts, benefits, and "how-to" steps of engaging in technology transfer and industry research partnerships. "Storytelling" interludes, success stories given by faculty members who have been involved in this activity, are significant contributions in these forums. In benchmarking studies conducted by the authors, these "success stories" tended to serve as a "best practice" within the most productive universities.[15]

Maximizing Extrinsic Motivation

While some members of the academic community pursue fundamental knowledge and the gain of scholarly insight, they feed their families and credit card bills via salaries, promotions, and the security of lifetime employment.

While nominally outside the sphere of the research administration function, it is important, nonetheless, that the CRO and his or her staff contribute to considerations regarding a system of rewards and incentives promoting research entrepreneurship. These are generally expressed in an institution's system of processes and criteria for promotion and tenure.

Regarding these criteria, based on normative practice among research universities,[16] systems which unambiguously encourage research productivity consider:

- They are transparent to participants in the system. The rules and procedures are operationally described and are adhered to.
- The locus of power in promotion and tenure decisions is closest to where the professor lives and works—the department, the institute, the

school—and not highly centralized for the entire institution.

- The criteria are grounded in explicit, often quantitative, metrics of research excellence.
- Faculty members have a say in the structure and operation of review procedures and practices for their department, school, and the overall institution.
- Performance reviews are rationally scheduled and timed to consider the academic "career lifecycle." A periodic performance review should not be scheduled at a time when a faculty member is preparing for or undergoing a major review such as tenure review or a promotion review. There should be policies that consider these issues when performance review systems are being set up.

Brokering Action

There are several areas in which the enabling role of research administration needs to go beyond information dissemination, and should extend to brokering relationships between units, people, and academic entrepreneurs. Most prominent of these are research funding opportunities that call for:

- Inter-disciplinary or multidisciplinary approaches to an area of inquiry,
- Partnerships with other institutions,
- Partnerships with industry or other third parties, and
- Sequenced activity that spans the R&D spectrum from basic inquiry through to technology commercialization (e.g., an ATP project).

Each of these types of research funding opportunities is likely to be looked at by the typical chairperson or the faculty member (not among the Lotka 15% group) as something that is not considered "normal" process. However, in the opinion of the academic entrepreneur, such determination is considered destructive to purpose of the research.

Every CRO should have the list of 20 to 50 individuals whose qualifications span the disciplines and levels of seniority who will respond favorably to these kinds of challenges (they are usually mutually known). The role of the CRO is to convene and to facilitate one or more meetings, if needed, which should have the following objectives:

- To decide, based on a free-and-frank exchange of views, whether the institution will make a pitch
- To decide who is in and who is not
- To forge a first pass research vision

- To assign roles and responsibilities to draft a proposal

This kind of brokering role is much more aligned to sponsorship opportunities that might be classified as ORUs (discussed earlier). Nonetheless, the campus that can tap into (and enable) the informal network of creative academic entrepreneurs to pull these things off is likely to look very good on their NSF research expenditures numbers.[ii]

Influencing Personnel Policies and Actions

While there may be protracted debate about whether academic entrepreneurs are made or born, often lost is the fact that academic entrepreneurs are more easily bought; while over the decades, the relative rankings of US research institutions generally stay the same in terms of measures (such as gross research expenditures). There are notable exceptions, however: for example, cases in which an institution rises several notches over a fairly brief period of time (within 10 to 20 years), and often that climb can be traced to very focused and aggressive efforts to hire senior, highly productive faculty from other schools to build critical mass. For example, in the early 1980s, the University of Texas at Austin (UTA) created over 30 endowed professorial chairs in engineering and the natural sciences. In engineering, 16 of these appointments were concentrated in microelectronics, computer engineering, material sciences, and manufacturing. Very soon after, UTA became a national player in these disciplines. Many have identified these appointments as a major contributor to the growth of the Austin technology economy (the landing of Microelectronics and Computing Center and Sematech, etc.).

More recently, in Atlanta, the Georgia Research Alliance (GRA) has pursued a similar strategy.[17] GRA operates as a consortium of state government, the private sector, and the Georgia-based universities. GRA has helped to endow nearly 40 eminent scholars, as well as to make major investments in laboratories and facilities to support their work. Each of these endowed positions is focused on a discipline or field that is aligned with a small number of strategic areas that are seen as the best bets to expand the Georgia technology economy. Of interest are the appointments of prominent scientists. There

[ii]The National Science Foundation's annual *Survey of Academic Research and Development Expenditures* captures information by institution of expenditures (not awards), by source, and by scientific field. It is an excellent benchmark of overall research performance.

is a definite tilt, overall, in the selection process, which identifies candidates who have industrial and/or business entrepreneurial experience.

While these examples of university action are among the more prominent regarding these recent developments, there are a number of other initiatives that have been designed and implemented by universities to "leapfrog" the academic research standing of state universities and, presumably, with impact on economic development, several other examples lend notable credence to this trend. In recent years, Kentucky has started a "bucks for brains" initiative; while Ohio State University is a few years into its "2010 program" (with the mission to get ten programs ranked nationally in the top 10 within ten years, and twenty other programs in the top 20). Relentless recruitment of top-flight professors is a prominent vehicle. It is difficult to pick up an issue of *The Chronicle of Higher Education* and not note similar initiatives within the job listings or within news articles. Obviously, not all such efforts work; there have been endowed chairs filled with little impact on a university's bottom line of research productivity. In order to achieve success in these areas, the following criteria should be considered as major ingredients for success:

Strategic Focus. Most initiatives that have had long-term effects and success in these areas tend to be clustered in a few fields or disciplines within an institution. The selection of these fields is typically the result of a lengthy (and often painful) strategic planning process. In general, it can help if state government and industry are part of that planning process. If the choice of fields is aligned with industry trends in the technology sector, it is easier to maintain financial and political support. We call this "technology match." Endowed chair appointments that are scattered across the campus tend not to have impact past the incumbency of the initial appointment. However, if appointments are grouped into complimentary disciplines or fields, the incumbents are likely to build connections and partnerships with one another, thus gaining leverage from the program investments.

Hire Active Academic Entrepreneurs. Appointments should be made not only on the basis of a candidate's past accomplishments, but also should be made to reflect the faculty and institution's current and future aspirations. In other words, a "retired-in-place" endowed professor will not serve the purposes of the institution. Similarly, in our opinion, the preferred candidate should be one who is "entrepreneurial," a person who works across disciplinary boundaries; is interested in the whole life cycle or science and technology; is inclined to partner with external organizations; and who is always pushing the methodological, epistemological, and theoretical boundaries of a field.

Fill Upholstered Chairs. In order to practice his/her field of science an incumbent in an endowed chair must have access to world-class laboratory facilities. One of the strengths of programs such as the Georgia Research Alliance is that investment in facilities has gone hand-in-hand with investment in people. In fact, the former makes luring the latter that much easier.

Maintain Longitudinal Continuity. One way to dilute the potential impact of endowed chairs is to utilize them as if they are fungible, sharable assets. For example, if a chair becomes vacant, it is often "rotated" to another discipline or field in the spirit of fairness or political correctness. However, what is lost by such practice and the ultimate loss of chain of command is the long-term continuity of investment that is necessary to build and maintain critical mass. In effect, the resource is frittered away.

The chief research officer (CRO) needs to be an active participant in all the above decisions. Decisions about very senior appointments (particularly handsomely funded endowed chairs) is perhaps the second-most significant tool that a university has to build research productivity, prominence, and academic entrepreneurship.

Building Cultural Support

What is the most significant tool, albeit, difficult to operationalize? Simply put, it is in the culture of the institution. The subtle and not-so-subtle messages that pervade an institution about what is laudatory, valued, and encouraged are often much more important than the official, written policies that seek to encourage faculty productivity and entrepreneurship. Despite the external appearance of universities as bureaucratic, formal organizations, at their hearts, they are governed more by the informal values and by the beliefs of those who work there.

This is also the venue in which leadership, often maligned, can have significant influence. This is particularly so in the many symbolic acts and behaviors that academic leaders can display. Some examples:

An academic administrator, chairperson, dean, vice president for research or provost, who continues to conduct an active (and externally funded) research program, despite the heavy weight of administrative dues, and who sends powerful messages to the community about what is important.

The amount of space devoted in university alumni magazines, or the institution's Web site, to research accomplishments of faculty is an interesting indicator of cultural support of these activities, as is the space given to acknowledge major patents or the launch of a spin-off company (if one is also trying to encourage technology entrepreneurship).

Every research university should employ a system of highly visible and remunerative formal awards to acknowledge research accomplishments.

The frequency of unit-level talks, workshops, or colloquia on research topics is also an indicator of a supportive culture.

Devoting time at departmental faculty meetings to acknowledge research accomplishments (getting a new grant, publishing an important article or book, being invited to a prestigious conference) offers opportunity to acknowledge and celebrate the research craft.

"Good hires" can positively "tip" and inspire a university culture. Adding two or three productive, charismatic, talented senior faculty to a unit almost inevitably results in elevating productivity standards New hires can become powerful advocates for new values and new priorities.

Concluding Comments

In summary, we believe that the goals of research leadership (to increase the quality and quantity of the research enterprise) can only be reached via ways beyond administration, per se. The CRO and his staff need to venture beyond the walls of their offices, beyond the orderly policies and practices, and travel into the fray of organizational renewal and change. This journey includes having focus on the best and brightest, serving as an advocate for smart hires of the extraordinarily talented, brokering partnerships between talented people and key units, and insuring that both formal extrinsic rewards, as well as the informal culture, are aligned with those goals.

• • • Endnotes

1. Lotka, Alfred J. "The Frequency Distribution of Scientific Productivity." *Journal of the Washington Academy of Sciences* 16, no. 12 (1926): 317–323.

2. David, Paul A. "Positive Feedbacks and Research Productivity in Science: Another Black Box." In *Economics and Technology*, edited by O. Grandstrand. Amsterdam: Elsevier, 1994: 65-89.

3. National Science Foundation. *Academic Research and Development Expenditures*, FY 2001 and FY 1994. Washington, DC: NSF, 1996 and 2003. Percentages of the total expenditures for each level were calculated from the basic data for this comparison.

4. National Science Foundation. *Science and Engineering Indicators 2002*. Washington, DC: NSF, 2002 (NSB-02-1). Comparisons were calculated from Appendix Tables 5-1, 5-2, and 5-8.

5. State Science and Technology Institute: Technology-Based Economic Development Resource Center, http://www.tbedresourcecenter.org/ (accessed September 19, 2005).

6. Boyer, Ernest L. *Scholarship Reconsidered: Priorities for the Professorate*. Princeton, NJ: Carnegie Advancement for the Advancement of Teaching, 1990.

7. National Association of State Universities and Land-Grant Colleges. *Renewing the Covenant: Learning, Discovery, and Engagement in a New Age and Different World*. Washington, DC. Kellogg Commission on the Future of the State and Land-Grant Universities, March 2000.

8. Tornatzky, L. G., P. G. Waugaman, and D.O. Gray. *Innovation U: New University Roles in the Knowledge Economy*. Research Triangle Park, NC: Southern Growth Policies Board, 2002.

9. NSF. "National Science Foundation FY 2004 Budget Request to Congress," http://www.nsf.gov/about/budget/fy2004/toc.htm (accessed September 13, 2005).

   NIH. "National Institutes of Health: Summary of the FY 2004 President's Budget," 2003, http://www.nih.gov/about/almanac/appropriations/index.htm (accessed September 13, 2005).

10. Gray, D. O., and S. G. Walters. *Managing the Industry/University Cooperative Research Center: A Guide for Directors and Other Stakeholders*. Columbus, OH: Battelle Press, 1998.

11. Tornatzky, L. G., P. G. Waugaman, and D. O. Gray. *Industry-University Technology Transfer: Models of Alternative Practice, Policy and Program*. Research Triangle Park, NC: Southern Growth Policies Board, 1999.

    Tornatzky, L. G., P. G. Waugaman, and D. O. Gray. *Innovation U: New University Roles in the Knowledge Economy*. Research Triangle Park, NC: Southern Growth Policies Board, 2002.

12. Waugaman, P. G., L. Tornatzky, and B. Vickery. *Best Practices for University-Industry Technology Transfer: Working with External Patent Counsel.* Research Triangle Park, NC: Southern Growth Policies Board, 1994.

Tornatzky, L. G., P. G. Waugaman, and L. Casson. *Benchmarking University-Industry Technology Transfer in the South: 1993–1994 Data.* Research Triangle Park, NC: Southern Growth Policies Board, 1995.

Tornatzky, L. G., P. G. Waugaman, and J. Bauman. *Benchmarking University-Industry Technology Transfer in the South: 1995–1996 Data.* Research Triangle Park, NC: Southern Growth Policies Board, 1997.

Waugaman, P. G., and L. G. Tornatzky. *Benchmarking University-Industry Technology Transfer in the South and the EPSCoR States: 1997–1998 Data.* Research Triangle Park, NC: Southern Growth Policies Board, 2001.

13. Blumenthal, D., E. G. Campbell, N. Causino, and K. S. Louis. "Participation of Life-Science Faculty in Research Relationships with Industry." *The New England Journal of Medicine* 335 (1996): 1734–1738.

14. Kirby, W. S., and P. G. Waugaman. "Performance Benchmarking in Sponsored Programs Administration: Selected Preliminary Practice Data from the 2002 SRA-BearingPoint Nationwide Survey." Paper presented at the SRA annual meeting, Pittsburgh, PA, October, 2003.

15. Tornatzky, L. G., and J. Bauman. *Outlaws or Heroes? Issues of Faculty Rewards, Organizational Culture, and University-Industry Technology Transfer.* Research Triangle Park, NC: Southern Growth Policies Board, 1997.

16. Tornatzky, L. G., J. Judd, D. Wilke, and P. G. Waugaman. *Leistungsbegutachtungssysteme an Staaatlichen US-Universitaten—Survey of Faculty Performance Review Practices.* Bonn, Germany: Bundesministerium fur Bildung und Forschung, 2001.

17. Tornatzky, L. G. "Technology-based Economic Development in Atlanta and Georgia: The Role of University Partnerships." *Industry and Higher Education* 16, no. 1 (February 2002): 19–26.

24

National and International Research Councils, Professional Associations, Accreditations, and Memberships

Lynne U. Chronister, MPA

Higher education and professional associations provide varying levels of support, training and education, science, and education advocacy; influence national and international policy; provide accreditation and credentialing and promotion of networking among peers. There are three general types of associations that support the research enterprise, most of which are 501(c)(3) or (c)(6) organizations and include professional associations that consist of individual memberships, institutional memberships, and memberships of organizations that provide accreditation or credentialing. Most of research-related organizations were formed in the later part of the 1960s or early 1970s as the concept of function and profession of research administration was first developing.

Professional associations can provide critical training, development, and networking for less experienced, as well as senior administrators. They are the primary vehicles for training outside of the employee's home institution. Annual and regional meetings offered by these associations offer breadth and depth of information and can offer credentialing and accreditation. When considering membership to such organizations, the value added of membership as a good return on investment should be considered. An individual who has committed to a career in research administration may benefit from volunteering in his/her chosen association and eventually assuming a leadership position. The support of the CRO and immediate supervisor is critical because the time demanded of the position of research administrator can be significant, especially if involved with associations. Aside from personal benefits of friendships, peer-recognition, and career advancement, there are other institutional benefits from an individual's involvement as a result of networking, developing critical contacts, and recognition for support of professional advancement.

Membership in some associations is institutional-based and may be restricted to types of institutions or function for a specific purpose. Associations like the National Association of State Universities and Land Grant Colleges focus membership eligibility primarily on the basis of land-grant and larger state university affiliation, while the American Association of State Colleges and Universities (AASCU) focuses on memberships from smaller and regional universities and the Council on Governmental Relations (COGR), the lead advocacy association for higher education, focuses on issues with government that impact universities. Cost for institutional memberships vary widely, as do the services offered.

The associations listed under the category of Accreditation and Credentialing in this text are both institutional and individual. The three organizations that review institutional human and animal subjects programs accredit those programs, while the Research Administrator Certification Council accredits individual members. Some programs like the Association of Clinical Research Professionals function as both a professional association and provide certification and a clinical research professional.

Categories of Associations

Following are selected associations that have direct or indirect relevance to the university research enterprise. This list does not include all associations that support the research function but does represent those that have a primary function in support of some aspect relevant to research at higher education and not-for-profit institutions.

Professional Associations

Association of Clinical Research Professionals (ACRP)

The 17,000 ACRP members include nurses and other clinical research professionals, and the organization focuses on clinical investigations from private research institutes, hospitals, and academic medical centers. ACRP helps professionals through seminars and conferences and offers a certification program. The organization offers continuing medical education hours covering a range of good clinical practices and human subjects protection topics.

Association of University Technology Managers (AUTM)

The AUTM is a nonprofit organization created to function as a professional and educational society for academic technology transfer professionals involved with the management of intellectual property.

AUTM measures success of the university technology transfer process through its contribution to public benefit and the impact it has on our daily lives. The ultimate benefits of the process are the products that achieve significant public improvement and affect the way we live now and in the future. Some of the leading pharmaceutical, information technology, biotechnology, and health-care products were the result of the patenting and licensing of innovations to the public from universities and nonprofit research institutions.

AUTM records the results of the transfer of academic research for commercial application through the annual AUTM licensing survey. The survey serves as a measure of success in technology transfer and offers university technology managers an opportunity to showcase product vignettes and new discoveries from their offices. Ten years of data successfully demonstrates that investments in academic research advance scientific knowledge and contribute to education, and also yield new products that would not exist but for the process of technology transfer.

Licensing Executives Society (LES)

LES operates in both Canada and the United States and is a profes-sional society "with members who are engaged in the transfer, use, development, marketing, and manufacture of intellectual property."[1] Membership is broad and includes individuals from the private sector and academia who are executives, scientists, lawyers, and government employees. LES provides educational opportunities as well as formal and informal networking.

National Association of State Universities and Land-Grant Colleges (NASULGC)

"Founded in 1887, the National Association of State Universities and Land-Grant Colleges (NASULGC) is the nation's oldest higher education association. A voluntary association of public universities, land-grant institutions, and many of the nation's public university systems, NASULGC campuses are located in all 50 states, the US territories and the District of Columbia. Dedicated to supporting excellence in teaching, research, and public service, NASULGC has been in the forefront of educational leadership nationally for over a century."[2] The association's membership stands at 211 institutions. This includes 76 land-grant universities, of which 17 are the historically black public institutions created by the Second Morrill Act of 1890 and 27 public higher education systems. In addition, tribal colleges became land-grant institutions in 1994 and 31 are represented in NASULGC through the membership of the American Indian Higher Education Consortium (AIHEC).

National Association of College and University Attorneys (NACUA)

"The NACUA was founded in 1960-61 by a small group of attorneys who regularly provided legal services to colleges and universities; they were the first such specialists in the United States."[3] Nearly 1,400 campuses (about 660 institutions), represented by over 3,000 attorneys, comprise the membership today. The association's purpose is to enhance legal assistance to colleges and universities by educating attorneys and administrators to the nature of campus legal issues. It has an equally important role to play in the continuing legal education of university counsel. "In addition, NACUA produces publications, sponsors seminars, maintains its own bulletin board (NACUANET) and home page (www.nacua.org), and operates a clearinghouse through which attorneys on campuses are able to share resources, knowledge, and work products on current legal concerns and interests."[3]

National Council of University Research Administrators (NCURA)

NCURA, founded in 1959, is an organization of individuals with professional interests in the administration of sponsored programs (research, education, and training), primarily at colleges and universities, with a common desire to:

- Promote the development of more effective policies and procedures relative to the administration of sponsored programs to assure the achievement of the maximum potential in academic programs.
- Provide a forum through national and regional meetings for the discussion and exchange of information and experiences related to sponsored programs in colleges and universities.
- Provide for the dissemination of current information and exchange of views on mutual concerns.
- Promote the development of college and university research administration and the administration of other sponsored programs as a professional field and stimulate the personal growth of the members of the council.

Public Responsibility in Medicine and Research (PRIM&R) and Applied Research Ethics National Association (ARENA) PRIM&R and ARENA "are peer organizations. PRIM&R is dedicated to creating, implementing, and advancing the highest ethical standards in the conduct of research."[4] ARENA is the membership division of PRIM&R and supports professionals involved with the protection of animal and human research subjects. The mission for ARENA is to enhance human and animal subject protection and the responsible conduct of research through the education and professional development of its members.

Society of Research Administrators International (SRA) "Founded in 1967, the SRA is a nonprofit association dedicated to the education and the professional development of research administrators, as well as the enhancement of public understanding of the importance of research and its administration."[5] The society fulfills its mission by means of the education of research administrators, professionals in related fields, and the public through the exchange of information, individual contacts, professional presentations, formal and informal meetings and publications; and the improvement of communications among researchers, host institutions and organizations, the sponsors of research administrators, and the general public.

"Through innovative programs and a wide variety of outreach programs, SRA continuously seeks to broaden and diversify its membership base. With over 3,000 members around the world, the Society is the premier international organization for research administrators in all settings, on all levels, and in all fields."[5] SRA's mission and objectives reflect the demands of a growing profession. Whether a research administrator works for a university, a business corporation, a health care facility, a government agency, or a not-for-profit organization, SRA offers everything needed to enhance professional growth, foster personal and professional connections, and explore the possibilities of the future.

Institutional Memberships

American Association for the Advancement of Science (AAAS) The AAAS is an international nonprofit organization dedicated to advancing science around the world by serving as an educator, leader, spokesperson, and professional association. In addition to organizing membership activities, AAAS publishes the journal, *Science*, as well as many scientific newsletters, books, and reports, and spearheads programs that raise the bar of understanding for science worldwide "Founded in 1848, AAAS serves 262 affiliated societies and academies of science, serving 10 million individuals. *Science* has the largest paid circulation of any peer-reviewed general science journal in the world, with an estimated total readership of one million."[6] The nonprofit AAAS is open to all and fulfills its mission to "advance science and serve society" through initiatives in science policy, international programs, and science education.

Association of American State Colleges and Universities (AASCU) "The AASCU represents more than 400 public colleges, universities, and systems of higher education throughout the United States and its territories."[7] The association has a fourfold purpose: to promote appreciation and support for public higher education and the distinctive contributions of the member colleges and universities; to analyze public policy; to advocate for member institutions and the students they serve; to provide policy leadership and program support to strengthen academic quality, promote access and inclusion, and facilitate educational innovation; and to create professional development opportunities for institutional leaders, especially presidents, chancellors, and their spouses. Membership is open to any regionally accredited institution of higher education offering programs leading to bachelor, master, or doctoral degrees and wholly or partially state supported or state controlled.

Association of American Universities (AAU) The AAU was founded in 1900 by a group of fourteen universities offering the PhD degree. The AAU currently consists of sixty American universities and two Canadian universities. The association serves its members in two major ways. It assists members in developing national policy positions on issues that relate to academic research and graduate and professional education. It also provides them with a forum for discussing a broad range of other institutional issues, such as undergraduate education.

Association of University Research Parks (AURP) A university research park or technology incubator is defined by AURP as a property-based venture which has existing or planned land and buildings designed primarily for private and public research and development facilities, high technology and science based companies, and support services. A contractual and/or formal ownership or operational relationship with one or more universities or other institutions of higher education, and science research is the foundation for building a park. There should be a role in promoting research and development by the university in partnership with industry, assisting in the growth of new ventures, and promoting economic development. Also important is the park's role in aiding the transfer of technology and business skills between the university and industry tenants. "The park or incubator may be a not-for-profit or for-profit entity owned wholly or partially by a university or a university-related entity. Alternatively, the Park or Incubator may be owned by a nonuniversity entity but have a contractual or other formal relationship with a university, including joint or cooperative ventures between a privately developed research park and a university."[8]

Council on Governmental Relations (COGR) The Council on Governmental Relations is an association of research universities. Since its inception in 1948, COGR has been continuously involved in the development of all major financial and administrative aspects of federally funded research. COGR's primary function is to provide advice and information to its membership and to make certain that federal agencies understand academic operations and the impact of proposed regulations on colleges and universities. COGR helps to develop policies and practices that reflect fairly the mutual interests and separate obligations of federal agencies and universities in research and graduate education.

National Association of College and University Business Officers (NACUBO) The NACUBO membership includes over 2,500 colleges and universities in the United States. Its representatives are chief administrative and financial officers and it offers a professional network and development opportunities for members. Its vision is to define excellence in higher education business and financial management. It has a monthly publication, *Business Officer,* and provides advocacy for university business functions.

The National Research Council (NRC) "The National Research Council is part of the National Academies, which also comprises the National Academy of Sciences, National Academy of Engineering, and Institute of Medicine. They are private, nonprofit institutions that provide science, technology, and health policy advised under a congressional charter."[9] The council was organized by the National Academy of Sciences in 1916 to associate the broad community of science and technology with the Academy's purposes of furthering knowledge and advising the federal government. Functioning in accordance with general policies determined by the Academy, the National Research Council has become the principal operating agency of both the National Academy of Sciences and the National Academy of Engineering in providing services to the government, the public, and the scientific and engineering communities. The Research Council is administered jointly by both Academies and the Institute of Medicine through the National Research Council Governing Board.

Research America Research America is an advocacy and outreach organization founded for the purpose of advancing funding for medical and health research in the public and private sectors. Among Research America's goals is to inform the public of the benefits of medical and health research and the institutions that perform the research. The organization also carries out activities to motivate the public and the research community to support research and to empower the public to take a more active role in promoting science.

Accrediting Organizations

Association for the Accreditation of Human Research Protection Programs, Inc. (AAHRPP) Incorporated in April 2001, the AAHRPP is a nonprofit organization that offers accreditation to institutions engaged in research involving human participants. The AAHRPP accreditation program uses a voluntary, peer-driven educational model. Responding to increased public and political scrutiny, AAHRPP seeks not only to ensure compliance, but to raise the bar in human research protection by helping institutions reach performance standards that surpass the threshold of state and federal requirements. By establishing a "gold seal" signifying adherence to a rigorous set of human protection standards, accreditation by AAHRPP helps ensure consistency and uniformity among all institutions conducting biomedical, behavioral, and social sciences research.

Association for Assessment and Accreditation of Laboratory Animal Care (AAALAC)   AAALAC promotes the humane treatment of animals through a voluntary accreditation program and endorses the use of animals to advance medicine and science when there are no nonanimal alternatives and when the research is done in an ethical and humane way. Research programs that are accredited must meet the minimums required by law but also must demonstrate excellence in animal care and use. Most major research programs in academia, nonprofit research institutes, and industry are accredited by AAALAC.

Research Administrator Certification Council (RACC) "The RACC was formed under the auspices of the Society of Research Administrators in 1993 and is an independent, nonprofit credentialing association."[10] The role of the RACC is to certify that an individual, through experience and testing, has the fundamental knowledge necessary to be a professional research or sponsored programs administrator. The individual who becomes certified receives a CRA or Certified Research Administrator designation.

Summary

The associations described also have Web sites providing additional information on membership, mission, and membership benefits and activities. In the past few years, it has become common for the research-related associations to partner for purposes of training and education as well as research advocacy. Some associations partner with groups such as COGR to respond to concerns over research policy and legislation. In 2004, two associations, NCURA and SRA, began a partnership with Drexel University and Cleveland State, respectively, to establish an academic program in research administration. The collaboration among asso-

ciations mirrors the trend within academic research to collaborate with researchers across disciplines and at other public and private research groups.

• • • Association Web Sites

University:
Association for Assessment and Accreditation of Laboratory Animal Care (AAALAC)
www.aaalac.org
American Association for the Advancement of Science (AAAS)
www.aaas.org
Association of American State Colleges and Universities (AASCU)
www.aascu.org
Association of American Universities (AAU)
www.aau.edu
Association of University Research Parks (AURP)
www.aurp.net
Council on Governmental Relations (COGR)
www.cogr.edu
The Joint Commission on Accreditation of Healthcare Organizations (JCAHO)
www.jcaho.org
National Association of Colleges and University Attorneys (NACUA)
www.nacua.org
National Association of College and University Business Officers (NACUBO)
www.nacubo.org
National Association of State Universities and Land-Grant Colleges (NASULGC)
www.nasulgc.org
The National Research Council (NRC)
www.nationalacademies.org/nrc
Research America
www.researchamerica.org

IRB:
Association for the Accreditation of Human Research Protection Programs (AAHRPP)
www.aahrpp.org
Association of Clinical Research Professionals (ACRP)
www.acrpnet.org
National Committee on Quality Assurance (NCQA)
www.ncqa.org
Public Responsibility in Medicine and Research (PRIM&R) and Applied Research Ethics National Association (ARENA)
www.primr.org

Technology Transfer:

Association of University Technology Managers (AUTM)

www.autm.net

Licensing Executives Society (LES)

www.usa-canada.les.org

Sponsored Programs:

National Council of University Research Administrators (NCURA)

www.ncura.edu

Research Administrators Certification Council (RACC)

www.cra-cert.org

Society of Research Administrators International (SRA)

www.srainternational.org

• • • References

1. Licensing Executives Society (LES), www.usa-canada.les.org (accessed September 5, 2005).

2. National Association of State Universities and Land-Grant Colleges (NASULGC), www.nasulgc.org (accessed September 5, 2005).

3. National Council of University Research Administrators (NCURA), www.ncura.edu (accessed September 5, 2005).

4. Public Responsibility in Medicine and Research (PRIM&R) and Applied Research Ethics National Association (ARENA), www.primr.org (accessed September 5, 2005).

5. Society of Research Administrators International (SRA), www.srainternational.org (accessed September 5, 2005).

6. American Association for the Advancement of Science (AAAS), www.aaas.org (accessed September 5, 2005).

7. Association of American State Colleges and Universities (AASCU), www.aascu.org (accessed September 5, 2005).

8. Association of University Research Parks (AURP), www.aurp.net (accessed September 5, 2005).

9. The National Research Council (NRC), www.nationalacademies.org/nrc (accessed September 5, 2005).

10. Research Administrator Certification Council (RACC), www.cra-cert.org (accessed September 5, 2005).

III

PART

Pre-Award Administration

Fundamentals of Sponsored Programs: An Overview

Dorothy Yates

The term "sponsored programs administration" encompasses both pre-award and post-award activities. This chapter focuses on the fundamentals of sponsored programs that occur in the typical pre-award office. The pre-award offices are normally responsible for assisting faculty in pursuing and administering external funds for their research and creative activities. Subsequent chapters provide additional detail for these functions.

The role of the sponsored programs office is to provide administration *for* research, not *of* research. The distinction reflects the symbiotic relationship between the researchers, the sponsors, and the research administrators. Sponsored programs offices facilitate the research enterprise while mitigating risk to the organization.

First and foremost, an office of sponsored programs should perform an evaluation of its organization to develop a clear understanding of the organization and the types of activities in which it is engaged. It is important to understand the resources, constraints, and culture of an organization in order to facilitate the process of seeking external funds. Researcher interests and expertise should be documented in a searchable database. Care should be taken to understand the relative experience of the researcher, e.g., is he/she at the beginning, middle, or end of his/her career? Researchers at different levels also require different services. For example, a senior researcher may require little or no assistance in identifying a possible funding source, while a new researcher may require significant assistance.

While the focus of the pre-award office is to facilitate the proposal development and the award negotiation process, the staff must have an understanding of the process from idea to close-out—often referred to as "cradle to grave." The broad categories of activities include:

- Proposal development
- Award receipt, negotiation, and administration
- Regulatory environment
- Expending funds
- Close-out

Proposal Development and Submission

The proposal development process begins in one of two ways: when an individual (typically a faculty member when in a higher education organization) has an idea or a sponsor has a specific need. In either case, it is important to match the proposed project with the sponsor's needs.

Many organizations subscribe to online subscription services with searchable data bases to locate funding sources. Sponsored programs' pre-award offices often monitor funding opportunities and notify researchers of opportunities in particular areas of interest and expertise. Typical sponsors are federal agencies, state agencies, foundations, associations, and industry.

Once a funding source is identified, the development of the proposal can begin. There are three types of proposals: pre-proposals, solicited proposals, and unsolicited proposals. Pre-proposals are a shortened version of a full proposal and usually do not require the same level of technical or financial information (actual requirements are determined by the sponsor). Solicited proposals are those in response to a particular announcement or request for proposal, often referred to as an RFP. Unsolicited proposals are those that are not in response to a specific announcement, but are related to an area of interest to the sponsor.

Typically, the researcher focuses on the technical aspects of the proposal, while the research administrator focuses on the logistics of the process. The first step for each is to become familiar with the sponsor's guidelines, both the general requirements and the program-specific requirements. This helps reduce the last-minute chaos that can occur on the deadline day.

Either the researcher or the research administrator completes the sponsor's forms. Assistance for this process is often found in the pre-award office. There is a certain amount of organizational information that is standard to all proposals: legal name, federal tax identification number, DUNS number, administrative contact, financial point of contact, and the name of the person authorized to sign for the organization (the authorized official). Additional information requested by federal sponsors includes the federal-wide assurance number for human subjects' approval, the assurance number for animal care and use, the CFDA (catalog of federal domestic assistance) number, the CAGE code, and the congressional district. It is helpful to summarize this information on "institutional data sheets" that are most often electronically available.

An integral part of the proposal development process is the development of the budget. In this book there is a subsequent chapter devoted to this process, so details are not provided here. However, it is important for the research administrator to understand the basic components of a budget, budget justification, and the regulatory issues in order to provide an appropriate level of assistance to the researcher.

Sponsors generally provide very specific guidelines for proposal development and submission. In addition to the technical aspects of the proposals, the guidelines include: acceptable margins; font size; page limits; formats for budgets and curriculum vitae; whether or not appendices are acceptable; when and how to submit; and a multitude of other requirements. It is extremely important to follow the instructions to the letter; the proposal will likely be rejected if it deviates from the sponsor's requirements.

In addition to the agency requirements, organizations also have their own processes for review and approval before a proposal can be submitted. As an example, at a higher education institution, a typical review and approval process and form (also referred to as the "routing" of a proposal) includes signatures from the researcher, his/her department head, his/her dean, and the person authorized to commit the organization. This process might also include questions about cost-share requirements, the use of human subjects, animal subjects, facilities, biohazards, and the like. Organizations generally use the approval process to gather additional information they might need for reporting and other purposes. In order to affect the process, organizations develop a routing form that documents the information detailed above as well as information about the researcher (name, phone number, department, etc.), the sponsor (name, address, contact information, etc.), title of the project, a budget summary, reductions or waivers of the facilities and administrative cost rate, and the project period. It is important that there is an approval process in place to prevent individuals from committing to projects that are outside the scope of the organization or that over-commit organization resources.

Once the internal review and approval process is complete, the proposal can be submitted. The key to a successful proposal submission is for the research administrator to be involved as early in the process as possible and to act as a facilitator in order to keep the researcher on track.

Award Receipt and Administration

A proposal will either be rejected or accepted. If rejected, the researcher will typically receive comments from the reviewers. He/she will often have the opportunity to resubmit the proposal for a subsequent competition. The research administrator should encourage and facilitate the resubmission.

If accepted, the sponsor initiates an award document that is sent to the organization. Negotiation as to the terms of the award and the budget then occurs. The administrative contact for the organization typically negotiates the terms and conditions, and the researcher negotiates the budget as it impacts the scope of work.

An award can be a grant, a cooperative agreement, a contract, or a subcontract. A grant is an award that has few strings attached. Generally, it incorporates the sponsor's guidelines, but allows significant flexibility in carrying out the project with little or no oversight from the sponsor. A cooperative agreement is a grant with ongoing oversight from the sponsor and involves a partnership-type relationship between sponsor and researcher to achieve the goals of the project. A contract is a very descriptive and restrictive award that provides specifics for the activities of the project. Typically, any deviations from the proposed project must be approved prior to execution under a contract award. A subcontract is an award made to one organization from another; the "prime" organization receives, negotiates, and accepts the award and subcontracts out a portion of the activity.

Once an award is received, negotiated, and accepted, it is set up in the organization's accounting system and expenditure of funds can begin. The pre-award office documents the award details for reporting purposes and then forwards the award to post-award for processing. Many pre-award offices summarize the award information for post-award set-up. The information summarized is similar to that included on the proposal routing form (described above), but may also include additional information as required by the organization.

While the post-award office focuses on accounting, financial reporting, and financial compliance, there are additional post-award activities that occur that are often handled by the pre-award office. Generally, the pre-award office remains the liaison with the sponsor for any changes to the project that require sponsor approval. These might include a change of researcher, a change in the scope of the project, a significant modification to the budget, purchase of equipment not in the original budget, or other changes as determined by the sponsor's requirements.

The Regulatory Environment

It is important that the pre-award research administrator have a solid understanding of the regulatory environment of sponsored programs administration. Depending on the type of organization, the levels of regulations differ. (For the sake of this discussion, the regulations that would apply to a public institution of higher education that is part of a statewide system are described.) The regulation levels include:

- Office of Management and Budget Circulars (OMB Circulars)
- Sponsor Policies
- State Policies and Procedures

- Regents' (or Trustees') Policies and Procedures
- Campus Policies and Procedures

There are three OMB circulars that outline compliance issues for public institutions of higher education. These include OMB Circular A-21, OMB Circular A-110, and OMB Circular A-133. OMB Circular A-21, "Cost Principles for Educational Institutions," outlines allowable and unallowable costs and prescribes the manner in which universities must determine their facilities and administrative cost rate. OMB Circular A-110, "Uniform Administrative Requirements for Grants and Other Agreements with Institutions of Higher Education, Hospitals, and Other Non-Profit Organizations," sets forth administrative procedures, such as financial reporting, the handling of program income, payment requirements, standards for financial management, federal requirements for cost-sharing, rebudgeting, and prior approvals. OMB Circular A-133, "Audits of Institutions of Higher Education and Other Non-profit Institutions," outlines audit requirements for universities and other nonprofit institutions that receive federal funds. In order to serve the research community effectively, the pre-award research administrator must have a deep understanding of Circulars A-21 and A-110 and be cognizant of Circular A-133. More detail on the circulars can be found in Part IV of this book.

Sponsors also have their own requirements that must be met by the recipient organization. These policies and guidance documents are typically available on the sponsor's Web site, or are part of the award document itself. The pre-award research administrator needs to have in-depth knowledge of the sponsor requirements so he/she can convey the requirements to the researcher to assist in ensuring compliance. Please note that specific programs within a sponsoring agency may have additional requirements.

In this public institution example, state policies and procedures must also be followed. The two primary policies that affect the research enterprise are fiscal and procurement. Again, the research administrator needs to have an understanding of the policies and also where to go to get answers if specific questions arise.

Since this public institution example is also part of a state system, another layer of policies and procedures must be followed. These are determined by the Board of Regents (or Trustees) and provide an umbrella under which all other institutional policies operate, and apply to all activities regardless of sponsor or source of funds.

The final level is at the campus itself. While the Regents (or Trustees) have established some general principles, the campus administration develops its own policies and procedures which guide the activities of the research enterprise.

In addition to the levels listed above, further rules may be imposed. For example, if the funding is through a contract from a federal agency, Federal Acquisition Regulations (FAR) may apply. It is imperative that the research administrator understand the complexity of the regulatory environment for the research enterprise. It is not expected that the research administrator know every regulation, but that he/she knows where to find the answers when asked.

Additional areas of compliance that impact sponsored programs are outlined in Parts IV and V of this book (human subjects, animal care and use, research misconduct, conflict of interest, technology transfer, etc.).

Expending Funds

While research administrators in the pre-award office do not generally get involved with the accounting aspects of the expenditure of funds, it is important to understand the issues surrounding those expenditures. The research administrator must know the rules guiding expenditures at the time the budget is being developed. At that point, he/she has the opportunity to guide the researcher in developing appropriate budget categories. Sponsors may reduce the budget by eliminating unacceptable categories.

Close-Out

The post-award offices of sponsored programs generally take care of the financial close-out of grants and contracts. However, the pre-award offices may also play a role. For example, the pre-award office may facilitate the submission of the final technical report by the research team. In addition, patent and property reports are often completed by the pre-award office.

Summary

Sponsored programs administration requires knowledge and skills in many areas, including funding source identification, proposal development, sponsor liaison activities, faculty encouragement, and compliance issues. Expertise is generally gained

in a "hands-on" fashion, and most research administrators have a basic working knowledge within a year or two of tenure. It takes many years, however, to gain real expertise in research administration, and even the most seasoned administrators are routinely required to learn new aspects of this field. Serving both the researchers by facilitating their research experience and the institution by mitigating risk are the two main dual functions of a research administrator, but the very nature of these divergent functions makes for a complex work day.

• • • Suggested Reading

Cole, Julie, John Terry Manns, Pam Miller, and Mary Watson. "Starting a Sponsored Projects Operation from Scratch." Society of Research Administrators International workshop, Salt Lake City, UT, October 2004.

Introduction to Basic Grant Management. Fairbanks, AK: Innovation Consulting, Inc.

The Journal of Research Administration, *Journal of the Society of Research Administrators International*, http://www.srainternational.org/newweb/publications/journal.

National Council of University Research Administrators/National Association of College and University Business Officers. *A Guide to Managing Federal Grants for Colleges and Universities.* Washington, DC: NCURA/NACUBO, 1999.

"RAPID—Research Administration Professional and Institutional Development." FIPSE proposal, Society of Research Administrators International, 2002.

Research at Carolina, University of North Carolina at Chapel Hill, NC. "Policies and Guidelines," http://php.unc.edu/services/policies.php (accessed October 13, 2005).

"Research Management Review." *Journal of the National Council of University Research Administrators*, http://www.ncura.edu/rmr/

Society of Research Administrators International. "SRA International Topical Outline," http://www.srainternational.org/newweb/Publications/topicaloutline/index.cfm (accessed: August 5, 2005).

University of California, Office of the President, Research Administration Office. "Contract and Grant Manual," 1996, http://www.ucop.edu/raohome/cgmanual/ (accessed August 4, 2005).

University of Michigan Research. "Sponsored Projects," http://www.research.umich.edu/sprojects.html (accessed August 5, 2005).

University of Washington, Office of Sponsored Programs. "Researchers Guide," http://www.washington.edu/research/guide/ (accessed August 4, 2005).

Yates, Dorothy. "Grants & Contracts—Cradle to Grave," Training module, University of Colorado at Denver, Denver, CO, 1999.

Yates, Dorothy. "Strategies for Success," Training module, University of Colorado at Denver, Denver, CO, 2000.

26

Special Issues of Departmental Administration

Tim Quigg, PhD

Before World War II, federal funding for research at US colleges and universities was rather limited with the notable exception of support for agriculture research (dating from the late 19th century). Before World War II, most research activity was funded through charitable contributions or from internal sources. The advent of the war spurred a mobilization of university science and engineering expertise as part of the war effort. Near the end of WWII, the federal Office of Scientific Research and Development (OSRD), under the leadership of Dr. Vannevar Bush, published an important report entitled *Science: The Endless Frontier*. Soon after, the National Science Foundation was established, signifying the federal government's formal and active involvement in the sponsorship of scientific research and development. With the subsequent rapid growth of federal funding and public investment of university research came the demand for research accountability—requiring proof of prudent funding management and management of programs that produced cutting-edge results: hence, was the creation of a new class of professionals called *research administrators*.

Even before institutional designation of this new professional area, department and laboratory staff were engaged in support of the scientific enterprise. Department chairs, financial managers, secretaries, and lab managers allocated space, ordered equipment, complied with safety requirements, posted work schedules, supervised employees, kept track of funding, disposed of dangerous chemicals, and performed the numerous essential support tasks later overseen by formal research administration. Thus, it can be argued that research administration began at the department level. Today, in research-intensive institutions, whether universities, private nonprofit research institutes, hospitals, or government labs, the success and the integrity of the research enterprise depends largely upon the quality of research administration at the department level.

Growth of Departmental Administration

As the size of sponsored research portfolios has increased dramatically at many institutions, it has become necessary to segment the work of research administration into components and to assign focused tasks to suboffices within the institution. Staff within these various suboffices have the opportunity to develop expertise in a limited range of issues. For example, Institutional Review Boards (IRBs) serve to guarantee proper protection for human subjects engaged in research, while pre-award staff review proposals for compliance with both agency and institutional requirements prior to submission to the funding agency. Similarly, accounting managers collect and organize financial data in preparation for negotiating a Facilities and Administrative (F&A) Rate Agreement with the institution's cognizant federal agency.

In contrast to this push toward specialization at the central institution level is the enduring importance of the generalist department research administrator. It is important to define the term *department* in this context. Department refers to any subunit of an institution charged with the dual responsibility of:

1. Providing quality support services to those employees working directly on achieving the institution's mission, e.g., in a university the faculty work directly on achieving the university's mission, research and education, and;
2. Complying with a wide range of institutional and agency-specific rules, policies, and expectations.

In other words, departments and department administrators are "in the middle" and assist the researcher by providing the proper resources at the required time to further the research objectives, and they insure that all relevant institutional and agency rules are being followed to protect the researcher, the institution, and the integrity of the scientific enterprise from recrimination. By this definition, many subunits with names other than their departments qualify, including centers, institutes, and schools. In some cases, even small research institutions that are not large enough to be subdivided into departments nor sophisticated enough to specialize at the central level may be properly considered as single departments.

An unavoidable reality of the job of research administration is the concern raised when support needs appear to be in conflict with the rules—the very condition that makes the job of department administrator so exciting! To be successful, the department administrator must have a basic understanding of the rules, but even more importantly, must know where to go to obtain guidance when present circumstances exceed his or her knowledge base. Maintaining strong relationships with staff in central research offices is essential. Not knowing an answer is acceptable, but not knowing where to find an answer is not.

Role of the Departmental Administrator

The department administrator must have enough familiarity with the content of the research to understand and appreciate the requests coming from the researcher, and in time will be able to anticipate and address many needs before the researcher asks. A flat "no" to a request is not an appropriate response, nor should the administrator comply with a flawed request simply to curry favor. The administrator should not be viewed as an obstacle in progress of research, but rather as a facilitator. The researchers do, however, expect the guidance of a department administrator in order to comply with the rules of the institution. In many cases, difficulty originates with an initial question (often an attempt by the researcher to propose a solution to a problem) that has not been clearly defined by the researcher. In these cases, the department administrator must guide the researcher's focus by asking a series of detailed questions. Only when the real issue is identified can the administrator use his or her knowledge and problem-solving skills to propose a creative solution to meet the needs of the researcher.

Range of Topic in Departmental Administration

A typical day in a department administration office illustrates the wide range of topics that are addressed and, by inference, the breadth of knowledge required for successful department administration. A day may begin with a purchase request of equipment to be charged to a particular grant account. This event raises the issues of *allowability*:

> *Are there any rules prohibiting the purchase from this account?*
>
> *Is there an equipment line item in the grant budget? If so, are there adequate funds available in this equipment line?*

and *allocability*:

> *Is the equipment needed to fulfill the work of the project?*
>
> *Does the total value of the equipment purchase accrue to that project?*

These questions require a fundamental knowledge of the relevant federal cost principles (A-21 or A-122) and a detailed knowledge of institution rules (for example, it may be possible to create an equipment line if none exists through an institution prior approval system request or, if there are inadequate funds in the equipment line, the department administrator may initiate a budget revision to move funds from another line, e.g., supplies to equipment). Once these issues are resolved, the purchasing process must be initiated following appropriate institution procurement procedures.

Skill Development in Multi-Tasking

The department administrator must be able to juggle multiple tasks at once; remain calm in situations when others are not; perform ongoing triage to determine which issues require immediate attention and which can be logged to be handled later; delegate tasks to staff and maintain an effective system for being kept apprised of progress toward task completion; and exhibit a keen understanding of how today's issues and decisions have an impact on the future direction of the department. While the duality of support and compliance objectives previously discussed informs much of the intent of research administration at the department level, there is an unmistakable reality concerning department administrators: they are first and foremost managers! They allocate resources; supervise staff; receive and act on requests; negotiate solutions to problems; and comply with various rules and policies set by others. They do these things in support of a research enterprise, but failing to see department administrators as managers is to miss the fundamental purpose of the job.

An operational definition of department management is to direct the process and to provide guidance in a research organization to achieve its mission with given sets of environmental constraints. This definition contains four primary concepts about the duties of department management:

- Understanding and supporting organization mission
- Intentionality in management
- Operation within certain environmental constraints
- Setting and achieving objectives that support the mission

Organization Mission

What is organization mission? How should it be understood? The proceeding story illustrates the important relationship between the success of an organization and the extent to which the members of the organization have a clear understanding of and agreement with its mission.

In 1954, a student graduated from a large southern university and was admitted to the business school of a prestigious Ivy League university to pursue his graduate education. Among his classmates, he found that there was only one other student who would also be attending that same university. The two young men soon became friends and agreed to be roommates; one of these friends was paralyzed from the waist down.

The day finally came for these two new graduates to begin their long trek and their van, specially equipped with hand controls replacing the foot petals, was loaded with all of their personal items. This was in the day before the creation of the interstate highway system, so the trip to New England was a substantial undertaking. After many hours on the road, the two weary, but enthusiastic travelers finally reached their destination. A quick survey of the campus led them to the dorm that would be their home for the next few years. They attempted to locate a parking place close to the dorm. None was to be found; however, there was a paved area close to the front door that would be a suitable stopping place while they unloaded. After bringing the first load to the room, the student returned to the van to get another load, and he saw a campus police officer standing by the van. Assuming that the police officer would write him a ticket, and fearful of getting in trouble on his first day at his new school, the student quickly offered an explanation. Upon hearing of the long trip and the special circumstances of his roommate's condition, the officer gave permission to keep the van in its location until the unloading was complete.

After several additional trips, the student came out of the front door and again saw the officer. Only this time, the officer seemed to be giving instructions to a workman in front of the van. The student feared the worst, but as he got closer he saw that the worker was painting a line on the ground. A sign had already been installed beside the van marking the place "Reserved." When the officer saw him, he said, "As long as you and your roommate remain students in good standing, this parking place is yours." The absolutely marvelous message behind this story is that the campus police officer knew precisely the mission of the university. It was to support the educational activities of students! Furthermore, the officer understood he had a role to play in the primary mission of the institution, and he felt empowered to make a decision that furthered this mission. In many organizations the officer would have been taught that his primary duty was to enforce parking regulations. Thus, he might not have been inclined to grant much leeway when the students were unloading their van. After all, they were breaking the rules! And he certainly would not have considered creating a special parking place. Yet, in this situation, the officer had a keen understanding of organization mission that guided his actions.

Healthy, successful organizations are ones that understand their mission and have developed methods for effectively sharing their mission with employees and other important interest groups. Indeed, this task is the challenge of all department administrators: *know the mission of your department, be enthusiastically committed to it, and be able to share it with others in a way that leads them to become committed to it as well!*

Intentionality in Management

The department administrator must be available and responsive to his clientele, i.e., the researchers and support staff at both the department and institution levels. Requests come into the office by telephone, e-mail, snail mail, and personal visits. The volume can be overwhelming and, if he or she is not careful, the job of the department administrator can easily devolve into that of a reactor to outside stimuli only. While it is important to address these needs, it is also important to periodically take stock of the organization to measure the extent to which it is accomplishing its mission.

In the midst of this chaotic environment, how does the department administrator find time to step back and look at the big picture? One way is through effective delegation, but he or she must never delegate responsibility without also delegating the appropriate level of authority. And this delegation must be made publicly so that everyone who needs to know of the delegation knows. Effective delegation can result in many benefits to the department including an increase in staff morale. This occurs when the supervisor willingly delegates some of the "good stuff," rather than simply delegating the tedious tasks that he or she doesn't like to do. Greater involvement in the important decisions within the department will lead to greater investment in the outcome, more enthusiastic commitment to the department's mission, and a corresponding increase in the morale of the staff.

Whenever important tasks are delegated by the department administrator, there is always the chance that something will go wrong. The employee may make the wrong decision, and the negative consequences of the decision may become known outside of the department. In this case, the old adage of "delegating credit, but never delegating blame" needs to be remembered. A good department administrator needs broad shoulders to assume the blame in these cases. Did he or she ask the employee to assume too much responsibility before the employee was ready to assume it? Should the administrator have required more reporting of progress before the employee took action? Or, in retrospect, does he or she now have information that indicates a limitation in the employee's ability to handle certain tasks? In any case, the department administrator now has additional important information that can help him or her be a more effective supervisor for that particular employee in the future.

As previously stated, the department administrator is first and foremost a manager. And one of the primary functions of management is to be a supervisor of staff. Many department administration offices experience a plethora of operational problems because many department administrators have little training or experience as supervisors. Frequently, they start their careers as content specialists in one aspect of research administration or finance, and through demonstrated competency in this area, they are promoted into department administrator positions. These administrators may believe their primary task is to teach their staff the rules and policies of research administration and fail to recognize that their role as supervisor requires so much more.

The primary role of supervision can be expressed by three simple, but extremely powerful tasks: set expectations, motivate performance, and evaluate performance. Most staff performance problems can be explained by a breakdown in one aspect of this simple formula.

First, the supervisor must set clear expectations for performance and indicate how success will be measured. Many supervisors like to involve the employee in setting some of the expectations and some of the performance metrics. This approach is fine as long as the final outcome is accepted by the supervisor and the employee's performance expectations are tied to the department mission. Once performance measures are established, they should not be modified unless there is agreement between both parties that they no longer represent a fair measure of success.

Second, the supervisor should not simply set expectations and then walk away only to return at some point in the future to measure success or failure. Instead, the supervisor should remain involved, asking for periodic progress reports, and offering advice and counsel along the way. This allows the supervisor to provide needed midcourse correction in a way that minimizes lost time and effort when an employee has gotten side-tracked. It also demonstrates to the employee that the supervisor is committed to a partnership designed to insure the employee's success.

Third, if the first two steps in the process are done correctly, the evaluation of performance should be the easiest step of all. There should be no surprises because both parties know the expectations, the measures for evaluating performance, and the work that has been done to achieve the expectations. If there are any major surprises, it is an indication that something likely went wrong earlier in the process, e.g., a communication problem resulting in a fundamental misunderstanding of expectations. One way to minimize this occurrence is to commit all agreements to writing and have both parties sign acknowledging agreement.

Environmental Constraints

Perhaps it is obvious and should require no explanation, but department administrators operate in an environment of externally imposed constraints. While it is important to be aware of these constraints, it is equally important that the department administrator not become "hostage" to them. Perhaps trite, but nonetheless true, the department administrator must find a way to succeed in supporting the mission of the department despite the constraints. But to ignore them is to proceed foolishly and can result in failure to support the mission adequately!

The important constraints may be divided into three categories: *resources*, *rules*, and *culture*. The most important resources available to the department administrator are money, people, time, and facilities. Each is rarely perceived to be adequate to get the job done. Indeed, the size of administrative budgets is actually shrinking at many institutions as state governments and private endowments struggle with the realities of limited resources. Hiring additional people or replacing an existing staff with new people who have all the talents currently required for the job is simply not feasible. The department administrator can try to work 24/7 for a while, but the limits of human endurance make this approach unrealistic. And you can't work 25/8!

Resources

Doing more with less is a mantra that reverberates throughout many institutions. While smart department administrators recognize the practical limitations for growth in their administrative budgets, they also recognize that through better delineated work assignments, more targeted staff training, and the elimination of unnecessary duplication, they may increase overall efficiency, for a while. However, there comes a point where no more work can be "squeezed from the turnip"! This is the point at which the department administrator must ask the all-important question: What can we stop doing without having a severe negative impact on supporting the mission of the department? It is only through carefully considered redefinition of the most vital support services that a wise department administrator can find an equilibrium between the resources available and the essential task of supporting the mission of the department. To fail to redefine tasks in light of resource limitations is to ensure mediocrity. A mediocre approach to the provision of department administration support services will only reduce the quality of the research output and ultimately have a negative impact on achieving the department's mission.

Rules

Rules are constraints that color the canvas of daily activity within a department administration office. Institution rules, laws, OMB circulars, agency rules—there is never a shortage of rules that tell the department administrator what he or she cannot do. While it is important to understand these rules and be certain to seek full compliance, the administrator must never stop at the first no, especially when the vital interests of the research enterprise are at stake. Sometimes a "no" simply creates an inconvenience, and all experienced department administrators learn to have a high tolerance for inconvenience. Other times a single "no" can bring an important research project to a dead stop. In these cases, the department administrator must persevere and consider:

- Is there a procedure for granting an exception?
- Was the initial question too broadly framed?
- Would a more targeted question have resulted in a different response?
- Was the no response associated with a relatively unimportant aspect of the request that can be modified without seriously impeding research progress?

The job of the department administrator is to find a way to support the research mission of the department, and when faced with a conflict between the legitimate needs of the researcher and the applicable regulations, he or she must persist until an acceptable solution is found.

Culture

The third category of constraint is *organizational culture*. Individual departments within an institution each have their own established methods for decision-making, preferred means of communication, and many idiosyncratic nuances that must be understood if the department administrator is to be successful. Success in one department does not automatically translate into success in another if the culture is dramatically different. These factors serve to constrain the actions of the department administrator every bit as much as resources and rules; however, these factors are rarely written down and can only be identified through experience. In truth, what is written down, e.g., formal organization charts, often confuses the matter when there is substantial dissonance between the formal and informal systems. Usually experience, either the department administrator's or the advice of a trusted colleague who has been through the wars and learned from it, is the only real teacher. New department administrators should tread lightly, ask many questions, keep their eyes open and their antennae up, test the waters with small initiatives first, and observe how the decisions are really made and by whom before initiating any major projects.

Setting and Achieving Objectives that Support the Mission

The department administrator must determine which objectives are most directly correlated with the department's mission, and then must determine how to achieve those objectives. Caution should be taken, however, as the obvious objectives may not be the ones that have the most impact on achieving the department's mission. For instance, a department administrator may initiate a policy that all proposals will be reviewed, signed and sent through the institution review process within 24 hours of receipt. This objective maximizes the value of efficiency, i.e., time spent on task. But it says nothing about the quality of the review. If the review occurs rapidly, but a large number of the proposals are returned to the department by the sponsored programs office to have errors corrected, the actual total review time may be increased. And then there is the matter of proposals that fail to be funded because of something that could have been caught during a more thorough

department review process. So, a more cogent objective may be one that measures the extent to which the department review minimizes the number of proposals returned to the department for error correction and maximizes the percentage of proposals that are actually funded. The key is to focus careful attention on the intended result, rather than being seduced by procedural issues that have marginal impact on the desired outcomes.

In order to build a system for achieving results, there are five key points that need to be considered:

1. Objectives should always be stated in positive, not negative, terms and should always be tied to the department mission. The key is to focus attention on what needs to be accomplished, not what needs to be avoided.

2. Write the objectives down on paper. This helps to crystallize thinking and can help to identify contradictory objectives. In addition, there is something magic about the increase in commitment that occurs when objectives are actually written down. Spoken objectives are easily forgotten or modified. Written ones are more lasting.

3. Quantify the objectives. It is important to know how to measure success. Too much effort can be expended on objectives that have actually been achieved, when the proper action is to declare success and move on to the next topic.

4. Make the objectives time-specific. One of the most powerful of all management techniques is to create deadlines that spur people to action.

5. Review the objectives regularly. Each department administrator needs to adopt his own approach, perhaps a formal periodic review or something considerably more casual. One idea is to write the objectives for the coming year on a sheet of paper, put it in a clear plastic cover for protection, and then place it somewhere visited regularly, perhaps on a bulletin board or in an office drawer that is opened frequently. Simply looking at the sheet, even without focusing on its contents, will bring the objectives to mind regularly and increase the likelihood of success.

Departmental Administrator as Financial Manager

No discussion of department administration would be complete without a review of the department administrator's role in financial management. Indeed, much of his or her effort is focused on managing money—spending, reporting, and projecting—and nothing will get him or her into trouble more quickly than to "mess up the money." Principal investigators are concerned with the financial aspects of their grants, lab managers with the budgets that support their labs, directors of graduate studies with the resources that fund their programs; but only one person in the department has responsibility for all the subbudgets as well as the consolidated department budget—the department administrator!

Performing at a level of excellence in this area is critically important to achieving the mission of the department. Poor financial management can cause research projects to slow down or even stop prematurely if the project runs out of money. It is not unusual for a piece of equipment or a person with a particular skill to be needed at a specific time in a research project, and it is the responsibility of the department administrator to deliver the needed resource at the proper time. To do so, the department administrator needs to back off the delivery date by an appropriate amount of time and initiate the transaction, e.g., the purchase requisition for the equipment or the hiring process for the employee, at the proper time to insure the resource will be available when needed. Failure to do so may result in unnecessary downtime in the research project, a waste of limited resources, and it can even have a negative impact on achieving the research goals.

Expenditure Rates

If the department administrator allows the expenditure rate within a project to be too rapid, there may not be adequate resources to last through the project period. If too slow, it may jeopardize receipt of a future funding increment. And if there are questionable expenses charged to a project, the department administrator can open the project, department, and institution to audit exposure. For all these reasons, the department administrator must implement a sophisticated financial management system that meets the three requirements discussed in the following sections.

The system must insure timely and accurate transaction processing Questions of staffing and transaction sequencing are important and must be addressed. Do you organize your accounting staff around transaction type, e.g., travel, equipment requisitions, personnel actions? Or do you organize around funding agencies, e.g., one person does all of the NSF and another all of the NIH? Or do you organize around logical subunits within the department, e.g., groups of labs or programs? Each approach has strengths and limitations. The first two provide greater opportunity for specialization,

and the third approach provides the opportunity to more closely integrate the accounting staff with the functional work units of the department. However, the department administrator must also consider the size of the accounting staff, the impact of staff vacancies, the need for cross-training, as well as the individual talents of the staff, when making these decisions.

Most department accounting offices use some version of first-in first-out (or FIFO) as a way to manage the orderly sequencing of transactions. However, the wise department administrator recognizes the importance of having the ability to "flag" transactions requiring special attention or prioritized processing. One approach is to have a certain class of transaction automatically routed to a supervisor or even to the department administrator based upon clearly stated, written guidelines. Perhaps those in excess of a certain dollar figure or that have an unusually short processing time requirement would receive this special attention.

The system must insure compliance with all applicable rules and policies Indeed, while most institutions implement various pre-approval and post-processing audit checks to measure compliance, it can be argued that the department administrator has the toughest job of all in the policy hierarchy because he or she has to make real-life policy interpretations at the cutting edge of the compliance system. The administrator knows what is needed by the researcher and also knows what is allowed under the rules. These critical judgments, made multiple times daily at the department level, greatly impact the integrity of the institution's compliance system. Poor decisions cascade through the system and can lead to significant audit exposure.

The department financial accounting system must insure proper expense classification consistent with the terms of the award Is the expense charged to the proper account (and the proper activity)? Is there a clear demarcation between direct and indirect costs? Are like costs being charged consistently without regard to fund type? Has the department captured and properly documented all cost sharing on a project? Did the expense occur within the project period? Is there adequate budget to support the expense? Is there an appropriate line item in the budget for the expense? These are some of the many issues that must be addressed at the department level. For it is only at the department level that the required information exists to make these important decisions.

Finally, while much energy at the department level goes into effectively managing the expenditure of money, the wise department administrator also assesses the impact of current trends on the department's finances one, two, or more years into the future. Based upon knowledge of projects that are ending and of the pipeline of proposals that have been submitted (which must be adjusted using historic success rates), the administrator must project future rates of growth or contraction. Some aspects of the department's research portfolio may be on the ascent, while others may be on the descent. Advanced knowledge of these trends and their impact on space, personnel, and equipment needs help the department administrator plan for the future. This ability to be proactive—to project future needs for department-supplied support services based upon an analysis of significant changes in the size and composition of the department—is perhaps the most important single function of professional department administration.

27

Representations and Certifications for Federal Grants and Contracts

Sandra Nordahl, CRA

Representations and certifications for proposals and awards can be extremely intimidating. This portion of an application or award is typically written in legalese with references to guides, notices, and law citations. Often the first thoughts when reviewing this portion of the document are, *What does all of this mean? Who needs to sign these documents? What trouble can signing these documents cause?* Each funding source may vary the requirements for completing representations and certifications or assurances and certifications (commonly referred to as "reps" and "certs"). Some funding sources, typically private funding entities, may not require any documentation of this nature. Contracts issued from state and federal agencies generally have the most extensive and comprehensive documentation to complete. Proposal submissions may often state on the cover page of an application that by signing the face page, the individual or organization agrees to comply with the assurances, certifications, policies, and representations (or a combination thereof). Most often, the individual that has authorized signature authority for the institution is the person who is charged with executing these documents on behalf of the organization.

Once a thorough understanding is gained, boilerplate documentation can and should be developed. This can save valuable proposal preparation time, as well as shorten the response time when finalizing the award documentation. It is important to periodically review boilerplate documents to ensure that changes (even minor) have not been introduced by the agencies. All changes to existing boilerplate documentation should be thoroughly reviewed to ensure that the grantee agrees and can comply with any revised language that has been introduced.

Sources of Information

The US Department of Health and Human Services (DHHS), Public Health Service PHS 398 grant application provides one of the most comprehensive listings of representations and certifications that are required to be completed at the proposal stage. Nineteen different statements must be reviewed and completed as a part of the proposal submission.[1] Below is a listing of the assurances, certifications, and policies that a grantee "certifies" they comply with when accepting funding from DHHS.

1. Assurance of Compliance (Civil Rights, Handicapped Individuals, Sex Discrimination, Age Discrimination)
2. Debarment and Suspension
3. Drug-Free Workplace
4. Financial Conflict of Interest
5. Human Subjects
6. Lobbying
7. NIH Policy on Inclusion of Children
8. NIH Policy on the Inclusion of Women and Minorities in Clinical Research
9. Nondelinquency on Federal Debt
10. PHS Metric Program
11. Prohibited Research
12. Prohibition on Awards to 501(c)4 Organizations That Lobby

13. Research Involving Recombinant DNA, including Human Gene Transfer Research
14. Research Misconduct
15. Research Using Human Embryonic Stem Cells
16. Research on Transplantation of Human Fetal Tissue
17. Select Agents and Toxins
18. Smoke-Free Workplace
19. Vertebrate Animals

Typically, Section K in the Request for Proposal (RFP) document addresses representations and certifications. This portion of an RFP is commonly entitled, "Representations, Certifications and Other Statements of Offerors." Depending on the agency soliciting the work, Federal Acquisition Regulations (FAR) clauses and Department of Defense Acquisition Regulations (DFAR) may be cited. Contract representations and certifications are generally more explicit by nature than clauses cited in grant applications and/or awards. Clauses that may be found in an RFP[2] in response to a contract solicitation could be:

52.222-25	Affirmative Action Compliance (APR 1984)
52.203-11	Certification and Disclosure Regarding Payments to Influence Certain Federal Transactions (APR 1991)
52.223-13	Certification of Toxic Chemical Release Reporting (OCT 2000)
52.209-05	Certification Regarding Debarment, Suspension, Proposed Debarment, and Other Responsibility Matters (DEC 2001)
52.222-38	Compliance with Veteran's Employment Reporting Requirements (DEC 2001)
52.230-01	Cost Accounting Standards Notices and Certification (JUN 2000)
252.209-7001	Disclosure of Ownership or Control by the Government of a Terrorist Country (MAR 1998)
52.226-02	Historically Black College or University and Minority Institution Representation (MAY 2001)
252.227-7017	Identification and Assertion of Use, Release, or Disclosure Restrictions (JUN 1995)
52.215-06	Place of Performance (OCT 1997)
52.222-22	Previous Contracts and Compliance Reports (FEB 1999)

252.247-7022	Representation of Extent of Transportation by Sea (AUG 1992)
52.219-01	Small Business Program Representations (APR 2001)—Alternate I (APR 2002)
52.204-03	Taxpayer Identification (OCT 1998)
252.227-7028	Technical Data or Computer Software Previously Delivered to the Government (JUN 1995)
52.204-05	Women-Owned Business (Other than Small Business)

These listings are not all inclusive. Depending on the work to be performed, other clauses may be incorporated into the solicitation, proposal guidelines, or an award document as appropriate. A complete listing of FAR clauses can be found at the Federal Acquisition Regulation Web site.[3] Clauses that begin with "52" can be located and reviewed in the Federal Acquisition Regulations, Part 52—Solicitation Provisions and Contract Clauses.[4] Clauses beginning with "252" can be reviewed by accessing Defense Federal Acquisition Regulations Supplement, Part 252—Solicitation Provisions and Contract Clauses.[5] A complete listing of DFAR clauses can be found at the Defense Procurement and Acquisition Policy Web site.[6]

Determining Applicability

Determining whether or not a clause is applicable to the institution and the work to be performed is the next step of the evaluation process. For example, 52.204-05 is the FAR clause citation "Women-Owned Business (Other than Small Business) (MAY 1999)." The clause as presented in a RFP[7] stated:

52.204-5 Women-Owned Business (Other Than Small Business) (MAY 1999)

(a) Definition. "Women-owned business concern," as used in this provision, means a concern that is at least 51 percent owned by one or more women; or in the case of any publicly owned business, at least 51 percent of its stock is owned by one or more women; and whose management and daily business operations are controlled by one or more women.

(b) Representation. (Complete only if the offeror is a women-owned business concern and has not represented itself as a small business concern in paragraph (b)(1) of FAR 52.219-1, Small Business Program Representations, of this solicitation.) The offeror represents that it [ ] is, [ ] is not a women-owned business concern.

(End of provision)

In the above clause, the offeror is requested to declare whether or not the organization is a Women-Owned Business by selecting one of the boxes at the conclusion of the clause. Typically, an institution of higher education would normally indicate that it is not a Women-Owned Business. For other organizations, such as nonprofit, commercial, and others, the choice may not be as clear, and a thorough review of the clause and additional citations should be performed.

Start the review process by obtaining the citation(s) pertaining to the clause. Review the documentation to determine the clause's applicability to the institution and the scope of work. For the above clause, reference is made to FAR 52.219-1, Small Business Program Representation, that states:[8]

52.219-1 Small Business Program Representations

As prescribed in 19.308(a)(1), insert the following provision:

Small Business Program Representations
(May 2004)

(a) (1) The North American Industry Classification System (NAICS) code for this acquisition is _____ [insert NAICS code].

(2) The small business size standard is _____ [insert size standard].

(3) The small business size standard for a concern which submits an offer in its own name, other than on a construction or service contract, but which proposes to furnish a product which it did not itself manufacture, is 500 employees.

(b) Representations.

(1) The offeror represents as part of its offer that it [ ] is, [ ] is not a small business concern.

(2) [Complete only if the offeror represented itself as a small business concern in paragraph (b)(1) of this provision.] The offeror represents, for general statistical purposes, that it [ ] is, [ ] is not, a small disadvantaged business concern as defined in 13 CFR 124.1002.

(3) [Complete only if the offeror represented itself as a small business concern in para-

graph (b)(1) of this provision.] The offeror represents as part of its offer that it [ ] is, [ ] is not a women-owned small business concern.

(4) [Complete only if the offeror represented itself as a small business concern in paragraph (b)(1) of this provision.] The offeror represents as part of its offer that it [ ] is, [ ] is not a veteran-owned small business concern.

(5) [Complete only if the offeror represented itself as a veteran-owned small business concern in paragraph (b)(4) of this provision.] The offeror represents as part of its offer that it [ ] is, [ ] is not a service-disabled veteran-owned small business concern.

(6) [Complete only if the offeror represented itself as a small business concern in paragraph (b)(1) of this provision.] The offeror represents, as part of its offer, that-

(i) It [ ] is, [ ] is not a HUBZone small business concern listed, on the date of this representation, on the List of Qualified HUBZone Small Business Concerns maintained by the Small Business Administration, and no material change in ownership and control, principal office, or HUBZone employee percentage has occurred since it was certified by the Small Business Administration in accordance with 13 CFR part 126; and

(ii) It [ ] is, [ ] is not a joint venture that complies with the requirements of 13 CFR part 126, and the representation in paragraph (b)(6)(i) of this provision is accurate for the HUBZone small business concern or concerns that are participating in the joint venture. [The offeror shall enter the name or names of the HUBZone small business concern or concerns that are participating in the joint venture: _____.] Each HUBZone small business concern participating in the joint venture shall submit a separate signed copy of the HUBZone representation.

(c) Definitions. As used in this provision-

"Service-disabled veteran-owned small business concern"-

(1) Means a small business concern-

    (i) Not less than 51 percent of which is owned by one or more service-disabled veterans or, in the case of any publicly owned business, not less than 51 percent of the stock of which is owned by one or more service-disabled veterans; and

    (ii) The management and daily business operations of which are controlled by one or more service-disabled veterans or, in the case of a service-disabled veteran with permanent and severe disability, the spouse or permanent caregiver of such veteran.

(2) Service-disabled veteran means a veteran, as defined in 38 U.S.C. 101(2), with a disability that is service-connected, as defined in 38 U.S.C. 101(16).

"Small business concern" means a concern, including its affiliates, that is independently owned and operated, not dominant in the field of operation in which it is bidding on Government contracts, and qualified as a small business under the criteria in 13 CFR part 121 and the size standard in paragraph (a) of this provision.

"Veteran-owned small business concern" means a small business concern-

(1) Not less than 51 percent of which is owned by one or more veterans (as defined at 38 U.S.C. 101(2)) or, in the case of any publicly owned business, not less than 51 percent of the stock of which is owned by one or more veterans; and

(2) The management and daily business operations of which are controlled by one or more veterans.

"Women-owned small business concern" means a small business concern-

(1) That is at least 51 percent owned by one or more women; or, in the case of any publicly owned business, at least 51 percent of the stock of which is owned by one or more women; and

(2) Whose management and daily business operations are controlled by one or more women.

(d) *Notice.*

    (1) If this solicitation is for supplies and has been set aside, in whole or in part, for

small business concerns, then the clause in this solicitation providing notice of the set-aside contains restrictions on the source of the end items to be furnished.

(2) Under 15 U.S.C. 645(d), any person who misrepresents a firm's status as a small, HUBZone small, small disadvantaged, or women-owned small business concern in order to obtain a contract to be awarded under the preference programs established pursuant to section 8(a), 8(d), 9, or 15 of the Small Business Act or any other provision of Federal law that specifically references section 8(d) for a definition of program eligibility, shall-

    (i) Be punished by imposition of fine, imprisonment, or both;

    (ii) Be subject to administrative remedies, including suspension and debarment; and

    (iii) Be ineligible for participation in programs conducted under the authority of the Act.

    (End of provision)

FAR clause "19.308—Solicitation provisions"[9] gives the solicitor the direction on when to place clause "52.219-1—Small Business Program Representations" into a solicitation. The offeror should review the solicitation provisions or prescription clause to determine whether or not it has been properly applied to the solicitation. There is the possibility of clauses being applied in the wrong circumstances. For instance, FAR clause 19.308[10] states:

(a) (1) Insert the provision at 52.219-1, Small Business Program Representations, in solicitations exceeding the micro-purchase threshold when the contract will be performed in the United States or its outlying areas.

If the solicitation were for work to be performed in an area that were outside of the United States and the outlying areas, a dialogue should begin with the agency to review and determine whether or not the clause has been properly inserted into the solicitation. The offeror needs to take care in addressing the situation ensuring that the agency understands that it is a point of discussion and not construed as taking exception to a clause. In certain circumstances taking exception to clauses may be expressly prohibited in the solicitation.[11] For example:

> Your offer must communicate your unconditional assent to the terms and conditions in this RFP, including any attachments and documents incorporated by reference. Our acceptance of your offer will create a binding contract between us. Your failure or refusal to assent to any of the terms and conditions of this RFP or your imposition of additional conditions or any material omission in your offer, may constitute a deficiency which will make your offer unacceptable to us.

Remaining silent on the issue is not advised. Once an award has been made, the agency does not have an obligation to the offeror to address the issue. The offeror is now required to abide by the conditions agreed upon in the award document.

If the clause has been applied appropriately, the offeror would move forward with the evaluation process. Offerors intending to represent that the organization qualifies as one or more type of small business must be able to meet one or more of the criteria to qualify as a small business entity.

Falsely representing or certifying an organization can lead to serious ramifications. Most representations and certifications list the penalties that can be imposed should an organization and/or an individual misrepresent their qualifications and/or standing. The penalties can be applied to individuals and/or the institution and can include jail, debarment, and suspension. For example, in clause 52.219, Small Business Program Representations, Section (d) Notice, Item (2) cites 15 U.S.C. 645(d).[12] 15 U.S.C. Section 645 is entitled, "Offenses and Penalties. This section of the US Code describes (see below) in detail the different offenses that can be considered, as well as the penalties that may occur:

-Cite-
> *15* USC Sec. 645
> -EXPCITE-
> TITLE *15* - COMMERCE AND TRADE
> CHAPTER 14A - AID TO SMALL BUSINESS
> -HEAD-
> Sec. 645. Offenses and penalties
> -STATUTE-
> (a) False statements; overvaluation of securities
>> Whoever makes any statement knowing it to be false, or whoever willfully overvalues any security, for the purpose of obtaining for himself or for any applicant any loan, or extension thereof by renewal, deferment of action, or otherwise, or the acceptance, release, or substitution of security therefore, or for the purpose of influencing in any way the action of the Administration, or for the purpose of obtaining money, property, or anything of value, under this chapter, shall be punished by a fine of not more than $5,000 or by imprisonment for not more than two years, or both.
> (b) Embezzlement, etc.
>> Whoever, being connected in any capacity with the Administration, (1) embezzles, abstracts, purloins, or willfully misapplies any moneys, funds, securities, or other things of value, whether belonging to it or pledged or otherwise entrusted to it, or (2) with intent to defraud the Administration or any other body politic or corporate, or any individual, or to deceive any officer, auditor, or examiner of the Administration, makes any false entry in any book, report, or statement of or to the Administration, or, without being duly authorized, draws any order or issues, puts forth, or assigns any note, debenture, bond, or other obligation, or draft, bill of exchange, mortgage, judgment, or decree thereof, or (3) with intent to defraud participates or shares in or receives directly or indirectly any money, profit, property, or benefit through any transaction, loan, commission, contract, or any other act of the Administration, or (4) gives any unauthorized information concerning any future action or plan of the Administration which might affect the value of securities, or, having such knowledge, invests or speculates, directly or indirectly, in the securities or property of any company or corporation receiving loans or other assistance from the Administration, shall be punished by a fine of not more than $10,000 or by imprisonment for not more than five years, or both.
> (c) Concealment, etc.
>> Whoever, with intent to defraud, knowingly conceals, removes, disposes of, or converts to his own use or to that of another, any property mortgaged or pledged to, or held by, the Administration, shall be fined not more than $5,000 or imprisoned not more than five years, or both; but if the value of such property does not exceed $100, he shall

be fined not more than $1,000 or imprisoned not more than one year, or both.

(d) Misrepresentation, etc.

(1) Whoever misrepresents the status of any concern or person as "small business concern," "qualified HUBZone small business concern," "small business concern owned and controlled by socially and economically disadvantaged individuals," or "small business concern owned and controlled by women," in order to obtain for oneself or another a–y -

(A) prime contract to be awarded pursuant to section 638, 644, or 657a of this title;

(B) subcontract to be awarded pursuant to section 637(a) of this title;

(C) subcontract that is to be included as part or all of a goal contained in a subcontracting plan required pursuant to section 637(d) of this title; or

(D) prime or subcontract to be awarded as a result, or in furtherance, of any other provision of Federal law that specifically references section 637(d) of this title for a definition of program eligibility, shall be subject to the penalties and remedies described in paragraph (2).

(2) Any person who violates paragraph (1) shall-

(A) be punished by a fine of not more than $500,000 or by imprisonment for not more than 10 years, or both;

(B) be subject to the administrative remedies prescribed by the Program Fraud Civil Remedies Act of 1986 (31 *U.S.C.* 3801-3812);

(C) be subject to suspension and debarment as specified in subpart 9.4 of title 48, Code of Federal Regulations (or any successor regulation) on the basis that such misrepresentation indicates a lack of business integrity that seriously and directly affects the present responsibility to perform any contract awarded by the Federal Government or a subcontract under such a contract; and

(D) be ineligible for participation in any program or activity conducted under the authority of this chapter or the Small

Business Investment Act of 1958 (*15 U.S.C.* 661 et seq.) for a period not to exceed 3 years.

(E) Representations under subsection (d) of this section to be in writing

Any representation of the status of any concern or person as a "small business concern", a "HUBZone small business concern", a "small business concern owned and controlled by socially and economically disadvantaged individuals," or a "small business concern owned and controlled by women" in order to obtain any prime contract or subcontract enumerated in subsection (d) of this section shall be in writing.

(F) Misrepresentation of compliance with section 636(j)(10)(I)

Whoever falsely certifies past compliance with the requirements of section 636(j)(10)(I) of this title shall be subject to the penalties prescribed in subsection (d) of this section.

Source

(Pub. L. 85-536, Sec. 2(16), July 18, 1958, 72 Stat. 395; Pub. L. 88-264, Sec. 2, Feb. 5, 1964, 78 Stat. 8; Pub. L. 99-272, title XVIII, Sec. 18009, Apr. 7, 1986, 100 Stat. 368; Pub. L. 100-656, title IV, Sec. 405, Nov. *15*, 1988, 102 Stat. 3875; Pub. L. 103-355, title VII, Sec. 7106(c), Oct. 13, 1994, 108 Stat. 3376; Pub. L. 105-85, div. A, title X, Sec. 1073(g)(4), Nov. 18, 1997, 111 Stat. 1906; Pub. L. 105-135, title VI, Sec. 603(c), Dec. 2, 1997, 111 Stat. 2632.)

References in Text

The Program Fraud Civil Remedies Act of 1986 (31 *U.S.C.* 3801-3812), referred to in subsec. (d)(2)(B), is subtitle B of title VI of Pub. L. 99-509, Oct. 21, 1986, 100 Stat. 1934, as amended, which is classified generally to chapter 38 (Sec. 3801 et seq.) of Title 31, Money and Finance. For complete classification of this Act to the Code, see Short Title note set out under section 3801 of Title 31 and Tables.

The Small Business Investment Act of 1958, referred to in subsec. (d)(2)(D), is Pub. L. 85-699, Aug. 21, 1958, 72 Stat. 689, as amended, which is classified principally to chapter 14B (Sec. 661 et seq.) of this title. For complete classification of this Act to the Code, see Short Title note set out under section 661 of this title and Tables.

Prior Provisions

Prior similar provisions were contained in section 209 of act July 30, 1953, ch. 282, title II, 67 Stat. 237, which was previously classified to section 638 of this title. The provisions of section 216 of act July 30, 1953, formerly classified to this section, were transferred to section 2(8) of Pub. L. 85-536, which was classified to section 637(c) of this title prior to repeal by Pub. L. 102-191. See section 656 of this title.

Amendments

1997 - Subsec. (d)(1). Pub. L. 105-135, Sec. 603(c)(1)(A), inserted ", a 'qualified HUBZone small business concern'," after " 'small business concern',".

Pub. L. 105-85 substituted "concern owned and controlled by women" for "concerns owned and controlled by women".

Subsec. (d)(1)(A). Pub. L. 105-135, Sec. 603(c)(1)(B), substituted "section 638, 644, or 657a" for "section 638 or 644".

Subsec. (e). Pub. L. 105-135, Sec. 603(c)(2), inserted ", a 'HUBZone small business concern'," after " 'small business concern',".

Pub. L. 105-85 substituted "concern owned and controlled by women" for "concerns owned and controlled by women".

1994 - Subsec. (d)(1). Pub. L. 103-355, Sec. 7106(c)(1), substituted ", a 'small business concern owned and controlled by socially and economically disadvantaged individuals', or a 'small business concerns owned and controlled by women' " for "or 'small business concern owned and controlled by socially and economically disadvantaged individuals' ".

Subsec. (e). Pub. L. 103-355, Sec. 7106(c)(2), substituted ", a 'small business concern owned and controlled by socially and economically disadvantaged individuals', or a 'small business concerns owned and controlled by women' " for "or 'small business concern owned and controlled by socially and economically disadvantaged individuals' ".

1988 - Subsec. (d). Pub. L. 100-656, Sec. 405(a), amended subsec. (d) generally, designating existing provisions as par. (1), redesignating former pars. (1) to (4) as subpars. (A) to (D), respectively, and in subpar. (D), substituting "subject to the penalties and remedies described in paragraph (2)" for "punished by a fine of not more than $50,000 or by imprisonment for not more than five years, or both", and adding par. (2).

Subsec. (f). Pub. L. 100-656, Sec. 405(b), added subsec. (f).

1986 - Subsecs. (d), (e). Pub. L. 99-272 added subsecs. (d) and (e).

1964 - Subsec. (c). Pub. L. 88-264 added subsec. (c).

Effective Date of 1997 Amendment

Amendment by Pub. L. 105-135 effective Oct. 1, 1997, see section 3 of Pub. L. 105-135, set out as a note under section 631 of this title.

Effective Date of 1994 Amendment

For effective date and applicability of amendment by Pub. L. 103-355, see section 10001 of Pub. L. 103-355, set out as a note under section 251 of Title 41, Public Contracts.

Section Referred to in Other Sections

This section is referred to in sections 636, 637, 657a, 687 of this title; title 12 section 1833a.

While representations and certifications are not the most exciting aspect of research administration, it is important to take the time and effort to ensure that all of the responses are accurate. The initial evaluation process for each of the representations or certifications should be performed with diligence to ensure the individual and/or the organization have met the qualifications of the article. Future application and award processes can be accomplished in a more expeditious manner with a review of each representation and certification to ensure that the clause has not changed from the previously accepted format, while fully reviewing all new representations and certifications not previously presented. Once the initial evaluation process has been completed, resource documentation should be compiled and kept on file for future use.

• • • References

1. U.S. Department of Health and Human Services, Public Health Service, Grant Application PHS 398 (revised September, 2004), Part III.

2. Space and Naval Warfare Systems Center, "Solicitation and Offer—Negotiated Acquisition, N66001-03-R-0004," *Theoretical Analysis, Exploratory Studies and Technical Services* (March 3, 2003): 36–47. Washington, DC.

3. Federal Acquisition Regulations, http://www. arnet.gov/far/ (accessed November 4, 2004).

4. Federal Acquisition Regulations, "Part 52—Solicitation Provisions and Contract Clauses," http://www.arnet.gov/far/current/html/FARTOCP52.html#wp340130 (accessed August 4, 2005).

5. Defense Federal Acquisition Regulations Supplement, Revision 20041101, "Subpart 252.1—Instructions for Using Provisions and Clauses," http://www.acq.osd.mil/dpap/dfars/html/current/252_1.htm (accessed November 1, 2004).

6. Office of the Under Secretary of Defense for Acquisition Technology and Logistics, Defense Procurement and Acquisition Policy, http://www.acq.osd.mil/dpap/dfars/index.htm (accessed November 1, 2004).

7. Space and Naval Warfare Systems Center, 37.

8. Federal Acquisition Regulations, "Part 52.219-1, Small Business Program Representations," http://www.arnet.gov/far/current/html/52_217_221.html#wp1135900 (accessed August 4, 2005).

9. Federal Acquisition Regulation, "Subpart 19.3—Determination of Small Business Status for Small Business Programs," http://www.arnet.gov/far/current/html/Subpart%2019_3.html#wp1099293 (accessed August 4, 2005).

10. Ibid.

11. Space and Naval Warfare Systems Center, 50.

12. Office of the Law Revision Counsel, U.S. House of Representatives, 15 USC Sec. 645, http://uscode.house.gov/uscode-cgi/fastweb.exe?getdoc+uscview+t13t16+1195+21++%2815%20U.S. (accessed January 6, 2003).

28

Elements of a Successful Proposal

Victoria J. Molfese, PhD, and Karen S. Karp, MS, DEd

Introduction

Proposal writers and research administrators share a common bond: both are invested in obtaining grant funding. Increasingly, it seems that performance evaluation of proposal writers (faculty, scientists, physicians, administrative professional staff, as well as research administrators) includes the measure of writers' success in obtaining grant funding. Therefore, information about how to improve proposals is greatly important to many. The purpose of this chapter is to identify the elements of successful proposals; to describe the proposal reviewing process; to consider proposal writing from the perspective of the reviewer; and to describe all of this information so that it can be effectively used during proposal writing. The ultimate success of a proposal after its acceptance occurs when funding is allocated. Proposals must be submitted to suitable funding agencies, and proposals must be written so that the goal of the project is clearly communicated to the reviewers. Success of a proposal often hinges on avoiding common mistakes.

Identifying and Understanding Funding Sources

There are many sources of grant funds available for a variety of different activities including big and small biomedical research, education and training activities, arts and humanities projects, sabbatical leaves and travel activities, and conferences and career development experiences. Funding for all of these activities is subsumed under the rubric of "grant." There are many different types of funding agencies and these agencies fund a variety of project activities. Some agencies, such as the National Institutes of Health (NIH), have funding programs (called "mechanisms") for research, training, career development, and conference activities on topics relevant to biomedical sciences. Other agencies have more narrowly defined funding programs. For example, the US Department of Education funds projects on a variety of topics related to education (e.g., grants for academic improvement, distance education, student learning, and technical assistance). The National Science Foundation (NSF) funds research and education projects in mathematics, science, and engineering, with many grants for basic science research. The Sloan Foundation provides funding for projects in science and technology, standards of living and economic performance, selected national issues, and civic programs. It is critical that the agency, funding program, and project all be aligned so that proposals are not submitted to agencies or funding programs that are not suited to the purpose of the funding agency. It is unlikely that misaligned proposals will be funded, and these often will not even be reviewed.

The easiest way to get information on funding agencies is from their Web sites. These Web sites (see Table 28-1 for examples), as well as other sites accessible through general search engines, contain information on funding programs and often include the actual forms needed to apply for grant funds. Additional information, including tips on proposal

TABLE 28-1	Web Sites for Selected Funding Agencies	
Agency	**Web Address**	**Types of Information**
US Department of Education	www.ed.gov/index.jsp Look for "Grants and Contracts"	- Overview - Finding & Applying - Awards, Accounts & Reporting
National Institutes of Health	www.Grants.NIH.gov/grants/oer.htm Look for "Grants Policy"	- Funding Opportunities - Grants Policy & Guidance - Forms & Applications
National Science Foundation	www.nsf.gov/funding/research-edu_ community.jsp	- Overview of Grants & Awards - What's New - Funding Opportunities - Proposal Preparation
The Alfred P. Sloan Foundation	www.sloan.org/grant/index.shtml Look for "How To Apply For A Grant"	- General information on types of grants & application process

preparation, is often available through the search option at specific sites. For example, the NIH offers "Answers to Frequently Asked Questions About Grants," an eight-page guide on proposal preparation. The US Department of Education has a Web site titled, "What Should I Know About ED Grants?"[1] The NSF has a link covering a variety of topics that are important for grant writing (though the link is misleadingly identified as related to Behavioral and Cognitive Sciences).[2] Further, there are books and Web sites specifically written about proposal writing. Indeed, one search engine found 239,000 links to Web sites in response to the key words "proposal writing tips." Information on these books can be accessed at booksellers' Web sites and by using the popular search engines. Journal articles can also be found dealing with proposal writing (for example, Molfese, Karp, & Siegel, 2002).

Contacting the funding agency directly is also a good approach, although some agencies (especially private agencies) do not allow direct contact. For agencies that are directly accessible (i.e., most publicly funded agencies), contact information is contained on the agency Web sites. While proposal writers are sometimes reluctant to contact agencies, it is a good strategy to call the person in charge of the specific funding program (often called the "program officer") and talk about the project. Such a phone call requires some preparation but here are some ideas:

[1] www.ed.gov/pubs/KnowAbtGrants/. Note: This link was developed in 1998, but is still active at the time this chapter was written.

[2] http://www.nsf.gov/sbe/bcs/ling/gdlns2.htm.

1. Check on the recent awards given by the funding agency. What are they funding and how large are most grants? This information is important to determine if the project topic is one that the funding agency might be interested in and whether the funds needed for such a project are in the ballpark of what the funding agency normally provides.

2. During the telephone call, talk about the project. It helps to have a concept paper, or a one- to three-page draft, already prepared with essential information about the goals of the project, the approach to be taken, and the scope and importance of the project (e.g., number of years needed to complete the project, approximate level of funds needed, the knowledge gap that the proposal will address, etc.). The development of a concept paper helps to formulate ideas and helps to keep the key points in mind during a brief presentation.

3. If the agency asks for information to be sent, it is important to immediately follow through by sending the requested information since the telephone call is intended to build a working relationship with the program officer.

4. If there seems to be disinterest or an indifference to the proposal topic or approach, the program officer can be asked to recommend another possible agency or funding source where the topic or approach might work. Most program officers try hard to be helpful, and many program officers are networked with colleagues at other agencies.

There are commonalities across funding programs within and across agencies:

- All funding programs require some sort of application or proposal.

- All funding programs have at least some information detailing what the application must include, how many pages the application can contain, and who is eligible to apply.
- All funding agencies use a review process for the applications. This review may be carried out by a large or small group of people, but often multiple readers are involved in the review.

These three common areas comprise the nuts and bolts of the proposal application process. Understanding these three areas is critical to proposal success.

The Application Procedure

Regardless of where information on funding programs is obtained, there is always specific information included on the purpose of the programs. Understanding the purpose of the funding program and determining if the project is a match for that purpose is of key importance. For example, the purpose of the program may be to create a new program of research that combines two areas of study. Therefore, the proposal must entail research that combines at least two areas of study. Efforts to force a fit between a project that may involve research within one area of study and a program that clearly expects two areas of study will not be successful. Successful proposals include not only activities that align with the purpose of the program but that also fit with an agency's high priority funding areas. If the agency is the US Department of Education, for example, proposing research that has nothing to do with educational practices will not be successful. Information about an agency's priority areas for funding can be derived from the title of the projects they have funded in the past. These titles often are contained in agency annual reports or on Web sites, Information about an agency's priority areas can also be found in the agency's mission statement. It is important to keep current on agency priorities because agencies sometimes change their priorities.

Funding agencies typically have information in hard-copy and/or electronic format on what forms and documentation are needed for a complete application. It is important to follow the directions provided by the funding agency and to provide complete documentation. Some agencies are flexible in their requirements and provide only general guidelines, such as requiring a cover letter, a brief description of the project, and a budget for the project. Other agencies are very strict about every aspect of the proposal from the font, text size, and line spacing used, to specific page limits for each section of the proposal, to the specification of each form needed and which forms need specific signatures from the applicant organization. For the proposal to be accepted by the agency and reviewed, it must be complete, mailed to the correct agency address, and received by the due date.

The Application or Proposal

At the heart of the proposal is the text that details the project's purpose and activities. Most funding agencies provide detailed information on the different sections of the proposal that are needed, such as an abstract, literature review, project design, project personnel, and budget narrative. It is important to use section headers with the agency's labels (e.g., "Project Narrative") so that it is clear that each section is included and to make it easier for the agency and proposal reviewers to find each section. It is common for proposal reviews to be linked to specific proposal sections. Reviewers are looking for certain key sections or proposal elements either because they are going to have to write a review that critiques those sections because these are key pieces of the proposal that they have been told to keep an eye out for, or because they are using a rubric with these headings. For example, the reviewers may be evaluating the proposal for "Significance: importance of the addressed problem, contribution of project to solution of the problem." Including a section labeled "Significance" and providing information about the significance of the project within that section will facilitate the reviewers' search for this key information.

Accurate references to sections of the text and to figures and tables within the text are important. Page numbers can facilitate the ease of finding key information in the proposal. Care must be taken so that references in the text to information in the proposal are actually located on that page or within that section. Sometimes proposal writers submit disorganized proposals with misdirected page references and missing tables, figures, and literature citations. Such "misdirections" in the text can result from the multiple revisions that most proposals undergo during the writing process. However, disorganized proposals do not help a proposal's chances of a positive review and a good funding score.

Because most agencies limit the number of pages that the proposal narrative can contain, it is important to maximize how each page is used by clearly and consistently presenting information, avoiding redundancy and the inconsistent use of terminology, and carefully using supporting materials (tables, figures, or charts) and references to enhance critical information. The goal is to keep the reader interested and focused on the underlying reasoning behind the project, and to enable the reader to follow the logic and rationale of the entire project.

Finally, it is important to choose the proposal title so that it conveys accurate information about the project. The title is important. It should establish in the reader's mind what the project is about. To do so, the title should include the most important or key descriptors for the project (e.g., who the participants are, or what leading-edge technology is involved, or what intervention program will be used). Efforts to craft words around an acronym or around a catchy phrase, or using only the name of the funding program (e.g., "Small Instrumentation Grant") do not make the title work to enhance the understanding of the project. Some agencies have a limit on the number of characters (letters and punctuation) the title can contain, so it is important to choose the words for the title carefully. Because agencies publicly list the projects they fund by title, it is important to think about how the project title will reflect on the project personnel and the institution(s). A "cute" project title may not seem cute if it appears on a national or hometown newspaper's front page.

The Abstract: Idea in a Nutshell

The central idea of the proposal must connect with the agency and the reviewers. The proposal must present a new idea, approach, method, or tool, or must address a critical issue that has not been studied (or adequately studied) in the past. There must be a reason why the agency and the reviewers should care enough about this project to fund it. The abstract is the introduction to the proposal, and it needs to be free of jargon or acronyms, since those, if used, should be defined or explained in the proposal text, and the abstract needs to convey the specific goals of the project within the space limitation allotted for the abstract. It is important to include information on why the project is important, how the project findings are expected to fit into the existing body of knowledge already accumulated in the field, and what the project activities will entail. Hypotheses, research questions, project

aims, or the issues to be resolved if the project is conducted as proposed should be clearly stated in the abstract.

It is not unusual for agencies to use a review process for proposals where some reviewers are given primary responsibility for the review of a group of proposals, including writing critiques of those proposals, and other reviewers are not required to read that group's proposals in their entirety. Indeed, these reviewers may only read the abstract of the proposals for which they do not have primary responsibility and listen to the discussion of those proposals by the primary reviewers. Therefore, it is important that the abstract be written so that reviewers who may score the proposal but who may have not read the entire proposal have the information they need on which to base their scoring. The abstract is the hook that can draw reviewers' attention favorably to the proposal.

The Literature Review

Every proposal should fit into a context of work already done on the topic and, for most proposals, there is a published literature base. A thorough but focused literature review is important to establish the importance and novelty of the project as well to establish that the author is knowledgeable about the topic. The works of other people in the field, as well as the author's relevant work, are important to describe and to critique in the literature review so that key ideas, findings, and approaches to the topic are established. Controversies as well as alternative or conflicting hypotheses should be included in the literature review section along with the approach to be taken by the project to establish that a breadth of information has been considered in planning the project. Incomplete or limited literature reviews may result in a project that is not current with the field, or that does not include key components found by other researchers to influence projects such as the one proposed. It is unusual for there to be nothing published on a particular topic, and contentions of proposal writers that there is "no published literature" are red flags to readers to prove otherwise. With the ready availability of search engines linked to book, chapter, and journal publications, it is likely that reviewers will search for literature on the topic, especially when the proposal writer contends there is nothing published on the topic.

Reviewers of the proposal are often experts in a field relevant to the project and they are looking for certain key publications to be cited (or for their own work to be cited). These reviewers may be particularly critical of a proposal that has an incomplete literature review because this could be interpreted as reflecting the author's lack of knowledge or expertise.

The literature review must also be written so that this review section leads up to the design of the project in a step-by-step logical progression. Therefore, the literature review must include information about what is known in the field, what needs to be known, and what the best approach is for bridging the gap between what is known and what needs to be known. Good literature reviews convince the reader that the proposed project will move the state of the art in the field forward.

Project Design: The Most Critical Section

Reviewers often single out the quality of the project design as the main reason a proposal makes or misses the funding cut. Many proposal writers focus on the literature review, and some writers appear to attend less to the many details needed for a high quality project design. The design must fit the project goals and be methodologically sound; that is, the project can be executed as described to achieve the project goals. Regardless of the type of project, the methods and techniques to be used, the procedures for evaluating the project's goals, hypotheses or research questions, and the time line for completing the project must be carefully described and logical. The reviewers are often experts in project design, and they can be counted upon to spend much of their reviewing time examining the project's design. It is critical, therefore, that the reviewers be convinced that the project design will work and all the important details about the project are included in the proposal.

Because the project design is so important, proposal writers need to get all the help they can in writing this section. Proposal writers should consider having their proposals reviewed by colleagues or, when relevant, by having local compliance committees review the proposal before it is submitted. By submitting the proposal to colleagues or a committee such as the Human Studies Committee, proposal writers can get helpful information on how the project might be "debugged" as well as how the methods can be clarified. The feedback may be

helpful in identifying a fatal flaw that makes the project impossible to execute as proposed. For example, an experimental approach that the local Institutional Review Board (IRB) finds unacceptable is likely to be noted as problematic by agency reviewers, as well. Changing the proposal to include an approach that is acceptable to the local IRB can result in a proposal that is more successful during the agency review and easier to obtain IRB approval when the project is funded. There are also frequent changes in compliance regulations, and asking the relevant compliance committee to review the proposal may help to make sure that the proposed plan is in line with current regulations.

Complete information on each of the key sections of the project design (i.e., participants, measures, procedures, and analyses) is very important. For example, the participants in the project must be completely described. Information on why those particular individuals are the participants must be included along with descriptions of the key characteristics of the participants and the process used to protect the participants if the project entails research activities. Proposals also need to make clear what the participants will be doing, how much of their time will be needed, and whether or how they will be compensated. Any anticipated problems related to the participants also should be considered, for example:

- *What happens if not all participants complete the project?*
- *What if sufficient numbers of participants with key characteristics cannot be recruited?*

Information on the data (or "evidence") to be gathered to evaluate the hypotheses, research questions, or project goals is important since these data play a critical role in the evaluation of the project's success. Therefore, information on the measures to be used to obtain the data is important. The measures selected need to be valid (that is, well grounded and measuring what they are intended to measure) and reliable (that is, producing the same results repeatedly). Because there are measurement standards in every discipline, it is important to select measures that meet those standards. Proposals to develop a new measure often are met with skepticism by reviewers because the development process can be complicated and lengthy, and the validity and reliability of such measures can be uncertain. If the project rests on a measure that will need to be developed, the potential jeopardy to the project's success must be carefully considered and explained as must the need for the new measure. Ideally, an established measure can be used along with a newly developed measure so that if one measure is not successful the other measure can be used. Proposing a measure that is not yet developed and for which there are no data to establish even preliminary validity and reliability is not a good strategy.

If the project includes the use of a complex or leading-edge technique or measure, it may be critical for the proposal to substantiate that the PI (or one of the key project personnel) is knowledgeable about and expert in the use of the technique or measure. It is not likely that reviewers will simply trust that because the technique or measure is included the project personnel will be able to use it. Along with substantiating the expertise of key personnel in the use of a technique or measurement approach, it is also critical to justify the essential role the technique or measure plays in the project design. Sometimes an expensive and popular approach is proposed in an effort to enhance the appeal of the project to the funding agency. But such an approach may not be the best choice for the project. While it is true that reviewers often are looking for leading edge approaches to topics, reviewers may also worry about the leading edge approach not working as proposed or not yielding valid or reliable outcomes. If the proposal does not work out as planned, then what? A good strategy may be an approach in which the leading edge approach is combined with a more standard approach so that there is a fall-back position. If the technique or measure relies on large equipment (such as an MRI or a scanning electron microscope), it is critical to establish through letters of support or in "resources and environment" statements that the equipment essential to the project is available for use by the PI if the project is funded.

Finally, the use that will be made of the data also must be described. For research projects, the quantitative or qualitative analyses to be applied to the data must be included along with an explanation about why these analyses are the best choice for addressing the research questions or hypotheses under study. How the data will be examined to test the hypotheses or research questions must be made clear. In many disciplines, standards, or traditions, "best approaches" have been established for data treatment. For example, most research studies proposed to the National Institutes of Health are expected to include power analyses to establish that a sufficient number of participants are proposed in the project design so that analyses will have sufficient data to test for experimental effects. It is

important to know about and include these disciplinary standards. Often, it is also helpful to obtain help from statisticians or methodologists, or to include a statistician or methodologist as a consultant on the project, so that the statistical methods most appropriate for testing the hypotheses or research questions are used and can be actually executed as proposed.

Special Issues

There are special, sometimes unique, issues that accompany most projects. These special issues can raise red flags about the proposed work, for example:

- How demographic characteristics of personnel implementing the project might affect the recruitment of or interaction with participants;
- How the training and supervision of the project personnel will be accomplished, especially if team members are located at multiple sites;
- How random assignment of participants to classrooms or schools (i.e., "conditions") will be justified and acceptable to parents and teachers in a way that will enable them to participate;
- How project consultants are selected and what project-related qualifications they must have;
- How ethical issues of risks versus benefits of a procedure can be determined and justified.

The limitations and benefits of a project are also special issues to consider. These issues vary depending on the project, but both limitations and benefits need to be addressed. An awareness of the limitations of the project is important:

- *What are the possible barriers to the success of the project?*
- *What will be done to overcome these barriers?*

The expected benefits of the project should be stated explicitly, as well. These benefits should be linked to the project goals and the funding program's purpose so that it is clear that this is the project that will contribute important information to the knowledge base that is intended to benefit from this funding program.

Many agencies want to know how the results of the project will be disseminated. The agencies want "bang for their bucks." It is critical that the results of the project be disseminated to those who can benefit from the work, such as other researchers or scholars, teachers, policy makers, families, and children. Dissemination can include publications, presentations at professional meetings, public lectures and workshops to interest groups, and articles in popular media. The strategy to be used for dissemination needs to be described and appropriate to the project and agency. Some agencies specifically require that a dissemination plan be included in the text of the proposal, but other agencies are less directive. It is a good idea, regardless of the agency, to describe, even briefly, what the plans are for dissemination of information. Such a plan can be included as part of the project time line to reflect what and when dissemination activities will take place.

In every field and specialty area there are acronyms. Some of acronyms are well known (e.g., APA, the American Psychological Association; NIH, National Institutes of Health) but other acronyms may be less well known or are used to identify more than one referent (e.g., SRA is used by Society of Research Administrators International and by other organizations, such as the Society for Risk Analysis). It is critical that acronyms be defined the first time they are used in the text so that the reader can learn what they stand for, and that the text not be heavily laden with acronyms because these can be hard for the reader to keep in mind. The task of proposal writing is to communicate, and often acronyms are less effective than words in communicating.

Appendices

It is tempting to use the appendices to include important information that does not fit into the text of the proposal without exceeding the page limitations. However, many funding agencies now limit the number of pages and/or what can be included in the appendices. Critical information on the design and analysis of the project must be included in the proposal text because this information is specifically "scored" in most proposal reviews and because reviewers are not under any obligation to read the appendices. Indeed, many reviewers are so focused on reading the proposal text carefully and writing detailed reviews that they do not have the time or do not take time to read through the appendices. Therefore, the appendices should be used strategically to provide information that amplifies information contained in the text should the reviewers be looking for additional information. Ideal materials to include in the appendix vary according to the type of project being proposed but can include:

- Copies of relevant manuscripts by the author(s) that are accepted for publication, but which have not yet appeared in print;
- Details about new editions of measurement instruments or new instruments to be used in

the project with which the reviewers might be unfamiliar, and;
- Letters of support and cooperation from consultants and organizations indicating an intention to participate in the project.

Personnel

The success of the project depends on the personnel. Just as it is important to make clear that the proposed project will make a significant contribution to the field by solving an important problem, it is also important that the reviewers have information about the expertise of project personnel and why these personnel are the best qualified to do the work. Descriptions of the roles and responsibilities for each key staff, along with vitae to substantiate the qualifications and accomplishments for the project roles, are essential. Having unnamed (or TBA) positions for key staff roles is not a good idea because the success of the project may rely on someone who has not been recruited to the team. Reviewers should have information on who will participate in the project, and they must be convinced that the project personnel have the expertise to do the project. The best way to convince reviewers that project personnel can do the project is by providing evidence in their biographical sketches or vitae documenting their previous success(es) in a similar role.

Evidence to substantiate personnel qualifications and accomplishments can come in many forms. The most common way is through vitae with publication history or previous grant success. Publications history counts a great deal to reviewers and agencies who are trying to determine if they trust the personnel to be able to do the project as proposed. The project goals and design must relate to what the named personnel have done in the past. Both published and "in press" articles, chapters, and books as well as other peer-reviewed accomplishments are viewed as valid evidence if these directly relate to the proposed project and relate to the specific roles that personnel will perform on the project. The number of publications needed to support an application depends on the quality of the publications, where the publications appear, and the quality of the work published. For example, longitudinal studies of participants over several years, studies of participants with a rare disorder, or the use of a procedure that requires a great amount of processing time can take several years to yield a publication. Project personnel who have few publications may be able to show that publications they have are of a particularly high quality and reflect complicated methods or methods particularly relevant to those proposed in the application. Personnel with no publications to document their expertise may be able to show years of experience in the field, licensing, or other special credentials that establish their expertise. The most difficult case to make is for early-career project personnel who do not yet have much evidence of their research expertise or evidence of their abilities to function independently as project investigators. These "new investigators" may do best by applying for funding from programs set up for new investigators rather than trying to compete against investigators who have stronger qualifications.

The issue of teaming up or collaborating with others is important because many funding agencies encourage proposals for multi-disciplinary, multi-investigator projects. However, it is sometimes harder to work with other people than to work alone. Co-investigators or consultants should be included, however, if they are assets to the project and if the scope of work that can be included in the project is enhanced. There are very few single investigator projects that are complex and involve multiple work sites. It often "takes a village" to be able to get a project going. The contribution of each member of the team must be clearly described. Letters of support from personnel who will be involved in the project in which they describe their roles is important for documenting that these individuals are available and willing to participate in the project. In some proposals, the collaborators may not contribute much to the project, either because they have little or no time on the project or because their role is limited. With some experts, their time on a project is limited by necessity because they are consultants on several other projects. If the collaborator plays a key role on the project (e.g., executing statistical analyses or applying a specialized technique, or enabling access to participants) it is important to document how the amount of time devoted to the project is realistic and sufficient. Including people as personnel on a project for any reason other than those strictly related to project activities is not likely to get past the scrutiny of the agency and the reviewers.

Budget

The budget and its justification are as much a key part of the proposal as the text is in detailing the project's significance and design. The budget must have entries for all aspects of the project, from personnel (salaries, fringe benefits, and time commitments) to equipment, supplies, contractual services, and travel costs. Increasingly, reviewers are directed to examine actual budget numbers at only a superficial level, but budget justifications—that is, the text that explains budget costs—are still part of the documentation provided to reviewers by many funding agencies. Budgets and budget justifications should be realistic, including reasonable and expected costs for project activities and straightforward explanations. Costs that can be expected to come from the institution (e.g., routine office supplies and local phone calls as well as general secretarial support and other expenses that might be considered part of "Facilities and Administrative Costs") should not be included as costs the agency is asked to cover. However, costs for items that are critical and specific to project activities must be included. Reviewers often have knowledge of budgets from their own experiences with funded projects, and they use that frame of reference for considering project budgets during proposal reviews. Therefore, the reviewers look at budgets and/or budget justifications to determine if the project costs and type of costs are in line with their experiences and the budget items are central to project activities as proposed.

The amount of funds that is requested is an often debated aspect of proposal writing. Should writers ask for exactly what is needed for the project activities or should they try to develop a budget that is bare-bones in hopes that if a small amount of money is "left over" the project just might get a little bit of funding? Sometimes the bare-bones approach does work; other times, it is not worth thinking about if the bare-bones nature is such that the project's success is in jeopardy because key costs are not included. Similarly, inflating the budget on the belief that agencies always cut funds requested by projects is also not a good idea. Reviewers and agency personnel reviewing budgets can often detect when budgets are inflated. It also is important to think about the funding agency. What is a reasonable amount to ask for from the agency? What are the funding guidelines provided by the agency? Many agencies include in their program information about what the size of the average grant is expected to be. The size of the budget also depends on the complexity of the project, the length of the project, the types of personnel and equipment involved, and the costs of the other supports needed for the project. New investigators might be expected to propose less complex and, therefore, less

TABLE 28-2	Common Proposal Writing Problems and Possible Solutions	
Problem	**Descriptive Examples**	**Solution**
Budget Cost/Benefits are a Concern	The project total costs are high and number of participants is small, generalizability is uncertain, and some costs appear high (e.g., payments to participants).	Consider the cost per participant. Is the cost per participant to get the expected project outcomes reasonable? Is the budget justification convincing and reasonable/conservative?
Methods are Weak	Proposal includes measurement approaches that are undeveloped, or the PI has little experience using a technique, or "state of the art" instruments are hard to justify as the best approach for the work proposed.	The validity and reliability of the instruments must be specified and selections justified. Experts in techniques can be included if needed. Justify the "value added" of the methods selected to the work proposed.
Personnel is Unclear	Roles of investigators are clear, but other personnel may not have qualifications that are aligned with roles; percent time on the project for investigators is small/large.	Role and qualifications of personnel must be clearly documented, double-check time commitments and responsibilities, consider including only qualified people.
Proposal Guidelines are Ignored	The proposal submitted to NIH uses headings of "What do you intend to do?", "Why is the work important?", etc., rather than "Specific Aims", "Background and Significance", etc., creating redundancy across sections and uncertainty as to where key information is located.	Follow agency guidelines. Adhere to text headings and organization, page limits, and font size. Put creative elements in the text content, not the organizational style of the proposal.
Text is Difficult to Understand	The proposal includes unfamiliar acronyms, refers the reviewer to the Appendix for key details on the method, and uses specialized terms without definitions.	Proposal information must be clear to readers. Define terms, avoid acronyms, and include all critical information in the text.

expensive projects than more experienced investigators, and multi-site projects are generally more expensive than single-site projects. The budget must be appropriate to the proposed project. Reviewers and funding agencies are quick to note when budgets contain elements that are unrelated to the project (e.g., a massage therapist for a project that does not include massage therapy in the project design; trips for meetings with consultants that could be accomplished by teleconference), include colleagues as consultants who have no described role in the project, and show inflated costs for items such as computers or clinical or educational services when ball-park costs are well known.

Summary

Each section in the application or proposal narrative provides important information about the project. Understanding what information must be contained in each section is an important first element in writing a successful proposal. Understanding how to best present that information so that the writer's goal of obtaining funds to support an important project is clearly communicated to the reviewers also is critical. Proposal writers need the most help with this latter aspect of understanding proposal preparation. Table 28-2 contains examples of one approach that could be used by research administrators and others working with proposal writers in developing effective writing skills. Common problems encountered in proposal writing are identified, and other problems can be identified with the help of faculty and staff who have been successful in obtaining grant funding. The help of successful proposal writers in describing common proposal problems and the solutions they have used to overcome these problems can be used in working with other people who are seeking to improve their grant writing skills.

The Proposal Review

One of the accompanying "benefits" to receiving grant funds is being asked to review proposals for the funding agency providing the grant. And the opportunity to do a lot of work over a short period of time on top of all the other work grant-active people are already doing can be thought of as a benefit. Reviewing proposals is a benefit because the task is interesting, informative, and usually relevant to the reviewer's scholarly interests. However, the task is also time consuming and stressful because grant awards are of such vital importance to proposal writers, and the reviews reflect on the reviewer's scholarly expertise in the proposal topic area. Reviewers take the task seriously and spend a great deal of time in preparing their reviews. The types of people who are asked to be reviewers are hardworking, Type A, and caring individuals, although reviewers can also be malicious, vindictive, and self-serving. Thinking about the reviewers as individuals, however, can help the process of successful proposal writing. "Individualizing" the reviewers can be done by looking at the Web sites of the funding agency to learn who the members are of the review panels and study sections. Many agencies make this information public, although some federal agencies and most private funding agencies do not. Reviewing recent listings of who the recipients of grant funding from the agency are also will yield likely names of people who will be involved in proposal reviews. Knowing the names of people who are prominent in a field can also yield ideas about likely reviewers because experts in topic areas are often asked to be reviewers. Getting a general idea of who the reviewers of the proposal are likely to be provides a context for considering the reviewer's perspective. While it is not appropriate to contact reviewers for any purpose related to the proposal, either before or after the review takes place, it is helpful to consider the reviewer's perspective while writing the proposal.

Thinking about the possible composition of any particular review panel can influence how the proposal is prepared. For example, if mathematicians will be included on the review panel, the proposal should be written so that the word "math" is not used. "Math" is an abbreviation and it irritates mathematicians, so the word "mathematics" should be used throughout. The expertise of reviewers that is relevant to the proposal under review is a major reason why they were chosen as reviewers. Their work or their perspective should be considered (if appropriate) in writing the proposal because they may look for references to their work or for the proposal to address their theory, model, or findings. Finally, there may be differences of opinion between experts about theory, methods or approaches, and interpretations of findings. Knowing this, proposals should be written to consider these differences and to use evidence to justify the proposed approach rather than ignoring these differences. The reviewers may not change their opinions but at least they cannot fault the proposal for ignoring opposing views.

The Review Process

The specific process used to review proposals can vary from funding agency to funding agency and also can vary from one review session or from one funding program to another within funding agencies. However, the basic process is the same. Proposals are received by funding agencies and assigned to reviewers by linking proposal topics and approaches to the expertise of reviewers. Many funding agencies allow proposal writers to indicate in a cover letter or in conversation with the program officer or review administrator the names of possible reviewers with whom they have a personal or professional conflict, an unresolved difference of opinion, or some other reasonable basis for disqualification. If the proposal writer believes that certain potential reviewers should not review their proposal, it is worthwhile to make that belief known to the agency before the review. Similarly, reviewers also must indicate those proposals for which they may have a conflict of interest or any other real or perceived conflict that should disqualify them from the proposal's review. Once the proposals are assigned to reviewers, the process of formally reviewing the proposals begins.

Proposal reviews typically involve two phases: in the first phase reviewers read and write a critique of the proposal, and in the second phase reviewers orally present their review of the proposal during the proposal review meeting arranged by the funding agency. Most agencies provide a timeline (from several days to several weeks) for the first phase and a deadline at which the agency asks reviewers to provide electronic or hard copies of their written critiques. Some agencies also ask for preliminary scores on the proposals at the end of the first phase with the intention of determining if a triage process can be applied. Triage is intended to reduce the number of proposals actually discussed at review sessions; thus, only proposals whose preliminary scores are in the fundable range or are above some minimum score are discussed, and other proposals receive only written critiques.

The second phase involves a review session where reviewers meet face to face (or via a conference call) to discuss the proposals. In the discussion, the reviewers assigned to each proposal as primary, secondary, and sometimes tertiary or more reviewers, present a summary of the strengths and weaknesses of each proposal. In the case of more than two reviewers, the other reviewers often provide commentary about only specific aspects of the proposal, such as a specialized technique or intervention proposed for use. There are opportunities during the discussion for other reviewers to add information. The written reviews of each proposal are intended to convey both the reviewers' critiques and the discussion at the review session. The written reviews are sometimes amended to include additional information that the reviewers want to convey to the proposal writers arising from the discussion. It is advisable to talk with the program officer or his/her designate after the review session to ask for information on the discussion. Program officers usually attend the review sessions to gain information about each proposal submitted for their program. It is helpful to ask the program officer questions about the key strengths and weaknesses of the project, the enthusiasm of the reviewers for the project topic and approach, and what the preliminary scores are for the proposal. Final scores and the written reviews can take several months to be sent to the proposal writers, but even preliminary information is helpful feedback. The feedback can provide an indication of whether the proposal might be funded and whether the intention of the proposal (i.e., obtaining funds to support an important project) was successful.

All reviewers attending the review session as well as those who are participating via conference call provide scores for the proposals. The reviewers' scores are averaged to determine the final score for the proposal. It is not unusual for proposals to be unsuccessful (i.e., not funded) on their first submission. However, if the proposal is revised as suggested by the reviewers, a subsequent submission of the proposal should more likely be successful.

Who Shows Up Makes a Difference

For any given round of proposal submissions, whether the proposals are submitted in response to an agency's call for submissions, such as a Request for Proposals, or in response to standing application dates for the funding program, the reviewers can evaluate only those proposals that are received for review. In general, a proposal submitted during a review that has few other proposals submitted has a greater likelihood of success than a proposal in

competition with a large number of other proposals. While unsound proposals are unlikely to be funded regardless of the number of other proposals under consideration, proposals that are basically sound and address an important topic but which might be less competitive against a large pool of proposals may be funded if there are few other proposals in contention. Proposal writers sometimes agonize over what "the competition" is and whether to submit for a particular program. However, it is impossible to know exactly what the competition will be and whether a proposal will be funded. However, it is very clear that if the proposal is not submitted, it has no chance of being funded.

Aggravating the Reviewer

Just like everyone else, reviewers are busy people. On top of their every-day responsibilities, reviewers receive a pile of proposals to read and are required to produce written reviews for each proposal within a short period of time. Proposal writers can help the reviewers by submitting proposals that are carefully prepared, proofread, complete, and are clearly communicated. "Problem areas" cited by reviewers are discussed below.

Appearance Proposals should look professional with a consistent use of font type and size to make the text easier to read. While unusual, proposals have been submitted with a handwritten cover sheet and budget pages. These proposals do not look professional and influence the reviewers' initial impression of the proposals. Agencies and reviewers are familiar with attempts to fit as much information as possible into the limited number of pages allocated for the proposal text. Proposals that use small font sizes, narrow side margins and few paragraphs do not advantage the task of the reviewer because the text is hard to read. Use of figures and graphics that are confusing or not labeled or are too small to read easily are not helpful in conveying key information. In considering the appearance of a proposal, ask people to look at the proposal for "readability" (font type and size, layout of the text, use of figures and tables, labels and headings, etc.) so that the text is easy to read and information is presented clearly and effectively.

Reason and Logic The reviewer's job is more easily facilitated if there are no gaps and no inconsistencies in information. This means that the following information must be carefully included. All of the required or key sections of the proposal are included in the application and are easy to find using labels or lead-in sentences that contain key words. Important information is defined and described as well as backed up with references so that theories, hypotheses and research, questions and project aims, and the project design itself are grounded. The budget is realistic, linked to elements in the project design, and well justified. The proposal is submitted in complete form and adheres to limits on page length and contents. Page numbers, complete citations for all literature referenced in the text, and all attachments or figures and tables referenced in the text are included. Information provided throughout the proposal should be consistent across sections.

Datedness   The project proposed should be for new work that is designed to add to the knowledge base of the field. Reviewers are selected because they have expertise and are currently active in the field or topic area. Therefore, the proposal should include current references, leading-edge approaches, and up-to-date supporting materials (e.g., vitae, the assessment instruments selected, analysis approaches) that reflect a current project. Proposals containing only or mostly references that are a decade or older, assessment instruments that are not the most recently revised or re-normed versions, or statistical approaches that are simplistic compared to the statistics typically used in the field or topic area today are difficult to justify as "leading edge." Dusting off an old proposal and submitting it without updating or reworking it to fit with the funding program requirements and the state of the art in the field are not viewed positively by reviewers. Similarly, proposals that contain unsubstantiated statements or statements of belief without backing evidence or references are not likely to be viewed by experts as well grounded in the knowledge base of the field.

Summary

Reviewers play an important role in determining the success or failure of the proposal based on the merits of the proposal. It is important for proposal writers to consider the perspective of the reviewers so that the proposal is written to communicate to them. Making a list of common problems that create difficulties in reviewing the proposal or that often are identified by reviewers as fatal flaws is a useful tool that can lead to improvements in proposal writing. There are excellent sources of information on fatal flaws and errors in grant-writing that do not lead to grant-getting success (for example, Bailey, 1987; Barnett, 1995; Oetting, 1986).

Table 28-3 is an example of one approach that could be used when working with proposal writers on skill development that focuses on common reasons why some proposals receive lower scores during the review process.

We Did Not Get the Grant—Now What?

Proposal writers should not despair if the project is not approved for funding. In any round of proposal review, only a small percentage of proposals are actually funded. Many more proposals get scores from the reviewers that are not too far from a fundable score. Therefore, unfunded proposals should always be considered as a challenge rather than a defeat. The first step in dealing with an unfunded proposal is to ask the funding agency for the reviewers' comments. There are some agencies, especially private funding agencies, that do not provide feedback beyond general information on whether the proposal was funded or not. There also are some agencies that will only provide feedback if they are asked. Others automatically provide feedback. Regardless of the agency, it is important to get whatever comments are available and to seek as much information as possible by contacting the program officer or the funding agency. It is important to talk with the program officer about the proposal review. Sometimes what the reviewers intended as constructive or encouraging comments can be misinterpreted. For example, a professional organization submitted a proposal to a federal agency and the proposal got what the writers interpreted as a negative review. Based on the negative review, the organization decided not to resubmit the proposal. However, the funding agency called after the next deadline had passed asking, "Where is your proposal?" The writers said, "Well, we didn't resubmit it because we didn't think the comments about the proposal were very positive." The program officer said, "No, those comments were great and were intended to be constructive." Calling the program officer and clarifying the reviewers' comments might have been helpful in avoiding the misinterpretation.

Proposal writers also should work with research administrators or other people experienced in grant writing and grant reviewing to consider how to revise the proposal. These experienced readers should be asked to read the proposal and the reviews. It is natural for proposal writers to hide the reviews they receive because the writers may be focusing on the negative comments in the review

TABLE 28-3	Common Weaknesses Cited by Reviewers in Written Reviews and Possible Solutions	
Problem	**Description**	**Solution**
Methods and the hypotheses don't match.	The proposal hypotheses focus on changes in infancy but the methods and measures specify participation of school-age children and use assessments only useful for older children.	More careful proof reading is needed to make sure that the proposal is consistent throughout. Careful attention to methodological details in aligning participant ages with instruments selection is needed.
The research plan is too ambitious and complex.	Participants will be included in 20 hours of assessments, both qualitative and quantitative assessments are planned, and the data require multiple levels of coding.	The proposal may be overly ambitious. Reducing the scope of work and creating a time line to show the start and ending dates for each project element can help in considering time demands on participants, tasks, and analyses.
There is no backup or alternative approach.	The method includes the application of techniques that are untried or novel, and it is possible that the approach will not be successful.	The novel approach might be combined with another more standard approach. Using both approaches might still yield some results even if the novel approach is not completely successful.
There is insufficient information about data analyses and interpretation.	The hypotheses and statistics are listed in a table but there is no explanation.	More description should be provided on how the hypotheses are to be tested and what data are used in the tests, what statistics will be used and how.
There is no preliminary relevant data.	The proposal seems feasible but there is no evidence that the methods will yield the expected outcomes, that the PI can obtain results using the method, or that the participants can perform as expected.	Provide preliminary data, even if only for a few participants or with limited data, to show that the methods can work and that there is a need to scale up with a bigger project.

that sometimes are painful to read and disparaging of the project or the writer. However, proposal writers need help interpreting comments, determining the strengths relative to the weaknesses of the project, and thinking through how the weaknesses can be addressed so that those aspects of the proposal are strengthened. With all the work involved in preparing a proposal, writers should never give up on a proposal easily.

One rule of proposal success (and failures) appears to be that stoicism and teeth-gritting determinism can pay off. It helps to remember that a lot of the work in writing the proposal is already done and now the proposal writer has feedback about the project that can be used to his/her advantage. Some of the feedback that comes from the review process is useful and reasonable, but some feedback may be neither useful nor reasonable. Sometimes reviewers do not write good reviews, and sometimes they differ in their opinions on proposal strengths and weaknesses. It is not uncommon for reviews to pro-

vide mixed messages that arise sometimes due to the short time period allowed for proposal discussion during the review meeting. But the review feedback does provide guidance on what aspects of the proposal came to the attention of the reviewers to an extent sufficient for them to comment specifically on those aspects. The portions commented on must be changed in the proposal. Some agencies allow a "rebuttal" or "response to the previous review" to be included with a resubmitted revised proposal. In that section, proposal writers can indicate where and what changes were made in the proposal along with a rationale for changes made and not made. It is critical that very careful consideration be given to justifying not making changes as called for in the previous review. Proposals resubmitted that are essentially unchanged or only changed cosmetically do not usually fare any better during a second review than they did in the original review, due in part because the same reviewers are likely to be part of the second round of reviews and the likelihood that unaddressed weaknesses will be identified again during the second review.

Tips for Proposal Revisions

Listed below are some tips intended to be useful in revising proposals that were not successfully funded after an agency review. Proposal writing is like any skill: it is learned, it gets better with practice, and everyone can learn good writing skills.

Persistence   Practice and persistence are keys to successful proposal writing. Successful proposal writing is learned, and no one is successful all of the time. In proposal writing, it is helpful to the learning process to be a proposal reviewer even on panels for small grants. Seeing proposals written by other people and judging them against the review guidelines of a funding agency is informative and helps proposal writers to know what is present and what is missing in well and poorly written proposals. This information can be carried over into writing proposals in the future.

Additional Readers   It is helpful if additional readers are asked to review the revised proposal. These readers might be especially helpful in suggesting ways in which information can be added to strategic part(s) of the proposal or presented in ways that are more prominent. For example, critical information contained in the text might be represented in a table or a figure or highlighted in bold so that the information stands out. Or a figure or graph can be eliminated and described in the text using less space, thereby creating more room to add additional text containing critical additional information. Readers might be able to provide advice to the proposal writer about how important information is presented so that readers can interpret the information as intended. Sometimes on the review sheets reviewers will identify information that they claim is missing from the proposal, but proposal writers can point to the page and paragraph where that information is contained. In these cases, strategies for making that "overlooked" information more prominent are needed, and other readers might be helpful in determining how to make the information more readily apparent. Because over-use of bold and italicized font can be irritating or make text reading difficult, be cautious in using font to highlight critical information.

Make a List   Make a list of all the information identified by the reviewers as weaknesses, in the proposal and use this list as a focus in revising the proposal. Often the reviewers' comments are helpful in identifying methodological weaknesses, and the reviewers sometimes offer possible solutions. In some cases, the project is identified as too ambitious, and the proposal can be simplified. With each weakness listed, careful consideration should be given to how that weakness can be addressed so that the proposal, at least in the eyes of the reviewers, can be strengthened.

Using the Agency   Grant writers should consider contacting the program officer about the revisions planned for the proposal and share their ideas about modifications. Encouragement from the program officer about the planned revision can go a long way toward preparing a successful proposal. The program officer may also offer suggestions as to what might not be a useful revision or suggest other approaches to consider. Just like the comments from the reviewers, suggestions from program officers should be taken seriously.

We Got a Grant—Now What?

The majority of proposal writers spend a great deal of time and effort writing proposals that are not funded. When a proposal succeeds in getting funded, the grant writer may be unprepared for what to do. At a minimum, the grant writer needs to meet quickly with the appropriate research administrator at the organization to talk about the next steps. Often proposal budgets need to be revised and in the case of "Just in Time" agencies, compliance and final budget documentation need to be prepared and submitted to the funding agency. Research administrators are good at answering questions about what the next steps are and how to accomplish those steps. If the activities planned in the proposal have not yet undergone compliance review, those reviews will need to be completed and the project will need to be approved before grant funding can begin.

Other preparatory steps will also need to be set in motion, such as requesting a grant account, beginning the hiring procedures if staff will be hired on the grant, developing documents and materials or gathering assessment instrument, and notifying service providers that services will be needed. All of the goals and objectives that were described in detail in the project design will now need to be accomplished. While grants are awarded based on "best effort" policies and contracts are based on "deliverables," both types of funding mechanisms are fundamentally based on carrying out what was proposed in the application. Therefore, it is important in the proposal writing stage to think about whether what is proposed in the project design can actually be done by the project team and whether the team actually wants to conduct the project as proposed. Once a proposal is funded, the expectation of the funding agency is that the project will proceed as proposed and will yield the outcomes as described. Finally, it is also important at the beginning of the project to understand what types and frequency of reporting will be required by the agency and by the grantee institution. Knowing ahead of time what is needed will allow the necessary document to be obtained as the project proceeds.

Overall, it is important to do a good job on grant-funded work because the quality of the work and the accomplishments can influence future funding. If a grant is received and the project team does not follow through with what was proposed, or the project yields no or very few publications, the project team may find it difficult to obtain funding in the future. Reviewers and funding agencies look at accomplishments from previous grants in evaluating proposals to determine the impact of the project. There may also have been revisions to the project design suggested by the reviewers that are intended to enhance the outcomes of the project. Efforts to get continuation funding for a multi-year project or a competitive renewal of the project may be affected if revisions to the project design are not made by the project team when they execute the project. Reviewers have access to previous reviews of projects when reviewing resubmitted applications, so it is important to follow through with changes in project design recommended or requested by reviewers.

Conclusion

The road to proposal success—from its writing to acceptance—can be a long one. There are frequent disappointments: proposals that are ultimately unfunded, difficulties in putting together research teams, challenges in completing the writing of all proposal elements by the submission deadline, reviewers' comments that are contradictory or otherwise difficult to address, and a multitude of other aspects involved in proposal writing that do not work out as planned. Research administrators and proposal writers have the opportunity to help each other in the development and writing process by collecting tips and information from colleagues, from professional development seminars and workshops on grant writing, and from the numerous sources of information (hardcopy and electronic documents) on proposal writing. It helps to remember that good ideas, when expressed well and submitted to the right funding agency, do get funded.

••• References

Bailey, A. 1987. "Errors to avoid when seeking funds from foundations and corporations," *Chronicle of Higher Education* (35): January 14.

Barrett, E. "Hints for writing successful NIH grants, 1995." Available at: http://www2.uta.edu/sswgrants/Technical%20Assistance/hints_for_writing_successful_nih.htm (accessed August 24, 2005).

Oetting, E. 1986. "Ten fatal mistakes in grant writing," *Professional Psychology Research and Practice* (17):570–573.

Molfese, V., Karp, K., and L. Siegel. "Recommendations for writing successful proposals from the reviewer's perspective," *SRA Journal* (33):21–24.

29

Peer Review and Project Implementation and Evaluation

Pamela F. Miller, PhD

Peer Review

The peer review process—evaluation of new ideas, proposals, and findings by experts—is a common-sense approach that has been used for centuries. Even Queen Isabella of Spain reportedly sought the advice of experienced navigators, which fortunately she ignored, prior to deciding to provide Christopher Columbus with funding to find a new trade route to India. (1) By the 1700s, the Royal Society of London, founded in 1660 to promote the new or experimental philosophy of that time embodying the principles envisaged by Sir Francis Bacon, had initiated the use of peer review to evaluate the quality of scholarly papers submitted for publication in its scholarly journal, *Philosophical Transactions*. (2)

The Royal Society, like the publishing bodies of today's scholarly journals, used an *ex post* peer evaluation process, which judges the quality of a product retrospectively, i.e., after results have been obtained. Queen Isabella's approach was based on an *ex ante* peer evaluation model that makes judgments in advance of performance. (3) The *ex ante* peer review process is most commonly used by today's private and government funding agencies to evaluate applications for funding.

The *ex ante* model places an additional burden on the peer reviewer in that the reviewer must judge an applicant's future performance on the basis of past efforts—if any—and must judge the applicant's ability to articulate a set of goals and objectives, as well as a plan of operation that satisfies one or more criteria set by the funding agency. These crite-ria can vary considerably among funding agencies; even among the twelve federal agencies, there is no government-wide definition of peer review or a federal policy for conducting peer reviews. (4) Successful applicants must be aware of how the funding agency selects its peer reviewers; the judging criteria used to evaluate proposals; how the peer review is conducted; and how the agency interprets its mission, goals, and objectives.

Evaluation Criteria

Every funding agency, private or public, wants to see its funding used in a cost-effective manner. However, every funding agency has a field of interest, a stated mission, and goals that influence how the other elements of a proposal are reviewed. Each agency has a "culture" that influences its vocabulary and terminology and the types of people it hires to implement its agenda. Each agency has beliefs about what is important and the way it sees itself contributing to the greater good.

The characteristics of a funding agency can change over time depending on emerging problems, e.g., HIV or AIDS, and corresponding changes in funding agency priorities and funding patterns. In the case of governmental agencies, a new administration at the federal level can herald the end of a previously well-funded program, the beginning of a new initiative based on a different philosophy, or even the beginning (or end) of an entire funding agency. Private funding agencies can make equally drastic changes, often more quickly than the government sector. Such changes affect the type and availability of funding support, and the successful grant and contract seeker must always be attuned to such funding policy changes and how these changes will affect available funding dollars.

The challenge for any funding agency, governmental or private, is to identify worthy projects that match the funding agency's funding objectives—over time—and are likely to succeed if funded. The peer review process—although not always perfect—is one way to achieve this goal.

The Proposal Review Process

The proposal process is a common method of soliciting applications for funding from outside groups. Some funding agencies, usually private foundations, may require the applicant to submit a short letter proposal to be followed by a more complete description of the project if the funding agency is interested in learning more about the applicant's project. Governmental funding agencies typically require a full proposal to be prepared according to a specific format.

Some funding agencies, usually private foundations, allow proposals to be submitted at any time; these proposals are typically reviewed when a board of directors meets. Other funding agencies, usually government agencies, establish postmark or due dates for applications. Failure to submit the application by these dates can result in the application being returned without being reviewed. It is very important to understand the format, content, and submission requirements of the funding agency before submitting an application. Failure to pay attention to even the seemingly insignificant requirements, e.g., font size, may cause the proposal to be returned or rejected.

Evaluating Proposals

The reason that funding agencies establish and disseminate their guidelines for proposals is to ensure that the proposals that are submitted can all be reviewed according to the same criteria. It is certainly easier to compare "apples to apples" than it is to compare "apples to oranges." The successful applicant always considers the needs of the proposal reviewer when preparing a proposal. This chapter explains in detail the needs of the individual reviewing a proposal.

Who are the people who review proposals? How are reviewers chosen? What are their responsibilities? The basic peer review model is to ask individuals with expertise in a particular area to review the content of the proposal and rate the proposal according to a specific set of criteria. For example, federal agencies employ peer review for the following purposes:

1. To assess the merit of competitive and noncompetitive research proposals.
2. To determine whether to continue or renew research projects.
3. To evaluate the results of the research prior to the publication of those results.
4. To establish annual budget priorities for research programs.
5. To evaluate program and scientist performance. (4)

To accomplish these objectives, some federal agencies use standing review groups with ad hoc members brought in only when proposals require review by an expert outside the existing group. Other agencies select a different set of peer reviewers for each funding competition.

The way the peer reviewers are selected has ramifications for the applicant. A standing group has a collective "memory" that comes into play if the applicant decides to resubmit a proposal for review by the same group, whereas review panels chosen on an ad hoc basis will not know the good and bad points of a previously submitted proposal, although they may agree with their predecessors!

No matter how a peer review committee is established, it is important to know what is meant by the word "peer." In some cases the funding agency is primarily concerned with the scientific expertise of the peer review panel. When this is the case, the agency tries to find panelists within the same or related scientific discipline that have had peer-reviewed journal and book publications as well as external funding from recognized private or governmental funding agencies. Often a funding agency chooses reviewers whom the agency has supported with grant or contract funds in the past. In this way the agency can be sure that the reviewer not only understands the goals and objectives of the funding agency but also has demonstrated the ability to write a successful scientific proposal to this agency.

For training or service proposals, a funding agency may be more interested in the views of a broader group of peer reviewers. The agency may choose individuals who represent both the providers and consumers of the desired training and service. These mixed peer review groups can provide the agency with information on each applicant's experience and expertise as well as feedback on how the project will be viewed and supported by those it purports to serve. In recent years, agencies have become more concerned with the views of consumers, especially consumers from underrepresented groups. Sensitivity to the involvement "in" and the effect of a funded project "on" such individuals is a serious consideration for most funding agencies.

The program officer who is responsible for the proposal review process usually gives peer reviewers guidance on the proposal review process. This process varies across funding agencies. Some funding agencies may ask the peer reviewer to read a group of proposals at home and to send the proposal ratings to the program officer who will then use these ratings to make funding decisions. Other agencies will send a group of proposals to a peer reviewer, ask the peer viewer to rate the proposals at home, and then convene a meeting of the peer reviewers at a central location to discuss and rate the proposals again after the discussion. Unfortunately, some reviewers may read the proposals for the first time while flying on an airplane to the review meeting! To deal with this reality, a peer reviewer may be asked to be the primary, secondary, or tertiary reviewer for one or more proposals that will be discussed on site. This ensures that every proposal has had an in-depth review at some level. Finally, some agencies provide the peer reviewers with copies of the proposals after they arrive at the site of the proposal review. This presents a stamina challenge to any peer reviewer who must evaluate a large number of proposals in a short time while staying in a less-than-luxurious hotel room in Washington, DC.

The issue of conflict of interest is typically addressed prior to the peer review process. Program officers ask peer reviewers to excuse themselves from reviewing any proposal in which they have participated in or will benefit from if funded. Reviewers also should not be asked to review any proposal from their agencies of employment. Funding agencies will sometimes request or require applicants to submit a Letter of Intent (LOI) to apply so that the funding agency will know if a particular conflict of interest is likely.

Program officers should give peer reviewers guidance on how the funding agency interprets the objectives of the funding program. This is particularly important when a funding program is new and if the agency is not yet sure how applicants will

have responded to the proposal guidelines. Program officers also may address problems or issues that have emerged in previous review cycles. For example, they may direct a standing review peer committee to review each proposal as though it were a new submission. The program officer may remind reviewers not to discuss proposals outside the review committee process, that certain proposal budget requests are not allowed, or to ignore the proposal budget entirely.

However, biases do occur. Chronister, Kulakowski, and Molfese (5) state that the peer review process is often unduly affected by biases for or against specific theoretical frameworks, methodologies, investigators, and institutions. A peer reviewer may legitimately disagree with an application's scientific premise or a particular reviewer may have a personality conflict with a colleague included in the proposal, which may lead to a less than objective review of the applicant's proposal. Some funding agencies recognize the unfortunate results that professional and personal conflict can produce and offer applicants an opportunity at the proposal stage to ask that a specific reviewer not be asked to review the applicant's proposal. When this option is not available, the applicant can only hope that the other peer reviewers will counteract any unwarranted negative review from a biased reviewer. Ultimately the best defense is a good offense: in short, write a good proposal!

Once the peer reviewers have been given a group of proposals to review, they are also given review criteria to use to evaluate each proposal. These criteria are usually published in the information provided to applicants. The criteria may be obvious and actually listed in the proposal guidelines, or the information may be embedded in the discussion of what the agency wants to fund. If this is the case, the applicant should discuss this issue with the program officer, a previously successful applicant, or someone who has reviewed proposals for this agency in the past. Under the federal Freedom of Information Act (FOIA), many agencies will provide novice applicants with copies of successful proposals to be used as a guide (not to be copied verbatim) that illustrate the agency's proposal criteria. (6)

When the agency's funding criteria are explicit, the criteria may be given different values in the evaluation of the proposal. For example, the section of the proposal that addresses the project objectives may be worth 25 points out of 100 points or 25% of the proposal's score, while project evaluation may only be worth 5 points or 5%. Or, the evaluation section may be worth more than any other section of the proposal depending on the agency's objectives. The point is for the applicant to know what the agency is looking for in response to these criteria. In today's competitive funding environment, all aspects of a proposal are important when one or more percentage points can make the difference between a funded proposal and one that is denied.

It also is important for previously funded applicants to stay "tuned in" to how a funding agency states and interprets their eligibility and funding criteria. For example, in recent years the National Science Foundation (NSF) introduced two equally important review criteria to the proposal review process, merit and impact. This was a signal from the NSF that how the applicant's research would impact the development of future scientists and consumers of science was just as important as the scientific merit of any NSF-funded project. Applicants that fail to recognize this shift are not likely to receive NSF support. Similarly, if an agency drops a focus area from a long-standing funding program, applicants need to notice this fact and respond to it, because the peer reviewers will be told to notice applicants that fail to pay attention to the funding criteria.

Learning about the Peer Review Process

Some applicants might wish that they could be flies on the wall when their proposals are being reviewed by a group of peer viewers. (This author cannot imagine a more painful experience!) Chapter 28 presents an excellent discussion of what peer reviewers do and do not want to see in a proposal, and how an unsuccessful applicant can use the comments of peer reviewers to prepare a subsequent and undoubtedly more successful proposal.

An alternative to the fly-on-the-wall approach is to actually become a peer reviewer. This is more easily accomplished with some funding agencies than others. However, it is worth pursuing for the educational value it provides. As mentioned earlier, funding agencies are interested in selecting peer reviewers who can help them make good funding decisions. Funding agencies notice potential peer reviewers who are "noticeable." The question of how to get noticed, if one is a researcher, has one good answer: publish, publish, and publish! Another good answer is to present papers at professional conferences where your work is likely to be noticed by program officers in attendance. There is also a social-interpersonal dimension to this: if a program officer or an

agency representative wants to talk about your research, make yourself available! It also works the other way: go to other conference sessions, especially those that indicate that the research was funded by an external agency. The presenter is likely to be a peer reviewer, and there may be an agency representative in the audience. Pay attention to what is presented and ask interesting questions! After the presentation, go up and introduce yourself and talk about what you have in common. You might learn something or meet someone who can give you guidance on your next proposal.

If such social-interpersonal interactions fill you with terror, a more straightforward way to become known to a funding agency is by making an appointment with a program officer, in person or via phone, to discuss your work and your ideas for future funding. In such a meeting, you might ask the program officer how the agency chooses its peer reviewers. If this is an agency that routinely selects people from the field and likes to recruit new people with new perspectives to participate on review panels, the program officer may encourage you to submit your name and vitae to a peer reviewer pool for consideration. Overall, talking to an agency program officer can help you better prepare a proposal, and provides the opportunity for the agency and its officers to know more about you and your work.

Individuals who are interested in serving as peer reviewers for federal agencies should also monitor the Federal Register for opportunities to comment on proposed agency guidelines. Published by the Office of the Federal Register, National Archives and Records Administration (NARA), the Federal Register is the official daily publication for rules, proposed rules, and notices of federal agencies and organizations, as well as executive orders and other presidential documents. Submission of well-thought-out suggestions can give your name recognition. Some agencies have a process for soliciting applications from individuals who would like to serve as peer reviewers for the agency; attention should be paid to such announcements when they appear in the Federal Register. Federal agencies in particular are sensitive to the need for geographical representation and the participation of underrepresented groups in the peer review process.

Alternatives to Peer Review

Although most funding agencies make every attempt to optimize the value of the peer review process, the process is not without its problems and its critics. The intent of the peer review process is to ensure that the merit of a proposal wins out over cronyism. Unfortunately, cronyism and the results of academic inbreeding can be subtle and difficult to detect. It can even be so subtle that a reviewer is not even aware that he or she is participating in it. For example, if a reviewer knows of a researcher's work, has seen the researcher's lab, and has met the people involved in the researcher's studies, the reviewer has undoubtedly formed either a positive or negative view of the researcher that could bias the way the researcher's proposal is reviewed. If the researcher does not address an important point in the proposal, the reviewer may unintentionally fill in this proposal "gap" with what he or she already knows about the research. During the panel review, the reviewer may offer this inside information to the other reviewers, and the proposal may get a higher score than it deserves on its own merit. Program officers try to keep this from happening, but if the program officer is moving between four or five panels, he or she may miss unintentional bias when it occurs.

Unintentional bias can also occur when peer reviewers compare research being conducted at an institution with substantial human and fiscal resources to that being conducted at a less well-funded organization. The competition for external support does not occur on a level playing field. Thus, some institutions and even some states may find it difficult to benefit from the federal funding scene. When federal dollars generated by US taxpayers are involved this disparity becomes a problem. It is easy to see how wealthier institutions will be more likely to garner more external resources over time under this system (representing the "rich get richer" syndrome).

Legislators from states that have had limited success in attracting federal agency funding support have raised such concerns with the funding agencies in recent years. This has led a number of federal agencies' participation in the Experimental Program to Stimulate Competitive Research (EPSCoR) program, which is designed especially to help underfunded states. The agency does use a peer review process as the basis for making funding decisions.

The growing use of federally earmarked funds to support specific projects in a particular state is a threat to the peer review process. These "pork" projects—worthy or not—are not subjected to any peer review. Instead, a member of Congress places language to fund a particular project within his or her state as a line item in the budget of a federal agency. The federal agency then requests the recipi-

ent agency to submit a proposal for the funds, but the funding is virtually guaranteed as long as the proposal reflects the purpose specified by Congress. Typically, the federal agency retains a portion of the allocated funds for internal administrative costs.

The tension between the peer review and the earmarking grant-making process is ultimately philosophical in nature: Which is better, funding decisions made by experts in a particular field or funding opportunities created by members of Congress who believe that it is their responsibility to obtain federal funding for their state? This is an issue beyond the scope of this short chapter. However, the way we ultimately answer this question is likely to affect our future as a county.

Project Implementation

"Don't panic!" should be written at the top of every award document. A proposal is written with the goal to describe how the project can unfold under the best of all circumstances. When the funding decision has been made and the award received, the project director faces real-world issues, including the reality that making use of the award involves working through a bureaucracy, since external awards usually are not made to individuals. People must be hired, equipment must be purchased, space must be allocated for the project, and the project budget must be administered. In addition, all of this must be done according to funding and home agency policies. The project director soon discovers that running a sponsored project may be more time-consuming than writing the winning proposal.

Every project director should understand that the grant or contract is between the funding agency and the organization that submitted the proposal. The people who wrote the proposal are responsible for carrying out the project, but the funding does not come directly to them, except in the cases of a fellowship or a prize. Therefore, the agency that receives the award has a vested interest to make sure that the project is carried out in a manner that conforms to the funding agency's terms and conditions that are outlined in the award document. The project director must fully understand these terms and conditions and administer the project accordingly; failure to do so can result in serious legal ramifications for the recipient agency, as well as for the project director.

Some major compliance issues for the federal funding agencies concern research involving human subjects, animal care and use, the handling of biological and radiological substances, and the scientific misconduct and conflicts of interest of key project personnel. A funding agency's award document may, in addition, cite a variety of governmental regulations to guide how the project is carried out. These regulations are often difficult to understand within the context of a project document, and so it is advisable that the research administrator obtain copies of these regulations and review them thoroughly to clarify their meanings.

The form of the award, e.g., a grant or contract, is also an important factor to consider. If, for example, the award is in the form of a grant, the recipient agency must make a reasonable effort to carry out the project according to the scope of work within the specified timelines. If all objectives are not realized (despite every effort to accomplish the tasks outlined in the proposal), the funding agency will generally award all of the funding promised, but likely will request that the project director report the problems encountered, the steps that were made to remedy the problems, and the outcomes that were realized. In cases indicating project mismanagement, the funding agency typically will not fund subsequent years of the project or award a continuation grant.

When the award is received in the form of a contract, the recipient agency must deliver the services or product specified according to timelines as listed in the contract in order to receive payment. Contracts are constructed to ensure that the funding agency is protected against project mismanagement. Before a contract is signed by the recipient organization, the project director, administration, and legal counsel should review the contract deliverables, terms, and conditions carefully. No work should commence or funds be spent until the contract has been fully negotiated and signed.

Each funding agency has a policy on making such changes. For example, most federal agencies operate under "Expanded Authorities" that allow the recipient agency more latitude in the administration of sponsored projects, while other funding agencies require that agency approval be obtained even for the smallest budget revision. Again, it is important that the project director follow specific agency guidelines carefully.

Post-Award Implementation

Project implementation involves planning and foresight. Often months have passed between the time

the proposal was submitted and the award received, and so it is important that before a project commences, the project objectives and timelines be examined, as proposed in the original application:

- *Are the project objectives still viable, or have circumstances changed?*
- *Do the timelines still work for the project?*
- *Are the people you had hoped to hire still available?*

Most often there are changes in circumstances that occur between the time the proposal was submitted and the time of the award; therefore, the project director is required to make some adjustments. When adjustments are minor and will not affect the project timelines, deliverables, or budget, prior agency approval of changes is not usually required. However, even minor changes should be communicated via required project reports submitted to the funding agency.

Changes in the scope of work, key project personnel, and significant budgetary needs may require prior funding agency approval.

The following barriers to project implementation can occur in any sponsored project—but hopefully not at the same time!

Hiring Qualified Project Personnel Each funding agency has a fiscal year, one which may not coincide with that of the recipient agency. Thus, the award may arrive after most agency positions have already been filled and the most appropriate people to work on the project have already been hired. Often, this can delay the hiring process for several months. If the award arrives at a time that is incompatible with the project's overall timelines (e.g., an award for a project that needs to take place during the school year, but arrives just before the school year is over), the funding agency may delay the project start date a few months to allow the project to start at a more opportune time. This also allows time to hire project personnel. Similarly, under Expanded Authorities, federal agencies can allow a project to start 90 days before the formal award is made. This allows the project director to hire personnel a little earlier, if necessary.

Personnel Turnover Since externally funded positions tend to be short-term employment, funded by what often is called "soft" money, project personnel may decide to leave for something more permanent. Turnover in project personnel can slow progress, especially since it takes time to recruit and train new employees. Thus, it is important for the project director to maintain good relationships with human resources personnel and understand the agency hiring procedures and policies, including affirmative action requirements, so that delays in hiring replacement personnel can be kept at a minimum.

Purchasing Personnel Services Often a sponsored project requires the contributions of individuals on an intermittent basis for the completion of a specific task. Such individuals, who are not employed by the recipient institution, can serve as consultants and independent contractors. These individuals are not considered employees, therefore, the project director may specify the outcomes but not the way these outcomes are achieved. It is important to understand that employees are eligible for fringe benefits, whereas consultants and independent contractors are not. Project directors at universities and colleges must also be sure not to use faculty consultants from within the same department as the project director. Federal regulations prohibit such interdepartmental consulting.

Subcontracts To avoid delays, any subcontract(s) established between the recipient agency and a lower-tier partner should be included as part of the proposal. Typically, in the proposal budget a letter of cooperation, along with a budget for the subcontract, should be included in the proposal, as well as the total cost of the subcontract. When the proposal is approved, the subcontract also is considered approved by some (but not all) agencies. If the subcontract was not included in the proposal, the project director will need to obtain funding agency approval for this expense.

A formal subcontract will need to be developed between the prime recipient and the subcontractor(s). This subcontract agreement should "flow down" all of the requirements of the prime agreement to the lower-tier partner, unless it is not feasible to do so (e.g., a foreign subcontractor). The project director of the recipient agency is responsible for monitoring the progress of the subcontract. In all cases, privity exists between the funding agency and the prime recipient only. The subcontractor has privity with the prime recipient.

Purchasing Equipment The federal definition of equipment is a unit costing at least $5,000 or more or the recipient's equipment threshold level, whichever is less. The equipment must have an expected service life of at least one year. Many agencies exclude equipment from their F&A cost calculation when using a modified total direct cost

base (MTDC), so this definition is important for budgeting purposes. Should funds that are budgeted for equipment be moved into another cost line, the project director should anticipate F&A charges on these expenditures.

Rebudgeting If the agency requires that prior approval be obtained for every budget adjustment, it is wise to carefully plan what is needed at the proposal stage. However, unanticipated events always occur during the life of a sponsored project. Costs go up and down. Delays cause unexpected expenses. Key project personnel find new positions at other agencies. Part-time employees become full-time employees and have different fringe benefits. In short, rebudgeting is often necessary.

The project director should estimate the changes needed in the overall budget and request approval for these changes all at once, rather than making a number of separate requests for approval from the funding agency. Even when operating under the federal project guideline of Expanded Authorities (allowing project directors to move money between and among budget categories as needed without specific agency approval), it is a good idea to make a comprehensive budget adjustment rather than a series of smaller modifications. Further, this will be appreciated by the post-award side of the recipient agency!

If by the end of the project period the project objectives have not been realized, the project director has two options. He or she may request a *no-cost extension*. Many funding agencies will allow the project to continue, without additional funding, so that all of the proposed tasks can be accomplished. This is a viable option only if funds are still remaining in the sponsored project account. The second option is to request a *funding supplement*. This request should be made only when the agency feels that the request is justified due to circumstances beyond the control of the project director. An important word of caution: if the project fails to meet its objectives, the costs and scope of the project were poorly estimated from the beginning, and the project director is forced to make one of these choices. A fixed contract presents a fiscal danger for the recipient agency. Under the terms of a fixed contract, should the actual costs of the project exceed those specified in the contract, the recipient agency will have to provide the additional support for the project—something it may or may not be able to do. Worse, should the recipient agency default, all of the contract funds may have to be returned.

Reporting Each funding agency expects something for its funding of a project. Project directors are expected to keep the agency informed of progress on a regular basis. Failure to provide reports in a timely fashion puts the recipient agency, as well as the project director, in a bad light. In years past, agencies were not as assiduous as they are today about tracking project reports, but with the advent of computer database systems, a funding agency is more readily able to identify those agencies that (and project directors who) have failed to turn in project reports. In some cases, the agency may determine not to provide additional funding without timely reporting of progress.

Cost-Sharing and Matching Funds Many agencies or programs require applicants to share the cost of the proposed project, while others do not. However, when cost-share is contributed on any federal project (required or not), it becomes a requirement if an award is made. When cost-share is required, it must be tracked. That is, there must be evidence that the recipient agency contributed to the project. Cost-share can be obtained by contributing agency personnel time, the fringe benefits associated with that time, and any F&A costs that apply. When personnel time is contributed, the recipient agency must keep effort report records for project personnel to document this contribution. When other than agency personnel time is used, the project director must keep accurate records of the expenditures made on the project from the recipient agency's funds. When other agency contributions are included as part of the project's cost-share, the project director of the prime agency must obtain documentation of this contribution should the project be audited.

Project Evaluation and Dissemination

Program officers cite the project evaluation section as the weakest in most proposals. It is easy to understand why this should be the case: most of the proposal is devoted to explaining why the funding agency would want to fund someone's innovative idea for research, training, or service. The evaluation section of a proposal asks the applicant to consider the possibility that the project might not turn out exactly as planned. Most applicants have a hard time thinking about—much less describing—the potential limitations of their project while writing a proposal to obtain external funding. Therefore, many applicants rely on an outside project evaluator to help design the evaluation section of a proposal.

The addition of an external project evaluator with well-known expertise in the field of study also can strengthen the project team and result in a higher overall proposal rating from the peer reviewers.

Proposals to obtain funding for research usually do not require a separate section on project evaluation. By definition, research is self-correcting. Good science will distinguish between significant and insignificant outcomes, and replication studies can identify spurious or atypical results. However, to analyze the importance of the findings, the research community does need to have information about the research subjects: the sampling or selection process, the treatment(s) used; the method of analysis; the quantitative and/or qualitative outcomes; and the limitations of the study. Good recordkeeping is critical. The ultimate evaluation of the contribution of the research occurs when the research community has an opportunity to evaluate the research findings in peer-reviewed journals.

Proposals for sponsored projects that have training or service goals are often required to include a special section on project evaluation. The funding agency will be interested in not only the outcome of the project (should it be funded), but also in the procedures that have been used to carry out the training or service activities with a particular population or within a specific setting. A comprehensive evaluation plan includes both process and outcome evaluation techniques.

Process evaluation looks at the objectives and activities of the project in relationship to timelines and anticipated outcomes. This enables project staff to determine if their strategies are working and if their timelines are realistic. Midcourse adjustments based on a clear understanding of the status of the project at a particular point in time can make the project more successful in the long run. Measurable project objectives can be used as the basis of a process evaluation, including, for example, information on *who* is responsible, *what* is to be done, *when* it is to occur, and *how* project personnel will know if they have been successful. When project personnel meet regularly to examine progress, changes in personnel assignments, project strategies, timelines, and success criteria can be made as needed.

Process evaluation is best carried out at short-term intervals by project personnel since they are involved in the day-to-day implementation of the project. The project director can bring key project personnel together on a weekly, monthly, or quarterly basis—depending on the needs of the project—

to discuss the progress of the project and any need for change or midcourse correction. An external project evaluator, project funds permitting, can also be of assistance in a process evaluation by helping in the beginning to identify ways to easily collect information as the project is being implemented and to help interpret the information collected.

Outcome evaluation focuses on the final results of the project. The types of questions that should be addressed by an outcome evaluation include:

- *Were products developed?*
- *Were these products effective or useful?*
- *Did anticipated changes in people and/or the environment occur?*
- *To what degree were the strategies used successful?*
- *Were outcomes significant?*
- *What did not work/succeed and why?*
- *What now needs to be done?*

Outcome evaluation requires that someone take an objective look at what the project has actually accomplished during the funding period. An outcome evaluation usually occurs at the end of each funding period and when the project concludes. This is when an external project evaluator can be of the most assistance. Project personnel still must be involved to provide data and other information on outcomes, but it is the job of the external evaluator to organize, interpret, and report this information for the project director. The project director can then use the information provided to prepare required reports to the funding agency.

Both forms of evaluation can be made easier at the proposal stage by setting clear goals (or research questions), "measurable objectives," and specific activities that support these objectives. Establishing a criterion for success for each objective will also be beneficial. Peer reviewers can easily identify projects with vague operational plans, and these proposals are rated lower as a result. Applicants who manage to line up project goals, objectives, and activities make project evaluation easier and are rewarded with higher application scores.

The objective of every funding agency is to make a positive difference in the agency's field of interest. The recipient agency is expected to report the results of their activities to the sponsoring agency and to disseminate these results to a wider audience. Post-award activities should include project reporting and presentation of results through conferences, journal articles,

media coverage, and, of course, project reports themselves are also valuable dissemination vehicles.

Such failure to report can also affect congressional funding. In 1993, Congress passed the Government Performance and Results Act, requiring that federal agencies produce strategic performance plans that include annual targets and performance reports explaining whether targets have been met. The federal agencies now ask that recipients of awards help provide this information to Congress. Thus, it is in everyone's best interest to provide high-quality reporting and evaluation of sponsored projects.

Summary

Those who have not engaged in the process of proposal submission or project administration may not understand:

> *Why proposals must often be submitted more than once;*
>
> *How anyone could submit an incomplete proposal;*
>
> *Why proposals so often are submitted at the last minute;*
>
> *Why sponsored projects cause so many post-award problems;*
>
> *Why sponsored project reports are so hard to obtain from researchers.*

The process of developing a proposal that satisfies a group of peer reviewers is difficult; the administration of an external award is time-consuming and sometimes frustrating; and the evaluation of a funded project requires foresight, attention to detail, and willingness to share what was learned—even if the project is unsuccessful. Those who engage in sponsored project activity and those who attempt to help them clearly deserve, at minimum, a "pat on the back" for attempting to surmount these challenges!

• • • References

1. Boorstin, D. J. *The Discoverers.* New York: Random House, 1983.
2. Kronick, D.A. "Peer Review in 18th-century Scientific Journalism." *Journal of the American Medical Association* 263, no. 10 (1990): 1321–1322.
3. Thornley, R., M. W. Spence, M. Taylor, and J. Magnan. "New Decision Tool to Evaluate

Award Selection Process." *The Journal of Research Administration* 33, nos. 2 and 3 (2002): 49–56.

4. United States General Accounting Office. *Report to Congressional Requesters: Federal Research Peer Review Practices at Federal Science Agencies Vary*, Report Number GAO/RCED-99-99, March 1999.

5. Chronister, L., E. Kulakowski, and V. J. Molfese. "Priorities for Federal Innovation and Reform: An SRA Perspective." *The Journal of Research Administration* 2, no. 1 (2001): 5–10.

6. Riggle, D. T., and P. F. Harrel. "FOIA and Sponsored Project Administration." *The Journal of Research Administration* 33, no. 1 (2002): 31–35.

30

Electronic Research Administration (ERA) Commencement, Practice, and Future

John A. Rodman, MBA, and Brad Stanford

Introduction

Implemention and subsequent use of computer systems have become standard responsibilities for research administrators. Electronic Research Administration (ERA) is loosely defined as improving administrative processes through the application of technology, particularly computer technology. ERA is one of several factors that is intended to help reduce costs in research organizations and to speed the movement of research ideas from the laboratory into products. This chapter provides a historical perspective on ERA and a roadmap for future improvements that is expected to aid research administrators who will have responsibility for implementation.

The Beginnings

A vision of paperless grants (electronic proposals, awards, progress reports) was inspired by the rapid evolution of the Internet and electronic commerce across many industries. Electronic commerce, the process of conducting business transactions through electronic means, began in the Department of Defense (DoD) in the 1960s as a technique for passing logistics data. This technique was adopted by private industry, where it was first used to track transportation assets, such as railcars and containers.

To facilitate the exchange of electronic information among different organizations, a common "language" was needed. In the mid-1970s the American National Standards Institute (ANSI) formed a committee to develop a national standard called Electronic Data Interchange (EDI), a common language by which various organizations could electronically exchange information. The X12 Accredited Standards Committees (ASC) created a national standard for EDI that was rapidly adopted among many diverse industries (banking, automotive, and grocery).

Organizational use of EDI in these industries helped speed up delivery of goods and services, while simultaneously reducing paperwork errors. For example, manufacturers transmitted electronic purchase orders to suppliers. Without the delay of the paper mail system, manufacturers received the materials faster from their suppliers. Suppliers transmitted electronic invoices to the manufacturers and received payment by electronic funds transfer (EFT). The result was a much faster turnaround of goods and services for the manufacturer and improved cash flow for the supplier.

Early electronic commerce was initially conducted using private networks between businesses and their suppliers. The very beginning of the Internet revolved around the electronic exchange of research information.

In 1969, four universities supported by DoD's Advanced Research Programs Agency (ARPA) established a program, ARPANET, to exchange data among their campuses to explore computer networking and communication technology. Based on the ARPANET protocols that evolved from this project, the National Science Foundation (NSF) created NSFNET in 1985 enabling five university supercomputer centers to exchange research data and leverage their combined computing power. In 1986 the first readily-available Web browser, "Mosaic," was created by one of the supercomputing centers on NSFNET, the National Center for Supercomputing Applications (NCSA) at the University of Illinois, Urbana-Champaign.

The development of Mosaic led to the development of a standard language for delivering information to the browser in the form of an electronic document. Called Hyper Text Markup Language (HTML), this standard allowed scientists, or anyone else with information, to publish the information on the Internet—information that could be retrieved using the Web browser. Web browsers, like Mosaic, and the HTML electronic document standard for publishing were widely and publicly available because of their scientific beginnings. Mosaic, developed with federal grant support, was free to anyone who wanted to use it, and any organization that had information available could publish it electronically using the HTTP standard. The resulting explosion of information, in the form of electronic documents, became known as the World Wide Web. (1)

Tim Berners-Lee and Robert Caillau both worked at CERN, an international high energy physics research center near Geneva. In 1989 they collaborated on ideas for a linked information system that would be accessible across the wide range of different computer systems in use at CERN. At that time many people were using *TeX* and *Post-Script* for their documents. A few were using *SGML*. Tim realized that something simpler was needed that would cope with dumb terminals through high-end graphical X Window workstations. HTML was conceived as a very simple solution and matched with a very simple network protocol HTTP.

CERN launched the Web in 1991 along with a mailing list called www-talk. Other people thinking along the same lines soon joined and helped to grow the Web by setting up Web sites and implementing browsers, such as Cello, Viola, and MidasWWW. The breakthrough came when the National Center for Supercomputer Applications (NCSA) at Urbana-Champaign encouraged Marc Andreessen and Eric Bina to develop the X Window *Mosaic* browser. It was later ported to PCs and Macs and became a runaway success story. The Web grew exponentially, eclipsing other Internet-based information systems such as WAIS, Hytelnet, Gopher, and UseNet.

The Web browser and electronic mail unlocked access to data and information that had been trapped inside organizations. It was first made available mostly over interconnected government and campus networks that later became the public Internet. Private business quickly understood that this speed of electronic communication could enable it to consider new ways to work not just with suppliers, as it had with EDI, but also with customers. IBM grasped the potential of the Web saying that the Internet was not about "browsing" but about "business." (2) What they meant was that by taking electronic commerce out of the realm of private networks and using it to connect business suppliers, customers, and partners, a whole new set of possibilities existed.

The potential for improving business processes among organizations and their "business partners" using the Internet returned to the research environment: this time in the management and administration of the research enterprise.

Early Federal ERA Systems

By the late 1980s federal agencies and universities had already been using technology to improve the administration, relationship, and communication among grantors and grantees. Two primary objectives of these projects were to:

1. Provide more efficient administrative services that saved the scientist time;
2. Show appropriate stewardship of the grant funds and protect the institution's integrity.

In the early 1990s, both the National Science Foundation (NSF) and the National Institutes of Health (NIH) had decided that receiving research proposals electronically would have significant benefit, although each chose a different approach to the solution. The potential benefit to each organization was tremendous. For every proposal deadline, the organizations were processing mountains of paper, literally thousands of boxes, each containing many copies of each grant application. These would continue to arrive by overnight delivery trucks within a day or two of the deadline.

Grant applications were prepared electronically by scientists using word processors, then printed and mailed to NIH or NSF—sometimes as many as twenty copies of each application. NSF and NIH received the applications and entered information into their proposal receiving computer systems. The paper was then sorted and mailed back out to scientific reviewers. The critiques supplied by these reviewers had to be collated with the proposals in preparation for review meetings that met face-to-face to decide which applications were the most meritorious. This process commonly took at least nine months, and each process would involve five to seven electronic-to-paper conversions (and back).

The cost savings from reducing paper processing and re-keying data alone was enough to justify major investments in electronic grant applications at both NIH and NSF. ERA offered a new process that was simple, economical, responsive, dependable, and versatile, and it allowed scientists to spend less time on administration and more time in their labs. (3)

In the area of grant management, the Office of Naval Research (ONR) developed an electronic payment process for their grantees. In the early 1990s ONR had implemented an electronic commerce process that allowed grant recipients to electronically send invoices for research work performed under a grant and receive payment electronically, directly delivered to their accounts. Once begun, this system processed over half of ONR's research business electronically and, for grantees, reduced the average time from invoice to receipt of payment from sixty to merely five days. (3)

At the time when DoD declared EDI the standard for conducting electronic business electronically with DoD (and that transactions would conform to ANSI X12 EDI standards), ONR's electronic grant payment system did not use the Internet. (3) Instead, a grantee would set up a specialized workstation to access a private Value Added Network (VAN) and would then send the invoice in an EDI standard format. This extra effort and cost of a specialized system for the grantee was offset by the improved payment cash flow.

To conform with the Bayh-Dole Act of 1980, NIH developed another electronic system in 1994 for research administration called EDISON, an invention reporting system. As a result of its success, the system was soon adopted by many other federal research agencies with similar invention reporting requirements for their grantees.

> iEdison (which stands for Interagency Edison) helps government grantees and contractors comply with a federal law, the Bayh-Dole Act. Bayh-Dole regulations require that government funded inventions be reported to the federal agency who made the award.
>
> iEdison is interagency because it provides a single interface for grantees and contractors to interact with any participating agency.
>
> iEdison makes it easy to learn about the law and its regulations and report an invention or patent funded by any of the agencies listed on the right. [on the iEdison.gov home page] (4)

Early ERA Effort at Research Universities

Pioneering research universities also saw the benefits of ERA, but from a different perspective than the grantors. The Massachusetts Institute of Technology (MIT) developed COEUS to streamline the processing of grant proposals and awards. At the same time, a consortium of six primarily state universities, lead by North Carolina State University, worked with IBM and USC Software Systems to design and implement the Grant Application and Management Software (GAMS). Other universities, including UCLA and Duke, also implemented grant management systems to help streamline their internal processes. (5)

These research universities made significant investments in their ERA systems early on, which enabled their researchers to quickly prepare proposals using online tools, electronically route proposals through the institution's approval process, and easily set up new projects when award notifications were received. The research administrators at MIT and the universities of the GAMS consortium participated in early pilots with federal agencies to provide the data from their internal systems to those federal agencies evolving ERA systems. While the early pilots were successful, agreement on a standardized approach was still a long way away.

There were several companies (small and large) who were early pioneers in the move to ERA. The companies, which sought to provide software and services to the grantee and grantor organizations, included SAP (which worked with MIT on COEUS), IBM (which managed the development of the software for the GAMS consortium), and USC Software Solutions and AMS (which worked with Duke University), and smaller companies, Research and Management System (RAMS) and INFOED International.

Governance and Policy for ERA

As ERA systems proliferated among federal agencies, one problem became apparent: the various electronic granting systems of NIH, NSF, ONR, and other large federal agencies placed a large burden on scientists and research administrators. Each system required different technologies, in turn requiring that grantee institutions employ a wide range of expertise in order to use the systems. Despite pressure from grantees to agree on a common approach to grant applications, the NIH Commons and NSF FastLane electronic grant application projects continued along separate paths under a "let many flowers grow" philosophy. However, three notable efforts were underway to provide a governance structure and more consistent approach to ERA that would alleviate this burden on the grantees:

1. Research and Management Systems, Inc. (or RAMS)

DOE funded a cooperative agreement proposed by Federal Information Exchange, Inc. (known as Research and Management Systems, Inc. or RAMS) to bring grantors and grantees together to develop a mutually beneficial approach to electronic research administration:

> DOE *has entered into an agreement with RAMS to establish a pilot project for the electronic transmission and processing of grant proposals for the Nation's colleges and universities. The purpose of the two-year project is to establish the system whereby an academic organization can receive, process and submit an application for federal funds, and whereby DOE can process and ultimately award the grant electronically. RAMS President, John Rodman called this process "electronic research administration (ERA)" to describe both the submission and the processing of the grant application.* (6)

Based on the success of an initial 1992 feasibility study, a three-year multi-agency cooperative agreement entitled, "Electronic Research Administration (ERA) Demonstration Project" (NewERA) was funded in 1994. On the agency side, the effort was lead by DOE and supported by other agencies interested in an improved grant application process including ONR, NIH, ARO, AFOSR, Army Medical Command, and the US Treasury. Participating grantees included well-known research universities that also saw the advantage of electronic research administration including Penn State, MIT, Notre Dame, Southern University, Duke, UCLA, Baylor Medical, Fred Hutchinson Cancer Research Center, Florida A&M, and North Carolina State University. (5)

The NewERA Project assisted in the development and testing of the 194 grant application standard and 850 award notification; promoted cooperative development; assisted in testing and involvement of all interested stakeholders in ERA; provided guidelines for streamlining grant management processes and paperwork; and implemented the first pilot submission of a secure electronic grant application to DOE and ONR (using RAMS grant management software from some of the pilot institutions).

2. Federal Demonstration Partnership (FDP) (7)

Another cooperative effort among grantors and grantees was established under the Federal Demonstration Partnership (FDP). The FDP, first started as the Florida Demonstration Project in 1985, had successfully established uniform federal procedures among the participating federal agencies. These uniform procedures helped reduce the administrative burden that grantees were experiencing when trying to remain compliant with policy rules that were different for every agency. The FDP began as an effort among five federal agencies and the Florida State University System and the University of Miami. The significant success of this effort led to the program's expansion in 1989 to the Federal Demonstration Project, involving eleven federal agencies and 21 institutions and consortia across the country. The 1993 NPR report also cited the FDP, in cooperation with the Office of Management and Budget (OMB), as the organizational model and demonstration focus for looking at ways to reduce administrative burden.

In 1996 the FDP entered its third phase involving the same federal agencies, sixty-five institutions, and six affiliate members, with the goal of guiding the developments in ERA to continue the improvement of the administrative process. Significantly, the FDP effort included research investigators, not just administrators, in their deliberations to keep the focus on allowing the researchers to spend less time on administration and more time on their research. This phase of the FDP broadened its original scope and focus to include electronic research administration (ERA) reengineered systems and procedures with increased productivity and decreased administrative burden. This phase formed five task forces studying specific aspects of ERA, including:

1. Electronic Notification of Awards: To design a standard electronic dataset to transmit award information.
2. Professional Profiles: To design an electronic dataset for static professional data.
3. Institutional Profiles: To design an electronic dataset for static institutional information.
4. Electronic Routing and Approval Systems: To investigate, design, test, and distribute alternative solutions for routing and approval systems.

5. Integrated Performance Standards: To identify opportunities to standardize and simplify business rules and performance standards associated with Federal Research Assistance.

3. Electronic Commerce Committee (ECC)

The third governance effort was strictly on the grantor side. The Electronic Commerce Committee (ECC) evolved from the disparate efforts of the various federal research agencies as a means of establishing a coordinated effort. The ECC attracted representatives from thirteen federal agencies and organizations (including several non-research entities). Together they pursued the following three goals: (8)

1. Establish consistency in the exchange of federal grant data.
2. Ensure that electronic commerce efforts in grants are conducted in a manner that uses fiscal and human resources effectively.
3. Improve information sharing among the agencies.

The ECC successfully gained agreement among the participating agencies for a common set of data elements that would support electronic grant proposals for all participating agencies. The ECC was able to get this data set approved and published as "The ANSI ASC X12 EDI Transaction Set 194 (194 TS)" in December 1995. The implementation convention for the 194 TS was subsequently drawn up and approved in January 1997. This common set of data elements for grant applications formed the basis for today's current ERA standards used by the federal government.

Crossing the ERA Technology Chasm (1997 to 2001)

This period was a critical one for two sectors, universities and government, both which played major roles in the establishment of standard electronic processes for grants.

The end of the early years left much hope and some frustration for the participants. Significant progress had been made toward the guiding principals of ERA:

• A data standard for the grant application had been approved by ANSI.
• The NewERA pilot project successfully demonstrated electronic grant applications to DOE and ONR using the new EDI standard.

• The FDP had streamlined grant policies and improved communication between government and universities.

In 1997 leaders, such as the NIH's Geoff Grant, Brad Stanford of ONR, and Jean Morrow at the DOE, predicted that the government grant operations would be completely electronic by the year 2000. *Crossing the Chasm* pioneers on both sides of the grant-making equation agreed that what was soon to be called electronic research administration (ERA) was expected to have a ten-year span, from 1990 to 2000. (10) One can see in Figure 30-1 the revised Technology Adoption Life Cycle for the adoption of the ERA Life Cycle. Ten years later ERA was and continues to take longer for adoption and success than any of the pioneers and innovators had ever thought it would take. (9)

In 1997 the momentum and direction of ERA became unclear. Several agencies had implemented their own initiatives (notably NSF's Fastlane) that were agency-specific, and that did not integrate with other government solutions. At the same time, the Office of Science and Technology Policy (OSTP) and the Office of Management and Budget (OMB) did not fully accept the business case for ERA, and university pioneers felt it was taking too long for the government to move toward cohesive approval. Pioneers had built a solid foundation for ERA with many of the early concepts on technology, standards, and security having been embraced by the early ERA adopters. As with many pioneering endeavors, the ideas and enthusiasm were ahead of the technical capability, marketplace, and the human factor of change acceptance.

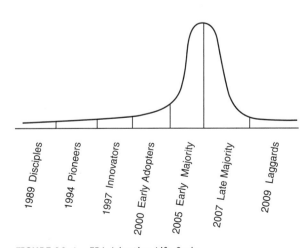

FIGURE 30-1 ERA Adoption Life Cycle.

Universities Stalled at the Early Adopter Stage

During this time period the university early adopters were affected by the federal reinvention effort in two ways:

1. *Regulatory requirements from the federal agencies increased significantly.* The increase in regulations required more complex processes, more skilled personnel, and enhanced information systems at the grantee organization.

2. *A growing number of federal ERA systems were not following the standards approach that would allow an ERA system at a grantee institution to send the data directly to the agency's ERA system.* Instead, these new ERA systems were requiring the researchers and their administrators to interact directly with the agency's own Web-based system.

MIT had licensed COEUS to many other institutions. The GAMS Consortium had grown to include NC State, Ohio State University Research Foundation, the University of Michigan, Oklahoma State University, and the University of Massachusetts. PeopleSoft and Oracle, prominent providers of enterprise software (e.g., finance, human resources) to academic institutions, had developed ERA modules in their products.

Because of the nonstandard ERA approach by federal agencies, grantees with these internal ERA systems had to do double work: interact with their own institution's ERA system and re-enter the same information on the agency's ERA system. These early adopters believed they did not receive the support from the government agencies regarding electronic application standards and the implementation of ERA to make returns on their early investments.

At this time, a major frustration among participants was that the federal government was not yet able to accept electronic grant applications on a system-to-system basis. NSF, the only agency that required submission of all applications electronically through its FastLane system, required a scientist to submit his or her application to NSF via an online Web-based application form in FastLane. FastLane was not developed using the ANSI standard for grant data, and NSF was not concerned with the effect this approach was having on the universities that had ERA systems.

Following the NSF model, other federal agencies like ONR, NASA, and the Department of Education were developing and testing their own Web-based ERA solutions. The proliferation of government electronic application systems was more time and work at the grantee organizations than the old paper process. One major goal of ERA in the early years was for the grantees to have one face to the government, a "one-stop shop" approach. This was not happening despite the promises and the governance efforts of the ECC and the FDP.

In addition, even though electronic commerce promised tremendous value to universities and the sponsors they served, research administrators were finding it difficult to obtain the needed financial and IT support required to implement ERA systems. During this time, university IT organizations were also consumed with projects to replace core systems (e.g., finance, human resources, and student administration).

Most of ERA efforts during the mid-1990's were being led by the pre-award offices at universities. Research administrators understood the benefits of ERA and spoke of the need to stay competitive in the implementation and use of such technology. However, research administrators frequently found university leadership hard to convince regarding the benefits of ERA; therefore, university adoption of ERA remained slow.

More widespread adoption by the "early majority" and "late majority" (as described in Moore's *Crossing the Chasm*) was slowed by the investment required, the lack of firm direction at the federal agencies, and the troubling experience of the early adopters. To be effective, the new federal ERA systems required comparable software and technology at the grantee organizations with which to interact and exchange data. Faculty and university administrators were dependent on the research organization to enable their institution to capitalize on electronic commerce.

Research administrators were expected to invest in information technology and the skills to manage them. Under the paper system, budgets of research administration organizations consisted primarily of personnel salaries and did not accommodate capital investments of this magnitude. This was a fundamental change for a research administration organization that had traditionally relied on paper systems and received little support from the university's IT organizations.

The Commons Approach Starts

In March 1998, the NIH's Geoff Grant proposed the idea of a Federal ERA Commons. This idea was first proposed to the Electronic Commerce Committee (ECC), and then to the Federal Demonstration Partnership (FDP). Geoff saw this as a way for the federal government to provide a common face to the grants community, as desired by many grantees in the FDP and other forums. The Government Services Administration (GSA), which had responsibility for government-wide IT projects, requested that the Federal ERA Commons idea be enlarged to include all grants, not just research grants. GSA agreed to help fund a broadened initial demonstration.

A group, formed under the ECC to design such a system, later became the Federal Commons Subcommittee. The proposed Federal Commons system would act as a single broker for the federal agencies and the grantees. The broker would handle standard electronic transactions and technologies from grantees and pass the information to each agency in its required format.

For the university ERA systems to send their proposal information through the broker, the standard information that would be requested by the agency, collected in the institution's ERA system and sent electronically, had to be specified. In the case of grant applications, this standard had already been established (the ANSI EDI 194 TS for grant applications).

The Federal Commons approach would provide substantial benefits to universities that needed to submit proposals to many different federal agencies and programs. The institution's ERA system would only have to connect to one electronic proposal system (the Federal Commons), eliminating the need to learn how to interface and manage dozens of proprietary systems.

By the end of the 1990s, large private health foundations were also implementing ERA systems. A group of these foundations (lead by the American Cancer Society, the Alzheimer's Association, and the Cystic Fibrosis Foundation) proposed a common application system: the Foundation Commons, akin to the Federal Commons effort. The group worked with Research and Management Systems (RAMS) to develop and implement a common electronic system that would reflect the review systems already shared by many foundations. After initial success, the Arthritis Foundation and many other foundations quickly joined the Foundation Commons, renamed proposalCENTRAL, which in 2004 was processing applications for twenty-two foundations and more than 6,000 applicants through a single Web site.

In November 1999, the *Federal Financial Assistance Management Improvement Act of 1999*, more commonly known as *Public Law 106-107*, was signed into law and in 11 short sections sought to:

1. improve the effectiveness and performance of federal financial assistance programs;
2. simplify federal financial assistance application and reporting requirements;
3. improve the delivery of services to the public; and
4. facilitate greater coordination among those responsible for delivering such services.

Congress established an 18-month time frame to carry out these actions (May 20, 2001). While the President signed this bill into law and thus shared the responsibility, it should be noted that he did so reluctantly, citing the short time frame for implementation and the lack of funding.

According to the law, the use of a "common application and reporting system" is mandated. As previously noted, one of the objectives of the Federal Commons was to provide the common face to federal research-related grant making, thus becoming an umbrella system for submission technology alternatives available to the research community. Hence, the Federal Commons was the logical system of choice for the 106-107 mandate.

With respect to implementation, it is also essential to note that OMB notified Congress that the 18-month deadline specified in the law would be interpreted to be the deadline for the submission of agency plans, not the deadline for the implementation of those plans.

On December 17, 1999, the President released "Electronic Government," a memorandum for the heads of executive departments and agencies. The directive of the memorandum was for executive departments and agencies, in conjunction with the private sector, as appropriate, to help citizens gain one-stop access to existing government information and services, and to provide better, more efficient government services and increased government accountability.

In the summer of 2002, GSA appointed the Department of Health and Human Services (DHHS) as the lead agency for a government-wide ERA effort, e-Grants. As part of President Bush's efforts to streamline government costs, the e-Grants effort received a significant boost in support. Within the first 18 months, e-Grants developed the Find and Apply portions of the grants management cycle. The e-Grants project was rebranded as Grants.gov in the summer of 2003. For fiscal year 2004–2005, the Grants.gov budget was scheduled to be $11.3m. (10)

The Grants.gov Web site defines itself as a simple, unified "storefront" for all customers of federal programs, providing a single, streamlined process for over 900 grant programs offered by twenty-six federal agencies. Collectively, Grants.gov processes have a potential to award over $350 billion grant resources annually to state and local governments, academia, not-for-profits, and other organizations. Grants.gov is one of the twenty-four federal cross-agency e-Government initiatives.

The charter of Grants.gov, one of 24 President's Management Agenda E-Government initiatives, is to provide a simple, unified electronic storefront for interactions between grant applicants and the Federal agencies that manage grant funds. There are 26 Federal grant-making agencies and over 900 individual grant programs that award over $350 billion in grants each year. The grant community, including state, local and tribal governments, academia and research institutions, and not-for-profits, need only visit one website, Grants.gov, to access the annual grant funds available across the Federal government. For an overview of Grants.gov, please review our Vision and Goals (.pdf). In short, Grants.gov provides:

- A single source for finding grant opportunities.
- A standardized manner of locating and learning more about funding opportunities.
- A single, secure, and reliable source for applying for Federal grants online.
- A simplified grant application process with reduction of paperwork.
- A unified interface for all agencies to announce their grant opportunities, and for all grant applicants to find and apply for those opportunities.

In addition to simplifying the grant application process, Grants.gov also creates avenues for consolidation and best practices within each grant-making agency. Grant-making Agencies and Grants.gov Partners (.pdf) provides a list of Grant-making agencies and Grants.gov partners. (11)

As part of its Phase II (from February 2004 to February 2006), Grants.gov plans:

1. Integration of the Find and Apply mechanisms;
2. Deployment of enhancements to Find and Apply mechanisms;
3. Definition of data standards for reporting;
4. Deployment of reporting functionality;

5. Definition of data standards for mandatory grant applications;
6. Deployment of mandatory grant application functionality;
7. Definition of Version 2 core data standards.

Plans for phase III (from February 2006 to September 2007) include: (12)

1. Implementation of further enhancements to Find and Apply mechanisms;
2. Implementation of enhanced reporting mechanisms and mandatory grants application mechanisms;
3. Identification of Version 3 core data standards;
4. Development of closeout data standards;
5. Deployment of closeout functionality;
6. Development of awards data standards;
7. Deployment award functionality.

NIH Pioneer a New Model for Implementing ERA with Grantees

In September 2001 as part of the first major federal effort to help fund small businesses that provide ERA software and services to the grantee organizations, NIH awarded six Small Business Innovation Research (SBIR) grants for ERA to the six companies: RAMS, eRA Solutions, Formatta, InfoEd, Cayuse, and Clinical Tools.

The paperless transfer of extramural research grant application and administrative data was and still is NIH's vision for the 21st century. Now, consistent with the government-wide mandate to migrate from paper-based to electronic systems ("e-Gov"), the NIH had undertaken an enterprise-wide ERA Project. ERA integrates two parallel systems: NIH Commons and IMPAC II. NIH Commons is the external grantee customer interface and IMPAC II is the internal NIH customer interface.

Scope & Purpose

Commons, n. A meeting place used by a community as a whole, especially for the exchange of information. For the purposes of exchanging research grants administration information, the NIH provides this "Commons." The Electronic Research Administration (ERA) Commons is a virtual meeting place where NIH extramural grantee organizations, grantees, and the public can receive and transmit information about the administration of biomedical and behavioral research. (13)

Early on, NIH recognized that a large number of grantee organizations might not independently develop all of the capabilities needed to interact fully with the NIH Commons. While midsize and smaller organizations account for fewer than 20% of overall NIH applications, more than 2,100 of these size organizations submit and obtain funds from the NIH—overall, a significant number. NIH, to meet the needs of these organizations, works with small business to develop ERA tools for purchase by their grantee organizations. (14)

Much of the ERA focus had and continues to be on the pre-award electronic development and submission of grant applications, status checking and award notification. However, in the *NCURA RMR Journal* (Winter/Spring 2001) William Irving of PricewaterhouseCoopers LLP (15) says that the ERA solution needs to be a system of records, secure and auditable by the federal government. This is an important ERA function that will have to be addressed more fully in the coming years to ensure ERA success.

Comparing Alternative ERA Models

Table 30-1 summarizes the comparison of various characteristics and capabilities that would exist in the local (one-stop shopping) and the agency-based models (e.g., NIH ERA Commons, Grants. gov, NSF FastLane).

In interviews and surveys done by Mr. Bill Kirby, Consultant, Bearing Point, and Dr. Michael Dingerson, Professor, Higher Education, Old Dominion University, in Winter 2003 and Spring 2004, researchers and institutional officials were asked about the characteristics and capabilities of ERA systems. Cited by officials as most important were:

Local control of profiles. Researchers and institutional officials preferred a single system to facilitate management of proposal information, including profile information, and did not support the mantenance of profile information on an agency-based system (e.g., NIH Commons), while also maintaining other proposal-related information in a locally housed system. Researchers and institutional officials believe that the profile data should be integrated with the proposal development process.

A "one-stop shopping" model. Institutional officials do not want a proliferation of different systems accommodating different sponsors or required for different processes. They want a single system from which requirements for mul-

tiple sponsors and all aspects of the grant "life cycle" can be generated. In order for commercial software products to be acceptable and viable, they must be designed to accommodate multiple sponsors. A commercial system that is designed just to NIH ERA requirements *only* is not a viable option.

ERA systems as management systems. Almost all officials interviewed used local databases and software to track proposals and help in award management. Most officials envisaged an effective ERA system as the engine to create such databases: for example, the creation of a CGAP 398 NIH or other proposals will populate local database tables, which will be used to generate management information and automate tasks. Agency-based systems (NIH ERA Commons, NSF FastLane, the proposed e-grants initiative, for example) do not provide this kind of capability, but do supply reporting agency-specific information. Still, the institution must assemble information across hundreds of agencies and organizations that support them through sponsored projects. In a model where the application information originates under institution control, this problem is eliminated. This issue has driven large grant recipients, like MIT, to invest in substantial ERA systems. Smaller institutions have similar needs, but not the resources to develop, implement, and maintain a system as complex as MIT's. While not all institutions have these needs, it is an important requirement for institutions considering an investment in ERA software. This finding also buttresses the need for locally based systems to handle ERA tasks.

Integration with institutional workflow and approvals. Similarly, almost all institutions envisage some form of internal workflow and approval automation as a by-product of an ERA system. Again, agency-based systems do not provide this capability. Frequently mentioned capabilities included:

- Proposal routing and approval.
- Electronic notifications of award.
- Work schedules and ticklers.
- Automated alerts to principle investigators and department administrators for deadlines, closeouts, and renewal dates.
- Automated process to facilitate initial accounting entries in the account set-up process. This would require some level of integration with the institutional accounting system.

The real definition and success of ERA remains an open question. While there have been many

TABLE 30-1	A Comparison of Key Characteristics of a Local Institutional ERA Software Model with Various Federal ERA Models

Local Model	Agency-Based Model	Federal E-Grants Model
One-stop shopping for multiple sponsors	Separate systems for each sponsor	One stop shopping for multiple sponsors
Integrates institutional workflow, approvals	Limited workflow capability	Limited workflow capability
Interfaces with local data sources (HR, financial)	No data interface	No data interface
Requires investment in software	No software investment required	No software investment required
Requires database, software maintenance	No maintenance required	No maintenance required
Provides control of and custom reporting	Limited reporting options	Limited reporting options
Local control of information dissemination	Limited control of dissemination	Limited control of dissemination
Profile information can be used for multiple sponsors or local institutional purposes	Profile information developed for single sponsor requirements	Unknown
Training required on single system	Training required on multiple systems	Training required on single system
Requires network access	Universal access (browser only requirement)	Universal access (browser only requirement)
Local security and privacy	Agency security; multiple access requirements (ID/passwords)	Security controlled at central source; presumably single password access

advances with cooperation between all parties involved in the research process, there are still challenges of technology implementation, security, regulations, and grantee acceptance of a paperless process.

Toward the Future (2005 to 2010)

In regard to the technology adoption life cycle as discussed at the beginning of this chapter, we estimate that the group defined as "laggards" (the last adopters of the technology) will participate in ERA by 2009, some twenty years after the first disciples of ERA. We believe that the majority of grantee organizations will have adapted electronic business processes by 2008. We anticipate that the federal government will have fully adopted electronic proposal submission, electronic notification, and electronic reporting by 2009, and federal agencies will no longer accept paper submissions (grant or other data) to process an estimated $400 billion dollars in grant funds for 2010.

Grantee Organizations

In coming years, all grantee organizations will be driven to change to comply with the federal govern-

ment ERA processes. But we believe, more importantly, that they will be driven more by need to develop better proposal and award management capabilities, including integration with local financial and human resource systems.

By the end of the decade, grantee organizations will have in-house systems (either developed or purchased from vendors) to provide seamless interface with federal government and private foundations. Universities will have the capability of a "one stop electronic shop" for federal government grants: a system that will include electronic grant opportunities, submission, award notification, status, compliance, annual financial and project reporting, and award closeout. Auditing of ERA systems will exist as part of an organization-wide audit system that will examine the record-keeping requirements and security of ERA practices.

In addition, products developed by major and boutique software vendors will provide tailored applications to grantee organizations for ERA processes. These products will include a sophisticated proposal development application (budget development tools, rules-based data checking, prefilled forms from legacy databases); capability to allow investigators to tailor professional profiles for each application; collaboration with colleagues from other institutions; integration with financial, payroll, and human resource databases; and workflow capability including institutional routing and approval of grant applications. Also, a compliance module will share protocol documents among committee members. Functions will include online discussions by reviewers, Web meeting agendas, Web meeting minutes, automatic notification via Web for committee members and the PI regarding deliverables and interface with clinical trial modules, and compliance with the Health Insurance Portability and Accountability Act (HIPAA). Finally, the post-award module will provide deliverables, status, and subcontracting capability and a transfer file to the legacy accounting system. There may also be a module that provides Web reports to the PI, office of sponsored programs, and dean, showing budget to expenditure by account, "hit rate," science trends, etc. As the technology progresses, this information will be available via wireless handheld devices, and push technology will provide the latest information to investigators and grantee organizations. For the small and micro grantee organizations, application service providers (ASP) will provide the same grant management functionality and services that we discussed above, based on a fee-for-transaction model.

By 2010, we envision that the PI will be able to develop a proposal via the Web from anywhere in the world. His/her home institution will route and approve the application, submit it electronically to the appropriate federal agency or foundation program, and obtain assurance the proposal was received. Application information standards will be implemented, and the information collected for each grant program will be similar if not exact. The PI and institutional profile data will not have to be entered with each application. The authenticated institutional profile will be centralized and accepted by the federal, state, local, and foundation agencies. The detailed investigator profile, including detailed publication information, will be kept in one place (locally) and made available to the sponsors with appropriate security. The investigator will have the ability to tailor his/her bio-sketch for each specific application submitted. In addition, the PI or organization will be able to electronically check the status of the application as it goes through the review process; obtain the award notification or rejection along with reviewers' comments; request continuations, renewals, and extensions; provide all reporting requirements—financial, technical, and compliance; and close out the account. ERA, when fully implemented, will provide major benefits to the PIs and allow them to concentrate on research and not administration.

Government Organizations

By 2010, agencies will begin reaping the benefits of electronic grants by more effective staffing, paper savings, and process efficiencies. Common costing algorithms will allow spreading of systems maintenance and improvement costs throughout the grant community, supporting the extension of interoperating systems, and discouraging the instigation of agency-specific ones. In addition, usage-based transaction charges will be formulated to share the costs of electronic development and transmission of documents by the grantee community, taking the place of previous paper, postal, and package delivery charges. Enhanced collaboration with the state components of federal programs should enforce the interoperability of common federal systems with those of the states and endorse state funding allocations for use on common systems development. Advanced business cases covering the total cost of ownership will prove the efficacy of common, interconnected government systems compared to suboptimized, individual agency, and program systems.

Success of streamlining legislation such as the Government Paperwork Elimination Act (GPEA) and PL 106-107 will lead to extension or renewal of legislation that carries forward the principles of grant process simplification and burden reduction, and strengthens the influence of the Office of Management and Budget in supporting their implementation. In particular, the GAO audit of PL 106-107[1] in 2006 should give good marks to its implementation effort and recommend continuation for the next five years or so. By 2010 progress on grants automation and interagency collaboration should be a routine part of agency reporting under the GPRA, and interoperation of IT systems for grants a routine requirement.

Innovations in Internet protocols and improved reliability of their capabilities will, by the end of this decade, lead to new concepts for exchange of grant information. For example, the concept of a proposal submission may change from the physical passing of a weighty paper document to a simple coded notification. The proposing institution will

---

[1]The Federal Financial Assistance Management Improvement Act of 1999, also known as Public Law 106-107, is the statute that underlies the agencies' efforts to streamline and simplify the grants and cooperative agreements administrative process.

retain possession of all the proposal information (profiles, descriptive text, pictures, graphs, holograms or other electronic media) in an escrowed part of its Web site. The institution will then use a certified protocol to notify the potential granting agency of the proposal availability, giving the agency permission to view that information for purposes of screening and review. The agency can use this view itself or automatically transfer its permission to selected reviewers based on reviewer restrictions and eligibilities. Automated collection of review comments, scoring algorithms, and agency funding constraints will speed and simplify the decision-making and approval process. All issues of format, appearance, changes during transmission, security, or storage in transit will be eliminated. Such ideas are only the beginning of the potential for improving the overall research administration process.

Nonprofit Organizations

By the end of this decade, foundations that provide peer-reviewed research funding to scientists at universities, colleges, research institutes, and hospitals will have a robust ERA system. These private foundations, similar to the federal government, will provide for electronic submission of applications, electronic peer review, status checking, award notification, reporting, and final close out.

Many of the health research foundations are currently working together via proposalCENTRAL and are developing a "common application" within the 194 transaction set, with a few specific foundation exemptions. Some pioneering foundations have already implemented mandatory electronic grant application, peer review, and award notification. These implementations seem to have been much easier for private foundations than their government agency counterparts. The major efficiencies and savings brought about by electronic commerce will speed ERA implementation at private foundations.

Researchers who receive funding from both federal agencies and foundations will come to demand a one-stop-shop approach for ERA. In response, foundations will work with the federal government to share institutional and professional profile information. By 2009 ERA systems and service providers will be available to offer researchers and institutions a common interface with federal and foundation grantors.

State and Local Agencies

Implementation of ERA at the state and local level will become active in 2006 after early successful ERA implementation by federal agencies and private foundations. The same state and local government organizations are major players in the grant business (as both grantors and grantees) and are essential for successful implementation of ERA. By 2010, state and local governments will also be integrated with the federal ERA efforts.

Summary

ERA has come a long way in the last decade, but within the next five years its real value will come to fruition, as was promised by its early proponents and participants. The growth in electronic grants systems at both grantor and grantee organizations will have a tremendous impact on staffing, training, technology, and organizational development. Within the next several years, ERA focus will shift from the technology to the use of the electronic grant information for more strategic purposes. The integrated grant information based on early ERA systems will help provide a basis for knowledge in management, community identification, development of "big science," and a more efficient and effective research enterprise in the United States and abroad.

Like any major cultural change, the transition from a paper system to ERA has taken much longer than the pioneers and the early adopters had hoped. It has been ten years since the first pilot electronic grant submission via the Internet was demonstrated by the RAMS consortium. Since then, development and advances in standards, technology, and engineering ensure successful, universal implementation of ERA by the end of this decade.

Authors' Note: The authors want to express their thanks and recognize James McKee, Michael Dingerson, and Bill Kirby for their insights and contributions.

• • • References

1. Weber, Marc et al. *Making of the World Wide Web.* 1997. http://www.webhistory.org/project/book.html (accessed September 29, 2005).
2. Gersner, L. V. Unpublished remarks made at the IBM Higher Education Executive Forum. Jamie McKee, IBM Consultant attended, now working with RAMS, Inc. Germantown MD.
3. Stanford, Brad. ERA Update Presentation, national meeting of NCURA, Washington, DC, November 10, 1993.

4. National Institutes of Health, U.S. Department of Health and Human Services. iEdison home page, https://s-edison.info.nih.gov/iEdison (accessed August 6, 2005).

5. Rodman, John. *New ERA Project*, funded by U.S. Department of Energy, 1994–1996. Germantown, MD.

6. *Electronic Public Information Newsletter* 4, No. 16 (August 12, 1994).

7. Federal Demonstration Partnership. "About FDP—History," http://www.thefdp.org/About_FDP.html (accessed August 6, 2005).

8. Logistics Management Institute. "EC Project Plan," *Federal Support Electronic Commerce Committee*. LMI: Washington DC, May 1996, 17–23.

9. Moore, Geoffrey A. "The Technology Adoption Life Cycle." *Crossing the Chasm*. New York: HarperBusiness, 1991.

10. Springer, Linda. *Memorandum*. Office of Management and the Budget, June 18, 2004.

11. Grants.gov. "About Us," http://www.grants.gov/AboutUs (accessed August 6, 2005).

12. Havekost, Charles. Grants.gov Planning Presentation, Grants.gov stakeholder meeting, September 24, 2003. Washington, DC.

13. National Institutes of Health, ERA Commons. "Scope and Purpose," https://commons.era.nih.gov/commons/scopeAndPurpose.jsp (accessed August 6, 2005).

14. SRA Newsletter (electronic publication), Volume 34, No. 4, Sept 2002

15. Irving, William S. "Electronic Research Administration—Forward View: Auditing, Record Keeping, and Security," *NCURA RMR Journal* 12, No. 1 (Winter/Spring 2001), http://www.ncura.edu/data/rmrd/pdf/v12n1.pdf (accessed September 29, 2005).

CHAPTER

31

Preparing a Budget for a Research Project

William H. Caskey, MS, PhD

Introduction

A budget for a research project is a funding plan that itemizes specific cost categories related to the goals as stated in the project's proposal. The budget should flow logically from the proposal narrative. It is important to remember that a budget is an estimate of the costs to be incurred during the performance of the project. The development of a comprehensive and accurate budget is crucial to the success of a proposal, as sponsors and their reviewers are trained to discern inappropriate budgets.

Sponsors often have very specific guidelines for the preparation of budgets. The guidelines may limit the maximum costs or exclude a specific category, such as equipment. Such guidelines should be followed explicitly during proposal development. However, the general principles discussed in the following sections are separated into universal categories and agency guidelines that typically include these categories. This chapter focuses on research budget preparation, but the basic principles discussed apply to other types of projects as well (including construction, demonstration, equipment, training, or service projects).

Multi-Year Projects

For multi-year proposals, a cumulative project budget and a budget for each year is usually prepared. The initial annual budget is prepared in detail and subsequent annual budgets are based on the anticipated flow of work and cost increases

(e.g., inflation and salary adjustments). Inflation factors can be related, at least to some extent, to the Consumer Price Index[1] or Biomedical Research and Development Price Index.[2] Sponsors often publish the inflation factors that should be used.

Regulations Regarding Project Costs

Budgets must be prepared in accordance with well-established, applicable cost principles. In the absence of specific sponsor or program guidelines, the applicant institution should adhere to the relevant federal document establishing cost principles for consistency. Discussion of these documents is beyond the scope of this article, but the documents are listed in Table 31-1.

All of these policies and principles are codified for each federal agency by department.[3] Of these documents, those specifying cost principles are the most relevant to budget preparation. And, each federal agency implements the regulations in grant preparation or policy publications. The National Institutes of Health (NIH) offers the *Grants Policy Statement*[4] and the National Science Foundation publishes the *Grant Proposal Guide*[5] and the *Grant Policy Manual*[6]; other agencies publish similar documents. For proposals that result in a contract, the Federal Acquisition Regulations (FARS)[7] will become applicable, imposing additional regulations. Under these principles, allowable costs for research projects must:

- *Be reasonable.* A reasonable cost requires "the nature of the goods or services acquired or applied, and the amount involved therefore,

TABLE 31-1	Documents Establishing Cost Principles and Administrative and Audit Requirements for Federally Funded Projects by Type of Institution
States, local governments, and Indian tribes	OMB A-87 for cost principles[8] OMB A-102 for administrative requirements[9] OMB A-133 for audit requirements[10]
Educational Institutions (including state colleges and universities)	OMB A-21 for cost principles[11] OMB A-110 for administrative requirements[12] OMB A-133 for audit requirements[10]
Non-profit organizations	OMB A-122 for cost principles[13] OMB A-110 for administrative requirements[12] OMB A-133 for audit requirements[10]
Hospitals	45 CFR 74, Appendix E (OASC-3) for cost principles[14] OMB A-110 for administrative requirements[12] OMB A-133 for audit requirements[10]

reflect the action that a prudent person would have taken under the circumstances prevailing at the time the decision to incur the cost was made (OMB A-21, Section C.3)."[11] The estimate should be consistent with the cost for the same or similar goods or services in the area in which they are acquired at the time of acquisition.

- *Be allocable.* A cost is allocable if "the goods or services involved are chargeable or assignable to such cost objective in accordance with the relative benefits received or other equitable relationship" (OMB A-21, C.4).[11] The cost of goods or services must clearly be identifiable as related to the research effort.

- *Be given consistent treatment* through the application of generally accepted accounting principles.

- *Conform to any limitations or exclusions* set forth by the document or those of the sponsor.

Two general types of costs are associated with research projects: *direct costs* and *facilities and administrative costs* (these are defined in the relevant documents establishing cost principles). Direct costs are those that "can be identified specifically with a particular sponsored project, an instructional activity, or any other institutional activity, or that can be directly assigned to such activities relatively easily with a high degree of accuracy" (OMB A-21, Section D.1).[11] Facilities and administrative (F&A) costs are those that "are incurred for common or joint objectives and, therefore, cannot be identified readily or specifically with a particular sponsored project, an instructional activity, or any other institutional activity."[11] F&A costs are nego-

tiated by institutional officials with their cognizant agency and applied using the formula established in the current rate agreement. Therefore, the focus of budget preparation is on estimation of direct costs.

Direct costs fall into one of nine general categories: (NOTE: F&A is not a direct cost, so the number of categories equals nine.)

1. *Personnel.* Salaries and fringe benefits of employees of the applicant institution constitute this category. The budget should include compensation only for those persons involved in the conduct of the project and the charges should be proportional to their effort. Generally, the name, role on the project, and percentage effort should be specified. Charges are based on the appropriate percentage of their institutional base salary and applicable fringe benefit rate. Calculations for persons on annual appointments are straight-forward, but, for those on other types of appointments (e.g., academic year), the salary should be calculated accordingly. For example, research technicians are often on annual appointments, so a 50% effort would translate into a charge of one-half of their annual salary. A faculty member on an academic year appointment might devote 25% effort during the academic year and 50% during the summer, so the requested salary should be itemized accordingly and should reflect the different fringe benefit rates as well.

   Institutional base salaries must be in compliance with standard institutional policies. If the personnel are current employees, then current salaries should be used. If new positions are to be created, then the salaries should be consistent with other similar positions within the institution. Human resources departments should be contacted for assistance in determining current base salaries or establishing an appropriate salary for a new position.

Fringe benefits are based on a number of factors that vary by class of employee and by institution. Again, human resources departments should be consulted to determine the applicable rates.

2. *Consultants*. A consultant is an individual or firm retained to provide professional advice or services on a project for a fee. Limitations on consultants are imposed by sponsors and vary greatly. Generally, institutions must have written policies governing their use of consultants that are consistently applied regardless of the source of support. A consultant is usually not an employee of the applicant institution, but unusual circumstances may permit an employee who works as a consultant. Such circumstances must be defined by written policies. All costs associated with the consultant should be itemized in this category, including travel, subsistence, and honorarium and designated as the fee, which may be a per-unit fee. OMB Circular A-21 does not limit consultant costs, but requires the costs be reasonable in relation to the services rendered and consistent with past practice. However, some agencies, such as the National Science Foundation, limit costs to a published daily fee excluding travel and other expenses if services or advice provided by consultants do not constitute a substantial or significant portion of the proposed work. If the portion of work to be conducted is determined to be substantial or significant, then a consortium or contractual agreement must be established with the institution and a principal investigator identified.

3. *Equipment*. These are nonexpendable articles having a useful life of more than one year and costing less than $5,000 (or other amount specified by the applicant organization). The equipment must be required for the performance of the research and must not otherwise be available at the applicant institution. Clearly defined specifications of the equipment should be provided to prospective vendors in order to estimate purchase costs. Since the equipment is required for the conduct of the research, maintenance should be a consideration. Maintenance agreements may be charged as direct costs for the duration of a project but should be included in the budget in the category of other expenses. If the equipment is to be used for more than one project, then the portion charged for each project for both the purchase and maintenance agreement should be proportional to the use for that project.

4. *Supplies*. Supplies are tangible items with a useful life of less than one year. Only those items to be consumed during the conduct of the pro-

posed project should be listed. Grouping the individual supplies by categories, such as "plastic ware and glassware" or "tissue culture supplies," simplifies the presentation. If animals are to be used in the project, purchase of animals should be listed in this category specifying the species and number to be purchased. If office supplies or similar items are included, care must be taken to ensure the costs are allocable, that is, that the supplies purchased are consumed solely for the purposes of the funded research.

5. *Travel*. Most sponsors provide funding for travel, but some do not. If travel funds are requested, the purpose, destination, and number of individuals traveling should be specified for each trip. Travel to foreign destinations is usually scrutinized more closely by sponsors and reviewers. Investigators should be encouraged to include travel costs to attend scientific meetings to disseminate results from the project. Since the destination of meetings in the later years of a project may not be known, average costs for domestic or foreign sites, whichever is applicable, may be used.

6. *Patient Care*. Costs associated with patient care should be separated into two categories: inpatient and outpatient. However, the details for each category should be developed in the same manner. Patient care costs are those specifically related to treatment or interventions directly related to or required for the research. Reimbursement to patients for travel and subsistence and stipends should be included in the category of other expenses. Details should include the frequency and number of times each procedure is performed for each patient and the number of patients to be enrolled. The budget justification should include an explanation of the charges and an estimate of the rate of patient accrual.

If "Other Support" for patient care is anticipated, details of that support should be included in the budget justification. Such support can be provided by a pharmaceutical sponsor or third-party payer. And, when a General Clinical Research Center (GCRC) funded by the NIH is sponsoring the trial, details of the GCRC budget requirements need to be included in the budget justification.

7. *Alterations and Renovations*. Alterations and renovation charges include any capital expenditures but must be directly related to the conduct of the project. Examples of allowable charges are laboratory repairs, special installation of equipment, shielding, air conditioning or filtering, and limited remodeling. If applicable, details should include the square feet affected and the unit cost. Inclusion of alterations and

renovations charges in a budget needs to be considered carefully, not only for need, but also for effect on the performance of the project and the timeline adjusted accordingly.

8. *Consortium and Contractual.* A consortium or contractual agreement permits a portion of a research project to be conducted by an institution that is not the applicant institution and is a separate legal entity. Essentially, the applicant contracts for the performance of a substantial or significant portion of the activities to be performed. Such an agreement involves a measurable effort by the contracting organization's principal investigator and requires a categorical itemization of costs using the same general principles and categories described for the applicant institution. Both the direct and F&A costs of consortium and contractual costs are direct costs for the applicant institution.

9. *Other expenses.* These include other less general cost areas—nontangible articles including rent and lease fees; communication, publication, and technical service charges; tuition remission in lieu of salary; costs related to research involving human subjects other than patient care (e.g., patient stipends and reimbursement for travel and subsistence); and animal care costs—usually based on average census and a unit cost.

10. *Facilities and Administrative (F&A).* Costs are incurred by the institution during the conduct of a project, but are not readily identifiable as benefiting a specific project. Examples of facilities costs include: plant operations, utilities, custodial services, and maintenance. Examples of administrative costs include: payroll and accounting services, sponsored projects administration, and departmental administration. The F&A rate is a negotiated agreement between an institution and its cognizant agency, the federal agency from which the institution receives the greatest amount of funding. The rate is based on costs incurred in prior years and is an average rate. A specific project may incur more or less expense for these costs, but having a large number of rates is impractical. Larger institutions frequently have more than one rate. These multiple rates typically include rates for sponsored research, instruction, patient care, and other sponsored activities. There also may be both on-campus and off-campus rates for each project type. The F&A rate agreement defines the rate and the basis on which it can be applied. Typically, the rate is applied on Modified Total Direct Costs—total project costs less equipment, other capital expenditures, patient care, tuition remission, and that portion of each subcontract in excess of $25,000. The negotiated rate for each institution is unique and the agreement should be consulted for details on

the appropriate rate and its application. Some sponsors do not permit recovery of F&A costs. Others limit the recovery to less than the negotiated rate. Clearly, the budgets should reflect such restrictions.

Tips for Budget Preparation

The foremost guide for preparation of the budget is the research narrative itself. A well-prepared budget is consistent with the proposal's outline and details and should reflect all necessary cost components required to complete the proposed work. The budget should not be under- or over-estimated.

Budget preparation should begin with an analysis of each specific aim or objective and activity necessary to determine the specific cost. For example, analysis of blood for specific compounds related to the administration of a pharmaceutical would require collection of the blood sample, preparation of the sample, and analysis of the sample. These activities would involve personnel time, supplies (e.g., sample collection tubes, needles, and skin disinfectants), and storage or transportation costs. Listing activities and breakdowns of their associated costs provides a clear, detailed outline for budget justification. Stating costs in "lump sum" categories (e.g., supplies, $3,000) is a practice that should be avoided. Detailing specific costs of each component of a study demonstrates a thorough planning effort to reviewers.

Budget Guidelines

In budget planning, one must follow agency guidelines and keep updated on any program announcements or changes. Guideline deviations may result in rejection of a proposal and can certainly affect reviewer recommendations for funding. Some of the more common restrictions found within guidelines include limits or exclusions of equipment purchases, personnel requirements (e.g., per cent effort, travel, and qualifications), or cost ceilings for (direct or total costs).

Exceptions to Detailed Budgets

Some sponsors for some programs do not require detailed budgets to be included with the research proposal or pre-proposal. Most notable among sponsors not requiring detailed budgets are the NIH. Proposals requesting $250,000 or less in each project year of a proposed project should be prepared using Modular Grant guidelines.[15] These guidelines require total direct costs requested in modules of $25,000, so the budget should reflect the total annual amount requested rounded to the nearest $25,000.

Budget Justification

The budget justification or narrative is an integral part of the budget and should present clear rationale for each requested charge in sufficient detail. The budget justification should correspond with details in the overall research narrative.

Unless specific instructions for the preparation of the budget justification are provided, it should be written using the major categories used for the budget itself. Explanations should be concise and clearly stated. A brief discussion of the elements for a good budget justification separated by budget categories follows:

1. *Personnel.* The role on the project, effort dedicated to the project, and responsibilities for the conduct of the project should be described. A salary request should be explained as a percentage of the appropriate institutional base salary. Calculation of fringe benefits should be explained, either as a percentage or as a fixed amount depending on how the applicant institution specifies the fringe benefits rates.

2. *Consultants.* Provide the names and institutional affiliations of each consultant and describe the services that each will perform. Explain the basis of the fees including honorarium, travel, per diem, and any other included costs.

3. *Equipment.* For each piece of equipment requested, describe the specific capabilities, include a vendor estimate, and discuss the need as related to the conduct of the proposed research.

4. *Supplies.* Separate the supplies requested into general categories and describe the category, the costs of individual items, and their use in the research project.

5. *Travel.* Requests should distinguish between domestic and foreign destinations, the purpose and frequency of the travel, and its relevance to the project. The basis for estimating the costs including details of fares and per diem should be described.

6. *Patient Care Costs.* Explanations should be separated into inpatient and outpatient categories. For each cost, describe the basis for its calculation including the treatment or intervention and frequency. Include information about accrual rates for each year of multi-year projects.

7. *Alterations and Renovations.* Detailed costs should be included based on contractor or institutional estimates. Specifically describe the relevance of the planned renovations to the proposed research.

8. *Consortium and Contractual.* A detailed budget for each consortium or contractual agreement should be included with a budget justification. Reference to the budgets and justifications prepared by each institution are sufficient.

9. *Other Expenses.* Separate the items included in this category into general groups and describe the groups, the costs of individual items, and their use in the research project.

10. *Facilities and Administrative (F&A).* Explain the rate applied and the basis for calculation. If a negotiated patient care rate agreement is used in addition to the standard rate, provide information about that rate. If not requested elsewhere, the date of the agreement and the cognizant agency should be listed.

When the Sponsor Does Not Require Detailed Budgets

Recent changes in policy and guidelines by the National Institutes of Health allow proposal budgets to be requested in modules of $25,000 up to $250,000 per year with no details either in the budget itself or the budget narrative. However, to determine the applicable number of modules to request, preparation of a detailed budget using the principles outlined above is strongly recommended.

Such modular budgets similarly should not include details in the budget narrative. As an example, for the National Institutes of Health, only personnel and consortium and contractual costs need justification, plus an explanation when the number of modules per year varies. For personnel, the role, effort on the project, and responsibilities should be described, but no salary details should be included. Consortium and contractual agreements should be briefly explained, should indicate whether the institution is a domestic or foreign entity, and should round the amount of the budget to the nearest $1,000.

Formatting for Specific Agency Sponsor

Sponsors most often provide budget forms or a template for budget presentation. In the absence of forms or templates, a format that is well-known or widely accepted within the subject area of the proposal should be used (e.g., for disease study, use NIH format; for sciences and engineering, use that of the NSF).

The foregoing discussion can really be summarized in two axioms for budget preparation:

- Prepare a budget that is logically related to and supported by the research narrative.
- Follow the guidelines and instructions of the sponsor exactly.

• • • References

1. U.S. Department of Labor, Bureau of Labor Statistics. "Consumer Price Indexes," http://www.bls.gov/cpi (accessed August 13, 2005).

2. National Institutes of Health. "Biomedical Research and Development Price Index (BRDPI)," http://ospp.od.nih.gov/ecostudies/brdpi.asp (accessed August 13, 2005).

3. Office of Management and Budget, The Executive Office of the President. "Codification of Governmentwide Grants Requirements by Department," http://www.whitehouse.gov/omb/grants/chart.html (accessed August 13, 2005).

4. National Institutes of Health. "NIH Grants Policy Statement," December 2003, http://grants2.nih.gov/grants/policy/nihgps_2003/index.htm (accessed August 13, 2005).

5. National Science Foundation. "Grant Proposal Guide: NSF 04-2," September 2003, http://www.nsf.gov/pubs/2004/nsf042/start.htm (accessed August 13, 2005).

6. National Science Foundation. "Grant Policy Manual: NSF 02-151, July 2002," http://www.nsf.gov/pubs/2002/nsf02151/index.jsp (accessed August 13, 2005).

7. "Federal Acquisition Regulations System," Title 48 Code of Federal Regulations, 2005.

8. U.S. Office of Management and Budget. "OMB Circular A-87, Cost Principles for State, Local and Indian Tribal Governments." OMB, 1997 (available from http://www.whitehouse.gov/OMB/circulars/).

9. U.S. Office of Management and Budget. "OMB Circular A-102 Grants and Cooperative Agreements with State and Local Governments." OMB, 1997 (available from http://www.whitehouse.gov/OMB/circulars/).

10. U.S. Office of Management and Budget. "OMB Circular A-133, Audits of States, Local Governments, and Non-Profit Organizations." OMB, 2003 (available from http://www.whitehouse.gov/OMB/circulars/).

11. U.S. Office of Management and Budget. "OMB Circular A-21, Cost Principles for Educational Institutions." OMB, 2000 (available from http://www.whitehouse.gov/OMB/circulars/).

12. U.S. Office of Management and Budget. "OMB Circular A-110, Uniform Administrative Requirements for Grants and Other Agreements with Institutions of Higher Education, Hospitals, and Other Non-Profit Organizations." OMB, 1999 (available from http://www.whitehouse.gov/OMB/circulars/).

13. U.S. Office of Management and Budget. "OMB Circular A-122, Cost Principles for Non-Profit Organizations." OMB, 1998 (available from http://www.whitehouse.gov/OMB/circulars/).

14. "Principles for Determining Costs Applicable to Research and Development under Grants and Contracts with Hospitals," Title 45 Code of Federal Regulations Part 74, Appendix E (also known as Office of Assistant Secretary Comptroller-3 [OASC-3]), 1991.

15. National Institutes of Health. "Modular Grant Application and Award," December 18, 1998, http://grants2.nih.gov/grants/guide/noticefiles/not98-178.html (accessed August 13, 2005).

CHAPTER

32

The Challenges and Opportunities of International Research

John D. Sites Jr., CRA

Introduction

International projects can offer an exciting and rewarding addition to the research activities of educational and nonprofit institutions. With proper planning, preparation, and support, the opportunity for growth on the part of research professionals, students, administrative personnel, and the institution can be uniquely rewarding

Local Customs and Traditions

When working in the international arena, it is important to consider possibly differing points of view, traditions, and expectations of the customer and end user of the services or products while developing a proposal. Methodologies used successfully at home may not apply to international interests; therefore, understanding the culture and traditions of the customer can sometimes be more important than the content of the proposal itself. In many cultures, the relationship between the customer and the institution is more important than the details or facts associated with the actual negotiations. Once the proper trust and respect have been established, the formal procedures of contract negotiation may proceed with a greater level of confidence. Wearing proper business attire and using correct forms of address according to a particular culture and its customs can also have an impact on the international customer relationship. Arriving at a meeting dressed in semi-casual attire can be interpreted as disrespectful, arrogant, and can portray a lack of

authority or commitment on the part of the institution. In some countries business attire is very formal, while in others, it tends to be more casual.

Using proper titles and forms of address can be as important as selection of business attire. Levels and forms of proper address vary from country to country, sometimes within a particular country itself. These differences can be confusing and can be easily misused. For example in many Latin American cultures, physicians, lawyers and dentists are often addressed as "Doctor," while an engineer may be addressed as "Engineer Smith" in a formal setting, but by his or her first name during informal meetings. Unintentional mistakes often go unnoticed by those trying to operate in foreign cultures, but such mistakes can send the wrong message to the customer. Therefore, it is important to take the time to learn about the local customs and to pay attention and be generally aware of such potential cultural gaffes when working with customer and local partners.

Preparing a proposal for an international project can present another set of unusual expectations and realities that can have an impact on the negotiations. Proper proposal preparation cannot be done easily from afar: the complexities of proposal development changes from country to country, from sponsor to sponsor, and from culture to culture. It is essential to identify and use local resources, knowledge, and expertise. While our offices are equipped with the most modern computers, printers, copiers, and scanners, offices in other countries may not have the same resources; something as basic as the quality and availability of electricity can be major factors in other countries. For example, the government in one Caribbean country during a summer energy shortage ordered a power shut down at 2:00 p.m. while one institution was in the midst of contract negotiation. Fortunately, in this case, the institution's local office was equipped with a back-up generator. However, unfortunately, the sponsor was not available during this time, which prolonged the time necessary to complete the negotiations.

In the United States in most metropolitan centers it is possible to go to a local office supply store or copy center in the middle of the night; not so in most other countries, where there also lesser chance of availability of high-speed copiers or speedy network access. While working on a proposal in Central America, one team stayed up until 3:00 a.m. making copies of a large proposal. While they had access to a copier, it was an older model that had to be hand-fed and collated one page at a time. If it had not been for the wonderful office staff of a local team member, they never would have been able to complete the task of numbering the pages, making three copies of 600 pages each, conduct the final review, and meet an 8:00 a.m. deadline later that morning.

The compilation, verification, and submission of a proposal can be accomplished from afar, but doing so restricts the amount of local knowledge that can often make the difference. While it may require some additional planning, it is often best if it can be accomplished in the country itself, even if requiring extra effort. In addition, proposal submissions must often be conducted in person, in the presence of the other bidders and sponsor representatives. The preparation of a proposal in the country of the program makes attendance of the official opening of proposals much easier.

Local Language and Translation Services

From the beginning of the solicitation process to the completion of the project itself, it is not uncommon for all correspondence, meetings, documents, and negotiations to be conducted in a language other than English. In some countries, this may be a legal requirement, especially when working with a government agency. The ability to work effectively in a foreign language may very well determine the success or failure of the proposal or project.

The official opportunity or expression of interest on the part of the sponsor is generally the solicitation. This is generally preceded by much informal communication between interested parties and the sponsor. Official documentation is almost always written in the native language of the sponsor and often contains a requirement that all correspondence and offers be written in that language. In the case of some international funding, the language used must generally be one of a limited few in order to be acceptable. These languages generally reflect the members of the bank, for example. Depending on the sources of funds being used by the sponsor, the solicitation package may include a copy of the intended award document, which may also be in a foreign language. The ability to adequately and accurately respond to the solicitation and to identify areas of concern prior to negotiation is dependent on the proper translation of documents.

Identifying an appropriate point of contact for correspondence between the institution and the sponsor is also very important. This individual must have the ability to understand the information, coordinate the needed response, and provide it to the sponsor in the proper language and in a timely manner. It is not uncommon for the sponsor to contact bidders requesting additional information for consideration by the reviewers during the review process, or request a meeting with the institution. These requests generally have a limited response period associated with them. Responses that occur outside of this period are generally not allowed for consideration.

While it is preferable for the institution to have representatives who are fluent in a foreign language, institutions may look to hire domestic or international translation services. These organizations generally offer experienced professionals who can assist in the drafting of correspondence, in the translation of solicitation and contract language, and with on-site meetings and negotiations. These services can be very expensive, however, and an organization must weigh the cost with the anticipated benefits of a successful proposal, especially when these expenses are generally classified as unallowable costs during the proposal preparation and negotiation phase (and, as such, represent an unrecoverable cost to the institution).

Often proposal criteria demand that senior project and field personnel be fluent in the local language. Under these circumstances, the use of translation services and assistance merely during proposal negotiations may not be an option, and the need for these services may very well continue throughout the life of the project; this should be considered, as should inclusion of cost for such services, during the development of the proposal.

There are a number of software packages available that can assist with much of the translation processes. These packages can be configured to recognize regional and cultural variations of some languages. Institutions should keep track of upgrade versions to keep up-to-date or add additional languages as needs arise; however, these programs are not perfect. Their translations can often be very literal and require review and modification by someone who is familiar with both the original and target languages. Imbedding these programs within many of the popular spreadsheet, presentation, word processing and e-mail packages makes it easy to work and translate written work.

In-Country Authority

When working in international settings, it is important to have the proper, locally recognized authority. This is especially important as the authority of the institutional representative may not always be recognized by the laws of the host country. Questions concerning authority and/or validity can also extend to the execution of formal documents on behalf of the organization, the type of visa held by an individual, and teaming agreements identifying a consortium of interested parties participating in the bidding process. Without this authority, months of hard work and effort can become null and void with little or no chance of solving the problem in time to participate.

When preparing to respond to a solicitation, it is important to contact an attorney or knowledgeable individual who is familiar with the laws of the country. Embassy or foreign consulate personnel can also provide valuable assistance and knowledge. In order for institutional authority to be valid outside of the United States, it is common for a power of attorney recognized by the host country, on behalf of the institution, to be required. Without this official documentation, the ability of the representative to legally execute documents in the country may be null and void within the host country. When representing a consortium of organizations, the ability to represent the other organizations within the consortium must also be established and recognized in a similar manner.

In the case of one program in South America, it was learned that despite possession of letters from the provost, university president, and board of trustees granting the authority necessary to obligate the institution, the instruction's representative was not legally qualified as an authorized

representative to sign the contract. In addition to having questions about the legal authority of the individual, it was learned that the institution's representative did not have the necessary business visa. The tourist visa (issued through customs at the airport) did not allow the individual to conduct business within the country. The need for local legal counsel or a knowledgeable agent to guide the institution through the maze of ever-changing regulations is immeasurable. It is often better to spend a little money on such legal counsel up front to avoid sending a team overseas for negotiations, only to learn of the difficulties upon arrival (or worse yet, during the negotiations). Trying to identify adequate, affordable legal counsel or knowledgeable agents within an extremely tight schedule is close to impossible. Under these unfortunate circumstances, it is not unusual to pay an exorbitant amount of money. These unfortunate events also typically place additional burdens upon the sponsor, since they must spend additional time and money to begin negotiations with the next qualified bidder. This can result in reducing the confidence level of the sponsor in your organization, affecting future interactions and opportunities.

Once the proper authority has been established and properly documented, it is important that the authorized institutional representative coordinate and supervise interactions with the sponsor. Many times, separate technical and administrative negotiations are held simultaneously to save time. It should be established with the sponsor that all promises and obligations agreed to by other members of the team must be reviewed and approved by the team leader. Learning of a previously unknown obligation made by a member of the team in the middle of final negotiations can present countless difficulties. When possible, it is recommended that the official representative attend all meetings to learn the technical and administrative needs of the project. This will help the official to accurately represent the needs of the entire project and to find mutually beneficial solutions to technical and administrative problems during development and contract negotiations.

This multifaceted approach may take more time and resources than traditional domestic proposal development and negotiation, but will serve to increase the potential for success. Regardless, these efforts will improve confidence levels created with the sponsor, which can only serve to increase the probability of working with the sponsor in the future.

Contract Language

Just as solicitations identify unique and important aspects of the proposal process, the contract should provide information that serves to ensure the success of a negotiation and even later over the course of a project's implementation. One of the most important and influential parts of contract language relates to invoicing. Many foreign countries use loans from international banks to fund their projects, which are often designed to create future revenue streams to be used to assist in repayment of the debt. The initial advance, payment schedule, and invoicing terms have an impact on the future cash needs of the project. While many institutions dealing with US sponsors may be accustomed to 60- to 90-day payment cycles, it is not uncommon for the cycles associated with international projects to extend as much as 180 days or more. A thorough understanding of these terms within the contract allows the institution to conduct an analysis of the anticipated financial needs of the project and to determine whether or not the project will operate with a positive or negative cash flow. This information will assist in determining the proper advance and amortization values for invoicing. On large projects, the problem of negative cash flow can literally determine the success or failure of the work. In the case of some state institutions, approval from the board of trustees or state legislature may be required before the organization can agree to float the project. In the case of some smaller institutions, the amount of money required may be too great and require securing additional cash reserves in order to operate the project.

In addition to requirements related to deliverables, governing law, termination and dispute resolution, the contract will often address tax and personnel issues. Many times educational and nonprofit institutions begin the proposal process under the assumption that their nonprofit status will be recognized in a foreign country, which is not usually the case. For example, during a lengthy negotiation in South America, a team discovered that the sponsor would be deducting 30% from each invoice for income taxes and another 18% for applicable sales tax. Taxes had not been included in the proposal by the bidder, and the institution was faced with the prospect of signing a cost-reimbursable contract and, depending on costs incurred, receiving payment for 52% of the invoice amount. It is important to note, however, that very few institutions are able or willing to share 48% of the costs.

Fringe benefits associated with foreign nationals can present another area of concern. It is not uncommon for the laws of another country to make certain types of benefits mandatory. This information is often found within the contract, but not in the solicitation. These benefits may include bonus pay for holiday periods, resulting in 13 or 14 months pay for 12 months worked. Local laws may require the institution to make contributions to a pension fund or retirement plan. These benefits can add substantially to a proposal budget.

Obtaining a copy of contracts the sponsor has with the lender or subcontractors can provide additional information that can be helpful to the institution during proposal preparation and contract negotiation. The source(s) of funds identified in the lending agreement can help the institution identify the appropriate terms and conditions associated with a particular lender, particularly important when faced with contract language or terms and conditions related to tax liability. The contract language found in the lending agreement should also be examined. During one negotiation process in the Caribbean, a contract from the sponsor included language placing certain tax liability provisions on the bidder. Upon requesting a copy of the subcontract with another company working under the same program and reviewing the terms and conditions, it was found that the agreement clearly stated taxes were not an allowable cost. It also stated that in the event that they were required by an authorized tax authority, the sponsor would immediately reimburse the subcontractor upon presentation of the invoice. The institution was able to use this information to negotiate more favorable language in its own contract.

Lastly, the schedule parameters identified in the contract are no less important. The amount of time needed to establish the institution in the country, to obtain necessary work visas, to identify and hire local personnel, and to mobilize equipment can take a great deal of time. If the contract has a start date of January 1 and the negotiations are completed December 15, and the mobilization requires 45 days, the start of the project will be 30 days late, assuming there are no complications along the way. If the government offices, required to assist in the mobilization, are closed for the holiday season, the mobilization process can be delayed an additional 15 days. The start of the project is delayed at least 45 days. If performance of the project is tied to a particular growing or rainy season or contractor, the institution's ability to meet its obligations can be seriously jeopardized. When combined with the usual optimism of the research staff, a difficult schedule can quickly turn into an impossible one.

Import and Export Considerations

Over the course of the project it is not unusual for the institution to purchase vehicles, computers, office furniture, special test equipment and other large purchases. Often, these items are not available in the host country and must be purchased abroad and imported. The costs associated with the procurement of these items can be substantial. The lead time required can affect the project schedule and must be taken into consideration as well. Not only must the official lead time be factored into the schedule, but the unofficial lead time must be estimated.

In one case, during the performance of a water-related project, the contractor needed to purchase some special test equipment that was available only in the United States through a distributor located in the intermountain west. The purchase of the equipment was very straightforward, but transporting the equipment to the country was terribly complicated. The trip from manufacturer to the job site involved multiple customs offices in various countries along the way. Upon arrival in the country, there were unofficial delays at the docks. While the institution had done everything possible to ensure delivery, the sponsor was concerned about the delay. In the end, the government sponsor had to use its influence to make things happen.

Regional conflicts are fairly common in many areas of the world. These conflicts can result in the establishment of trade restrictions between neighboring countries or trade agreements between allies. Understanding the nature of these regional arrangements is imperative to successfully obtaining and delivering needed equipment. In addition to these regional considerations, US institutions need to be aware of export restrictions regarding dual-use equipment and software. Dual-use equipment generally refers to those items generally used for science or engineering but have the potential for military purposes. For example, many people are alarmed to learn that something as simple as an electronic handheld game or laptop computer can be subject to certain export restrictions.

A number of years ago an educational institution entered into an agreement with a nation from the former soviet block of nations. The two countries had been working for a few years on space-related research and development. When the deliverable was completed and sent to the sponsor, it was held up in US Customs. The institution was surprised to learn that it did not have the proper authority or license allowing it to transfer the technology out of the country. The issue was complicated even more by the fact that the delivery schedule was planned in conjunction with a planned space launch. Launch opportunities are not easily changed. In those few instances where it is possible, the associated costs are substantial.

In order to take advantage of the most advanced technology available and avoid complications generally associated with export/import restrictions, the lease/buy decision may provide an alternative worthy of consideration. This can be particularly appealing for those projects where needed vehicles and office equipment are available within the host country. Items that can be purchased in the country are usually configured to function in the conditions found at the jobsite. These conditions may include unique fuel types or voltages. They may function better due to a configuration designed to recognize the unique infrastructure, fuel availability, or power grid found within a particular country. Purchasing these items outside the country would require a certain level of specific knowledge in order to request that the items match a particular configuration to ensure functionality upon delivery.

Nonprofit Status

Educational and nonprofit institutions are structured very differently from commercial counterparts: these differences can affect the terms and conditions institutions are willing to accept as they relate to cost structures of nonprofit organizations. If a foreign sponsor is unable to recognize these differences, it can seriously jeopardize the likelihood of success and dramatically increase the level of risk.

Many foreign sponsors require that the institution agree to be bound by the laws of the host country, including tax and business laws. The structures associated with these laws often require a tax identification number issued by the local IRS (or equivalent) within the country to verify that the institution is legally established in the country and, as an authorized representative, able to sign an agreement. While this is not always a requirement in order to enter into a contract, the requirement does alleviate some of the more difficult legal issues that can arise without such measures.

Taxation can be one of the most frustrating problems. If the institution decides not to establish itself in the host country, then a thorough understanding of local tax law must be considered in the development of a realistic proposal budget. Most countries have two kinds of taxation, income and sales, which, in many cases, can add as much as 30% to 50% to a budget. These costs must be included within the proposal: failure to do so can create a financial disaster for the institution upon award. This is often complicated by a performance bond requirement during the proposal stage, a requirement that penalizes the institution if it refuses to sign a contract after being selected as the winning bidder.

If the institution does decide to establish a nonprofit entity recognized by the host country, there are a few additional decisions that must be made:

- First, will the organization establish a local office or run the program remotely from the main campus?
- Second, will the new entity be a local office of the institution or a new entity all together, governed by or reporting to the main office?
- Third, who will represent the organization in the host country? Will it be a local person living in the country, as may be required, or will someone from the United States be responsible and, if so, will local law allow this?
- Fourth, has the institution taken into account the legal obligations of the new entity or office and made arrangements for them to be met? Will these obligations be handled locally or remotely?

The process of establishing a new office or gaining local recognition for the institution can become overwhelming if these issues are not addressed early on. Competent legal counsel within the host country is essential. To identify this help, it may be useful to learn about the process from another US-based entity established in the country. Yet, this process can take a great deal of time and money: the process can take up to one year and cost $10,000 or more. The costs of meeting additional legal obligations, once the entity is established, can also add additional costs to the process, especially if the organization is required to maintain a local legal representation.

The establishment of a teaming agreement with a local organization that can operate as a subcontractor under the prime agreement is worth consideration and can provide a process by which the institution can work in a foreign country and benefit from the unique opportunities it offers.

Project Travel/Visas

Getting people, supplies, and resources to the job site can truly be challenging. Recognizing the unique aspects of foreign travel helps minimize these challenges and delays that can seriously affect the success of the project.

When involved in international project work, institutions can struggle to get the right people to the right place at the right time: one or two delays along the way can create a much bigger problem at the destination.

Many airlines have a limited number of flights to countries outside of the United States. A missed connection flight may land someone in a strange city or airport overnight. It is recommended to plan at least one or two extra travel days each way to minimize the impact of such a scenario. While en route to a negotiation in the Caribbean, fog in one city caused the negotiation team to miss all of its connections, making it impossible to get to the final destination that day. The airline sent them instead to Puerto Rico for a connecting flight the next day to the final destination. However, the following morning, the airline experienced three mechanical failures prior to departure and the negotiators arrived one hour before the start of the negotiations. The combination of little or no sleep, general travel fatigue, and newness of culture and foreign language can make the actual conduct of business extremely trying.

Prior to departing the United States, institutions should make sure that everyone has the proper visa to accomplish the tasks. Many countries require technical personnel to have special work visas (different from the standard tourist or business visa). Similar requirements may apply to administrative personnel and negotiators. While negotiating in South America, for example, despite having been in the country for over two weeks negotiating the contract, one institution representative learned that he did not have the necessary visa and could not act as an authorized representative to sign the negotiated contract. Instead, the sponsor was going to be forced to send the final contract to one of its consulates in the United States, and the representative was forced to travel back to finalize the contract.

In most foreign cultures, scheduled time is not as rigid as in the United States; therefore, in a culture where meeting schedules are frequently changed, stiff adherence to travel schedules can give a wrong impression and affect negotiation. When making travel arrangements, plan on frequent changes to the meeting schedules and subsequent changes to arrival and departure dates. Whenever possible, purchase fully refundable and changeable tickets. Discount tickets, though cheaper in the beginning, can end up being more expensive.

Health and Safety Issues

Outside industrialized Europe and the United States, food, water, transportation, and medical service can be much different and far less reliable. Taking the necessary precautions and planning accordingly can make the difference between a successful trip and disastrous one.

"Do Not Drink the Water": this tried and true saying cannot be reinforced enough. Regardless of the assurances by the hotel staff, if it is not bottled, sealed, and provided by a recognized vendor, leave it alone and drink soda, coffee, or spirits. Use bottled water to brush your teeth, and when eating in restaurants, ask for the can or bottle and drinks without ice. Purchase a few extra bottles of water at the airport before leaving the United States and place them in a carry-on bag. If at all possible, bring a portable water filter that is small enough to fit in a case.

Prior to leaving, talk with a physician about the country to learn of any health concerns particular to its region and get any necessary immunizations.

Bring along medication and include a little extra, just in case, as it may not be possible to obtain some medications overseas. Check with your health insurance provider to learn about coverage while traveling abroad: if the provider does not cover foreign travel, secure additional coverage. Lastly, you should obtain emergency medical evacuation insurance, which, in the event of a medical emergency, will provide assistance and coordination of medical personnel and, if necessary, return you to your personal physician via air ambulance.

The US State Department Web site is a wonderful resource that should be consulted for preparations. The site contains information about traveling abroad, and it covers everything from health and safety recommendations to political and economic conditions by country.

Closing Thoughts

International projects can provide some wonderful and exciting opportunities for any institution. Opportunities to exchange cultural, scientific, and other knowledge increase our level of understanding and encourage future projects. The opportunity to study and observe science, administration, and culture in another country can only serve to increase the unique and beneficial results of our efforts.

33

Federal Research Contracts

J. Michael Slocum, JD

The Supreme Court has said that "Men must turn square corners when they deal with the government."[1] In research contracts, as in all other dealings with the government, this means that almost every aspect of the contracting process is covered in great detail by laws and regulations that must be observed by all the parties involved. Through legislation, judicial decisions, and administrative regulations, each branch of government has played a role in creating an extremely complex regulatory environment that exposes participating contractors to hidden traps and pitfalls that may result in penalties ranging from diminution of profits to criminal sanctions. Congress has declared its procurement policy to be that of promoting "economy, efficiency, and effectiveness in the procurement of property and services . . . ."[2] In these efforts, methods for such achievement include:

- Full and open competition.
- Policies to require acquisition of goods and services of the quality actually needed at the lowest reasonable cost.
- Elimination of fraud and waste.
- Avoidance of duplication or overlapping in procurement related activities.
- Elimination of redundant or unnecessary requirements on both contractor and government personnel.
- Greater uniformity and simplicity in procurement procedures.
- Intradepartmental or agency coordination of procurement activities.

- Promotion of understanding of procurement laws and policies by organizations and individuals doing business with the government.
- Fair dealing between the government and contractors.

Numerous pieces of legislation have been passed and several executive orders issued to attempt to carry out the intent of the Office of Federal Procurement Policy Act. These, in turn are implemented by "regulations" issued by the Executive Branch Departments.

Rules and Rulemaking

The Code of Federal Regulations

The Code of Federal Regulations is a codification of the general, permanent rules published in the *Federal Register* by the executive departments and agencies of the federal government. The code is divided into fifty titles that represent broad areas subject to federal regulation. Each title is divided into chapters that usually bear the name of the issuing agency. Each chapter is further subdivided into parts covering specific regulatory areas. Each volume is revised at least once a year on a quarterly basis. The code is considered a special edition of the *Federal Register* and is supplemented and updated by individual daily issues of the *Register*. The two publications are to be used together to determine the latest version of a given rule. The Federal Acquisition Regulations

and the individual agencies' supplementing contracting regulations are usually codified in Title 48 of the
Code of Federal Regulations.

The Administrative Procedure Act (APA)

The APA[3] provides the general principles, requirements, and governing procedures of most federal
agencies. The APA was passed in 1946 and established the basic framework of administrative law
for agency action, including rulemaking. For grant
administration, this applies across the board to all
agencies. However, for most procurement actions,
such methods are discretionary.

The Office of Management and Budget (OMB)

The office issues its own regulations, known as
"circulars." OMB circulars give *general* policy
direction to government agencies. They apply to a
broad range of government activity, and directly
affect persons participating in government programs. Circulars are published in the *Federal Register*, with the invitation for comments from
interested parties.[4] The promulgation of circulars is
not a rulemaking governed by the Administrative
Procedures Act, but the public comment process
used is similar. Numbers are assigned to circulars,
but are not sequential or subject-matter related.
The "A" designation is merely a prefix OMB
adopted in the 1950s for use with the identifying
number of a circular.

How does a circular compare to a regulation? A
circular gives general guidance, expressing overall
government policy. A regulation is the product of a
rulemaking conducted by an individual agency. In
terms of practical effect, differentiation may be difficult. Agency regulations can also define policy and
give general guidance. The crucial difference is the
rulemaking *proceeding* required of agencies by
the APA.

In listing federal assistance programs, the *Catalog of Federal Domestic Assistance* emphasizes that
applicants must be familiar with the requirements
of these government-wide circulars. The catalog
identifies those circulars that apply to a specific
program and summarizes their requirements.
Although circulars often parallel regulations issued
by individual agencies, they are typically not considered "binding" unless *adopted* by agencies. Most
of the circulars have now been implemented by government-wide "common rules." As with contracting regulations, individual agencies have issued
regulations that supplement the "common rule."

Although the common rule language is the same for
each agency, individual agency adoptions must be
carefully reviewed to identify:

- Agency-unique information or deviation requirements.
- Statutory requirements not addressed by the
  common rule.

Additions and Exceptions to Programs Covered by Common Rules

Federal agencies may not impose additional administrative requirements affecting classes of grants and
grantees unless those requirements are authorized and
published in the *Federal Register*. These additional
requirements can be found in the agencies' individual
Code of Federal Regulations (CFR) compilations.

OMB Circular A-21. Establishes principles for
determining costs applicable to grants, contracts, and other agreements with educational
institutions. All federal agencies that sponsor
research and development, training, and other
work at educational institutions are to apply the
circular's provisions in determining the costs
incurred for such work. The same principles are
to be used as a guide in pricing fixed-price
or lump-sum agreements. Additionally, when
Federally Funded Research and Development
Centers (FFRDCs) associated with educational
institutions are subject to cost accounting standards (CAS) under defense-related contracts,
they will be required to comply with such standards and the rules and regulations issued by
the Cost Accounting Standards Board set forth
in 48 CFR.

OMB Circular A-122. "Cost Principles for
Nonprofit Organizations" sets out the principles for determining costs of grants, contracts,
and other agreements with nonprofit organizations. In drafting the circular, OMB sought to
make the language consistent with cost principles for educational institutions provided in
Circular A-21, and those for state and local
governments in Circular A-74-4.

OMB Circular A-128. "Single Audits of State
and Local Governments" established the audit
requirements for state and local governments
that receive federal aid. It also defines federal
responsibilities for monitoring those requirements.

OMB Circular A-133. Provides guidance to federal agencies for establishing uniform requirements for audits of awards to institutions of
higher education and other nonprofit institutions.

Critical Topics

Many topics in the CFR are important to researchers, including:

1. *Care of Laboratory Animals and Protection of Human Subjects in Research Activities.* The government's policies and procedures used when contracts involve live vertebrate animals are provided in the CFR. Similarly, whenever individuals may be involved as subjects in research activities under a contract, the policy and procedures to be followed are found in the regulations on the Protection of Human Subjects in the CFR. Most of the agencies, such as the Department of Health and Human Services, the Department of Defense, the Department of Energy, and the Food and Drug Administration, have similar regulations.

2. *Labor and Wage Rate Determination of Minimum Wages for Federal and Federally Assisted Construction.* General wage determinations by the Secretary of Labor of prevailing basic hourly wage rates and fringe benefits are made in accordance with 29 CFR. These rates and fringe benefits, in accordance with those statutes, constitute minimum wages payable on federal and federally assisted construction projects and on service contracts.

3. *Bid Protests Made to the Comptroller General.* The regulations governing protests made to the Comptroller General concerning solicitations for bids or proposals for procurement by a federal agency, or to proposed awards or awards of contracts are contained in 4 CFR 21.0-21.12.

4. *Export of Technical Data Involved in Research.* Universities and other organizations using or employing foreign students or researchers in conducting research, experimentation, or development could be unwittingly violating federal export laws and acting contrary to policies concerning the export of "technical data" from the United States. This might occur when such a student or researcher carries home technical data in his memory or notebooks. Under both the Export Administration Act of 1979 (administered by the Department of Commerce) and the Arms Export Control Act (administered by the State Department), it is unlawful to export commodities or articles, and technical data pertaining to them without obtaining an export license. Under Commerce Department regulations, the "export" of technical data includes the release of such data in the United States with knowledge that it will be shipped or transmitted to a foreign country. The statutes have heavy criminal penalties as well as civil sanctions; thus, institutions remain wary.

Legal Framework for Contracts

For most of the 20th century, the two basic laws that governed government contracting (also called "procurement") were the 1947 Armed Services Procurement Act (ASPA) and the 1949 Federal Property and Administrative Services Act (FPASA). These statutes provided the basis for contracting practices for almost forty years, until 1984, when, in a sudden turn of interest, Congress began to pass a stream of significant contracting legislation. Some of these have been in the form of amendments to Competition in Contracting Act (CICA); others have been concerned with specific topics, such as disputes, technology transfer, and small business problems. The US government has established the Federal Acquisition Regulation system to implement these laws and to establish uniform policies and procedures for acquisition by all executive agencies. This system is intended to produce a uniform procedure for procurement within the federal government.

The Federal Acquisition Regulations System

The Federal Acquisition Regulation System was established to codify and publish uniform policies and procedures for acquisition by all executive agencies. The system consists of the Federal Acquisition Regulation (FAR) and agency acquisition regulations that implement or supplement FAR. The FAR system is developed in accordance with the requirements of the Office of Federal Procurement Policy (OFPP) Act, as amended, and Office of Federal Procurement Policy Letter 85-1, dated August 19, 1985. The FAR system is prescribed and maintained jointly by the Secretary of Defense, the Administrator of General Services, and the Administrator, National Aeronautics and Space Administration (NASA) under their several statutory authorities. Subject to these statutes, the FAR is revised through the coordinated actions of two councils, the Defense Acquisition Council (DAR Council) and the Civilian Agency Acquisition Council (CAA Council). Each council has primary responsibility for processing revisions to specified parts or subparts of the FAR. Proposed revisions are initially processed by joint FAR committees as cases to be considered by the DAR Council or CAA Council. Case preparation includes an initial analysis, recommendation, and draft coverage, which is then transmitted to the councils.

A FAR Secretariat, established and operated by the General Services Administration, prints, publishes, and distributes the FAR through the Code of Federal Regulations (CFR) System. The Secretariat also provides the two councils with centralized services relating to the FAR and performs administrative tasks pertaining to its maintenance. The Administrator of General Services has the responsibility for compliance of civilian agencies with the FAR. The Secretary of Defense has the responsibility for compliance by the military departments and defense agencies, and the Administrator of NASA has that responsibility for NASA activities. The authority of agency heads to issue regulations is limited to those that concern policies, procedures, solicitation provisions, or contract clauses that supplement the FAR and satisfy the specific needs of the agency.

A Federal Acquisition Regulatory Council (consisting of the Administrator for Federal Procurement Policy, the Secretary of Defense, the Administrator of NASA, and the Administrator of General Services) was created in 1988 to assist in the direction and coordination of government-wide procurement policy and regulatory activity. In consultation with the council, the Administrator of OFPP is to ensure that procurement regulations promulgated by agencies are consistent with the FAR and the policies expressed in the OFPP Act. Under the FAR, responsibility for implementation in civilian agencies is vested in the General Services Administration. The other regulatory agencies are the Department of Defense and NASA. Each has primary responsibility for specific parts/subparts of the regulations.

The provisions of the Competition in Contracting Act have been incorporated into the FAR. CICA amended both the Armed Services Procurement Act and the Federal Property and Services Act. Earlier, sealed bidding was mandated as the preferred method of procurement. This mandate had become an anachronism, and in reality only about six percent of government contracting was being affected by formal advertising. Until the decade of the 1970s, negotiation had been perceived as noncompetitive. Idea followed action and CICA specified full and open competition, but placed competitive proposals on a par with sealed bidding, limiting other than competitive procedures to specific circumstances and requiring written justification for circumstances of less than full and open competition.

FAR procedures contain unique and complex requirements for soliciting contract bids, contract performance, and contract management. Further, this procurement system employs dispute resolution procedures that are unique within the US judicial system. To complicate matters, the federal system of procurement varies slightly from agency to agency depending on the specific needs and functions to be served. These procedures vary in some significant ways from what is familiar to international contractors or contractors with no federal contracting experience. FAR and its agency supplements serve as implementing regulations for more general laws related to procurement enacted by Congress. The FAR regulations govern each of the issues outlined below in great detail. Individual agencies, including especially the Department of Defense, then provide even greater detail in their Supplements.

Solicitations

FAR Part 5, Publicizing Contract Actions, sets out the policies and procedures for publicizing contracting opportunities and award information. Agencies are required to publicize proposed contract actions through publication of synopses in Federal Business Opportunities.[5]

Competition Requirements, Method of Contract Award

The Competition in Contracting Act requires "full and open competition" for all government contracts. These requirements are implemented in "FAR Part 6, Competition Requirements and DFARS Subchapter B, Competition and Acquisition Planning." These regulations set out the policies and procedures that promote the basic goal: All contracts should be awarded using full and open competition in the acquisition process unless a specific rationale is provided for making awards without full competition.

- Sealed Bid Contracts: FAR Part 14, Sealed Bidding sets out the details for this bidding process. It requires that sealed bids be submitted, opened in public, and evaluated without discussions before award of the contract. The contract will be awarded to the party with the bid that both conforms to the invitation and is the most advantageous to the government, considering price and price-related factors only. This methodology is not appropriate for almost any research contract, but it is the "traditional" way that government contracts have been awarded since the Civil War.

- Competitive Proposal Contracts: When appropriate, Contracting Officers may require that contractor candidates submit to a competitive proposal process rather than submitting sealed bids. This process is initiated by a Request for Proposal (RFP). The RFP sets forth the government's requirements for the contract. The contract(s) are awarded based on an announced set of factors including quality of the proposal, the contractor's experience and proposed staffing, and the estimated cost or price.

Exemptions from Competition

Justification for not obtaining competition must be cited if the government does not use the "full and open" methods. The permissible exemptions are:

- Single source of supply: Only one source of the product or services exists.
- Unusual or Compelling urgency, as in time of war.
- Industrial mobilization in time of national emergency; establishing engineering or development services for federal educational or research facilities; acquisition of expert witness testimony.
- When international agreements may supercede the requirement for full and open competition.
- When otherwise authorized or required by statute.
- When in the interest of national security.
- When doing so serves the public interest.

Contract Types

Contract types are specified by the FAR. The type of contract utilized can drastically alter the risks to the contractor. The contract "type" can refer to how the contract is awarded, the type or method of payment associated with the contract, what the government is buying, the method of bidding, or the size of the contract. The FAR provides for:

- Fixed-Price Contracts: Utilized when contract specifications and requirements are sufficiently definite and precise to fairly enforce a bid.
- Cost-Reimbursable Contracts: Utilized when the contract specifications are uncertain or the need is urgent. Cost-plus percentage contracts are forbidden. Cost-sharing, straight costs, or cost-plus fee contracts are permissible and used.
- Incentive Fee Contracts: Can include guaranteed maximum price contracts under which the government and contractor share in cost savings achieved by the contractor.

- Indefinite Delivery Contracts: Utilized when the quantity of the product or services being purchased is unknown.
- Task Orders: Can be fixed price or cost reimbursable.
- Time and Materials: Rarely used; utilizes a set rate to pay for labor and reimbursement for actual material costs.

Various types of contracts create different financial relationships between the government and the contractor. Cost-reimbursement contracts require some administrative activity that is not applicable to fixed-price contracts, e.g., audit of the contractor's books to determine allowable and allocable costs. This administrative task is directly related to the financial arrangements in the contract. The different fixed-price types of contracts also have certain administrative aspects that are related to financial arrangements. Some of the differences in financial arrangements and the time and method of payment are outlined here.

Fixed-Price Contracts. Although fixed-price contracts always require the contractor to deliver some item or complete some defined task as a condition for payment under the contract, this does not mean that no money is paid until the work is done. Payments under a fixed-price contract may be made as:

1. A lump sum upon completion;
2. Partial payments for delivery of some but not all of the items due;
3. Progress payments based on percentage or stage of completion or costs incurred; or,
4. Advance payments.

Cost-Reimbursement Contracts. Cost-reimbursement contract types do not require delivery of items or the completion of work as a condition for payment; under these contracts, payment is made upon submission of invoices showing the costs incurred in performance regardless of the degree of success achieved. Payment of a fee may be conditioned upon acceptance of end items or otherwise successful completion of the work, but in general, disbursements will be made as originally agreed, subject only to the expenditure of effort by the contractor. If additional money is needed above and beyond the original estimated cost to complete the work of the contract, the government may choose to increase its financial obligation.

Contract Funding. The government is legally prohibited from making any contract expenditures or commitments to expend that are not appropriated by Congress. Thus, all types of contracts and contract modifications must be coordinated with budget personnel to assure that the agency's appropriation is sufficient to cover the specific work desired in addition to all other work that has been approved. When the contract is to have a fixed price, this procedure is fairly simple. The amount needed is either completely or substantially known at the outset. But when the contract is to be cost-reimbursable, the situation is quite different. In that case, the amount of money needed to complete the task is not known with any precision; there is only an estimate. If the government is to finish such work within the constraints of the law, it must be prepared to obligate additional funds to contracts that are considered valuable but that cost more than was initially estimated. This is the problem of contract funding.

Limitation of Cost. Although the government is obligated under the Allowable Cost, Fee, and Payment clause to pay the contractor's allowable costs regardless of dollar amount, the Limitation of Cost clause provides that the government is not obligated to pay a larger amount than the estimated cost of performance set forth in the contract schedule. The purpose of the Limitation of Cost clause is to avoid violation of the Anti-Deficiency Act that prohibits government personnel from obligating the government to pay amounts that exceed appropriated funds.

All cost-reimbursement types of contracts contain a Limitation of Cost (or similar) clause. The basic provision of the clause is that the contractor agrees to use its best efforts to perform the work within the cost estimate originally negotiated (exclusive of any applicable fee). The contractor is not obligated to perform any work that exceeds the cost estimate in the contract, nor is the government obligated to pay for any work in excess of the estimate. The government may, however, make a determination to increase the amount of funds committed to the contract, thus facilitating completion of the work. Whenever it has reason to believe that the aggregate of all costs expected to be incurred on the contract will, within the next 60 days, exceed 75% of the estimated amount in the contract, the contractor must notify the contracting officer. The contractor must also make such a notification if it believes that the total cost of performance will be substantially greater or less than the estimated costs.

The clause authorizes the contracting officer to notify the contractor in writing when the estimated cost of the contract is increased. The revised cost stated in the notice becomes the estimated cost of performing the contract and the contractor's obligation to continue performance is revived. Any costs incurred in excess of the previous estimated cost and within the new estimated cost are reimbursable. Note that the Limitation of Cost clause also provides that a change order under the Changes clause is *not* an authorization to exceed the contract estimated cost. If a contractor under a cost-reimbursement contract happens to incur liability to a third person for personal injury or otherwise in the course of performing the contract, the Insurance-Liability to Third Persons clause provides for government reimbursement for the liability (to the extent not covered by insurance) despite the Limitation of Cost clause.

Modifications. The exigencies of funding require that the contract manager be fully aware of the progress on cost-reimbursement contracts. If the funds obligated are not sufficient, that is, if the estimated cost of the work is below the actual or likely costs, the government has only three options:

1. Obligate additional money;
2. Scale down the scope of the work; or,
3. Allow the contract to lapse or be terminated prior to completion of the desired work.

To make such a decision in light of budget limitations and the competing claims on resources made by various projects, the contracting officer must be able to assess the cost benefits of the work being performed. Program or project officers play a significant role in whether additional funds should be committed to a particular contract since they determine the need. Nonetheless, the contracting officer is the central point for information on the contractor's progress and analysis of information obtained through monitoring of technical progress, financial reports, and other data gathered in administering the contract.

When a decision is made to modify the contract by increasing funding to cover increased estimated costs (e.g., issuance of a change order), the contracting officer must obtain a certificate of availability of funds from financial personnel. This requires coordination among the government officials involved.

Form of Government Contracts

Government contracts follow a defined format and use many similar or standard clauses. The Uniform Contract Format (UCF) is used for most contracts and solicitations. However, many specialized research contracts do not necessarily utilize this standard format. Most contracts are organized into four basic sections:

1. Schedule: Generally organized as Sections A through H of the contract. Addresses special contract requirements, inspection and acceptance, marking and packaging, deliveries or performance, contract administration, supplies or services, and price or costs.

2. Contract Clauses: Generally found in Section I of the contract.

3. List of Documents, Exhibits, and Attachments: Generally found in Section J of the contract.

4. Representations, Certifications, and Instructions: Sections L and M of the contract.

Socio-Economic Provisions

The federal government utilizes procurement policies, in some instances, to effect socio-economic change. Some of the legislation designed for this purpose has such a long history that it has almost become second nature in the area of government contracting. Contractors should never take for granted that they are familiar with the requirements of this type of legislation or regulation, however, but should read carefully and adhere strictly to those stipulations contained in the clauses included with the Request for Proposal, Invitation for Bid, or the contract. Some of these are:

- *The Davis-Bacon Act.* Applies to all contracts for the construction, alteration, and repair of public buildings involving the services of laborers or mechanics. The Act requires the payment of prevailing wage rates.
- *The Walsh-Healey Public Contracts Act.* Makes similar provisions for supply type employees of contractors and subcontractors with contracts in excess of $10,000.
- *The Fair Labor Standards Act.* Covers minimum wages, maximum hours (with overtime pay provisions), and child labor restrictions.
- *The Contract Work Hours and Safety Standards Act.* Consolidates work hour standards into one comprehensive statute.

- *The Buy American Act.* Gives preference in procurement to domestically made products.
- *Environmental protection resulting from the Clean Air Act, the Clean Water Act, the Noise Control Act, and the Resource Conservation and Recovery Act of 1976.*
- *Non-discrimination clauses.* These include Equal Employment Opportunity clauses and clauses to provide special contracting consideration for organizations owned by individuals, socially and economically disadvantaged or by women, and for potential contractors located in labor surplus areas.

Small Business Development

Public Law 97-219, the Small Business Innovation Development Act of 1982 (reauthorized in 1986), created the Small Business Innovation Research (SBIR) Program to stimulate technological innovation and the commercialization of such innovations by increasing the role of small business in federally supported research and development (R&D). The SBIR Program consists of three phases, the first two of which involve federal funding. The objectives of Phase I are to establish the technical merit and feasibility of a proposed research or R&D effort that may ultimately lead to a commercial product or technology, and to determine the quality of performance of the small business awardee organization.

Phase II aims to continue the research or R&D efforts initiated in Phase I, which are likely to result in commercial products or technologies. Funding is based on the results of Phase I and the scientific and technical merit of the Phase II application. (Only Phase I awardees are eligible to apply for Phase II funding.) The objective of Phase III is for the small business organization to pursue with non-federal funds the commercialization of the results of the research funded in Phases I and II. Occasionally Phase III may involve non-SBIR-funded follow-on contracts with a federal agency for products or technologies intended for use by the US government.

The SBIR Program makes use of both grants and contracts as funding mechanisms. Program solicitations, issued annually, describe the program, provide guidelines and instructions, and suggest topics on which small businesses may propose research. Organizations and investigators seeking SBIR funding must meet specific eligibility requirements stated in the solicitation. If funded, the research must be performed in the United States.

SBIR grant applications and contract proposals undergo the same review processes as regular research and grant applications and R&D contract proposals.

Environment, Conservation, Occupational Safety, and Drug-Free Workplace

FAR Part 23 prescribes acquisition policies and procedures supporting the government's program for ensuring a drug-free workplace and for protecting and improving the quality of the environment through pollution control, energy conservation, identification of hazardous material, and use of recovered materials. Agency activities are to conduct their acquisitions in a manner that will result in enforcement of the Clean Air Act and the Clean Water Act and cooperate with the Environmental Protection Agency to that end. Similarly, FAR Subpart 23.3 concerns hazardous material. The Occupational Safety and Health Administration (OSHA) issues and administers regulations that require government activities to apprise their employees of hazards, conditions, and precautions for safe use and exposure to those hazards, and information on symptoms and treatment for exposure. Contractors must submit data about hazardous material when the contract requires the delivery of hazardous material; the FAR requires a clause in the contract concerning exposure to that material in the performance of the work, use, handling, manufacturing, packaging, transportation, storage, inspection, or disposal incident to that contract.

In addition, the Environmental Protection Agency has issued regulations concerning hazardous waste. 40 CFR Part 260 contains the regulations on the hazardous waste management systems in general. Part 261 provides for the identification and listing of hazardous waste. Part 262 sets out the standards applicable to persons who generate hazardous waste, and Part 263 covers the transportation of that waste. Disposal methods and disposal sites are the subject of detailed regulations.

Legislation That Limits Competition

Although the general policy of the government is "full and open competition," some procurement statutes actually have the effect of limiting competition. In addition to the Buy American Act and statutes and executive orders that require contractors to prove nondiscriminatory employment practices, the Federal Acquisition Regulation (FAR) provides "set-asides" for various categories of small businesses. The FAR encourages agencies to accept unsolicited research proposals for unique or innovative projects if such proposals have scientific, technical, or socio-economic merit and would make a contribution to the agency's specific mission. Such proposals could be the basis of a contract award through the process of negotiation without competition.

Determining Allowable Costs

To determine whether costs the contractor claims for reimbursement are allowable, the contracting officer must refer to the principles set forth in FAR Part 31 (referencing OMB Circulars including, for instance, A-21 for universities). Under these principles, the government will pay costs incurred by the contractor only if they are *reasonable* and *allocable*. Costs excluded or limited by provisions in Part 31 or by provisions in the contract are not allowable. This quotation from the decision in the case of *Louisiana State University*, IBCA No. 2057, 86-2 BCA ¶18,854 (March 21, 1986), illustrates how the requirement that costs be reasonable and allocable is applied:

> "There are different accounting principles for educational institutions as opposed to those for commercial organizations. These principles recognize that the purpose and organization of educational institutions differ from commercial firms, and that the differences warrant special rules for accounting for costs. The lack of provision for profit in contracts with colleges and the variety of duties of the faculty that militates against precision of timekeeping are among the reasons for different cost principles."

Educational institutions must maintain cost records in accordance with their contractual obligations and, where required, provide documentation in support of transactions. A failure to conform to federal procurement regulations outlining applicable cost accounting standards will bar the recovery of costs (*Washington State University*, IBCA No. 1228-11-78 [1980], 80-1 BCA ¶14,297). In the *Louisiana State University* decision, the Board, in discussing the record-keeping errors at issue in the case and the evidence supplied in support of the costs, stated that a contracting officer must use his own judgment to determine whether the evidence available is persuasive that the costs were properly expended on the project.

Reasonable Costs

Reasonable costs are those that are of an amount and type that would be incurred by a prudent person in a competitive business. Costs must generally be recognized as necessary for operation of the organization. They must be incurred in accordance with sound business practices, such as arms-length bargaining, and must be consistent with the normal practices of the contractor.

Allocable Costs

Allocable costs include:

1. Direct costs or expenses incurred specifically for performance, for example:
   - Salaries of personnel performing a specific portion of the contract work.
   - Costs of materials or supplies used for the contract.
   - Costs of subcontracts entered into solely for performance of the contract.
2. Indirect costs that benefit both the contract and other work of the contractor and that can be distributed between the contract and the other work based on relative benefit or another equitable basis, for example:
   - Depreciation on buildings and equipment used partially for the contract and partially for other work.
   - Fringe benefits of employees charged directly to the contract.
   - Supervisory salaries, if time is not charged directly to the contract.
3. Indirect costs that are necessary to the overall operation of the contractor but that cannot be distributed to projects in accordance with relative benefit, for example:
   - Office supplies.
   - Bid and proposal costs.
   - Salary of an accountant.

Predetermined Indirect Cost Rates

FAR16.307(i) provides that when a cost-reimbursement research and development contract with an educational institution is contemplated and predetermined indirect cost rates are to be used, the contracting officer shall insert the clause set forth in FAR 52.216-15 in solicitations and contracts. This is the clause describing how predetermined indirect cost rates are to be obtained and applied in the contract. FAR 42.703-3 states that OMB Circular A-88 assigns each educational institution to a single government agency for the negotiation of indirect cost rates, and provides that those rates shall be accepted by all federal agencies. The section further states that predetermined final indirect cost rates may provide the basis for payment for reimbursable indirect costs.

Use of Accounting Principles to Determine Allowability

Costs that the contractor claims for reimbursement must be compiled according to generally accepted accounting principles and practices or, if applicable, according to the accounting standards of the Cost Accounting Standards Board. Costs may be found to be in accordance with generally accepted accounting principles even though the contractor uses an accounting system different than that of other contractors. However, if the contract is more than $100,000, some uniformity of accounting treatment may be required by the Cost Accounting Standards Board.

Costs Specifically Limited or Excluded

Certain costs are specifically limited or excluded by the FAR:

- Entertainment costs are not allowable.
- Interest expenses are not allowable.
- Advertising expenses are limited to certain purposes.
- Depreciation on government-owned property is not allowable.

Costs may also be limited or excluded by specific provisions in the contract. The contracting officer cannot agree in the contract to allow a cost that is specifically disallowed by FAR Part 31, but can agree to limit or exclude costs allowable under the FAR.

Pre-Contract Costs

Special treatment of costs is sometimes provided for in *advance agreements* included in the contract. For example, a clause may be included in order to clarify and limit the allowability of pre-contract costs. Note that costs incurred in expectation of an award may be allowable, but only if an advance agreement concerning those costs is negotiated. The costs so allowed must be otherwise allowable and must be incurred *after* the date specified in the advance agreement. If for some reason a contract is *not* awarded, the government is *not* obligated to pay for those costs. Incurrence of a pre-award cost, even under an advance agreement, is at the contractor's risk.

Contract Modifications

The authority for the government to modify a contract is contained in FAR Part 43, which defines a contract modification as any written change in the terms of the contract.

Methods of Modification

There are two kinds of modification: *unilateral* and *bilateral*. In the first, a one-sided change, the contracting officer makes a change without the consent of the contractor. This change must be "within the scope" of the contract. However, in a bilateral or two-sided modification, the consent and agreement of both sides are needed to make a change in the contract.

Unilateral Modification A change order is a unilateral modification that may derive from:

User-Agency Changes. During the performance of a contract, the user agency or department may have a dramatic change in staffing or mission that necessitates a rethinking of needs. This may require a change in delivery time or scope of work and could require a suspension of work or stop work order while the redesign takes place. In some rare instances, it may require termination of the contract.

Other Changes. Other factors beyond the control of either party (late delivery of government-furnished equipment or unavailability of site, unusually severe weather, or strikes) may cause delays in the contract. These may require a change in contract price or completion time. The intent of the "changes" clause is to allow necessary changes within the originally contemplated scope of work. It is not intended to be used to make "cardinal" changes to avoid the requirements of competition such as adding another facility's work or conducting new research not originally contemplated. Cardinal changes should be accomplished by a separate contract or (when noncompetitive contracting is justified) by a supplemental agreement. Boards and courts have held that attempts to use the "changes" clause to make cardinal changes are a basis for claims of breach of contract. A change order must be distinguished from an excusable delay. Facts and circumstances that do not give rise to a claim for a

price increase under the "changes" clauses may constitute grounds for an excusable delay under the default clause. Issuance of a change order is a right reserved to the government. The government need not give the contractor consideration for the change at the time it is issued, but the contractor might later be entitled to equitable relief, called *equitable adjustment*, in the contract price or in terms of performance, or both.

Bilateral Modification A bilateral modification is called a *supplemental agreement*. A supplemental agreement is essentially a new, negotiated contract entered into by the parties and is an addendum to the existing contract. Supplemental agreements are used rather than change orders whenever the parties can agree to the need for a change, the cost effect of a change, or both. However, supplemental agreements need not be made by any specific authority in the contract. As long as the parties agree and the rules on sole-source procurement are followed, even a "cardinal" change can be made by agreement. But since the contractor has not agreed in advance to perform this work, such work cannot be ordered without the contractor's consent. As noted, supplemental agreements that are not just substitutes for change orders are tantamount to sole-source procurements and must be justified by a contracting officer's findings and determination not to procure by competitive methods. The following circumstances may justify the use of such a supplemental agreement:

- The work that is to be accomplished is so interrelated with that being presently accomplished as to make utilization of a separate contract impractical.
- The site is so remote and the amount of work so small that obtaining an offer from a contractor other than the contractor presently on-site is impractical.
- Public exigency.

Supplemental agreements are used to:

- Finalize change orders,
- Accommodate decisions of the boards of contract appeals,
- Finalize equitable adjustments in connection with other contract clauses,
- Finalize a termination for convenience,
- Allow a contractor to complete a contract after non-excusable delay, change contract price, or,
- Make major changes in delivery schedule, quantity, quality, or other terms, since the

"changes" clause does not permit these types of changes without the consent of the contractor.

A bilateral modification or supplemental agreement is preferred and should be used rather than a unilateral change order whenever possible. The advantages of supplemental agreements over change orders are:

- The parties are in a better bargaining position before rather than after the work is done.
- The government and the contractor may better plan the change.
- The supplemental agreement reduces the possibility of a claim by the contractor that the government has issued an illegal change.

A supplemental agreement should be deemed to be "generally beyond the scope of the contract" if one or more of the following circumstances occur:

- The nature of the proposed work under the modification is generally different than that under the original contract.
- The quantities of materials and work called for under the modification are substantially beyond those required under the original contract.
- The time required for performance of the modification is such that the overall performance time of the contract will need to be substantially lengthened.
- The conditions of performance of the proposed modification are materially and substantially different than those of the original contract, in terms such as degree of risk or market conditions.

Limitations on Supplemental Agreements Since a supplemental agreement is essentially a new contract, it must be founded upon offer, consideration, and acceptance. The contractor promises to perform certain work in return for the government's promise to pay a certain sum upon completion. There are times, however, when other circumstances require attention. A contract may be modified only when it is found to be in the best interests of the government. If a supplemental agreement lessens a contractor's original obligation or in any way improves its bargain, the government must receive beneficial consideration, such as reduction in price or better end product.

Authority Under and Scope of the Changes Clause

Contracting Officer Authority The contractor must realize that not every government officer is an authorized representative of the contracting officer—i.e., a person able to direct changes. If a con-tract manager discovers that an agreement has been made with an unauthorized person, he or she should speak to the contracting officer authorized to make the change or agreement. The contracting officer should be asked to take the necessary steps to ratify the unauthorized act. Contracting officers are not required, however, to take any steps to ratify any order or agreement made by an unauthorized representative.

Oral versus Written Changes. Although the "changes" clause requires change orders to be in writing, the claims court has held that the clause will not prevent a contractor from getting an equitable adjustment when the contracting officer verbally orders a change and accepts the benefits of the work performed [*W. H. Armstrong and Company v. United States*, 98 Ct.Cl. 519 (1947)]. The appeals boards have also followed this theory (*C.A. Logeman Company*, ASBCA 5692, 61-2 BCA ¶3232; *A. L. Harding, Inc.*, DCAB PR-44, 65-2 BCA ¶5261, *Lincoln Construction Company*, 1 BCA 438-5-64, 65-2 BCA ¶5234). In these cases, the court and the appeals boards have decided that in issuing an oral instruction, the contracting officer had, in fact, issued a change order, and that not putting it in writing was an administrative error that could be corrected. These boards have also said that they will regard as done that which should have been done. Application of this principle, which is sometimes referred to as the "constructive changes doctrine," can give an oral order the effect of a written order. FAR 52.243-4(b) recognizes the existence of oral constructive changes but continues to require ordered changes to be written.

General Scope of the Contract

A section of the changes clause reads, "Make changes in the work within the general scope of the contract." The general scope of the contract has been defined by the Supreme Court in *Freund v. United States*, 260 U.S.C. 60 (1922) as what was "fairly and reasonably within the contemplation of the parties when the contract was entered into." Determination of scope is difficult and often depends on the circumstances of the individual contract. A change involving a relatively large increase in cost may still be within the scope of the contract. In *Axel Electronics, Inc.*, ASBCA 18990, 74-4 BCA ¶10,471, the board found no change beyond the scope of the contract where Axel sought equitable adjustment of 170 percent of the contract price because of alleged over-interpretation of the specifications. If the change order is written within the scope of the contract, it is a change contemplated by the parties and thus binding on the contractor. If the change is not within the scope of the contract, however, it is extra work that the contractor could legally decline to perform. Another court guideline provides that the number of changes may not matter. In *Coley Properties Corp.*, PSBCA 291, 75-2 BCA ¶11,514, the board found that approximately 100 change orders to a contract for construction of a post office and tower were not beyond the general scope of the contract.

When time allows, it is better to use a supplemental agreement rather than a change order. Under a change order, the contractor must proceed; afterwards, the contractor and the contracting officer negotiate an equitable adjustment. With a supplemental agreement, these decisions are reached in advance and both parties know the cost of the proposed change.

Causation: Causation refers to what has caused the change to come about. It means "cause and effect." The claims court held that to be entitled to equitable relief, the contractor must establish that its increased costs were caused by the changes, and not by something else [*Electronic and Missile Facilities v. United States*, 189 Ct.Cl. 237, 416 F.2d 1345 (1969)].

Failure to Agree: The changes clause states that the contractor may assert a claim for an equitable adjustment under this clause if the parties fail to agree; however, the contractor is legally required by the contract to proceed with the work as changed and to negotiate an equitable adjustment later. If the contractor fails to do this, it may be terminated for default.

Equitable Adjustments: If any change causes an increase or decrease in the contractor's cost or the time required for the performance of any part of the work under the contract, an equitable adjustment should be made. This adjustment should encompass the effect of the change on any part of the contract work, including delay expense. If contract documents are defective (e.g., plans or specifications) and the government is responsible, the equitable adjustment should include any increased cost reasonably incurred by the contractor when trying to comply with the defective documents. Equitable adjustment means fair adjustment. The government is expected to do whatever is fair, right, or reasonable if the contractor can prove entitlement. Contemplated remedies are adjust-

ment in price, delivery schedule, or both. The purpose of equitable adjustment is to keep both parties (government and contractor) in relatively the same position after the change as before the change.

Pricing Techniques for Equitable Adjustments of Fixed Price Contracts

Basically, there are five pricing techniques for measuring equitable adjustments. They are commonly referred to as:

- The Subjective Method (or *actual cost method*)
- The Objective Method (also the *reasonable value* or *market pricing method*)
- The Jury Verdict Method
- The Total Cost Method
- The Bruce Case Rule

1. The Subjective Method   The subjective method of computing equitable adjustments attempts to measure the actual cost impact of the change on the contractor. It is based upon the use of available historical cost data and supportable estimates as to future costs.

A case often used as an example of the subjective technique is the *Ensign-Bickford Company*, ASBCA 6214, 60-2 BCA ¶2817. In this case, two identical contracts were awarded to two different contractors for identical quantities and at identical prices. The contracts were administered by different government offices, with no coordination. Early in the performance of both contracts, identical change orders were issued to each of the contractors (A and B). A's change order was negotiated prospectively, and the amount was based on a negotiated subcontract price of $42,000 for the contemplated work (the subcontract happened to be with contractor B). In the case of contractor B's prime contract, the change order was issued without prior coordination and was ultimately negotiated on the basis of actual costs at $16,500. When the government office administering A's contract heard about the price that B had negotiated on the contract, they attempted to reduce A's contract amendment to $16,500, rather than the $42,000 previously agreed to. Contractor A, of course, insisted on $42,000. The case went to appeal and the board found in favor of the contractor and awarded $42,000. The basis for the ruling was:

- A's price was prospectively priced (estimated) and considered reasonable by both parties at the time they negotiated.

- B's price was based on actual cost data verified, after the fact, and therefore had no bearing on the reasonableness of A's price.
- It is the intent of the language of the changes clause to make equitable adjustments prospectively, based on estimates before the work is done, or retroactively, based on actual costs incurred. In addition, A's actual cost of performance for the change was $42,000 vis-à-vis its firm subcontract commitment to B.

2. The Objective Method The objective method, also known as "the reasonable value" or "market pricing" method, is used for pricing adjustments before performance under the change order occurs. The rule is that remuneration to the contractor should be equated with the reasonable or fair market value of the goods or services, rather than the actual cost. In the case above, contractor A's price was calculated by the objective method.

3. The Jury Verdict Method Where costs cannot be segregated and identified, both the government and the contractor may have to approach an equitable adjustment on the basis of estimates alone. In cases where meaningful comparisons cannot be made from the available cost data, the court and the boards have permitted the use of expert opinion to estimate the cost of a change. Based on all the evidence, including the opinions of qualified experts (e.g., estimators, cost and price analysts, auditors, etc.), the court or board can determine what should be paid in the same manner as a jury. This method has become known as the "jury verdict" method. First advanced by the claims court in *Western Contracting Corporation v. United States*, 144 Ct.Cl. 318 (1958), the method was later adopted in similar situations by the boards [see *Fishbach & Moore International Corporation*, ASBCA 18146, 77-1 BCA ¶12,300]. In *Western Contracting*, supra, since the contractor's costs could not be verified by records, the court considered the opinions of qualified estimators regarding the reasonableness of the claimed costs and determined the equitable adjustment on the basis of a "jury verdict." The circumstances under which this method may be employed are limited to situations where:

- Actual costs cannot be segregated and identified.
- Both parties rely on the opinion of qualified experts to estimate the costs incurred.
- There is a dispute relating to conflicting estimates by the parties.

The final amount of price adjustment is thus a judgment call, based on an evaluation of the conflicting positions of the parties, careful examination of all available data, and weighing of those data. Despite the name of this method, a "jury" is not actually used. The expert testimony of both sides is weighed by the court or the board, and the evidence is weighed as if by a trier of fact (i.e., the jury).

4. The Total Cost Method Normally the contractor must prove the actual costs *of the change*. If the contractor fails to prove this, but does show entitlement to an equitable adjustment, a determination on amount can nevertheless be made by the "total cost" method. The total cost method is the determination of the difference between the original contract price (unchanged) and the actual cost of performing the contract as changed. Simply stated, it is actual cost versus originally expected cost. This method is universally criticized as being the least preferable approach to an equitable adjustment on at least two grounds:

- The total costs include not only the costs properly attributable to the change but also those that were incurred through the fault of the contractor.
- The cost of performing the unchanged contract is frequently based on unrealistically low bid "buy-ins."

This method has been used, however, when there is no better method available. The claims court, for instance, has stated that the total cost approach should be used only as a last resort. To overcome the serious objections to this approach, courts have been careful to ascertain the contractor's actual costs incurred as a result of the change and have reduced those costs by deducting those amounts attributable to the fault of the contractor. This eliminates the first major criticism. The court attempts to avoid the second major criticism by using an average estimate, derived from the estimates of the government and the other bidders, in order to preclude the possibility of "getting well" on changes after a buy-in. While reiterating its distaste for the approach, the court has conceded that the total cost basis may be used under appropriate circumstances and when no other method is available. The General Services Board of Contract Appeals has indicated that it will follow the criteria for considering a total cost claim enumerated by the claims court in *WRB Corporation v. United States*, 183 Ct.Cl. 4909:

It may be used when no other method is available and the reliability of supporting evidence is substantiated and depends on proof that:

1) The nature of the particular losses make it impossible or highly impracticable to determine them with a reasonable degree of accuracy,

2) The original bid or estimate is realistic,

3) The actual costs are reasonable, and

4) The contractor is not responsible for the added expenses. (1968)

5. The "Bruce Case" Rule The basis for most determinations of equitable adjustment is the series of decisions involving the Bruce Construction Company. The rule emanating from these cases is that the proper measure of value of an equitable adjustment is the contractor's costs, reasonably incurred. The rule is, in effect, a compromise between the objective and subjective concepts. The rule gives weight to the objective standard in that the costs must be reasonably incurred, but does not otherwise disturb the subjective fundamental of the contractor's costs. The Bruce case involved a fixed-price construction contract for a number of buildings at Homestead Air Force Base, Florida. A fine-textured building block was required by the original specifications. After the contractor had ordered the building block, the requirement was changed to sand block. The sand block was more brittle than the concrete masonry block generally produced in that area, requiring a higher degree of care in its handling and entailing a higher production cost. However, the contractor's supplier furnished the sand block at the same price as the originally required concrete block.

The issue arose when the contractor claimed, among other things, $42,415.98 as the difference between the value of the sand block furnished and the value of the block originally specified on the grounds that the fair market value of the sand block was greater than the purchase price and that the government should not benefit from the contractor's bargain. The ASBCA accepted the fair market value measure but denied the claim on the basis of failure of proof, i.e., the contractor had failed to prove that the price paid for the original concrete block was not also the fair market value of the substituted sand block at the time of the transaction. The Board held that the fair market value at the time of purchase, not at some subsequent time, is to be used in considering the validity of the equitable adjustment, and that the fair market value at the time of purchase was not different from that of the substituted block. Upon further appeal, the Court of Claims resolved the issue in *Bruce Construction Corporation v. United States*, 324 F.2d 516. The court held:

. . . But fair market value is not the measure of damages in this case. This is not to say that in all cases, historical cost is to be the gauge. The more proper measure would seem to be a 'reasonable cost.' The concept of a 'reasonable cost' is not new. Indeed it has been defined in the following manner:

A cost is reasonable if, in its nature or amount, it does not exceed that which would be incurred by an ordinary prudent person in the conduct of competitive business.

Use of the 'reasonable cost' measure does not constitute 'an objective and universal procedure,' involving the determination of the reasonable value (or reasonable cost of any contractor similarly situated) of the work involved; but determination of reasonable cost required, is in and of itself, an objective test. The particular situation in which a contractor found himself at the time his cost was incurred . . . and the exercise of the contractor's business judgment . . . are but two of the elements that may be examined before ascertaining whether or not a cost was reasonable. (Ct. Cl. 1963)

The court rejected the purely objective method, and substituted a new test of "modified subjective," of "actual costs, reasonably incurred." This new test requires the application of an objective standard of "reasonableness," to the actual or historical costs experienced by the contractor in the particular circumstances (subjective). The court held further that the contractor's "historical" costs are presumed reasonable. Since the presumption is that a contractor's claimed cost is reasonable, the government must carry the heavy burden of showing that the claimed cost was of such a nature that it should not have been expended, or that the contractor's costs were more than were justified in the particular circumstance.

Considered Costs

In negotiating the price of a modification, the basic objective is an equitable adjustment in the contract price for increases or decreases in cost and/or time resulting from the modification with an appropriate upward or downward allowance for profit. Under the present "Changes" and "Differing Site Conditions" clauses, an equitable adjustment clearly encompasses the effect of a change order upon any part of the work, including delayed expense, provided, of course, that such effect was the necessary, reasonable, and foreseeable result of the change. The "impact" of the change must be considered, computed, and negotiated. Assuming that a change was ordered that will extend the performance time of the contract, consideration will include numerous types of costs such as the following:

- Additional compensation for performance of unchanged work because of extended performance time caused by the change, including extended time on extended supervision, overhead, and bonding.
- Increased wage rates for labor on unchanged work, when the contractor is thrown into a period of higher labor costs by the extended performance time.
- Additional costs for materials required to be used in unchanged work deferred due to changes, including storage, protection, trucking and rehandling.
- Heating costs incurred during the extended performance period in order to permit plastering, painting, and other unchanged work originally scheduled for accomplishment in summer months.
- Inefficiency resulting from changes in the planned sequence of contract activity.
- Increased costs for rental of equipment for affected work necessarily deferred due to changes.

In summary, the most common elements of cost involved in equitable adjustment are:

- Added supervision costs.
- Added direct labor costs.
- Resulting labor inefficiency costs.
- Added materials costs.
- Added indirect (overhead) costs.

Disputes and Appeals

During the course of contract performance, a number of adjustments can be made to the contract for example:

- Change order may be issued;
- The contract may be wholly or partially terminated for convenience or default;
- The contractor may deliver nonconforming services; or,
- The government may fail to deliver government property as called for in the schedule.

Each of these occurrences requires some type of adjustment to either the price or the schedule. The contracting officer is authorized to make this adjustment. Although negotiations with the contractor for an equitable adjustment or settlement of claims nor-

mally run smoothly (i.e., both parties agree that the proposed settlement or adjustment is fair, and both go on to other things), sometimes there are problems. If the parties cannot reach agreement, the contracting officer, after conferring with counsel, may issue a unilateral decision on the claim by applying the principle of equitable adjustment. Following this decision, the parties may enter into the disputes process. As with all other aspects of federal contracting, the process is subject to the FAR.

Role of the Contracting Officer in Contract Adjustments

The contracting officer is the primary agent of the government in attempting to meet procurement objectives and must represent the interests of the government in dealing with the contractor. Whenever any adjustment is called for or is claimed by the contractor, the contracting officer must decide whether it is in the best interest of the government to take a specific action. Thus, when a change order has been issued, for example, the contracting officer must decide whether to pay what the contractor claims is an equitable adjustment or to continue negotiating for a lower figure. The process of reaching the decision will involve the contracting officer in fact-finding, analysis, and negotiations for the government. But when a final decision on a dispute that cannot be settled by agreement must be rendered, the contracting officer must render it impartially and independently.

This change in role is a difficult one. How can the same person be an advocate for the government's position and then, on a moment's notice, be transformed into an impartial judge? The conflict, however, is more apparent than real. Even when acting as a party to the disagreement, the contracting officer is supposed to be seeking an equitable adjustment or settlement that takes into account the valid claims of the contractor. In the effort to reach an equitable solution, the change from the role of a party to the dispute to that of impartial arbiter is hardly a change at all for the contracting officer since the goal of equity is the same.

Final Decision of the Contracting Officer

The Act requires timely issuance of the contracting officer's final decision. Decisions on claims for $50,000 or less *must* be issued within 60 days after a request is made by the contractor. Decisions on claims that exceed $50,000 should be issued within 60 days or within a reasonable time after the contractor is notified a decision is pending.

Appeal of the Contracting Officer's Decision Two routes are available to the contractor who wants to contest the contracting officer's decision. The contractor may appeal to the Board of Contract Appeals within 90 days of the decision or may appeal the decision to the Court of Federal Claims within twelve months of the contracting officer's decision. If the contractor is not satisfied with the remedies proposed by the Board or Court of Federal Claims, it may thereafter obtain a review by the Circuit Court of Appeals for the Federal Circuit unless the claim was processed under small claims procedures. The Circuit Court of Appeals for the Federal Circuit will consider the board's or court's decision on questions of fact as final unless such decisions are fraudulent, arbitrary, capricious, or so grossly erroneous as to imply bad faith. Decisions of the board on questions of law are not final nor conclusive.

Disputes (Far Subpart 33.2, Disputes and Appeals) If the contracting officer and the contractor cannot agree regarding a claim, they must turn to the disputes clause of the contract (FAR 52.233-1). This clause requires the contracting officer to make a final written decision on remaining issues. FAR 33.211 provides guidance on the content and format of a final decision. Establishing the date of receipt by the contractor of a final decision is important. Regulations require that the decision be delivered by certified mail or by other means which provide a dated receipt for delivery. The disputes procedure is governed by the Contract Disputes Act of 1978 (41 U.S.C. 601, et seq.). Procedures have been implemented through publication of the Uniform Rules of Procedure for Boards of Contract Appeals. Set forth below is a summary of the revised disputes clause and the actions that are now taken to process disputes.

Board of Contract Appeals Section 8(a)(1) of the act permits an agency board of contract appeals to be established when there are sufficient contract claims to justify a full-time board of at least three members. Board members are empowered to administer oaths, to authorize discovery, and to issue subpoenas. A party failing to honor such a subpoena may be ordered to do so by any US district court under threat of contempt proceedings. A contractor with a claim related to a contract must submit the claim in writing to the contracting officer. Usually these claims are initially submitted for negotiation and settlement. If no settlement can be reached, the contractor then requests a final decision from the contracting officer. The disputes clause defines a claim as:

1. A written request submitted to the contracting officer,
2. For payment of money, adjustment of contract terms, or other relief,
3. That which is in dispute or which remains unresolved after a reasonable passage of time,
4. That for which a final decision is requested.

This definition of claim allows for the current practice of negotiating a "claim" with accrual of interest.

The disputes clause requires the contractor to proceed diligently with performance pending a final decision. The section can be interpreted as altering a contractor's right to work stoppage as permitted prior to the act (e.g., in case of government failure to make payment when due). The board's jurisdiction is maintained over appeals from the contracting officer's final decision, and jurisdiction is extended to the deciding of "all claims" by the parties "relating to the contract." This grant replaces the "arising under" jurisdiction provided by the former disputes clause contained in almost all government contracts. The act makes it clear that the boards have the power to decide breach of contract claims that were previously excluded under the old disputes clause. A contractor who claims breach of contract is no longer left to legal remedies in court but may also approach the board for a decision. A board's jurisdiction over disputes is now equal to that of the Court of Federal Claims.

The act, in attempting to streamline the disputes process for claims of $10,000 or less, requires each board to provide for "expedited disposition of the claim." The contractor may invoke the informal and expedited small claims procedure within 20 days of docketing the claim, with the issue decided by a single board member within 120 days. These decisions are not valuable as precedents in subsequent cases but, in the absence of fraud, are final and nonappealable by either party. A motion for reconsideration may still be filed, however. Section 8(f) of the act establishes a procedure for "accelerated disposition" of any appeal of a contracting officer's final decision for claims of $50,000 or less. This procedure is at the election of the contractor, with the appeal being resolved "whenever possible" within 180 days. Under the Uniform Rules and Procedures for Boards of Contract Appeals, the board member hearing the appeal will arrange an informal meeting with the appropriate parties to assure that all the issues are identified and simplified. Decisions are rendered by the board member with the concurrence of the chairman or vice chairman. A motion for reconsideration may also be filed in this case, although it need not be decided within the 180-day limit.

Under the act, the government as well as the contractor can now appeal an adverse board decision to the Court of Appeals for the Federal Circuit. The government may appeal an adverse decision only with the concurrence of the Attorney General. An appeal by either party must be made within 120 days from the date of receipt of a copy of the board's decision. The court exercises appellate jurisdiction under the Wunderlich Act, which provides that administrative findings of facts and decisions made pursuant to the disputes clause by the contracting agency or a board are "final and conclusive." These findings cannot be set aside unless the decision is fraudulent, capricious, arbitrary, so grossly erroneous as to imply bad faith, or not supported by substantial evidence. The act gives the court the discretion to remand the case for further factual findings or to retain it and take additional evidence. A board's decision on a question of law is not final.

The contractor also has direct access to the Court of Federal Claims. Under the act a suit may be initiated by filing a petition with the court within 12 months from the date of receipt of the contracting officer's final decision. As a practical matter, it is rare that the contractor will file an action in the Court of Federal Claims unless the case is for a substantial amount of money. Proceedings in the court are complex and time-consuming and can take years to be resolved.

Disputes Provisions in Subcontracts   There is no privity of contract between the government and a subcontractor. They are not parties to the same agreement. Therefore, the subcontractor may not directly appeal a decision of the contracting officer under the disputes clause of the contract.

Comparison between the Legal Framework for Contracts and Federal Grants

Grant programs support or stimulate public purposes defined in statutes authorizing those programs. In the late 1800s, federal grants took the form of land grants for the development of agricultural colleges, railroad construction, and other pub-

lic purposes. Federal grants of cash were made to assist programs such as aid to the blind and agricultural experimental stations. There was a steady increase in use of grants, and in 1922 grant expenditures for highway construction amounted to almost 80% of $118,000,000 expended for grants that year. During the 1930s' depression period, the government used grant-enabling statutes such as the Social Security Act to stimulate the economy and create jobs. This reliance on grants continued through the 1940s and 1950s. During the periods outlined above, most grants were awarded to states. The states participated on a voluntary basis, and there was a federal recognition of autonomy on the part of the states in developing and administering grant programs. From 1960 through 1980, there was a marked increase in reliance on grants, along with a change in approach. The Congress passed laws that imposed national standards on grantees, and state and local governments lost some of the autonomy they had previously held. Many of these grant programs were created to implement broad national goals. There was an increase in grants to colleges and universities, hospitals, and other nonprofit organizations. In 1981, payment to the private sector for grant activity amounted to 30% of the grant payments made to state and local governments. The terms of the grant, together with applicable laws and regulations, determine the obligations, rights, and relationships of the parties to a grant agreement. The general purpose of a grant program is usually stated in laws authorizing the grants and their implementing regulations. The grant agreement itself will detail how the money can be expended.

One may ask, "What difference does it make whether we call an agreement a grant, a license, or contract?" The answer lies in the tortuous history of the law. While the basic purpose of contract law is enforcement of mutual promises, the grant brings the entire body of law related to gifts to the table. Further, statutory and common law relating to intellectual property add unique twists when a license is at issue. While grants, contracts, licenses, and partnerships are all agreements, each has its own language, its own underlying legal principles, and its own place in the "tool chest" of research administration. If the parties focus on the purpose of the agreement and strive to maintain the distinction in drafting the terms, there will be fewer misunderstandings and conflicting expectations during performance.

Grants cannot be described as contracts, although there is a temptation to characterize the money paid and the assurances made in connection with a grant as a mutual consideration pointing to that conclusion. The first distinction between grants and contracts is the means for enforcement. The central element of a contractual agreement is that it is "enforceable" with damages being provided to the injured party who does not receive the promised performance. The Federal Grant and Cooperative Agreement Act requires agencies to clearly distinguish between grants and procurement contracts. Since grants do not fall in the second category, they are not governed by Title 41 of the United States Code and the Federal Acquisition Regulation (FAR). A grant is better viewed as a "gift in trust." When called upon to rule on a grantee's use of interest earned on grant funds, the Comptroller General held that the grantee had to return the interest earned since the underlying grant funds were held "in trust" for the United States and any profit inured to the benefit of the United States. The distinction is most important in two areas. Grants have been compared to a trust in the enforcement situation because in the course of trust administration, the grantor has little right to complain so long as the trustee acts in good faith to accomplish the purposes of the trust. In fact, in the grant situation the grantor has even less to say about the actions of grant recipients. This lack of enforcement mechanism is evident in most grant relationships. It is not until after an initial period of performance that a sponsor may decide not to fund the project. In some cases, a sponsor can retain the right to disallow costs in certain categories. Still, the failure of a university research administration organization to carefully control costs or the inefficiency of the sponsored investigator provides no basis for contractual remedy or legal action. Only in the exceedingly rare case of bad faith or actions amounting to fraud does a legal remedy exist.

In summary, a federal grant and a federal contract serve different purposes. Each is entered into through different procedures and carries different conditions. They are enforced differently, with different remedies permitted for each type of relationship. Grants and contracts are generally administered by separate groups of people and in different ways.

The Commission on Government Procurement

During the late 1960s, Congress became increasingly concerned with the procurement processes of

the federal government and recognized that statutory and regulatory changes were needed to improve the way the government carried out its contracting responsibilities. Consequently, in 1969, Congress established the Commission on Government Procurement and charged the Commission with the task of evaluating the government's contracting practices and recommending to Congress ways to improve the efficiency and effectiveness of government contracting. Also crucial were clearer definitions of "grant," "contract," and "cooperative agreement." Somewhat as an afterthought, but because of the increasing volume of federal grants, the commission established a Grants Task Force to perform a rudimentary analysis of grants. The original purpose of the review undertaken by this task force was to gain an understanding of the significance of the use of grants and contracts, and the extent to which procurement rules and regulations might be applied to grant-type assistance. As data on federal grant-type programs were examined, the focus of the grants task force study was enlarged to include such questions as:

- What is the nature of the relationships that exist between the government and a grantee?
- Can and should grant-type assistance be distinguished from procurement?

The task force efforts led to the commission's development of two recommendations, the first of which is as follows:

> Enact legislation to (a) distinguish assistance relationships as a class from procurement relationships by restricting the term 'contract' to procurement relationships and the terms 'grant,' 'grant-in-aid,' and 'cooperative agreement' to assistance relationships, and (b) authorize the general use of instruments reflecting the foregoing types of relationships.

The Federal Grant and Cooperative Agreement Act (41 U.S.C. 6301-6308)

The Federal Grant and Cooperative Agreement Act (FGCAA) establishes criteria for selecting the appropriate kind of contract or assistance instrument when agencies wish to award either grants, cooperative agreements, or contracts. Not only did the FGCAA seek to distinguish the appropriate use of each instrument, but the act encourages a uniform approach to developing contract and grant award instruments. The act does not dictate the specific terms or conditions that should be placed on types of contracts, grants, or cooperative agreements, but it does require that the choice and use of these legal instruments reflect the type of basic relationship expected between the federal and nonfederal parties. Sections 6303, 6304, and 6305 of the act set forth the criteria that require the use of either a procurement contract, a grant, or a cooperative agreement. These sections require that the legal instruments employed in transactions between federal agencies and nonfederal recipients of awards reflect the basic character of the relationships established.

Assistance and Contract Relationships The following are the basic relationships found in transactions between federal agencies and recipients of contracts and federal assistance awards:

- A *procurement contract* is used when the principal purpose of the relationship is the acquisition, by purchase, lease, or barter, of property or services for the direct benefit or use of the federal government.
- A *grant agreement* is used when the principal purpose of the relationship is the transfer of money, property, services, or anything of value to the recipient in order to accomplish a public purpose of support or stimulation; there is no substantial involvement between the federal agency and the recipient during performance of the activity.
- A *cooperative agreement* is used when the principal purpose of the relationship is the transfer of money, property, services, or anything of value to the recipient to accomplish a public purpose of support or stimulation; there is substantial involvement between the federal agency and the recipient during performance of the activity.

Legally, the only difference between a grant and a cooperative agreement is the extent of federal involvement. The act itself does not give an agency the authority to make grants, contracts, or cooperative agreements. Grant-making authority flows from authorizing legislation. The FGCAA is merely steerage for agencies to properly define the business relationship with grantees and contractors. If an agency has authority to use one or more of the instruments and is not specifically prohibited from using any of them, then it may use any of them provided they are used in the correct circumstances as described in Sections 6303, 6304, and 6305 of the FGCAA Act.

Choosing the Appropriate Contract Instrument Using the definitions appearing in the act, one must first deter-

mine whether a particular award is for acquisition or assistance purposes. Procurement contracts would usually be used in the following circumstances:

- Items of hardware acquired.
- Evaluation of the performance of a grantee or contractor initiated by an agency when the results of the evaluation are to be provided to the agency for action.
- Consulting or professional services.
- Training projects where the agency selects the trainers and specifies the content of the curriculum.
- Production of publications or audio-visual materials.
- Conferences conducted for the agency's benefit.
- Research reports are developed, surveys or studies are done, and the work is provided to the agency for its use or to disseminate to others.

Choosing the Appropriate Grant Instrument Grant or cooperative agreements would normally be used in the following circumstances:

- Research where the purpose of the award is to augment the scope of knowledge and publish the results for public consumption.
- Provision of services for the general public or some segment of the public.
- Stimulation of an organization to provide services to the general public or some segment of the public, or develop an organization for a similar purpose.
- Evaluation, where the results of the evaluation are provided to a grantee for its benefit.
- Training projects where the recipient selects the trainees and develops the curriculum.
- Production or publication of audio-visual materials necessary to carry out a grant and for showing to the general public or a segment thereof.
- Conferences conducted for the benefit of grantees.

Using Cooperative Agreements: Substantial Involvement

Although differentiating between grants and cooperative agreements is important, the instruments are very similar. What really distinguishes a cooperative agreement from a grant is the concept of substantial involvement. Substantial programmatic involvement means that after the award, the awarding office staff provide technical assistance and guidance to, or coordinate or participate in, certain programmatic activities of award recipients to a degree beyond their normal responsibilities in the administration of grants. This participation may include, but is not limited to, the following:

- Participating in the design or direction of activities to devise a research protocol or a training or service delivery model.
- Assisting in the selection of contractors.
- Coordinating the collection and analysis of data.
- Providing training of project staff in the participating institution.
- Reviewing and approving each stage of a clinical trial before subsequent stages may be started.
- Participating in selection of project staff or trainees.
- Participating in the presentation of results in publications.

When an Agency Might Select a Cooperative Agreement
Examples of the types of circumstances where an agency might opt for a cooperative agreement rather than a grant are as follows:

- The government wants to review and approve one stage or phase of performance before allowing the recipient to carry on with the next stage or phase.
- Government program personnel collaborate in the performance of the project.
- The government participates in selecting or gives prior approval to the selection of subrecipients under an award.
- The agency participates in selecting key recipient personnel and reserves the right to approve changes in those personnel.
- The agency reserves the right to direct or redirect the recipient's efforts or methodology.

Management of the Federal Contract Process

Contract management involves enforcing, from inception throughout performance, the specific promises or agreements that make a contract. The government and the contractor are concerned with three essential aspects—quality, time, and cost. Quality and time are so intertwined that they should not be separated in the minds of contract managers and administrators. Meaningful or useful research or services produced under contract may be less valuable if not delivered to the government when needed; but substandard research or services may also cause problems. A contractor must also

balance concerns for quality and time with the costs of performance. These concerns are faced in every contract, public or private. However, where private contracts are primarily a matter of private agreements and informal bargaining, public contracts are bound on every side by rules, regulations, and formality. Proper management of a federal contract requires knowledge and skills well beyond private contract management.

Award of a government contract begins a lengthy and complicated administrative process. Throughout the life of the contract, information must be collected, organized, communicated, and evaluated as a basis for decision making. A significant part of the administrative process is directed at enforcing the government's comprehensive and complex contract clauses and requirements. Most administrative actions are pursuant to rights and obligations defined in the General Provisions clauses of a contract. Substantial administrative effort must also be devoted to compliance with contract clauses that further social and economic objectives, often unrelated to the objectives of the contract.

Statement of the Requirement

The portion of a contract that produces the most administrative activities and problems is the statement of the requirement—i.e., the statement of work, specification, or purchase description. These describe what the government wants the contractor to do. Much of the contract manager's effort results directly from the failure of these descriptions to define adequately what is required. Problems also arise when parties to the contract do not have the same understanding of the requirement. Sometimes the statement of the requirement may be ambiguous or defective and at other times it may be quite precise, yet either case may still produce difficulty simply because the contractor and the contracting officer interpret it differently. Parties to contracts view difficulties or problems encountered during performance from opposite points of view. The contractor sees problems and ambiguities in the statement of the requirement, whereas the contract manager for the government sees problems and deficiencies in the contractor's performance. Making accommodation between these two points of view, or establishing one as correct, is a major task of contract management.

Pride of authorship and the human tendency not to want to admit error are further sources of contract difficulties. Government specification writers are slow to admit that their documents are ambiguous or defective. Similarly, the contractor is slow to recognize poor management decisions, erroneous interpretations of the requirement, or poor quality assurance procedures. In a contractual relationship, it is necessary to determine responsibility for the problem. This is a crucial yet often overemphasized aspect of contract management. Contract management should not be a fault-finding exercise. Instead, successful and timely completion of the contract should be the primary objective of all parties.

A large percentage of contract problems are created before the contract is awarded, and many of them are in the statement of work or specifications. Some are generated by ambiguous or defective terms and conditions written specifically for the contract. A few are founded upon some general term or condition included in the contract because of regulatory requirements. Clauses imposed by regulation are seldom the source of contract difficulties. But in combination with the statement of the requirement, the clauses may create problems. Over-optimism concerning the requirement is another source of difficulties; the government may be in a hurry to get the work started, or the contractor may be anxious to begin work even though the requirements have not been adequately reviewed and analyzed.

Solving Administrative Problems

There is no simple solution to all problems of contract management. Many problems could be mitigated or even eliminated, however, if the government reviewed technical requirements more carefully before issuing solicitations and its contractors reviewed them carefully before submitting offers. Excellence in the specifications is one half of the package; the other half is contractors who have the know-how, facilities, manpower, motivation, and financing to perform the job successfully. Government contracts frequently last many months and, in some cases, several years. Complex relationships develop over time. These relationships must be adaptable to changes in requirements and in the various contract environments. The contract should facilitate the work, not hinder it; it must therefore be capable of revision that will reflect ongoing demands and relationships. Effective contract administration includes management of such changing circumstances. The process of contract management must also be discussed in terms of:

- People involved.
- Time at which they become involved.

- Manner in which they work.
- Parameters within which they operate.

Each of these topics is covered in the sections that follow. The basic objective of contract management (i.e., meeting the government's needs for quality goods and services in a timely manner and at a profit) must be kept in mind. In addition, one should never lose sight of the fact that *contract* management is being discussed. The basic definition of a contract is a legally enforceable agreement of competent parties to do or refrain from doing certain specified actions in pursuit of a legal objective. Both the contracting officer and the contractor must always operate within the framework of the contract and of the governing procurement regulations toward the objective of a timely, acceptable product.

Ordinary versus Problem-Solving Functions

One informal distinction, maintained throughout this book, is that between *ordinary* administrative activities and *problem-solving* activities. Activities involving inspection and acceptance, payments, and handling of government property are among the typical, *ordinary* administrative activities. Terminations, changes, and delays, on the other hand, are related to problems that occur on some, but not all contracts. Mechanisms for handling them are written into the agreement—but in the hope that they will never be needed. These are *problem-solving* activities.

> *Teamwork.* It is important not to lose sight of the need for teamwork in the process of contracting. During the contract administration phase of the procurement cycle, the need for teamwork may intensify. The contract manager is charged with directing the course of the contract, but will rarely have expertise in all areas necessary for successful performance. Decisions must, therefore, be based upon the input of many people.
>
> *Personnel Involved.* Depending upon the complexity of the contract, some or all of the following people may become involved in contract management: administrative support personnel, legal counsel, property administrators, cost estimators, accountants, technical specialists, and on-site personnel. Of particular importance are those employees responsible for technical oversight of the work. These employees and their staff must supply their expertise and knowledge of the project in actual performance and in defining and controlling the nature of

the work. Other specialists must provide their input as called upon.

Management Responsibility. The government contractor must be a contract manager who organizes and coordinates the efforts and team of the functional specialists. The members of this team may shift constantly as various people are called from other tasks to work on the specific contract. Effective contract management then is more than the application of expertise to specific problems; it is also leadership to ensure that personnel from many areas and with various kinds of skill and knowledge work together as a team. Based upon information and advice supplied by this interdisciplinary team, the contract manager assures enforcement of the contractor's *and* the government's rights under the contract, ensures timely delivery under the contract, and, in essence, manages the overall business relationship. The contract manager is responsible for implementing diverse contract terms and conditions, controlling costs, and keeping the contractor's books and records. The nature of the legal relationship between the government and the contractor is also a part of the contract manager's responsibility.

Contractual Authority of Governmental Officials. The federal government, like private organizations, must exercise its power to contract through employees with varying degrees of authority and responsibility. These employees are legally called "agents." An agent can be defined as one who represents another person, a principal, in contractual matters. The relationship created by the association of a principal and agent is called "agency." This agency relationship is created when the principal authorizes the agent to act for him or her for a business or contractual negotiation with a third person, and the agent consents to so act. The concept of "authority" is the link that binds third parties to the principal. Authority is the power of the agent to affect the legal relationships of the principal by acts done with the principal's consent. Ultimately, the authority of persons who act on behalf of the government stems from the US Constitution or a federal statute. Of prime importance to the ultimate success of a contract are two government officials charged with administration of the government's side of a contract. These officials with whom the contractor must work, the contracting officer (CO) and the contracting officer's representative(s) (COR), are the persons who can create or resolve most contract problems.

Contracting Officers. These are official representatives of the government who are authorized to enter into and modify contracts that bind the government. This authority may also include the signing of the determinations and findings and other internal documents that are necessary in the contracting process: for example, the contractor's right to seek relief before the Board of Contract Appeals under the standard Disputes clause requires a contracting officer's final decision. The contracting officer may delegate some powers to other authorized agents; however, these agents do not generally have the same authority to bind the government. Their duties are specialized and they are subordinate to the contracting officer. There are other government employees who deal directly with contractors as part of their duties but have no formal status.

Designated Contracting Officers. As a general rule, the designation of a government official as a contracting officer invests that person with authority to make contracts for the United States within legal limits, and the authority expressly delegated to the individual in the designating document, i.e., the "warrant." FAR 1.603-3 states that contracting officers shall be appointed in writing on a "Certificate of Appointment," which shall list any limitations on their scope of authority, other than limitations listed in applicable laws or regulations. In addition to these limitations of authority, agencies may impose additional limitations prescribing methods or procedures by which contracting officers are to exercise their authority. The courts have consistently held that persons dealing with a government contracting officer are presumed to have notice of the limitations on the officer's authority, even though the contracting officer may personally have been unaware of them. The risk of lack of authority is on the contractor.

Implied Authority

Authorized Representatives. Although acts by its agents will not bind the government under the doctrine of apparent authority, the courts and boards have frequently granted contractors relief on the basis of "implied authority." Such authority is generally implied when it is considered to be an integral part of the duties assigned to a government employee. For example, the government will be bound by the actions of inspectors, engineers, or other technical personnel acting within the scope of their authority. Although such persons lack authority to issue change orders, if they give instructions or issue interpretations that induce the contractor to perform work beyond actual contract requirements, the courts and boards will frequently hold the government to a constructive change.

Contractors should bring to the attention of the contracting officer any interpretation or instruction issued by an official who lacks formal contracting authority. Simply relying on the supposed "implied authority" of government employees who administer day-to-day performance may result in the denial of a contractor claim. In *Singer Company, Librascope Division v. United States*, 215 Ct.Cl. 281, 568 F.2d 695 (1977), the court denied a constructive change claim based upon interpretations issued by a technical coordinating group. The contractor was aware that the group lacked formal contracting authority, but failed to bring the interpretations to the attention of the contracting officer.

Designated Contracting Officers. The courts and boards are less willing to find "implied authority" to bind the government in cases involving designated contracting officers. The rationale of the rulings is that the contractor can verify the limits of the contracting officer's authority by examining the Certificate of Appointment and applicable regulations. In *Strick Corporation*, ASBCA 15921, 73-2 BCA ¶10,077 (1973), the administrative contracting officer (ACO) had been delegated administrative responsibility for the contract, but no authority to execute contract modifications. When the ACO inadvertently included a change order on a list of "no cost" modifications, the agency canceled the modification. The board held that the ACO did not have implied authority to execute a contract modification and that the contractor had reason to know this from: (a) the delegation, (b) previous practices involving administration of the contract, and (c) discussions with the government.

Notification of Limits upon Authority. The government sometimes informs the contractor of limitations on the authority of particular government personnel. The method of notification is frequently a contract clause (see FAR 52.243-7 and 52.202-1). By expressly informing the contractor, the government hopes to preclude any implied authority for the unauthorized acts of its personnel.

Imputed Knowledge. Generally, the relationship between a principal and agent is a fiduciary one, requiring good faith and loyalty on the part of the agent in the performance of duties for the principal. A primary characteristic of the relationship as it affects third parties is the imputation of knowledge acquired by the agent within the scope of its agency to the principal. A principal will be bound by knowledge of its agent concerning information that the agent had a duty to deliver to the principal. The rationale is that, in reality, the agent is the principal for purposes falling within the scope of the agent's duties. There are several exceptions to the rule that will relieve the principal of liability for knowledge not disclosed to the principal by the agent. The courts will not impute the agent's knowledge to the principal in the following situations:

1. Where an agent acquires knowledge from a source that requires that it be kept confidential,
2. Where the agent and the third party conspire to cheat or injure the principal, and;
3. Where the agent acquires knowledge in some capacity other than his or her agency.

The basic rule of "imputed knowledge" is applicable in government contracts. In some situations, a court may charge a contracting officer with knowledge of information delivered to other government officials. The government will be bound by that knowledge even though the contracting officer lacked actual notice and the government official who received the information lacked authority to make formal contract changes. The knowledge is "imputed" to the contracting officer through the basic principle of agency discussed above.

Ratification An agent's act that is not binding on the principal solely because the agent lacked authority may become binding upon the principal's adoption of the act. In such cases, the principal is said to have "ratified" the actions of the authorized agent. The principal must have been able to authorize the act at the time it was performed and still have the power to do so at the time of ratification. Generally, ratification occurs only with acts that the principal could have authorized at the time the contract was entered into. The principal of ratification is applicable in government contracts. Government officials who have the authority to bind the government may adopt actions of unauthorized personnel. However, the courts and boards will find ratification only if the government official had actual or constructive notice and expressly or implicitly adopted the acts of the unauthorized agent. Ratification may also be inferred from the contracting officer's silence or inaction if he or she has actual knowledge of the subordinate's actions. In *Lox Equipment Company*, ASBCA 8985, 1964 BCA ¶4463, the contractor sought compensation for additional work ordered by government inspectors. The board held that even though the resident inspector had no authority to issue directives, the chief of the contract administration branch in effect ratified them when he knew of the directives and failed to take corrective action.

Government Bound by Acts of Its Authorized Agents

When government officers, agents, and employees carry out their duties properly, the government will be bound. However, in performing their duties, government personnel cannot be expected to act only in ways favorable to the United States. Because of mistakes, negligence, or poor judgment, their statements, acts, or omissions are sometimes prejudicial to the government. In such cases, the government may attempt to avoid the consequences by repudiating or countermanding the agent's acts. There are two major concepts that the courts will invoke to prevent the government from disowning the agent's acts or agreement, thereby making them binding on the government. The concepts of "finality" and "estoppel" will make the agent's actions binding on the government. These concepts have particular applicability to actions of contracting officials.

Finality Since the government can act only through its agents and employees, their actions within the scope of employment are the actions of the government itself. Once an authorized agent has performed a contractual act on behalf of the government, the government is bound like any other contractual party. Contractual acts may be final and binding as a result of either the application of a provision in the contract that defines when finality attaches or the operation of a legal rule. A contract clause that the courts have interpreted as creating finality is the allowable cost, fixed-fee, and payment clause. In *Chrysler Corp.*, ASBCA 17259, 75-1 BCA ¶11,236, affirmed 76-1 BCA ¶11,665, the board held that this clause should be interpreted to bar the government from contesting payments after it had made the final contract payment. The courts have also interpreted the limitation of cost clause as creating finality when a contracting officer decides to fund a cost overrun. Neither the allowable cost, fixed-fee, and payment clause nor the limitation of cost clause contains express language stating that decisions or actions of the contracting officer will be final. However, courts and boards have interpreted the clauses as having the effect of finality. The best example of a legal rule creating finality is the binding effect on the government created by an authorized official's acceptance of an offer. In *United States v. Purcell Envelope Company*, 249 U.S. 313 (1919), the court held that the government was bound when the Postmaster Gen-

eral accepted the offer of a company in a sealed bid procurement. Similarly, the government will be bound if an authorized official enters into a contract price modification after a change has been ordered.

Estoppel The second concept invoked to prevent the government from escaping liability for an agent's acts or statements is the doctrine of *estoppel*, which prohibits a party from escaping liability for statements, actions, or inactions if the other party has relied on them. The doctrine is applicable in private as well as government contracts. It accomplishes the same result as "finality," and because of this, the two concepts are often confused. However, there are two important differences between estoppel and finality. Estoppel requires a detrimental reliance by the party invoking it, while reliance is not an element of finality. The other difference is that a "final" action is by its very nature contractually binding upon the government through the operation of legal principles, such as offer and acceptance, acceptance of goods, etc. In contrast, the government is held bound by estoppel simply because it would be "unfair" not to do so, even though the statement, action, or inaction would not be contractually binding on the government.

Waiver The concept of waiver is sometimes used interchangeably with estoppel. Like estoppel, the government will be bound by a waiver if the contractor relies upon it to its detriment. The term "waiver" is frequently used when the government fails to promptly terminate a delinquent contractor and that contractor relies on the government's inaction to continue performance with the government's implied consent. In such cases, the government will have waived its right to terminate the contractor for default. The term is also used when the government allows the contractor to deviate from the contract requirements. Government officials generally do not have the authority to waive statutory requirements. Contractors should not assume recovery under either estoppel or finality. Litigation of contract claims is time-consuming and expensive. The wise course of action is to confirm the authority of any individual other than the contracting officer and to notify the contracting officer of *any* questionable direction received from any other governmental agent.

Policies and Procedures Governing the Contracting Officer's Activities

Federal statutes and regulations require that no contract be entered into unless all requirements of law, executive orders, and regulations are met. In this context, agency and service regulations and those of any other regulatory agency are included. Of these requirements, funding limits are perhaps the most critical. The availability of funds must be ascertained prior to obligating those funds by contract. Contract officers (COs) must justify the use of negotiated procurement procedures or the use of certain types of contracts. COs must obtain competition between sources, determine that the proposed contractor is responsible, and obtain any administrative approval required by the agency. In negotiated procurements, COs must obtain from the contractor any required certification of current cost and pricing data and must perform price or cost analysis.

Agency regulations specify that procurement contracts shall conform to all laws and regulations applicable to the agency, with the policies and procedures set forth in internal regulations, and with any applicable policies and procedures otherwise announced or prescribed. Clearly a CO must continually review the policies and procedures required by the agency as well as applicable laws and executive orders. The complexity and detail of contract administration responsibilities have resulted in a separation of duties related to procurement. Accordingly, a CO for the purchasing office is frequently labeled the procuring contracting officer (PCO) and a contracting officer at a contract administration office as an administrative contracting officer (ACO). Additionally, a CO responsible for settlement of terminated contracts is referred to as the termination contracting officer (TCO). The ACO and TCO normally are subordinate to the PCO and are essentially assistant contracting officers.

Contractor's Officer's Representative The term "contracting officer" not only means the person executing the contract on behalf of the government but includes, except as otherwise provided in the contract, the authorized representatives of the contracting officer acting *within the limits* of their authority. These officials may also be called contracting officer's technical representatives, project officers, resident engineers, or other titles. For this text and as a matter of law, all are contracting officer's representatives. Occupying a unique position in the administration of government contracts, the contracting officer's representative (COR) serves as technical advisor to the CO. Through physical observation, the COR ensures that work under the contract is performed in *exact* compliance with the requirements of the contractual agreement. It is the COR who makes many of the decisions or recommendations incident to the day-to-day administration of a

contracted project, and the CO relies heavily on the judgment exercised by the COR since the COR is usually experienced with the type of work being contracted for and possesses the technical background needed to evaluate performance.

Limitations of the Contracting Officer's Authority The responsibilities of the COR are established in the COR's designation. Specific limitations are included in such designations. The letter of designation normally reserves for the CO the right to decide disputed facts and to amend or modify contract prices and times. It further states that the COR will be directly responsible to the contracting officer for the administration of the contract within the authorities and limitations prescribed in the letter of designation issued by the CO. A sample memo to a COR listing the specific responsibilities and duties of the COR follows.

Responsibilities and Duties of the Contracting Officer's Representative

1. Thoroughly familiarize yourself with the terms and conditions of the contract and all related documents.
2. Establish specific due dates for contract submittal required under the Statement of Work (SOW) and establish an appropriate suspense or "tickler" file.
3. Verify the availability of any government-furnished property, services, or facilities that are to be provided in accordance with the SOW.
4. Arrange for the conduct of a post-award conference if appropriate. During such meeting be prepared to discuss with the contractor:
   a. Specific requirements of the SOW.
   b. Special requirements and restrictions, if any.
   c. Access clearances.
   d. Material and equipment approval requirements.
   e. Emergency service requirements.
   f. Inspection procedures.
   g. Contract report and data submittal requirements.
   h. Roles, responsibilities, and authorities of key government and contractor personnel.
5. In the case of some service and construction contracts, inspect the work site with the contractor's representative prior to the contractor's start of work and obtain:
   a. A list of all persons scheduled to work on-site.
   b. Contractor's operating instructions and procedures.

c. Contractor's schedule of work to be performed.

d. A list of materials and equipment to be used.

e. Assurance that applicable wage rate determinations are properly posted and that the contractor has a satisfactory system for preparation of required reports.

6. Perform or cause designated contract monitors to perform during the life of the contract the following functions:

a. Coordinate with the contractor all matters affecting the work to be performed under the contract.

b. Make inspections as necessary to ensure that required work is being done satisfactorily.

c. Ensure that the contract complies with all terms and conditions set forth in the contract.

d. Verify the contractor's invoices for payment.

7. Inform the CO of any contractual problems or disagreements which could result in a claim against the government.

8. Maintain a complete record of inspections rendered on the contractor and advise the CO of the progress noted. In the event the contract contains any incentive provisions, report monthly to the CO on the contractor's performance so that appropriate consideration is given to the payment of incentive fees.

9. Maintain a record of items of government property furnished to the contractor, if any.

10. If contract is for service or construction:

a. Ensure that the contractor establishes and maintains a contractor's employee sign-in/sign-out log.

b. Ensure that when any emergency occurs the contractor diverts the force from their normal assigned duties to take care of the emergency.

c. Obtain a certified copy of the contractor's record for each employee at the end of each work week, showing employee's name and daily hours worked on-site.

Obligations of the Government

Just as the government pays extra for special requirements, it pays less when it undertakes certain responsibilities. Determining the obligations of the government is important. For example, the contract may state that government will provide property [government-furnished property (GFP)] or data to the contractor. If the property or data are not provided within the time frame stated in the contract, the contractor often has an excuse for delay-

ing performance and may even have a basis for a monetary claim against the government.

Suggested Government Contracts Internet Resources

Statutes, Regulations (including the FAR), and Decisional Law

- Thomas

  http://thomas.loc.gov/

  This site is maintained by the Library of Congress and is excellent for bill tracking and for conducting legislative history. Content includes bill texts and links to committee reports and to relevant portions of the Congressional Record. Contains data back to 93rd Congress (1973-74).

- GPO Access

  http://www.gpoaccess.gov/index.html

  This site is maintained by the Government Printing Office (GPO). The site links to all three branches of government as well as to a variety of agencies. The site is valuable as a starting point for researching the federal government and specifically for searching the Federal Register and CFR. However, the content goes back only as far as 1994-1995.

- Legal Information Institute (Cornell)

  http://www.law.cornell.edu

  Good all-purpose site includes statutes, regulations, and short explanatory articles on a variety of legal topics with helpful links.

- FAR Sites

  http://farsite.hill.af.mil

  Provides links to the FAR and to several defense-related FAR supplements (Army, Navy, Air Force, etc.) and to the NASA FAR. This site also has archived versions of the FAR, FAR supplements, and forms. Updates are prompt.

- General Services Administration Acquisition Network (Acqnet)

  http://www.acqnet.gov/far/

  This site, among other things, has the current FAR and archived versions available in text and PDF formats. The archives go back to 1995.

- Defense Acquisition Regulation Directorate

  http://www.acq.osd.mil/dpap/dars/dfars.index.htm

This site obviously caters only to the Defense FAR supplement. The site includes not only the DFAR in a variety of formats, but also has information on class deviations, the Defense Acquisition Deskbook, information on costs and pricing, change notices to the DFAR, and other DFAR specific information.

- United States Court of Appeals for the Federal Circuit

  http://www.fedcir.gov

- United States Court of Federal Claims

  http://www.uscfc.uscourts.gov

- Armed Services Board of Contract Appeals

  http://www.law.gwu.edu/ASBCA/

- Comptroller General Decisions

  http://www.gpoaccess.gov/gaodecisions/index.html

  The GAO Comptroller General Decisions database contains decisions made by the Comptroller General in areas of federal law such as appropriations, bid protests, civilian and military personnel pay and allowances, household goods and freight loss damage, and transportation rates. It is sponsored by the US General Accounting Office (GAO) and accessed through GPO Access. The database contains decisions from October 1995 to the present. The database is updated within two business days after decisions have been released. Documents are available in text and PDF formats.

Agency and Procurement Sites

- Library of Congress: Official US Executive Branch Web Sites

  http://www.loc.gov/rr/news/fedgov.html

  This site, created and maintained by the Library of Congress lists the home pages of executive branch agencies.

- Office of Federal Procurement Policy (OFPP)

  http://www.whitehouse.gov/omb/procurement/index.html

  This is the official site of the OFPP, which is responsible for providing guidance to and writing policies for federal procurement. Several OFPP publications are available on this site while others are linked via the Acqnet Web site. The site contains (or links to) OFPP documents located in a virtual library and links to agency homepages as well as information on opportunities, procurement forecasts, and small business information.

- Federal Acquisition Jumpstation

  http://prod.nais.nasa.gov/pub/fedproc/home.html

  This site, maintained by NASA, links to executive agencies and to agencies' internal offices having to do with procurement issues and contracting opportunities of the agency. Some agencies have more links than others. For example, the Defense Department agencies have extensive links; HUD has only two.

- FirstGov

  http://www.firstgov.gov/

  This site is the US Government's official Web portal.

- FedBizOpps

  http://www.fedbizopps.gov/

  FedBizOpps.gov is the single government point-of-entry for federal government procurement opportunities over $25,000. Government buyers post business opportunities directly to this site. Commercial vendors can search, monitor, and retrieve opportunities solicited by the entire federal contracting community.

- Gov.Com

  http://www.gov.com

  "GOV.com is a partnership of private enterprise and public-sector government news and information bureaus, with the goal of delivering official information from official government sources, preserving the highest level of information integrity." This site has links to many agency offices that have their own Web sites. Also includes lists of links to the Executive, Judicial, Defense, Congress, and Senate. The author does not know why there is no link to the House.

- Govcon

  http://www.govcon.com/content/homepage/default.asp

  This site is "the premier information source for the government contracting industry. Find products and suppliers, read current headlines, and keep up with the latest information in your professional community."

Gateway Sites: Providing Links to Related Sites

- Federal Acquisition Jumpstation

  http://prod.nais.nasa.gov/pub/fedproc/home.html

  See above.

- U.S. Army Robert Morris Acquisition Center Library

  http://w3.arl.army.mil/contracts/library.htm

  This site has links that include all the FAR supplements and links to other military acquisition related sites.

- Cyrus E. Phillips IV, Attorney at Law

  http://www.procurement-lawyer.com

  This site is maintained by Cyrus E. Phillips IV, an attorney in private practice who has put together extensive links to items such as court sites, agency documents, agency regulations, procurement reform documents, international procurement information, and his own newsletter (which is not up to date).

- General Services Administration Acquisition Network (Acqnet)

  http://www.acqnet.gov

  This site provides links to the Office of Federal Procurement Policy (OFPP), FAR links, a virtual library that is organized to correspond to the procurement process, business opportunity links, links to training sites (both governmental and private), and a page on E-Government Initiatives.

- Professor Steven Schooner's Government Contract Law Site

  http://docs.law.gwu.edu/facweb/sschooner/links.html

  Professor Schooner's site provides links of interest to George Washington University Law School J.D. and L.L.M. students, as well as links arranged by topical headings including "Research," "ADR," "Environmental," "International," and "State Procurement."

- FirstGov

  http://www.firstgov.gov/

  The US Government's official Web portal. When dealing with the federal government, sometimes it is best to start at the beginning.

Miscellaneous

- AT & L Knowledge Sharing System

  http://akss.dau.mil/jsp/default.jsp

  The Acquisition, Technology & Logistics (AT & L) Knowledge Sharing System (AKSS) has replaced the Defense Acquisition Deskbook. This Web site is the central point for accessing all acquisition, technology, and logistics resources and information. This site is a reference center for those working in defense procurement.

- Government Contracts Research Guide

  http://www.law.gwu.edu/burns/guides/govcont.pdf

  This is our handy research guide. Always the good place to start when you are lost.

- Federal Acquisition Institute Online University

  http://www.fai.gov

  A complete online university devoted to federal procurement. Registration is required, but they offer a free tour (no registration required) that allows you to look around.

- Federal Procurement Data System

  http://www.fpds.gov

  The Federal Procurement Data System (FPDS) is part of the US General Services Administration. The FPDS is the central repository of statistical information on Federal contracting. The system contains detailed information contract actions over $25,000 and summary data on procurements of less than $25,000. The Executive departments and agencies award over $200 billion annually for goods and services. The system can identify who bought what, from whom, for how much, when, and where.

- Where in Federal Contracting?

  http://www.wifcon.com

  A commercial site that is aimed at the contractor side. Very interesting links and worth a look.

- Defense Acquisition University Glossary of Terms

  http://www.dau.mil/pubs/glossary/preface.asp

  Downloadable PDF document providing the meaning of defense acquisition acronyms and Terms.

- Doing Business with the DoD

  http://www.defenselink.mil/other_info/business.html

  Specialized site dealing with Department of Defense.

- PubKLaw

  http://www.pubklaw.com/

  This is a private site run by a former Commerce Department attorney. This site is very valuable for keeping up to date on the latest happenings in the world of federal procurement.

- Procurement Reference Center
http://ec.msfc.nasa.gov/msfc/procref.html
Another excellent site run by NASA with links to agency procurement related Web sites and information for contractors.

• • • Endnotes

1. *Rock Island, A. & L. R. Co. v. United States*, 254 U.S. 141 (1920).

2. *Office of Federal Procurement Policy Act*, P.L. 93-400, 41 U.S. Code (1974) § 403(a). For full classification of this Act, consult USCS Tables volumes. P.L. 93-400, § 4[3][4], 88 Stat. 797, October 10, 1979. P.L. 96-83, § 3, 93 Stat. 649; December 1, 1983. P.L. 98-191, § 4, 97 Stat. 1326; July 18, 1984. P.L. 98-369, Division B, Title VII, Subtitle C, § 2731, 98 Stat. 1195; October 30, 1984. P.L. 98-577, Title I, § 102, 98 Stat. 3067; November 17, 1988. P.L. 100-679, § 3(c), 102 Stat. 4056; November 5, 1990. P.L. 101-510, Division A, Title VIII, Part A, § 806(a) (1), 104 Stat. 1592; October 13, 1994. P.L. 103-355, Title IV, Subtitle A, § 4001, Title VIII, Subtitle A, § 8001, 108 Stat. 3338, 3384; February 10, 1996. P.L. 104-106, Division D, Title XLII, § 4204, 110 Stat. 655; October 5, 1999. P.L. 106-65, Division A, Title VIII, Subtitle A, § 805, 113 Stat. 705; November 24, 2003. P.L. 108-136, Division A, Title XIV, Subtitle A, § 1411, Subtitle C, § 1433, 117 Stat. 1663, 1673, as amended October 28, 2004. P.L. 108-375, Division A, Title VIII, Subtitle A, § 807(b), 118 Stat. 2011.

3. The APA is codified at U.S. Code Title 5 (1966) § 551 through 559 and 701 through 706. P.L. 89-554, § 1, 80 Stat. 381; Sept. 13, 1976. P.L. 94-409, § 4(b), 90 Stat. 1247, as amended July 5, 1994. P.L. 103-272, § 5(a), 108 Stat. 1373.

4. Circulars are available free of charge from the Executive Office of the President, telephone (202)395-7332.

5. Federal Business Opportunities is found at www.fedbizopps.gov.

34

Research Contracts with Industry

J. Michael Slocum, JD

Types of Research Activities Engaged in by Industry

Most countries acknowledge a symbiotic relationship between investment in science and technology and success in the marketplace. Science and technology are essential for countries to remain competitive in international trade and to attain commercial success in the global marketplace. At any given time, these same governments are usually striving to support industries seen as high-technology (science-based industries whose products involve above-average levels of R&D). However, every industry provides opportunity for research activity. The most mundane activities are often the most ripe for research advances.

Enabling Technologies

Much of industrial research is aimed at development of *enabling technology*—technology that enhances the creation and delivery processes of products and services. While industry conducts much of this research itself, it also relies on the use of engineering firms and engineering-oriented academic institutions.

Educational institutions are often the source of the ideas and fundamental research surrounding new and existing enabling technologies. Industrial research organizations are involved most often at the technology development stage because development of these technologies is often of relatively high cost for any one company, and sometimes hard to justify when compared to

shorter-term company product goals. Many times the final stages of this kind of research are conducted internally, because of competitive issues that arise with the intellectual property being developed.

Problem-Solving

Universities and nonprofit research organizations are seen by industry as a problem-solving resource. Many collaborative efforts are initiated by industry for a specific purpose to help with a step in a process that is not working, is not efficient, or is affecting the quality of the product. Most often, this type of project is initiated by a company contacting the organization based on "word-of-mouth" relationships established by faculty members with industry personnel.

Developing Value-Added Technologies

Many times it is the academic or nonprofit organization or individual who approaches industry. This happens most often with "value-added" research activity. Value-added technologies are anything that can be added to an existing product that allows industry to charge more for that product. Examples include "bioceuticals" (i.e., foods with pharmaceutical properties), materials research that may transform commodities or waste into more valuable products, and "nanotechnology" projects that seek to develop molecular-sized machines.

In certain technological areas such research is often welcomed by industry. Individual companies welcome the approach by universities and non-profit organizations with ideas to sponsor value-added research. In other industries there is a reluctance to use outside resources, although the various companies may well conduct value-added research within the company.

International Trends in Industrial R&D

In high-wage countries such as the United States, industries stay competitive through innovation. Innovation leads to better production processes and higher quality products, thereby providing the competitive advantage high-wage countries need when competing against low-wage nations. R&D activities serve as incubators for the new ideas that can lead to new products, processes, and industries.

Industries that traditionally conduct large amounts of R&D have met with greater success than those that are less R&D intensive. The United States, the European Union (EU), and Japan represent the three largest economies in the industrialized world and are competitors in the international marketplace. These countries and regions are serving as the model for other countries moving from a manufacturing focus to the "post-industrial" economy. However, each has approached research in somewhat different ways.

United States

R&D performance by the US service-sector industries (i.e., contract research organizations and academic and nonprofit organizations providing services to industry) underwent explosive growth in the last decades of the 20th century, driven primarily by computer software firms and firms performing R&D on a contract basis. The US aerospace industry performed the largest amount of R&D in the late 1980s. During the mid-1990s, however, the nation's R&D emphasis shifted; the aerospace industry's share declined, and the share for the industry manufacturing communications equipment increased. At the end of the century, the communications and other electronics equipment industry was the top R&D sector in the United States. As the new century began, there was a further shift to biotechnology and an apparent push into materials science and "nanotechnology." In each case, government encouraged the research emphasis, but the research was primarily a matter of private capital investment.

Japan

Unlike the United States, Japan has not traditionally used service providers for R&D. Japan's industrial

R&D performance continues to be dominated by the individual manufacturers conducting the work internally. This reflects that country's long-standing emphasis on electronics technology (including consumer electronics and audiovisual equipment), motor vehicles, and electrical machinery. However, Japanese companies have begun to exhibit an interest in acquiring technology from academic institutions in the United States and elsewhere.

European Union

As in Japan and the United States, manufacturing industries perform the bulk of industrial R&D in the 15-nation EU. The EU's industrial R&D appears to be somewhat less concentrated than that in the United States but more so than that in Japan. Large increases in R&D performed by service providers are apparent in many EU countries, but especially in the United Kingdom, Italy, and France. In keeping with their histories, much of the research is performed in collaboration with government institutions.

The Industry and University Research Model

In the United States, and increasingly in the other advanced economies, the industry/ university agreement has emerged as a model for effective and cost-efficient research. In biology, chemistry, computer science, and even education and psychology, the lure of increased research support has tempted the "ivory tower" to come to the marketplace while the potential for "revolutionary" profits has brought the entrepreneur to academia's ivy-covered halls. The resulting, sometimes prickly, collaboration has driven waves of innovation that in turn have driven the economy of the United States and the world. Several versions of research support have been developed to accomplish the varying objectives of the funding corporations while satisfying the academic purposes of the universities and other nonprofit institutions.

There is a continuous examination of the roles of the different sectors in the overall R&D enterprise by both academics, the government, and by the sectors themselves. Many of the earlier relationships that stressed "contract research"—even when applied within the confines of a single corporate entity—can be expected to continue in a classical mode. However, a greater emphasis has been placed on strategic alliances or "partnering," even across corporate lines during the last decades.

Choosing the Type of Agreement

The types of agreements that may exist between industry and university fall into the broad categories of:

- Philanthropy.
- Agreements with individuals.
- Agreements with university for university research.
- Contracts for supplies and services in support of research activities.
- Agreements for exploitation of research findings.

There is often a blurring between the categories. For instance, a company may enter into a contract for research and simultaneously make a grant of equipment, facilities, or other property to a university. Similarly, many research agreements include license provisions relating to commercial exploitation of any resulting research findings.

The reasons for undertaking any one type of agreement differ for universities and industry. Further, statutory and policy considerations affect the direction in which a given company or university may go. For instance, many universities have defined generally the types of research for which they will accept funding. Typically, universities are not interested in accepting research that is too routine in nature (basically, as service function) or that is so narrow in scope as to limit basic scientific endeavors, the primary thrust of university research. Also, some universities have refused to accept funding for certain projects related to the defense industry, for example, chemical or biological warfare research.

Some corporations require that universities utilize their equipment in conducting research for them. Acceptance of such a stipulation could be both counter to the university's philosophy and also be very expensive. For instance, assume that a university accepts a research contract from the XYZ Computer Corporation for the development of a new type of microchip. The contract includes a clause requiring that all computer equipment purchased on the contract be XYZ equipment. Several of the university researchers involved feel strongly that ABC Co. equipment is more appropriate for several applications. Also, the university has a major investment in computer equipment that is not compatible with the XYZ equipment. Thus, acceptance of the contract would result in the university's acquiring equipment that is not optimal for the task, is not compatible with the university's equipment of choice, and would require a rather expensive maintenance outlay after the conclusion of the contract.

However, aside from these kinds of issues, the choice of agreement should be a matter of purpose. A basic decision matrix can be developed to help negotiators and administrators make a choice as to the form of agreement most appropriate to a given joint endeavor.

The selection of the form of agreement is not an issue faced solely in industry-university relations. The United States Federal Grant and Cooperative Agreement Act makes the purpose of the agreement the deciding factor in the selection of a particular form of agreement. The distinctions made in that Act are useful in the private arena as well. The government looks first at the primary beneficiary. If the purpose of the agreement is to fulfill a societal need or to advance the basic level of knowledge, an assistance document is used. If the purpose of the agreement is to acquire goods or services (including the

TABLE 34-1 Matrix of Agreement Types	
Factor/Situation	**Type of Agreement**
Specific research objective to be accomplished by one party for other party's use	Research contract
Guidance or advice needed from one party for other party to proceed with in-house project	Consulting agreement
Supplies or services needed to support research effort	Contract/subcontract
Joint effort to conduct on-going research	Partnership
Joint effort to conduct on-going research where passive investors will be involved	Limited partnership
Joint effort to undertake specific research project	Joint venture
Research of research by one party to be used by other party	License agreement

knowledge necessary to produce goods or services) then a contractual instrument is used. Within the assistance area a further distinction is drawn. If no continuing relationship is intended, the instrument of choice is the grant. Where facilities, personnel, or other results will be shared or where the sponsor will exercise continuing involvement in the project, the Act calls for a cooperative agreement.

For industry-university agreements, the category of contractual agreements can be further subdivided. When the purpose of the agreement is a one-time end result, a research contract is appropriate. When the purpose instead is the overall development and commercialization of a research endeavor, the research partnership or a consulting agreement is likely to be the vehicle.

Under any of the primary agreements, two contractual actions are common. For completed research to be properly exploited, license agreements may be needed. And, of course, both the corporation and the university often enter into purchase agreements and subcontracts for goods and services.

Areas of the Law Affecting Research Contracts

Practitioners handling industry/university and other private research contracts must be familiar with a broad range of legal issues, most importantly, the basics of contract law. However, the research administrator must also be familiar with the law related to business entities. For instance, a partnership is a contract between business owners. Similarly, the research administrator must have some understanding of intellectual property and licensing laws (a license agreement is a contract to use certain property). Since the institution may face claims based on product liability, malpractice, or environmental abuse, the research manager must be aware of these legal arenas. The drafter and administrator of a research contract may deal with issues from bankruptcy to torts and from choice of law to warranty. This text cannot begin to provide the legal underpinnings for a contract negotiator working with complex agreements. While this section identifies the areas that require study, a competent research manager will assure that he or she has access to competent counsel.

The primary areas of the law to be concerned with in negotiating research contracts include:

- Basic contract law.
- Agency.

- Business organizations (corporate and partnership law).
- Negligence–product liability and insurance law.
- Intellectual property law.
- Public contract law and administrative procedures.
- Bankruptcy.
- Anti-trust.
- Civil procedure.

The clauses of even a simple contract for research services are molded by the complex interplay of each legal area listed above. These legal areas dictate the particular clauses to be used, the rights of the contracting parties and others under those clauses, the role of governmental entities in private contracts, and the value of the end results to the contracting parties.

Types of Contractual Agreements

One reason so many areas of the law apply to contracts is that there are many types of contractual agreements. As discussed earlier, consulting agreements, partnerships, subcontracts, and purchase orders for supplies all fall into this category. The common element in each is a reasonably specific purpose and the concept of mutuality of enforceable promises. The particular aspects of the arrangement then dictate the form of agreement most appropriate.

Anatomy of Research Contracts

A review of the literature concerning industry-university research indicates a set of very common problems faced in almost every research field. These problems arise because the organizations have different goals, different "cultures," and different governing rules. Many of the problems arise, however, simply because one party is paying and the other is performing. These problems as well as the institutional variations must be addressed if successful agreements are to be reached.

Tradition and function dictate a somewhat standardized format for research contracts. This is not a matter of style or convention. Research (and other) contracts tend to look alike because the same topics must be covered.

Every contract should include provisions concerning the following:

- Identification of the parties.
- Work to be done or property to be transferred.
- Period of performance.
- Consideration/financial arrangement.

- Control of the work/interface provisions.
- Use of other party's property, name, data, (including patents), etc.
- Extra-contractual liability (including issues relating to insurance and to third parties).
- Provisions relating to disputes resolution.

If a central topic is not covered, the parties run the risk of a court inserting language into the agreement to cover the issue or even declaring the agreement to be null. In many cases, there may be statutory or case-derived "language" that will be applied to "fill the gap" in a contract that does not cover a particular topic. On the other hand, the parties may well want to incorporate such language, or they may intentionally not cover a subject that is unlikely to become the subject of dispute.

The contract may well include additional provisions covering a multitude of other topics, but the topics set out above are what define the species within the contract genus. In addition, many contracts include "recitals" or statements of intent and explanation. These, however, do not usually have the legal force of actual contract clauses.

Some of the contract clauses to be used in each section are discussed below. However, it is imperative that research administrators remember that the protocol or statement of work to be done is a part of the contract even when it is "incorporated by reference" (stated to be included even though it is not physically inserted). If a contract has been chosen as the form of agreement, the statement of work should be reasonably precise. If broad exploratory research with no firm objective is being funded, an assistance document might be the better vehicle of agreement.

The particular issues to be addressed in a work statement will vary with the nature, purpose, size, and complexity of the work to be performed. At a minimum, however, every work statement should:

- Give a precise statement of objectives.
- Identify the work to be performed.
- Set parameters by which the desired scope of work can be defined and by which progress and results can be measured.
- Require some defined "end product" and some tangible form of progress/compliance reporting.

A work statement for a level-of-effort type requirement should specify:

- Kind of personnel (labor categories) required to perform the work and any qualification requirements (e.g., education, experience, and certification).
- Nature of work.

- Required deliverables.

In writing the final version of the statement, elements may need to be combined or rearranged in individual sections to fit particular circumstances. The main objective should be to arrange and present the elements in a manner that:

- Is logical and readable.
- Emphasizes the most important elements.
- Conveys exactly what is required of the contractor.

Special Types of Contracts

While consulting agreements, partnerships and joint ventures, and license agreements all conform to the basic anatomy of contract, each has special attributes related to the peculiar nature of the relationship that is created. These attributes may involve additional sections or particular "twists" to the basic contractual language.

Agreements with Individuals

Most commonly, agreements with individuals are consulting arrangements. However, such agreements might also arise when a university needs advice on the organization of a research foundation or on the tax consequences of a proposed research partnership. In any of these or other agreements with individuals, the basic contractual structure may be modified substantially because of the problem of avoiding the creation of an employment situation. Employers and employees are subject to a series of tax and work protection laws. While these laws are not meant to apply to independent consultants, companies and individuals have repeatedly tried to use the consulting arrangement to avoid withholding, overtime, or unemployment compensation requirements. As a result, legislators and regulators in the United States and elsewhere have defined employment in the broadest possible way, making even legitimate consulting arrangements more difficult to establish.

The difficulty is compounded by governmental or university restrictions on noncivil service employment for government employees or university faculty, by government conflict of interest restrictions, and by the objective held by many companies to assure the "loyalty" of consultants. To address these problems, the drafter of a consulting agreement should include specific language, crafted in light of governmental labor laws (and conflict provisions, where applicable) that preserves the independent status of the consultant (see, in particular, for the United States, Section 1706 of the Tax Reform Act of 1986).

Partnerships and Consortia

Organizations of all sizes and all around the world conduct research activities through partnerships, collaborations, and outsourcing. Many organizations will pursue multiple relationships, each for a specific technological or business goal. These relationships have had many names:

1. **Alliance.** A generally long-term agreement between two or more organizations to cooperate in the development of future products and technologies. Members are generally all within the same industry. This relationship provides for a mutually planned approach to solving a specific technical problem or sets of problems. An alliance is not a defined legal entity, *per se*, but alliances are often structured as a partnership or joint venture

2. **Strategic alliance.** Collaboration between two or more organizations designed to achieve some specific corporate objective. This relationship is usually structured as a partnership, but may also include international licensing agreements, management contracts, or joint ventures.

3. **Collaboration.** Generally two organizations, not necessarily with common products or technologies, that agree to cooperate to develop a new product through the combination of mutually complementary expertise. Both organizations share in the profits of the resulting products.

4. **Consortium.** A group of organizations with generally common products who cooperate and share resources in order to achieve a common objective. The US National Science Foundation defines these as "partnerships of multiple institutions, which can be academic and/or nonprofit, which are formed for the expressed purpose of carrying out research activities."

5. **Cooperative.** A form of collaboration in which two or more, usually nonprofit, organizations join forces, primarily for cost-sharing benefits.

6. **CRADA** (Cooperative Research And Development Agreement): An agreement formed typically between two government agencies or one government agency and a private corporation or university to develop a specific set of technologies or prototype products.

7. **Joint venture.** An agreement between two or more organizations to undertake the same business strategy and plan of action. Joint ventures may be structured as partnerships, co-owned corporate bodies, or other forms of business collaborations.

8. **Outsourcing relationship.** A situation where one party sends out (work, for example) to an outside provider, usually to cut costs. Basically contracting for research, but also often for research management.

9. **Partnership.** Business relationships in which two or more organizations carry on a business together with a shared ownership. Partners are each fully liable for all the debts of the enterprise, but they also share the profits exclusively.

10. **R&D limited partnership.** A partnership whose investors put up money to finance new product R&D in return for profits generated from the products. The investors are said to have limited liability in that they have a limitation of loss to what has already been invested. Other legal variations include a general partnership and a master limited partnership. General partners have unlimited liabilities for the obligations of the partnership. A general partnership is a partnership in which all participants are general partners.

R&D limited partnerships and limited liability companies are often vehicles for funding research while obtaining tax benefits. Investors provide the funds, a research institution gets the funding to do major projects, and new products and processes tumble out without a company being forced to mortgage its assets for an uncertain future. Similarly, governmental economic development entities and entrepreneurial university managers often establish consortia to join multiple research institutions with complementary capabilities that may attract additional research funds not available to any of the individual organizations. Sometimes universities or nonprofits are even members of joint ventures.

The R&D limited partnership scenario sounds perfect for industry-university cooperation; however, the actual story is a bit more complicated. All of these conjoined entities are partnerships of one sort or another. However, partnership law is complex, tax law (which is a primary consideration in R&D partnerships) is horrendously complex, and securities law (i.e., the law dealing with the ownership of fractional interest in the conjoined entities) is a gordian knot made of hardened steel cable. To a great extent, partnership law derives from agency law. Each partner is considered an agent of every other partner. Thus, the agency concepts of imputed knowledge and responsibility for acts done within the scope of the partnership relationship will apply.

Partnership law is distinct from agency law in an important way. A partnership is based upon a voluntary contract between two or more competent persons who agree to place some or all of their money, effects, labor, and skill in business with the understanding that there will be a proportional sharing of the profits and losses among them. An agent can be compensated from business profits but does not agree to bear the ordinary business losses and has no ownership interest in the business.

In the past, attempts to formulate a concrete definition of the term partnership have caused endless controversy among judges, lawyers, and members of the business community. Partnership is defined by the Uniform Partnership Act (passed by most states) as "an association of two or more persons to carry on as co-owners a business for profit." Therefore, two essential elements of a partnership are (1) a common ownership interest in a business and (2) sharing profits and losses of the business. (University administrators may cringe at this, seeing challenges to the university's tax exempt status if it enters into such a relationship.[1])

R&D partnerships are often a special kind of organization called a limited partnership. The limited partnership is a creature of statute. Most states in the United States have adopted some form of the Uniform Limited Partnership Act (UPLA), which codifies the law of limited partnerships. Limited partnerships are frequently used in the context of commercial investment. A person willing to purchase the financial interest in a business might not want any management responsibility or personal liability for partnership debts. The limited partnership form meets this need since only the general partner(s) must have unlimited liability. In this case, the general partner assumes management responsibility of the partnership and takes full personal liability for all its debts. A limited partner contributes cash (or other property) and owns an interest in the firm but undertakes no management responsibilities and is not personally liable for partnership debts beyond the amount of his or her investment.

Finally, to the extent that a wide range of limited partner investors will be solicited, state and federal securities laws may apply and will produce an exponential increase in complexity. A recent "simple," publicly traded R&D partnership has been reported to have taken over a year to structure, with several very high-priced lawyers and accountants working on the deal continuously.

This is not to say that a university or nonprofit may not undertake research work using the partnership format. Outside the tax-based R&D partnership arena, partnerships are a common form of business organization. They are long-term working relationships built on mutual trust and commitment between partners with complementary capabilities and shared goals and risks. Partnerships serve to achieve goals that may be difficult or impossible for either party to accomplish alone.

Research Consortia

A common form of partnership seen in the academic research environment is the research consortium. Consortia may also be structured as separate corporate entities and sometimes as loose alliances with only contractual arrangements to serve as the structural framework.

Research consortia could take the form of public-public arrangements (government agencies and public providers), private-public partnerships, or a private-private consortium. Research consortia come together around a wide and diverse range of issues and take many different forms:

- Focused around a single industry sector on common user needs.
- Involving research and technology cutting across sectors.
- Involving discrete joint ventures within an industry or supply chain.

Research consortia are often focused on achieving tangible and specific objectives. These include new platforms leading to new products, services, or processes, or solving focused and difficult research problems needed to transform existing services, products and processes. There are, for example, consortia related to nanotechnology, waste disposal, marine mammals, and structural genomics, to name only a very few. Each of these is a unique entity, with its own structure, defining and controlling documentation, and membership.

Most consortia have a single governance entity, which could be a separate company (with its own management structure), a partnership management committee, a joint venture (again with multiple forms possible), or a cooperative. Whatever the consortium's legal structure, the governance entity needs to:

- Enable user-leadership in setting and managing evolving research directions.
- Sufficiently bind the collaborating parties around the achievement of the consortia objectives.
- Manage the necessary adjustments and realignments of research effort and priorities between the parties as circumstances change.

- Provide an intellectual property policy that encourages innovation by collaborating parties, promotes research use or commercialization, and protects the individual members' separate interests.
- Create the management disciplines and capabilities needed to monitor and enforce performance by the members and by third parties with whom the consortia interacts.

The most important issue to be addressed in establishing a consortium is the allocation of control (e.g., voting rights) over the consortium. This should be carefully documented in the organizing documents, along with a mechanism for altering the control at later stages. The initial organizing documents are the "constitution" on which the consortium government is based.

Additionally, consortium agreements must provide for management of research priorities between consortium parties as circumstances change and establish the role of the consortium in negotiating with third parties, managing individual research contracts, and coordinating commercialization and technology management.

Organizations establishing consortia need to establish just how much freedom the consortium will have to take risks and redirect research as circumstances change in order to achieve the consortium objectives. Consortium partners should identify the research priorities and projects and programs for which the consortium will have responsibility. They will need to determine if the consortia will act as an agent for the members, working within specified principles and parameters, or if the consortium will be more of a clearinghouse, simply transferring work and results among the members and third parties?

Consortia should have either wind-up or grow strategies, or have critical milestone points where exit or growth may be evaluated. Exit may include attracting venture capital for commercialization or even stock market listing. Consortia might instead wind themselves up following the spin-off of new ventures or transfer of the research results to the members or to third parties. An Intellectual Property (IP) agreement should be agreed upon between consortium parties before the venture begins. This should detail the IP that each party brings with them, who will own the IP that arises, and what access rights the parties will have. It should reflect the inputs, contributions, and risks of each party. The consortium should have a method for evaluation against milestones and objectives. Methods include:

- Audit assurance that governance and management systems are in place and operating appropriately.
- Financial and progress reviews.
- Full outcome evaluation of objectives achieved by the funding or participating members or users.

Having review points at specific points during the planned consortium life provides the opportunity for parties in a consortium to reassess funding needs and directions. The consortia agreement should fully discuss the amounts and nature of investments and contributors. Members may contribute investment funds, staff effort and time, and existing IP. In other cases, time and effort and IP may be provided in return for compensation. This should be clearly delineated in advance.

Joint Ventures

In some cases, joint ventures provide the best partner-like form of business activity. Joint ventures are used in a wide variety of manufacturing, mining, and service industries and frequently also involve technology licensing (discussed below) by one or more of the parties to the joint venture. In the business world, the term joint venture usually relates to an organizational format where companies come together to pool their resources and expertise to pursue common opportunities.

While often established as a partnership, it is increasingly common to see joint venture corporations. That is an activity that includes the creation of a new organization to further specific ends of two or more organizations. Partner organizations share governance of the new organization. For example, organizations might initiate a joint venture whose mission is to develop and service software developed by one organization which is to be sold by another organization with access to distribution channels. The partners would name agents/designees to sit on the joint venture corporation's board, and perhaps would even name the individual officers.

For international deals, the host country's laws may require that a certain percentage (often 51 percent or more) of a business activity be owned by nationals of that country, thereby limiting the ability of a foreign entity to operate independently. In addition to such legal requirements, research institutions, and even commercial firms, may find it desirable to enter into a joint venture with a foreign firm to help spread the high costs and risks frequently associated with foreign operations or a newly developed technology. The partners in a joint venture normally bring to the joint venture their knowledge of the technology, manufacturing, perhaps a distribution network, and valuable business and political contacts. For international deals, a joint venture with a local partner may also lessen the "foreigner" image of the outside institution or company, and thus may provide some protection against discrimination or expropriation if conditions change.

The obvious disadvantage to using joint ventures is the loss of effective managerial control. This can result in reduced profits, increased operating costs, inferior product quality, exposure to product liability, and environmental litigation and fines. The issue of control and governance will be normally the most important topic in negotiations with the prospective joint venture partner. Joint ventures can raise anti-trust issues in certain circumstances, particularly when the prospective joint venture partners are major existing or potential competitors in the affected national markets.

Alliances and Strategic Alliances

The terms "alliance" or "strategic alliance" are widely-used but loosely-defined terms that encompass a wide range of collaborative business activities. Alliances may take any number of forms, including equity investments, exclusive supply arrangements, joint research and development, joint production, joint purchasing, and joint marketing through copromotion, cobranding, and other similar arrangements. Strategic alliance has been broadly defined as including "any form of inter-firm cooperative arrangement beyond contracts completed in the ordinary course of business."[2] Alliances have become increasingly popular. This is, to some extent, because of the flexible and often not fully defined nature of the term. Organizations are often parties to multiple alliances, of many different sorts. Several factors have contributed to this proliferation of more or less structured alliances.[3]

These include:

- *Globalization.* Well-positioned local firms, different cost structures, local customs and preferences, restrictive national laws, and the sheer complexity of global operations make it difficult for individual firms to operate alone.
- *Specialization.* At the same time as the economies of scale and scope increase, firms are recognizing the difficulty with trying to do

everything alone. This is the impetus for outsourcing and for creating alliances with the outsourcing activity.

- *Technical complexity.* Many key technologies have grown so complex that companies look for partners who can provide the expertise they themselves lack.
- *Pace of technological change.* R&D alliances respond to rapidly changing markets, flexible enough to adapt to changing market conditions, with comparatively low entry and exit costs.
- *Network effects.* In technology-driven markets, the network effects make it critical that a firm capture the first mover advantage so that its technology becomes the industry standard. Alliances between new technology firms and established manufacturers are often used as a way to get off the starting block more quickly in order to capture these network effects.

All of these forces drive organizations to rely on other firms to perform functions that are critical to their success or failure. This, in turn, confronts them with all the problems Oliver Williamson identified in his groundbreaking work on transactions costs, notably, on bounded rationality and opportunism.[4]

Firms are naturally reluctant to make investments specific to arms-length transactions with another firm because the other firm may become opportunistic and try to capture all of the gains from that investment. The combination of opportunism and bounded rationality makes arms-length contracting inefficient. Alliances can reduce transaction costs among firms by aligning the organizations and interests.[5]

This may be accomplished through exclusivity and reciprocity agreements, through joint ownership of productive assets, or through equity investments in each other and through governance structures that coordinate some or all of the activities of the individual members of the alliance.

Alliances are usually distinguished from joint ventures and partnerships by the continuing independence of the partners. Often an alliance provides for the acquisition of a minority, noncontrolling investment by one of the parties in their alliance partner, together with some sort of undertaking to work on a cooperative basis in a particular area. The alliance normally allows the parties to independently pursue interests outside of the alliance. However, even the most informal strategic alliances differ from regular contracts because the partners make some attempt to align their longer-term interests.

Alliances may also act as a mechanism for transferring technology and even the skills and relationships of employees within participating members of the alliance. They generally involve swaps, trades, or barter, rather than the exchange of goods and/or services for money. Each party has something the other wants, involving either tangible or intangible assets.

As with joint ventures, alliances almost always involve the loss of some managerial control. Alliances also can raise antitrust issues, particularly when the prospective alliance members are competitors or when there is an effective "integration" of the market, beyond that which is considered reasonable.

Outsourcing of R&D

Outsourcing, or transferring an entire function to another organization, has been common for many years, with much of this activity directed toward individual departments within an organization or individual projects conducted by an institution or company. Since the 1990s, the practice has become much more widespread, covering a broader range of activities, a growing set of partners, and usually, relationships that are longer term.

Sporadic case-by-case outsourcing is being replaced by more intimate partnering, even to the point where major industrial concerns will essentially turn over the entire R&D process to an external performer or research management institution. In many cases there is a close collaboration between the industrial concern and the research management organization to the point where the research management activity becomes involved in the internal R&D planning process. The arrangements tend to incorporate aspects of the alliance or joint venture, the standalone research contract, and the license agreement.

License Agreements

When technology is sold or assigned, the ownership rights for the technology pass from seller to buyer. Much more often, however, only the right to use technology is passed from the technology owner to the licensor to the user to the licensee. The manner in which the technology will be used, for how long, and in what region or area will be determined by the terms negotiated in the licensing agreement. Unlike a sale, the licensor continues to own the technology and may maintain some control over further development, manufacture, sales, and use. The licensor in many cases may even license the technology to additional licensees. In some ways a licensing agreement is like a partnership because it establishes a continuing relationship, and usually the licensor and licensee work together to maximize

their mutual profit. Assuming that the relationship is successful, both parties will profit from the product's success in the market.

Licensing agreements often enable nonprofits to profit from technology developed by them, and pose fewer financial and legal risks than owning and operating a manufacturing facility or participating in a partnership or joint venture with a for-profit company. Licensing also permits firms and nonprofits to overcome many of the barriers that frequently hamper international exploitation of technology. Technology licensing can also be used to deal with multiple holders of complementary technology. Organizations can use licenses such as cross-licensing agreements (or grant back clauses in licenses) to transfer rights to improved technology developed by a licensee back to the licensor.

One negative aspect of licensing is that control over the technology is lessened when it has been transferred to an unaffiliated firm. That firm may not use the technology properly, may not pay over the payments (royalties) due to the licensor, and may avoid payment completely through the use of the bankruptcy laws of the licensee's jurisdiction. Additionally, licensing usually produces fewer profits than actually manufacturing the actual goods or services. There also may be problems in adequately protecting the licensed technology from unauthorized use by third parties. Licensees may use the licensed technology to compete with the licensor or its other licensees. In international transactions, it is important to investigate not only the prospective licensee but both the licensor's and the licensee's countries as well. The government of the host country often must approve the licensing agreement before it goes into effect. Some governments prohibit royalty payments that exceed a certain rate. In many cases, particular technologies may be subject to restrictions on licensing in any form.

The prospective licensing parties must always take into account that both countries have:

- Patent, trademark, and copyright laws.
- Exchange controls.
- Product liability laws.
- Possible countertrading or barter requirements.
- Antitrust and tax laws.
- Government attitudes toward repatriation of royalties and dividends.
- The existence of a tax treaty or bilateral investment treaty.

Licensing parties always need to consider whether there are any issues concerning the unlawful restraint of trade (i.e., antitrust) that will arise from the license agreement. Some restraints may be per se unreasonable (for instance, patent licenses that extend beyond the life of the patent). Most of the time, the issue is whether any restraint on free use of the technology is reasonable. Whether or not a restraint is reasonable is a fact-specific determination that is made after consideration of the availability of:

- Competing goods or technology.
- Market shares.
- Barriers to entry.
- The business justifications for and the duration of contractual restraints.
- Valid patents, trademarks, and copyrights.

The United States and other countries, particularly the European Union, have strict antitrust laws that affect technology licensing. The European Union has issued detailed regulations known as a block exemption, governing patent and know-how licensing agreements, as well as ancillary provisions relating to other intellectual property rights.*

Just as partnership law involves agency and contract law, the law of license agreements also intertwines contract law with the law of "intellectual property." This thorny issue must be addressed if technology transfer is to occur.

Additionally, persons dealing with license agreements must be concerned with the Uniform Commercial Code. Changes in this model law may drastically affect the transactions in information products, including copyrighted works, databases, and computer software. The Uniform Commercial Code is a model act drafted by committees of attorneys associated with the American Law Institute (ALI) and the National Conference of Commissioners on Uniform State Laws (NCCUSL). Those organizations, acting together, propose to the states the model for implementation of a "virtual" national law on various aspects of commercial transactions. Adopting a model law helps to facilitate interstate commerce because all parties across the many jurisdictions can be confident that they are operating under a similar body of law.

The various players in the Uniform Laws bureaucracy began with an effort to standardize software licenses. However, the effort has expanded and contracted over time to cover more or less of the law

of licensing generally. At present, only a few states have adopted any part of the Uniform Law, but students should maintain an awareness of this effort.

Licensing agreements cover as many elements as the parties wish. The payment structure (the form and rate of royalty, time frame, and incentives for maximizing profits), geographical area in which the licensee may operate, exclusivity of licensee, rights to improvements to the technology, etc., are among many factors that should be discussed. Because the license agreement may cover many kinds of intellectual property, deal with many different uses, and entail almost limitless types of relationships, the variation among agreements is practically infinite. The parties will need to work through checklists and previously drafted agreements to help identify necessary coverage in their particular situation. Some of the topics to be covered are discussed below.

The parties will need to discuss what is licensed. The subject of the license might be discoveries, concepts, or ideas, whether or not patentable, processes, methods, software, tangible research products, formulas and techniques, improvements thereto, and know-how. Copyrighted works, trademarks and trade Dress, derivatives, and background rights may be licensed, as can parking spaces, air rights, and waste disposal sites. Essentially, any kind of property that could be transferred by one party to another can be licensed instead.

What rights are gained and given by the license? Licenses normally cover not only existing rights, but also previously discovered or developed property or rights. Often licenses also cover rights to discoveries or works not yet developed. The licenses may preserve certain preexisting interests in intellectual property as unaffected by the activities to be carried out under terms of the agreement.

Intellectual Property Basics[6]

Intellectual property (IP) is a concept encompassing all forms of creativity that are protected either under statutes or by common law. It includes inventions, discoveries, know-how, show-how, processes, unique materials, copyrightable works, original data, and other creative or artistic works. IP also includes the physical embodiment of intellectual effort. For example, IP can sometimes include the actual models, machines, devices, apparatus, instrumentation, circuits, computer programs and visualizations, biological materials, chemicals, other

---

*Commission Regulation (EC) No. 240/96 of 31 January 1997 on the Application of Article 85(3) of the Treaty [of Rome]

compositions of matter, plans, and records of research. Some IP is protected by statute or legislation, such as patent, copyright, trademark, service mark, or mask work, or by plant variety protection certificate and confidentiality agreements. Often a specific technology is protected using multiple mechanisms. For example, some computer software can be protected by copyright, patent, trade secret, trademark, and contracts.

Ownership of Intellectual Property

Ownership of intellectual property arises as a question with research in three ways. The first is the nature of ownership between the researcher and his or her employer, the second is between the research institution and the external funding body, and the third is in relation to a student's intellectual property. In many countries, the employer is given statutory ownership of the IP developed by employees. In the United States, there is a distinction made between patent ownership, and the ownership of copyrights and other intellectual property under the various statutes. Because of the variations in law, almost every organization developing IP has established policies and contractual understandings to control ownership. Under these policies and contracts:

1. the employer owns those inventions created by its employees and consultants;
2. nonacademic employers own copyrights and other IP created by its employees, but academic employers often allow academics such as professors and researchers to own copyrights in scientific materials meant for publication;
3. IP developed outside the employment relationship but used in the conduct of employment is often subject to noncompensated license or even assignment to the employer;
4. employees are often provided with compensation for IP, such as a share of income obtained by the employer; however, in most for-profit situations, this compensation may be minimal.

IP Created by Independent Contractors

Consultants, subcontractors, and other independent contractors often create a wide variety of original or new materials for research institutions and for other research sponsors. The IP created ranges from actual research results, prototypes, and research material to ancillary materials such as business plans, marketing plans, training manuals, information manuals, technical guides, software, a Web site, designs, drawings, research reports, databases, and even trademarks and logos.

Inventions

In most countries, an independent contractor hired to develop a new product or process owns all rights to the invention unless specifically stated otherwise. This means that unless the contractor has a written agreement assigning the invention to the funding organization (whether sponsor or prime contractor/principal research institution), in general the funding organization will have no ownership rights in what is developed, even though it paid for the development.

Copyright

In most countries, a freelance creator owns the copyright unless a written agreement is executed providing that the material created is to be a "work for hire." If, and only if, there is such a written agreement in place, then the entity that commissioned the job will normally own the intellectual property; even then, the "moral rights" usually remain in principle with the author. In the absence of such an agreement, the entity that paid for the work is generally entitled to use the work only for the purposes for which it was created. Different rules or exceptions may apply, such as in the case of commissioned photographs, films, and sound recordings.

Industrial Designs

If a freelance designer is contracted to produce a specific design, in many cases the intellectual property rights will not pass automatically to the commissioning party, but will remain with the freelance designer. In some countries, the commissioning party owns the rights in a design only if reward has been paid for that design.

The Bayh-Dole Act

In the United States, ownership may be statutorily established to be held by the independent contractor by a law called the Bayh-Dole Act.[7] Passed in the 1980s, the Act permitted universities and small businesses to elect ownership of inventions made under federal funding and to become directly involved in the commercialization process. This new policy also permitted exclusive licensing of the inventions.

The Act applies to all inventions conceived or first actually reduced to practice in the performance of a project that is fully or partially funded by a federal agency. In almost every case, ownership of IP between employee and employer, research institution and its contractors, and research institution and funding entity can be established by contractual provision. However, it must be specifically established and cannot be presumed. The inventor (or employer of the inventor), whether a subcontractor, consultant, or prime awardee or contractor, is granted the right to patent the invention. The contract clauses implementing the Act specifically direct the IP owner to file for the patent for the invention. The coverage for copyrights is less explicit, but the Act has been held to cover copyrights that are similar in purpose to patents (e.g., for software).

The federal government is provided a non-exclusive, irrevocable, paid-up license to practice the invention (or have it practiced on behalf of the United States) throughout the world. In some circumstances, the government can require the university to grant a license to a third party. This might occur if the invention was not brought to practical use within a reasonable time, if health or safety issues arose, if public use of the invention was in jeopardy, or if other legal requirements were not satisfied. The higher-tier contractor or grant awardee is given no rights in the invention. The inventor may not assign its rights to third parties, except to a patent management organization; so the higher-tier contractor or awardee is prohibited from obtaining the rights in that way.

The employer of the person who actually developed the invention must share with the inventor any income collected on the invention. Any remaining income, after expenses, must be used to support scientific research or education. The employer/IP owner must also produce a written IP policy that covers all developments subject to the act. Each prime contractor or grant awardee must include the clauses that implement the act in all subcontracts and subawards under which an invention might result.

License Agreement Issues

Current, Anticipated, and Background IP

In most cases the process of IP development is incremental. There may have been IP developed in the past that must be the subject of licensing. Normally, the agreement will deal with IP developed under the current agreement. Sometimes (and often for copyright) the agreement will need to cover later (or derivative) work.

Level of Information Sharing

The patent laws require disclosure of inventions in order to obtain patent protection. However, the level of confidentiality for IP not yet covered by a filing and for IP that will not be dealt with under the patent or copyright laws (i.e., trade secret IP) should be addressed.

Cross-Licensing

It is common that each party will come to the table with IP. In such cases, and where additional development may be done by the licensee after the execution of the license, there should be an agreement on the use of licensing of such IP back to the original inventor.

Exclusivity, Royalties, and Geographic Scope of License

Licenses may be more or less exclusive, may require the payment of royalties for use, and may allow the practice of the IP in only one country, region, or worldwide. The amount of time and money required to bring most IP to market is most likely to be rewarded by exclusive marketing rights; non-exclusive rights often do not offer the proper incentives for development in this area.

Joint Ownership Issues

Purely joint owners probably do not require a license to commercialize and have no obligation to account to other owners for profits. However, more often each party has or will contribute IP to a common development effort. This may be dealt with by cross-licensing, allocation of fields of use, etc. However, this area is fraught with legal peril. Issues, such as antitrust law, far beyond the scope of this text, are raised.

Time Limits

IP licenses should contain reasonable time limits for disclosure, exercise of rights under the license, commercialization, payment, etc. Where the license is for patent rights or copyright, the failure to set limits on exclusivity may again bring in the specter of antitrust violations.

Administrative Costs and Procedures

The license should deal with which party will pay associated patent (or copyright, etc.) filing and maintenance costs. These can be very substantial, especially when worldwide rights are at issue. A related issue to be covered is who will file the patent applications, choose counsel, litigate infringements, and maintain records.

Sublicenses, etc.

The agreement should cover the right to grant sublicenses, the rights of the IP developer to step into the shoes of the sublicensor, sharing or other payment of royalties or other proceeds received under such sublicenses; commitments by sublicense, terms that do not exceed any limits imposed by the prime license or law; audit rights of the prime licensor; reservation of the rights of the US or other government, if applicable; and any indemnification from liability arising from development, marketing, and use of the IP.

Common Issues in Research Agreements between Industry and Academia

Who Controls the Research?

For many years, the primary issue in industry-university relations has been the control of the research activity. In his 1984 study, Donald Fowler identified one of the significant issues in industry-university agreements as industry attempts to "control what research the university does in the field of the proposed university-industry relationship."[8,9] This issue has not, and will not, abate, since it is the defining core of the relationship. There are several ways to "control" the research, beginning with the statement of work (SOW) itself. Dr. Alfonza Atkinson, D.V.M., M.P.H., Ph.D., and Dean, College of Veterinary Medicine, Nursing and Allied Health, was both an accomplished research administrator and a much published principal investigator who wrote specifically on this issue.

As Dr. Atkinson points out, both parties may have reason to want a broad SOW and also to want a narrow one. The narrow SOW holds the university scientist "in check" but also limits the scope of any company rights to discoveries. A broad SOW gives the university leeway but also gives the company great rights to any discoveries made.

Going beyond the statement of work, there are several "standard" contract clauses that may be used to:

1. Limit industrial control;
2. Assure the right to industry technical direction;
3. Define the extent of financial control given to industry.

The research institution is almost always given "independent contractor" status. Under almost all circumstances, both parties will not want to establish an agency relationship where one party can act in the other's name. Therefore, except in partnership/joint venture arrangements, a clause such as the following should be used:

Independent Parties

The parties agree that each is independent, and not a partner, joint venturer, or agent of the other. The employees of each party shall not be deemed the employees of the other party for any reason whatsoever. Neither party shall have any right or authority to commit the other, incur any obligation on behalf of the other, or represent to any person or entity that any such authority exists.

This clause, or one of the many similar clauses, should cause no controversy in any grant or contract, or even in consulting agreements. In cooperative agreements that resemble partnerships, the parties should specifically set out any exceptions under which one party might commit the other. More of a problem is the acceptable extent of "technical direction." Normally, when technical direction by the company is provided for in the contract, the course of the work is made subject to the guidance of a technical representative of the company. "Technical direction" usually is defined to mean directives that approve approaches, solutions, designs, or refinements; fill in details or otherwise complete the SOW; or allow the company to shift emphasis among work areas.

Usually the technical representative does not have the authority to issue any instruction that:

1. Constitutes an assignment of additional work outside the statement of work;
2. Constitutes a material change;
3. Constitutes a basis for any increase or decrease in the total estimated contract cost, the fixed fee (if any), or the time required for contract performance;
4. Changes any of the expressed terms, conditions, or specifications of the contract;
5. Interferes with the contractor's rights to perform the terms and conditions of the contract.

The university is normally required to proceed with technical direction, even if it disagrees with the directive. If the university disagrees with the direction, it is required to notify the company. If the parties do not agree, the issue is usually made subject to a formal mediation or dispute resolution clause in the contract. Even where a company may provide technical direction, the parties remain independent. Other clauses often seen in contracts with substantial company control include anti-assignment clauses (that prohibit the university from turning the work over to others) and key personnel clauses (that limit the personnel to those initially assigned or otherwise approved by the company).

The primary driver in selecting the extent of technical direction should be the same as in selecting the basic form of agreement. That is, in grants there should be little, if any, right of direction; in contracts for basic research only, only minimal direction; and in contracts for applied research and development of actual products, more comprehensive company rights. In cooperative agreements, the best method of assuring satisfactory direction is joint selection of a project manager or management team to provide ongoing coordination/supervision.

Who Obtains Patent and Other Intellectual Property Rights

Commentators have routinely identified patent issues as one of the most problematic in industry-university relationships. Robert Killoren, Assistant Vice President for Research, Pennsylvania State University, and Susan B. Butts, Director, External Technology, The Dow Chemical Company, summarize these issues well in a white paper, "Industry-University Research In Our Times."[10] In their 2003 paper, the authors set out the history of industry and university intellectual property "discussions"; issues regarding the ultimate ownership of intellectual property; "background" rights; publication, copyright, and confidentiality concerns; worries about foreign access; and graduate student involvement.

Killoren and Butts note, however, that as the consequence of extensive federal funding of university research, the US government is a strong presence within the university-industry relationship and its presence influences related issues pertaining to intellectual property rights. The authors identify the early 1980s as the watershed period of industry-university research, during which time three major changes occurred that changed the nature of the industry-university relationship, particularly by two government-based events:

1. The 1984 passage of the Bay-Dole Act.
2. Many companies abandoned their stand-alone

basic research laboratories and "outsourced" research to universities, research institutes, and federal laboratories.
3. The federal government pushed industry to support more of the cost of the nation's fundamental research. IRS rules regarding tax-exempt bonds limited the universities' ability to negotiate with companies on intellectual property issues.

Publication Rights

Directly related to the patent issue is the question of publication of research results. The importance of this issue to universities is widely recognized, even in industry. Agreements must balance the university's right to publish with the need to delay publication when needed to obtain patent protection. The International Committee of Medical Journal editors have stated their position and enforce that balance by refusing to publish unless the balance, as they see it, is maintained. The editors strongly oppose contractual agreements that deny investigators the right to examine the data independently or to submit a manuscript for publication without first obtaining the consent of the sponsor. They take the position that such arrangements not only erode the fabric of intellectual inquiry that has fostered so much high-quality clinical research but also make medical journals party to potential misrepresentation, since the published manuscript may not reveal the extent to which the authors were powerless to control the conduct of a study that bears their names. The editors therefore require authors to disclose details of their own and the sponsor's role in the study. Many of the editors ask the responsible author to sign a statement indicating that he or she accepts full responsibility for the conduct of the trial, had access to the data, and controlled the decision to publish.

The editors' position is that a sponsor should have the right to review a manuscript for a defined period (for example, 30 to 60 days) before publication to allow for the filing of additional patent protection, if required. When the sponsor employs some of the authors, these authors' contributions and perspective should be reflected in the final paper, as are those of the other authors, but the sponsor must impose no impediment, direct or indirect, on the publication of the study's full results, including data perceived to be detrimental to the product. The editors require that a submitted manuscript be the intellectual property of its authors, not the study sponsor. They will not review or publish articles based on studies that are conducted under conditions that allow the sponsor to have sole control of the data or to withhold publication.

Confidentiality Agreements

Almost every agreement between universities and government or industry discusses confidential information. Some agreements solely address confidential information—commonly called nondisclosure agreements, confidentiality agreements, or secrecy agreements. More comprehensive and complicated contracts between the parties, such as research agreements, almost always require at least some confidentiality. The common elements in these agreements include a definition of just what is covered, the terms by which confidential information may be transferred, and exceptions to the requirements for confidentiality.

Nondisclosure agreements, confidentiality agreements, or secrecy agreements are often presented to individual researchers for their signature. These persons should always ask their employer to review such agreements. In many cases the individual researchers should not be parties to these agreements, although they may sign the document to acknowledge the terms of the arrangement. Even when researchers are acting as independent consultants, they should make sure that they have counsel review any agreements. For confidentiality agreements between institutions, such as between a university and a funding party, the persons who normally sign contracts should be the authorized signing authorities. As with preresearch confidentiality agreements, university researchers are not parties to these agreements, although they may be required to consent to the terms before the document is accepted by the university.

What Is Confidential Information?

Confidential or proprietary information can exist in many different forms. It may consist of notes, testing procedures, trade secrets, formulae, test data, specifications, "know-how," software, etc. An important attribute of such information is its unavailability and inaccessibility to the public. It is this shroud of restricted use that imputes the confidential nature to the information in the eyes of the law. The agreement on confidential information should clearly define the confidential information, or, in the alternative, contain terms that allow for both parties to subsequently agree in writing as to what constitutes confidential information. It is

important to remember that in some cases, a signatory can agree not to disclose information that has otherwise been disclosed. All agreements should make information that is otherwise available to the public available for disclosure by the parties.

In determining what information is to be kept confidential, it is important to distinguish between information provided by the parties and that which arises from the research. Most universities require that results of research undertaken at the university be fully publishable at the discretion of the researcher, subject to limited and mutually agreed upon publications delays. This rule does not apply in some cases when clinical research is at issue. Agreements on the transfer of confidential information should almost always exclude information that is:

- Already known by the recipient;
- Independently developed by the recipient;
- Disclosed to the recipient by a third party without an obligation of confidentiality;
- In the public domain (at the time of disclosure or during term of agreement); or
- Disclosed pursuant to judicial or administrative order.

For clinical research, it is also important to except information necessary to treat the patients. Some negotiate to except information needed by a party for its own legal defense, since one cannot subpoena oneself to obtain the information for use in litigation.

The language or clauses covering confidential information should specify how the information may be used. The clause(s) might restrict the use of the information to a specific research purpose, and require that it only be disclosed to those employees of the parties or those researchers who agree to acknowledge the confidential nature of the information and be bound by terms similar to those in the parties' agreement.

The research agreement normally binds only the university and the company or companies that are signatories. However, the group of persons who may have access to company confidential information includes faculty members, university administrative staff, technicians, and graduate (and perhaps even undergraduate) students. These persons may not have any legal (as opposed to moral) obligation to preserve confidentiality unless they sign specific agreements. While asking the principal investigator to enter into a nondisclosure agreement does not present major problems, similar requirements for support staff and graduate students may be the cause of vociferous protests and, as a practical matter, unenforceable. Instead of trying to require such arrangements, universities should consider instituting a university-wide policy requiring nondisclosure of confidential information generally. The violation of university policy and the resulting academic- or employment-related sanctions that may be imposed are often of greater concern to those staff members and students than a contractual agreement with a "faceless corporation." Also, the parties can use the policy to support civil or criminal enforcement of the confidentiality requirements. (See, for example, Carmen McCutcheon's *Fairplay or Greed: Mandating University Responsibility Toward Student Inventors*, Duke Law & Technology Review 0026, 2003.)

Financial Arrangements

Because the federal government dictates detailed payment and financial administration terms and procedures for universities, there is a tendency to mimic these procedures in industry-university agreements, even though industrial sponsors are not used to them and may not even care about the minutiae of the university's finances. On the other hand, many industry sponsors apparently balk at payment of the entire university overhead burden. Federal policy on the appropriate type of contract is logical and provides a good guide for private agreements. The Federal Acquisition Regulations note that the absence of precise specifications and difficulties in estimating costs with accuracy normally precludes using fixed-price contracting for R&D. Therefore, it is common to use cost-reimbursement contracts in both basic research and development work. When levels of effort can be specified in advance, a short-duration fixed-price contract may be useful for developing system design concepts, providing ongoing consulting, and well-defined testing activities.

Projects having engineering requirements as a follow-on to R&D efforts normally should progress from cost-reimbursement contracts to fixed-price contracts as designs become more firmly established, risks are reduced, and processes move into prototyping and production consulting. Similar considerations suggest that cost-reimbursement procedures are normally appropriate for grants, although a pure best-effort type statement of work will be customary. The federal government also prescribes detailed accounting procedures and cost principles (see OMB Circular A-21) and payment provisions for its research grants and contracts. For many universities, the payments are made by letter of credit drawdowns since most universities cannot borrow working capital or charge loan interest as an expense. A similar procedure may be advantageous for private agreements, providing quick payment to the university without tying up corporate funds in advance payments.

Audit Rights

Related to many of the financially oriented clauses is the question of audit. Under government agreements the sponsoring agency, specialized audit agencies such as the General Accounting Office, the Defense Contract Audit Agency, and even congressional investigators have substantial rights to audit not only for expenditures, but also internal management systems, patent administration, personnel actions, and property management. For the most part, both parties in private agreements will balk at such broad powers being granted to anyone, including private accounting firms. Further, few companies want to become involved in the internal details of a university's accounting system.

In many cases the pervasive nature of the federal grant and contract process provides a simple solution to any question of cost accounting or allocations. Since most universities do undergo federal audit, the results of the federal auditor's work can be used for private agreement purposes. For example, in payment related clauses, the allowable overhead may be set at the same level allowed by the federal government, which is determined by audit. For most purposes, this kind of reference to a federal standard removes any need for private audit rights. Occasionally, where the parties are dealing with sensitive information, such as patient data or proprietary software, there will be a need to provide for audit of the records.

Disputes Resolution

Fortunately, disputes, which rise to the level of legal action, are very rare in research agreements. However, one of the functions of any agreement is to cover the "what ifs" of the relationship. Unlike the federal system, there are many dispute resolution schemes available to private parties. Of course, the particular dispute resolution procedures available are bounded by the circumstances of the parties. For instance, many state institutions are required by law to use state dispute procedures or forums. In the absence of state or federal mandates, the choice of procedures is essentially between arbitration, either binding or nonbinding, and litigation in a court. (As noted by William W. Park in "Arbitration of International Contract Disputes" [The Business Lawyer, Vol. 39, p. 1783, August, 1984], arbitration may be the only mutually acceptable procedure in international contracts.)

Many non-lawyers are enamored of arbitration because it is allegedly quicker and less expensive than litigation. However, arbitration's speed and money-saving features may be gained at the expense of completeness of the decision. In addition, there are indications that arbitration has evolved into a more complicated process that parallels litigation in cost and time.

Whether or not arbitration is chosen, certain choices must still be made. The first of these is the "choice of law." The governing law for a contract or grant can vary tremendously. For example, where a contract was made between a Texas company and a Mississippi company for performance in Louisiana, the governing law could be that of any of the three states. In addition, the parties can agree to have the law of another state or country applied if there is a rational basis for the selection. For instance, the companies might agree to use New York law if both companies were subsidiaries of New York companies. As a practical matter, the choice of law is often intentionally not made explicit. Each party wants their own jurisdiction and neither will accept the other's choice. Therefore, the choice is left to the arguments of litigators.

The forum is also often specified in agreements. If arbitration is used, the rules of an arbitral institution (e.g., the American Arbitration Association or the International Chamber of Commerce) should be specified, or a detailed discussion of procedural ground rules should be included for ad hoc arbitration. If the courts will be used, the parties should specify the court(s) that will be available. The parties may have to consider waiver of sovereign immunity (not an easy decision for a state institution) or a "direct action" clause under which insurers may be sued instead of the sovereign (and therefore immune) organization. Where any part of an arbitration award may be payable by the federal government, the parties should agree to require detailed findings of fact and conclusions of law to support the decision when arbitration is used. Otherwise, government officials may require that the case be relitigated under federal disputes procedures. Where the parties are in the position of prime and subcontractor under a federal contract, generally arbitration should not be used for claims related to the federal contract. Instead, disputes can "flow through" the prime to the contracting officer and the board of contract appeals. If this procedure

is not used, the prime faces the possibility of owing the subcontractor but not being able to collect from the government.

Insurance, Liability, and Indemnification

Part of any agreement today, and as a practical matter, part of almost any activity is the risk of a lawsuit. A consumer may allege that a product has injured person or property. A competitor may allege patent infringement. A patient may allege negligent medical treatment. The list can virtually go on forever. The immediate result of such allegations is usually legal fees and court costs. Ultimately, if accepted by a jury or court, the cost of such an allegation may be a multi-million dollar judgment that can bankrupt a company or strain the resources of a university. The standard response to such risk is to obtain insurance against liability. However, as the costs of liability insurance skyrocket, a second response is usually to try to shift liability to other parties. The allocation of risks can be one of the most difficult areas of negotiation in any agreement. When the agreement is with a public institution or even a private not-for-profit university, the issues become even more complex. Clauses in this area cover several topics. Many clauses require that the parties follow particular safety, health, manufacturing, or other risk prevention procedures. These clauses may aid an "innocent" party in shifting blame.

Clauses requiring specific insurance coverage are commonly used to assure that everyday risks are covered. In the industry-university setting, the costs of such coverage for the university should be specifically dealt with since many institutions are "self-insurers" and insurance costs may not be fully recoverable as indirect costs under federal contracts. (The federal government limits insurance costs since it indemnifies cost-reimbursement contractors for some losses.) Many agreements will need to cover procedures for obtaining liability waivers from third parties (e.g., patients in drug testing and experimental subjects). In other cases, it will be important to make sure that all parties agree that no waivers are allowed (e.g., in clinical trials, patients generally cannot be made to waive their legal rights).

Each of the parties will usually want indemnification against certain risks. Indemnification clauses allow a party to shift some or its entire share of the damages to another party. Indemnification is normally quite contentious and negotiation can be complex. Clauses may provide individual and company indemnity arising from any, or only certain, claims. Rights and obligations may be triggered if the claim is made regardless of when or if the occurrence, accident, or event took place. In some cases, not only does the claim have to be made, but it must be reported by the indemnified party to the indemnitor within a certain period. The more friendly form does not require that the claim be reported during the specified period. Instead, it simply requires that the reporting take place "as soon as practicable" or similar language. Many clauses fail to define the term "claim." This may lead to confusion and litigation battles between the parties. A clause might define the term "claim" to include a "written demand for money" and a "civil proceeding." It goes without saying that the broader the definition of the term "claim," the broader the coverage that is afforded by the clause. Some of the "claims" that may need to be specified include:

- Written demands for monetary, nonmonetary, and injunctive relief;
- Civil proceedings for monetary, nonmonetary, and injunctive relief;
- Criminal proceedings;
- Administrative/regulatory proceedings;
- Arbitration proceedings;
- Civil, criminal, administrative, or regulatory investigations;
- Securities investigations;
- Administrative and regulatory proceedings against the entity on a codefendant basis.

The indemnity clause usually covers not only the parties, but also directors and officers, employees, agents, and representatives. In appropriate circumstances, the following might also be specified:

- Trustees and governors of the corporate entity
- Management of joint ventures
- Members of limited liability companies affiliated with the corporate entities
- Executives of the company serving as executives on specifically covered "outside entity" companies
- Counsel, accountants, etc.
- Students
- Consultants

Corporate entities might include the following:

- Subsidiaries of the corporate entity
- Subcontractors, vendors, and suppliers

Under most indemnity clauses the indemnitor promises to pay some or all of the "loss" arising from a claim. Usually the definition of "loss" will include the following:

- Damages
- Judgments
- Settlements
- Defense costs

It often explicitly excludes the following:

- Civil or criminal fines or penalties
- Punitive or exemplary damages
- The multiplied portion of multiplied damages
- Taxes

Loss might also include the following:

- Punitive, exemplary, and multiple damages
- Civil fines.

However, in many states these types of losses may not be subject to indemnification if there is any "moral turpitude" or other "bad act" involved on the part of the indemnified party. Usually indemnity clauses obligate the indemnitor to defend the other party in connection with potentially covered litigation. Sometimes, the clause allows or requires the indemnified party to defend the litigation and only provides for reimbursement of defense costs. Usually, the indemnitor does have at least the "right" to associate in the defense. Under some state laws it may be necessary to specifically provide for "advancement" of defense costs. This means that the indemnitor will pay defense costs before the end of the litigation.

Under most indemnity clauses the indemnitor cannot settle a claim without first obtaining the written consent of the indemnified party. Some clauses include an additional provision that provides that if the indemnified party withholds consent to such a settlement, the indemnitor's liability will not exceed the amount for which the indemnitor could have settled. Alternatively, the indemnified party should seek to modify the language so that it applies only when that party "unreasonably" withholds consent to such a settlement. The exclusions in indemnity clauses vary tremendously. Some of the typical exclusions include the following:

1. The "Bad Conduct" Type Exclusions
   - Intentionally dishonest acts or omissions
   - Fraudulent acts or omissions
   - Criminal acts or omissions
   - Willful violations of any statute rule or law
   - Illegal profit
   - Illegal remuneration
2. The Internal Claims Exclusion

   Clauses may contain an exclusion for a claim brought either by an employee, officer or director, etc, of the indemnified corporation against the corporation. Thus, a nurse who brings a claim for an adverse reaction to a drug to which he or she was exposed as a part of the clinical trial could not be subject to indemnification. The research institution would have to deal with the claim under worker's compensation or similar procedures.

Some indemnity clauses contain a requirement for "alternative dispute resolution." It provides the mechanism by which disputes or differences under the policy must be resolved. The various ADR clauses include the following:

- Binding arbitration only
- Mediation and, if mediation is unsuccessful, then binding arbitration
- Election between mediation and arbitration, with one party or the other having veto power over the selection
- Mediation or binding arbitration with a waiting period before suit is filed (typically 120 days) if mediation is selected

All indemnification contains a "cooperation" obligation. While most clauses do not elaborate on the scope of cooperation, it is generally understood to require the indemnified party to cooperate in the handling and defense of the litigation. It may be necessary to modify this provision to deal with cases where the indemnified party may not have control over some of the players, such as students.

Competition and Conflicts

As awareness of the potential for profitable arrangements with universities has grown in the commercial world, so too have academics been drawn to the "filthy lucre" of Wall Street. Professors and even graduate students have taken equity positions in commercial organizations, often without considering all the issues that arise. However, as Laurie Garrett has said, "There are problems." (*SRA Journal*, Fall 1985). The problems are straightforward. First, to what extent should universities and faculty members compete with (1) their sponsors, and (2) private business generally? Second, how can the university avoid the loss of open debate and a free exchange of ideas while cooperating with sponsors to whom privacy is money?

Many times, the issue of competition has not been addressed squarely, even in very large research institutions. While the federal tax code and various state laws generally militate against competition by universities with for-profit organizations, there is

no federal law prohibiting such activities. Intra-university conflicts, while related to the issue of competition, have been a subject of much debate. Unfortunately, there has not emerged any real consensus as to a solution. One response has been to restrict faculty consulting—with the result that some of the most creative faculty members have simply left the university. Other universities and several states have required disclosure statements—a step in the right direction, but not the answer for individual agreements.

While covenants not to compete and warranties against organizational conflicts of interest are common in industry-to-industry agreements, it may be so difficult to reach agreement upon equivalent clauses that no language will be included in many industry-university agreements. Instead, industry will have to simply accept the bad with the good. The clauses below are crafted as compromises, but the authors expect less than a friendly response to even such diluted clauses. In fact, the more popular clause may be a disclaimer of any responsibility such as the last clause sets out below.

Disclosure of Conflicts

University shall use its best efforts to disclose activities by the university to sponsor which are determined to be detrimental to sponsor's present commercial interests in the following areas. The university shall not be liable for failure to disclose any detrimental activity, nor shall the disclosure (by the university or others) of such activity provide any basis for actions for breach of contract or for return of any funds paid under this agreement. However, sponsor shall have the right to discontinue its support upon receipt of such a disclosure by the university if the sponsor gives thirty (30) days' notice of discontinuance and pays for all work completed through the date of discontinuance of support. This clause does not apply and university makes no representation or warranty related to the independent consulting activities of faculty, staff, or students.

Competition

University as a public institution is not in competition with sponsor. However, the university reserves the right to engage in research, undertake sponsored research, and enter into agreements of any kind allowed under state law [and which do not generate unrelated business income as defined in the Internal Revenue Code] with any other organization whether or not said organization is in competition with sponsor. Sponsor acknowledges that it has reviewed the lists of university agreements and sponsors provided to it.

Organizational Conflicts of Interest (General)

The university warrants that, to the best of its knowledge and belief, and except as otherwise disclosed, there are no relevant facts that could give rise to organizational conflicts of interest. The university agrees that, if after award, an organizational conflict of interest with respect to this contract is discovered, an immediate and full disclosure in writing shall be made to sponsor that shall include a description of the action that the university has taken or proposes to take to avoid or mitigate such conflicts.

Disclaimer of Any Warranty Related to Conflicts of Interest

University specifically disclaims that it has made or is making any warranty that its activities are not in conflict with the interests or business of sponsor. Sponsor understands and agrees that the activities of the faculty, staff, and students of the university are not such that the university can represent that it, its faculty, staff, or student body is not in conflict. Accordingly, the university is not liable for any damage, loss, or competitive harm that may come to sponsor because of any activity by the university, its faculty, staff, or any student.

Changes in the Agreement

When a contract is formed, certain rights and responsibilities become legally binding between the parties. Normally, neither party has an inherent right to change a contract in any way that affects the other party's rights and obligations. However, because there is no inherent right to make changes, one (or both parties) almost always wants to incorporate a changes clause in all but the simplest agreements. The "buyer" (i.e., the sponsor) usually wants a clause that allows it to unilaterally alter a contractor's work so long as the change is within the general scope of the contract. In this way, a sponsor may rapidly react to unanticipated changes or conditions that alter the original plan for the research.

Most changes clauses require that changes be reduced to writing. A written change order protects both parties—the sponsor from having to pay for unwanted work, and it also protects a research institution by evidencing changes that require an adjustment of contract price and or completion time.

Sometimes a research institution, as opposed to a sponsor, will request a change order. Under most clauses the research institution is required to provide formal, written notice of the anticipated changed work. This written notification, which is separate from the actual change order, allows the other party to investigate, correct, and accommodate a change in an effective manner, minimizing its impact upon project costs and schedule. The party affected should always provide formal notice when events have occurred that may constitute a change to the contract, irrespective of whether there has been a formal change. Such events are called "constructive changes" and are usually treated as a change for compensation purposes, especially in connection with US federal government contracts and subcontracts. When notice of such "constructive changes" is followed by written confirmation, such as a letter or meeting minutes, the courts may avoid forfeiture of compensation claims and consider them on their merits. Absent a written memorial, though, the likelihood of prevailing in a subsequent lawsuit is drastically reduced.

Of course, the parties to a contract may always agree to have additional or different work to be done outside their contract or alter the provisions of the written agreement. The course of conduct between the parties may evidence a modification of the contract terms where formal written notice is no longer required. If a party has actual notice of the events giving rise to a claim, and there was no prejudice by the absence of written formal notice, then a court may consider the merits of the claim for changed work. Nevertheless, absent proof of waiver, notice provisions will normally be enforced.

Disputes regarding scope of work are often the reason for claims. Scope of work is defined as the extent of the responsibility to perform certain contract work. To determine the scope of work, the parties may have to look to other contract documents—specifications, contracts with others—and to "industry" standards (good clinical practices, etc.). Questions regarding scope of work should be resolved in the written contract. Scope of work references should be detailed in contract.

Changes clauses should always address the scope of the changed work, the measure of the adjustment in price, and the procedure to be followed to perform the work and price the adjustment. Under the typical changed work provision, the owner may direct changes and the contractor must perform changes even if there is no agreement as to price. Extra work is work not usually contemplated by contract. Changed work is work contemplated by contract but where the scope of the work has changed.

Termination of Contracts

Normally contracts are concluded by full performance by all parties. However, sometimes parties cannot or will not complete their obligations under the contract. Therefore, contracts may be terminated by reasons of rescission, breach, or impossibility of performance. In research contracts, it is also common for one or both parties to have the right to simply terminate upon notice to the other party.

Impossibility of Performance

Normally, each party to the contract must perform its obligations, completing the exchange of promises and receiving what has been bargained for. Impossibility of performance can terminate a contract if an unforeseen contingency prevents the performance of the contract. While in most cases, the law allows either party to avoid its obligations if those obligations are actually rendered impossible to perform, that rule is not universal. Therefore, most contracts contain what is called a "*force majeure*" clause. *Force majeure* literally means "greater force." These clauses excuse a party from liability if some unforeseen event beyond the control of that party prevents it from performing its obligations under the contract. Typically, *force majeure* clauses cover natural disasters or other "Acts of God," war, or the failure of third parties—such as suppliers and subcontractors—to perform their obligations to the contracting party. It is important to remember that *force majeure* clauses are intended to excuse a party only if the failure to perform could not be avoided by the exercise of due care by that party. *Force majeure* clauses normally apply equally to all parties to the agreement. Usually, the clause sets forth some specific examples of acts that will excuse performance under the clause, such as wars, natural disasters, and other major events that are clearly outside a party's control. Inclusion of examples will help to make clear the parties' intent that such clauses are not intended to apply to excuse failures to perform for reasons within the control of the parties.

A *force majeure* clause might read as follows:

Neither party shall be liable in damages or have the right to terminate this Agreement for any delay or default in performing hereunder if such delay or default is caused by conditions beyond its control including, but not limited to Acts of God, Government restrictions (including the denial or cancellation of any export or other necessary license), wars, insurrections and/or any other cause beyond the reasonable control of the party whose performance is affected.

Rescission

Rescission may terminate the obligations of a contract in a variety of circumstances. One party may have the legal right to rescind the contract, or the parties together agree to terminate the contract. Normally, rescission is not considered termination, but a "rolling back" of the contract to the situation existing before it ever began. For instance, a minor may be able to rescind a contract to buy a car and get all of his or her money back, even if he or she has wrecked the car. Normally rescission is a legal right and not covered by contract clauses.

Breach of Contract

Breach of a contract may terminate the obligations of the contract. Either one party or both parties have failed to perform an obligation as expected under the contract. A breach may occur when a party refuses to perform the contract, does something that the contract prohibits, or prevents the other party from performing its obligations. It is important to note that there is a distinction between material and immaterial breaches of contract. A material breach is a serious one; it is a breach that goes to the heart of the contract. The injured party can seek "damages," that is, a money payment to cover losses resulting from the breach. An immaterial breach of contract is a trivial breach of contract and does not give rise to any rights under the contract. Many actions or inactions might be technical breaches but will not be recognized as cause for litigation. Terminations for breach need not be pursuant to a contract clause, but there usually will be such clauses in almost any contract.

Termination Clauses

Termination clauses describe when the parties may stop performing their obligations prior to the end of the contract. Most provisions permit termination only for serious breaches of the agreement such as failure to actually do the work, failure to pay money owed, breaches of warranty such as the warranty that a product will not infringe another's IP, or failure to limit access to confidential materials. Additionally, the parties may specify the breaches they consider material. That way, the agreement cannot be terminated for a breach that only one party thought was serious.

Termination on Notice and Termination for Convenience

Some agreements permit either party to terminate the agreement for any reason, or no reason at all, provided adequate notice is given to the other party. Usually either party may terminate by giving timely notice to the other. Although this sounds equitable and convenient, it can lead to inequitable results. Therefore, most termination clauses provide for payment by the terminating party of the costs of performance and the costs that cannot be avoided after termination. This type of clause is mandatory in all US federal government contracts. However, only the government is given the right to "terminate for convenience." The university or other contractor must perform its obligations or be subject to "termination for default" (i.e., for breach of its duty to perform).

Notice of Termination and Termination Procedures

Notice of the termination of a contract may be given according to the terms of the contract. For example, the parties may agree in a contract that it can be terminated in a particular way. In such cases it is important to follow the required procedures to the letter. After receipt of a notice of termination the parties should normally stop work as specified in the notice, and stop any subcontracts except as necessary to complete the continued portion of the contract. They will need to determine the need to terminate subcontracts and cancel or divert applicable personnel, including student assignments that extend beyond the effective date of termination. The parties will need to determine who has what rights and interest in the "work in progress" and any tangible and intangible (e.g., IP) property acquired or developed under the terminated contract. One or both parties will need to settle all outstanding liabilities and termination settlement proposals arising from the termination of subcontracts. The parties

will have to deliver any confidential information and items that, if the contract had been completed, would have been required to be returned. Normally, the contractor will need to submit a termination settlement proposal. In most cases, the university and the sponsor will negotiate and agree on the amount to be paid because of the termination. The parties may want to use the cost principles and procedures in Part 31 of the Federal Acquisition Regulation (FAR) to govern which costs can be claimed and how such costs are measured.

Contract and Grant Administration: Responsibilities and Duties

The contract and grant administration function is broad and complex, often involving many persons with expertise in varied subject areas. Many of the responsibilities and duties in contract and grant administration flow from the specific terms and conditions of the particular agreements, but others are a matter of internal organization and the delegations of authority within the organizations of the parties. Senior management, principal investigators, other officials, project administrators, and appropriate or participating administrative offices should be advised of and understand the commitments they are undertaking under accepted or executed agreements. The contract administration functions are many. The persons who negotiated and executed the contract or grants often delegate many of these functions. Some of the primary activities that may need to be done include:

1. Conducting post-award orientation conferences internally and coordinating activities between the parties.
2. Resolving issues in controversy.
3. Determining the adequacy of performance as it occurs and when delivery of the "end product" is made.
4. Preparing, reviewing, and approving or disapproving the requests for payments under the progress payments or other payments clauses.
5. Making payments and allocating the payments in financial records of the parties.
6. Ensuring timely notifications under the contractor.
7. Monitoring the financial activities under the contract.
8. Dealing with tax and tax exemption issues.
9. Processing import and export documents such as duty-free entry certificates.

10. For classified contracts, administering those portions of the applicable industrial security program.
11. Negotiating and administering individual task requests under master contracts.
12. Negotiating prices and executing supplemental agreements.
13. Negotiating and executing contractual documents for settlement of partial and complete contract terminations.
14. Negotiating and executing contractual documents related to multiyear contracts (e.g., options, cancellations, renewals, etc.).
15. Processing and executing novation, assignments, and change-of-name agreements.
16. Handling administration of property purchased under the agreements or used in connection with performance.
17. Administering acquisition or fabrication of special test equipment, laboratory animals, biological materials, radioactive or hazardous substances, etc.
18. Performing necessary screening, redistribution, and disposal of equipment, inventory, supplies, etc.
19. Ensuring compliance with socioeconomic requirements imposed by government programs or contractual commitments.
20. Administering subcontracts.
21. Accomplishing administrative closeout procedures.
22. Administering continuing obligations concerning IP, records management, and audit.

It is important to reiterate that the mutual obligations of the parties are established by, and limited to, the written stipulations in the contract. The parties should assure that both know just which persons are responsible for assuring compliance with the different aspects of the contract, especially any statutory, legal, business, and regulatory provisions. This should be established in either a post-award conference or a letter (if not already stipulated by contract provisions).

• • • Endnotes

1. *National Conference on Commissioners on Uniform State Laws*, "Uniform Partnership Act," 1997, http://www.law.upenn.edu/bll/ulc/ulc_frame.htm (accessed September 27, 2005).

2. *Canadian Competition Bureau*, Director of Investigation and Research, Minister of Supply and Services, "Strategic Alliances Under the 'Competition Act,'" 1995, http://strategis.ic.gc.ca/pics/ct/alliance_e.pdf (accessed August 5, 2005).

3. See, e.g., Thomas Keil, "Strategic Alliances—A Review of the State of the Art," Helsinki University of Technology Institute of Strategy and International Business, Working Paper Series 2000 | 10, Espoo, Finland, 2000, http://www.tuta.hut.fi/units/Isib/publications/working_papers/tk.reviewallianceliterature_2000.pdf (accessed August 5, 2005); Niki Hynes and Diane A. Mollenkopf, "Strategic Alliance Formation: Developing a Framework for Research," 1998, http://130.195.95.71:8081/www/ANZMAC1998/Cd_rom/Hynes3.pdf (accessed August 5, 2005).

4. O. E. Williamson, *The Economic Institutions of Capitalism*, New York: Free Press, 1985.

5. Ibid.

6. Refer to Thomas G. Field Jr.'s "Intellectual Property: The Practical and Legal Fundamentals" at http://www.piercelaw.edu/tfield/pLfip.htm (accessed August 8, 2005) for more information. Article adapted from Field Jr., "Intellectual Property: Some Practical and Legal Fundamentals," originally published in *IDEA*, 34 (1994): 79–128.

7. Technically, the act is entitled "The Patent and Trademark Laws Amendments of 1980, as Amended" (in Chapter 18 of title 35 of the U.S. Code). Regulations implementing federal patent and licensing policy regarding "Rights to Inventions Made by Nonprofit Organizations and Small Business Firms" are codified at 37 CFR Part 401.

8. Donald Fowler, "University-Industry Relationships," *Research Management* 27 (January–February 1984):35–41.

9. Also see S. Atkinson, "University Industry Research Agreements: Major Negotiation Issues," *SRA Journal* 17 (Fall 1985):67.

10. Robert Killoren and Susan Butts, "Industry-University Research in Our Times," white paper organized by the Government-University-Industry Reasearch roundtable, the Industrial Research Institute, and the National Council of University Research Administrators, June 23, 2003.

35

Contracts: Form, Function, and Issue Spotting

Cindy Kiel, JD, CRA

Introduction

This chapter focuses on the formation of a contract, the different types of contracts one might come across in research administration, and specific contractual terms that a research administrator for a nonprofit entity should consider during negotiation. To start, the definition of a contract is an agreement between two or more persons that creates an obligation to perform. A contract is a promise, legally recognized, which, if the terms of it are breached, gives one party rights to seek legal remedy from the other for failure to comply with the duties of the contract. A contract is not a gift: there are terms attached. In a legal sense, all grants, cooperatives, and other agreements are contracts, though a true governmental contract is treated under different codes and guidelines than grants, cooperative agreements, and other agreements.

Contract Formation

Contract formation is nothing more than a simple equation. If you take the above definition and divide it up into key points, the equation looks like this:

Offer + Acceptance + Consideration = CONTRACT

This section addresses each element of a contract and breaks it down into comprehensible terms.

The Offer: An offer is a statement or communication about what someone will do if the offer is accepted by another party. The offer must be communicated to the other party, contain definite terms, and show the intent to enter into a contract by the one offering. The definite terms and intent are the elements that distinguish offers from advertising. Requests for proposals, requests for applications, or requests for bids are not offers. Rather, they are invitations for entities to submit an offer to a sponsoring or contracting entity.

Acceptance: Acceptance must also be communicated to the one offering in the manner specified by the one offering, or by any reasonable means if the method was not specified and the acceptance must (as common law) mirror the terms of the offer in order for a contract to be formed. Under the Uniform Commercial Code, the acceptance does not have to perfectly mirror the offer, but the material or key elements of the offer must be accepted without modifications.

Consideration: In the world of legal contracts, consideration does not mean being kind or nice or considerate. Rather, consideration can be defined as "something bargained for and given in exchange for a promise." Other terms used for consideration can be *quid pro quo*, "give and take," or "you scratch my back and I'll scratch yours." This is the essence of the contractual relationship. In the world of research administration, you see consideration at work in a proposal and award. The proposal might say, "Institution promises to perform the following scope of work and provide Agency with annual reports if Agency promises to provide funding in the amount of 1 million dollars." The consideration from the institution is research work and reports and the consideration from the agency is money.

Different Forms of Contracts and a Discussion on Signature Authority

In the world of contracts, you will hear terminology including the following: unilateral and bilateral agreements; parol versus written; express versus implied; fixed price; cost reimbursable; and conditional or absolute agreements. Meanings of these terms are described in this section.

Unilateral versus Bilateral: There is a popular notion among research administrators that a unilateral agreement is an agreement that is signed by only one party and a bilateral agreement is signed by both parties, and that you can turn an agreement into a unilateral one simply by stating that it must be signed only by one party. This is not entirely true. The mode of acceptance and terms of consideration are determined by whether an agreement is unilateral or bilateral.

A unilateral agreement is one where the means of acceptance of the offer is based on actual performance measure and funds are not payable until actual performance is rendered. This would occur, for example, when the sponsor states that it will pay $1 million dollars to the first entity that comes up with a cure for cancer: the only means of acceptance is to provide the cure for cancer.

A bilateral agreement occurs where acceptance comes in the form of a promise to provide the consideration or to perform in the future. This would be the case when, for example, the sponsor states that it will reimburse a company for expenses of research incurred toward finding a cure for cancer, where the center, then, would provide annual reports of progress.

Parol versus Written: Agreements can be either verbal (parol) or written in nature. While this can seem pretty straightforward, people fail to understand that verbal agreements are as contractually binding as written documents. If the agreement is specific enough in its terms, the court will readily uphold the terms of a verbal agreement if challenged. However, there are some agreements that must be in writing under a law, the "Statute of Frauds," which was developed in order to prevent fraud. Contracts that are subject under this law include contracts for real property, sureties, executor's agreements to pay for estate debts, sales of commercial goods for $500.00 or more between merchants, or agreements that cannot be performed in one year. The above agreements must be in writing to be enforceable or the parties must admit, in court, that there was an agreement in order to satisfy the statute of frauds.

Conditional vs. Absolute: An absolute agreement is where one party performs, as does the other party. A retail transaction is a great example of an absolute contract: the customer pays for merchandise and the retail entity gives it to the customer to take. A conditional contract is one where the very existence and performance depends on some contingency or condition happening before the parties have met their contractual obligations, for example, a pre-award agreement where the obligations of the parties are contingent upon receipt of a governmental award.

Express vs. Implied: An express contract is an actual agreement of the parties where the contract terms are spoken openly or are written in distinct and explicit language. The implied contract is one that is not created by an explicit agreement of the parties but is, instead, inferred by law because of the conduct of the parties. For example, if a scientist started performing work for an industry sponsor and it appears that the scientist expected to be reimbursed for his/her costs associated with the project, an institution may make a claim for reimbursement under an implied contract theory, even though no official contract exists. Some terms of agreements are always "implied at law" even if an express agreement does not include these provisions. An example of this is the implied condition that each party will put forth reasonable efforts to complete the terms of the agreement.

Actual and Apparent Authority: In the corporate world, employees must act on behalf of companies or organizations in order to enter into a contract. Every organization should determine which employees have the authority to contractually bind the corporation. If someone without authority attempts to enter into an agreement on the company's behalf, the company should immediately notify the contracting party and the employee that the employee did not have authority. Negligence in not immediately handling this situation could result in an organization being held responsible for a contract under the notion of "apparent" authority. There are some legal cases that stand for the idea that there is no such thing as "apparent" authority when it comes to contracting with state governmental entities, but this is not true in all states.

Defenses to Formation of a Contract

Defenses to formation of a contract can include:

- Mistake by both parties

- Ambiguity of Terms
- Misrepresentation and Fraud
- No Consideration
- Illegal Subject Matter
- Contrary to Public Policy
- Restraint of Trade (noncompete clauses that are overly broad)
- Unconscionable Contracts
- Lack of Capacity of a Party (infant, insane, intoxicated, under duress, or no signature authority)

Special Issues in Research Administration Contracts
Titles and Recitals

The title and recital sections of an agreement are the first items seen by the contractual parties. They also give clues to auditors, lawyers, and others regarding the nature of the agreement (research, service, testing, work for hire, output, etc.) and the types of parties involved in the agreement (merchant, commercial, research, nonprofit, public, etc.). There typically is a general statement of consideration for the agreement. The recitals and nicknames adopted in the initial paragraphs of a contract are important because interpretation of other clauses in the agreement can be impacted by these initial statements.

The title should use the legal name of the parties and give some indication of the type of agreement that will follow. Types of agreements include:

- Service
- Professional Service
- Testing
- Work for Hire
- Subcontract
- Inter-local
- Memorandum of Understanding
- Teaming
- License
- Material Transfer

Nonprofit, 501c3 organizations should avoid title language that appears to apply to commercial or merchant work-for-hire agreements; these types of activities would fall outside the nonprofit mission. There have been IRS cases involving clinical studies where testing agreements have been determined to fall outside a research and educational mission and therefore may be subject to IRS Unrelated Business Income Tax (UBIT) provisions; likewise, when setting up names for the parties of the agreement, try to avoid language that appears to make the agreement commercial or profit-oriented.

Instead, it is recommended to choose terms such as *University*, *Nonprofit*, *Organization*, or *Institution*, instead of terms like *Contractor*, *Vendor*, *Provider*, or *Business Associate*.

The research institution's mission and its commitment that the work to be performed fits within the institution's nonprofit status should be spelled out in the contract's title and recital sections, stating, for example, "Whereas the research institution has determined that the scope of work identified herein falls within its mission as a nonprofit entity . . .".

Payment and Compensation

These terms specify the financial terms of agreements. In research administration agreements, an administrator should look for forms, invoicing processes, or paperwork requirements that the institution cannot agree with. If the administrator knows that the financial system cannot send out final invoices within 60 days, the agreement should not state that the final invoice is due in 45 days. If the invoice instructions request original receipts or if the institution is large, the agreement should be renegotiated to allow for copies to be sent instead, allowing originals to reside with the institution. In international agreements, it is important to be cognizant of any charges that might be incurred for wire transfers and to know how these fees will be paid (and adjust payment schedules to reduce the number of transfers, and thus, the amount of transfer fees).

> *Fixed Price:* A fixed price agreement is one where payment is contingent upon completion of the scope of work and all deliverables as required in the agreement. The benefit to this approach is that, if the project comes in under the cost estimated in the agreement, the institution can keep the remaining funds and use them as unrestricted funds for other purposes. However, if the project comes in over budget, the deliverables must still be met in order to receive payment and the cost of any such overruns will have to be borne by the institution. Fixed price agreements should generally not be used for research-related activities because the nature of research activities often entails unforeseen delays. A fixed price agreement is risky for the institution performing the work: if the terms are not met, the sponsor can legally withhold payment even if the work has been substantially completed. Additional problems can occur if either of the parties terminates the

agreement prior to the specified termination date. If a fixed price method of compensation is chosen for services, the contract negotiator must be careful to make sure the terms of the work are precisely detailed and the contract does not leave the institution open for liability if there are changes in the project's scope. Project milestones (with payment required for reaching each milestone) should be designated within the agreement. It is also important to be aware that any significant difference between the compensation received and the actual costs for the work performed can cause UBIT issues for the institution.

Fee-For-Service: In this type of arrangement, a fee is charged based on a task or activity. Contract language could state, for example, "Sponsor shall pay $100 for each sample processed up to $1,000.00," or "Sponsor shall pay $500.00 for each patient enrolled in the study," or "It is anticipated that Sponsor will enroll a minimum of 100 patients." The institution could bill as the samples are processed or as patients are enrolled, but the billing would not be based on the actual costs associated with doing the analysis or the patient enrollment. This type of activity is also susceptible to UBIT issues if the fees are significantly higher than the actual cost of doing the work. There is less risk in getting payment for services, because payment becomes due upon completion of each individual task instead of upon completion of the entire scope of work as in the fixed price compensation method.

Cost Reimbursable: This type of agreement, which is the most common in research administration, allows an entity to invoice for actual costs incurred in performing the research or service. It is less risky because compensation is earned as costs are incurred. An institution is required to perform only on the scope of work up to the point where funding under the agreement is exhausted. The agreement will specify a cost reimbursable agreement with language similar to the following: "Sponsor shall pay contractor up to $1 million. Any unspent funds remaining at the end of the project shall be reimbursed to Sponsor."

Scope of Work

The scope of work defines what a party to an agreement must do for the duration of the contract. The scope of work should be definitive enough that in the event a sponsor or contractor refuses to pay amounts specified in the agreement due to incom-

plete work or a failure to perform, such failure or incompleteness could be verified or disputed based on the work identified in the agreement. The scope of work should set forth any milestones, deliverables, reporting requirements, or end products that are expected to be provided to the other party and the time frame for these deliverables.

Standard of Care

In medical, legal, and professional malpractice cases, a standard of care is applied to measure the competence of the professional. The traditional standard for doctors is that he or she exercise the "average degree of skill, care, and diligence exercised by members of the same profession, practicing in the same or a similar locality in light of the present state of medical and surgical science." With increased specialization, however, certain courts have disregarded geographical considerations holding that in the practice of a board-certified specialty, the standard should be that of a specialist practicing in the same field in the same area.

Reasonable Care: This is the standard that one must observe to avoid liability for negligence under all circumstances, including foreseeing of harm to a foreseeable plaintiff. The standard implies fair, proper, just, moderate, and suitable actions under the circumstances. It requires the institution to take such acts as may be fairly, justly, and reasonably required—that degree of care which a reasonably prudent person should exercise in the same or similar circumstances.

Best Efforts: This requires the institution to take "ALL reasonable means" to avoid foreseeable harm to a foreseeable plaintiff. Even if the institution acts reasonably, if it does not use the "best" or most effective reasonable means of avoiding injury, it can be held liable for damages (e.g., meeting delivery schedule). If the institution does not deliver on time, then the institution is liable unless it has done everything possible despite the cost to meet the schedule. A best-efforts standard of care places onerous and burdensome obligations upon the institution to fulfill the agreement's obligations. For instance, a clinical sponsor might have requested that an institution "use best efforts" to meet patient enrollment numbers by a specific date, and by using this phrase, the sponsor requires an institution to use all means regardless of expense to achieve the patient enrollment numbers by the specific date. The sponsor, however, is not adequately compensating the institution to use such extreme measures. If the sponsor resists the reasonable care standard, then it may be acceptable to allow this phrase to remain *except* if the phrase is used in the context of meeting patient enrollment or meeting a specific deliverables schedule in a research agreement.

Highest Professional Care or Expert Standard of Care: This standard commits the institution to something more than the "reasonable man" negligence standard of care. This language can place the institution at risk for liability even if the institution is not negligent in its duties. It is in its best interest that the institution delete the phrase "highest professional efforts" from any contract and, instead, use "reasonable efforts" in all research and service agreements. If it is not possible to use the "reasonable efforts" standard of care, the contractor might agree to a "prevailing local" standard of care for professional level work (MDs, JDs, or other professionally licensed individuals), if such individuals are covered by institutional professional liability insurance. Any liability under the standard should be limited to the institution's applicable insurance limits, for example, "PI shall conduct the Study as outlined in the Protocol and shall use his/her highest professional efforts according to *prevailing local* professional standards to complete the planned enrollment of patients by date."

Industry Standard of Care: This language is usually used in commercial agreements, purchase orders, and the like. This commits the institution to provide the same level of care as commercial entities when performing similar work. This may or may not be the reasonable man standard depending on the industry involved. It is recommended that an institution try to delete any reference to an "Industry Standard of Care" and request that this language be replaced with the reasonable person standard. The main argument against this language is that research institutions are not industry, and they do not engage in commercial activities, thus, such activities cannot be legally compared with commercial entities providing similar work. Research and service from a university/nonprofit perspective is different than industry and commercial work and service. Nonprofit entities are unique and this is why industry often wishes to team up with nonprofits on projects because they have something that standard industry cannot provide.

Strict Liability: Strict liability is simply liability without fault. An institution could be held liable for any and all defective or hazardous outcomes of service, or providing goods under a sponsored agreement regardless of whether the institution was actually negligent or did anything wrong. Note that the term "standard of care" is also used in reference to insurance and patient care. Generally, standard of care in this context is what a patient of the same disease type in the same situation would receive if he or she chose to receive treatment (often referred to as "patient care"). In this case, the costs associated with standard-of-care procedures are billed to a patient's insurance carrier, and a research hospital would not be reimbursed by the sponsor for this particular standard-of-care cost. Thus, whenever a standard-of-care clause is included in an agreement, request the "reasonable" efforts standard to be included in the clause.

Warranties

It is important to note that there are different kinds of warranties covering different types of situations (e.g., for fitness of a product for a particular use; general warranties of condition of goods and services; those regarding title to or infringement of property including intellectual property). Implied warranties are warranties granted by law but not written or verbalized within the context of an agreement. Express warranties are written or verbalized within the context of an agreement. If a commercial contract is involved, even if warranty provisions are not included in the text of the agreement, a court could imply that Uniform Commercial Code ("UCC") warranties were applicable to the agreement. In law, a warranty can give rise to a separate cause of legal action from breach of the contract itself. For example, the institution could be in full compliance with the terms and conditions of an agreement, yet be in violation of an implied warranty. Also, a breach of warranty could be considered to be a breach of a contract agreement. Depending on the nature of the warranty provision included in an agreement and the nature of the contract itself, inclusion of a warranty provision may or may not be a deal breaker. Some of the different types of warranties are discussed in more detail below.

Negotiating Warranty Provisions

An administrator should attempt to delete any warranty provisions requiring an institution to warranty the results of research. In research agreements, for instance, there may be occasions when a sponsor asks the institution to make an express warranty about the research to be done and warrant that the results will be as expected. If the sponsor is merely providing funds to do research, such warranty provisions would not be appropriate because the institution should not warrant its research work that, by its very nature, is unpredictable. More importantly, you may want to add the following provision to a sponsor's research agreement: "The Materials provided under this agreement are provided 'as is' without any warrantees of any kind including warranties of merchantability, fitness for a particular purpose, or noninfringement of intellectual property rights."

Warranties and the Uniform Commercial Code (UCC): Most states have adopted the UCC in one form or another. However, nonprofit research institutions are not commercial entities and should not want to appear as if they are commercial entities by including warranty provisions in their agreements, especially when the warranties are regarding research-related work. Warranties in a clinical study or service agreement should be avoided because such language may infer that the institution is acting outside of its research and education mission as a 501c3 organization giving rise to UBIT issues. Warranty language may also give the other party an argument that the agreement is covered by the UCC and that the institution is, indeed, doing commercial-type work in spite of its nonprofit, public agency status.

Warranties and Governmental Immunity: Including warranty language in agreements may give rise to the argument that the institution is involved in commercial activities outside the scope of its nonprofit, research, and education mission. Institutions that are state governmental agencies also should consider the governmental immunity provisions of their state statutes. Most immunity acts only protect a state agency from suit and/or limits indemnification if it is involved in a "governmental function." If the institution is deemed to be performing a commercial rather than a governmental function, there is an argument that it loses its governmental immunity in the event it is sued for something that went wrong involving the agreement. There is also an argument that a warranty may create a waiver situation regarding indemnification within an immunity act. This argument is unique depending on each state's immunity law provisions. It is important to review these issues with legal counsel.

Warranties and the Inherent Nature of Research: For research contracts, an institution should rarely, if ever, agree to warrant the results of research. A sponsor's insistence that there be a warranty of the scope of work should break any deal. As one professor has put it, "The world of research is fraught with incidental failure." The nature of research is that one cannot predict the final outcome of the research, nor can the actual timing of events or failures be predicted. In fact, we should probably be adding language (such as referenced prior) specifying that there are no express or implied warranties for the work to be accomplished.

Sponsor or Subcontractor Attempts to Waive All Warranties: Generally, any sponsor or subcontractor warranty provision (often it is a paragraph in all caps and bolded) should be taken out of an agreement, as well as any language that limits implied and express warranties and/or that waives rights to claim warranties against them. However, inclusion of such language should be determined on a case-by-case basis depending on the negotiation demands and nature of the work. If the sponsor insists on such language, the warranty waiver should be mutual, if appropriate. The institution should not accept any sponsor warranty provision that limits future claims of human subjects. This matter should be reviewed with the institution's internal review board, to insure that human subject rights are protected and that the negotiated agreement does not waive a participant's legal claims against a company or manufacturer.

Indemnification and Insurance

Indemnification is an undertaking whereby one agrees to restore the victim of a loss in whole or in part by payment, repair, or replacement upon the occurrence of a loss. This is a contractual or equitable right under which the entire loss is shifted from a tortfeasor who is only technically or passively at fault to another who is primarily or actively responsible. If this language is not included in a contractual arrangement, it could open the institution up for unnecessary liability.

Most state institutions are protected by governmental immunity laws that limit indemnification rights, i.e., place limits on liability. These rights should always be inserted into an indemnification provision when they can be used in accordance with state laws. It is wise to consult with legal counsel to determine the appropriate language for insertion. Avoid language that requires the institution to indemnify for the wrongful acts or failure to act of the other party. When reviewing indemnification provisions, mutual indemnification provisions should be included in any contract. Any attempts by industry or nongovernmental partners to limit liability to the levels that the institution has under its legal governmental immunity laws should be avoided for the following reasons:

1. The Governmental Immunity Act is designed to protect taxpayers from lawsuits with certain exceptions. It is not appropriate to use the governmental, nonprofit, taxpayer umbrella to protect private, profit corporations.

2. Due to the provisions and exceptions listed in the Immunity Act, the institution cannot insure that the company would have the same or different status as a governmental entity and, depending on legal claims, there may be no limits to indemnification available under the Act.

3. The Act covers not only indemnification limitations, but also statute of limitations, procedural notification issues, and other clauses that are not applicable to the private sector in any way.

Review insurance requirements to make sure they do not exceed the level of the institution's current policies and/or governmental immunity limitations. If a company requires additional insurance, consider taking on a rider policy if the company is willing to pay for the additional premiums (consult the institution's risk management offices for additional details regarding the institution's flexibility in this area). Often, professional liability limits may differ from general liability limits. Workers' compensation and unemployment should be limited to those amounts "as required by law." Most insurance provisions will not protect an institution or its officers or employees from acts that are willful, wanton, fraudulent, or intentional.

Publication and Confidentiality

Reasons for Retaining Publication Rights

Most educational institutions and nonprofit organizations have a tax status based on an identified nonprofit-related mission. Depending on the mission of the organization, most 501c3 organizations with goals of education, research, and community outreach must retain publication rights to their work without external influence in order to avoid Unrelated Business Income Tax (UBIT) on the sponsored work. Publication rights should also be maintained due to potential student theses and/or adverse events in clinical investigations where the public should be informed of potential hazards of a particular product or invention. A possible solution to the publication negotiation dilemma is to allow a sponsor for a period of time (six months) to review a publication and give the sponsor the right to request removal of any trade secrets or proprietary information owned by the sponsor, and/or to allow a period of time for intellectual property to be protected via patent or copyright. Limitations on publication rights also pose a risk if there are any foreign national researchers, students, or consultants on a project. Depending on the nature of the work, proprietary restrictions in an agreement may bring export and trade regulation issues.

Nondisclosure agreements should be limited in scope and duration, and for governmental institutions may be limited by state records access statutes and/or the federal sunshine laws: Federal Open Information Access Act (FOIAA). The Health Insurance Portability and Accountability Act (HIPAA) is also a new concern in clinical study agreements.

Ownership of Intellectual Property

Intellectual property (IP) refers to intangible property that is the result of research, invention, or creative endeavors. It covers ideas and designs that are patentable, as well as copyrightable works. IP also encompasses the world of trade secrets, trademarks, and service marks. All institutions should develop an internal policy regarding how to deal with their intellectual properties. Some non-profit entities with their own publishing abilities are quite strict about ownership of copyright; others allow students or professors to retain rights to what they create. All contractual terms and conditions should be negotiated in order to comply with an institution's particular intellectual property policy.

Termination and Remedies for Breach

Actual or Compensatory: These are real, substantial, and just damages for an individual's actual and real loss or injury. They compensate the injured party solely for the injury sustained (and nothing more). The rationale is to restore the injured party to the position he/she was in prior to the injury

Consequential or Incidental: This is damage, loss, or injury that does not flow directly and immediately from the act of the party sued, but only from some of the consequences or results of such act. They include damages arising from intervention of special circumstances not ordinarily predictable and losses or injuries that are the result of an act, but not direct and immediate. Consequential breach of contract claims can include any loss resulting from general or particular requirements and needs of which the seller at the time of contracting had reason to know and which could not reasonably be prevented and any injury to person or property caused by a breach of warranty. Costs incurred due to acts of a breaching party are also included.

Punitive, Exemplary, or Presumptive: This is an award of damages above what will compensate an individual for his or her loss, where the wrong was aggravated by circumstances of violence, malice, fraud, or wanton disregard for the other party's rights. These damages are designed to punish the wrongdoer, to make an example of the wrongdoer, and/or to provide incentive for a wrongdoer to change future behavior. These damages are normally not awarded for a breach of contract claim.

Expectancy or Loss of Profits: These are awarded in actions for nonperformance of contract calculated by subtracting the injured party's actual dollar position as a result of the breach from that party's projected dollar position had performance occurred. The goal is to determine the dollar amount necessary to ensure that the aggrieved party's position will be the same as if the other party had actually performed under the agreement.

Nominal: This is a trifling sum awarded to a plaintiff in an action where there is no substantial loss or injury to be compensated, but the law recognizes a technical invasion of the plaintiff's rights or a breach of the defendant's duty.

Prospective or Speculative: These are damages anticipated from the same acts, but those that depend upon future developments that are contingent, conjectural, or improbable. Damages that have not yet accrued at the time of the trial, but that, in the nature of things, may result from the complained upon acts of facts may also be included.

Injunctive or Specific Performance: This requires that a breach result in irreparable harm to an injured party or damages for which no certain pecuniary standard exists for measurement or that are not easily ascertainable at law. A court uses injunctions to enjoin a party from taking an action or to require a party to perform an action.

Liquidated Damages: This is a specified amount of funds required in the contract itself in the event of a breach of contract. This method is used in a contract when the difficulties of proof of loss, inconvenience, or unfeasibility of other methods of compensation are unable to obtain an adequate remedy. Damages that are set unreasonably high in the agreement in light of the actual damage occurred after breach will be voided as a penalty.

Legal Matters and Resolution

Jurisdiction is the court's authority to decide a matter in controversy and presupposes the existence of a duly constituted court with control over the subject matter and the parties to inquire into facts, apply law, make decisions, and declare judgment. Again, governmental entities usually prefer to leave this provision silent or have jurisdiction named as the state or governmental entity of which they are a part due to sovereignty issues. When negotiating jurisdiction, note that industry partners and nonprofits have much more flexibility in agreeing to a different jurisdiction than do governmental parties.

Venue is the geographical location where a lawsuit or arbitration will take place. For example, it is possible that under a particular contract, governing law could be Delaware, jurisdiction in Florida, with venue in Orlando.

Choice of law is the set-up laws under which a contractual arrangement shall be governed. These are the laws and rules that control the actions or conduct of parties and that can determine processes and rights or obligations of the parties. The agreement may define federal law or a particular state's law as governing the agreement. Most, if not all, governmental institutions will not agree to be governed by the laws of another sovereign. In the event this clause is disputed, attempt to leave the choice of law provision silent or leave the choice of law to be determined by a court of competent jurisdiction. In the absence of a choice of law clause, courts look at several factors to determine the applicable law, including place of contracting, place of performance, and public policy factors. Application of these factors can lead to inconsistent results, so although contract law is fairly uniform throughout the United States, parties can use this clause to try and shop around for the law they think would give them the best deal or that would be the most convenient for them or their lawyers.

Conflict Resolution

When conflict arises in the conduct of the research or other activity defined by the contractual agreement, the method for resolving the conflict must be defined. Mediation and arbitration are the most common forms of conflict resolution outside of the court of law. Some state laws do not allow a state entity to give up sovereignty and mandatory binding arbitration clauses must be deleted. Other states allow arbitration, but only if it follows state laws. Arbitration may be the best choice of dispute resolution in international contracts due to treaties involving enforcement of judicial awards from one country to another.

Mediation is a private informal dispute resolution process in which a neutral third person, the mediator, helps disputing parties reach an agreement. The mediator has no power to impose a decision on the parties.

Arbitration is a process of dispute resolution in which a neutral third party, the arbitrator, renders a decision after a hearing at which both parties have an opportunity to be heard. Where arbitration is voluntary, the disputing parties select the arbitrator who has the power to render a binding decision. In binding arbitration, the parties must abide by the decision of the arbitrator and a judgment can be entered as legally binding by a court of competent jurisdiction. The majority of states have now adopted the Uniform Arbitration Act. However, due to sovereignty issues, many governmental entities will not allow binding arbitration in their agreements. In the event such a clause is agreed to, it should define what arbitration panel will be used, the venue of the arbitration, and the language that will be used during arbitration. The purpose of this clause is to avoid costly litigation in the event that the parties can not mutually agree to terms of a dispute.

Litigation is a lawsuit. It is a contest in a court of law for the purpose of enforcing a right or seeking a remedy.

Signature Authority:

Actual: the power of an agent to bind its principal where such power derives from express or implied agreement between the principal and the agent.

Apparent: When actual authority does not exist, but the actions between an individual and a third party lead the third party to rely on apparent authority to his or her detriment, and the principal failed to take reasonable action to avoid the misrepresentation.

Express: Agency delegated to an agent by words that expressly authorize him/her to act on behalf of the principal.

Implied: Authority created by act of the parties and deduced from proof of other facts.

36

Legal Perspective of Government Representations and Certifications

J. Michael Slocum, JD

The Federal government, as a study sponsor, and other sponsors often require that organizations competing or applying for contracts or grants provide written affirmation of compliance with a variety of federal, state, local, and internal policies, whether or not these policies may be directly applicable to the proposed project. Sponsors of all sorts also require the supplicant organizations to "warrant" or represent that the organizations meet certain standards, are owned by certain types of individuals, will use only certain supplies or services, etc. These are called "representations and certifications."

Contracts and grants are governed by various federal regulations that mandate specific contract or grant award mechanisms, particular contract and grant structures and clauses, and much more. The Federal Acquisition Regulations System was established for the codification and publication of uniform policies and procedures for acquisition (contracting) by all executive agencies. The Federal Acquisition Regulations System consists of the Federal Acquisition Regulation (FAR), Title 48 of the Code of Federal Regulations (CFR), which is the primary document, and agency acquisition regulations that implement or supplement the FAR. The Office of Management and Budget (OMB) established Title 2 in the Code of Federal Regulations for grants and other financial assistance and nonprocurement agreements. Title 2 consists of two subtitles, Subtitles A and B. In Subtitle A, OMB publishes government-wide guidance to federal agencies for grants and agreements—guidance that currently is in seven separate OMB circulars and other OMB policy documents. Subtitle B is for supplementary material and material that does not apply government-wide. Representations, certifications, and assurances are mandated by these regulations.

One agency has defined these representations and certifications as:

> Required statements by an offeror or contractor that must accompany federal contracts and *proposals*, such as details of its accounting procedures and compliance with *small business* and trade agreements. [1]

In many cases these statements are similar to or duplicative with the organization's required "assurances" that are also made to sponsors, including the federal government.

Among the common topics covered by these required statements are the following:

Human Subjects. In accordance with federal regulations, research institutions may be required to make a representation or have an *Assurance Agreement* with the federal government, which affirms the existence of policies and procedures for the protection of human subjects in research.

Laboratory Animals. As with human subjects, research organizations often must make representations, certifications, and assurances concerning their compliance with the regulations mandating humane care and use of animals for research and/or teaching.

Radiation Safety. Those organizations with research that may involve radioactive materials will find that there are several representations to be made concerning compliance with the procedures for radiation safety.

Recombinant DNA. As with radioactive materials there are certifications, representations, and assurances to be made if there is any possibility of the use of recombinant DNA in an organization's research.

Environmental Health and Safety. There are many environmental representations and certifications required under various federal and state programs. Even private sponsors often require certification of compliance with the major federal environmental laws.

Debt, Debarment, and Suspension. Potential contractors and grantees must certify that they are not delinquent on the repayment of any federal debt before an award can be made. In addition, both the organizations and their key personnel (e.g., the principal investigators, officers, and directors) are required to certify that they are neither debarred nor suspended from doing business with the federal government and that they are not contracting with any such organizations or persons.

Drug-free Workplace. Federal prime contractors and grantees are required by federal regulation to maintain both a drug-free workplace and formal drug and alcohol abuse prevention programs. There are certifications and representations to assure that all contractors and grantees warrant their compliance as a precondition to obtaining any federal funds.

Lobbying. Federal rules severely restrict the use of federal funds to influence officials of Congress and Executive Branch agencies in connection with a specific award. There are several representations and certifications that must be made to assure compliance with these restrictions.

Misconduct in Science. Several federal agencies require potential contractors and applicant organizations to certify that the institution has established appropriate administrative policies for dealing with and reporting possible scientific misconduct.

Conflict of Interest. Many federal agencies, including the Public Health Service (PHS) and the National Science Foundation (NSF), now require applicant organizations to certify that the institution has written and enforced administrative policies for identifying, managing, and reporting the significant outside financial interests of principal project staff. Agencies also require certifications concerning organizational conflicts of interest and "conceptual" conflicts that may harm the requirements for objectivity in science.

Civil Rights, Handicapped Individuals, Sex Discrimination, Age Discrimination. With most proposals, sponsors also require the offerors and applicants to certify that they comply with various federal, state, and local nondiscrimination statutes and that they are undertaking affirmative action to promote employment of persons within various groups that have suffered discrimination.

Inventions and Patents. Organizations are required to certify that they are in compliance with the patent reporting and disclosure requirements imposed by the federal government.

Many of the representations and certifications required in federal research contracts are "housekeeping" provisions and others relate to enforcement of socio-economic policies mandated for government contractors. As shown in Table 36-1, the National Institutes of Health (NIH) lists many of these "by reference."[2]

Many agencies are converting to electronic versions of the representations and certifications. For instance, the primary agency in charge of federal procurement policy, the General Services Administration, has developed the Online Representations and Certifications Application (ORCA), an Internet-based system[3] and e-Government initiative to replace the paper-based Representations and Certifications ("Reps and Certs") process. That system is now mandated in the Federal Acquisition Regulation (FAR). Under the system, potential contractors provide most information just once, but then must supplement ORCA information by providing contract specific representations and certifications and updates in response to a specific solicitation.

Similarly, many granting agencies are moving to electronic versions of the required "assurances." For instance, the NIH provides for an Institution Profile File (IPF) as a part of its "eRA Commons" system, a Web-based system that allows NIH extramural grantee organizations, grantees, and the public to receive and transmit information electronically about the administration of biomedical and behavioral research. Grantee institutions verify that they are in compliance with specified assurances and certifications by completing the IPF Assurances and Certifications.

Much of the effort in this area is based on a federal law mandating more coordination of grant-making activity to bring it into line with the unified

TABLE 36-1	NIH List of FAR Representations and Certifications
1. FAR 52.203-2	Certification of Independent Price Determination
2. FAR 52.203-11	Certification and Disclosure Regarding Payments to Influence Certain Federal Transactions (DEVIATION)
3. FAR 52.204-3	Taxpayer Identification
4. FAR 52.204-5	Women-Owned Business (Other Than Small Business)
5. FAR 52.204-6	Data Universal Numbering System (DUNS) Number
6. FAR 52.209-5	Certification Regarding Debarment, Suspension, Proposed Debarment and Other Responsibility Matters
7. FAR 52.215-6	Place of Performance
8. FAR 52.219-1	Small Business Program Representations
9. FAR 52.219-19	Small Business Concern Representation for the Small Business Competitiveness Demonstration Program
10. FAR 52.219-21	Small Business Size Representation for Targeted Industry Categories Under the Small Business Competitiveness Demonstration Program
11. FAR 52.219-22	Small Disadvantaged Business Status
12. FAR 52.222-18	Certification Regarding Knowledge of Child Labor for Listed End Products
13. FAR 52.222-21	Certification of Nonsegregated Facilities
14. FAR 52.222-22	Previous Contracts and Compliance Reports
15. FAR 52.222-25	Affirmative Action Compliance
16. FAR 52.222-38	Compliance with Veterans' Employment Reporting Requirements
17. FAR 52.222-48	Exemption From Application of Service Contract Act Provisions
18. FAR 52.223-4	Recovered Material Certification
19. FAR 52.223-13	Certification of Toxic Chemical Release Reporting
20. FAR 52.225-2	Buy American Act Certificate
21. FAR 52.225-4	Buy American Act—North American Free Trade Agreement—Israeli Trade Act Certificate
22. FAR 52.225-6	Trade Agreements Certificate
23. FAR 52.226-2	Historically Black College or University and Minority Institution Representation
24. FAR 52.227-6	Royalty Information
25. FAR 52.230-1	Cost Accounting Standards Notices and Certification
26. FAR 15.406-2	Certificate of Current Cost or Pricing Data

Source: National Cancer Institute, Research Contracts Branch, http://rcb.cancer.gov/rcb-internet/forms/rcneg.pdf (accessed August 2, 2005).

procurement system. In 1999 Congress passed the Federal Financial Assistance Management Improvement Act requiring federal agencies to develop common grant application and reporting procedures. The Act (P.L. 106-107) covers all domestic "federal financial assistance" programs, including all programs (including entitlements) that provide resources (e.g., grants, contracts, loans, in-kind contributions) to states, localities, organizations, or individuals. Since it is limited to domestic programs, the act does not apply to foreign aid or assistance used in nondomestic situations. The law requires the Office of Management and Budget

(OMB) to work with other federal agencies to establish:

- A uniform application for financial assistance (e.g., grant applications) from multiple programs across multiple federal agencies;
- Ways to simplify reporting requirements and administrative procedures, including uniformity and standardization of rules affecting funding from multiple programs;
- Electronic methods for applying for, managing, and reporting of financial assistance funds;
- Improved approaches for the collection and sharing of data pertaining to financial assis-

tance programs, and efforts to strengthen the information management capacity of state, local, and tribal government and nonprofit organizations.

Most recently, the agencies have begun to collaborate on a single system for submission of grant applications, including representations, certifications, and assurances. Central to this effort, the federal Grants.gov program was developed to simplify and centralize all federal grants management and applications process. The site lists over 900 grant programs of twenty-six federal grant-making agencies that award hundreds of billions of dollars annually. As a part of that effort, OMB and the participating agencies are working on standardizing the representations, certifications, and assurances required, and establishing a single file containing all of the generally required items for an applicant institution or researcher.

As part of the effort to move to online system processes, as of January 1, 2005 FAR requires that the Online Representations and Certifications Applications (ORCA), a Web-based management system, must be used in federal solicitations as part of the proposal submission process. ORCA allows centralized and standard collection, and storage and viewing of FAR-required "reps and certs." That allows government contracting officers to readily access and evaluate FAR compliance that must be federally certified on an annual basis.

Summary

The federal government relies upon the certifications made by an institution's authorized official

that it is in compliance with all of the assurances required of any entity submitting to the federal government. The applicable assurances are provided for in the Grants Regulations and the Federal Acquisition Regulations. The number of assurances increases annually and at times are viewed merely as unfunded mandates that increase the cost of research. Generally, these certifications and representations have been designed to protect our research subjects, the general public, and our environment as well as ensure fiscal and fiduciary responsibility.

• • • Endnotes

1. See NIAID, "Glossary of Funding and Policy Terms and Acronyms," http://www.niaid.nih.gov/ncn/glossary/default6.htm (accessed August 2, 2005).

2. Full text of citations can be found in the Federal Acquisition Regulation (FAR), Regulation (FAR), "Representations, Certifications, and Other Statements of Offerors or Quoters (Negotiated)," http://www4.od.nih.gov/ocm/contracts/rfps/REPCERT.htm (accessed August 2, 2005).

3. Business Partner Network, "Online Representations and Certifications Application (ORCA)," http://www.bpn.gov (accessed August 2, 2005).

Post-Award and Financial Requirements

CHAPTER

37

Facilities and Administrative Costs

Paul Nacon

General Background

The concept of indirect costs, currently referred to as facilities and administrative (F&A) costs, goes back to 1958 when the then federal Bureau of the Budget issued a document called A-21. The circular contained the first set of formal guidelines for determining indirect costs associated with federally sponsored agreements conducted at educational institutions. While A-21 has been modified many times since its 1958 release, the basic methodology set out in the original document has not significantly changed.[1]

F&A costs are part of the total costs of a federally sponsored agreement. Unlike direct costs, F&A costs are those costs that cannot be easily assigned to specific projects. F&A costs include, but are not limited to, executive management, accounting, budgeting, payroll, and space related costs such as repair and maintenance, security, plant operations, and utilities. Because these administrative and facility costs are difficult to charge directly to federally sponsored agreements, the federal government reimburses F&A costs through the application of an F&A rate. The F&A rate is a ratio expressed as a percentage of F&A costs (the numerator) and a modified total direct cost (MTDC) base (the denominator).

The general cost principles for establishing F&A rates are contained in three different Office of Management and Budget (OMB) Circulars:

1. Circular A-21 pertains to educational institutions;[1]
2. Circular A-122 pertains to nonprofit organizations, and;[2]

3. Circular A-87 pertains to state, local, and Indian tribal governments.[3]

The US Department of Health and Human Services (DHHS) also publishes a document, Office of the Assistant Secretary Comptroller (OASC) –3, Revised, a guide for hospitals that contains the cost principles and procedures for establishing indirect costs and patient care rates for grants and contracts with DHHS.

All institutions that wish to be reimbursed for F&A costs must periodically, sometimes annually, prepare and submit an F&A rate proposal to the federal government for review and negotiation. The two primary federal departments responsible for review and negotiation of F&A rates are the US Department of Health and Human Services (DHHS) and the US Department of Defense (DoD). Within DHHS, this review and negotiation process falls to the Program Support Center, Division of Cost Allocation (DCA). Within DoD, it falls to the Office of Naval Research (ONR), University Business Affairs. DCA offices are located in Washington, DC, New York City, Dallas, and San Francisco. The ONR office is located in Arlington, Virginia.

The F&A rate is usually prepared using fiscal year-end financial data reconciled to audited financial statements. Not all costs are allowable or allocable to federally sponsored programs. Section J of A-21, Attachment B of A-122, and Attachment B of A-87 address the allowability of selected items of cost as both direct and indirect.[1,2,3] Institutions should become familiar with these cost items and their treatment. Some costs may only be charged to federal programs as direct costs; some may not be charged as either direct or indirect costs; other costs need to be reclassified from indirect costs to direct costs for calculating the indirect cost rate; and others should be eliminated from the rate calculation in total. This process is usually referred to as a screening of accounts or a scrubbing of object codes. Applicable credits must also be considered. Applicable credits are receipts or negative expenditures that reduce or offset expenses that are allocable to federal awards as either direct or indirect costs. They include, but are not limited to purchase discounts, rebates, and adjustments to expenditures. An explanation of applicable credits can be found in Section C.5 of A-21, Attachment A.5 of A-122, and Attachment A, Section C of A-87.[1,2,3]

The F&A rate submitted to the federal government should represent what the institution believes accurately reflects the administrative and facility costs associated with conducting federal sponsored programs, taking into account the limitations and restrictions set forth in the OMB Circulars.

Although this chapter will make references to the organized research F&A rate, which is the most common, other F&A rates that may be negotiated include other sponsored programs and instruction.

OMB Circular A-21: Principles for Determining Costs Applicable to Grants, Contracts, and Other Agreements with Educational Institutions

Educational institutions that wish to be reimbursed for administrative and facility costs associated with conducting federally sponsored agreements must periodically prepare an F&A rate proposal using one of two methods set forth in OMB Circular A-21.[1] Educational institutions receiving $10 million or less in total direct work covered by A-21 may use the simplified method that is covered in Section H of the circular. Educational institutions receiving federal awards over $10 million must use the long form method unless agreed to with the federal cognizant agency to use the short form methodology. The two methods are very different and are explained in the following sections.

The Simplified Method

Section H of Circular A-21 addresses the simplified method for preparing an F&A rate proposal at

small educational institutions. Section H applies to those institutions where the direct cost of work covered by the circular does not exceed $10 million in a fiscal year. The institution's annual financial report and immediately available supporting information are used as the basis for calculating the F&A rate.

The simplified method employs the concept of one indirect cost pool (the numerator) and one direct cost base (the denominator). The direct cost distribution base may be direct salaries and wages or modified total direct costs. Modified total direct costs (MTDC), as described in A-21, Section G.2, consist of salaries and wages, associated fringe benefits, materials and supplies, services, travel, and subgrants and subcontracts up to the first $25,000 of each subgrant or subcontract. Costs of equipment and other capital expenditures, patient care costs, tuition remission, rental costs, scholarships and fellowships, as well as the portion of subgrants and subcontracts in excess of $25,000 are excluded from modified total direct costs. The MTDC base is used in the development of F&A rates at all institutions where considered appropriate. The simplified method results in a single institutional-wide rate that is applicable to all sponsored agreements. In some cases, an off-campus rate may also be developed. The cap on administrative costs that is applicable using the long form method is not applicable to the simplified method. However, there are other restrictions associated with both administrative and facility costs that prevent the institution from proposing full costs. These restrictions relate to the calculation of departmental administration, building and equipment depreciation, and operations and maintenance.

Institutions that are not heavily involved with sponsored research or other sponsored programs that reimburse full F&A costs should consider the simplified method. Overall, an F&A rate proposal using the simplified method is relatively inexpensive and easy to prepare, requires little documentation, and can usually be negotiated in a short period of time.

The Long Form

Developing an F&A rate using the long form method is a complicated and time-consuming process.[4] It requires an institution to identify and accumulate certain types of costs into common cost pools and allocate or distribute the costs to benefiting activities using an allocation statistic common to the benefiting activities. There are two major categories to the F&A rate.

The "F" in F&A stands for "facilities," and the costs included in the facilities category include building depreciation, equipment depreciation, interest on debt associated with certain buildings, equipment and capital improvements, operation and maintenance (O&M), and library operations. The "A" in F&A stands for "administration," and the costs included in the administration category include general administration and general expenses (GA), departmental administration (DA), sponsored projects administration (SPA), and student administrative and services (SAS). The changes to Circular A-21 in 1991 placed a cap or limit on the administrative category at 26 points. This administrative cap prohibits an institution from recovering all of the administrative costs associated with the conduct of federally sponsored agreements. The cap on administrative costs has caused a lot of controversy from its original effective date to today. The federal government has placed a lot of additional administrative burdens on colleges and universities that conduct federally sponsored programs, but the cap on administrative costs has not been adjusted or rescinded.

Section F of A-21, "Identification and Assignment of F&A Costs" generally describes the costs that should be included in each of the cost pools as well as describing the preferred allocation or distribution method.

The Facility Cost Pools The facility costs pools have become the most important cost pools in the F&A rate development process since the administrative components were capped at 26 points in October 1991. Institutions wishing to increase the F&A rate must look to the facility components to accomplish this increase. Likewise, the government has taken steps to devote more time and energy reviewing the facility components. The space use study has become one of the most important steps in developing the F&A rate. Building and equipment depreciation, interest, operations, and maintenance are allocated to benefiting functions (activities) primarily on square feet occupied, and these space-related costs can account for as much as 50 percent or more of the total F&A rate.

In order to determine the amount of square feet that activities occupy, it is necessary to perform a space use survey. The space use survey is not an inventory; rather, it identifies how space is used within the institution (i.e., general administrative, facilities, instruction, organized research, other institutional activity, student services, other sponsored programs, etc.). The square feet assigned to each activity are used to allocate the space-related

cost pools mentioned above to the various activities. The government focuses heavily on the space use survey because they know that more space coded as organized research results in more space-related costs being allocated to organized research. Space identified as organized research must be matched with financial accounts that support the activity in that space. The process of matching organized research space with MTDC organized research base accounts is a critical part of the space use survey. If a space survey is not conducted, the A-21 default allocation for space costs is full-time equivalents or salaries and wages of those individuals benefiting from the use of the space.

Each facility cost pool and allocation base is briefly discussed below.

Building Depreciation: A-21 Section F2

Cost pool accumulation. The building depreciation cost pool includes depreciation on buildings and improvements to land and buildings calculated in accordance with Section J.12. An entire building may be depreciated as a single asset and depreciated over its estimated useful life, or the building may be separated into multiple components and each component may be depreciated over different useful lives. A-21 identifies three general components—building shell, building service systems, and fixed equipment. Institutions that depreciate buildings using the component method must use the same method for financial statement purposes and F&A proposal purposes.

Cost pool distribution. Building depreciation is generally allocated to benefit activities based on square feet. The square feet assigned to particular activities such as organized research are subject to scrutiny by the federal negotiators and auditors during the F&A review process. The manner in which space is assigned to functions is called a space use survey discussed earlier in this chapter.

Equipment Depreciation: A-21 Section F2

Cost pool accumulation. The equipment depreciation cost pool includes depreciation on equipment. A-21, Section J.16 defines equipment as "an article of nonexpendable, tangible, personal property having a useful life of more than one year and an acquisition cost which equals or exceeds the lesser of the capitalization level established by the organization for financial statement purposes or $5,000." Equipment may be assigned to an asset class and each asset class may be depreciated using estimated useful lives based on the historical use of the asset class at a particular institution.

Cost pool distribution. Equipment depreciation is allocated to benefiting activities based on square feet. Some institutions use university-wide square feet; others allocate on a department basis, and the most common allocation basis is room-by-room. Allocating equipment depreciation room-by-room is the most beneficial to an institution for increasing their F&A rate because research equipment usually has a higher purchase value than equipment purchased for administrative or instructional activities. However, if room-by-room allocation is used, the institution must assure that an accurate asset management system is in place to track the moving of equipment.

Interest: A-21 Section F3

Cost pool accumulation. Interest incurred on borrowed funds associated with certain buildings, equipment, and capital improvements may be identified and assigned to the buildings, equipment, and land improvements to which the interest relates. There are a number of conditions associated with claiming capital interest and the conditions are discussed in Section J.22.f. This section should be reviewed thoroughly before allocating interest costs to federally sponsored programs.

Cost pool distribution. The interest is further allocated to the major functions of the institution in the same manner as the depreciation on the buildings, equipment, and capital improvements to which the interest relates.

Operation and Maintenance (O&M): A-21 Section F4

Cost pool accumulation. The O&M pool includes costs associated with the operation of the physical plant. Costs generally associated with this activity include utilities, janitorial services, security, environmental safety, hazardous waste disposal, grounds maintenance, plant operations, repairs and ordinary maintenance of buildings, equipment and furniture, property, liability and all other insurance relating to property, facility planning and management, central receiving, and space and capital leasing. This cost pool may also include apportionments from previously allocated cost pools, including building and equipment depreciation and interest.

Cost pool distribution. The standard A-21 allocation base for the O&M cost pool is based on square feet. Costs are initially allocated to buildings and subsequently to the functions within a building based on the square feet each function occupies.

Multiple cost pools. Generally, A-21 refers to one O&M cost pool, but many institutions develop several cost pools (subpools) within O&M to more discretely accumulate and distribute O&M costs. For instance, an institution might establish separate cost pools for each utility and allocate each utility subpool on meter readings; or it might establish a separate cost pool for hazardous waste disposal and allocate the costs using the results of a special analysis that identifies the actual users of the service. It should be noted that the federal government usually spends more time reviewing the multi O&M cost pools versus one O&M cost pool. This is to assure that the costs accumulated in the O&M subpools are being allocated using statistics that most accurately allocate the costs to benefiting functions.

Library: A-21 Section F8

Cost pool accumulation. This cost pool is comprised of library expenses associated with library administration, circulation, cataloging, book and periodical purchases, other materials and supplies, and online access.

Cost pool distribution. Allocating library costs under A-21 is a two-step process. The initial step is to allocate allowable library costs to categories of primary library users using full-time equivalents. A-21 refers to students, professional employees, and other users that normally include outside users. The cost assigned to students is distributed 100 percent to instruction; the cost to other users is assigned to other institutional activities; and the cost to professional employees is further allocated to the major functions of the institution based on salaries of all faculty and professional staff associated with those functions. This standard allocation method does not result in a large portion of library costs being allocated to sponsored research.

Some institutions choose to conduct a library user survey at their specialized libraries to optimize the library costs that are allocated to federally sponsored programs. This study should be performed over a 12-month period, and statistical sampling is usually employed. The study is designed to identify who actually enters the library, who uses its many services and materials, and for what purpose. Library user surveys, if conducted properly, can result in additional costs being allocated to federal sponsored programs.

The Administrative Cost Pools

General Administration and General Expenses (GA): A-21 Section F5

Cost pool accumulation. A-21, Section F.5 defines GA as those expenses "incurred for the general executive and administrative offices of educational institutions and other expenses of a general character which do not relate solely to any major function of the institution...". The activities that are normally included in this cost pool include, but are not necessarily limited to, institutional executive and business management, finance and accounting, payroll, human resources, purchasing, risk management, and general counsel. Unallowable costs and non-allocable costs should be identified and be reclassified or excluded as appropriate. The GA pool can also include, when appropriate, costs allocated to the institution from a central university system administration, board of regents, or chancellor's office. Public institutions may also include costs allocated through a statewide cost allocation plan. The GA pool also includes apportionments from previously allocated cost pools including building and equipment depreciation, interest, and operations and maintenance.

Cost pool distribution. The GA cost pool is allocated to benefiting functions on modified total costs (MTC). This MTC base includes the same cost elements as described in Section G2 under modified total direct costs.

Multiple cost pools. Generally, A-21 refers to one GA cost pool, but many institutions develop more than one cost pool or subpools within GA to more discretely accumulate and distribute the costs. This is similar to the O&M subpooling discussed earlier. The most common GA subpools are university-wide administration and academic administration. University-wide administration would include activities such as the offices of the president, business affairs, and controller, as well as human resources, budgeting, and general accounting. Academic administration could include the provost, vice president for academic affairs, faculty senate, and other academic administrative activities. Each of these sub-pools is then allocated to benefiting functions using statistics that most accurately allocate the costs.

Departmental Administration (DA): A-21, Section F6

Cost pool accumulation. A-21, Section F.6 defines DA as costs "incurred for administrative and supporting services that benefit common or joint departmental activities or objectives...". DA is usu-ally incurred within academic deans' offices, academic departments and divisions, and organized research units. To qualify as DA, the expenses must be administrative in nature, not a direct cost of instruction, research, or other direct function that may be funded through the administrative unit. This happens frequently in deans' offices where discretionary money is used to fund direct instruction and/or research activity. The deans' accounts must be screened for nonadministrative and unallowable costs prior to classifying deans' cost to DA. The DA pool also includes apportionments from previously allocated cost pools including building and equipment depreciation, interest, operations and maintenance, and general administration.

DA is the most difficult cost pool to develop because it is not reconciled to a financial statement function or accounted for as a distinct organizational unit. The cost pool is fabricated through formulas that reclassify costs from other functions, especially instruction.

There are three limitations that affect the amount of DA that can be included in the A-21 F&A rate proposal. The first is the limit on the salaries and fringe benefits for performing administrative work by faculty and other professional personnel conducting research and/or instruction. DA for these positions is limited to 3.6 percent of a department's modified total direct cost. The second is the overall 26-point administrative cap that A-21 places on the administrative components of the F&A rate. The third is called the direct charge equivalent, referred to as the DCE. The DCE is a calculation that results in an adjustment to academic department unrestricted general funds. The DCE helps to compensate for certain types of costs that A-21 says, "should normally be treated as F&A costs," but those which have been charged directly to sponsored agreements. The most common reference is for secretarial and administrative salaries. The DCE calculation helps assure that there is a consistent charging pattern between sponsored agreements and instruction before assigning costs to DA. The calculation and adjustment is made department by department because charging patterns tend to be different among academic departments.

Cost pool distribution. DA is allocated to department functions using a two-step process. The initial step allocates the administrative expenses of a college or school dean's office to the academic departments within that college or school. The allocation is based on each department's modified total costs. The second step allocates administrative expenses of each academic department (as well as the department's share of the dean's office allocation) to department functions. The allocation is based on the modified total costs for the department functions.

Sponsored Projects Administration (SPA): A-21 Section F7

Cost pool accumulation. Costs assigned to this cost pool are usually associated with pre-award and post-award activities including, but not limited to, grant and contract administration, the vice president for research, and the office of research administration. Costs assigned to this cost pool are those that specifically provide a benefit to non-federal and federally sponsored programs.

Cost pool distribution. SPA costs should be allocated to the major functions of the institution based on the MTDC of sponsored programs within each function.

Student Administration and Services (SAS): A-21 Section F9

Cost pool accumulation. This cost pool includes the costs for activities related to the administration of student affairs and services to students. Examples of activities include admissions and records, student health services, placement services, counseling, and the dean of students. This cost pool can also include allocations from previously allocated cost pools such as building and equipment depreciation, interest, operations and maintenance, and general and administrative services.

Cost pool distribution. A-21 states that all student services costs, unless supported through a special study, shall be allocated to the instruction function. Although there are some types of student services costs that could be allocated to sponsored organized research, most institutions no longer try and claim the cost because of the administrative cap.

Rate Development and Application

Once the individual F&A cost pools have been fully allocated to the major functions, one of which is organized research, the sum of those allocated costs are combined into one cost pool. That pool (numerator) of costs represents the individual F&A cost pool allocations that benefit organized research. The base (denominator) will be the modified total direct costs of organized research programs. The costs included in this MTDC organized research base should include all sponsored grants and contracts (federal and nonfederal), institutionally

funded research projects that are separately budgeted and accounted for, and all mandatory and voluntary committed cost shared accounts and dollars that are used to support organized research programs. All funding sources used to support activity in organized research space should be coded to the organized research MTDC base. The resultant F&A rate is applied to all organized research MTDC dollars to recover F&A costs associated with the conduct of organized research.

According to data from the National Science Foundation, for example, the average F&A negotiated rate for the top 100 federally funded educational research and development institutions listed in 2001 was 51.4 percent of MTDC. The average rate for private institutions was 57.5 percent, while the rate for public institutions was 48.7 percent.

OMB Circular A-122: Cost Principles for Nonprofit Organizations

Developing an F&A rate proposal under OMB Circular A-122 is less complicated than A-21 and can be accomplished within a shorter time frame. Generally speaking, this is due to the less complicated organizational structures and diversity of major programs associated with nonprofit organizations rather than with educational institutions.

There are three methods described in A-122, Attachment A:

1. Simplified Allocation Method
2. Multiple Allocation Method
3. Direct Allocation Method

The method used by a nonprofit organization is usually determined by the activities or functions performed by the organization.

The Simplified Method

When an organization has one primary activity, or where multiple activities are performed but benefit from the F&A costs to a similar degree, the Simplified Method may be used. The Simplified Method results in a single rate that is applicable to all sponsored programs at the organization and is the most common method for A-122 nonprofit organizations. The distribution base may be modified total direct costs, similar to A-21, direct salaries and wages, or some other base that equitably distributes the costs. Reclassifications, unallowable costs, and excludable costs as described later in this chapter must be taken into account when developing both the indirect cost pool and the direct cost base.

Attachment B of A-122 should be reviewed prior to preparing the F&A rate.

Nonprofit organizations using the simplified method and receiving more than $10 million in federal direct funding during a fiscal year are required to separate the indirect costs into two broad categories: facilities and administration as defined in A-122. The indirect cost rate is presented as a facilities component and as an administrative component of the total rate. Nonprofit organizations receiving less than $10 million may submit the rate proposal as a single rate.

The Multiple Allocation Method

The Multiple Allocation Method is used for those nonprofit organizations where the indirect costs benefit the major functions in varying degrees. In this situation, the indirect costs must be classified as a "facilities" cost or an "administrative" cost. The costs assigned to the facilities component are the same as those under A-21, with the exception of library costs. They include building and equipment depreciation; interest associated with certain buildings, equipment, and capital improvements to buildings and land; and operations and maintenance costs. The costs that are assigned to the "administration" component are similar to those under A-21 except that library costs are treated as administration under A-122. Each of the costs pools must be allocated to the major functions of the organization using similar allocation statistics that have already been described in this chapter under Circular A-21.

The Direct Allocation Method

This method is used primarily by voluntary health and welfare organizations. The direct allocation method is used where an organization elects to charge every program directly for costs except for supporting services costs. The process allows for general supplies and telephone costs, operations and maintenance-type costs, and depreciation to be prorated to individual programs using an appropriate distribution base. An institution that uses this direct allocation method must assure that every program is treated consistently when prorating the costs. Costs should not be prorated to programs only because they have the budget to pay for them.

Normally there are three categories of costs: general administrative and general expenses (GA), fundraising, and the individual direct programs including those funded by the federal government. The costs prorated to GA become the F&A cost

pool (numerator) for developing the F&A rate. The costs prorated to fundraising and to the individual direct programs become the F&A base costs (denominator) for developing the F&A rate.

This method results in a lower rate than you would normally see for a nonprofit organization. The rate is lower because the costs assigned to the F&A pool are purely GA in nature, and all comparative costs associated with programs have previously been prorated to those programs and are included in the MTDC base.

OMB Circular A-87: Cost Principles for State, Local, and Indian Tribal Governments

State governments must follow a two-step process to recovery all F&A costs associated with conducting federal programs.[3,5] The first step is to develop a Statewide Central Service Cost Allocation Plan (SWCAP). Each state is required to prepare and submit a SWCAP to DHHS-DCA every year. The DCA is responsible for reviewing and negotiating a SWCAP for each of the fifty states. This SWCAP identifies and allocates statewide central service administrative and support costs to every state department and agency. A SWCAP can have three variations, allocating:

1. All statewide costs to its operating departments and agencies through Section I, Exhibit A;
2. Some statewide costs through Section I, Exhibit A; other costs may be charged directly to operating departments and agencies through Section II; or,
3. All statewide costs directly to operating departments and agencies through Section II.

Once the SWCAP is approved, each state department or agency that wishes to be reimbursed for F&A costs must prepare an F&A rate proposal. The proposal identifies the individual department or agency indirect costs as well as costs that are allocated to or directly charged to the department or agency through the SWCAP. OMB Circular A-87, Attachment E identifies two specific methods that government department or agencies may use. The method chosen should be the one that results in the equitable distribution of costs to the direct cost activities of the department or agency.

The same concept is applied to counties and cities, except if the plan is referred to as a Countywide or Citywide Central Service Cost Allocation Plan. Although these central service plans must be prepared annually to make central service costs allowable, only the largest counties and cities are required to submit them for review and negotiation. All others must prepare a central service plan and keep it on hand for possible future audit.

OASC-3—A Guide for Hospitals: Cost Principles and Procedures for Establishing Indirect Costs and Patient Care Rates for Grants and Contracts with the Department of Health, Education, and Welfare

The cost principles for hospitals have not been revised to keep pace with the many changes that have taken place in the other cost principles. In addition, the hospital cost principles are contained in a DHHS publication, not in an OMB circular as the other cost principles. Originally published in 1967, OASC–3 has not been revised since 1974.[6] The publication has recently gone through a major revision, but that revision has not been formally published to date. This badly needed revision includes many changes that will make it more consistent with the other cost principles.

The method used to develop F&A rates for hospitals is based on the Medicare Cost Report (MCR). A separate cost center is established on the MCR for organized research, and costs are stepped down to this research cost center similar to all the other hospital cost centers on the MCR. As with the other cost principles, reclassifications, adjustments and exclusions for unallowable and non-allocable costs, and applicable credits must be made before the administrative and facility costs pools are allocated to the organized research cost center. These reclassifications and adjustments are usually made through the MCR worksheets A-6, Reclassification of Costs, and A-8, Adjustments. The direct cost base can be direct salaries and wages or modified total direct costs, which is similar to that discussed under A-21.

OASC-3, Section VIII also provides for a Simplified Method for Small Institutions. This method may be used to develop an initial F&A rate or when the amount of sponsored programs is minimal. The formula is extremely rigid, however, and does not result in an equitable recovery of costs.

Unallowable Costs, Excludable Costs, and Unallowable Activities in an F&A Rate Proposal

Unallowable costs, excludable costs, and unallowable activities are identified through a process referred to as screening of accounts or scrubbing of object codes. It involves a detailed review of organizational units and object code classifications to identify and code costs that are not allowable.

Unallowable Costs

An unallowable cost is a single cost item (object code) that the federal government identifies as not reimbursable under federal regulations. Therefore, these unallowable costs should not be charged directly to federal programs, nor should they be included in cost pools that will be allocated to federally sponsored programs. Examples of an unallowable cost include alcoholic beverages, entertainment, some forms of advertising, bad debt, commencement and convocation, contributions and donations made to other organizations, and losses on other sponsored agreements. Capital expenditures are unallowable as F&A costs. Unallowable costs are treated differently. Some unallowable costs must be reclassified from an administrative category to a direct cost category so they can be burdened with institutional administrative costs. These costs are usually associated with an unallowable activity such as fundraising and development. This assures that similar costs are treated in like circumstances. However, other unallowable costs are excluded from the rate calculation in total because their inclusion distorts the overall allocation of the F&A costs. The most common excludable costs include equipment and other capital expenditures. (Others are discussed in each of the applicable circulars.)

Excludable Costs

The difference between an excludable cost and an unallowable cost is that an excludable cost is taken out of the F&A rate calculation from both the numerator and the denominator. The cost is not included in the F&A rate calculation. The elimination is made to prevent a distortion in the allocation of administrative costs. The most common excludable costs include equipment and other capital expenditures, costs of goods sold, financial aid costs, patient related costs, and subgrant and subcontract costs over the first $25,000.

Unallowable Activities

There are certain activities an institution performs as part of the normal business environment that the federal government chooses not to reimburse. These unallowable activities usually have multiple cost elements, including salaries and wages and operating expenses. They also occupy institutional space and generate F&A costs. Some examples include public and community relations, fund raising and investment management, and certain types of lobbying. Although these activities are not allowable as F&A costs for federal reimbursement, they do generate F&A costs. Therefore, the federal cost principles require that the costs for these unallowable activities be reclassified from an administrative category to a direct cost category for developing the F&A rate.

The Review and Negotiation Process

Although last in the F&A process, it is by no means the least important. The review and negotiation process is initiated subsequent to submitting an F&A rate proposal to the federal government. The processes are distinctly different. The review process is performed by the government and may involve the grantee being asked to submit additional detailed information not provided in the F&A rate proposal. The grantee should be careful to submit only the information asked for, and not what the grantee thinks the government wants. It is important not to assume requirements, and the grantee must present clear details with the submission. The review may also involve the government visiting the institution to perform on-site work, especially where a space use survey has been performed to support the allocation of facility costs. The information submitted in the original proposal, the additional detail subsequently submitted based on the governments' request, and the information gathered during an on-site visit is analyzed by the government and used to develop their positions on costing issues and allocation methodologies.

The review process can vary with Department of Health and Human Services (DHHS), Divisions of Cost Allocation (DCA) from region to region, and negotiator by negotiator. It also varies between the DHHS and the Department of Defense (DoD), Office of Naval Research (ONR). DHHS-DCA negotiators usually conduct individual F&A proposal reviews prior to negotiations, and rarely has a rate proposal been audited by the DHHS, Office of the Inspector General. However, it is quite common for ONR to have the Defense Contract Audit Agency (DCAA) audit F&A rate proposals prior to ONR entering into negotiations.

The negotiation of the F&A rate is subsequent to the review and/or audit of the F&A rate proposal. Once the government formulates their position, they are ready to enter into negotiations. The

F&A rate negotiation is a process of settling on a rate (number) that is usually, but not always, lower than the proposed rate. Negotiations may be conducted over the telephone, conducted on-site at a particular institution, or on federal premises. They can be formal or informal in nature and can include one person from each side or a team of people.

Types of Rates

There are three types of F&A rates negotiated depending on the type of institution, the experience the government has with a particular institution, and the cognizant federal agency. The three rates are *predetermined, fixed with carry-forward*, and *provisional/final*.

Predetermined Rate

These are typically established for a two- to four-year period and do not change during the period for which they are established. Predetermined rates are beneficial to both the government and the grantees in that they facilitate budget preparation and permit more expeditious closeouts of grants and contracts. The predetermined rate also allows an institution to submit an F&A proposal every two to three years rather than annually.

Educational institutions are the predominant users of predetermined rates under Public Law 87-638 (76 Stat. 437). Predetermined F&A rates are generally not used for nonprofit organizations, hospitals, or state or local government agencies.

Fixed Rate with Carry-Forward

These are used primarily with state and local governments with some educational institutions under the Office of Naval Research. The fixed rate is not used much anymore; most rates are either predetermined or provisional/final. The fixed rate with carry-forward allows an institution to use a specific rate that does not change during the fiscal year for which the rate has been established. Any difference between the fixed rate and the actual rate in a particular year is carried forward to the next open year. One disadvantage is that the fixed rate requires annual submission of direct cost rate proposals. An advantage of fixed rate is that it allows an institution to either recover or pay back any under- or over-recoveries of F&A costs through the F&A rate process. Fixed rates are most commonly used today with fringe benefit rates where an institution uses a fringe benefit rate for both budgeting and charging to federal programs.

Provisional/Final Rate

These permit an institution to claim F&A cost reimbursement. The provisional rate is subject to adjustment at any time during the year, but normally is adjusted to a finalized rate based on an indirect cost rate proposal for each fiscal year end. Most non-profit organizations are on a provisional/final rate.

Within each of these three types of rates, an institution can negotiate on-site (on-campus) rates or off-site (off-campus) rates. The on-site rates include administrative and facility costs, while the off-site rates contain only administrative costs. When off-site rates are used, it is quite common to charge facility and other space-related costs directly to federal programs.

Code of Federal Regulations, Title 2, Government-wide Guidance for Grants and Agreements

In June 2003, OMB issued a notice of proposed rulemaking that relocates policy guidelines for grants and other agreements to make it easier for applicants and recipients to use. OMB also proposed to publish guidance to federal agencies for grants and agreements located in seven separate OMB Circulars and other policy documents in a single title in the Code of Federal Regulations (CFR). The new title would be 2 CFR Grants and Agreements.

OMB has begun to incorporate the OMB Circulars in 2 CFR. The first was OMB Circulars A-110 "Part 215-Uniform Administrative Requirements for Grants and Agreements with Institutions of Higher Education, Hospitals and Other Non-Profit Organizations" (OMB Circular A-110).[7] In addition, information about 2 CFR, a discussion of guidance for government-wide debarment and OMB Circulars A-21, A-87, and A-122 that address the costs that may be charged to federal awards for educational institutions, state and local and Indian tribal governments, and non-profit organizations, respectively, was published in the Federal Register on August 31, 2005.[8-12]

In the future 2 CRF is supposed to also include:

- OMB Circular A-102, which contains the administrative requirements for grants and cooperative agreements with state and local governments,[13]
- OMB Circular A-133, which contains the audit requirements for state and local governments and non-profit organizations,[14] and

- OMB Circular A-89, which contains the federal domestic assistance program information.[15]

• • • References

1. Office of Management and Budget. "Circular A-21, Cost Principles for Educational Institutions," revised May 10, 2004, http://www.whitehouse.gov/omb/circulars/a021/a21_2004.html (accessed August 17, 2005).
2. Office of Management and Budget. "Circular A-122, Cost Principles for Non-Profit Organizations," revised May 10, 2004, http://www.whitehouse.gov/omb/circulars/a122/a122_2004.html (accessed August 17, 2005).
3. Office of Management and Budget. "Circular A-87, Cost Principles for State, Local and Indian Tribal Governments," revised May 10, 2004, http://www.whitehouse.gov/omb/circulars/a087/a87_2004.html (accessed August 10, 2005).
4. US Department of Health and Human Services, Program Support Center, Division of Cost Allocation. "Review Guide for Long-Form University Facilities and Administrative Cost Proposals," June 2001, http://rates.psc.gov/lfrevugd1.pdf (accessed August 31, 2005).
5. Department of Health and Human Services. "ASMB C-10: DHHS Implementation Guide for OMB Circular A-87," April 1997, http://www.os.dhhs.gov/grantsnet/state/asmbc10.pdf (accessed August 31, 2005).
6. Department of Health and Human Services, Office of the Assistant Secretary Comptroller. "OASC-3, Revised: A Guide for Hospitals," 1974.
7. 2 CFR Grants and Agreements, http://www.access.gpo.gov/nara/cfr/waisidx_05/2cfrv1_05.html (accessed September 5, 2005).
8. Grants Policy Streamlining Overview and Guidance on Nonprocurement Debarment and Suspension and Cost Principles Guidance; Cost Principles for Educational Institutions (OMB Circular A-21), State, Local, and Indian Tribal Governments (OMB Circular A-87) and Non-Profit Organizations (OMB Circular A-122); Final Rules. *Federal Register* 70, no. 168 (2005):51861–51863, http://a257.g.akamaitech.net/7/257/2422/01jan20051800/edocket.access.gpo.gov/2005/05-16646.htm (accessed September 5, 2005).
9. Guidance for Government-wide Debarment and Suspension (Nonprocurement). *Federal Register* 70, no. 168 (2005):51863–51880, http://a257.g.akamaitech.net/7/257/2422/01jan20051800/edocket.access.gpo.gov/2005/05-16647.htm (accessed September 12, 2005).

10. Principles for Educational Institutions (OMB Circular A-21). *Federal Register* 70, no. 168 (2005):51880-51909, http://a257.g.akamaitech. net/7/257/2422/01jan20051800/edocket.access. gpo.gov/2005/05-16648.htm (accessed September 12, 2005).

11. Cost Principles for State, Local, and Indian Tribal Governments (OMB Circular A-87). *Federal Register* 70, no. 168 (2005): 51910–51927, http://a257.g.akamaitech.net/7/257/2422/01jan 20051800/edocket.access.gpo.gov/2005/05-16649.htm (accessed September 12, 2005).

12. Cost Principles for Non-Profit Organizations (OMB Circular A-122). *Federal Register* 70, no. 168 (2005):51927–51943, http://a257.g. akamaitech.net/7/257/2422/01jan20051800/ edocket.access.gpo.gov/2005/05-16650.htm (accessed September 12, 2005).

13. OMB Circular A-102, Grants and Cooperative Agreements with State and Local Governments, 1994, revised August 29 1997, http://www. whitehouse.gov/omb/circulars/a102/a102.html (accessed September 5, 2005).

14. OMB Circular A-133, Audits of States, Local Governments, and Non-Profit Organizations June 24, 1997, includes revisions published in *Federal Register*, June 27, 2003, http://www. whitehouse.gov/omb/circulars/a133/a133.html (accessed September 5, 2005).

15. OMB Circular A-89, Catalog of Federal Domestic Assistance, revised August 17, 1984, http://www.whitehouse.gov/omb/circulars/a08 9/a089.html (accessed September 5, 2005).

38

Compliance Toward the Disclosure Statement (DS) Required by Public Law 100-679

Amy J. Sikalis, MPA

Introduction

As stated in 48 CFR 9903, a Disclosure Statement (DS) is required for institutions who are selected to receive a Cost Accounting Standards (CAS) (specified in part 9905) covered contract or subcontract of $25 million (or more), or which are reporting $25 million (or more) in the most recent cost accounting period. The DS is a written description of a contractor's cost accounting practices and procedures. The requirement for this disclosure from Public Law 100-679 (41 USC 422) is the establishment of the Cost Accounting Standards Board within the Office of Federal Procurement Policy. Further, it is the recommendation of the Council on Governmental Relations (COGR) that institutions establish policies and practices to ensure compliance with mandated CAS (501, 502, 504, & 505) via:

- The DS filed with the institution's cognizant audit agency; and,
- Training (adequate and appropriate) to ensure affected units are adhering to the DS.

Establishment of Cost Accounting Standards Board

Because of perceptions that defense contractors had been manipulating costs of contracts, Congress enacted Public Law 91-379 (1970). Re-enacted as Public Law 100-679 in 1988, the establishment of

the Cost Accounting Standards Board came about as the result of defense pricing scandals of the 1980s. The impetus for Public Law 100-679 was, in part, to control fraud, waste, and abuse of federal contracts. The Bill S.2214, also known as the Office of Federal Procurement Policy Act Amendments of 1988, was introduced March 24, 1988 by Senator Chiles and revised October 19, 1988. In the October revision, the Senate agreed to a House amendment, with an additional amendment, and the act became Public Law: 100-679 on November 17, 1988. Major components of the bill include establishment of:

- The Federal Acquisition Regulatory Council, which provides permanent authorization of appropriations for the Office of Federal Procurement Policy,
- An independent board known as the Cost Accounting Standards Board within the Office of Federal Procurement Policy,
- Civil and criminal penalties for violations of this act,
- Requirement that the head of each federal agency establish procurement ethics programs,
- Amendment to the Federal Property and Administrative Services Act to expand the definition of architectural and engineering services, and
- The position of Advocate for the Acquisition of Commercial Products in the Office of Federal Procurement Policy.

As part of Public Law 100-679, codified at 41 USC 422 (1988), the establishment of the Cost

Accounting Standards Board, Section (f) of 41 USC 422 provides executive authority to:

(1) Make, promulgate, amend, and rescind cost accounting standards and interpretations thereof designed to achieve uniformity and consistency in the accounting standards governing measurement, assignment, and allocation of costs to contracts in the United States, (2) cost accounting standards mandatory by all executive agencies and by contractors and subcontractors in estimating, accumulating, and reporting costs in connection with pricing and administration of, and settlement of disputes concerning all negotiated prime contracts and subcontract procurements with the United States over $500,000.

Proposed Cost Accounting Standards (CAS) rules and regulations for contracts were published in the Federal Register, 59 FR 55756 (November 8, 1994) with the final regulation found in the Code of Federal Regulations (CFR), 48 CFR 9903. For grants, the proposed rule reference published in the Federal Register is 59 FR 43760 (August 25, 1994) and the final rule is found in 45 CFR 74.

Code of Federal Regulations (CRFs)

What do the CFRs say? According to Section 9903.302 of the CFR, cost accounting practice, they are:

Any disclosed or estimated method or technique used for allocation of cost to cost object, assign of cost to cost object, assign of cost to cost accounting periods or measurement of cost.

Section 9903.303, Effect of Filing, states:

(a) Disclosure of a cost accounting practice does not determine allowability of particular items of cost; (b) Disclosure Statements may be used in audits of contracts (or grants) or in negotiation of price leading to award.

Section 9903.202, disclosure requirements, states:

Any institution selected to receive a CAS covered contract or subcontract of $25 million or more shall submit before award.

After January 1, 1996, any business unit of an educational institution that has been selected to

receive contracts or subcontracts greater than $500,000 and is part of a college or university located in Exhibit A of Office of Management and Budget (OMB) Circular A-21 is required to file a Disclosure Statement (DS). Disclosure is not required if the institution can demonstrate that federal awards in the preceding accounting period were less than $25 million. Disclosure must be on form no. CASB DS-1 or CASB DS-2, as applicable. (These are forms obtained from a federal agency or cognizant federal audit agency.) Prime recipients are responsible for disclosure requirements of all affected subrecipients. OMB A-21 regulation also contains the disclosure requirement in Section (c)(14) Disclosure statement:

(a) Educational institutions that received aggregate sponsored agreements totaling $25 million or more subject to this Circular during their most recent completed fiscal year shall disclose their cost accounting practices by filing a Disclosure Statement (DS-2), reproduced in Appendix B.

Compliance with Regulations

When receiving contracts or grants with federal agencies, an institution must be compliant with applicable regulations and CAS and related OMB circulars. Section J of OMB A-21 provides: "General provisions of selected items of cost" lists, by name, allowable direct cost, and indirect (facilities and administrative) (F&A) cost. Applicable CAS regulations are: Sections 99005.501 (consistency in estimating, accumulating, and reporting costs), 99005.502 (consistency in allocating costs incurred for the same purpose), 9905.505 (accounting for unallowable costs), and 9905.506 (accounting period). To ensure compliance, institutions must be familiar with all federal cost principles and regulations, their related disclosure statement (with amendments), provide adequate review of proposal budgets (prior to submission), and appropriate post-award administration of grants and contracts received (including appropriate subrecipient monitoring).

The Public Health Service (PHS) Guide contains the following statement:

The fact that a cost requested in a budget is awarded, as requested, does not ensure a determination of allowability.... The organization is responsible for presenting costs consistently and must not include costs associated with their Facilities and Administrative (F & A) rate as direct costs.

This statement underscores that the recipient institution is primarily responsible to ensure allowability of all costs proposed. If subject to a DS, the institution can find its determination of direct, indirect, and unallowable costs (for grants and contracts) in its filed DS.

Institutional Disclosure Statement

In general, the DS is broken down into parts. Part I is a statement of general information regarding each reporting unit. Parts II through VI define the types of costs generally incurred by the segment of each reporting unit directly performing under federally sponsored agreements (contracts and grants). Part VII details types of costs that are generally incurred by a central or group office and are allocated to one or more segments performing under federally sponsored agreements. Part VII also describes costs related to sponsored research and how those costs (direct and indirect) are treated and allocated:

It is expected that the disclosed cost accounting practices (48 CFR 9903.302-1) for classifying costs either as direct or indirect costs will be consistently applied to all costs incurred by the reporting unit...For all major categories of cost under each major function or activity such, as instruction, organized research, other sponsored activities and other institutional activities, described on a continuation sheet, your criteria for determining when costs incurred for the same purpose, in like circumstances, are treated either as direct costs only or as indirect costs only with respect to final cost objectives.

Examples of these costs are those for personnel (including fringe benefits), material, and supplies. Institutions must carefully consider all activities and appropriately disclose and justify where indirect costs may be charged as direct costs within their institutions. If not disclosed appropriately, such costs could be deemed unallowable under audit, which could create penalties and grounds for further audit investigation. Finally, by appendix to the DS, institutions should provide institutional guidelines and/or established institutional policies for special items of cost or circumstances (e.g., policies and guidelines for effort reporting, cost sharing, foundation funding, and recharge center activities).

Costs associated with these activities and others, as may be applicable, could be unique in circumstance and application; therefore, disclosure is necessary to ensure allowability of costs applied (both direct and indirect).

Prior Approvals

All proposals should require institutional approval prior to proposal submission. It is important to insist on detailed budget and budget justifications as part of the approval process and to identify costs requiring additional justification per the content of a DS. If a budget is not required as part of the application, budget for "internal purposes" should be required prior to proposal submission. If proposals contain costs for subrecipients or third parties, those budgets and costs must be approved by administration (provided in writing to the prime institution) prior to submission. If a subrecipient, a detailed budget must be prepared, appropriate backup justification be provided, along with documentation (with a written approval to the prime institution making the application), even if it is not requested. At post-award, a detailed budget review must be provided with approval for all continuation funding and changes in scope of work. Levels of spending must also be closely monitored; principal investigators and departmental administrators should be trained and encouraged to review financial reports on a monthly basis and to make corrections in a timely manner for costs charged in error. Appropriate subaward agreements should be generated that reference mandatory cost principles to all subrecipients. Agreements should detail required cost documentation, the routing of invoices, technical reports, and proof of audit for the prime institution. Corrective action of misallocations and appropriate notification where notification may be required (by and to prime agencies) must be promptly managed. It is important that effective award closeout (technical and financial) of all sponsored activity be encouraged and facilitated by all responsible parties.

For institutions subject to CAS regulations, implementation of training and education is critical in order to ensure compliance. Institutions should create curriculums for all levels of administration, including principal investigators and departmental administrators. While financial officers are expected to know the cost accounting regulations, vice presidents, deans, chairs, and financial and nonfinancial sponsored project administrators also need training about the content and application of regulations and the content of the DS. Resources for information should be readily accessible to all. The DS should contain the following certification:

> I certify that to the best of my knowledge and belief this Statement, as amended in the case of a Revision, is the complete and accurate disclosure as of the date of certification shown below by the above-named organization of its cost accounting practices, as required by the Disclosure Regulations (48 CFR 9903.202) of the Cost Accounting Standards Board under 41.U.S.C. § 422.

Below the signature line should note:

> The penalty for making a false statement in this disclosure is prescribed in 18 U.S.C. § 1001.

Compliance toward cost accounting practices and policies disclosed is critical to institutions.

In June 2004, Health and Human Services (HHS) announced plans to resume audits of CAS Disclosure Statements (DS-2s). These audits are to be conducted by the Defense Contract Audit Agency (DCA) under contract with HHS. Letters to 80 to 90 institutions under the cognizance of HHS and which had not had prior DS audit, "ask institutions to tell DCA whether their DS-2s on file with HHS are up-to-date (i.e., whether they accurately reflect the institution's current cost accounting practices)." Due to these changes in auditing practice and regulations, it is ever more important that institutions review their DS to determine whether any changes are needed.

Summary

In summary, the impact of PL 100-679 to institutions is that they must assure consistency in:

- Estimating, accumulating, and reporting costs (CAS 501).
- Allocating costs incurred for the same purpose (CAS 502).

The required CAS Disclosure Statement is a detailed and comprehensive documentation of all cost accounting practices and policies from institutions subject to CAS. For institutions engaged in federal funding, this document should be considered the "Bible" or the "rulebook" for any auditor investigating cases of fraud, waste, or abuse. The CAS DS is a certified statement; there are real penalties for noncompliance. However, changes to disclosed cost accounting practices require a "cost impact study." These studies are very involved and difficult for institutions to complete because there is scarce or no guidance on conducting such studies.

• • • **References**

Public Law:
Office of Federal Procurement Policy Act Amendments of 1988, Pub. L. no. 100-679, Nov. 17, 1988, 100th Congress, 1402 Stat 4055.

United State Code:
41 U.S.C. Sec. 422 (1988).

Federal Register:
Cost Accounting Standards (CAS) Final Rule, 59 FR 55756, November 8, 1994 (to be codified at 48 CFR 9903 for contracts).

Cost Accounting Standards (CAS) Final Rule, 59 FR 43760, August 25, 1994 (to be codified at 45 CFR 74 for grants).

Code of Federal Regulations:
CAS Rules and Regulations, 48 CFR 99.

CAS Rules and Regulations, 45 CFR 74.

Agency Regulations:
Office of Management and Budget Circular A-21 Cost Principles for Educational Institutions, revised May 10, 2004, http://www.whitehouse.gov/omb/circulars/a021/a21_2004.html (accessed August 28, 2005).

NIH Grants Policy Statement Part II: Terms and Conditions of NIH Grant Awards, revised December 2003, http://grants.nih.gov/grants/policy/nihgps_2003/index.htm (accessed August 28, 2005).

CHAPTER

39

Financial Reporting for the Research Administrator

Cary E. Thomas, MBA, CMA

Of all the responsibilities to be met by the research administrator, the development, production, and reporting of financial information is at the top of the list. This chapter:

- Describes the foundations necessary for a quality financial reporting system;
- Classifies financial reports for the various target audiences;
- Discusses special considerations for handling cost-sharing budgets and expenditures;
- For those research administrators responsible for the control and management of F&A ("indirect") costs, Section 4 provides some special considerations for this complex working environment; and,
- Includes appendices showing the details of financial reporting requirements for selected granting agencies.

Foundations of a Quality Financial Reporting System

A quality financial reporting system is one that delivers timely, accurate, relevant, and useful information. It is unlikely that the research administrator can develop such a system alone; instead, the savvy research administrator will seek out the people, systems, and tools to provide the foundation for his or her reporting system.

People

The research administrator, in all but the smallest nonprofit organizations, is able to rely on a finan-

cial management officer or senior financial executive for support, advice, and direction. Every research enterprise benefits when there is a mutual, informed, regular, and cooperative relationship between the research administrator and the financial professional(s) of the organization. Each party brings expertise to the partnership, and the conduct of research is more orderly and compliant when the parties are mutually supportive. One of the best ways to exhibit such mutual support is in the design and preparation of financial reports.

The savvy research administrator establishes good working relationships with accounting and financial professionals and learns as much as possible about the financial accounting system on which they all rely. Table 39-1 highlights topics of mutual interest and the interaction between the research administrator and the financial professional.

Systems

The research administrator in most organizations can rely on the assurance that the organization's financial management system meets at least the minimal requirements of Federal Circular A-133 for auditability and Circular A-110 for record keeping. Financial systems can be complex, arcane—or both. Compounding these problems, most financial accounting systems at organizations for which the mission includes teaching and public service in addition to research, tend to support fund accounting needs to the detriment of research needs. A quality financial reporting system can be created only when the research administrator understands fully how the financial system works, when and how financial

TABLE 39-1	Interaction between the Research Administrator and the Financial Professional	
Topic	**Role of the Financial Professional**	**Role of the Research Administrator**
Understanding expense classifications	Provides a clear set of object (or expense) codes. Informs the research administrator as codes are added or changed.	Understands the coding structure and how the various cost categories are to be represented in financial reports.
Differentiating between those costs subject to F&A and those exempt from F&A	Provides clear guidance on how to handle transactions involving equipment, large subcontracts, facilities costs, patient care, etc.	Understands the special treatment accorded equipment, large subcontracts, facilities costs, patient care, etc.
Differentiating between those costs which are recurring and those that are one-time or nonrecurring	Provides guidance to departments on specialized transactions (e.g., tuition charges, vacation accrual, severance payments, retroactive cost allocations, etc.).	Has an acute awareness of when one-time transactions are likely to be posted to accounts; plans for and reserves funds to cover one-time transactions.
Clarity in how transactions are handled during the fiscal year-end closing process.	Provides a closing schedule with orderly procedures on specifying which costs are *old year* versus *new year*.	Monitors expenditures carefully at fiscal year-end, assures an orderly close-out of purchase orders, codes transactions for proper accrual.

TABLE 39-2	Elements of the Financial System	
Topic	**Information Systems Professional**	**Research Administrator**
Understanding the monthly processing cycle	Provides a clear guidance to users regarding which transactions are updated *real-time* versus *batch* versus *periodically*.	Understands the accounting cycle, when transactions are updated, and the overall timeliness of data.
On-Line access	Provides easy-to-use tools for on-line access to financial data.	Is an adept user of online system access protocols.
Generating reports	Creates standard reports that are useful to users of financial systems, including documentation describing the contents of report fields.	Can generate reports as needed.
Downloading accounting data	Provides tools that support the extraction of user's data and the transmittal to user's personal computers.	Is skilled at using tools to extract data in a format that is suitable for manipulation with personal computer tools.

records are updated and archived, and where and how data are stored in the system.

Table 39-2 provides guidance on elements of the financial system that the research administrator must fully understand. If the financial professionals in the organization cannot provide clear guidance on these elements, then the research administrator should turn to financial systems professionals for support.

Tools

The ideal situation for the research administrator is that the financial accounting system automatically produces every report needed on demand. The reality is, however, that this ideal system seldom exists. Many systems, however, do have standard reporting tools that can automatically generate common standard monthly reports produced for each research agreement that list budget, to-date expenditures, and remaining balance.

Standard Reports

The financial system on which the grant accounting relies will have a series of standard reports. The savvy research administrator meets with the people who are knowledgeable about the standard reports, understands how many reports there are and the content and timing of each, and also learns how to produce these reports.

Report Writers and Specialized Report Generators

Since many financial systems are designed for purposes other than grant accounting, frequently the standard reports are not fully useful to the research administrator. This problem can be overcome by using a report writer or report generator to produce financial data in a format that is more useful than the standard reports. For the research administrator to gain access to such tools, it is necessary to secure authority to access the data and attend training classes on the proper methods to use with such programs.

Data Extraction or Downloading

While report writers and generators are of great value, but for the computationally adept research administrator, it is best to extract financial data using tools such as Microsoft Excel or Microsoft Access to sort, arrange, and summarize data into useful information. The protocol for extracting data varies from one institution to another, but the basic goals are essentially the same: to obtain permission to access the data, learn to use the data extraction tool, learn to load the extracted data (into either Microsoft Access or Microsoft Excel), and become skilled at manipulating the data to best use. The author encourages research administrators to take training courses in Microsoft Excel, particularly in the use of "pivot tables," or to learn to use the database tool, Microsoft Access, for more complex data manipulations.

The Right Financial Reports for the Right Audience

A variety of audiences look to the research administrator for quality financial reports. The target audiences include the sponsor of the research; the principal investigator ("PI") responsible for the orderly conduct of a specific research agreement; laboratory heads, department chairs, deans, or center managers responsible for a collection of research projects; institutional officials responsible for overall research management; internal and external auditors; and, in some cases, the CEOs and Boards of Directors or Boards of Trustees. Obviously,

financial reports that are relevant and useful to one audience can be of limited or no use to others.

Sponsor Reporting

Many sponsors of research prescribe the format and timing of reports on the expenditure of sponsor funds. Some examples are covered below, supplemented by the appendices at the end of this chapter.

- The National Institutes of Health (NIH) require grant recipients to submit financial status reports (FSR) on prescribed forms. The most common form is the FS-269 (used when a grant has program income) or the FS-269A (used when there is no program income). The timing of reports varies but is specified on the Notice of Grant Award. Electronic submission of FSRs is becoming more common, thus research administrators should check with the NIH policy manual for guidance. The grantee is required to assure that the information on the FSR is "...accurate, complete, and consistent with the grantee's accounting system."
- For domestic NIH grants issued under the Streamlined Non-competing Award Process ("SNAP"), NIH requires the quarterly Federal Cash Transactions Report ("FCTR") to be utilizing standard form SF 272 (in lieu of the annual FSR) and to be submitted to Payment Management System (PMS) to monitor the financial aspects of grants.
- The National Science Foundation (NSF) utilizes a computer system called "Fastlane" for the electronic administration of grants. NSF also employs the FCTR system for quarterly reporting of financial transactions (refer to the NSF Grants Policy Manual for details).
- The Department of Defense (DoD) submission process has not been standardized, but most offices within DoD accept electronic proposals. The DoD uses Standard Form (SF) 272, Federal Cash Transactions Report (www.usamraa.army.mil) for financial reporting.

Principal Investigator Reporting

Financial reports provided to the PI should focus on the conduct of the science: these describe the total financial resources available to the sponsored agreement, how those resources have been expended, the balance of resources available, and the period over which these resources can be applied. Providing these basic elements within a financial report is easily within the grasp of any well-managed institution. The typical tool used to provide PI reporting is a monthly summary of each award showing:

- The expense categories for each category.

- The amount of money budgeted.
- The amount of money expended in the most recent month.
- Cumulative expenditures.
- Encumbered funds (e.g., known salary commitments).
- Purchase orders issued but not yet paid.
- The resulting remaining budget balance.

Supplementing this summary information with reports of detailed transactions is essential if the PI is to review expenditures for accuracy and reasonableness.

Some research administrators develop specialized tools to enhance the standard monthly report to the PI to include:

- Forecasts of the expenditures expected through the end of the award.
- An estimation as to whether the funds remaining are sufficient to see the conduct of the science to the award end date (or if there will be a short-fall in funding).
- The identification of significant budget variances.

The financial status of each award must be considered separately. It is very common for a scientist to have multiple awards, however, and for there to be some similarity in the statement of work among the awards. In these cases, it is reasonable for the research administrator to prepare financial reports that provide an overall picture of all of the funding resources for a PI.

Laboratory/Department/School/Center Reporting The well-managed research institution will have financial reports that use the basic award-centered financial reporting described above, but aggregated into reports showing the financial state of groups of PIs. Such reports could represent a laboratory of PIs engaged in similar research areas, a department of faculty members, or a school within a large institution or organized research center. In any of these aggregated cases, the financial status of a collection of awards alone does not represent interesting or informative data. These reports are much more useful when they are compared to similar reports of prior years or periods and answer critical questions:

- Is our research volume increasing or decreasing? Is our funding profile more or less diversified than in prior years?
- Are our new faculty recruits ramping up in research funding as expected?

- What projections can be made about future funding based on grant application trends at current and projected funding levels?
- Assuming a consistent level of cost sharing, are there funds sufficient to meet cost-sharing obligations?

Institutional Reporting While research administrators in academic departments need reports that are project specific, administrators in central offices typically produce and use reports that provide broad measures of research activity and productivity. However, there are important issues for centralized research administrators to consider as they develop these reports, such as annual reports of awards and expenditures. The financial statements should support decision making on these issues. Examples of questions to consider are:

- Is the research funding profile of the institution increasing in volume or declining?
- Is the success rate of grant applications changing, and in what ways?
- What is the relationship between federal and nonfederal awards, and is the funding pattern changing?
- Are institutional investments in new areas of science or recruiting programs yielding the number and volume of research awards that were expected?
- What is the current and projected recovery of facilities and administration costs, and are cost recoveries sufficient to meet actual expenses?
- Are institutional cost-sharing obligations being met in an orderly way?
- Are new funding sources being identified and secured, or is diversification of funding an issue of concern?

Questions such as these can never be answered from standardized reports, and custom reports will be necessary to address such issues.

Special Considerations for Reporting Cost Sharing

This section describes some of the best practices for cost sharing and associated "matching funds" in financial reporting systems. (Cost sharing and the importance of budgeting and accounting for these costs are discussed elsewhere in this book.)

When a sponsored agreement is awarded and a condition of the award requires that the recipient institution provide for some of the direct or indirect costs of the award, a cost-sharing obligation has been created (e.g., when an agency makes an award to the institution for $100,000 under the condition that the institution provide an additional $50,000 for a total award of $150,000).

The research administrator responsible for receiving, accepting, and implementing the award should take the responsibility of clarifying the obligation in budget terms. The amount of cost sharing should be specified as to the amount for each fiscal year for the full award period and indicating any special cost categories for the obligation. Special care should be exercised to differentiate between direct cost versus indirect costs, and special cost categories (equipment or large subcontracts) should be clearly identified.

The most common way to document the magnitude and timing of the cost-sharing obligation in financial records is to establish a "companion account," an account number with an appropriate set of cost subaccount categories, created explicitly for the cost-sharing portion of the total award. If, for example, it is assumed that a $150,000 award was for a two-year period, then the award account budget and the cost-sharing budget should be reflected (e.g., a dollar-for-dollar matching or cost-sharing requirement for equipment purchases, and a $10,000 salary matching requirement). Assuming that budgeted funds are spent equally in the two years, the budget may look like the one in Table 39-3.

One of the important postaward obligations of the research administrator is to monitor both the award and companion accounts throughout the conduct of the award to ensure that the cost-sharing obligations are met as incurred. As a best practice, the research administrator must ensure that the reporting system for any awards that have a cost-sharing obligation meets budget expectations and clearly measures expenditures against that obligation.

A significant issue surrounding cost sharing is the impact that it has on the calculation of F&A rates and F&A recovery. In an especially notorious case, for a number of years a major research institution failed to classify its cost-sharing expenses as part of its research base. This resulted in an F&A rate that was significantly higher than it would have been if the cost-sharing expenses had been properly reported. Once this error was reported, the institution agreed that it had recovered funds from federal agencies in excess of its allowable recovery. Subsequently, a multimillion dollar settlement was reached. As another example of best practice, the postaward research administrator must ensure that the companion account is classified in the institution's accounting records in a manner that assures that these research expenditures are properly classified as part of the institution's research base.

Complexities Associated with Control and Management of Facilities and Administration Costs

Most research administrators work in an environment where the scientists are responsible for the direct cost portions of the financial conduct of the science. In other words, most scientists and their research administrators are insulated from the F&A costs associated with sponsored agreements. By contrast, there are some research administrators who have budget and fiscal control responsibilities for both the direct costs and the F&A costs—a complex issue.

There are essentially two things that can go wrong with financial management of F&A costs: expenditure of direct costs can lag budget expectations or expenditure of F&A costs can be in excess of F&A recovery income.

TABLE 39-3	Cost Sharing Budgeted over a Two-Year Period					
	Award from Agency (Award Account)			**Cost-Sharing Obligation (Companion Account)**		
	Year 1	Year 2	Total	Year 1	Year 2	Total
Salaries	25,000	25,000	50,000	5,000	5,000	10,000
Supplies	5,000	5,000	10,000			
Equipment	20,000	20,000	40,000	20,000	20,000	40,000
Total	$50,000	$50,000	$100,000	$25,000	$25,000	$50,000

Expenditure of Direct Costs Lag Budget Expectations

F&A rates are awarded to institutions based on a review by the cognizant audit agency and a calculation of the expected research direct expenditures (the "base") and the anticipated cost of facilities and administrative expenses ("F&A"). The F&A rate, then, is a "budgeted" rate, and as every research administrator knows, sometimes budgets go sour.

Suppose that in determining the F&A rate for the new fiscal year, the institution had planned that the research base was going to grow by 10%. What happens if this planned growth fails to materialize?

As Table 39-4 demonstrates, if the actual research base lags the budget figure, in this case by $5 million, the F&A recovery will be less than the budgeted expenditures. For the research administrator responsible for solving such issues, the choices for budget control are grim: reduce F&A costs (which can be quite difficult as these costs tend to be semifixed), rebudget funds from direct to F&A (which will anger the faculty), or cover the deficit from other funds (no easy trick).

To avoid these situations, the research administrator should take care to set the research base amount in rate negotiations to a level that can be confidently achieved.

F&A Costs Exceed F&A Recovery

The next issue for the research administrator to consider is the monitoring of the actual level of facilities and administrative costs and to contrast these to the recovery of F&A income to pay for them.

Typically, facilities costs are fixed or semifixed and are not easily controlled in the short run (e.g., the costs of buildings and/or leases are commitments made over many years). Similarly, the consumption of utilities, communication infrastructures, and other scientific support costs are fixed in nature. To a lesser extent, but nearly as fixed, are the administrative costs of running a fully compliant research organization. Therefore, moderating or adjusting these F&A costs quickly is normally an unattainable goal.

Table 39-5 below demonstrates a comparison of budgeted F&A costs to actual cost of operations.

Even if F&A income is greater than the amount budgeted (as listed in Table 39-5), increases in F&A costs can create a budget crisis. The research administrator must monitor both F&A recovery income and F&A costs closely, track monthly income and expenses, and consistently update fiscal

TABLE 39-4	Impact of Budget Variations of F&A Recovery	
Item	**Budget**	**Actual**
Research Expenditures, Prior Year	$100,000,000	$95,000,000
Anticipated Growth in Research Base @ 10%	$10,000,000	$5,000,000
Total Research Expenditures (or "Base")	$110,000,000	$100,000,000
Facilities and Administrative Costs	$55,000,000	$55,000,000
F&A Rate	50%	50%
F&A Recovery (F&A rate times total research expenditures)	$55,000,000	$50,000,000
Shortfall in F&A Recovery (F&A costs, less F&A recovery)	-0-	$5,000,000

TABLE 39-5	Budgeted F&A Cost versus Actual Cost	
Item	**Budget**	**Actual**
Facilities Costs	$30,000,000	$31,000,000
Utilities	$5,000,000	$5,600,000
Voice and Data Communications	$1,000,000	$1,500,000
Administrative Costs	$14,000,000	$15,200,000
Total F&A Costs	$50,000,000	$53,300,000
F&A Recovery	$50,000,000	$51,000,000
Shortfall in F&A Recovery (F&A costs, less F&A recovery)	-0-	$2,300,000

year projections. Corrective actions can be taken during the course of any fiscal year, but only if it is recognized that corrective actions are needed.

Research administrators must also be aware whether F&A costs are increasing as research is expanded or whether they are remaining relatively constant in a time of stable or declining research volume. The research administrator should note the fact that one year's increased costs are typically adjusted in the establishment of the next year's provisional rate, but that good financial managers avoid constantly playing "catch up" by assuring that the F&A rate for the following year adequately provides for rising costs.

Appendices

A few appendices, current as of the date of publication, are provided for a full picture of the similarities and differences in reporting requirements among agencies.

Appendix 39–A is from the National Institutes of Health (NIH) and describes due dates for financial status reports, the use of the proper forms, use of unobligated balances, and how to submit corrected financial reports.

Appendix 39–B is from the National Science Foundation (NSF). It should be noted that NSF uses an electronic communication system between its agency and its funding recipients. The appendix contains a synopsis from the NSF Grants Policy Manual, and provides information particular to financial reporting and cost reimbursement.

Appendix 39–C is from the Department of Defense (DoD). All DoD forms are available at their Web site. All forms are available at www.usamraa.army.mil. While many of the DoD forms and procedures are similar to NSF, the appendix highlights DoD-specific reporting procedures for inventions, equipment, and other specifics.

Appendix 39–A

From the NIH Policy Statement.

Financial Reports

Reports of expenditures are required as documentation of the financial status of grants according to the official accounting records of the grantee organization. Financial or expenditure reporting is accomplished using the FSR (SF 269 or SF-269 A; the SF-269 is the "long form" and is required when a grantee is accountable for the use of program income).

Except for those awards under SNAP and awards requiring more frequent reporting, the FSR is required on an annual basis. An annual FSR is required for awards to foreign organizations and Federal institutions, whether or not they under SNAP. When required on an annual basis, the report must be submitted for each budget period no later than 90 days after the close of the budget period. The report also must cover any authorized extension in time of the budget period. If more frequent reporting is required, the NGA will specify both the frequency and due date.

For domestic awards under SNAP, in lieu of the annual FSR, NIH will use the quarterly FCTR (SF 272), submitted to PMS, to monitor the financial aspects of grants. The GMO may review the report for patterns of cash expenditures, including accelerated or delayed draw-downs, and to assess whether there are possible performance or financial management problems. For these awards, an FSR is required only at the end of a competitive segment. It must be submitted within 90 days after the end of the competitive segment and must report on the cumulative support awarded for the entire segment. An FSR must be submitted at this time whether or not a competing continuation award is made. If no further award is made, this report will serve as the final FSR (see "Administrative Requirements-Closeout").

FSRs may be transmitted electronically to OFM, NIH, which, for this purpose, is equivalent to submission to the GMO. Prior to submitting FSRs to NIH, grantees must ensure that the information submitted is accurate, complete, and consistent with the grantee's accounting system. The signature of the authorized organizational official on the FSR certifies that the information in the FSR is correct and complete and that all outlays and obligations are for the purposes set forth in grant documents, and represents a claim to the Federal Government. Filing a false claim may result in the imposition of civil or criminal penalties.

Unobligated Balances and Actual Expenditures

Disposition of unobligated balances is determined in accordance with the terms and conditions of award. (See "Administrative Requirements-Changes in Project and Budget" for NIH approval authorities for unobligated balances.)

Upon receipt of the annual FSR for awards other than those under expanded authorities, the GMO will compare the total of any unobligated balance shown and the funds awarded for the current budget with the NIH share of the approved budget for the current budget period. If the funds available exceed the NIH share of the approved budget for the current budget period, the GMO may select one of the following options:

* In response to a written request from the grantee, revise the current NGA to authorize the grantee to spend the excess funds for additional approved purposes;
* Offset the current award or a subsequent award by an amount representing some or all of the excess; or
* Restrict from use some or all of the excess funds in the current budget period and take that amount into account when making a subsequent award.

There may be instances where the grantee is required to revise or amend a previously submitted FSR. When the revision results in a balance due to NIH, the grantee must submit a revised FSR whenever the overcharge is discovered, no matter how long the lapse of time since the original due date of the report. Revised expenditure reports representing additional expenditures by the grantee that were not reported to NIH within the 90-day time frame may be submitted to the GMO with an explanation. **This should be done as promptly as possible, but no later than 1 year from the due date of the original report, i.e., 15 months following the end of the budget period (or competitive segment for awards under SNAP).** If an adjustment is to be made, the NIH awarding office will advise the grantee of actions it will take to reflect the adjustment. NIH will not accept any revised report received after that date and will return it to the grantee.

Appendix 39–B

From the NSF Grants Policy Manual.

450 Grant Financial Reporting Requirement

451 Quarterly Disbursement Reporting—Federal Cash Transactions Report (FCTR)

Shortly (usually within twelve days) after the end of each calendar quarter, NSF will create and make the FCTR available to grantees on FastLane. E-mail notices are sent to each grantee announcing the reports availability and its due date. Grantees are required to update, certify, and submit the FCTR to NSF by the due date even if funds have not been drawn during the reporting period. Grantees certify to its truthfulness as stated in the Certification, Save and Submission page of the FCTR. The report elements are in compliance with the uniform Federal standards applicable to financial reporting by grantees.

Failure to submit the FCTR to NSF in a timely manner can result in one or more of the following actions:

a. suspension of all future payments;
b. closeout of expired awards based on previously reported disbursements;
c. suspension of unexpired awards; and
d. suspension of review and processing of new proposals.

Additional information on electronic submission of FCTRs and passwords for the FastLane Financial Administration functions may be obtained by calling the cognizant accountant at (703) 292-8280.

452 Final Disbursement Reporting

NSF does not require grantees to submit individual SF 269, Financial Status Reports, for purposes of final grant accountability. NSF procedures have been designed to extract the final financial data from the entries in the FCTR. This reporting is accomplished as follows:

a. For any grant listed on the FCTR that expired prior to the beginning of the quarter covered by the FCTR, the grantee will enter the final disbursement amount in the "Net Disbursement Reporting Quarter" column.
b. If there are valid unpaid obligations outstanding at the time final disbursements are due, the obligations must be charged against the NSF cash advance and reported in the "Net Disbursement Reporting Quarter" column as if they had actually been paid. If subsequent disbursements differ by $300 or more from the amount previously reported, the grantee must report the amount as an "Adjustments to Financially Closed Awards" and specify the reason for the adjustment under the remarks section of the FCTR. The Cost Analysis/Audit Resolution Branch, CPO may request additional documentation. Adjustments will not be approved for amounts less than $300.

c. If by law, regulation, and/or accounting system limitations, valid unpaid obligations cannot be charged against the NSF advance and reported as disbursed in accordance with b. above, closeout by NSF will be deferred provided that:

1. the grantee identifies grants with "unpaid obligations" in the Remarks section of the FCTR;
2. the grantee submits the FCTR before the quarterly financial closeout procedure is run; and
3. the appropriation that funds the grant has not lapsed as noted under Public Law 101-510.

d. The final disbursement amount may not exceed the amount of the award.

e. When the final disbursements have been recorded by NSF, the award will be financially closed and no additional disbursements shall be shown by the grantee in subsequent reports. When all final reporting requirements have been met, the award will be deleted from the FCTR. When this is done, the award will be shown in the next "Schedule of Awards Purged and Subsequent Adjustments During the Quarter," Part IV of the FCTR.

Appendix 39–C

From the USAMRAA (DOD-Army) Grants Policy Administration Manual.

7. Award Close Out with Advance Payments (NOV 2000) (USAMRAA)

a. The recipient shall submit an original SF 272, Federal Cash Transactions Report (forms are available at web site www.usamraa.army.mil) within 30 calendar days following the end of the final quarter.

The following documents shall be submitted within 30 calendar daysfollowing the research ending date:

(1) Final Scientific Report, as listed in Paragraph 7.
(2) Patent Report (DD Form 882, Report of Inventions and Subcontracts) submit as specified in Paragraph 16. (Forms are available at web site www.usamraa.army.mil.)
(3) Cumulative listing of only the nonexpendable personal property acquired with award funds for which title has not been vested to your institution. (This may be submitted on your institution's letterhead.)
(4) (4) Volunteer Registry Data Sheet, USAMRDC Form 60-R (forms are available at web site www.usamraa.army.mil). The Principal Investigator shall be directed to complete a form for each subject enrolled in this study and forwarded in accordance with the clause entitled "Use of Human Subjects."

c. In the event a final audit has not been performed prior to the closeout of the award, the sponsoring agency will retain the right to recover an appropriate amount after fully considering the recommendations on disallowed costs resulting from the final audit.

8. Award Close Out with Cost Reimbursement Payments (NOV 2000) (USAMRAA)

a. The recipient shall submit a final SF 270, Request for Advance or Reimbursement (forms are available at web site www.usamraa.army.milil), within 30 calendar days following the end of the final quarter.

The following documents shall be submitted within 30 calendar days following the research ending date:

(1) Final Scientific Report, as listed in Paragraph 7.
(2) Patent Report (DD Form 882, Report of Inventions and Subcontracts) submit as specified in Paragraph 16. (Forms are available at web site www.usamraa.army.mil.)
(3) Cumulative listing of only the nonexpendable personal property acquired with award funds for which title has not been vested to your institution. (This may be submitted on your institution's letterhead.)
(4) Volunteer Registry Data Sheet, USAMRDC Form 60-R (forms are available at web site www.usamraa.army.mil). The Principal Investigator shall complete a form for each subject enrolled in this study and forwarded in accordance with the clause entitled "Use of Human Subjects."

c. In the event a final audit has not been performed prior to the closeout of the award, the sponsoring agency will retain the right to recover an appropriate amount after fully considering the recommendations on disallowed costs resulting from the final audit.

40

Working with Internal and External Auditors

Abby Zubov

As a recipient of federal and other sponsor funds, universities are subject to a variety of audits and reviews. The purpose of these activities is to provide evidence that proper stewardship of sponsor funds is in place, assure compliance with laws and regulations, and safeguard animal and human subjects.[1] While these would seem to be fairly straightforward goals, they are not always easily accomplished, and noncompliance may have significant ramifications.[2]

Research sponsors, both public and private, place the responsibility of "stewardship," compliance, and protection on the principal investigator (researcher). As expected, the primary focus of a principal investigator in research is the science of research. Doing research right is an important, but secondary obligation, and one that often appears to the researcher as impeding the ability to conduct the science. It is the responsibility of research administrators to see to it that principal investigators do research right, while smoothing the way for streamlined processes to allow the science to proceed unfettered by perceived cumbersome, overly complex, and ever-changing regulatory requirements.[3]

The role of audit, both internal and external, can assist research administrators in achieving their seemingly dichotomous responsibilities. In working with internal and external auditors, research administrators should recognize that successful audits contribute to solutions: approaching audits, reviews, or other monitoring activities from this perspective will elicit an outcome that is positive for the institution as well as value-added for the research administrator.[4]

Regardless of who conducts a review, understanding the audit process, types of reviews and related objectives, what triggers a review, and knowing how to work collaboratively with the auditors will foster successful outcomes. Even in the most egregious cases, such as a for-cause investigation, the audit process should support a mutual need to promote compliance.[5]

The Audit Process

Auditing is a simple concept: the auditor determines whether activities conform or comply with requirements. To that end the audit process consists of a determination of how activities occur, assessment of whether procedures described comply with regulations and/or requirements, and tests of systems or transactions to determine whether activities or operations are really proceeding as described. Understanding the concept of audit is fundamental to promoting successful audit outcomes: describing a perfect process in compliance with all regulations will do no good, if, in fact, the actual conduct of activity is different than described, as this will become evident during audit testing.

While all entities, whether internal or external, have slightly different audit procedures, all will follow a similar process: entrance, survey, fieldwork, exit.

For example, all reviews commence with some sort of advance notice. The receipt of the notice may vary depending on the type of review, with routine reviews providing the most advance notice while investigations may serve notice as the auditors/investigators arrive. The notice will usually state the purpose, scope, and timing of the review. The purpose is the general objective of the review, while the scope is usually expressed as the period of transactions or specific projects to be included in the review.

Once notice is served, a meeting usually occurs to discuss the audit process and timing. The timing of the review varies from days to weeks depending on the nature and purpose of the review. At the time the meeting occurs, the auditors begin obtaining information to identify and set specific focused procedures related to the purpose and scope of the review. In audit parlance this is sometimes called an "opening conference" or "engagement conference."

The discussion is usually followed by an audit survey where detailed information is collected and compiled by the audit team. This information is used to determine and assess polices, procedures, and practices related to the particular objectives of the review and may entail review of policies, departmental procedures, interviews, and/or a walk-through of a particular process. The information obtained is recorded in the audit team's working papers (official notes and records of data collected subject to documentation requirements promulgated by the audit entity's professional affiliation), and fieldwork begins to assess procedures and determine conformance or compliance with regulations or stated requirements. It is at this point that testing occurs. Typically, testing involves looking at specific documents or transactions such as IRB or proposal documents and records, accounting records (cost-transfers, time cards, effort reports, invoices, or other specific original input documents), and status reports, and can even include scientific research documents such as lab notebooks. Auditors use this information to determine whether actual operational practices conform to procedures and policy or regulatory requirements as stated.

The results of this work are then discussed and reported to institution management during a meeting termed a closing or exit conference. Typically, observations are communicated first verbally and followed later with a draft report. Verbal communication and draft reports provide an opportunity to address any perceived deficiencies, provide additional information, and clarify practices that the audit team may have misinterpreted or not clearly understood.

Draft reports are the institution's opportunity to assure that the report accurately reflects the audit observations (findings), facts, and position of the institution. Typically, the burden of proof for factual accuracy resides with the audited entity. To that end, every effort should be made by the institution to assure that changes in procedures or corrective actions taken based on the preliminary findings of the review are reflected by the auditors in the report, and the observation is removed from inclusion in the report or acknowledgement of actions taken is made in any final reports.

In some cases an audit response, generally in the form of management actions or action plans, may be requested or required depending on the audit entity and the severity of the audit observations. Action plans may be and often are subject to negotiation, as at times an audit finding can be an area of potential but acceptable vulnerability. For most reviews the responses and actions are typically included or attached to the report.

It is important to bear in mind that final audit reports conducted by government agencies and public institutions are normally considered public documents (unless they contain classified data) and are often considered newsworthy depending on the type of review or severity of audit observations. It is not uncommon for audit reports to be featured in newspaper articles, published on an agency Web site, or subject to release through the Freedom of Information Act (FOIA), or a comparable state public records act, to the general public.

Types of Reviews

To a certain extent, the type of audit or review conducted dictates how formal or informal in nature the audit process will be and also affects the number and sequence of audit steps performed. Although each type of audit has specific objectives, all follow standard audit procedures and requirements as promulgated by the auditing entities' sponsoring affiliation. Underlying all audits are sound accounting practices known as Generally Accepted Accounting Practices (GAAP), Government Accounting Standards (GAS), and/or Cost Accounting Standards (CAS).

Typically, audits and reviews are of three basic types:

- Routine scheduled inspections and reviews
- Directed reviews
- For-cause reviews (investigations)

Each type of review may have a specific focused objective: financial, compliance, or performance/

operational; or contain components of all three objectives within the scope of the review.[6]

In general, financial reviews assess the accuracy of the financial information, whether for formal financial statements or for reporting of costs; compliance oriented reviews determine whether the entity is complying with laws and regulations, policies, or other contractual requirements either internal or external; and performance/operational based reviews focus on achieving programmatic objectives and/or assuring the efficiency and effectiveness of operations.

Routine Scheduled Inspections and Reviews

Routine reviews and inspections may be conducted by either internal or external auditors. These are scheduled in advance and usually based on some planned methodology: in the case of internal reviews, a risk assessment or annual audit plan; in the case of an external review, a recurring schedule or annual audit plan. Notification is usually well in advance of the audit engagement; and the objective of such reviews is usually more comprehensive, containing financial, compliance, and performance components.

The most common routine scheduled review is the OMB Circular A-133 audit conducted annually for each higher education research institution by independent auditors paid by the institution. Such reviews are reported to the institution's cognizant audit entity. The intent of this review is to ascertain whether weaknesses in control and compliance practices exist that could give rise to fraud, waste, or abuse; and on a test basis, confirm that funds are expended consistent with purposes stated in the contracts and/or grants. The A-133 review (Single Audit Act) is accepted by research sponsors as an overall opinion on the state of controls for the research institution, providing confidence that the institution will conduct research in a financially responsible manner by exercising its fiduciary responsibilities for handling and use of research funds. Another routine, periodic review of note is the Division of Cost Allocation (DCA) Disclosure Statement (DS-2) review for establishing a clear understanding of the practices and accounting principles that an educational institution follows or proposes to follow for compliance with Cost Accounting Standards and the Office of Management and Budget (OMB) Circulars A-21, Cost Principals for Education Institutions, and A-110, Grants and Agreements with Institutions of Higher Education, Hospitals, and Other Non-Profit Organizations.[7]

Periodic, comprehensive reviews are also conducted by the Office of Human Research Protection (OHRP) for institutions conducting clinical studies or other research involving human participants, and the Food and Drug Administration (FDA) or United States Department of Agriculture (USDA) for institutions conducting human and/or animal research. For national laboratory and defense research institutions, the Department of Energy (DOE) conducts periodic assessments such as the Controller's Compliance Review and the Contractor Procurement System Review (COSR).

Such periodic, comprehensive reviews are an opportunity for research administrators to showcase best practices, clarify ambiguous institutional or regulatory requirements, and establish a collaborative relationship with internal and external audit professionals. As the rapport established during routine reviews is fundamental to positive audit outcomes that transform research administrative problems into solutions, this aspect of a routine audit engagement should not be undervalued.

Directed Reviews

Directed reviews are program and management evaluations that may be conducted by internal or external auditors that focus on a specific issue or concern. These reviews may be requested by department or institutional management, be the result of random selection, or may be triggered by specific congressional request. Other triggers for a directed review are significant expenditures of funds and services, failure to submit timely interim or final status reports, or significant management or financial concerns that have surfaced at other research institutions.

Notification of directed reviews typically occurs within a week to several weeks in advance of the commencement of the review. The notice may not state the specific objective of the review, but indicates the scope of the review, i.e., to include particular research project(s) and/or time period(s). Rapport established during routine reviews can assist the institution in determining the nature and scope of any directed reviews.

Directed reviews may be conducted by any public or private entity that has awarded sponsored research to the institution, including the institution's internal auditors, internal monitoring functions (such as institutional compliance officers or functions), and peer groups and programs; or by external audit entities (both public and private) such as the General Accounting Office (GAO) which is the audit arm of the US Congress, CPA firms, the Bureaus of State Audits, the National Institutes of Health (NIH), Department of Health and Human Services (DHHS), Office of Naval Research (ONR), private foundations, and/or charitable trusts that have awarded research grants or contracts to the institution.

The objective of directed reviews is usually focused on one particular component, such as compliance with regulatory or contractual requirements, financial management, or programmatic performance, to assure the institution is achieving the mission or objectives of the program funded. The scope of the review is typically narrower than that of a routine review or inspection, and most likely has been scheduled to answer a specific question or concern. Internal monitoring functions are primarily concerned with assuring compliance of existing practices to institutional polices and procedures, and regulatory requirements. External entity directed reviews are most concerned with compliance regarding contractual obligations, although specific practices or financial performance reviews can occur. Peer reviews primarily focus on programmatic goals. Regardless of the entity conducting a directed review, the audit process itself is fairly straightforward and standard; and, again, a collaborative approach influences a positive, successful audit outcome, as the audit entity is usually seeking assurance that contractual or programmatic obligations are being met.

For-Cause Reviews

For-cause reviews are in reality investigations conducted by either internal or external investigators. Such reviews are usually the result of a specific complaint and may even have been triggered by a news or press report of a problem. Typically, little or no advance warning of the review is provided. The investigators arrive with notice in hand.

A for-cause review notice does not typically identify the purpose or scope of the review, but must provide the provision granting the authority to conduct the review. The review commences immediately and continues until it is completed. The institution may first be made aware of the impending investigation via a subpoena for records, or a cease-and-desist notice to discontinue research. For-cause investigation may be conducted by the institution's

internal audit function, police, external CPA firms, the Bureau of State Audits (BSA), the GAO, the FDA, HHS, Federal Bureau of Investigations (FBI), or the Office of Inspector General (OIG). Private investigators typically do not and should not conduct investigations at research institutions.

The objective of a for-cause review is usually to address specific allegations of financial or research misconduct. The allegations may stem from a whistleblower complaint, a subcontractor complaint, or a notification to the research sponsor indicating an egregious problem of some sort, such as a failure to notify FDA of a significant adverse event in a human subject study. In some cases, such complaints may originate for a disgruntled employee, an animal rights activist, or an individual who has previously reported a problem that has not been adequately addressed. In all cases, there must be sufficient evidence to support the claim prior to the commencement of a formal for-cause review or investigation. Such reviews are serious matters and should immediately involve notifying the appropriate institutional officials and leadership.

Proactive Site Visits

Site visits promote collaboration with research sponsors and recipient institutions. This relatively new format of proactive research compliance visits was implemented in 2000 by the Department of Health and Human Services, National Institute of Health (NIH). These reviews are conducted by the Division of Grants Compliance and Oversight in partnership with the institution to foster research compliance on current and future NIH-supported research activities. The proactive site visit is not an audit nor investigation and does not result in a written report. Rather, it is a mutual information exchange with an emphasis on partnership.[8]

When the Auditors Arrive: Dos and Don'ts

No matter what type of review is being conducted, make every effort to be prepared for the review. For internal reviews, coordination is usually not required. For external reviews, once a notice letter is received, contact the designated institutional coordinator (in some cases this is the internal audit office, in others it is the office of sponsored research or research compliance office). The role of the "coordinator" is to act as liaison to the audit entity on behalf of the institution. If no "coordinator" has been identified for your institution, contact the internal audit office/function for assistance. This office understands your institution, audit procedures, and how to present and package information to facilitate the audit process.

Clarify the Scope

If it is not immediately clear in the notice letter, contact the entity and request clarification of the scope and timing of the review. The more information obtained on the exact project(s), transactions, and intent of the review gained at an early stage allows the greatest amount of preparation.

Try to determine how many auditors will be working on the review and ask about specific needs of the audit team when they arrive. Will workspace be needed? If so, for how many? What equipment needs will there be (telephone, computer printer, internet access, etc.)? Not only do the answers to these questions give some indication of the depth and extent of the review, but asking the questions sets the stage for a collaborative audit process and allows the opportunity to arrange the best workspace for the arriving audit team, preferably nearby, but away from the mainstream of daily operations to minimize disruptions to ongoing business and to prevent the potential for misinterpretation of activities and/or conversations the auditors may see or overhear that do not pertain to the scope of the review.

Be Prepared

If at all possible, do a pre-review of the project(s) or transactions identified in the notice letter. The pre-review can solidify the knowledge and understanding of current practices and regulatory and policy requirements. Knowing ahead of time what vulnerabilities and weaknesses in policies exist, and where practices diverge from requirements, greatly assists in turning potential problems into solutions. Remember the audit process: it is counterproductive to indicate practices exactly follow policy if they do not. Inaccurate representations do more harm than good and become apparent in the audit testing. The discrepancy and resultant skepticism generated can influence and taint any other representation or information provided to the audit team, regardless of how accurate or truthful. It is much better to describe what is actually done and work with the auditor to understand what needs to be corrected to comply with requirements. Auditors are reasonable people. If the actual practice meets the intent of the requirement

or policy and the explanation for the deviance is logical, it is very likely to be accepted, or accepted with minor modifications. If the practice or policy is materially divergent from requirements, clarify with the auditor exactly what is needed and begin discussion with the auditors to facilitate development of a revised practice or process that complies with regulations. This is how potential problems turn into solutions and result in successful audit outcomes.

Be Responsive

One of the primary benefits of a pre-review is to coordinate and ready any and all pertinent backup documentation and other records the audit team will likely request. Excessive delays in producing requested documents raise questions about both the ability to adequately manage research projects and whether documents are not being produced because of what they illustrate/indicate. If requested records do not exist, communicate this fact as soon as possible to the audit team and begin working with them to identify an alternative source of evidentiary information to satisfy the audit test requirements. For example, if manual time records do not exist at the institution, ascertain the audit purpose of the time record review. If the intent is to verify effort charged to a project, it is possible that a job description with a specific percent of effort identified for a specific project in conjunction with a monthly payroll report indicating the percent of the pay charged to that fund source will suffice for the audit purpose. This type of collaborative exchange increases the research administrator's understanding and knowledge of regulatory requirements and costing policy, adding value to the audit engagement from an institutional perspective.

Be Forthright

Answer all audit questions honestly and concisely. It is not necessary to provide information beyond the question asked, unless elaboration is requested or provides insight into a best practice related to the question asked. Do not make up answers, or try to hide or obfuscate known problems. Research administration is complex and regulations continually change. The complexity of financial and management systems utilized in pre- and post-award administration make it virtually impossible to know the answer to every process question asked. If the answer is not immediately known first-hand, acknowledge what you do not know. Commit to finding the answer to bring back to the audit team, and then do so. This simple act instills confidence in audit team members that any corrective actions necessary are likely to be handled in the same responsive and committed manner.

Be Professional

In the event information provided or practices and procedures in place do not meet requirements, ask the audit team what should occur. Be respectful of the auditor's experience and opinions. Auditors have seen many different research institutions and a multitude of methods for complying with requirements, and have a sound basis for opining on what methods work well and which don't. Remember, at all times, that research administrators and auditors have a common goal: to promote effective and efficient research compliance.

Listen to how other institutions handle similar requirements. This exchange can be extremely helpful in establishing new policies or adapting existing procedures going forward, and may open the door for negotiating a compromise position. Remember, also, that an audit observation or finding identifies a potential vulnerability, and the ideal solution is to mitigate the likelihood of the risk occurring at an acceptable cost. Aggressive confrontation on why a policy or procedure cannot be enacted is not likely to result in a compromise solution. An adaptation of an existing process or a suggested practice has much more possibility of turning a potential problem into a solution that is amenable to both the institution and the audit entity, assuring a successful audit outcome.

• • • Endnotes

1. For an overview of research compliance requirements see the text of Diane Dean and Cheryl Chick's presentation, "A Federal Perspective on Compliance" (Society of Research Administrators regional seminar, Palo Alto, CA, April 2003); and the text of Diane Dean and Susan Sherman's presentation, "Compliance Perspectives" (Society of Research Administrators annual meeting, Orlando, FL, October 2002), http://grants1.nih.gov/grants/compliance/compliance.htm (accessed September 10, 2005).

2. Donald Koenig Jr., "Proposed Federal Sentencing Guidelines Amendments Signal Future Direction for Compliance Programs," *Journal of Health Care Compliance* 6, no. 3 (May–June 2004).

3. See Stephen Hansen and Kim Moreland, "The Janus Face of Research Administration," *Research Management Review* 14, no. 1, (2004): 43–53.

4. See Mike Egan, "The Auditor—Partner or Adversary?" *Local Government Auditing Quarterly* (September 2003), www.nalga.org/qrtly/art0903d.html (accessed September 10, 2005).

5. For an excellent overview of the audit process, types of reviews and how what to expect, see "Audit & Oversight Department, Lawrence Livermore National Laboratory, What to Expect in an Audit, Appraisal, or Review," unpublished guidelines, UCRL-AR-11373, Rev 1.

6. Department of Health and Human Services, Office of Inspector General, "Work Plan Fiscal Year 2003," pp. 1–2, http://oig.hhs.gov/reading/workplan/2003/Work%20Plan%202003.pdf (accessed August 2, 2005).

7. All OMB circulars can be accessed in their entireties at www.whitehouse.gov/omb/circulars (accessed August 2, 2005).

8. See National Institutes of Health, Office of Extramural Research, "Proactive Compliance Site Visits FY 2000-FY 2002: A Compendium of Findings and Observations," November 7, 2002, http://grants1.nih.gov/grants/compliance/compendium_2002.htm (accessed September 12, 2005).

41

Fundamentals of Post-Award Administration

Jerry Fife

Introduction

When an organization receives a new grant, many believe that the most difficult work is over. However, those experienced in the post-award world understand that the real work, possibly the hardest, has just begun. Post-award responsibilities of financial offices include many highly-detailed activities, including account establishment, billings/cash management, transaction monitoring/testing, closeout and audit processes, effort reporting, cost-sharing, cost transfers and general cost accounting standards.

During my 30 years in sponsored program administration in both pre- and post-award environments, in each environment I have heard talk from staff about which office is more needed. In truth, both are needed to facilitate research and to ensure compliance with applicable regulations.

Account Establishment

When a new award is received, it is not unusual for the principal investigator (PI) to immediately request an account number to begin charging project-related expenses to the proper source. In fact, so much attention has been given to this activity, I have given this priority in all post-award offices that I have directed. Unfortunately, sponsors often do not provide awards at the beginning of a project, and many times awards arrive only after the beginning date of the project. Unless the grantee has a mechanism to allow the assignment of an account number prior to the receipt of the award

(often referred to as an advance account), the project team is forced to either delay start-up of the project or, more likely, the project will begin with expenses being charged to the wrong account. If this occurs, these expenses are transferred to the project account when it is established. This is not desirable because in accounting all cost transfers are viewed as highly suspect. It is especially problematic if the PI houses these expenses on another federal project that are most likely considered unallowable.

Account establishment is the process of setting up an account in the grantee's accounting system. Although organizations differ on whether the pre-award or post-award office performs this function, since it occurs after the award, for purposes of this chapter I am directing this as a post-award function. Regardless, in order for this process to be operated successfully, there must be clear roles and responsibilities and clear communications between the two offices. This process includes:

- Establishing the sponsor-approved project budget in the accounting system
- Placing the sponsor restrictions on the budget
- Placing the correct facilities and administrative costs, also called indirect cost (F&A) rate, on the project
- Establishing the account in the proper fund grouping for financial statement and F&A purposes
- Placing the correct attributes in the accounting system. These include but are not limited to:
  - Name of principal investigator(s)

- Project period
- Agency
- Letter of credit number/grouping or billing frequency
- Cost-sharing amount
- Administrative contact (sometimes referred to as "department responsible person")
- Reporting requirements (financial and technical)

Organizations vary on how new account information is communicated to principal investigators and research teams. Some send account briefs (either in written or electronic form) that summarize the award and any applicable restrictions while others meet with investigators and review this information. This may include a copy of the sponsor award. In either event, the key is to communicate clearly and completely so as to avoid misunderstanding and get the project kicked off successfully.

Expense Monitoring

I began my career in research administration in 1974. At that time, many research organizations lacked today's sophisticated systems and were highly centralized. Virtually all sponsored project expenses were pre-audited prior to permitting payment. Over time most post-award offices have adopted varying levels of post-auditing where expenses are reviewed after payment or sampling is performed on a limited number of transactions. This has occurred for a number of reasons including:

- Increasing sophistication of systems that permits blocking or alerting post-award staff of questionable expenditures
- Continued growth in sponsored-program awards
- Delegation of responsibilities to the unit level
- Failure of post-award staffing to keep up with higher level of awards

At the early stages of this transformation many of us in post-award offices were skeptical and thought this would increase audit risk. Over time, I came to realize that with proper after-the-fact monitoring, this permitted me to focus reviews on areas and expense items with the most risk rather than simply reviewing the thousands of documents that would arrive in my office.

A good post-audit process includes a system that identifies higher-risk expenditures that are of a questionable nature. It also includes a well-trained, qualified, and persistent staff that quickly follows up on questionable expenditures; and either affects the transfer of the expenditure to an appropriate source or documents the appropriateness of the expenditure in the event of a future audit. An ideal situation implemented by some organizations is to empower the post-audit staff to make the transfer to the unit source rather than relying on unit administration to make the transfer. This permits more timely disposition of questionable expenditures; however, this will work only in organizations where units have trust in the post-award staff to transfer only unallowable expenses.

Billing

Producing bills or requesting funds is one of the primary responsibilities of post-award offices. The office is expected to produce correct bills/requests in a timely manner so funds can be obtained as quickly as possible. This billing failure forces the organization to needlessly subsidize the sponsored-program enterprise by diverting scarce organizational funds to cover project expenses while awaiting reimbursement. Thus, this area is one that should be carefully managed to ensure that it is performed efficiently.

There are multiple methods for which funds are obtained from sponsors, as discussed separately in the following sections.

Advanced Payments and Letter of Credit

The guidance for advanced payments for federal grants is contained in OMB Circular A-110 and applies to institutions of higher education, hospitals, and other nonprofit organizations.[1] Similar guidance is contained in OMB Circular A-102 for state and local governments.[2] The federal government normally provides advance payment on grants provided that the organization maintains the following:

- Written procedures that minimize the time elapsing between the transfer of funds and disbursement by the recipient.
- Financial management systems that meet the standards for fund control and accountability as established in the circular. Cash advances are to be limited to the minimum amount needed and timed to meet immediate cash needs in carrying out the purpose of the project. The timing and amount of cash advances shall be as close

as is administratively feasible to the actual disbursements by the recipient for project direct and applicable F&A costs.

Whenever possible, federal agencies are to consolidate advances to cover all awards made by a single federal agency. This situation is often in the form of a letter of credit (LOC). Each agency has a different dollar threshold for initiating a LOC with an organization. If the organization has a system that supports the requirements needed to maintain a LOC, then it provides the best opportunity to minimize cash deficits for the organization and requires less administrative effort to obtain reimbursement for the organization's grants. Pooling all grants from a single agency makes one request for all grants as often as there is an immediate cash need. The US Department of Education is an exception to this as they require organizations to identify the cash need for each grant and then issue a single payment for all Department of Education grants. This requires more effort to make a request than other agencies where this is not a requirement. It is important to note that while most letters of credit do not require identification of grant expenditures when requesting funds, there is a quarterly expenditure report that requires a reconciliation of funds drawn with project expenditures. With the advent of electronic funds transfer (EFT), requests made one day often result in funds in your organization's bank account the next day. There are varying levels of sophistication among organizations in projecting cash needs. For instance, some organizations know when a payroll posts and can project the amount of the payroll and request these funds the day before the payroll posts. These organizations may also do the same with large equipment purchases and subcontract payments. In any event, the government has written A-110 to permit some imperfection in the process. If a cash advance or LOC is over-projected, then the funds must be kept in an interest-bearing account and returned with the interest to the federal government on an annual basis. An organization is allowed to keep $250 per year for administrative expenses. There are other requirements in A-110 regarding banking and payment forms that should be reviewed.[1]

Many organizations also request scheduled cash advances when negotiating contracts with industry: these can help to balance an organization's cash position.

In summary, cash advances or LOCs are a preferred method of receiving funds and minimizing staff time and overall cash deficits within your organization.

Scheduled Payments

Scheduled payments are payments that occur on an agreed upon frequency and may or may not be tied to expenditures. These payments can be used in fixed-price agreements or for cost reimbursement agreements. Scheduled payments may take the form of progress payments tied to project milestones or may occur at certain times during the project with an amount withheld until all deliverables have been provided. Often scheduled payments are negotiated for industry contracts with the first scheduled payment occurring at the beginning and subsequent payments occurring on a schedule that maintains a positive cash balance throughout the life of the project. This form of payment is also a desirable form of payment if an upfront payment (advance) can be negotiated.

Cost Reimbursement Billings

Cost reimbursement billings are used in conjunction with federal contracts and other sponsored grants and contracts when a cash advance cannot be negotiated. These bills provide an accounting of expenditures on the project for the billing period and some provide a summary of the expenditures. Most cost reimbursement billings are prepared on a monthly basis because to bill less frequently can create an unacceptable time lag for payment. Most grants and contracts that are invoiced on a cost reimbursement basis carry a minimum 30- to 45-day time lag between the time the bill is mailed and payment is received. This lag is due to the time spent for invoice preparation, mailing, invoice review and approval, and the time it takes to return an invoice payment by mail. Cost reimbursement bills at some universities are generated electronically, while at other universities they are generated manually. Federal cost reimbursement bills use standard form 1034/1035. For nonfederal cost reimbursement agreements, it is imperative that the office responsible for negotiating agreements be sensitive to the format that the post-award office can accommodate; for example, often the efficiency of an electronic billing system can be negated by the time it takes to prepare a custom billing to use such a service.

As later discussed in more detail, cost reimbursement billings are the least desirable billing arrangement (from an accounts receivable perspective), as accounts operating in this fashion always operate at a cash deficit.

Accounts Receivables

Accounts receivables are an area of priority for post-award offices: failure to maintain an overall zero accounts receivable balance means that the organization is subsidizing the sponsored program enterprise by diverting organizational funds to cover project expenses while awaiting reimbursement. Does this mean that every organization should strive for a zero fund balance? The answer is, "No": each institution has its own unique culture, and some choose to operate their letter of credit systems as a form of cost reimbursement, rather than as a zero balance system. However, there are some necessary steps to be taken in managing accounts receivables in order to minimize institutional risk:

- Develop a system that provides information regarding payrolls and fringe benefits that have not posted, but will pay within the next few days. A similar system is needed for subcontract payments and encumbrances that might be in the payment process. This accommodates more precise letter-of-credit draws.
- Develop, implement, and maintain a process document for follow-up on cost reimbursement billings, which should include:
  - A clear statement of roles and responsibilities or, simply, a statement of who does what when.
  - A standard time period for sending a second notice (e.g., 60 days from the date of first invoice).
  - A time period for making a follow-up call (e.g., within 90 days).
  - Documentation standards to ensure that all collection attempts are recorded.
  - A communication process that identifies all parties to be informed of each attempt to collect. This typically includes the PI, department head, pre-award office, management in the post-award office, and possibly others (depending on the institution).
  - Notice of legal counsel during this process signifying when it is appropriate for them to take over. In some instances, the sponsor should be notified when a matter is to be turned over to legal counsel for collection.
- Develop goals for accounts receivable. This is crucial for effective cash management. There are benchmarks that can be used for this purpose that are often discussed at meetings for research administrators sponsored by national associations.
- Develop a strategy for which accounts should be pursued first. (As a general rule, I would recommend that small start-up businesses be pursued first as they can represent a higher risk than government agencies.)

Industry-Sponsored Payment Arrangements

Billings and management of accounts receivables is one of the primary functions of the post-award office. Like other responsibilities in the office, the management of accounts receivables requires resources, systems, competent personnel, and effective management to operate successfully. There is specific guidance available for federally sponsored agreements (grants and cooperative agreements are covered in one of the OMB circulars—A-110 for colleges and universities, and A-102 for state and local governments) and within the Federal Acquisition Regulations (FAR) for all federally sponsored programs.[3] There are no specific guidelines available, however, when dealing with industry; thus, many universities must attempt negotiation of advanced payment for industry-sponsored projects in order to minimize risk.

Project Close-Out

Project close-out is yet another of the primary duties of the post-award office and is also an area where A-133 audit findings are cause for late financial reporting.[4] This section examines the keys for success in project close-out: the duties surrounding close-out and strategies to avoid late financial reporting.

In order to achieve and sustain success at the point of the close-out, there are some key points that should be understood, which include:

- Good communication between departmental personnel and close-out staff. This is likely the most important item to ensure a good close-out process.
- An early alert system. This consists of an effective advanced notice sent to the department so that they can begin close-out activities.
- A "do it right the first time" philosophy. With the workload in post-award offices, there is simply not the time to do work more than once.

- A management reporting system that permits planning to anticipate the reporting workload. Unfortunately, the reporting workload does not report evenly on a month-to-month basis, so in order to avoid late reports, the office must anticipate the upcoming workload so proper planning can take place to accommodate the workload.
- A strategy for prioritizing the reporting workload. Which report comes first? To answer this question, one should consider the penalty imposed by the sponsor if the report is late. Some sponsors withhold further funding if reports are late, while others may hold the final invoice or a specified amount until all reports are submitted. As a general rule, it is advisable to prioritize federal sponsors first, then corporate sponsors last.
- Proper wording in subcontract agreements is another area where communication is key. The post-award office must have effective communications with the pre-award office so that subcontract agreements have a reporting requirement that provides at least 30 days for the primary institution to complete the report.
- A strategy for dealing with trailing charges, those charges which have not been charged to the account by the termination date. The post-award staff must be instructed as to how to deal with these post-accounting charges.

When a project terminates, staff in the post-award office must work with departmental staff to clear the account so a final financial report can be prepared. This coordinated effort intensifies when the final financial report is being prepared. There are many different ways in which post-award offices accomplish final financial reports with departments. Final reporting methods range from the department clearing of any charges that must be removed, to the moving of charges to a departmental account. Some universities use both methods when the department has a set number of days to move charges or when the post-award office has the authority to move them to the department's general fund account.

Reviews that take place during final financial report preparation vary depending upon how closely the project has been monitored during the life of the project. If reviews are not performed during the life of the project, they should be performed during close-out; however, they can affect administrative ability to complete all close-outs in a timely fashion. Such reviews include:

- Review to determine that any unallowable costs are removed from the project.

- Review to determine that all cost-sharing commitments have been met and have been properly recorded within the institution's accounting records.
- Review to determine that the NIH salary cap has been properly applied.
- Review to determine that the proper F&A rate has been applied.
- Review to determine that the Cost Accounting Standards (CAS) have been properly followed.
- Review to determine that any special project restrictions have been followed.

Other matters to deal with during financial report preparation include:

- Removing encumbrances from the project.
- Dealing with cost overruns. If the overrun consists of allowable costs, then they should be recorded as cost-sharing; otherwise, overrun costs should be transferred to another allowable source such as a general fund account.
- Ensuring that all close-out documents are received from any subcontracts so that they can be incorporated in the close-out.
- Making sure that the proper accounting entries are made to zero in the account or multiple accounts, in the event of a multiple account project (e.g., an NIH program project or center grant).
- Ensuring that other required reports are complete and are incorporated in the close-out packet. These may include property reports, patent reports, and other required close-out documents.

Once the close-out packet has been submitted, the file should be prepared for long-term storage, which includes marking the file so that it is retained for a proper period of time. (Most federal projects require that records be retained for three years after the date of final report submission, although some programs require a longer time period.) It is always best to check the specific guidelines of the project. In the case of record retention, more is not better: if records are retained past the required time, they may be included in the event of an audit.

Audits

In today's funding environment, most can anticipate an annual audit as part of OMB A-133 compliance.[4] These audits are performed by independent auditors hired by the institution or, in the case of state organizations, conducted by state auditors. In general, audits review management of sponsored programs at a high level, although they do review larger sponsored programs and specific areas, including subrecipient monitoring, effort reporting, and NIH salary cap compliance. Other possible grounds for audits can occur, including desk audits, contract close audits, random audits, desk audits, and audits performed in connection with the institution's F&A proposal. Some audits are performed in connection with whistleblower allegations. Regardless of their nature, audits are conducted with some general guidelines, so there are some general practices to follow to ensure the best possible outcome.

When notified of an audit, the project file should immediately be reviewed. It is also critical to identify an audit liaison as a central point of contact to communicate all requests for information. Below are some tips to ensure that audits conclude with the best possible outcome.

- Always request an entrance and exit interview. This helps to anticipate outcomes.
- Brief departmental personnel in advance of interviews so that they can be prepared.
- Provide only information that is requested. Providing additional information can lengthen the audit process and provide opportunity for the auditor to expand the audit scope.
- Answer questions concisely.
- Be truthful.
- Accept that there may be differences with the auditors; know avenues for appeal.
- It's OK not to know all the answers. If answers are unknown, agree upon a future date to provide the answers or information.
- Keep leadership informed.

Special Topics

Effort Reporting

The models for where effort reporting responsibilities reside vary between organizations; however, the post-award area will inevitably end up with some level of responsibility for this function. Regardless of where responsibility lies, effort has and will represent the single largest area of vulnerability for federally sponsored programs because salaries represent the largest portion of sponsored program expenditures. Problems in this area have ranged from A-133 audit findings to false claims suits and large settlements with the federal government.

Effort reporting is the means of ensuring that appropriate salary/wage expenses are charged to sponsored programs, that cost-sharing commit-

ments are met, and that labor costs are appropriately classified for facilities and administrative (F&A) rate purposes. Organizations may also use effort reporting to segregate costs between organizational functions and for other management reporting functions.

Most organizations design effort reporting systems to meet federal requirements. Guidance for universities is provided in the Office of Management and Budget (OMB) Circular A-21.[5] Universities account for faculty and professional effort based on a percentage of the person's total effort, with 100% effort being the maximum allowable for reimbursement in all but the most exceptional circumstances. Hourly paid employees certify effort via their time sheets. Under A-21 (Section J.8), universities can choose one of three alternatives—plan confirmation, after-the-fact activity reports, or multiple confirmation records for faculty and professional employees. Effort certification is accomplished by a certification by the person performing the effort or by someone that has firsthand knowledge of the activities of the person performing the effort. The frequency of effort reporting varies depending on the type of system and the culture and risk tolerance of the university. A-21 permits effort reporting frequency from monthly to yearly, with most universities reporting each academic term. Universities willing to accept more risk may choose to have only those employees charged directly to federally sponsored programs to complete effort certifications. These universities may also permit individuals other than the person performing the work to certify and may rely on an annual certification. OMB A-122 governs nonprofit organizations; industrial organizations are governed by the Cost Accounting Standards. Nonprofits may record effort on either an hourly or percentage of total hours for professional employees or may report on an hourly basis. Industrial organizations report effort for all employees on an hourly basis via timesheets.

There has always been audit attention given to effort reporting; however, recently there has been an increased audit interest in this area due to problems revealed at some institutions. In many whistleblower allegations, effort arises as an area of review. Some of the issues that have surfaced relate to the salary base used for budgeting versus the salary base used for charging effort to projects. Universities with medical schools, clinical practice plans, and Veterans Administration Hospitals have experienced the most problems in this area. What do auditors look for when reviewing effort reports?

Certainly they expect the existence of a signed effort report or timesheet signed on a timely basis by the person performing the effort or by someone who has firsthand knowledge of the work performed. They also expect that those performing the effort will affirm that the effort charged to the project is equal to the time spent on the project. Some common issues that universities and nonprofits experience in this area include effort reports certified by someone without firsthand knowledge of the effort performed, effort certified according to the amount budgeted rather than the actual effort performed, effort reports not completed or retained for the proper period, and instances where the effort reports do not agree with the amounts shown in the payroll system.

Organizations that wish to avoid effort reporting problems begin with support from top administrators. This support includes a clear compliance focus and good policies that include clear roles and responsibilities. Training of all individuals involved in effort reporting is a necessity. This should include faculty, departmental administrators, and others required to complete effort reports. Training in this area should be repeated both as a refresher to current staff and to train new employees. It is also critical that a monitoring system be developed and used to ensure compliance. The system should cover all common issues identified above.

Cost Transfers

Cost transfers are another area where auditors focus. This occurs because they are easily identified, often are questionable, and in large numbers might represent a symptom of poor internal controls in an organization's financial system. Late cost transfers, those occurring more than 90 days after the original charge, are especially suspect and can be expected to receive a higher level of audit scrutiny.

Cost transfers are defined as transfers of expenses to or from a federally funded sponsored account that was previously recorded elsewhere. They are of particular concern when:

- Transferring costs to or between federally sponsored programs.
- Transferring to federal projects occurring at the end of the project.
- Cost transferring where the charges are greater than 90 days old.
- Transferring with an inadequate explanation such as to correct error or to charge correct project.

- Transferring between federal projects that clears an overdraft on one of the projects.
- Cost transferring that has the effect of using unspent funds on a federally funded project that is ending.

The guidance for cost transfers cannot be found in the OMB cost circulars or grants administration circulars. They can be found in the compliance supplement to OMB A-133 that provides audit guidance to federal auditors. Guidance can also be found in other audit guidance such as the DHHS Guide to F&A Proposal Review.[6] Done properly, they represent a reassignment of costs to the proper account. All cost transfers should include a written justification providing the reason for the cost transfer and should include necessary administrative review and approval.

Organizations that are in compliance regarding cost transfers have an updated policy that is widely distributed to all of those individuals that are responsible for assigning costs to federally sponsored programs. They have a monitoring system in place to test the adequacy of cost transfer policy compliance and provide periodic training in the area. All cost transfers that include the transfer of costs greater than 90 days old include a higher level of administrative review and approval.

Cost-Sharing

Cost-sharing or the provision of matching funding represents those costs of a sponsored project borne by the organization rather than by the sponsor. Cost-sharing normally occurs on federal grants rather than federal contracts or those projects sponsored by industrial organizations. In a university setting, cost-sharing often takes place within academic year faculty salaries, although costs can also include travel, supplies and equipment, or any other cost category allowable on the grant. Under the provisions of the Cost Accounting Standards, cost-sharing also occurs when allowable costs exceed available federal funding. Many universities also treat the applicable amount over the NIH salary cap as cost-sharing.[7] Guidance for cost-sharing on federal grants can be found in OMB circular A-110 for universities and nonprofits and in A-102 for state and local governments.[1,2]

Cost-sharing can be in one of two forms. Mandatory cost-sharing is required by the sponsor as a condition for making an award. For example, the National Science Foundation (NSF) has a mandatory cost-sharing requirement for its grantees of 1% of each award or 1% on the aggregate total costs of all NSF projects requiring cost-sharing. The grantee can choose either of the two methods to satisfy the requirement.[8]

In 2001 OMB issued a cost-sharing clarification that added the terms "voluntary committed cost-sharing" and "voluntary uncommitted cost-sharing."[9] The clarification also indicates that most projects should have some level of effort charged either in the form of charges to the project or as cost-sharing. This effort can occur any time during the year.

Voluntary cost-sharing is not required as a condition of the award; however, for universities and nonprofits, voluntary cost-sharing becomes legally binding if it is reflected in the proposal leading to the award. Cost-sharing reflected in the proposal is referred to as "committed cost-sharing." There is a difference of opinion on how much cost-sharing can be mentioned in a proposal before it is considered committed cost-sharing. It is clear that if voluntary cost-sharing is included in a proposal budget, it is considered committed. However, if it is mentioned in the body of the proposal without a dollar number associated with it, it is questionable whether it should be considered committed cost-sharing. The danger here is that federal auditors' interpretation may differ from the organization's.

Cost-sharing that occurs without mention in a proposal is termed "voluntary uncommitted cost-sharing" and is not required to be tracked as cost-sharing. Voluntary uncommitted cost-sharing occurs when a faculty member spends more time on a project than budgeted for without mentioning it in the proposal.

In order for cost-sharing to be allowable it must meet the following criteria:

- Must be verifiable in the grantee's accounting system.
- Must meet all allowability criteria as per the applicable federal cost principles.
- Reasonable and necessary for project purposes.
- Allocable to the project (provide benefit to the project in proportion to the amount charged to the project).
- Is given consistent treatment through application of those generally accepted accounting principles appropriate to the circumstances.
- Must conform to any limitations or exclusions in applicable federal cost principles or in the sponsored agreement as to types or amounts of cost items.

- Is not counted as cost-sharing toward more than one federal program.
- Is not funded by other federal funds unless specifically approved in advance.

So how do organizations ensure that cost-sharing is verifiable in their accounting records? Many organizations create a cost-sharing entry that reflects the cost-sharing within the sponsored program account. This entry is designed so that it does not have any cost impact on the sponsored program account but ties cost-sharing to the account where the cost-sharing occurs, thus meeting the verification standard for cost-sharing.

Cost-sharing has both positive and negative dimensions. On the positive side, it can assist investigators in meeting agency requirements and add to the funds available for the project. On the negative side, it can consume scarce financial resources in an organization and can reduce an organization's F&A rate. Cost-sharing increases the F&A base, thus reducing the F&A rate.

In order to ensure cost-sharing compliance, organizations should develop a cost-sharing policy that defines mandatory, voluntary committed cost-sharing and voluntary uncommitted cost-sharing. The policy should also define which expenses can be considered cost-sharing and who is authorized and expected to approve cost-sharing. Once the policy is developed, it should be distributed to all individuals involved in the cost-sharing process and followed by training of these same individuals. Compliant organizations also have an established method to capture cost-sharing in their accounting system and include instructions on this process in their policy. Finally, compliant organizations manage their cost-sharing by monitoring systems that allow detection of projects where cost-sharing commitments are not being met and where units are committing large amounts of cost-sharing where it is not required.

• • • References

1. Office of Management and Budget, "Circular A-110, Uniform Administrative Requirements for Grants and Agreements with Institutions of Higher Education, Hospitals, and Other Non-Profit Organizations," amended September 30, 1999, http://www.whitehouse.gov/omb/circulars/a110/a110.html (accessed August 15, 2005).

2. Office of Management and Budget, "Circular A-102, Grants and Cooperative Agreements with State and Local Governments," amended

August 29, 1997, http://www.whitehouse.gov/omb/circulars/a102/a102.html (accessed August 15, 2005).

3. AcqNet, "Federal Acquisition Regulation," http://www.arnet.gov/far/ (accessed August 15, 2005).

4. Office of Management and Budget, "Circular A-133, Audits of States, Local Governments, and Non-Profit Organizations," revised June 27, 2003, http://www.whitehouse.gov/omb/circulars/a133/a133.html (accessed August 15, 2005).

5. Office of Management and Budget, "Circular A-21, Cost Principles for Educational Institutions," revised May 10, 2004, http://www.whitehouse.gov/omb/circulars/a021/a21_2004.html (accessed August 15, 2005).

6. U.S. Department of Health and Human Services Program Support Center, Division of Cost Allocation, "Review Guide for Long-Form University Facilities and Administrative Cost Proposals," June 2001, http://rates.psc.gov/fms/dca/frevugd1.pdf (accessed August 29, 2005).

7. National Institutes of Health, *Grants Policy Statement*, December 2003, http://grants1.nih.gov/grants/policy/nihgps_2003/index.htm (accessed August 15, 2005).

8. National Science Foundation, *Grant Policy Manual*, July 2005, http://www.nsf.gov/pubs/manuals/gpm05_131/gpm05_131.pdf (accessed August 15, 2005).

9. Office of Management and Budget, "Clarification of OMB A-21, Treatment of Voluntary Uncommitted Cost Sharing and Tuition Remission Costs," January 5, 2001, http://www.whitehouse.gov/omb/memoranda/m01-06.html (accessed August 15, 2005).

CHAPTER

42

Cost Sharing and Matching Funds

Elliott C. Kulakowski, PhD, FAHA, and Vincent Bogdanski, MBA

Introduction

The implications of cost sharing or matching funds in a proposal and the requirements for accounting for these funds during an award are frequently misunderstood by faculty and administration alike. Some investigators believe that if an institution provides additional, not-required, specified internal or other external support in a grant application, the sponsor will perceive a greater commitment from the institution to the project. They conclude that the sponsor is more likely to support the project over another, possibly one that is more meritorious. There have been no definitive studies conducted to support or disprove this hypothesis. However, major grant funding agencies have stated that cost sharing is not a factor in merit review. For example, the National Science Foundation (NSF) has actually implemented procedures to eliminate cost share from proposal review.

Additional funds to support the project from the institution or from a third party that are included can be included in the proposal to support the entire cost of the project, but not without a "cost" to the institution. Regardless of the outcome of whether a particular project is or is not funded because of cost sharing or matching funding, offering such funding can have a negative impact on future facilities and administrative (F&A) rates for the institution.[1] Sometimes this impact can be nearly as great or greater than if the institution itself provided the funds directly without applying for external support.

This chapter defines the different types of cost sharing (providing examples of each) and discusses the difference between mandatory and voluntary cost sharing models. The chapter also discusses when cost sharing is required and how an institution can minimize the impact of the effects of the additional contributory support. Included in the chapter discussion is a comprehensive example demonstrating the impact of cost sharing on the F&A rate.

Cost Sharing

Office of Management and Budget (OMB) Circular A-110, Uniform Administrative Requirements for Grants and Agreements with Institutions of Higher Education, Hospitals, and Other Non-Profit Organizations, defines cost sharing and matching as interchangeable terms as defined below.[2] However, some institutions interpret the two terms differently. For example, Duke University has its own specific definition for matching funds, citing that:

> Some agencies have programs which will 'match' funds raised by Duke from third parties. The match is given in addition to the basic award. ORS (Office of Research Services) is required to certify the award of the third party funds before the agency will provide the matching award.[3]

Cost sharing is that part of the budgeted cost of a project that is provided by some entity or person other

437

than the sponsor to support the sponsored activity. The federal government is the sponsor most likely to require cost sharing because in supporting projects, it would like to get the biggest return for its investment.[4] Industry generally does not want to share the cost of a project because it may dilute their rights and competitive edge in the market.

If the ultimate sponsor of the award is the federal government, other federal funds cannot be used as cost share. In certain rare instances federal flow-through funds are allowable as cost sharing, but require the approval of both the federal sponsor and the flow-through sponsor.[4] Cost sharing commitments generally come from the institution submitting the proposal or from a third party that provides the cost share to the institution. Normally, funds or other cost shared assets can only be used once as cost share or matching. For example, an institutional intramural grant awarded to a department for a piece of equipment cannot be used by the principal investigator as cost share for a Department of Energy award and by the same or another investigator for a NSF instrumentation award.

As noted in the OMB Circular A-110 regulations, cost sharing is not as simple as the term implies:

(a) All contributions, including cash and third party in-kind, shall be accepted as part of the recipient's cost sharing or matching when such contributions meet all of the following criteria.

(1) Are verifiable from the recipient's records.

(2) Are not included as contributions for any other federally-assisted project or program.

(3) Are necessary and reasonable for proper and efficient accomplishment of project or program objectives.

(4) Are allowable under the applicable cost principles.

(5) Are not paid by the Federal Government under another award, except where authorized by Federal statute to be used for cost sharing or matching.

(6) Are provided for in the approved budget when required by the Federal awarding agency.

(7) Conform to other provisions of this Circular, as applicable.

(b) Unrecovered indirect costs may be included as part of cost sharing or matching only with the prior approval of the Federal awarding agency.

(c) Values for recipient contributions of services and property shall be established in accordance with the applicable cost principles. If a Federal awarding agency authorizes recipients to donate buildings or land for construction/facilities acquisition projects or long-term use, the value of the donated property for cost sharing or matching shall be the lesser of (1) or (2).

(1) The certified value of the remaining life of the property recorded in the recipient's accounting records at the time of donation.

(2) The current fair market value. However, when there is sufficient justification, the Federal awarding agency may approve the use of the current fair market value of the donated property, even if it exceeds the certified value at the time of donation to the project.

(d) Volunteer services furnished by professional and technical personnel, consultants, and other skilled and unskilled labor may be counted as cost sharing or matching if the service is an integral and necessary part of an approved project or program. Rates for volunteer services shall be consistent with those paid for similar work in the recipient's organization. In those instances in which the required skills are not found in the recipient organization, rates shall be consistent with those paid for similar work in the labor market in which the recipient competes for the kind of services involved. In either case, paid fringe benefits that are reasonable, allowable, and allocable may be included in the valuation.

(e) When an employer other than the recipient furnishes the services of an employee, these services shall be valued at the employee's regular rate of pay (plus an amount of fringe benefits that are reasonable, allowable, and allocable, but exclusive of overhead costs), provided these services are in the same skill for which the employee is normally paid.

(f) Donated supplies may include such items as expendable equipment, office supplies, laboratory supplies or workshop and classroom supplies. Value assessed to donated supplies included in the cost sharing or matching share shall be reasonable and shall not exceed the fair market value of the property at the time of the donation.

(g) The method used for determining cost sharing or matching for donated equipment, buildings and land for which title passes to the recipient may differ according to the purpose of the award, if (1) or (2) apply.

(1) If the purpose of the award is to assist the recipient in the acquisition of equipment, buildings or land, the total value of the donated property may be claimed as cost sharing or matching.

(2) If the purpose of the award is to support activities that require the use of equipment, buildings or land, normally only depreciation or use charges for equipment and buildings may be made. However, the full value of equipment or other capital assets and fair rental charges for land may be allowed, provided that the Federal awarding agency has approved the charges.

(h) The value of donated property shall be determined in accordance with the usual accounting policies of the recipient, with the following qualifications.

(1) The value of donated land and buildings shall not exceed its fair market value at the time of donation to the recipient as established by an independent appraiser (e.g., certified real property appraiser or General Services Administration representative) and certified by a responsible official of the recipient.

(2) The value of donated equipment shall not exceed the fair market value of equipment of the same age and condition at the time of donation.

(3) The value of donated space shall not exceed the fair rental value of comparable space as established by an independent appraisal of comparable space and facilities in a privately-owned building in the same locality.

(4) The value of loaned equipment shall not exceed its fair rental value.

(5) The following requirements pertain to the recipient's supporting records for in-kind contributions from third parties.

(i) Volunteer services shall be documented and, to the extent feasible, supported by the same methods used by the recipient for its own employees.

(ii) The basis for determining the valuation for personal service, material, equipment, buildings and land shall be documented.[2]

Cost sharing must take place during the time of the award, if it does not, then it cannot be counted against the project. For example, the price of a donated piece of equipment currently being used in a department cannot qualify for cost share because cost sharing expenditures must take place concurrent with the start and end date of an award.

Mandatory Cost Sharing

An agency requires in a proposal or by policy that the respondent provide a certain amount of funding to support the budget of a particular project. Among the more common ways that sponsors require cost sharing:

- A flat amount such as $50,000 in cost sharing.
- Two dollars of cost sharing for each dollar awarded
- Fixed percentage such as 30% cost share and 70 percent awarded funding.[4]

The sponsor also may require increasing or decreasing amounts of cost sharing based on the dollar amount of the award. The cost sharing may be based on the total amount of the award, total allowable costs of the entire project, or total direct cost.

While each federal agency determines whether a particular program is to be required, there is only one easily identifiable unique instance of Congressionally-mandated cost sharing:

In accordance with Congressional requirements, NSF requires that each grantee share in the cost of NSF research projects resulting from unsolicited proposals. These requirements may be met by the recipient through cost sharing a minimum of one percent on the project or by cost sharing a minimum of one percent on the aggregate costs of all NSF-supported projects subject to the statutory requirements.[5]

Usually, this particular 1% cost share is provided directly to NSF cumulatively on an annual basis by the institution's accounting or government office. There is no need to provide the 1% in each proposal. These conditions should be verified with the appropriate office at your organization.

Voluntary Committed Cost Sharing

Voluntary cost sharing occurs when an investigator proposes cost sharing when it is not required or when the amount is in excess of the required cost share, and the institution agrees to the cost share in the proposal or in the subsequent award. The OMB has determined that voluntary cost sharing proposed in a budget or budget justification must be treated as mandatory cost share if the award is made and the voluntary cost share becomes a required term or condition of the award.[2] This is not "funny money" that is revocable at the wish of investigator or the institution if it cannot make the match. Only the awarding business officer can withdraw the requirement. For example, a principal investigator (PI) proposes a certain percentage of effort but requests no compensation for him/her self in the proposal, but by definition, the PI must expend effort on that award. If no compensation is requested from the sponsor, the compensation (appropriate commensurate salary and fringe benefits) must come from another source and is, therefore, considered cost sharing.

Because of the potential negative impact on an institution's F&A rate, institutions tend to discourage voluntary cost sharing.[4,6] Voluntary cost sharing should only be used under exceptional circumstances that suit the best interest of the institution.

For example, if an institution undertakes a community project to support the development of senior housing, voluntary cost sharing may be a suitable option. An application may be submitted to the Department of Housing and Urban Development that could benefit the institution's community and could also provide for long-lasting goodwill from the local area. The institution may submit the proposal, with not only community, city, and/or state political letters of support, but also with committed support in terms of money or in-kind contributions from neighborhood groups, churches, and the institution itself. While not required for funding, these voluntary contributions by the local groups not only demonstrate the local support, but it is considered cost sharing.

While institutions sometimes identify salary cap cost sharing in their policies as a separate category of cost sharing, the OMB recognizes salary cap as a form of voluntary committed cost sharing. For example, the National Institutes of Health (NIH) places a salary cap on the salary that an investigator can receive on a grant (limited to the level of pay at federal executive level I can be paid annually).[7] Policies at some institutions (e.g., Virginia Commonwealth University) also include another internal category of "cost sharing which occurs when the University proposes (or later assigns), effort by individuals whose salary exceeds a sponsor-imposed limit for individual salaries."[8]

Voluntary Uncommitted Cost Sharing

According to the OMB, voluntary uncommitted cost sharing is faculty-donated additional time above that agreed to as part of the award or additional effort actually worked above the effort committed to within the proposal.[2] Voluntary uncommitted cost share does not have to be tracked and accounted for like mandatory or voluntary committed cost share.[9]

Methods of Providing Cost Sharing

Cost sharing can be in cash or in-kind. Cost sharing can be derived from a number of sources, as discussed in the following sections.

Uncollected or Reduced F&A

When a proposal that requires cost sharing is funded at less than the full and appropriate F&A level, the institution, depending on the sponsor, may include the uncollected F&A as part of the required match. Many institutions require that uncollected F&A costs be calculated on faculty effort and other normally F&A eligible contributed resources, and included in the cost sharing totals. Because cost sharing is part of the overall project budget, the uncollected F&A on the institution's contribution is a legitimate claimed cost. Some sponsors, such as the Department of Education, do not allow uncollected F&A as cost share; therefore, it is important to read and know each sponsor's policy. Uncollected F&A cannot be claimed on third party in-kind contributions.

Certain sponsors may limit the amount of F&A that they provide for a project. The reduced F&A level can be considered cost sharing. The institution may not be required to cost share the project, but when it does not get the appropriate amount of F&A, it is, in fact, cost sharing.

Investigator and Staff Efforts

When full salary and benefits commensurate with the level of effort of an investigator or other staff working on a project is not fully requested in the budget to the sponsor and the institution is to make up the difference, this is considered cost sharing. This also can include any amount above any salary cap by the sponsor. For proposals in which there is mandatory or voluntary cost sharing, the level of effort must be tracked and reported accordingly to the institution's guidelines for time and effort reporting.

Other Institutional Resources

Reductions in F&A and donated time by the investigator or other personnel on a project are common methods of cost sharing: other sources can include the purchase of supplies, equipment, travel, or other expenses. These items must be related to the project and procured and used during the project period. In the case of equipment, the equipment must be purchased during the project period and the extent of its use can be cost shared.

Third Party Contributions

Third party contributions can be determined according to the same guidelines above for the institution receiving the award. Dealing with third parties can be difficult if the third party contributor is not familiar with the sponsor requirements and the management and record keeping necessary to ensure that it is appropriately tracked and reported. It is especially difficult if the contributor does not have a contractual relation with your organization.

Generally if there is a sub-award contemplated, the recipient is expected to provide a proportionate amount of any cost share. After the award to the institution, the resulting sub-award should allow for payment of invoice only, to the extent that accurate, verified and proportional cost share documentation is provided with the invoice.

For in-kind contributions where there is no contractual relation with the institution for the award, the institution must develop a method to collect not only the cost share amounts but also the verifiable and auditable records that will be necessary to later validate that all cost sharing has been met.

Procedures for Processing Proposals with Cost Sharing

Every institution has its own procedures and generally a form for handling cost sharing issues.[3,4,8,10] Following is an example of how a proposal involving cost sharing can be handled.

In the very early planning stages of a proposal, the PI should read the guidelines from the sponsor to determine if cost sharing is required. If cost sharing is mandatory or there is a compelling reason to provide voluntary cost sharing, the PI or administrator should determine the appropriate amount of cost sharing needed. The institutional cost sharing forms should be completed as early as possible and circulated for approval to the appropriate individuals who can make the commitment.

Some institutions have different signature requirements based on the amount and source of the cost share. For example, in an academic institution, if cost sharing is less than $50,000, the department chair may be able to commit the funds from the operating budget or from developmental funds. If the required cost share is between $50,000 and $100,000, the dean of the investigator's college or school must approve the cost share; and if the cost share is greater than $100,000, approval of the provost, vice president for research or president may be necessary. In certain instances (e.g., construction or renovation projects), the size of the cost sharing may demand that the institution raise money to meet its obligation, which may conflict with other institutional fundraising priorities. In these instances, the development office should be brought into the discussion. It is often helpful for senior administrators (department chairs, deans, vice presidents, and the president), when contacted to provide cost sharing, to discuss the issue with the sponsored projects office (SPO) to determine if there is an unforeseen impact on the institution and to verify the cost sharing proposal. These discussions should also discuss other possibly more effective means to achieve the cost sharing requirements.

When cost sharing is to be provided by a third party (e.g., a nonprofit or a for-profit), the external contributor or collaborator should be contacted as early as possible and be made aware of the requirements. In addition, the PI should always obtain letters of commitment from the third party who is cost sharing the project.

The cost sharing forms and letters of commitment should be forwarded to SPO along with the proposal. The SPO is responsible for review of the proposal and to determine the appropriateness of the cost sharing.

Once an award is made, SPO works with grant and contract accounting to establish the institutional account for the award. Grant and contract accounting may want to establish another account to track the cost sharing. If there is contribution of institutional personal effort, the institution's accounting office tracks the effort reporting. The office of grant and contract accounting verifies any purchases and provides for the appropriate distribution between the sponsored activity account and the cost sharing account. Detailed records are needed for these accounting purposes. This process continues for the life of the project until the office of grant and contract accounting does the final closeout.

It is practical to remember that all cost sharing, regardless of the source, gains federal identity during the award. This means that for a federal project if cost sharing is included in the terms of the award, the institution must treat it just the same as if the cost shared or in-kind funds were from the federal government. Therefore, the cost sharing is subject to federal rules, requirements, and regulations included within the award.

Impact of Cost Sharing

The economic impact of cost sharing by an institution can be considerable. The administration time for cost share can be both time consuming and complicated, especially if there is in-kind third party involved.

Cost sharing also has the potential to impact the federal negotiated facilities and administrative cost rate of an institution. In this example, we examine the period from fiscal year (FY) 1991 to FY 2003, described in Table 42-1.

Cost Share Budget Definitions

Before we begin this example, let us define a couple terms.

Base. For a university, this includes the direct costs less items defined in OMB Circular A-21 to be excluded, such as subcontracts greater than $25,000, scholarships, and equipment, of the missions of the university (research, instruction, and other organized activities) which includes cost share if the funds are provided from the institution.

Pool. Allowable costs associated with eight major expense functions as defined by OMB Circular A-21, which cannot be directly allocated to an individual sponsored activity. The eight categories are:

1. Depreciation and use allowance
2. Interest
3. Operations and maintenance
4. General administration and general expenses
5. Sponsored projects administration
6. Department administration
7. Student services
8. Library

Expenditures. Actual expenses for the fiscal year as accumulated in the university accounting system. The expenses will be different from the booked sponsored activity yearly gross funds.

Research, Instruction and Other Sponsored Activities. These are the three most common components of sponsored activities associated with the negotiated F&A agreement. Combined with the on-campus (for activities that occur on institutional or institutional designated space) and off-campus (for activities that occur at a site other than institutional space) components, there can be a total of six negotiated rates.

Assumptions

We have made two assumptions in the calculations in Table 42-1. First, the base and pool increase at the same relative rate over the period from FY 1991 and FY 2003. Second, the spending rates versus booked sponsored activity gross awards remain constant. The percentages for research, instruction and other sponsored activities in relation to gross awarded dollars, spending and F&A recovery also remain constant.

Method Used

We began by looking at the base and pool amounts for FY 1991 and these amounts that were used to negotiate an agreement. The FY 1991 base and pool were increased by the percentage increase in sponsored project funding from July 1, 1999 through June 30, 2003 for research instruction and other sponsored activities. This represents the actual base and pool for FY 2003, ending June 30, 2003.

The actual F&A recovery amount was calculated for research and other sponsored activities based on the percentage of actual sponsored project funding for FY 2003. This represents the amount of F&A money collected.

In the example, we calculated the FY 2003 base for research and other sponsored activities by $1 million to represent cost sharing. The F&A reduction was calculated based on the $1 million cost sharing.

Finally, the actual rate and the reduced rate were multiplied by the estimated F&A recovery to show the loss of recovery in one year.

TABLE 42-1	Calculating the Impact of $1 Million Cost Sharing on F&A Rate						
	Other Sponsored Activities (escalated from 1991 to 2003)				**Research Activities (escalated from 1991 to 2003)**		
	Base ($ in millions)	**Pool** ($ in thousands)	**Perentage**		**Base** ($ in millions)	**Pool** ($ in thousands)	**Perentage**
ORIGINAL							
Buildings and Improvements Depreciation	$160.9	$1,126	0.70		$115.6	$3,656	3.16
Equipment Depreciation	$160.9	$2,809	1.75		$115.6	$5,542	4.79
Operation and Maintenance of Plant	$160.9	$5,814	3.61		$115.6	$16,318	14.12
General Administration	$160.9	$8,010	4.98		$125.0	$6,224	4.98
College Administration	$160.9	$3,619	2.25		$125.0	$3,958	3.17
Department Administration	$160.9	$15,465	9.61		$125.0	$20,565	16.45
Sponsored Projects Administration	$33.4	$925	2.77		$125.0	$3,432	2.75
Library	$160.9	$1,363	0.85		$115.6	$1,447	1.25
TOTAL			26.51*				50.67
BASE INCREASED BY $1 MILLION DUE TO MATCHING							
Buildings and Improvements Depreciation	$162.0	$1,126	0.69		$116.6	$3,656	3.14
Equipment Depreciation	$162.0	$2,809	1.73		$116.6	$5,542	4.75
Operation and Maintenance of Plant	$162.0	$5,814	3.59		$116.6	$16,318	13.99
General Administration	$162.0	$8,010	4.94		$126.0	$6,224	4.94
College Administration	$162.0	$3,619	2.23		$126.0	$3,958	3.14
Department Administration	$162.0	$15,465	9.55		$126.0	$20,565	16.32
Sponsored Projects Administration	$34.4	$925	2.69		$126.0	$3,432	2.72
Library	$162.0	$1,363	0.84		$116.6	$1,447	1.24
TOTAL			26.27*				50.25

*NOTE—Decrease is about 0.25% in F&A rate

Errors in rounding

Impact

Using the data from Table 42-1 it is shown that one million dollars in cost sharing decreases the institution's F&A rate by 0.25%. The result of this decreased F&A rate in this example is $400,000 in unrecovered F&A per year for research and $66,000 of unrecovered F&A per year for other sponsored activities (Table 42-2).

Example of When Not to Cost Share

Let us see examine how the impact of cost sharing translates into an example that is summarized in Table 42-3.

In our example, a faculty member proposes to submit a three-year proposal for a social science service project seeking to obtain $399,702 from the federal sponsor over three years. By the time the faculty member discusses the proposal with the SPO, the faculty member obtained several cost sharing commitments from the institution and from local organizations to support the project. The faculty member believes that the project will be more successful with the more cost sharing that can be shown in the application for the project. Two departments, a center and an institute at the institution, agreed to provide support to the project for $676,994. The faculty member also received commitments from the provost to waive all F&A by the institution, for an additional $86,210 of cost sharing. Overall, the institution also stands to lose $209,881 in uncollected overhead on its match that it counts as cost sharing. The faculty member also had approached city government and county government, and they agreed to provide an additional $51,055 in cost sharing. The school district and a neighborhood community group also agreed to cost share the project. Finally, a management company agreed to provide free space for the project; that

also is considered cost sharing of the project. Combined, the external organizations agreed to cost share the project for a total of $265,876. The total three-year project budget was $1,689,718, of which only $399,702 is from the sponsor. Therefore, there is a nearly three-to-one match, or for every dollar from the federal government, there are three dollars in cost sharing.

If we look at the impact of cost sharing in this example based on the calculations from Table 42-1 and Table 42-2, there is a potential loss of between $66,900 and $100,000 per year in unrecovered F&A in the other sponsored and research category for the institution, depending on how much of the third party matching is put into the base. Since most of the third party match is from government or quasi-government sources, that amount will be very large. Considering the F&A waivers in our example, the institution starts losing money in the second or third year of their negotiated F&A rate agreement. A more practical business decision would have been to fund the original $399,702 from the institution's own resources.

Conclusion

In general, institutions should be very select about cost sharing, as it can have a negative impact on the institution's F&A rate.

Institutions should limit programs that require mandatory cost sharing, only allowing them when the project is in the best interest of the institution and not the individual investigator. Mandatory cost sharing terms should be strictly kept to required levels.

Voluntary cost sharing should be discouraged and the SPO should make every effort to avoid such as a term of condition. However, if voluntary cost sharing is necessary, it should be accepted at only a minimum level and the institution must determine

TABLE 42-2	Financial Impact on Institution of $1 Million in Cost Sharing				
Activity	F&A Rate	F&A Collected	Lost Revenue (per year)	Comment
Research	49.50%	$43,740,000		Actual
	49.25%	$43,340,000	$400,000	Projected*
Other Sponsored Activity	27.50%	$6,107,400		Actual
	27.25%	$6,040,500	$66,000	Projected*

*Note: Projected lost revenue is based on $1 million matching funds that reduced the F&A rate by 0.25% as determined from Table 42-1.

TABLE 42-3

Funding Sources		Amount Requested	Subtotal by Category
Federal Agency		$399,702	$399,702
University			
	Department A	$146,340	
	Department B	$37,500	
	Center	$24,021	
	Institute	$469,133	
	Loss of F&A from Federal Agency Award (27.5%)	$86210	
	Loss of F&A from University Cost Sharing	$209,881	
			$973,085
Local Government			
	City	$23,920	
	County	$27,135	
			$51,055
Other Non-University Commitments			
	Management Group	$8,880	
	Neighborhood Group	$121,996	
	School District	$135,000	
			$265,876
TOTAL			$1,689,718

how to minimize the impact on future F&A rate negotiations. Failure to meet the required match or failure to have costs appropriately verified can force the institution to return sponsor funds.

Institutions must be fully aware of the sum total impact of all cost sharing activities: institutions must keep track of the total amount of these activities, while keeping them to a minimum. The impact of cost sharing can be considerable and can affect future F&A rate calculations and the amount of F&A funds collected can be reduced significantly.

Acknowledgments

The authors wish to thank Ms. Barbara Nielsen and Mr. William Ernest for useful comments and suggestions.

• • • References

1. The White House, Office of Management and Budget. "Circular No. A-21, Cost Principles for Educational Institutions," (revised 05/10/04). Available at http://www.whitehouse.gov/omb/circulars/a021/a21_2004.html (accessed on October 16, 2005).

2. The White House, Office of Management and Budget. "Circular A-110, Uniform Administrative Requirements for Grants and Agreements with Institutions of Higher Education, Hospitals, and Other Non-Profit Organizations," (revised 11/19/93, as Further Amended 9/30/99), "Subpart C—Post-Award Requirements Financial and Program Management _.23." Available at http://www.whitehouse.gov/omb/circulars/a110/a110.html#23 (accessed on October 16, 2005).

3. Duke University, Office of Research Support. "Cost Sharing and Matching." Available at: http://www.ors.duke.edu/ask/proposal/budget/costshare.html (accessed on October 16, 2005).

4. University of Washington, "Cost Sharing Overview." Available at http://www.washington.edu/research/gca/costshare/ (accessed on October 16, 2005).

5. National Science Foundation. "Important Notice: Implementation of the New NSF Cost sharing Policy." Available at http://www.nsf.gov/pubs/1999/iin124/iin124.htm (Accessed on October 16, 2005).

6. University of Utah. "Guidelines for Cost Sharing on Sponsored Agreements." Available at http://www.utah.edu/govacct/costshar.htm (accessed on October 16, 2005).

7. National Institutes of Health. "NIH NOT-OD-04-034, Change in 2004 Salary Limitations on Grants, Cooperative Agreements, and Contracts." Available at: http://grants2.nih.gov/grants/guide/notice-files/NOT-OD-04-034.html (accessed on October 16, 2005).

8. Virginia Commonwealth University. "Grants and Contracts Cost Sharing Policy." Available at: http://www.vcu.edu/finance/CostAccounting/policy.htm (accessed on October 16, 2005).

9. The White House, Office of Management and Budget. "M-01-06, Clarification of OMB A-21, Treatment of Voluntary Uncommitted Cost Sharing and Tuition Remission Costs." Available at http://www.whitehouse.gov/omb/memoranda/m01-06.html (accessed on October 16, 2005).

10. Harvard University, Office of Research Administration. "Cost Sharing." Available at http://vpfweb.harvard.edu/osr/proposal/prop_bud_sharing.shtml (accessed on October 16, 2005).

V

Responsible Conduct
of Research

43

Education in the Responsible Conduct of Research: Opportunities and Potential Impact on the Research Institution

Chris B. Pascal, JD

Introduction

In 2000, the US Office of Research Integrity (ORI) issued the "Public Health Service (PHS) Policy on Instruction in the Responsible Conduct of Research,"[1] (RCR) that would require PHS-funded research institutions to provide RCR education for all PHS-project research staff. In 2001, however, implementation of the policy was put on hold, following Congressional concerns over the need for formal rulemaking.[2] Following internal discussions within ORI and HHS, formal implementation of the RCR policy through a legal mandate was abandoned. In its place, ORI began a series of collaborations with the research community to stimulate RCR education efforts at scientific and academic societies, graduate schools, and individual research institutions. To emphasize the importance of the responsible conduct of research, the revised HHS research misconduct regulations state that each research institution must foster "a research environment that promotes the responsible conduct of research, research training, and activities related to that research or research training, discourages research misconduct, and deals promptly with allegations or evidence of possible research misconduct."[3] The preamble to this provision explains that "this is not a requirement for institutions to establish a new program for the responsible conduct of research." Rather, "(t)he new provision recognizes the continuing importance of the responsible conduct of research to competent research that is free of any research misconduct."[4]

This chapter discusses three issues relevant to the research institution and how research administrators can assist institutions in responding to concerns involving responsible research practices and education programs designed to address them:

1. What is RCR and how has it been defined by the research community and federal agencies?
2. What federal and institutional efforts have been made to implement RCR education programs?
3. What are the opportunities offered by RCR programs and the potential benefits to the research institutions, laboratories, and scientists in adopting and implementing RCR programs?

Historical and Philosophical Background

However important many people may think it is to include research ethics as part of graduate training in science and engineering, ... there is a substantial gulf between stated importance and activity levels. Explicit training in research ethics is only slowly becoming a recognized part of the 'tools' for doing scientific research. The reasons range from the pressures of time and crowded curricula to the view of some faculty that learning research ethics is not an integral part of doing science or being a 'good' scientist. Also, some believe that research ethics is too far outside their area of expertise to contemplate including it in the education of their students."[5]

This passage from a 1995 article by Swazey and Bird reflects the majority view of the recent past that, while important, education in responsible research practices is not a core part of science education. In short, good scientists need to learn the techniques for high quality research, but research integrity or ethics is innate or will be learned by watching others. Unethical scientists were considered to be beyond help.

Many academic leaders have argued against this view, and important developments in research integrity and misconduct, from high profile cases, proposed legislation, hearings, and research findings have called this attitude into serious question. A 2002 report from the Institute of Medicine (IOM) specifically disavows the prior view that research ethics and responsible conduct concerns are somehow separate and distinct from the actual conduct of the research. In the report, "Integrity in Scientific Research: Creating an Environment That Promotes Responsible Conduct," the IOM states that "the responsible conduct of research is not distinct from research; on the contrary, competency in research *encompasses* the responsible conduct of that research and the capacity for ethical decision making."[6] Some of the important antecedents for RCR education are discussed in this chapter.

Since 1990, the National Institutes of Health (NIH) has required applications for institutional national service award research training grants to include a component on instruction in the responsible conduct of research. Although the specific content of the instruction was left up to the institution, NIH recommended in 1994 that the RCR education program cover the following topics: conflict of interest, responsible authorship, policies for handling misconduct, policies regarding the use of human and animal subjects, and data management.[7] According to a survey of institutional RCR programs developed under NIH training grants, 68% covered four or five of the six topic areas recommended by NIH and the top five topic areas covered overall matched the NIH recommendations.[8]

During the period between announcement of the NIH policy requiring RCR instruction for training grants and the proposed PHS policy that expanded RCR education to all PHS funded research staff and expanded the topic areas of instruction from six to nine (adding mentor/trainee relationships, peer review, and collaborative science), there were a number of activities occurring related to RCR education.

In 1989, the Institute of Medicine issued a report, "The Responsible Conduct of Research in the Health Sciences," which included a number of recommendations intended to promote responsible research. Recommendation seven from the report states that "universities should provide formal instruction in good research practices."[9] In discussing the recommendation, the report further observed that while less formal methods of instruction were helpful, such as mentoring and guest lectures, "they were no longer adequate because of the size and complexity of the modern research environment."[10] The NIH policy requiring RCR education for research trainees was a start in addressing this recommendation.

In 1992, the National Academy of Sciences issued a report, "Responsible Science: Ensuring the Integrity of the Research Process," which reaffirmed the earlier IOM recommendation on RCR education that "scientists and research institutions should integrate into their curricula educational programs that foster faculty and student awareness of concerns related to integrity of the research process."[11] This recommendation expands on the prior IOM recommendation in two important ways. First, it recommended that individual scientists, as well as institutions, take action to foster RCR awareness. It also specifically mentions that the educational programs should foster faculty awareness of concerns related to integrity. The report further recommends that "scientists and their institutions should act to discourage questionable research practices through a broad range of formal and in formal methods in the research environment."[12] This recommendation is significant for RCR education since many potential areas of "questionable research practices," as defined by the report, cover areas that would be included in RCR education programs, such as conflict of interest, authorship issues, and handling of research data. For more detailed information on principles and philosophy behind the NAS recommendations on questionable research practices, see chapter 50.

In 1995, the statutory Commission on Research Integrity (CRI) made thirty-three recommendations to the Department of Health and Human Services intended to improve departmental policies on research misconduct and research integrity. One of the commission recommendations called for the department to "require that each institution applying for or receiving a grant, contract, or cooperative agreement under the Public Health Service Act for research or research training add to its existing misconduct in science assurance a third declaration, one certifying that the institution has an educational program on the responsible conduct of research."[13] This would mean that the NIH RCR program currently limited to research trainees would be applied to "all individuals supported by PHS research funds."[14]

This recommendation was endorsed by HHS in 1999 following a full review of the department's misconduct and research integrity policies. At that time, the HHS announced that, through ORI, the department would require research institutions to provide training in the responsible conduct of research to all staff engaged in research or research training with PHS funds. In discussing its recommendation, the commission stated that the "specific content of educational programs on the responsible conduct of research should be at the discretion of each institution, and tailored to that institution's configuration and culture. However, programs should include discussion of areas in which problems are known to arise, such as supervision of trainees; data management; publication practices; authorship; peer review of privileged information; conflicts of interest and commitment; integrity issues in clinical and epidemiological research; whistleblower rights and responsibilities, including their right to be protected from retaliation; and responsibilities and procedures for reporting suspected misconduct."[15]

This general approach proposed by the commission, providing flexibility for the institution in the specific content of instruction while identifying core areas of instruction was the path taken by PHS in its RCR policy. In fact, the subject areas of concern identified by the commission closely track the nine core areas identified by PHS, although with a few differences. In its background discussion for the policy, the commission stated that it "strongly believes that all of these individuals would benefit from participation. Providing such training is an important step in creating a positive research environment that stresses the achievement of research integrity more than the avoidance of research misconduct."[16] This, too, tracks the interest of ORI in promoting responsible research and research integrity instead of just responding to misconduct after it occurs or correcting questionable practices.

In its 2002 report, the IOM recommended five objectives for a successful RCR education program:

1. Emphasize that responsible conduct is central to conducting good science;
2. Maximize the likelihood that education in the responsible conduct of research influences individuals and institutions rather than merely satisfying an item on a "check-off" list for that institution;
3. Impart essential standards and guidelines regarding responsible conduct in one's discipline;
4. Enable participants in the educational programs to develop abilities that help them to effectively manage concerns related to responsible conduct of research as they arise in the future; and
5. Verify that the first four objectives have been met.[17]

In discussing objective four on enabling participants to develop RCR abilities, IOM makes additional observations regarding the importance of using RCR education to develop ethical reasoning skills and practical research skills (sometimes referred to as survival skills), such as how to present results at scientific meetings, defend methodologies and interpretations of data, including justifications for excluding data, prepare written reports, conduct peer review, etc.[18]

In addition to this very clear trend of recommendations supporting RCR education from the research community and pointing the way for research institutions to move forward with effective RCR education programs, evidence of problems with research practices during the past several years also provides impetus to move in this direction.

Research Findings Relevant to RCR

In understanding the relevant context for the PHS policy on RCR, it is important to note recent research literature suggesting that departures from accepted research practices may be more common than previously thought. Many research administrators and scientists are familiar with the high profile case exposes of the past few years. These include the gene therapy death at the University of Pennsylvania that involved a significant conflict of interest by the lead investigator and the several major research institutions that had their Federal Wide Assurance suspended for conducting studies on human subjects because of deficiencies in protecting the subjects from real or potential harm. However, few members of the research community are aware of recent studies suggesting that authorship disputes, conflicts of interest, misrepresentation of credentials, and other questionable research practices are more common than suspected.

In its 1992 report, "Responsible Science," the National Academy of Sciences (NAS) coined the concept of "questionable research practices" to describe actions by scientists that "violate the traditional values of the research enterprise"[19] but fall short of research misconduct. NAS further opined that these practices deserve attention "because they can erode confidence in the integrity of the research process, violate traditions associated with science, affect scientific conclusions, waste time and resources, and weaken the education of new scientists."[20] (For a more detailed discussion of this report, see Chapter 50.) The NAS report identified the following specific activities as questionable research practices:

1. Failing to retain significant research data for a reasonable period;

2. Maintaining inadequate research records, especially for results that are published or relied upon by others;

3. Conferring or requesting authorship on the basis of a specialized service or contribution that is not significantly related to the research reported in the paper;

4. Refusing to give peers reasonable access to unique research materials or data that support published papers;

5. Using inappropriate statistical or other methods of measurement to enhance the significance of research findings;

6. Inadequately supervising research subordinates or exploiting them; and,

7. Misrepresenting speculations as fact or releasing preliminary research results, especially in the public media, without providing sufficient data to allow peers to judge the validity of the results or to reproduce the experiments.[21]

There is a substantial overlap between the areas identified by the NAS as areas where questionable research practices may occur and the core areas in the PHS policy that warrant RCR education. These areas include: data management, mentor/trainee relationships, publication and authorship issues, and collaborative science. Unreported conflicts of interest, disclosure of confidential material obtained during peer review, and violations of rules covering human and animal subjects could also constitute questionable research practices. An important goal of RCR education is to promote the responsible conduct of research and discourage research misconduct and questionable research practices through education and awareness. The increasing complexity of research, including federal, state, and institutional policies and regulations on responsible research practices, make such education and awareness more important than ever.

A review of the scientific literature and case reports from ORI's database and that of other sources suggests that the incidence of questionable research practices may be greater than realized. Kalichman and Eastwood surveyed graduate students and postdoctorate fellows and found that, based on self reports, a significant number would select, modify, or omit data for a paper or grant application, or add honorary authors, to get published or funded (see Table 43-1).[22,23]

Several studies have shown that applicants for research fellowships would falsely represent the status of their publications in order to increase their chances of selection. The misrepresentation ranges from bogus articles to inflating author rank (see Table 43-2).[31,32,33,34,35]

Other studies suggest that duplicate publication may occur 5% to 10% of time. This may give a false impression of productivity and waste resources of reviewers, editors, and journals. In particular, such duplicate publication in clinical studies may lead to false conclusions about the efficacy of treatments or drugs by increasing the apparent size of successful studies (see Table 43-3).

A recent study published in Nature by Martinson et al., reported data on self-reports by early (postdoctorate) fellows and mid-career scientists (those who had already received their first R01 grants) on a variety of scientific behaviors, either

TABLE 43-1	Self-Reported Attitudes Toward Misconduct	
Action	1992 Kalichman[24]	1996 Eastwood[25]
Past misconduct (yes/no?)	15.1%	12%
Future misconduct (yes/no?)	14.8%	—
Modify data for paper	7.3%	15%
Fabricate data for a paper or grant application	1.3%	2%
Select or omit data for paper or grant application	14.2%	27%
List an undeserving author	—	41%

TABLE 43-2	Misrepresentation in Medical Resident Training Program Applications				
Author Speciality	1995 Sekas Gastro-Enterology[26]	1996 Gurudevan Emergency Medicine[27]	1997 Panicek Radiology[28]	1998 Bilge Pediatrics[29]	1999 Dale Orthopedic[30]
Total Applications	236	350	201	404	213
with citations	53 (22%)	113 (32%)	87 (43%)	147 (36%)	64 (30%)
misrepresented	16 (30%)	23 (20%)	14 (15%)	29 (20%)	11 (17%)
Total Citations	—	276	261	410	76
misrepresented	—	44 (16%)	39 (15%)	41 (10%)	14 (18%)
Research experience	138 (59%)	—	—	—	—
not confirmed	47 (34%)	—	—	—	—

actual research misconduct or questionable research practices that do not meet the normative behavior expected by the scientific community or the public. While some of the questions asked in the study can be criticized for ambiguity, thus raising doubts about the meaning or significance of the results, overall the results indicate that the rate of questionable scientific practice in areas such as dropping data points based on a "gut feeling" (15%), inappropriately assigning authorship credit (10%), inadequate record keeping (27%), publishing the same data in two or more publications (5%), also referred to as duplicate publication, and overlooking others' use of flawed data or questionable interpretation of data (13%) gives legitimate cause for concern. This suggests that improved graduate education in appropriate scientific practices and better training by principal investigators of young scientists in the lab, especially in the areas of data management, interpretation, and reporting, is warranted.[36]

Data from ORI case files and the Harvard Medical School ombuds program suggest that disputes over authorship, disputes over credit and intellectual property, and other research issues may be widespread in the research community. Since

ORI began operation in June 1992, it has reviewed over 2400 putative allegations of scientific misconduct. Approximately 25 percent of those allegations, or about 600, were found by ORI to constitute disputes over authorship, intellectual property, or credit that did not fall with the PHS definition of scientific misconduct. Based on ORI's experiences in reviewing these allegations and discussions with institutional officials, it is estimated that hundreds of additional disputes of similar kind arise at the research institutions annually without ever coming to ORI's attention.

In this regard, ORI notes that the Harvard ombuds program reported in its annual report for the year 2001 to 2002 that it handled 129 research issues brought by forward by the Harvard staff. Research issues are defined by the ombuds program as "issues related to intellectual property, proprietorship of work, authorship, conflict of interest, professional misconduct, misrepresentations of data, protocol error, plagiarism, etc."[37] Research issues constituted 19% of the issues brought to the ombuds program that year. The data for 2002–2003 were similar, with 130 research issues, also comprising 19% of the disputes brought forward. In 2003–2004, the total research issues

TABLE 43-3	Duplicate Publication		
Study	Journal	Articles	Duplicate %
Waldron (1992)	BMJ	354 published	6–12%
Barnard (1993)	NTvG	172 published	11%
Koene (1994)	NTvG	108 rejected	4%
Blancett (1995)	INJS	642 published	9%
Bloemenkamp (1999)	NTvG	148 published	7%
Rennie (1999)	JAMA	Case Study	23% over-estimate of research effect

Source: The three tables just presented are based largely on a literature review, "Assessing the Integrity of Publicly Funded Research," prepared for ORI by Nicholas H. Steneck, Ph.D.

brought forward was 134, constituting 18% of the total issues.

NIH also has an active ombuds program for dealing with scientific disputes as well as other matters. Due to a major database problem a few years back, NIH does not have specific statistics to provide. However, based on a direct communication with Howard Gadlin, who heads up the ombuds program, it is estimated that the NIH ombuds program handled 600 cases overall in the past year, with about 33% dealing with research-related issues. Estimated frequency of issue categories addressed are that about 50% involve mentoring issues, 30% relate to authorship, a smaller number reflect intellectual property issues (including sharing of biological materials), and potential misconduct issues are under 10%.[38] Overall, the evidence suggests that there are enough research integrity problems to warrant greater efforts by the research community in promoting responsible research practices both in the institution at large and in the individual labs.

Key Features of the Proposed PHS Policy and Current Status

Now that we have discussed the historical, philosophical, and evidentiary background for RCR education, we will briefly review some of the key features of the proposed PHS policy announced in 2000. While this policy is an historical document and not binding, it provides guidance for those research institutions that are considering adopting or modifying RCR education programs.

The policy includes a basic requirement that research institutions adopt and implement an education program for all research staff working on PHS-supported projects and that education programs for research staff be established to include nine core subject areas of RCR instruction (data acquisition, management, sharing, and ownership; mentor/trainee responsibilities; publication practices and responsible authorship; peer review; collaborative science; human subjects; research involving animals; research misconduct; and conflict of interest and commitment). While some institutions may decide to provide a basic level of instruction in all of these areas to research staff covered by the policy, they are not required to for any areas that are not applicable to their staff. For example, researchers working only on basic science would not be required to have instruction on human and animal subject issues. The PHS policy

also provides a brief description of subtopics under each core area, included as an appendix to this chapter. This list of topics is suggestive only; the institution retains discretion in determining the exact content of instruction in the core areas.

In addition to the areas of discretion discussed above, the PHS policy provides flexibility to the institution in implementing the policy in the following ways:

1. The policy requires only a basic level of instruction. The institution determines the exact content, length, level, and method of instruction consistent with the policy. A demonstration of competency by recipients of instruction is optional with the institution.

2. The institution determines the method of documenting that instruction has occurred.

3. While the policy recommends that institutions consider offering RCR instruction to all research staff at the institution, including those not supported by PHS support, this is optional.

4. The PHS policy recommends that the institution consider providing instruction to departmental and sponsored research/administrative staff and other support staff with instruction relevant to their jobs and roles in the research enterprise.[39]

While ORI recommends the use of case studies, hands-on experience and the active participation of principal investigators (PIs) to provide effective and meaningful RCR education that improves the capacity of the individual scientist, the lab, and the institution at large to conduct ethical, quality research, this level of effort is not required by the PHS policy. The policy provides that an acceptable educational activity includes reading a self-study guide; attending a lecture, formal course, workshop, or seminar; or working through a CD-ROM or Internet program.

ORI Resources for RCR

In order to ensure that adequate resources are available to those institutions that want to adopt RCR educational programs, ORI has developed its own "ORI Introduction to the Responsible Conduct of Research" for use by institutions as they deem appropriate. This booklet can be purchased from the Government Printing Office or downloaded from the ORI Web site; it is accessible at http://ori.hhs.gov/publications/ori_intro_text.shtml.[40] In addition, ORI has posted 20 educational programs on its Web site. They were developed by research institutions under the ORI RCR Development Program. All of the nine core areas of RCR are covered and some topics have two or more products each.

ORI established the RCR Development Program in 2002 to provide up to $25,000 in funding to research institutions to support development of RCR curricula materials at the institution. As a condition of funding, the institution must agree to make the curricula available to all PHS-funded research institutions free or at nominal charge. In the first four years, forty-nine contracts were made to support a variety of programs covering all nine core areas, such as human subject protections and conflicts of interest, case studies, and other topics in a variety of formats and approaches. Most of these materials are still under development. In year three of this program, ORI asked applicants to submit more ambitious proposals that focus on identifying, developing, and providing instruction on specific skills and abilities needed in the responsible conduct of research. Efforts to develop curricula materials on RCR that can be used in basic science courses (e.g., statistics, research design, methodology, and hypothesis development and testing) are also encouraged. ORI also established a cooperative agreement program with the Association of American Medical Colleges to provide funding to academic and scientific societies to undertake initiatives in research integrity and responsible research. The first year of funding was 2003 and thirty-two awards have been made to twenty-seven societies for projects ranging from meetings or conferences on research integrity and RCR to development of guidelines. The full list of awards and contracts made is on the ORI Web site under http://ori.dhhs.gov/education/rdp.shtml[42] and http://ori.dhhs.gov/education/pas.shtml.[43] ORI also funded a Web-based resource on RCR for several years through the University of California, San Diego, to provide instructional resources to RCR teachers and trainers. This educational resource can now be accessed at http://rcrec.org/r/index.php.[44] This site provides a variety of tools and resources on RCR topics, including the nine core areas from the PHS policy, case studies, research guidelines, and links to other resources. Originally designed to provide information that allows institutions to develop their own RCR courses, the site now also provides links to variety of existing RCR courses and resources that can be adopted by individual instructors or institutions.

Most recently, ORI has funded the Council of Graduate Schools to support RCR education programs at ten graduate schools. Twenty-five additional schools have affiliate programs.[45]

Activities by NIH and CDC

Following suspension of the PHS policy, both NIH and the Centers for Disease Control (CDC) decided to go ahead with implementation of RCR education for their thousands of intramural scientists. CDC had actually created an RCR education program entitled "Scientific Ethics" for its intramural scientists before announcement of the PHS policy. However, it did not cover all the nine core areas that ultimately ended up in the proposed policy. In 2003, CDC updated this program by adding modules on the remaining RCR core areas. The training is required for all intramural scientists submitting protocols for IRB review. Free copies of the CDC program are available in CD-ROM format from Fran Reid-Sanden, MS, CIP, PH Educator, CDC/OD/OCSO/OSRS, 1600 Clifton Road, N.E. (MSD-73), Atlanta, GA 30333; 404-371-5396; 404-371-5988 (fax); fsanden@cdc.gov.[46]

At this time, CDC continues to require training in human subjects protections for all new IRB members and administrative staff.

NIH began providing RCR instruction to its intramural scientists in 2001 by discussing case studies in a small group format. New case studies were used in subsequent years. See http://www1.od.nih.gov/oir/sourcebook/ResEthicsCases/nih-policy.htm. Later, NIH developed a Web-based overview of the nine core areas as required training for all intramural scientists. NIH has now made this program available to the extramural community, and it can be accessed at http://researchethics.od.nih.gov/.[47]

RCR Activity at Research Institutions

RCR activity at PHS-funded research institutions has increased considerably since the proposed PHS policy was announced in 2000. Based on a review of Web-based RCR programs at research institutions and numerous discussions with institutional officials, ORI believes that more institutions offer RCR programs to more scientists, students, and postdoctorate fellows than ever before. However, the number of institutions that provide mandatory training for PHS-supported researchers is still a small percentage of the approximately 4,000 PHS funded institutions. Nevertheless, a number of substantial RCR programs have been developed, and many institutions are willing to make them available to other PHS funded institutions without charge. Several of these programs are posted on the

ORI Web site and may be accessed by research institutions and other members of the public. These are not the only programs, nor necessarily the best. Inclusion on the list should not be considered an endorsement, but rather a sample of what is currently available.

Another important initiative related to RCR was the NIH's June 5, 2000 announcement that all human subject investigators submitting research grant applications or contract proposals to NIH beginning October 1, 2000, or receiving new or noncompeting awards would have to participate in an education program on protections for human subjects. The NIH policy provides that all "key personnel" (defined as all individuals responsible for the design and conduct of the study) involved in the proposed research have to receive training in human subjects protection and that the education received would have to be described in a cover letter. After October 1, 2000, investigators were required to include descriptions of such education in annual progress reports. The NIH requirement for human subjects protections training remains in effect and requires documentation of the education for each investigator involved in the design and conduct of NIH-funded human subjects research. That documentation must be provided prior to the award and applies to both nonexempt human subjects research and exempt human subjects research.[48]

Institutions and clinical researchers have been participating in human subjects education programs for a few years now, and many institutions have developed their own programs for such education or participated in programs developed by others, such as the CITI program developed by the University of Miami (www.Miami.Edu/Citireg).[49] In addition, NIH provided new resources to many of the larger research institutions to provide enhancements for human subject protections in 2002 and 2003. In the second year, institutions were required to collaborate with other institutions to share resources, expertise, and products developed under the award. New educational programs related to human subject protections were eligible for funding as part of this program.[50]

The Office of Human Research Protections also recommends training in human subjects protections for institutional "assurance" officials (the individual who signs the federal wide assurance for human subjects protections), institutional review board chairs, and IRB staff. Tutorials for these individuals are located on the OHRP website (www.hhs.gov/ohrp) and a CD-ROM tutorial for investigator training in human subjects protection is available free of charge to those institutions that have an assurance with OHRP.[51]

Issues and Opportunities for Institutions

Although there is substantial agreement in the research community that RCR education is important to provide a basic level of knowledge for all PHS-funded researchers on scientific norms, good research practices, and regulatory requirements, many institutions are not ready to endorse mandatory training for all research staff. This is particularly true for educating senior scientists, but in many cases also applies to training for postdoctorate fellows and graduate students that are not supported by training grants. In deciding whether to implement an RCR education program, institutions will have several important decisions to make, such as:

- Should the institution provide a basic education or a more detailed, comprehensive program? Should it create a customized program for its students, research trainees, faculty, and others or use an off-the-shelf program?
- Should RCR education be provided only to staff on PHS funded research projects or include researchers funded by all sources?
- Should the institution require RCR education only for defined research staff or all staff working on the research project?
- Should an RCR program be developed to meet the specialized needs of auxiliary staff, such as departmental and sponsored research/administrative staff and other support staff or just focus on the core research staff who have direct and substantive involvement in the research?
- Should students and research trainees receive the same RCR education provided to more experienced researchers, or should it be more detailed and comprehensive and perhaps different in other ways, as well?
- Should unique RCR resources be provided for unusual or unique programs at the institution where more generic approaches do not seem to fit?

The answers to these questions vary with the needs of the institution, the fiscal and staff resources of the institution, its educational philosophy, and other factors. Over time, ORI expects that multiple options for implementing RCR programs will develop at the several thousand institutions that receive PHS research support. ORI will continue to provide resources to support RCR tools, curricula, and other materials and will publicize them on the ORI Web site as they become available. Many institutions will choose to adopt existing resources to fulfill their RCR needs but others will create their own Web-based or didactic programs. Specialization and customization is expected to flourish over time as new resources and materials become available and institutions find that more unique approaches are needed to serve their interests.

RCR as a Quality Improvement Program

For those institutions with the fiscal and staffing capacity to mount a more ambitious effort, the author encourages institutions to think about RCR education in a more systemic and strategic way. Instead of just focusing on basic knowledge transfer of regulatory requirements and scientific norms related to RCR, the institution could consider ways that RCR education can be used to benefit the individual scientist in improving his or her skills, how it can improve the productivity of the lab, and improve the overall quality of research conducted by the institution. As mentioned earlier, the IOM recommends that RCR education be designed to develop skills and abilities of investigators to identify and respond to ethical conflicts in appropriate and ethical ways. In ORI's experience in discussing RCR issues with investigators, many researchers have not received formal instruction in certain research skills or techniques that are needed to conduct and report quality research but are also relevant to the responsible conduct of research and research integrity.

It is important to consider, for example, how a student, trainee, or young scientist can learn to determine which data can be legitimately excluded when interpreting and reporting research results. Some situations are relatively clear (e.g., the project fails when the wrong catalyst is added to the experiment and all the data is tossed out). However, what about dropping individual data points that conflict with the hypothesis? The temptation to develop a "ruse" for dropping the offending data may be too strong for some to resist (see Kalichman[52] and Eastwood,[53] who suggest that many researchers would change the data for the benefit of getting published or funded). How can lab chiefs, faculty, and other senior investigators educate developing scientists in fair, consistent, and logical decisions in making these determinations? Failure to learn these skills not only harms the individual scientist, but has the potential to harm the scientific community at large and under-

mine the quality of research that gets published and relied on by other scientists and the public.

Similar responsible conduct and research quality issues are raised by:

- Potential conflicts of interest that may bias interpretations but are not disclosed or managed.
- Use of statistical techniques that improve the significance of reported results but are not appropriate for the type of research conducted or the methodology used.
- Approval by IRBs or institutional officials of research designs that place human subjects at risk but are not likely to result in usable data because the design is inappropriate for the type of research conducted or the research protocol is seriously flawed.

Thus, in developing RCR education programs, ORI encourages institutions to consider the relationship between RCR, the development of important skills and abilities in investigators, and the quality of research conducted, reported, and supported by the institution. This is certainly not an easy job, but this approach should benefit the individual scientists, the labs, and the institution by improving effectiveness, quality, and morale and making RCR education really meaningful.

The author believes that over time, this type of skill based RCR education would improve research quality because it improves the interpretation and reporting of data, reduces bias in conducting and reporting research, reduces conflicts over authorship disputes, and raises the morale and productivity of lab members because of greater consensus concerning data practices, authorship, and other RCR matters.

Special Issues for Research Administrators

Research administrators of all levels of experience and seniority have an opportunity to play an important role in implementation of RCR programs at their institutions. Most institutions will ask senior research administrators to work with the research staff in designing and implementing the institution's RCR program, whether that program develops unique curricula materials and methods or selects existing resources to provide the RCR education. Furthermore, the institution often turns to the research administrative staff to monitor internal implementation of the RCR program and to make sure that key goals are met. The responsibility or coordinating role may be assigned to staff in the vice president for research office. Occasionally administrative staff at the college, school, departmental, and sometimes laboratory level are also asked to play a role in RCR education.

Research administrators can also get involved with the RCR education program in a variety of other ways. For example, administrators can help design and present curricula materials on RCR issues for administrative and support staff. Research administrators should be knowledgeable about federal requirements and institutional policies regarding RCR education to help the institution ensure that it is properly administering the RCR program. Research administrators may also be able to co-present with researchers and others on those topics and compliance issues that arise out of the federal requirements and institutional policies. In order to understand the needs and challenges of the researchers themselves, research administrators may want to participate in the RCR program for the regular research staff to ensure that they are aware of the RCR basics from the researchers' viewpoint.

By being involved in developing and implementing the RCR program and aware of the content of the institution's program, the research administrator will become knowledgeable about this important part of the research environment at the institution and better able to assist the institution and individual researchers to conduct high quality, productive, and responsible research.

Conclusion

Issuance of the proposed PHS policy has spurred many new institutional and academic efforts to establish and implement RCR education programs. However, many institutions are waiting for a consensus to develop in the research community before deciding whether to initiate or expand RCR efforts or make them mandatory for research staff. Whatever the final outcome of this process, the author encourages institutions, scientific associations and societies, and individual scientists to embrace RCR education as a core element of a quality education in good science and to move forward with implementation of RCR programs without further delay. A rare opportunity is upon us to create a more responsible and productive research enterprise for years to come. It is time to move forward.

Author's Note

The opinions expressed herein are those of the author and do not necessarily represent the views of the Office of Research Integrity, the US Department of Health and Human Services, or any other federal agency.

• • • References

1. "PHS Policy for Instruction in the Responsible Conduct of Research," notice of announcement of final, 65 *Federal Register* 76647, December 7, 2000.
2. "PHS Policy on Instruction of the Responsible Conduct of Research," notice of suspension of, 66 *Federal Register* 11032, February 21, 2001.
3. "PHS Policies on Research Misconduct," 42 *Code of Federal Regulations* 93.300(c), *Federal Register* 70, 28378, May 17, 2005.
4. 42 CFR 93.300(c), 2005.
5. Swazey, J. P., and Bird, S. J. "Teaching and Learning Research Ethics," *Professional Ethics* 4 (1995):155–178.
6. Institute of Medicine (IOM). "Integrity in Scientific Research: Creating an Environment that Promotes Responsible Conduct." Washington, D.C., National Research Council of the National Academics, 2002, p. 9.
7. National Institutes of Health. "Reminder and Update: Requirement for Instruction in the Responsible Conduct of Research for Institutional National Research Service Award (NRSA) Research Training Grants." *NIH Guide* 23, No. 23 (June 17, 1994): 2.
8. Mastroianni, A. C., and Kahn, J. P. "Encouraging Accountability in Research: A Pilot Assessment of Training Efforts." *Accountability in Research* 7 (1999): 85–100.
9. Institute of Medicine. "The Responsible Conduct of Research in the Health Sciences." 1989, p. 30.
10. Institute of Medicine, 1989.
11. National Academy of Sciences. *Responsible Science: Ensuring the Integrity of the Research Process.* Washington, DC: National Academy Press, 1992, p. 13.
12. National Academy of Sciences, 1992, p. 14.
13. U.S. Department of Health and Human Services. "Integrity and Misconduct in Research." Report of the Commission on Research Integrity, 1995, p. 18.
14. U.S. Department of Health and Human Services, 1995, p. 18.

15. U.S. Department of Health and Human Services, 1995, p. 18.
16. U.S. Department of Health and Human Services, 1995, p. 17.
17. Institute of Medicine, 2002, pp. 84–85.
18. Institute of Medicine, 2002, pp. 90, 96.
19. Institute of Medicine, 2002, p. 28.
20. Institute of Medicine, 2002, p. 28.
21. Institute of Medicine, 2002, p. 28.
22. Kalichman, M. W., and Friedman, P. J. "A Pilot Study of Biomedical Trainees' Perceptions Concerning Research Ethics." *Academic Medicine* 67 (1992): 769–775.
23. Eastwood, S. et al. "Ethical Issues in Biomedical Research: Perceptions and Practices of Post Doctoral Research Fellows Responding to a Survey." *Science and Engineering Ethics* 2 (1996): 89–106.
24. Eastwood et al., 1996.
25. Eastwood et al., 1996.
26. Sekas, G., and Hutson, W. R. "Misrepresentation of Academic Accomplishments by Applicants for Gastroenterology Fellowships." *Annals of Internal Medicine* 123 (1995): 38–41.
27. Gurudevan, S. V., and Mower, W. R. "Misrepresentation of Research Publications among Emergency Residency Applicants." *Annals of Emergency Medicine* 27 (1996): 327–330.
28. Panicek, D. M., Schwartz, L. H., Dershaw, D. D., et al. "Mispresentation of Publications by Applicants for Radiology Fellowships: Is It a Problem?" *Academic Medicine* 74 (1998): 221–230.
29. Bilge, A., Shugerman, R. P., and Robertson, W. O. "Mispresesentation of Authorship by Applicants to Pediatrics Training Programs." *Academic Medicine* 73 (1998): 532–533.
30. Dale, J. A., Schmitt, C. M., and Crosby, L. A. "Misrepresentation of Research Criteria by Orthopaedic Residency Applicants." *Journal of Bone and Joint Surgery* 81 (1999): 1679–1681.
31. Sekas and Hutson, 1995.
32. Gurudevan and Mower, 1996.
33. Panicek, Schwartz, Dershaw, et al., 1998.
34. Bilge, Shugerman, and Robertson, 1998.
35. Dale, Schmitt, and Crosby, 1999.
36. Martinson, B. C., Anderson, M. S., and DeVries, R. "Scientists Behaving Badly." *Nature* 435 (2005): 737–738.
37. Harvard Medical School Ombuds Office. "Annual Reports for 2001–2004," available from Linda Wilcox, Ombudsperson, at Linda Wilcox@hms.harvard.edu. (For more information, see http://www.hms.harvard.edu/ombuds/).
38. Gadlin, H., NIH Ombudsman. Personal communication to the author on June 21, 2005.
39. Public Health Service. "Policy on Instruction in the Responsible Conduct of Research (RCR)," December 1, 2000, available at http://ori.dhhs.gov/policies/RCR_Policy.shtml (accessed October 21, 2005).
40. Steneck, N. H., for the DHHS. "ORI Introduction to the Responsible Conduct of Research," 2004. Available at http://ori.dhhs.gov/ education/rcr_intro_text.shtml (accessed October 10, 2005).
41. ORI. "RCR Educational Resources," 2005. Available at http://ori.dhhs.gov/education/rcr_resources.shtml (accessed October 10, 2005).
42. ORI. "RCR Resource Development Program," 2005. Available at http://ori.dhhs.gov/education/rdp.shtml (accessed October 10, 2005).
43. ORI. "RCR Program for Academic Societies," 2005. Available at http://ori.dhhs.gov/education/pas.shtml (accessed October 10, 2005).
44. Kalichman, M. "Online Resource for RCR Instructors," 2004. Available at http://rcrec.org/r/index.php (accessed October 10, 2005).
45. ORI. "RCR Program with the Council of Graduate Schools." Available at http://www.cgsnet.org/ProgramsServices/conductresearch.htm (accessed October 10, 2005).
46. CDC. "Scientific Ethics: An RCR Education Program," 2003, available in CD-Rom format from Fran Reid-Sanden, MS, CIP, PH Educator, CDC, OD/OCSO/OSRS, 1600 Clifton Road, N.E. (MSD-73), Atlanta, GA 30333, 404-371-5396, 404-371-5988 (fax), fsanden@cdc.gov.
47. NIH. "RCR Education Program for Intramural Scientists," 2005. Accessible to the public at http://researchethics.od.nih.gov/ (accessed October 10, 2005).
48. NIH. "NIH Guide: Required Education in the Protection of Human Research Participants." June 5, 2000, revised August 25, 2000 (OD-00-039, revised August 25, 2000. http://grants2.nih.gov/grants/guide/notice-files/NOT-OD-00-039.html (accessed October 21, 2005).
49. University of Miami. "Collaborative IRB Training Initiative," 2005. Available at http://Miami.edu/citireg/ (accessed October 10, 2005).
50. NIH. "NIH Guide: Human Subjects Enhancements Program." RFA: OD-02-003, March 5, 2002.
51. OHRP. "Human Subjects Educational Materials," 2005. Accessible at http://www.hhs.gov/ohrp/education/#materials (accessed October 10, 2005).
52. Kalichman, 1992.
53. Eastwood et al., 1996

43-A

Description of Core Instructional Areas

---

1. Data Acquisition, Management, Sharing, and Ownership

   Accepted practices for acquiring and maintaining research data. Proper methods for record keeping and electronic data collection and storage in scientific research include defining what constitutes data, keeping data notebooks or electronic files, data privacy and confidentiality, data selection, retention, sharing, ownership, and analysis, and legal requirements affecting the collection and use of data.

2. Mentor and Trainee Relationships

   The responsibilities of mentors and trainees in predoctoral and postdoctoral research programs; this includes the selection, role, and responsibilities of a mentor, potential conflicts between mentor and trainee, collaboration and competition, and abusing the mentor and trainee relationship.

3. Collaborative Research

   Research collaborations and issues that may arise from such collaborations, including setting ground rules early in the collaboration, avoiding authorship disputes, and the sharing of materials and information with internal and external collaborating scientists.

4. Publication Practices and Responsible Authorship

   The purpose and importance of scientific publication and the responsibilities of the authors, which includes collaborative work and assigning appropriate credit, acknowledgments, appropriate citations, repetitive publications, fragmentary publication, sufficient description of methods, corrections, and retractions; conventions for deciding upon authors; author responsibilities; and the pressure to publish.

5. Peer Review

   The purpose of peer review in determining merit for research funding and publications, which includes how peer review works, editorial boards and ad hoc reviews, responsibilities of the reviewers, impartiality, confidentiality, and disclosure; and resolution of potential conflicts of interest.

6. Conflict of Interest and Conflict of Commitment

   Identifying, disclosing, managing, and resolving conflicts of interest and commitment. Types of conflicts encountered by researchers and institutions include those associated with collaborators, publication, financial conflicts, obligations to other constituencies, and other types of conflicts.

7. Research Misconduct

   The definition of research misconduct and the regulations, policies, and guidelines that govern the handling of research misconduct allegations involving researchers at PHS-funded institutions. These include: fabrication, falsification, and plagiarism; error vs. intentional misconduct; institutional misconduct policies; identifying misconduct, procedures for reporting misconduct; conducting misconduct inquiries and investigations; protection of whistleblowers; and institutional and federal responses to findings of misconduct.

8. Human Subjects

   Issues important in conducting research involving human subjects. Includes topics such as the definition of human subjects research, ethical principles for conducting human subjects research, informed consent, confidentiality and privacy of data and patient records, risks and benefits, preparation of a research protocol, institutional review boards, adherence to study protocol, proper conduct of the study, and special protections for targeted populations, e.g., children, minorities, and the elderly.

9. Research Involving Animals

Issues important to conducting research involving animals. These include: definition of research involving animals, ethical principles for conducting research on animals, federal regulations governing animal research, institutional animal care and use committees, and treatment of animals.

44

Developing a Research Compliance Program

Daniel Vasgird, PhD, CIP, and Ellen Hyman-Browne, JD, LLM, MPH

Introduction

Over the last decade, research compliance and the responsible conduct of research have received increasing attention and responsive action from the scientific community. The broad forces behind that heightened consideration are the increasing potential rewards that can be garnered from innovation and the changing scale of research. The more specific driving factors are an increase in regulatory requirements; the influence of publicized compliance breakdowns at institutions of higher education; and heightened scrutiny from the media, advocacy groups, and government. An added element is the idealistic desire of many scientists to attain a high ethical standard while practicing what many perceive as humanity's best hope for advancement to a more supportive and fulfilling existence, namely the scientific enterprise. The practical side of all this reflection and action can be summarized in a line from the recent National Academies publication *Integrity in Scientific Research*: "The public will support science only if it can trust the scientists and institutions that conduct research." [1]

With these basic motivating forces in mind, it is easy to understand why many academic research institutions are looking for effective ways to foster and promote a culture of research integrity. This is not to say that these institutions have not supported the ideal of research integrity in the past, but the transmission of standards was done more informally, for the most part through mentoring and routine administrative activity. The present, more formal approaches are simply an acknowledgement that the stakes are higher with today's high levels of funding, the intensity of competition, and the related increased levels of litigation and enforcement risk. Even in the past, mentoring could be inconsistent, but now the scale of research activities can make contact between researchers and their trainees very limited. What has emerged are two realizations: many researchers need and want assistance and research institutions themselves simply cannot afford to merely hope that in some indefinable way compliance and integrity are fostered within the institution's walls.

The Columbia Experience

The story of Columbia University's response to this changing compliance environment is an instructive one. The Columbia University Office for Responsible Conduct of Research (ORCR) evolved out of growing concern with compliance issues coupled with a new paradigm of oversight at Columbia. The objective was to have the individual schools and their research communities largely implement and oversee their own compliance activities. The philosophy was one of local support and problem-solving. Operational decisions would be made close to research activity, but ORCR was to offer central advisory and educational support to aid each school in this. Expected benefits from this collaborative approach were an increase in personal involvement with responsible research for those actually doing the work and avoidance of the sense of external policing that can undercut that kind of individual responsibility.

Although Columbia, like most institutions, had been attentive to issues of responsible conduct of research and federal enforcement for many years, the chain of events leading to the creation of the ORCR began with a comprehensive risk assessment exercise carried out by Columbia's internal audit office in collaboration with the university's external auditors. That risk assessment appropriately identified a range of regulatory compliance issues for attention in research administration and in other areas. The resulting development of a billing compliance program in the university's clinical practice plans provided an example of how a significant division of the university, the medical center, could mobilize itself to address existing compliance challenges. In that case, the mobilization involved the creation of a central compliance office for billing headed by an officer with a dotted-line reporting relationship to the chief financial officer of the university and, through him, to the audit committee of the trustees. The direct line of reporting was to the senior associate dean of the Columbia University Medical Center and through him to the dean of medicine. This structure demonstrated that a compliance structure could be locally based but responsive and accountable to direction from the center of the university.

Another example of a model for securing local compliance in a decentralized organization was the university's preparation for the Y2K transition. The challenge was to establish a standard of preparation for conversion to Y2K compliance that could both be carried forward by individual operating units and simultaneously monitored from the center. In addition, it was necessary to create a set of requirements that were flexible enough to accommodate the different operating styles and structures of different parts of the university in a way that would facilitate something getting done as opposed to wasting energy on battles over structure, all the while reaching an effective level of compliance or readiness.

In 1999 these two initiatives were the important background to a series of conversations in the university regarding achieving greater focus on research compliance issues and reassuring the leadership of the university and the trustees that research compliance issues were being addressed university-wide.

The research compliance working group assembled by the executive vice president for finance in consultation with the provost was composed of a dozen people, including outstanding researchers from chemistry and medicine, as well as the deans of schools with heavy research involvement. What emerged from the conversations was a model for activism, which basically matched a decentralized model of the university. It was agreed that the most useful form of support for researchers dealing with responsible conduct of research was to provide the support locally in a school. The dean of each school needed to be accountable for the progress of the school in addressing these concerns, and a central structure for support and monitoring of what was needed. The idea was to do this by having a central office with no operating role, but rather with the advocacy, educational, advisory and, to a certain extent, monitoring role necessary to interface with the responsible individuals identified with research in the schools. The deans, knowing local practice and culture, would best be able to devise structures that would work in each school.

The trustees were briefed as the process continued, and eventually they endorsed the creation of a central research compliance office which, when finally established, was called the Office for Responsible Conduct of Research. The philosophy of that central office was for it not to have an operating role but to serve as a critical resource and catalyst in encouraging the creation of appropriate structures and commitments regarding research in each school. These, in turn, would embody a major theme that emerged in the planning process: that compliance, if thought of as a rigid monitoring and enforcement activity, would be far less effective than if envisioned as a more collaborative venture in problem-solving at the local level, with involvement from the central university taking the form of advice and education. Therefore, a critical part of the philosophy that evolved was that the role for ORCR ought to be that of a supportive, central resource gaining credibility through partnering with local research communities.

The relationship between ORCR and internal audit needed to be addressed. On the one hand internal audit shouldn't be involved in advocacy and planning, because that would lead to a conflict in appraising university compliance structures, while on the other hand, the ORCR shouldn't play a monitoring role, since that would be better served by internal audit.

The demands on the ORCR in this model are multiple: remain abreast of research precedent and regulation, advise and collaborate with diverse individuals and groups, and find ways to provide palatable and effective education and support without seeming overregulatory. It must be remembered that ultimately ORCR's raison d'etre was to create an environment in which responsible research was standard practice. To that end ORCR has, as one of its governing tenets, the idea that responsibility is not just institutional but also local. Most important was creating contact with the practitioners, actively making a very visible and concerted effort to reach all individuals within the university who are involved with research. The objective is to insure that researchers have an ethical involvement in their own work. As many philosophers will state, the only successful ethical systems are those that the practitioners adopt as their own.

The General Planning Process for a Research Compliance Program

There is no generic, one-size-fits-all compliance program that every organization can adopt. The two main variables in research compliance programs are content and structure, which substantive areas the program will cover, and how the program will be organized and operate. Existing programs reflect so many different responses to these variables because of the distinctiveness of the institutional features that determine the nature of an effective program. To borrow a slightly revised favorite saying of Allan Shipp, Director of Outreach at the NIH Office of Biotechnology Activities, "When you've seen one research compliance program, you've seen *one* research compliance program."[2]

It is essential that the research compliance program be designed with attention to the *fit* of the program with the institution as the Columbia model illustrates. Care in the initial planning process is worth the investment of time, however, as the right approach can generate widespread support for the program and also thwart the kinds of problems that result in injury, litigation, enforcement actions, or bad press.

Every organization's history, culture, and existing structures and systems are unique. Organizations are likely to have in place numerous administrative departments and committees with varying degrees of responsibility for the research process. The culture of an organization may be conducive to highly centralized decision making, or it may favor local control within departments. It should be asked:

- Are existing policies and procedures institution-wide or specific to schools and departments? Is there a tradition of decentralized management?

- Are there venues that bring administrators together?

It is important to reflect on the circumstances unique to each institution, and it is crucial to keep in mind that effective compliance grows out of internalization of values.

Equally distinctive is the organization's impetus for establishing a program, and the priorities and justifications that the program is intended to address. Every program is developed in response to a certain state of affairs based on an institution's experience with regulatory problems, awareness of certain risks, motivation to be proactive, or tradition of institutional values. It follows that every program should be designed to address the key organizational issues and priorities: fulfilling the terms of an agency settlement, reducing financial risk, building and maintaining trust, and promoting core institutional values. The legal and regulatory context in which the organization operates will shape program decisions, as does the institutional context. Other determining factors include the size and complexity of the organization; the extent of available resources; the scope and volume of the research program; and how quickly the research program is growing (and in what directions).

The best way to ensure that the design of the program has taken all these factors into account is to employ a planning process that is inclusive of those most interested in and affected by these issues (senior level officials, administrators, and faculty including the general counsel, finance, internal audit, and the operational research units of the organization). It is critical in the planning process to articulate both the organization's priorities and the criteria for success, and to do so in a way that generates support while managing expectations and moving the agenda forward.

The Functional Elements of a Compliance Program

Aside from content and structure, a compliance program is defined by its functional elements. There is now broad acceptance of the minimum essential elements of any formal corporate or research compliance program, a consensus largely shaped by the guidance provided by the *Federal Sentencing Guidelines for Organizations* (FSGO), promulgated in 1991 by the United States Sentencing Commission. In fact, the motivation for the establishment of many compliance programs is the strategic legal advantage offered to organizations with effective compliance programs, as defined by the FSGO. Though the adoption of the FSGO by organizations is voluntary, they are taken into account in determining an organization's sentence in a criminal case and they have come to be accepted by many as the minimum standards for compliance programs.

The guidelines set forth seven steps that are necessary for an "effective program to prevent and detect violations of law" (the full text of relevant portions of the FSGO is in the *Resources* section of this chapter):

1. Established compliance standards and procedures;
2. High-level personnel responsible for compliance;
3. Due diligence in personnel assignment in high-risk areas;
4. Communication of the standards and procedures through dissemination or training;
5. Monitoring and auditing of the organization's activities, and a mechanism for employees and other agents to report wrongdoing without fear of retribution;
6. Enforcement of standards through appropriate mechanisms, including discipline of those failing to detect the offense;
7. Responding appropriately and acting to prevent further similar offenses, which includes modifying the program itself.

This seven-part definition of an effective compliance program has been adopted by the Department of Health and Human Services, Office of Inspector General (OIG). Specific compliance guidance to various segments of industry, for the avoidance of fraud and abuse in federal health care programs, recommend these steps. Since 1997, DHHS has issued eleven voluntary guidances, including one for the hospital industry.[3] In addition, all corporate integrity agreements which are executed as part of civil settlements between a health care provider and the government to resolve a case arising under the False Claims Act (FCA), including the *qui tam* provisions of the FCA, require that the organization maintain a compliance program consisting, at minimum, of the seven elements of the FSGO.

In September 2003, the DHHS Office of Inspector General gave its first indication of intent to develop compliance guidance for the recipients of extramural research grants and cooperative agreement awards from the NIH (i.e., applicable to most research entities). The OIG published a notice of "Solicitation of Information and Recommendations for Developing Compliance Program Guidance for Recipients of NIH Research Grants," (Federal Register, Vol. 68, No. 172). Further, the notice proposes that such guidance will contain the seven core elements of FSGO, and a possible eighth element, "Defining roles and responsibilities and assigning oversight responsibility." The OIG received some comments highly critical of the proposed guidance, some on the grounds that there is already much existing guidance from federal agencies for the research community, a great deal of which is overlapping and inconsistent. But it would appear that this is a clear sign that such compliance program guidance is forthcoming.

So in planning a research compliance program, institutions should determine that these basic elements are covered. Existing compliance standards and procedures should be reviewed and gaps addressed. There should be a clear assignment of responsibility, preferably at a high level, for all areas of compliance. In assigning responsibility in high risk areas, the institution must take care, to rely on individuals with known or clearly warranted expectations of competence. The standards and procedures must be communicated clearly and often, throughout the research community. This may include distributing codes and policies, conducting training sessions, making resources available on the Web, and encouraging dialogue within units of the organization. The organization's activities should be monitored, often through a combination of "for cause" and random review of research activities. It is crucial to have and promote reporting mechanisms that allow individuals to come forward with concerns, without fear of retribution, which means having an option for anonymous reporting. And there should be a means to enforce standards and a continuing assessment of the program to prevent future problems.

Experience within the research community, and in the wider corporate world, has shown that these principles can be implemented through a variety of methods and processes. The elements must be shaped into an overall program to support ethics and compliance in whatever design will most effectively put the principles into practice.

Structuring a Research Compliance Program

Due to the distinctiveness of institutional culture, history, and existing structures and systems, research compliance programs reflect a wide diversity of responses to structural questions such as:

- How will the program be organized?
- What will be the reporting relationships?
- What are the roles and responsibilities of the staff and of leadership?

- How much interaction should there be with other organizational functions?
- How will the program balance collaboration with autonomy, and centralization with local flexibility?
- What is the optimal format and content of internal codes and policies?
- Should there be an oversight committee?
- How will success be defined and what assessment techniques will be employed?

Organizations are likely to have in place numerous administrative departments, offices, and committees, including: office of sponsored projects, office of clinical trials, institutional review board, institutional animal care and use committee, conflict of interest committee, HIPAA privacy board, and biosafety office. The individuals who have a degree of responsibility in these matters include a broad range of administrators, managers, laboratory directors, principal investigators, research coordinators, graduate students, and post-doctoral fellows. Taking into account this tangle of roles and responsibilities, the program structure must clarify accountability and functions to ensure that all elements are in place.

A continuum can be seen running from a highly centralized compliance function at one end to decentralized structure on the other end. A centralized program typically has a director of compliance, reporting to a high level executive, such as a vice president for research. Responsibilities of the director would include overseeing the compliance function, collecting and analyzing relevant data, developing and interpreting policy, and developing and administering education and training materials. The advantages of a centralized program are found in the greater control that can be exercised over the program. There may be enhanced consistency in communications, materials, and training, and more precision in monitoring and auditing. Decision-making authority is clear.

On the other end of the continuum is a decentralized program, with delegation of substantial control to local units. This system employs policies and procedures that are applicable to discrete sections of the organization and assigns compliance responsibilities to each operating unit. A decentralized structure allows for greater tailoring of policies, communications, and training to local needs. There may also be an increased sense of program ownership among faculty and staff. The changing nature of research impacts this issue. A decentralized structure can work well when research is mostly conducted within discrete units of the organization. Today's research environment, however, promotes collaborations between different departments within the institution, between different institutions, and between academia and industry. In these situations, institution-wide policies and procedures may be necessary to avoid conflicts. Each institution should seek an ideal balance between centralized authority and local flexibility, and between collaboration and autonomy. These choices can affect the degree of support the community offers the program, the effectiveness of the program to anticipate and respond to problems, and the extent to which employees will seek out its guidance.

Even if compliance responsibilities are decentralized, however, it is necessary that some individual (preferably at a high level) be charged with oversight of the entire program. The eighth element added by the OIG in the proposed guidance described earlier, "Defining roles and responsibilities and assigning oversight responsibility," anticipates the existence of a decentralized arrangement, by stating the need to coordinate and provide oversight for the structural components. And whether the program is centralized or decentralized, there needs to be a clear assignment of responsibility in each area of concern for overseeing the compliance function, collecting and analyzing relevant data, developing related policy, developing and administering education and training materials, overseeing investigations, and auditing. One approach for the development of such a plan, to ensure that gaps in assigned accountability for compliance are identified and filled, specifies, and analyzes:

1. Each component of the compliance program (e.g., policies, communication, reporting),
2. The compliance areas (e.g., scientific misconduct, human/animal subjects, grant administration), and
3. The roles of those involved in research (e.g., deans, principle investigator, managers).

Content of a Research Compliance Program

The core priorities of a compliance program involve meeting legal and regulatory requirements, and minimizing risks of litigation and enforcement actions. Broadly then, the program should encompass all research-related content areas that are subject to legal and regulatory requirements, and those that expose the institution to risk. Depending on the actual scope of research activities, the organization may be subject to regulation in some or all of the following (nonexclusive) areas:

- Human subject protection
- Animal use protection
- Biosafety
- Select agents
- FDA
- Privacy
- Financial conflicts of interest
- Grants management
- Fraud and abuse
- Research misconduct
- Intellectual property
- Import/export

A logical allocation of resources among content areas follows upon an analysis of the *likelihood* and *impact* of the risks of noncompliance in each relevant area. For example, a new risk assessment at Learned University (L.U.) concludes that a high *likelihood* of risk exists in the areas of animal use protection, conflicts of interest, and environmental health and safety; while a medium *likelihood* of risk exists in the areas of faculty practices and research billing compliance, records management and retention, and HIPAA implementation. The *impact* of these various risks, if realized, can also range from low to high. For example, Learned University decides that, while the *likelihood* of risk from research billing compliance is medium because L.U. conducts very few clinical trials, that the *impact* of such noncompliance may be high due to the possible outcomes of a fraud and abuse charge. This analysis of relevant content areas and assessment of risk will be used as a basis for allocation of resources and development of a comprehensive plan to address priority areas.

Though a compliance program may be primarily concerned with following the laws and avoiding or minimizing the risk of litigation, the institution also may decide to make *compliance and ethics* the focus of its program. Formal ethics and compliance programs seek to promote awareness of legal and ethical concerns and to encourage ethical behavior among employees at work. There are many reasons to take this approach.

Clearly the responsible conduct of research goes beyond laws and regulations. The Office of Research Integrity of DHHS identifies nine core areas in the responsible conduct of research:

1. Data acquisition, management, sharing, and ownership
2. Mentor/trainee responsibilities
3. Publication practices and responsible authorship
4. Peer review
5. Collaborative science
6. Human subjects
7. Research involving animals
8. Research misconduct
9. Conflict of interest and commitment

Norms and standards in these areas exist in agency pronouncements (e.g., data sharing), professional codes, and in institutional policies and guidelines. A concern for ethics also extends to attention to human rights, the environment, and social responsibility. Many think of this broader focus as "doing the right thing while doing things right," and believe that compliance will more likely occur in a culture of integrity and ethics.

The Ethics Resource Center, Washington, D.C. (http://www.ethics.org/) is a nonprofit, nonpartisan educational organization whose mission it is to strengthen ethical leadership worldwide by providing leading-edge expertise and services through research, education, and partnerships. Their research shows that an *effective* integrity program goes beyond narrow compliance and integrates elements of organizational and individual integrity, determent to wrongdoing, satisfying legal requirements, as well as the organization's broader responsibilities to society.[4] Most institutions have a commitment to a core set of values, including historically transmitted values and norms that go beyond legal obligations. This moral culture of the institution sets the stage for all conduct.

It is widely believed that effective compliance grows out of the internalization of values. There is a concern that when behavior is motivated by external control and authoritarian means, people comply mainly if and when they are closely supervised and fear punishment. On the other hand, reliance on shared moral values and internal convictions means that people conduct themselves voluntarily in line with the values and because they subscribe to them. Merely knowing what is right is no assurance that we will do it. While external controls are needed to a point, if relied on excessively, they undermine the cultivation of self-discipline.

A compliance program needs to strike an effective balance between conveying, on the one hand, the detailed content of government regulations and, on the other, an appreciation of the more broad-based general principles that underpin those regulations. It is critical for an effective compliance program to have the goal of promoting a change of awareness and behavior in the workplace, such that decisions are made in reference to the full spectrum of legal and ethical concerns—with a desire to comply with external law and regulations, as well as organizational policies and procedures—and are guided by organizational and individual values. This can occur when there is a consistent message conveyed in the design and structure of the program, with the aim that the message becomes a central part of the *culture* of the institution.

Measuring Effectiveness

Outcomes of an effective compliance program are difficult to assess and can be quantitative or qualitative. The most typical methods of monitoring are surveys, individual and group interviews, observation, and audits. In a positive, ethical culture it can be expected that personnel will be willing to seek advice and report suspected violations. Research staff might report a sense that the compliance program contributes to ethical decision making. One hopes to see an increased awareness of ethics and compliance issues at all levels of the institution. In many institutions, the compliance officer reports assessment results directly to a committee of the board of trustees.

The Cost of Compliance

Although most of the focus of a compliance program will be on avoiding the costs of noncompliance and litigation, the financial expense of implementing such a program is considerable. Entities that engage in federally funded research and those with federal assurances already incur substantial expense in creating and maintaining the administrative support systems necessary to satisfy compliance requirements (which cannot be fully recovered due to the cap on F&A expenses). An effective compliance program will likely add staff and resources—auditing and monitoring, training, and internal reporting mechanisms—that will add considerably to the cost of conducting research.

In addition, these very activities, when carried out effectively, all create a real risk that the information and documentation created will be used by potential litigants to the detriment of the organization. This risk is often referred to as the "litigation dilemma," and it can be a major concern in developing an effective program. These issues must be discussed with top executives and general counsel with the goal of achieving a balanced approach—

one that weighs the risks of exposing and documenting problems against the costs and risks of an institution not being well informed.

Conclusion

In the beginning of this chapter we emphasized the importance of trust for the successful conduct of research; the value of trust has to be thought of in its broadest sense—not just applicable to the individual research practitioner. Research institutions will only flourish when those who support them and ultimately make use of their product (i.e., the public) have high regard for their ways and means. Many institutions have internalized this insight and have expanded their research compliance and integrity programs concomitantly to meet the needs of a more demanding era while others are just evidencing the glimmerings of awareness. What can be said for all is that the stakes are too high to place the hope for compliance and integrity on a wish and a prayer.

It is in the planning stages of a research compliance program that forethought, care, and inclusion can exponentially express their worth in the final product. The Columbia University experience underscores the importance of patiently considered ramifications and outreach to all who participate in the process to insure the content and structure are appropriate to the individual institution. The necessary functions of a reliable compliance program are delineated as the seven core elements in the "Federal Sentencing Guidelines for Organizations" and can be shaped into an overall program to support ethics and compliance with the objective of effectively putting principles into practice. Considering the complexity of most academic research institutions, designing the appropriate structure becomes essential to ensuring accountability and the inclusion of all elements.

The core of any compliance program will be evidenced by its depth and breadth of content. Many institutions choose to focus solely on compliance with the letter of law and regulation while others seek to integrate edict and ethics, implicitly believing that legal compliance itself will be more likely to occur in an environment that promotes the responsible conduct of research. The latter approach presumes that institutions can consciously possess and foster a moral culture that will act as the ethical foundation for all that occurs within its confines and under its rubric. Whichever approach is chosen, the test comes in spreading the word of compliance, whether narrow or broad in its focus. The final proof is always in the doing.

Resources

I. References

Ad Hoc Advisory Group for the United States Sentencing Commission. "Report of the Ad Hoc Advisory Group on the Organizational Sentencing Guidelines." United States Sentencing Commission, October 7, 2003.

http://www.ussc.gov/corp/advgrprpt/AG_FINAL.pdf (accessed June 2, 2005) (see p. 19 for compliance elements).

Council on Governmental Relations. "Report of the Working Group on the Cost of Doing Business," June 2, 2003.

http://rbm.nih.gov/fed_reg_20030906/FRNotice/Associations/AAU_A-21_CODB.pdf (accessed June 2, 2005).

Gilman S. C. "A Word from the President: Is Mere Legal Compliance Dangerous?" *Ethics Today Online* [serial online] 2, no. 4 (2003). http://ethics.org/today/et_v2n41203.html (accessed June 2, 2005).

Gunsalus, C. K. "Preventing the Need for Whistleblowing: Practical Advice for University Administrators." *Science and Engineering Ethics* 4, no. 1 (1998): 75–94.

Institute of Medicine and National Research Council of the National Academies. "*Integrity in Scientific Research.*" Washington, DC: The National Academies Press, 2002.

II. Web Sites of Selected Research Compliance Programs

Columbia University, Office for Responsible Conduct of Research
http://orcr.columbia.edu (accessed June 2, 2005).

Creighton University, Research Compliance Office
http://www.creighton.edu/researchcompliance/index.htm (accessed June 2, 2005).

Dartmouth College, Research Compliance
http://www.dartmouth.edu/~comply/rc_home.shtml (accessed June 2, 2005).

Kansas University Medical Center, Research Compliance Division
http://www2.kumc.edu/researchcompliance/ (accessed June 2, 2005).

Stanford University, Institutional Compliance Program
http://institutionalcompliance.stanford.edu (accessed June 2, 2005).

University of Arkansas, Research Support and Sponsored Programs
http://www.uark.edu/admin/rsspinfo/compliance/index.html (accessed June 2, 2005).

University of Pittsburgh, Research Conduct & Compliance Office
http://www.rcco.pitt.edu/ (accessed June 2, 2005).

University of Utah, Research Integrity and Compliance
http://www.research.utah.edu/integrity/index.html (accessed June 2, 2005).

III. 2002 Federal Sentencing Guidelines for Organizations, Chapter Eight – Part A – General Application Principles §8A1.2. Application Instructions—Organizations Available at: http://www.ussc.gov/2002guid/8a1_2.htm (accessed June 2, 2005).

(k) An "effective program to prevent and detect violations of law" means a program that has been reasonably designed, implemented, and enforced so that it generally will be effective in preventing and detecting criminal conduct. Failure to prevent or detect the instant offense, by itself, does not mean that the program was not effective. The hallmark of an effective program to prevent and detect violations of law is that the organization exercised due diligence in seeking to prevent and detect criminal conduct by its employees and other agents. Due diligence requires at a minimum that the organization must have taken the following types of steps:

(1) The organization must have established compliance standards and procedures to be followed by its employees and other agents that are reasonably capable of reducing the prospect of criminal conduct.

(2) Specific individual(s) within high-level personnel of the organization must have been assigned overall responsibility to oversee compliance with such standards and procedures.

(3) The organization must have used due care not to delegate substantial discretionary authority to individuals whom the organization knew, or should have known through the exercise of due diligence, had a propensity to engage in illegal activities.

(4) The organization must have taken steps to communicate effectively its standards and procedures to all employees and other agents, e.g., by requiring participation in training programs or by disseminating publications that explain in a practical manner what is required.

(5) The organization must have taken reasonable steps to achieve compliance with its standards, e.g., by utilizing monitoring and auditing systems reasonably designed to detect criminal conduct by its employees and other agents and by having in place and publicizing a reporting system whereby employees and other agents could report criminal conduct by others within the organization without fear of retribution.

(6) The standards must have been consistently enforced through appropriate disciplinary mechanisms, including, as appropriate, discipline of individuals responsible for the failure to detect an offense. Adequate discipline of individuals responsible for an offense is a necessary component of enforcement; however, the form of discipline that will be appropriate will be case specific.

(7) After an offense has been detected, the organization must have taken all reasonable steps to respond appropriately to the offense and to prevent further similar offenses—including any necessary modifications to its program to prevent and detect violations of law. The precise actions necessary for an effective program to prevent and detect violations of law will depend upon a number of factors. Among the relevant factors are:

(i) Size of the organization—The requisite degree of formality of a program to prevent and detect violations of law will vary with the size of the organization: the larger the organization, the more formal the program typically should be. A larger organization generally should have established written policies defining the standards and procedures to be followed by its employees and other agents.

(ii) Likelihood that certain offenses may occur because of the nature of its business—If because of the nature of an organization's business there is a substantial risk that certain types of offenses may occur, management must have taken steps to prevent and detect those types of offenses. For example, if an organization handles toxic substances, it must have established standards and procedures designed to ensure that those substances are properly handled at all times. If an organization employs sales personnel who have flexibility in setting prices, it must have established standards and procedures designed to prevent and detect price-fixing. If an organization employs sales personnel who have flexibility to represent the material characteristics of a product, it must have established standards and procedures designed to prevent fraud.

(iii) Prior history of the organization—An organization's prior history may indicate types of offenses that it should have taken actions to prevent. Recurrence of misconduct similar to that which an organization has previously committed casts doubt on whether it took all reasonable steps to prevent such misconduct. An organization's failure to incorporate and follow applicable industry practice or the standards called for by any applicable governmental regulation weighs against a finding of an effective program to prevent and detect violations of law.

Authors' Acknowledgment

We are grateful to John Masten of Columbia University for his invaluable editorial contributions to this chapter. We are also grateful to Michael Kalichman for useful discussions and insight. Finally, we want to thank Gesenia Alvarez-Lazauskas for her supportive contributions.

• • • Endnotes

1. Institute of Medicine and National Research Council. *Integrity in Scientific Research: Creating an Environment That Promotes Responsible Conduct.* Washington, DC: The National Academies Press, 2002, 1.

2. As Director of Outreach at the NIH Office of Biotechnology Activities, Mr. Shipp employs this phrase in the context of institutional biosafety committees.

3. "Publication of the OIG Compliance Program Guidance for Hospital," *Federal Register* 63, No. 35 (February 23, 1998): 8987–8998.

4. In Ethics Resource Center. *Ethics Today Online* 2, No. 4 (December 15, 2003), http://ethics.org/today/et_v2n41203.html (accessed August 16, 2005).

Belmont as Parable: Research Leadership and the Spirit of Integrity

Edward F. Gabriele, MDiv, DMin

Introduction: The Changing World of Research Administration

What can an academic theologian have to say to research administration? A good number of years ago I entered into the world of research administration and have, since that time, joined in the seemingly endless attempt among research administrators to understand how we started, why we remain, and where we might be headed on the course of research administration.

The first generations of research administrators were focused on the management of research and daily tasks required to ensure that the terms and conditions of sponsored projects were met successfully and on time.

Today, life is very different. Research administrators today are confronted with complex managerial tasks far more demanding than the simple reporting obligations of decades past. Today research administration serves as a leadership service for interdisciplinary and interagency initiatives that have wide implications and requirements, including the realm of research integrity. Since 2000, the Standards for the Responsible Conduct of Research (RCR) (issued by the Office of Research Integrity), have helped to reshape and redefine the intrinsic place of research administration in research enterprise. With this has come a concomitant understanding of the identity and role of research administrators within the communities they serve, as well as their interactions with sponsor agencies. While it is simpler to delineate the various

new challenges and areas of expertise that face research administrators in an ever-changing environment, this chapter discusses some of the fundamental leadership and integrity issues faced in research administration today.

As an academic theologian, my penchant has always been to look at the wider panorama of the meaning of things. It is no wonder that theologians have been closely allied with their academic kin, philosophers, and social scientists. As a research administrator with such an academic perspective, it is of great interest to me to ask, like Alice going through the looking glass: What is the meaning of all this? Do the inroads of standards for responsible and ethical research make a difference? If so, what are these differences? Most importantly, what does all this mean to my identity, self-understanding, and place as a research administrator within the context of the research culture I serve? The answers to these questions will be as diverse as those of us who ask them, and equally as diverse as are the missions of the institutions we serve.

Any and all of the answers and perspectives discussed in this chapter have something in common. The responsibilities we assume as research administrators are challenging to a point unforeseen by ourselves or our forebears. In addition, the service of contemporary research administration is far deeper and more substantive than the simple articulation of regulation and precept. Research administration has far greater importance and impact than simple compliance with terms and conditions of sponsored projects. It demands more than simple assurances of minimalist structures of prescriptive norms to institutions, investigators, project management procedures, and support services. In essence, the contemporary role of research administration, while continuing to ensure compliance and assurance, is deeply involved with the unfolding evolution of the identity and mission of the research enterprise itself, and the contributions that a research community makes to the human progress toward which all responsible research must be ordered. Ultimately, research administration is more clearly tied today to the growth of research as a culture of inquiry and not simply as a locus of industrial production. Research administrators under this rubric of today are intimately involved in the evolution, growth, deepening, and development of "the cultural soul of each corporate sole" that we call the research institution.

But how are these responsibilities captured and made understandable to ourselves, to our colleagues, staff members, and those we serve? The remainder of this chapter provides critical and challenging reflections.

As a research administrator whose efforts have been concentrated on the ethical protection of research subjects, it has been my increasing appreciation that The Belmont Report constitutes a philosophy of human research ethics. Over time, it has occurred to me that Belmont has an impact not just upon human research ethics but upon the entire gamut of service we call "research administration." While Belmont does not speak to the specifics of all aspects of the research administration science, it does speak to its art and its philosophy. Belmont articulates a vision of concern and challenge that goes far deeper than ethical compliance. It goes to the heart of creating an *ethos* of research: *a portrait of the fundamental character of the research culture*. From my perspective as an academic theologian, this has led me to appreciate The Belmont Report as a type of parable in the broad sociocultural understanding of parables as ancient literature. The remainder of this chapter, therefore, reflects upon Belmont as a parable to stretch the imagination regarding the identity and mission of research administration. First, we will review briefly the nature of parables as cultural literature. Second, we will examine the ethos of The Belmont Report and its fundamental hallmarks as cultural metaphor or parable-analogue. Finally, we will pose and summarize some of the challenges that The Bel-

mont Report poses for research administrators and for the research communities we serve.

The Parable Experience: Culture through the Looking Glass

For many Westerners, a parable may be a familiar literary genre from one's religious background. For those who are acquainted with Christian literature, these literary pieces appear to be important means by which a wandering rabbi named Jesus of Nazareth taught his followers and others. From the Christian gospels, many are familiar with the parable of the sheep and the goats, or the parable of the prodigal son, or the story of the good Samaritan. Sometimes these and other parables have made their way into nonreligious literature or educational forums not associated with the explicitly religious. In any event, the parables of Jesus of Nazareth are familiar to many and carry with them clear instructional value for defining human moral behavior.

But is that all there is to the parables of Jesus? Are parables merely ancient fables and stories that carry with them aphoristic value encouraging human morality or just common sense good behavior? Scholars strongly debate such ideas.

Parables are not simple stories or analogies that teach appropriate behavior. The parables found in the Bible are a cultural construct that were stinging and jarring for hearers and for the leadership of those times. They represented an in-breaking of a new order of existence. Sometimes this in-breaking was an abrupt challenge to the cultural mores and strictures of the time. For example, the parable of the prodigal son violated the economy of relationships, property, family, and commerce in the ancient Near East. The parable of the good Samaritan was a particularly prophetic and stinging rebuke to a society that made sharp distinctions regarding the culturally unclean as outcasts from the community of the self-appointed chosen.

The figure of a wandering rabbi teaching such things by common story is the picture of a social prophet empowering the dispossessed with new knowledge and unprecedented freedom by pressing their faces to a dangerous juncture of conscience and culture. The parables were and are a means by which the face of society and individuals are pressed from a present mode against a pane of meaning to see beyond the self into a world never envisioned or thought possible. As literary scholars would agree, the parables therefore are truly metaphors of power and meaning wherein wider vistas give new and sometimes radical reinterpretation to the meaning of human experience in the present.

This concept of the parable is not unique to the Bible or to religious literature. Rather it is a literary example of the wider experience of transformation in personal and cultural life. Cultural anthropologists have addressed rites of passage in the life of the young passing from childhood to adulthood. In various ways but within all cultures, individuals at the onset of puberty are separated and, in a period of liminality or shadows, begin to experiment and experience the behaviors and traditions of full adult life. At a time determined to be appropriate and after ritual celebration, they are reaggregated into the wider community and take their proper place and role as adults. This is not just a pattern found in so-called primitive societies. It is endemic to all cultures and societies. It is part of the process of human formation. Neither is this pattern limited to what we call adolescence. More deeply than an age-specific or culture-specific phenomenon, rites of passage comprise a type of moveable pattern that is repeated at various times differing in degree and intensity throughout the human development life cycle.

However, there are times that a rite of passage does not end with the expected. Sometimes what one sees, hears, and experiences is utterly different from the expected, ending with a complete change of identity, lifestyle, personal understanding, social role, etc. This is when a rite of passage mutates and becomes something utterly different. Religious reflection calls this conversion. It might also be called a rite of transformation. It can happen to the individual. It can happen to a group. It can happen to an entire community, culture, or enterprise. It ultimately is a quantum leap out of the ordinary into something completely unforeseen, though indeed most likely its elements were a long time in coming.

From a particular perspective, the parable experience is an invitation to an experience of transformation both personal and cultural. The reader or hearer of the parable is much like Alice in Wonderland. The white rabbit of a new and intriguing piece of knowledge passes by and one is caught up in the mad dash to something for which I know I dare not be late. My face gets pressed to a looking glass. I see things vastly different, almost backwards from what I have been taught. I eat and drink things that make me short or tall. There suddenly are unbirthdays to celebrate. And indeed, I am invited to strange games with loud royal personages who seem to want my head. Comfortable? No. Familiar? In no way. But something keeps me from resisting the fascination; and I pursue madly, blindly. Somehow, somewhere, what I am hearing and experiencing in the parable jars my senses and my thinking out of the past. It hits a space within me that has always desired to be filled. There is a price: change. Pain will be inevitable. But there is no way to resist truth. One can only surrender and succumb to the moment.

Such is the parable experience. Not something specifically religious unless we mean by that something specifically human. Theologians are those who are trained to reflect upon and understand human nature and human experience from particular vantage points. As a theologian, I propose that the new and expansive demands for research integrity are shaping, stretching, and redefining our understanding of who we are as professional research administrators and the service we are asked to provide for our research communities. We are undergoing a radical transformation in our identity and mission. But how do we understand who we are and what we do in these days of research integrity? Are we merely meant to articulate new regulations, new ethical parameters? I suggest that we, like Alice, are being invited to set out on a pathway to something far deeper, something that requires for us a parable or metaphor, a new image, if you will, of what it is we are all about. We need something that, like the parables of old, stretches our minds and hands to things unforeseen and strengthens us for tasks yet to come. We do not need a new set of ethical regulations. We need an "ethos": a fundamental character. But an ethos is elusive. It requires something to give it substance so that it is visible to the world. It requires something so that its voice is heard. That something I would suggest is grounded in The Belmont Report, not just as a philosophy hinge for human subject protections, but a touchstone for the phenomenology of research administration itself.

What follows is a reflection upon The Belmont Report as The Belmont "Parable." The materials to follow are adapted with permission from previous papers and articles I authored for the 2003 Symposium of the Society of Research Administrators International and The Journal of Research Administration. While Belmont itself and my original work are directed specifically toward human research subject protections, the reflections to follow are germane not only to human research ethics, but constitute foundational principles for research administration and the purpose of research as a process of inquiry, information, knowledge, wisdom, and human progress.

The Belmont Parable

On July 12, 1974, the National Research Act was signed into law, establishing the National Commission for the Protection of Human Subjects of Biomedical and Behavioral Research. Among other charges, the commission was directed to identify and articulate the ethical principles that must form the basis of all human subject protections in research. Over a four-year interval, the commission convened physicians, behavioral and biomedical researchers, academic theologians, ethicists, philosophers, and lawyers to discuss from a wide variety of perspectives the common bases from which could be articulated the fundamental ethical principles for protecting human participants in any form of research. In April 1979, the commission issued The Belmont Report and in it identified three principles that serve as the foundations for the protection of human research subjects: respect for persons and their autonomy, beneficence, and justice. In this, the commission unintentionally articulated what has become a fundamental philosophy for human subjects protections, shaping a type of metaphor or parable that remains the measuring rod for succeeding discussions, regulations, codes, and requirements for the protection of human subjects from research risks.

However, the work of the commission clearly stated the principles of respect, beneficence, and justice are not "ethical codes" as one might find in other documents. The Belmont Report and its foundational principles are far deeper. These principles and the report itself are a metaphor, an analytical framework, or "paradigm" best understood by the origin of the word "ethics" itself.

The term ethics comes from the Greek *ethos*, a term I have used previously. *Ethics* are sets of regulations or standards against which behaviors can be measured. *Ethos* is the fundamental character of a person, an institution, a society, or a culture. In the ideal, ethics or codes should be born from the originator's *ethos* (i.e., fundamental character). *Ethos* is something profoundly more fundamental than any set of regulations. The three principles articulated

in The Belmont Report are three fundamental markers of the *ethos* of human subjects' protections. However, these same principles form more broadly hallmarks of integrity for all forms of research and research administration.

Respect for Persons

Respect for persons is the first of the three foundational principles of The Belmont Report. For all who read The Belmont Report, the principle of respect for persons conjures up nostalgical values learned in education and home rearing. Respecting others is a basic principle, and one of the normative lessons of life in the ordinary family or school setting. Respect for others and their personhood is so basic that the nostalgia and ordinariness of this life lesson are what can anesthetize people from its significance in human subjects protections. While the principle of respect for persons is basic, it is far from commonplace and can never be presumed.

Respect for persons has two elementary parts. First, this principle refers to the inviolability of the autonomy of another person. Second, the Belmont Report indicates that respect for persons means special obligation to protect those who have a diminished capacity for making autonomous decisions and self-determination. In essence, each human being has a right to individual autonomy and self-determination that cannot be diminished by the will of another.

The principle of respect for persons as understood by the 18th century had sought to elevate the dignity and worth of the individual human person over tyranny. Evolving gradually over time, the rights of the individual were a crowning achievement in Western thought and formed part of the very cornerstone of the American experiment itself. The implications of this profound principle have not been exhausted and never will be. The cultural discussion regarding the protection of equal rights and individual autonomy is far from over. In each age and context, human beings must carefully and honestly look for the emergence of the darker side of human experience that is capable of exploitation, manipulation, bigotry, and power. Protecting individual autonomy and those with diminished capacity is as old as civilization itself and has been traditionally one of the major measures of the moral centeredness of a society and its leaders.

The impact of this foundational principle for research and research populations has grown and expanded in line with new insights regarding the inherent dignity and autonomy of women, men, and children. New experiences of what it means to be human and humane provide reinterpretation for this first of the three foundational principles of The Belmont Report.

To discover for ourselves what it means to revere this principle of respect for persons, one need only look at the origin of the term. *Respect* comes from Romance language roots that mean "to look back" or "to regard again." An image may prove helpful to understanding what is meant here. Assume you are riding at full gallop down a road. You come upon a country scene that simply takes away your breath. At full gallop you turn your attention away from the road to "look again" or "look back" simply because you cannot resist the scene. Sometimes, the price for being so transfixed is obvious. But the reality of what is seen cannot be resisted and ultimately seems to be worth the price of falling off one's horse.

Respect for persons occurs when the absolute worth of other human beings suddenly arrests one's attention away from mundane concerns of daily living. One suddenly becomes aware of an other and the magnitude of this other constitutes a manifestation of humanness itself. It invades the perceptions and senses. Strange how this occurs at the most inconvenient times and upends one's assumptions and one's activity. History is replete with stories and examples how the most inconvenient and unlikely of characters became themselves messages about the dignity of human nature to those who were too busy to see and remember. The lowly in these stories unexpectedly invaded the sensibilities of the busy making them stop and wonder and be amazed.

In the act of human subjects research, genius and industry meet in a relationship between researcher and enrollee. In that meeting there always must be something that arrests the attention and makes one wonder. For after all, to be in the presence of another woman or man or child who generously would give of themselves in research to benefit human welfare is certainly enough to make one look back or regard again.

For an institutional review board (IRB) whose mission is clearly the protection of the ethical rights and welfare of human subjects from research risks, the responsibility found in respect for persons is immense. That responsibility is to uphold the rights and dignity of individual persons in any culture as preeminent over the charging energies arising from the research enterprise. To uphold the autonomy and rights of persons is sometimes an inconvenient stop in the busyness of research. In the research culture where "produce or perish" can be the whisper heard by new investigators, an IRB has a moral obligation to voice more loudly a deeper wisdom: "protect or perish." While one must practically be concerned about what is produced in research for sponsors and for the public trust, to violate or leave unprotected the personhood and rights of human subjects, especially the vulnerable, is, as T.S. Eliot might image it, "the deepest treason of them all."

Beneficence

Beneficence, from the Latin phrase, "bene facere" or "to do the good," is the second of the principles articulated in The Belmont Report. For many, the meaning of beneficence seems rather immediate or familiar. The report clearly grounds beneficence, the "doing of the good," upon respect for persons, its first ethical principle. Respect for persons and their autonomy must necessarily give birth to doing the good. However, in the discussion of this second ethical principle, the report engages in a series of reflections that take the reader far deeper than a reminder to have the best interests of other people firmly in mind. In what can only be deemed an act of sheer wisdom, the report's discussion concerning beneficence draws the reader to consider the balance between "doing no harm" and "always doing the good."

There is always an element of risk in human research, regardless of discipline. As part of the inherent risk in research, it is not always easy to maintain a definitive difference between what constitutes the avoidance of harms and the embrace of doing the good. It is entirely possible that to do the good means to take risks that are above and beyond what is routinely met in daily life. A doctor certainly wants to heal a patient suffering from an infection. But the most effective and lifesaving therapy might require a needle stick and painful disinfection of a wound. Healing does not always guarantee freedom from pain. Medical research history is filled with examples of ingenious and lifesaving discoveries brought into being because someone, somewhere took a risk. Risk is at the very heart of human subjects research. Beneficence ensures that the risks of the act of research are kept within the essential context of the commitment to "do the good" for the benefit of others. But how does one approach this way of understanding beneficence? How does a researcher or an IRB itself understand the critical and delicate interplay between avoiding harm and doing the good?

Since 1991, the importance of human subjects protections has exploded into the world of research in a completely unanticipated way. Few could have realized, in light of such events as the Holocaust and Nuremberg Trials, that research tragedies and problems could occur in our own communities, including the atrocities that occurred during notorious research trials at Tuskegee, Willowbrook, Fernald, etc. Yet even in the face of these events, there still abides an unarticulated bias that IRB procedures have something to do with administration, or secondary scientific review, or institutional safeguards, or legal compliances. In its bold articulation that one must approach human subjects protections as a balance between risks and benefits, between avoiding harm and embracing the good, the principle of beneficence says something completely different regarding the purpose of an IRB and the mandate to protect the rights and welfare of human research participants.

IRBs are not about the business of administration or secondary scientific review. Their primary purpose is not about safeguarding institutions, institutional officials, or legal standards. Rather, IRBs are about the act of ethics: to make discernment of what is best for human participants who freely enroll in the act of research which itself has inherent risks. IRBs, therefore, do not engage in the facile world of simple black and white standards; they must delve into the gray fog that comes with human circumstance and perspective. IRB review is an act of both balance and beacon of beneficence and safety, despite inherent risks.

For human beings, learning how to balance things is a lifelong process, beginning with balancing ourselves and growing as we learn to carry objects or with the challenge of balancing a checkbook. Some of us first saw the beauty of balance, along with its dangers, when we held our breath during circus high wire acts. There we gaped and gasped as women, men, and children danced and twirled, caught between the free flight of air and the ever present possibility of harm and danger below. Somehow we learned that true balance comes about when one can juggle both: the high call of the ethers and the pull of gravity. Researchers, institutions, and IRBs are called to do exactly the same. In the spirit of beneficence, IRBs call researchers and the act of research itself to a deeper sense of balance between risks and benefits, between avoiding harm and doing the good, between the strong headiness of advancement and the looming practical ground of human welfare, safety, and goodness.

Justice

The third of the ethical principles articulated in The Belmont Report is *justice*, as philosophers say, a multiple "meaninged" term. Linguists remind us that language is absorbent. Words accrue and sop up diverse meanings over time. As human experience expands and unfolds, the words we use take on new, sometimes even ironic, or contradictory, meanings. For many people, the term "justice" conjures up an image of a blindfolded Greek woman bearing weighing scales. Courtrooms and legal briefs become the easy images that appear when the word "justice" is articulated. But is that the fundamental meaning of this critical term in human social experience? Does justice in the human protections sense refer to civil entitlements arising from a common consensus that is the assumed basis of democratic law?

To understand justice, it is important to appreciate its roots in the Greco-Roman and later traditions of philosophy. As Western society evolved in its understanding of human nature and the place of the individual in society, the concept of justice equally grew and developed. Philosophy, especially after it emerged from medieval neo-scholasticism, increasingly though slowly addressed the fundamental dignity and freedom of the human individual. This dignity and freedom eventually evolved into a deeper cultural understanding of inalienable human rights. These rights are part of one's fundamental nature and therefore are owed by society itself to each person under the virtue of justice. With the coming of the Renaissance, the Reformation, the emergence of nation states, and the beginnings of the scientific and industrial revolutions, women and men increasingly claimed life, liberty, and the pursuit of happiness as matters owed to them under the virtue of justice. Justice therefore is a virtue that admits that each woman, man, and child is, in the spirit of our American heritage, endowed with inalienable rights.

Justice as an ethical principal of The Belmont Report is something far deeper than simply a legal protection. As the human dignity and freedom of each volunteer must be protected indiscriminately above all things, Belmont's concept of justice means that the risks of research can never be made to sit unfairly on any one part of the population. Justice, in tandem with respect for persons as well as beneficence, requires that special attention be paid to vulnerable individuals who will be more prone to risks because of their age, incapacity, social status, or any other circumstance. Belmont's concept of justice also means that the benefits of research cannot be distributed unequally. The benefits of research cannot become the property of the privileged while others share risks with greater proportion.

Justice can be seen to challenge the mission and service of IRBs in a very different way. Respect for persons challenges the central vision of the research act. Beneficence challenges the means by which risks and benefits are to be calculated. One way of understanding justice is in its challenge to the telos, or end of research itself. In its search to assure that both the risks and benefits of research are distributed equitably, there is a question as to what is the final end of research and who owns it. In saying that the risks of research can never be borne inequitably by one part of a population and the benefits are not the privilege of an other, IRBs point investigators and their institutions to the reality that research itself in the final analysis can never belong to the scientist, the university, the industry, or the sponsor, alone, but it belongs to the public trust. Research, unlike alchemy of old, is not a secret industry hidden from human scrutiny and awareness; it belongs to the entire human community. Its telos is human progress, but never at the expense of human protections or the expense of the widest possible benefit to society. When an IRB weighs inclusion and exclusion criteria in a protocol, inherently, albeit, often unconsciously, an IRB challenges investigators to the proprietorship of research inquiry. In an age of consumerism, where simplistic and uncritical preoccupation with metrics and benchmarks can turn human subjects into data to be mined, this is an enormous challenge. In essence, the discernment of justice in human research leads one back full circle to the Belmont principles of respect for persons and beneficence. Justice poses the inherent question: Why are we doing this anyway? Are we doing it with integrity?

Like all three of the Belmont principles, *justice* is a process with a pervading and even disturbing energy. Assuring a level playing field regarding risks and benefits as part of the process of justice is not an easy task, especially in a day and age of increasing human rights and human equality sensitivities and initiatives. It is of paramount importance that researchers, IRBs, institutional officials, research associates, key personnel, and sponsors be keenly aware that justice requires careful ethical discernment of all factors that would affect research participants. Such factors go well beyond the physical or medical. Justice further requires critical reflection upon the ultimate purpose of the research act in question. Justice stings the researcher with the awe-filled responsibility that comes when asking others to take part in that fragile and vulnerable act of human inquiry we call "research."

And Finally . . .

In any principled society, there is always need to enact regulations and laws to keep people safe from harm and protect the heartbeat of human existence. As society progresses, however, we learn that pro-

tecting human life and making humane choices are measures that are not merely about complying with laws and regulations. Human life and human choices are more about the shades of gray that one finds in fog. Like travel through a fog, the journey of ethical decision making in human subjects protections is a matter of discernment, not merely a matter of compliance. But words do not come easy in fog. As Eugene O'Neill reminds us in *Long Day's Journey Into Night*, "Stammering is the strange eloquence of us fog people." The ethical discernment of human subject protections necessitates some stammering before we can articulate with precise eloquence any directions, judgments, decisions, and parameters for a protocol, an informed consent document, a continuing review, or even final report. The same is true for every act of research administration.

Research administration is ordered toward the stewardship, leadership, service, and support of the research process that, itself, must benefit human and humane living. Research administration, therefore, will never be a facile process. It entails responsibilities far deeper than simply punching the right tickets, making the administrative grade, or ensuring one has met the minimal requirements of a regulation or precept. Today, as research administrators, we are beginning to speak more and more about establishing not a culture of compliance or conscience, but a culture of integrity. This effort is highlighted in the quest to understand what it means to apply and practice the principles of The Belmont Parable. Principles in the report remind the world of research's commitment to render to the public trust and the human community what is their utter and inalienable due: the protection of life, of liberty, of freedom . . . the dignity that comes to mind whenever one utters the word "human." And when we ensure this foundation for any and all forms of human participation, then we are more surely on the pathway to real "progress" in any act of research.

Conclusion: The Research Administrator as Agent of Transformation

All parables and all paradigms are subject to the process of "hermeneutics," the act of interpretation. Under this process, the three principles of The Belmont Parable must undergo a hermeneutic and, thereby, be understood anew in each age and in each context so that research efforts are tempered and shaped by the principles of human dignity and integrity. Research is best preserved and protected in this manner as a humane pathway always leading investigators, institutions, human participants, and society toward the good and always away from anything less. But what does this mean for the identity and mission of research administrators?

A number of years ago, a mentor of mine spoke to me of the mission of the teacher or philosopher to be a "hermeneut." Drawing upon the work of other authors of the time, my mentor explained to me that this word has its origins in the Greek deity, Hermes, the winged messenger of the gods, whose vocation was to bring the message of the other gods, not his own, to mortals. To do so, he had to cross the waters of chaos and bear the message to the reality of human beings. However, Hermes brought the message not as a simple quid pro quo. Rather he would trick mortals to hear, to believe, and to obey. Hermes was a subversive character. He subverted the way that people would think and live. He undercut the usual and the ordinary. He was a herald of new things and new orders and new ways of behaving. It was uncomfortable to listen to him. I believe that this image of the hermeneut, coupled with the central present discussion concerning Belmont as parable are a powerful twinning that give an unprecedented future for the identity of research executives and the mission of research administration itself.

Since the early 1990s, the American research community increasingly has been confronted with the concept of research integrity and the emerging standards for the responsible conduct of research. More deeply than mere compliance with regulations, research administrators are being charged today to explore concepts and design educational strategies to promote the prophetic and often uncomfortable stretchings of integrity and ethics that are inherent in the fundamental act of research. Research integrity is not apart from research; it is a fundamental part of the research process, per se. Without the spirit of integrity, the structures of research lose their soul and make the genius of human and humane discovery a self-serving blood-feast for the vampires of greed, power, and self-serving pride.

Research administrators who are stung by the Belmont Parable and accept a role as hermeneuts in the research community effectively become agents of transformation and change. Such agents articulate not just strategies of institutional responsibility to comply with regulations, or strategies by which to ameliorate noncompliance and the ever possible legal regulatory violation. Research administrators who accept the challenge to be hermeneuts explore and strategize long range goals and opportunities by which the fundamental character of the research community is deepened as a humane process truly respectful of the human community that sponsors it, ordered toward the benefit of others more than the self, and centered such that the fruit of research labor enriches the public trust.

The community of research needs to beware, however. Since the 19th century, the scientific enterprise in America has come under the sway of the American industrial, technological, and information revolutions. Research communities often uncritically have adopted the language of commerce such that volunteers in clinical trials are no longer patients but customers or, worse yet, consumers. Young scientists are reminded that salary, bonus, and promotion depend on a "produce or perish" algorithm. Thus the research community itself has stood on the brink of becoming an industrial assembly line where a diagnostic assay draws more attention for its utility as "cost effective" than its ability to affect an accurate diagnosis to alleviate human pain and suffering. When those who lead and assist the executive shaping of the research community's life, process, and self-understanding take on a new and deeper sense of stewardship that calls the community itself to consider carefully what it is that it does, the uncritical aspects of the research institution's life must and will come under scrutiny, hopefully for the better.

However, this is not an easy place to be. It is not easy for those called to be agents of transformation in research communities. It is not easy for research communities either. Institutions always find it difficult to change and to listen to those who challenge the community understanding; while the very purpose of research is meant to support the common good, not the common wants. When the first research administrators began their careers, they supported the common good by meeting compliance and funding responsibilities by reporting time and effort. Today the challenge of research administration is to support the common good by calling our research colleagues beyond the self, beyond the regulation to a new sense of self and purpose and mission imbued with integrity and character imbued with a new sense of what our ancestors called "ethos."

46

Cultivating Interpretive Mentorship: A Role for Research Administrators

Melissa S. Anderson, PhD, Janet M. Holdsworth,
and Joseph B. Shultz, PhD

Mentorship poses a conundrum for research administrators in universities and colleges, while it is often touted as one of the most critical aspects of scholarly and professional preparation at advanced levels. A true mentor can be the single most important (and positive) influence on a graduate student's professional life, encompassing both academic and personal dimensions over a long period of time.(1) Given this, it would appear that universities should arrange for every student to have a mentor.

Administrators readily acknowledge, however, that they have little influence over the development of mentoring relationships. The power of mentoring derives from the personal nature of the relationship. It takes a wise, generous, and experienced person to exert a mentor's influence on the course of a student's professional life. The mentor and student are often closely bonded through shared work and other experiences. The quality of such close relationships is often linked to the mentor's personal qualities or, more likely, the fit between the mentor's and student's personalities. From this standpoint, mentoring is a highly personal and even idiosyncratic relationship that is clearly beyond the scope of administrative influence. The dilemma for research administrators, then, is how to develop these critically important mentoring relationships when the very nature of mentoring seems to put it out of administrative reach.

One response is to rely wholly on faculty to develop mentoring relationships. This approach puts the control and responsibility for mentoring in the hands of people who are best qualified to provide discipline-specific guidance in the context of close working relationships.

The problem with this approach is that it allows many students to fall through the cracks, so to speak. Not every faculty member is well-suited, either, by temperament or training, to serve as a mentor in the ideal sense. Left on their own, faculty members tend to mentor as they were mentored, which means that some faculty scarcely serve in the mentor role at all. Depending on individual faculty to provide all the guidance that students will need also ignores the vastness of the knowledge, both explicit and tacit, that students must acquire to become successful professionals in complex academic or other arenas. Even a student who is fortunate enough to have a diligent mentor is unlikely to get all the assistance and guidance he or she needs from a single mentor.(2,3)

A second response is to rely on the institution's instructional and advisement systems to ensure that students get the guidance they need. These formal systems are designed to ensure that graduate students and other early-career professionals acquire the knowledge and skills needed for advanced work in their fields. The foundation of this formal system is graduate programs' courses, research projects, and examination processes, with their respective faculty, supervisors, and graduate committees.(4) Through all these avenues, students learn not only the content of their fields of study but also what constitutes the tacit knowledge of the disciplines.(5) They typically learn, for example, how to work within the norms of professional relationships, how to present research at conferences and how to prepare their work for publication.(5) Mandatory courses or workshops on ethical issues in research are becoming common, as are optional programs for professional development or preparation for teaching.(6–8) Formal policies and regulations (departmental, institutional, or external) can, of course, prove notably instructive to young scholars.

The problems here, however, are that instructors are focused on course content rather than on career course and advisors typically see their primary responsibility in terms of guidance on degree requirements.(9,5,1) As important as the instructional and advising systems are, they do not necessarily provide the individual-level support that mentors do. Happy are those students who find a true mentor in an instructor or advisor, but the system is not designed to guarantee such an outcome.

In this chapter, we advocate a "mid-range" approach that university research administrators can use to develop programs or other initiatives to cultivate mentorship on their campuses. We recommend *interpretive mentorship* as a model that lends itself to programmatic development at the university, college, or department level. We focus on graduate students, but much of what we recommend could be extended to post-doctoral fellows, early-career academics, or even undergraduates.

In our description of interpretive mentorship, we emphasize distinctions between this model and the alternatives of advising and ideal mentorship. We realize, of course, that such distinctions overstate actual differences in approaches to mentoring, but we present the alternative models in caricature to clarify our argument. Also, the model is not entirely novel, in the sense that many faculty already exhibit this kind of mentoring with their students. We applaud those who are already engaged in this kind of mentorship, while recognizing that the caricatures all too often capture the reality of graduate student mentoring.

Interpretive Mentorship

The need for a new model of mentorship is related only incidentally to administrators' search for ways to provide support to graduate students. A more important impetus is found in changes in graduate education and in the context of research at academic institutions.

Recent studies of graduate education have highlighted the need for better preparation of graduate students for a wider array of careers. As a recent study notes, fewer than half of the PhDs in any of the 11 major fields studied ultimately end up in tenure-

track positions.(10) In some fields this proportion is even smaller. There are persistent calls for graduate education to recognize the complex employment markets and market conditions that their graduates will face; to prepare students better to make the transition from the academic research environment to business, industry, government, the nonprofit sector, other levels of education, entrepreneurial arenas, and other contexts; and to transform the curricula and requirements of graduate programs to make students and their work more adaptable to and successful in employment markets.(11) Even graduate students who plan to seek faculty positions face significant challenges in the academic market. Institutional shifts toward part-time and untenured positions increase recent graduates' competition for full-time, tenure-track positions. In short, graduate students need good advice. They often need more or better advice than their graduate advisors are prepared to give.

Advisors work closely with students, but their responsibilities formally and generally end with the completion of the students' graduate degree. An advisor might see mentorship in ideal terms as a major, possibly lifelong commitment and be unwilling to assume such a responsibility. Someone serving as a true mentor might, on the other hand, look with disdain on those who serve as mere advisors. Perhaps the most common division of effort between these models is a faculty member's commitment to be a mentor to those whose career paths most closely parallel the mentor's own, but a more cursory form of service as advisor to the rest. Professors who find kindred souls in their graduate students have been known to bring the students into their scholarly dynasties, with all the advantages and complications that implies.(12) Other faculty members, when confronted with graduate students whose experience or goals differ significantly from their own, too often assume that they can be of little assistance to such students. Herein lies a missed opportunity.

The Interpretive Mentorship Model

The view of mentorship presented here is an alternative way of thinking about mentorship. Its value lies in suggesting an approach less circumscribed than is advising, less encompassing than ideal-type mentoring, and more amenable to administrative development.

Interpretive mentoring can be contrasted with advising and ideal mentoring by analogy. If graduate students are thought of as travelers, preparing for and indeed beginning the long journey of their careers, then an uninspired advisor is like a travel agent: able to offer basic information about routes and alternatives. An ideal mentor, in caricature, would be someone who draws the student traveler into the professor's own culture, making the student a member of the family, so to speak. An interpretive mentor, by contrast, would be an experienced traveler who knows the general region well but who may not be on the same path as the student. As they travel together for awhile, the experienced traveler gets to know the student well enough to offer guidance tailored to the student traveler and to his or her journey to an intended destination, even if the mentor has never actually visited it.

Similarly, the student traveler needs help in interpreting the confusing signals picked up along the way. Making good choices involves making sense out of a cacophony of messages coming from the student's past experiences, preconceived ideas, current work, achievement, colleagues, heroes, fears, misunderstandings, opportunities, failures, academic aspirations, and career aims. An interpretive mentor is one who helps the student to interpret—as defined by Webster's, "to explain or tell the meaning of; present in understandable terms"(13)—these messages into useful information that will contribute to good decision making.

More to the point, Webster's distinction between "interpret" and "explain" reflects three important dimensions of interpretive mentorship: "*Interpret* adds to *explain* the need for imagination or sympathy or special knowledge in dealing with something." These three dimensions (imagination, sympathy, or special knowledge) distinguish interpretive mentorship from advising and from ideal mentorship.

First, *imagination* reflects a need for an interpretive mentor to extrapolate guidance beyond the bounds of his or her own direct experience. Many, if not most students will take career paths that differ from the mentor's own. When faculty members perceive mentorship in terms of only two alternatives (advising versus ideal mentorship), they will likely reserve true mentorship for only those students whose career paths align with their own; other students will have to settle for mere advising. The imagination dimension of interpretive mentorship suggests that university faculty members can be held responsible for providing substantial guidance to students, including those who are not likely to become university faculty members.

Students need help in imagining or envisioning how their work and abilities fit into the field. Many students float along with no clear goals or conception of how their academic work connects to work in other contexts, particularly in non-academic fields they are preparing to enter. Many students exhibit a striking myopia in terms of their own work, after spending necessary and lengthy focus on highly specialized research during their graduate study. It is the responsibility of the interpretive mentor to help students set their work in the context of the field and the career possibilities that it offers, inside or outside academia, and to offer this support and guidance in a proactive way.

Sympathy suggests that an interpretive role requires a kind of gut-level understanding between the faculty member and student. It reflects a need for mentors to know their mentees better than an advisor would typically know his or her students. An interpretive mentor is well connected to each mentee, and has extensive and current knowledge about each student's background, abilities, experiences, understanding of the field, goals, and aspirations. Without knowing a student well, a professor is likely to fall back on standard advice, which is unlikely to be appropriate for all.

Third, *field-specific expertise* indicates a need for interpretive mentorship to fall within the bounds of a faculty member's field of study. At advanced levels, students do not need career counselors: they need faculty members who can offer advice on research, projects, opportunities, networks, connections, and professional advancement in the context of the discipline, because all of these factors vary significantly by field.

Combining these three aspects of mentorship produces a model of interpretive mentoring in which faculty have a responsibility to help students to bridge the gap between general information (e.g., standards, requirements, and advice) and the students' own career aspirations, preparation, and choices. The faculty role is therefore that of *interpreter*. The interpretive mentor translates the vast and confusing information about academic and professional opportunities, requirements, qualifications, norms, regulations, and so on into terms that have meaning for the student in the context of his or her own specific goals. With years of accumulated experience and expertise, a faculty member can interpret all the general advice and requirements for a student who needs help in sorting through it all, in focusing attention on the most relevant parts, and in foreseeing how it all will be applied in a prospective career. What makes the role of interpretive mentor so potentially powerful is that the mentor can summon the weight of the discipline's and institution's general precepts, together with his or her own wisdom, to bear on an individual student's progress.

Such a vision goes beyond advising but falls somewhat short of ideal mentoring. It puts a lower limit on expectations and responsibilities of mentors, but higher than those of advisors. Similarly, this dynamic places a limit on what is expected of mentors, in contrast to the unbounded expectations associated with classical mentoring.

Programmatic Implications of the Interpretive Mentorship Model

This image of the interpretive mentor lends itself to programmatic development, partly because it admits administrative action (which ideal mentoring, as a personal, dyadic relationship, does not), and also because it raises expectations of faculty-student relationships beyond those of advisor-advisee relations. Most faculty would benefit from the support of a mentoring program, particularly in the imagination and sympathy dimensions of interpretive mentorship.

Table 46-1 displays some of the programmatic implications of interpretive mentorship. As it shows, advising is typically a formal, institutional system for the delivery of advice and guidance in the completion of graduate requirements and the graduate degree. Ideal mentorship is embedded in an informal relationship between a faculty member and a student. Interpretive mentorship lies between these extremes as a semiformal, programmatic initiative. Here, the mentoring program supports the student–faculty relationship, but not in directive or mandatory terms, as in advising.

An interpretive mentor focuses on the student as an individual with a unique academic profile and prospective career path. In contrast, an advisor, at least in our continuing caricature mode, sees the student as one of many who need the same basic advice. A mentor of the ideal type would likely see the student as an apprentice, training to do the mentor's own work: the student presumably emulates the mentor, whose role is that of hero or champion. The fundamental difference here is that the advising connection is impersonal, the ideal mentorship relationship is deeply personal, and the interpretive mentorship relation is individual without being especially personal.

Advising usually guarantees that students meet basic programmatic requirements, but mentoring goes beyond that minimum. One assumes that mentoring in its traditional concept is a highly positive experience, though the significantly personal nature of the relationship has been known to yield "toxic" effects over time. Interpretive mentorship is a way of extending the positive effects of ideal mentoring to all students, without demanding the level of involvement, commitment, or sacrifice typical of ideal mentoring.

The administrative role in interpretive mentorship is to provide active, programmatic support in the form of attention, resources, and coordination; to prepare faculty for the interpretive-mentor role; and to maintain some degree of administrative involvement in addressing issues that may arise in the context of expanded mentorship capacity at an institution. This programmatic role can help to assure that mentorship can make significant contributions to students' academic and professional lives, while mitigating some of the possible negative effects of mentoring relationships.

Programmatic Initiatives

Our concept of interpretive mentorship has implications for the kinds of mentoring programs that research administrators might develop. The model assumes that advisors can serve as interpretive mentors, with programmatic support. The existing system of matching students with advisors might therefore be adequate, if advisors can meet the higher expectations of interpretive mentoring. Research administrators would have to decide on a best approach for their own institution; it would presumably require some combination of encouragement, incentives and, in some cases, requirements. There might, of course, be faculty resistance to the idea that all advisors serve as mentors, particularly if faculty think of being an ideal mentor as exhausting work. Some institutions might, instead, choose to pair students with mentors through an alternative process, so that the mentor is someone in addition to the advisor. In this case, the administration would take over the matching function. In keeping with the principle of field-specific expertise above, the mentor should be of the student's department or in a closely aligned unit.

TABLE 46-1	Programmatic Implications of Advising and Mentoring Models		
	Advising System	**Interpretive Mentorship**	**Ideal Mentorship**
Nature of the model:	Systemic	Programmatic	Relational
Partners:	Institution/department, faculty member and student	Program, faculty member and student	Faculty member and student
Structure:	Formal	Semiformal	Informal
Administrative role:	Directive	Supportive	Virtually none
Role of the faculty member:	Formal advisor	Interpreter	Champion or hero
Role of the student:	One of many graduate students	Individual with a particular academic and career path	Apprentice
Orientation:	Impersonal	Individual	Personal
Positive potential:	Usually assures that student meets requirements appropriately	Usually makes a significant contribution to student's academic and professional lives	Usually produces life-altering, positive effects
Negative potential:	May provide only minimal guidance	May result in inadequate mentoring, but effects are mitigated by the program	May produce "toxic" effects
Bottom line:	Necessary	More effective than advising sytem; more feasible than ideal mentoring	Inestimably valuable, but rare

A program that supports interpretive mentoring should address the three aspects of interpretive mentoring. To support the *imagination* component, research administrators should find ways to help students and their mentors access information about opportunities in their fields. Some information at the level of specific specialties is needed, but should also include more information at a broader level. Faculty can help students interpret information related to academic and nonacademic labor markets, employment patterns, career opportunities, and prerequisite experiences that are needed for various professional roles. Most faculty do not have specialized knowledge about nonacademic areas, but most are able to provide critical advice to help students make decisions, provided both faculty and student have ready access to banks of related information. We do not mean to suggest that faculty provide all types of this information to their students, rather, students should be responsible for accessing the information and should consult their mentors on how to interpret information for professional development.

Mentoring programs should collect realistic case studies that illustrate graduate school experiences, as well stories that illustrate the path from graduate school to employment. Articles in the news and careers sections of the *Chronicle of Higher Education* are good sources for these case

studies, which can serve to launch valuable discussion between students and their mentors about opportunities and stumbling blocks in career development.

Mentoring programs can also increase students' connections with others in their fields by sponsoring projects, including online forums for exchange of information or brainstorming, virtual or in-person matches between students and alumni or others working in the field, and linkages between students and professionals who can expand students' sense of their own potential. These efforts can support students' successful transitions into a broad range of professional arenas (including, of course, academic arenas of all different kinds). The programmatic goal is to provide information to faculty–student pairs—information that helps faculty to help students to interpret and frame their career goals. We advocate online delivery of this information, when possible. Often mentoring programs benefit from face-to-face meetings or other in-person encounters, but much useful career information is offered on Web sites or through other electronic means. Programs that consist strictly of meetings, workshops, or other time-intensive methods can curb mentors' and students' willingness to participate.

A mentoring program can also support the *sympathy* dimension of interpretive mentoring, which emphasizes mentors knowing students well enough to tailor their advice to individual students. In some fields, students work very closely with faculty members, while in others, the connection is more tenuous. Electronic portfolios that record all of a student's academic and other relevant experience on an ongoing basis can keep mentors up-to-date on the student's work. Professional planning can also be included in portfolios so that both student and mentor together can keep track of the student's short-term plans (upcoming conference presentations, publications, contacts with other professionals) and long-term planning (career goals and related strategies). If an institution chooses to develop interpretive mentoring between students and faculty members who are not the students' advisors, then online communication forums, chat rooms, and electronic checklists that mentor-mentee pairs can also support the mentors' efforts can be consulted on a regular basis. A somewhat expanded form of the checklist can also function as a log of mentor-mentee interactions.

In support of the *field-specific expertise* aspect of interpretive mentoring, administrators can work with faculty in their departments or other field-based units to develop mentoring within those specific academic and intellectual contexts. Most faculty are good at most aspects of mentoring. Administrators or staff associated with a mentoring program can work with faculty to expand their skills in certain areas. If faculty are to be encouraged to expand the range of their mentoring, mentoring programs must find ways to help them to do so. Some will need help with academic mentoring, related to coursework, research, publication, scholarly independence, dissertation work, academic assessment, and management of the academic workload. Others will need support in becoming better career mentors, for example in addressing professional development, networking, contacts, employment, career opportunities, and hiring situations. While good at the basics, some faculty do not challenge their mentees to take a broader view in terms of long-range planning, career progression, the art of survival, institutional and disciplinary dynamics, and political aspects of careers. Others need practical guidance on how to work one-on-one with individual students (e.g., how to balance support and pressure, champion the student, provide realistic assessments of the student's abilities, cajole the stragglers, challenge the overconfident, enlighten the clueless, cope with failure, bridge cultural differences and misunderstandings, cultivate subscription to disciplinary norms, and squelch

misconduct). Again, disciplinary-specific approaches are likely to be most effective in these approaches.

A mentoring program cannot force faculty to be good mentors nor can a program coerce students into learning from faculty members' advice and example. A good mentoring program can, however, foster a sense of collective responsibility for students' development and heighten faculty members' awareness of the potential for and means of affecting students' academic and professional careers in positive ways.

Issues in the Management of an Interpretive Mentorship Program

The development of an interpretive mentoring program involves not only questions of overall orientation, as discussed, but also continuing discussion about the ongoing management of the program. Each institution will confront specific problems, but some issues can be anticipated, which we will discuss.

Scope of the Mentorship Program

We have so far addressed mentorship largely in the sense of the guidance of graduate or other advanced students by faculty members. Mentoring programs may focus on enriching existing relationships between graduate students and advisors, or they might instead seek to match students with other faculty members with compatible skills, interests, and capacity for interpretive mentoring.

Other forms of interpretive mentoring are possible, however, including peer mentoring, mentoring by individuals working outside of the university in research or clinical settings, mentoring by faculty members who are at other universities, and mentoring of students and others at different levels.(14) Mentoring programs can also address other groups who need expert guidance, such as newly appointed faculty or those preparing for tenure review.

Peer-to-peer mentoring may enhance a graduate student's psycho-social development during the graduate school experience. If a peer mentor is more advanced in the graduate program than the student, then support and development are maximized.(15) Mentoring programs can foster peer mentoring, sometimes in collaboration with student-run organizations. These organizations may be discipline-based or may cross disciplines; some may offer specific social, academic, and professional support for graduate students from historically underrepresented(16) or nontraditional groups.(17)

Mentoring programs may involve individuals from other organizations, academic or not, who serve as mentors of graduate students. Complementary mentoring relationships may form as the graduate student becomes more involved in professional associations, has research-oriented internships or clinical experiences, or is introduced to the mentor's professional network. Much of this type of mentoring can take place electronically, via e-mail.

Some mentoring initiatives are oriented to undergraduate students, while others match early-career faculty or other academic professionals with mentors. The same kinds of interpretive mentoring can, of course, take place in these situations as well, with adjustments to the needs of the mentored population. Mentor programs need to set parameters for the scope of the mentorship initiatives they will support, so that their programmatic strength is not diluted by too many disparate objectives.

No matter what group a mentoring program serves, it is important to note that the program and the mentors should not be held responsible for the delivery of instruction. A mentoring program should not be assumed to replace instruction in ethical issues or in research-project development. These topics belong explicitly in the graduate curriculum. It is the mentor's responsibility to interpret and clarify ethical norms and requirements that the student learns about elsewhere. Likewise, the graduate curriculum needs to address the processes of initiating, developing, funding, and managing research projects, though students can benefit from witnessing a mentor's methods of management of these processes.

Mentoring from the Mentor's Viewpoint

To become and remain engaged, faculty members must see mentorship initiatives as making positive contributions to their institutions' and their own professional goals. Intrinsic rewards and a sense of collective responsibility for students' progress can motivate faculty for awhile, but over the long term, more direct benefits of mentoring must be understood. Mentorship programs must find ways to acknowledge and reward participation. Awards that recognize outstanding mentorship may be more symbolic and inspirational than effective. More appropriate would be ways to include participation in mentorship initiatives in performance or salary reviews.

Other benefits can accrue directly from the mentoring experience itself. Mentors may find working closely with individuals with the support of a mentorship program to be highly stimulating and enjoyable. They may find their own work enhanced by discussions with students, and be able to use mentoring skills toward the advancement of their own careers. Mentoring programs can develop ways to help faculty track their own experiences and development as interpretive mentors, so they can capture and appreciate accumulated benefits.

From the faculty member's standpoint, assessment can be an important component of a mentorship program. Many mentors have no sense of the impact of their work on individuals. Informal and formal feedback and evaluations can help mentors and students track the progress of the mentoring relationship and lead to better understanding of the student's expectations and level of satisfaction. Periodic, informal assessments may be useful.

Stages in Mentoring Relationships

The course and duration of the mentor relationship are difficult to predict. When mentoring programs exist to support interpretive mentoring, stages of the relationship can be better anticipated and faculty can be given resources or other help specific to developmental steps.

A mentoring relationship begins with the selection or initiation process. An interpretive mentoring process depends less on personality or fit than do the more personal forms of mentoring. Reciprocity in the selection process and, ultimately, in the relationship's maintenance is significant for effective forms of mentoring. Promoting appropriate relationship boundaries and clarifying expectations of roles can help mentors and mentees to build a positive foundation early in the relationship. Patterns of interactions can be shaped and trust can be established in these early formative stages of the mentoring relationship through both formal and informal interactions.

A positive and effective mentoring relationship evolves over time as the graduate student moves closer to degree completion. Elasticity in the relationship enables the faculty–student form of interaction to transform into interactions that are more associated with colleagueship. At this later stage, the mentor can trigger an induction process for the mentee into professional roles and contexts. This transformation from a student–faculty to a colleague–faculty relationship may increase the student's success through graduation and into professional work.(18,19,20)

A positive mentoring process that evolves over time gains roots, effective communication, openness, and trust. This type of relationship may not end with the student's graduation. Instead, the mentoring relationship may be redefined. The mentor's interpretive role in relation to professional development can shift at this point to the mentee's establishment of professional networks, navigation through politics in work environments, and strategic presentation of work.

There are times when a mentoring relationship may need to end, a kind of divorce. Mentorship programs should offer support in these situations, supporting both student and faculty during the process of separation. Open, honest discussions about the state of the mentoring relationship are essential to avoid negative outcomes. If the mentoring relationship must end, neutral representatives at the mentorship program level can help the parties avoid further interpersonal conflict or threats to either party's established professional network, academic integrity, and professional credibility.

Problems in Mentoring

In its ideal, a symbiotic mentor relationship is close and enduring and it is assumed that the relationship can only benefit a student's growth and development. However, the nature of a close relationship can also lead to some negative experience for both the student and the mentor. Certainly it is common for both parties to make mistakes or to experience frustration with one another as the relationship develops. In extreme cases, the highly personal nature of traditional mentoring can produce highly damaging effects.

Of even greater concern, however, are those cases in which mentors have deleterious effects on students because of their inadequacies as mentors or because of their modeling of unethical or other inappropriate behavior. Such people have been termed "toxic mentors:"(21) these include "avoiders," who are never accessible to students; "dumpers," who let students sink or swim in new situations; "blockers," who stall students' development by failing to meet their needs or by supervising them too closely; and "criticizers," who tear students down constantly and publicly. In some cases, toxic mentoring takes the form of exploiting a student by demanding an inappropriate amount or type of work. Other overtly toxic mentoring behaviors include harassing the student; soliciting sexual relations with the student; engaging in angry or hostile behavior; or discriminating against the student based on gender, race, age, sexual orienta-

tion, or other characteristics. The potential for toxic mentoring behaviors can be demonstrated by mentors who are unsupportive, inflexible, unsympathetic, overbearing, or inconsiderate of the student's personal life. Possibly the most lethal form of mentoring, in terms of the student's eventual career prospects, is a mentor's advice or example that teaches a student to work or behave in unethical or inappropriate ways. The inherent power differential between students and faculty can make students hesitant to confront toxic mentors or take other steps to remove themselves from the relationship.

Mentoring programs can play a critically important role in identifying and addressing problems of poor mentoring, including cases of toxic mentoring. Programs can mitigate negative effects by providing recourse for students who are struggling with problematic mentoring. They can also develop and publicize standards and expectations for mentoring on campus, so that both students and faculty have a means of comparing and measuring their mentorship experiences against a norm. Mentor programs can set up grievance procedures for handling particularly outrageous violations. Without a system in place, toxic relationships can go undetected or ignored during a student's entire tenure at the institution. Training faculty and empowering students to challenge advice and behavior are important components of such systems.

While toxic mentoring is often associated with the mentor, it is important to recognize the possibility of toxic behavior by mentees and a variety of other improprieties that can occur within relationships. Mentoring programs should be prepared to help faculty members deal with situations in which students stalk mentors, damage their reputations, blame them for things they did not do, or violate personal boundaries.

Student Responsibility

Finally, it is important for students to have a sense of responsibility in the mentoring relationship. In the model we have proposed, students bear significant responsibility for their own development as scholars and professionals. Armed with current and valuable information about professional arenas and students' own goals, faculty can serve as interpreters through students' graduate study and their transition to their subsequent careers. It is up to the students, however, to bring their concerns and puzzlement to faculty.

Resources on Mentoring

Most current mentoring programs serve students in specific academic units. Few institutionally based mentoring programs exist, and virtually none are oriented to the kind of mid-range, interpretive mentorship program that we advocate.

There are, however, a variety of useful resources available online. At present, the following Web sites provide guidance on mentorship, particularly in terms of the scope of mentoring tasks:

- Yahner, R., and Goodstein, L., "Graduate Student Mentoring: Be More Than an Advisor," Penn State University http://www.gradsch.psu.edu/facstaff/practices/mentoring.html (accessed August 28, 2005).
- "Counseling and Educational Psychology Mentoring Policy," College of Education, Indiana University (www.indiana.edu/~soedean/edpsymentoring.html).
- "Resources on Faculty Mentoring," University of Michigan, Center for Research on Learning and Teaching (www.crlt.umich.edu/departments/deptfacment.html).

Award programs for mentors, including criteria used to identify excellence in mentoring, are described on a number of Web sites:

- "The Marsha L. Landott Distinguished Graduate Mentor Awards," University of Washington, (www.grad.washington.edu/mentor).
- "Distinguished Graduate Mentoring Award," University of California, Davis (www.mrak.ucdavis.edu/senate/dgma.htm).
- "Everett Mendelsohn Excellence in Mentoring Awards," Harvard University, School of Arts and Sciences' Graduate Student Council (hcs.harvard.edu/~gsc/awards).

We conclude that interpretive mentoring programs offer great promise for expanding and improving the support and guidance that graduate students and others receive at their universities. Graduate students stand to reap tremendous benefits from mentoring programs that successfully guide faculty from roles as basic advisors to roles as interpretive mentors.

• • • References

1. Weil, V. "Mentoring: Some Ethical Considerations." *Science and Engineering Ethics* 7 (2001): 471–482.

2. Swazey, J.P., M.S. Anderson, and K.S. Louis. "Ethical Problems in Academic Research." *American Scientist* 81 (1993): 542–553.

3. Anderson, M.S., E.C. Oju, and T.M.R. Falkner. "Help from Faculty: Findings from the Acadia Institute Graduate Education Study." *Science and Engineering Ethics* 7 (2001): 487–503.

4. Braxton, J.M., and L.L. Baird. "Preparation for Professional Self-Regulation." *Science and Engineering Ethics* 7 (2001): 593–610.

5. Bird, S.J. "Mentors, Advisors and Supervisors: Their Role in Teaching Responsible Research Conduct." *Science and Engineering Ethics* 7 (2001): 455–468.

6. Fischer, B.A., and M.J. Zigmond. "Survival Skills for Graduate School and Beyond." *New Directions for Higher Education* 101 (1998): 29–40.

7. Gaff, J.G., A.S. Pruitt-Logan, L.B. Sims, and D.D. Denecke. *Preparing Future Faculty in the Humanities and Social Sciences.* Washington, DC: Association of American Colleges and Universities, 2003.

8. Gaff, J.G., A.S. Pruitt-Logan, and J.E. Jentoft. *Preparing Future Faculty in the Sciences and Mathematics.* Washington, DC: Association of American Colleges and Universities, 2002.

9. Swazey, J.P., and M.S. Anderson. "Mentors, Advisors, and Role Models in Graduate and Professional Education." *Missing Management: A New Synthesis.* Edited by E.R. Rubin, 165–185. Vol. 2. Washington, DC: Association of Academic Health Centers, 1998.

10. Golde, C.M., and T.M. Dore. *At Cross Purposes: What the Experiences of Today's Doctoral Students Reveal about Doctoral Education.* Philadelphia: The Pew Charitable Trusts, 2001, www.phd-survey.org (accessed August 16, 2005).

11. Nyquist, J.D. "The PhD: A tapestry of Change for the 21st Century." *Change* 34 (2002): 12–20.

12. Kanigel, R. *Apprentice to Genius: The Making of a Scientific Dynasty.* Baltimore: Johns Hopkins University Press, 1993.

13. *Webster's Ninth New Collegiate Dictionary.* Springfield, MA: Merriam-Webster, 1984.

14. Eby, L.T. "Alternative Forms of Mentoring in Changing Organizational Environments: A Conceptual Extension of the Mentoring Literature." *Journal of Vocational Behavior* 51 (1997): 125–144.

15. Grant-Vallone, E.J., and E.A. Ensher. "Effects of Peer Mentoring on Types of Mentor Support, Program Satisfaction and Graduate Student

Stress: A Dyadic Perspective." *Journal of College Student Development* 41 (2000): 637–642.

16. Granados, R., and J.M. Lopez. "Student-Run Support Organizations for Underrepresented Graduate Students: Goals, Creation, Implementation, and Assessment." *Peabody Journal of Education* 74 (1999): 135–149.

17. Miller, M.T., and J.M. Dirkx. "Mentoring in Graduate Education: The Role of Graduate Student Organizations." *Journal of Adult Education* 23 (1995): 20–30.

18. Berg, H.M., and M.A. Ferber. "Men and Women Graduate Students: Who Succeeds and Why?" *Journal of Higher Education* 54 (1983): 629–648.

19. Boyle, P., and B. Boice. "Best Practices for Enculturation: Collegiality, Mentoring, and Structure." *New Directions for Higher Education* 101 (1998): 87–94.

20. Girves, G.E., and V. Wemmerus. "Developing Models of Graduate Student Degree Progress." *Journal of Higher Education* 59 (1988): 163–189.

21. Darling, L.W. "What to Do about Toxic Mentors." *Nurse Educator* 11, no. 2 (1986): 29–30.

47

Data Management

Michael Kalichman, PhD

Introduction

One of the hallmarks of a scholarly institution is the discovery of new knowledge. The credibility of such discovery is determined by the supporting data. Therefore, one of the most important considerations for effective research administration is the responsible conduct of data management.

For the purpose of this discussion, *data* are defined to be those products of research that are intended as a basis for reporting of research findings. By definition, the existence of such data is necessary to ensure the veracity of a research report. Before publication, the data are necessary to the researcher so that he or she can verify what has already been done, what has and has not worked, and whether or not the data can support a credible and reportable finding. After publication, the data may be important to the researcher or others to verify that analyses had been conducted correctly, to test alternate hypotheses, to support intellectual property claims, or to respond to allegations of research misconduct. Based on these diverse roles, numbers written in a lab notebook are an example of *data*, but are not the only example.

If *data* are the basis for assessing the veracity of a reported finding, then many different research products will fit the definition. As a minimum, any written measurements or observations are examples of data, whether recorded on paper or in computer files. Data might also be stored in the forms of photographs, video recordings, or audio recordings. Other kinds of data might include tissue or other physical samples, slides or other media upon which

such samples are mounted for making observations, gels for separating different molecular species, DNA sequences, or DNA libraries. Many specialized products of research can also be essential for assessing reported inferences or conclusions. These can include unique cell lines or reagents, transgenic animals, or even custom-made software or hardware. Taken together, it should be apparent that data can take many different forms.

Because *data* can take so many different forms, data management is governed by few if any regulations. It is simply not possible to envision meaningful regulations that would govern so many different types of data. However, despite this difficulty, it is reasonable to outline a variety of principles relevant to data collection and analysis, data sharing, publication, and data retention. These are the subjects of the remainder of this chapter.

Data Management

The central element of data management is the data records. The quality and value of those records depend on many factors. Effective data management begins with planning before data collection begins and ends with a decision to destroy or no longer maintain research records. An overview of data management is illustrated in Figure 47-1. In this section, each of these components of data management is briefly described.

Planning

A necessary first step for good data management is to plan. Because research takes many different

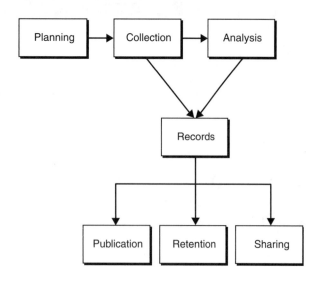

FIGURE 47-1 Components of Data Management

forms, it is not possible to provide a universally comprehensive planning list, but certain basic considerations are worth noting. Before data collection begins, questions to be addressed include, minimally, those listed in Table 47-1. The answers to these questions are important, but not likely to remain fixed. Much will change during the course of a research project, necessitating the need to reconsider many of these elements as the project progresses.

Collection

Any deficit in the quality of data collection will diminish the value of the research records. Minimally, the goal is that records will be accurate, unbiased, and retrievable.

Accuracy depends on personnel who are qualified by experience and training and on measurement instruments that are appropriate to the task, properly maintained, and correctly calibrated.

Elimination or minimization of bias depends on the design of the experimental study. In particular, unintentional bias is a risk if any element of the data collection allows for independent or subjective judgment that might shift the data set to favor a particular bias. To be biased is not a case of sloppy science; however, the failure to guard against bias is.

Retrievable records are produced by the recording of the accurate and unbiased data such that it is possible to extract those data long after the experiment has concluded. This goal can be met in many ways, but most commonly scientists are encouraged to enter all records chronologically, legibly, and in ink into a bound lab notebook with numbered pages. Because it is necessary to record not only the data, but also the methods of data collection, many types of research also warrant having a methods notebook. A methods notebook can be a reference for frequently used methods, and can serve as a

TABLE 47-1	Questions To Be Asked in Planning for Data Collection, Analysis, Sharing, Publication, and Retention.
Collection	What data will be collected?
	How will data be recorded?
	Who will collect the data?
Analysis	What criteria will be used for rejecting data?
	What criteria will be used for accepting data?
	What methods of analysis will be used?
Publication	Which results are to be published?
	When will the results be submitted for publication?
	Where will the results be submitted for publication?
Retention	Which research records are to be retained?
	How will the records be retained?
	How long will the records be retained?
	Who will be responsible for retaining records?
Sharing	Which research records might be shared?
	When can the records be shared?
	Who is responsible for making decisions about sharing records?

valuable aid when it is time to write up a report of a research study.

Analysis

Research reports, as a rule, are based on a presentation of only some of what was done and what was found. In practice, this is not a matter of deception, but is necessary to provide a clear and focused picture. To produce such a report, researchers must make choices about how data will be selected or rejected, what methods of statistical analysis will be used, and how those results are to be presented. These questions are all matters of uncertainty. The nature of published science is to balance the risks of reporting something to be true when it is false and to report something as false when it is in fact true. This seemingly simple requirement is not easily met and is in the realm of statistics and experimental design. Because many scientists do not have the necessary training, it is important that the necessary expertise be sought out. Responsible data management may necessitate consulting with statisticians to design experiments that will provide data suitable to test a clear hypothesis, to select endpoints and methods of analysis that are appropriate, to carry out data analyses, and to assist with interpretation of statistical findings.

Publication

Publications represent a specific example of public sharing of data. The process of publication includes many dimensions of responsibility (e.g., authorship, proper citation of the literature, or respect for copyright), but the focus of this discussion is only the responsible presentation of *data* in a publication. As noted above, reports of data will almost invariably be comprised only of some, not all, of the data collected. Therefore, one aspect of responsible publication must be that the material presented in the paper is adequate for a reader to understand what was done and neither the results nor the discussion should be a misrepresentation of what was found. Because a paper is a summary of what was found, it is also necessary that the methods of data selection, the statistical methods for data summary and comparisons, and the methods of data display are not used in such a way as to mislead the reader. Finally, a significant implication of publishing a paper is that the authors are in effect guaranteeing that the paper is adequately supported by data records. By extension, the authors should be prepared to present those data for review by a journal editor, a funding agency, or other scientists.

Retention

A published paper is the public summary of what was found in a research study, but those findings cannot be considered definitive if it is not possible to verify the information that supported the findings. In this respect, it could be argued that it is the obligation of a responsible researcher to indefinitely retain all data for all reported findings. Unfortunately, this is not always practical. Some data records are so massive that long-term storage would be economically, if not physically, impossible. Other kinds of original data may be in a form that will quickly degrade. In some cases it may be prohibitive in time, money, or skill to make a large set of data sufficiently accessible so that it could have value to future researchers. Given these concerns, it is appropriate to ask what criteria should be factors in determining how and how long a data set should be retained.

Some federal regulations provide specific guidance on retention of data in certain circumstances. However, more generally, other considerations may be cause for increasing the duration of retention. Some examples include data sets that are not easily reproduced and which may have significant secondary uses, data that are the basis for findings that are widely recognized as having unusual significance, and data that are easily retained and can serve as a verifiable source for published findings. In contrast, several factors might diminish the merits of retaining data. These include risks to the confidentiality of human subjects, excessive costs for storage, ample supportive evidence for the same or similar findings in other studies, and the existence of credible summary data or analyses that can serve in place of the raw data.

Sharing

Science is a communal enterprise. Even if one individual had the intellect to address all issues relevant to a field of science, no one individual can do all of the work. For this reason, it makes sense that the interest of science would be best served by rapid and unrestricted sharing of findings, insights, and ideas. On the other hand, personal interests of scientists may be best served by withholding information to protect priority for sole credit, for publication, for patent rights, or simply for being more sure of an interesting finding.

The tension between the interests of science and the individual is not easily resolved. As long as career success is defined more by personal credit than by willingness to share, it is hard to expect—much less require—that scientists readily share data other than in the form of published reports. However, despite this concern, some policies and guidelines require certain levels of sharing. Also, some scientists have made an affirmative decision to share even in the absence of requirements to do so. Presumably, scientists who choose to share do so because the perceived benefits of mutual sharing are greater than the hypothetical risk of losing credit to a competitor.

Regulations

Most elements of data management are not governed by regulations, and the few relevant regulations are easily met or exceeded simply by adhering to common sense and the responsible practice of science. The regulations most frequently relevant to research include those described below from the Food and Drug Administration (FDA), National Institutes of Health (NIH), National Science Foundation (NSF), and the Office of Management and Budget (OMB). The areas in which these regulations have a role are recordkeeping, sharing, access, and retention. However, it should be noted that many other aspects of research are governed by regulations (e.g., human subjects, animal subjects, intellectual property), but are beyond the scope of this discussion.

Recordkeeping

FDA regulations relevant to data management are found in Title 21 of the Code of Federal Regulations. Title 21 Part 58 covers "Good Laboratory Practice for Nonclinical Laboratory Studies." In Part 58.190, "Storage and retrieval of records and data," the standards for research records are described as follows: (1)

> There shall be archives for orderly storage and expedient retrieval of all raw data, documentation, protocols, specimens, and interim and final reports. Conditions of storage shall minimize deterioration of the documents or specimens in accordance with the requirements for the time period of their retention and the nature of the documents or specimens.

Title 21 Part 312 is titled "Investigational New Drug Application." These regulations include a number of specific expectations for research records, including Part 312.62: (2)

> Case histories. An investigator is required to prepare and maintain adequate and accurate case histories that record all observations and other data pertinent to the investigation on each individual administered the investigational drug or employed as a control in the investigation. Case histories include the case report forms and supporting data including, for example, signed and dated consent forms and medical records including, for example, progress notes of the physician, the individual's hospital chart(s), and the nurses' notes. The case history for each individual shall document that informed consent was obtained prior to participation in the study.

In addition to the above, the FDA has recognized the ongoing move toward electronic records and signatures, which are the subject of 21 CFR11. (3)

Sharing

The NIH recently published a Grants Policy Statement covering a wide range of issues, including the sharing of research data. (4) This policy makes clear that the grantees (the institutions), "own the data generated by or resulting from a grant-supported project." Relying in part on published guidelines, (5) the policy encourages reasonable dissemination of NIH-funded research:

> NIH expects recipients to determine the appropriate means of effecting prompt and effective access to research tools (including inventions for which patents and exclusive licenses are inappropriate) to further advance scientific research and discovery. If further research, development, and private investment are not necessary to realize the primary usefulness of a research tool, publication, deposit in an appropriate databank or repository, widespread non-exclusive licensing, or other dissemination techniques may be appropriate.

NIH has further emphasized sharing in a variety of documents (6) and a 2003 notice: (7)

> The NIH expects and supports the timely release and sharing of final research data from NIH-supported studies for use by other researchers. Starting with the October 1, 2003 receipt date, investigators submitting an NIH application seeking $500,000 or more in direct costs in any single

year are expected to include a plan for data sharing or state why data sharing is not possible. . . .

NIH recognizes that the investigators who collect the data have a legitimate interest in benefiting from their investment of time and effort. We have therefore revised our definition of "the timely release and sharing" to be no later than the acceptance for publication of the main findings from the final data set. NIH continues to expect that the initial investigators may benefit from first and continuing use but not from prolonged exclusive use.

Guidance on implementation of this policy has been developed by the Council on Governmental Relations (COGR). (8)

The NSF similarly expects sharing of data generated by NSF funding: (9)

NSF expects significant findings from research and education activities it supports to be promptly submitted for publication, with authorship that accurately reflects the contributions of those involved. It expects investigators to share with other researchers, at no more than incremental cost and within a reasonable time, the data, samples, physical collections and other supporting materials created or gathered in the course of the work. It also encourages awardees to share software and inventions or otherwise act to make the innovations they embody widely useful and usable.

Retention

Federal regulations outline the period of time and circumstances for retention of research records. The range of time in most cases varies between two and five years; however, much longer times are expected in some cases, such as patient records and patents. For the FDA, the retention periods are defined for investigational new drug applications as: (2)

Record retention. An investigator shall retain records required to be maintained under this part for a period of 2 years following the date a marketing application is approved for the drug for the indication for which it is being investigated; or, if no application is to be filed or if the application is not approved for such indication, until 2 years after the investigation is discontinued and FDA is notified.

In the case of nonclinical laboratory study results, the FDA requirements for record retention are: (10)

. . . documentation records, raw data and specimens pertaining to a nonclinical laboratory study and required to be made by this part shall be retained in the archive(s) for whichever of the following periods is shortest:

(1) A period of at least 2 years following the date on which an application for a research or marketing permit, in support of which the results of the nonclinical laboratory study were submitted, is approved by the Food and Drug Administration. . . .

(2) A period of at least 5 years following the date on which the results of the nonclinical laboratory study are submitted to the Food and Drug Administration in support of an application for a research or marketing permit.

(3) In other situations (e.g., where the nonclinical laboratory study does not result in the submission of the study in support of an application for a research or marketing permit), a period of at least 2 years following the date on which the study is completed, terminated, or discontinued.

Record retention under NIH regulations is set at three years after the final financial report: (4)

Grantees generally must retain financial and programmatic records, supporting documents, statistical records, and all other records that are required by the terms of a grant, or may reasonably be considered pertinent to a grant, for a period of 3 years from the date the annual FSR is submitted.

NSF regulations also call for records to be retained at least three years: (11)

Financial records, supporting documents, statistical records, and other records pertinent to this award shall be retained by the awardee for a period of three years from submission of the final reports specified in Article 16.

Access

Data records are of potential interest to many different entities, including colleagues, other researchers, the home research institution, funding agencies, professional societies and journals, the public, and the media. In some cases, such as a misconduct allegation, the institution has a right as owner of the data to review or sequester all relevant research records. In other cases, such as demands from a competitor to see unpublished data, a researcher may not have to release the requested information. However, researchers, especially those who are federally funded, should be aware that the OMB modified Circular A-110 to allow Freedom of Information Act (FOIA) requests to serve as a basis for forcing a release of at least some records: (12)

> ...in response to a Freedom of Information Act (FOIA) request for research data relating to published research findings produced under an award that were used by the Federal Government in developing an agency action that has the force and effect of law, the Federal awarding agency shall request, and the recipient shall provide, within a reasonable time, the research data so that they can be made available to the public through the procedures established under the FOIA.

OMB Circular A-110 defines *published* as: (12)

> ...either when:
>
> (A) Research findings are published in a peer-reviewed scientific or technical journal; or
>
> (B) A Federal agency publicly and officially cites the research findings in support of an agency action that has the force and effect of law.

Responsibilities

Promoting the integrity of research data is the responsibility of all of those involved.

Principle Investigators

As the leader of a research investigation, the principle investigator (PI) has primary responsibility for project planning and final decisions about methods of data collection and analysis, sharing of data (what, when, and with whom), publication (what, when, and where), and retention (what, how, and for how long). On an ongoing basis, the PI should also establish clear standards of conduct regarding data collection, recordkeeping, and reporting of problems. Such standards are ideally written and readily available and should be specific for the areas of research unique to the PI's research program.

Researchers (Students, Postdoctoral Fellows, Staff, and Others)

Those who carry out the research are responsible for collecting and recording data as requested. However, the integrity of the data also depends on the willingness of researchers to speak out about any problems that interfere with the performance of their role, including observations of questionable conduct or outright misconduct.

Research Institutions

The leadership of a research institution sets the tone for standards of conduct. The importance of responsible data management is emphasized by clear policies and guidelines, by effective communication through a variety of mechanisms (courses, workshops, mailings, Web sites, flyers) and by decisive responses if and when problems occur.

Departments and Other Groups of Researchers

Departments can do their part in promoting responsible data management by creating guidelines and policies that can be more specific than those established for a more diverse institution. As with the institution, those guidelines will have an impact only if it is clear both what is expected and that failures to meet those standards will have consequences. To make this clear, it is essential that departmental guidelines be as specific as practical, but that PIs be encouraged to meet their responsibilities by communication of expectations and by developing written policies for their individual research groups.

Journals

Journals have few resources to investigate alleged problems or to routinely review raw data for submitted publications, but they can still have a significant role in promoting responsible data management. Guidelines should lay out expectations that publications are based on clear research records; that original records will be retained for some minimal duration; that reasonable access will be granted to view data supporting the publication; and that other scientists will have reasonable access to unique materials. In the case that alleged misconduct must be addressed, such concerns should be presented to the home institution(s) of those involved.

Professional Societies

Because professional societies represent a collection of researchers with common interests, a minimal expectation is that such a group would create guidelines for the responsible conduct of research. A central component of such guidelines is the topic of data management. Society guidelines for the responsible conduct of research would be a valuable framework for promoting discussion and for resolving disputes among society members. In addition, societies should have a role in advocating good management practices on the part of PIs; good research practices on the part of researchers; and regulations, policies, and guidelines that are appropriate for institutions, research groups, journals, and regulating agencies.

Federal Agencies

Regulating agencies have a responsibility that must balance between defining a meaningful, minimum standard and avoiding counterproductive micromanagement. The danger of overly specific regulations has at least three dimensions. First, regulatory agencies could not possibly have the resources necessary to ensure compliance with every element of responsible data management. Second, the imposition of overly ambitious requirements, for which compliance cannot be assured, runs the risk of increasing cynicism of researchers about the merits of any regulatory controls. Finally, because research methods and environments are so diverse, it will rarely be possible to enact a regulation relevant to all. However, establishing minimal standards can have a role in fostering responsible data management practices. In addition to regulations that are already in place, it might be useful to require that investigators or institutions develop guidelines or education programs, but to set no or minimal specifications for what those guidelines or programs must look like.

Guidelines

Many institutions and organizations have published guidelines or policies which are intended to set a standard, but do not necessarily have the same weight as a law or regulation. Nonetheless, guidelines fill an essential role in defining the responsible

conduct of research. While some standards of conduct may be highly desirable, failing to meet those standards may not be justification for imposing sanctions or penalties. However a document that contains specific expectations for behavior can be a valuable tool for socializing new researchers into a culture that values integrity, for promoting discussion among researchers to better define acceptable and exemplary standards of conduct, and for serving as a framework for discussion when disputes arise. The following are representative examples of guidelines that address some or many of the dimensions of responsible data management.

University of California, San Francisco (UCSF)

The Brain Tumor Research Center (BTRC) of UCSF developed detailed guidelines for research data and manuscripts in 1989, followed by a revision in 2000. (13) These guidelines continue to be among the most comprehensive of institutional guidelines for responsible data management. Some of the key elements included in the BTRC guidelines are summarized in Table 47-2. Some other noteworthy institutional guidelines include documents on lab notebooks (14) and data ownership and retention. (15–18)

International Committee of Medical Journal Editors (ICMJE)

In 1978, a group of biomedical journal editors met in Vancouver and formulated a set of guidelines for submission of manuscripts to their journals. Those guidelines have been periodically revised over the years and are now subscribed to by over 500 biomedical journals. (19) The guidelines cover a wide range of issues in biomedical publication, but include several considerations for data management, including accurate description in the methods section of a paper about how the data were collected, descriptions of methods and statistics

TABLE 47-2	Selected Components of Data Management Guidelines of the Brain Tumor Research Center at the University of California, San Francisco(13)
Laboratory notebooks	Descriptions of two types of notebooks: experimental and methodological
Responsibilities	Outline of principal investigator responsibilities
Statistics	Emphasis on importance of obtaining expert statistical advice
Ownership	Verification of institutional ownership of data
Retention of records	Responsibilities of principal investigator for storing and retaining records for at least 5 years after ending of funding for study

sufficient for a knowledgeable reader to understand what was done, and how journals should handle disputes about how a given data set should be reported.

In addition to the general guidelines of the ICMJE, many individual journals now include specific guidance on questions of data sharing and depositing data in public databases. Based on a survey of the 56 most frequently cited journals in the life sciences, 39% included a policy on sharing materials and 41% included a policy on depositing data in a public database. (20)

National Institutes of Health (NIH)

The NIH has provided guidelines relevant to many aspects of the responsible conduct of data management. In addition to newly defined policies on sharing of data, NIH has produced a variety of documents that address the sharing of research data. (6) These guidelines and recommendations generally recognize both the value to science of open sharing of data and the need to protect intellectual property interests of institutions and individuals.

National Association of College and University Attorneys (NACUA)

The law profession provides a valuable perspective on the legal dimensions of data management. In association with the National Council of University Research Administrators, NACUA has addressed questions of data ownership and retention of data. (21) The purpose of this pamphlet is to assist academic institutions and the funders of research by clarifying issues relevant to data management.

American Statistical Association

Statistical analysis is or should be an important element of most published research. Because a misuse of statistics can easily mislead a reader about flawed data, and can easily lead to a misinterpretation of robust data, it is important to consider the ethical obligations of statisticians in assisting with data analysis. The American Statistical Association recently created a set of ethical guidelines for statisticians. (22)

Collaborative Electronic Notebook Systems Association (CENSA)

Researchers are increasingly dependent on computer-based storage of information. For this reason, it is important to keep apprised of options available for electronic records. CENSA is an organization dedicated to improving "the state of the art for electronic recordkeeping systems and collaborative technologies wherever they are used." (23)

Council on Governmental Relations (COGR)

COGR is a university association that closely monitors all dimensions of federally funded research, including the responsible conduct of data management. In this capacity, COGR has developed guidelines on a variety of aspects of data management, including data sharing, (8) material transfer agreements, (24) and retention of data. (25)

Office of Research Integrity (ORI)

The ORI's responsibilities include oversight for the handling of allegations of research misconduct by institutions funded by the Public Health Service (PHS). In this role, many of the cases seen by ORI, as well as the NIH ombudsmen, revolve around disputes about the handling of data. With the goal of decreasing the risk of misunderstandings, two NIH ombudsmen recommend that collaborators develop clear agreements about the collaboration before it starts. (26)

Creating Institutional Guidelines

Responsible data management is the subject of few regulations, but is an appropriate subject for guidelines. This distinction is important. The process of research takes many different forms. Therefore, it will rarely make sense to have a rule that would be meaningful or sensible for the many different types of research. However, data management is so fundamental to good research that it is desirable to have some basic guidelines to provide a meaningful framework for the responsible conduct of data management. A suggested checklist for an institutional policy on data management is included as Table 47-3.

Additional Resources

Several books on responsible conduct of research include additional material relevant to the topic of data management. (27–30)

References

1. Food and Drug Administration. "Storage and Retrieval of Records and Data." Part 58: Good Laboratory Practice for Nonclinical Laboratory Studies, Subpart J: Records and Reports. *Code of Federal Regulations*, title 21, sec. 58.190 (April 1, 2003).

TABLE 47-3	Suggested Components To Be Included in Institutional Guidelines or Policies on Responsible Data Management
__ Commitment	Statement of institutional commitment to integrity of research, including research records
__ Definitions	Definitions of data, data management, and who is covered by this policy
__ Recordkeeping	Minimal information that should be recorded:
	Name of researcher
	Date of experiment
	Title or brief description of experiment
	Methods or location where methods can be found
	Raw data or where data can be found
	Summary or interpretation of experiment
	Goals of recordkeeping:
	Accurate
	Retrievable
	Complete
	Reliable (e.g., ink, numbered pages, dated entries)
	Examples of acceptable records:
	Lab notebook
	3-ring binder
	Electronic/computer
__ Retention of Records	At least 5 years after final financial report, but list considerations that might favor keeping records for longer periods of time
__ Ownership	Institutional ownership of research records
	Researcher responsibility for planning, conducting, and reporting research
	Collaborators' agreements about responsibilities for jointly created research records prior to beginning research
__ Resources	Institutional resources: where to go with questions or problems
__ Disputes	Institutional committee or individuals with responsibility for hearing and resolving disputes about data ownership, sharing, retention, and publication

2. Food and Drug Administration. "Investigator Recordkeeping and Record Retention." Part 312: Investigational New Drug Application, Subpart D: Responsibilities of Sponsors and Investigators. *Code of Federal Regulations*, title 21, sec. 312.62 (April 1, 2003).

3. Food and Drug Administration. "Part 11: Electronic Records; Electronic Signatures." *Code of Federal Regulations*, title 21, sec. 11 (April 1, 2003).

4. National Institutes of Health. "NIH Grants Policy Statement, 2001," http://grants.nih.gov/grants/policy/nihgps_2001 (accessed September 30, 2003).

5. National Institutes of Health. "Principles and Guidelines for Recipients of NIH Research Grants and Contracts on Obtaining and Disseminating Biomedical Research Resources: Final Notice," *Federal Register* 64, no. 72090 (December 23, 1999), http://ott.od.nih.gov/ RTguide_final.html (accessed August 17, 2005).

6. National Institutes of Health. "NIH Data Sharing Policy, 2003," http://grants.nih.gov/grants/policy/data_sharing (accessed September 30, 2003).

7. National Institutes of Health. "Final NIH Statement on Sharing Research Data," Notice No. NOT-OD-03-032, February 26, 2003, http://grants.nih.gov/grants/guide/notice-files/NOT-OD-03-032.html (accessed September 30, 2003).

8. Council on Governmental Relations. "Guidance to Campuses on NIH: Principles and Guidelines for Recipients of NIH Research Grants and Contracts on Obtaining and Disseminating Biomedical Research Resources," February 2000,

http://www.cogr.edu/docs/ResearchTools.htm (accessed September 30, 2003).

9. National Science Foundation. "37. Sharing of Findings, Data, and Other Research Products." *National Science Foundation General Grant Conditions*, 2002, http://www.nsf.gov/pubs/2002/gc102/gc102.pdf (accessed August 17, 2005).

10. Food and Drug Administration. "Retention of Records," Part 58: Good Laboratory Practice for Nonclinical Laboratory Studies, Subpart J: Records and Reports, *Code of Federal Regulations*, title 21, sec. 58.195 (April 1, 2003).

11. National Science Foundation. "23. Audit and Records." *National Science Foundation General Grant Conditions*, 2002, http://www.nsf.gov/pubs/2002/gc102/gc102.pdf (accessed August 17, 2005).

12. Office of Management and Budget. "Circular A-110, Uniform Administrative Requirements for Grants and Agreements with Institutions of Higher Education, Hospitals, and Other Non-Profit Organizations," *Federal Register* 64 http://www.whitehouse.gov/omb/circulars/a110/a110.html (accessed August 29, 2005).

13. Eastwood, S., J.R. Fike, P.H. Cogen, H. Rosegay, and M. Berens. "BTRC Guidelines on Research Data and Manuscripts." University of California San Francisco: Brain Tumor Research Center, 1989. Revised and updated in 2000 and reprinted in *The Ethical Dimensions of the Biological Sciences*. 2nd ed. Edited by R.E. Bulger, E. Heitman, and S.J. Reiser, 236–243. New York: Cambridge University Press, 2001.

14. University of Minnesota. "Guidelines for Maintaining Laboratory Notebooks," 2003, http://www.ptm.umn.edu/v3/documents/labnotes.pdf (accessed August 30, 2005).

15. University of Pittsburgh. "Guidelines on Data Retention and Access," 1997, http://www.pitt.edu/~provost/retention.html (accessed September 30, 2003).

16. Henry M. Jackson Foundation. "Retention of and Access to Research Data." In *The Ethical Dimensions of the Biological Sciences*. 2nd ed. Edited by R.E. Bulger, E. Heitman, and S.J. Reiser, 231–235. New York: Cambridge University Press, 2002.

17. Michigan State University. "Data Control and Management Guidelines." *Research Integrity Newsletter* 4, no. 2 (Fall 2001): 2–4.

18. Wake Forest University. "Data Ownership Guidelines," 2003, http://www.wfubmc.edu/school/OurFacStaff/OPHandbook/SectionIV/DataOwnership.htm (accessed September 30, 2003).

19. International Committee of Medical Journal Editors. "Uniform Requirements for Manuscripts Submitted to Biomedical Journals." *JAMA* 277 (1997): 927–934. Also available at http://www.icmje.org (accessed September 30, 2003).

20. National Research Council. *Sharing Publication-Related Data and Materials: Responsibilities of Authorship in the Life Sciences. Committee on Responsibilities of Authorship in the Biological Sciences*, National Research Council. Washington, DC: National Academies Press, 2003.

21. Stevens, A.R. "Ownership and Retention of Data," National Association of College and University Attorneys, 1997, http://www.nacua.org/onlinepubs/ownership.html (accessed September 30, 2003).

22. American Statistical Association. "Ethical Guidelines for Statistical Practice." Prepared by the Committee on Professional Ethics, American Statistical Association, 1999, http://www.amstat.org/profession/index.cfm?fuseaction=ethicalstatistics (accessed August 17, 2005).

23. Collaborative Electronic Notebook Systems Association, 2003, http://www.censa.org (accessed September 12, 2005).

24. Council on Governmental Relations. "Materials Transfer in Academia," June 1997, http://www.cogr.edu/docs/MaterialsTransfer.pdf (accessed September 30, 2003).

25. Council on Governmental Relations. "Policy Considerations: Access to and Retention of Research Data," August 1995, http://www.cogr.edu/docs/RetentionData.pdf (accessed September 30, 2003).

26. Gadlin, H., and K. Jessar. "Preempting Discord: Prenuptial Agreements for Scientists," 2003, http://ori.hhs.gov/education/preempt_discord.shtml (accessed September 12, 2005).

27. Barnbaum, D.R., and M. Byron. *Research Ethics: Text and Readings*. Upper Saddle River, NJ: Prentice Hall, 2001, 45–47, 349–356.

28. Bulger, R.E., E. Heitman, and S.J. Reiser. *The Ethical Dimensions of the Biological and Health Sciences*. New York: Cambridge University Press, 2002, 221–243.

29. Macrina, F.L. *Scientific Integrity: An Introductory Text with Cases*. Washington, DC: American Society for Microbiology Press, 2000, 179–209, 231–256.

30. Resnick, D.B. *The Ethics of Science: An Introduction (Philosophical Issues in Science)*. New York: Routledge, 1998, 90–95.

48

Authorship: Credit, Responsibility, and Accountability

Bryan Benham, PhD, Dale Clark, and Leslie P. Francis, PhD, JD

Introduction

Reporting the findings of research and receiving credit for that work is critically important for scientific research. Publication of research plays an essential role in the stimulation and dissemination of scientific knowledge. Published research establishes priority of discovery and confers the benefits of prestige and recognition to the discoverers. Perhaps most importantly, for individual scientists, the prospects for securing jobs, promotions, and future funding are all crucially dependent on the researcher's publication record. In a phrase, publications are the "coin of the realm" when it comes to advancing careers in science.[1] So it is no surprise that attribution of authorship is a critical ethical issue in contemporary science.

The last several decades have seen a rise in disputes about authorship. In fact, many charges of scientific misconduct have to do with authorship issues.[2] The increase in complaints has to do in part with the parallel rise in the number of jointly or multiply authored papers.[3] Jones reports that in some disciplines, such as the humanities and mathematics, the tradition of single-authored and dual-authored papers remains relatively intact, whereas in other disciplines, such as high-energy physics, it is not unusual to have hundreds of authors on a single paper.[4] The biomedical sciences, especially medicine, display similar trends, though not reaching the extremes of high-energy physics. For example, Huth notes an "exponential rise" in the average number of authors for papers published in the *New England Journal of Medicine* and the *Annals of Internal Medicine* between the years 1915, in which the average was just over one, and 1985, in which the average was more than six.[5] The rise in the number of authors in scientific publications can be explained by any number of factors: the increased specialization of scientists, the move toward questions that require a more interdisciplinary approach, and ultimately the pressures of securing funding, jobs, and promotions. Whatever the reasons for the increase in multiple-authored papers, the result is an increase in problems relating to authorship.

Some problems are quite simple: it is wrong to take credit for the work of another. Others are far more complex: among the many contributors to a manuscript, who should receive primary credit? What should the order of authors be in multiple-authored papers? If errors are discovered in a work, who bears responsibility and what do these responsibilities involve? To add to these problems, conventions for attributing authorship vary across disciplines and different journals often have different criteria. Is there any way to provide a unified account of proper authorship?

In this chapter, we offer a principled approach to guide decisions about authorship, without providing yet another proposal for authorship criteria. Authorship may involve issues of trust, collegiality and, of course, prestige, but the underlying ethical principles that inform authorship are fairness (giving credit where credit is due) and responsibility (accountability for the work). Questions concerning fairness and responsibility can be treated separately but they are also interrelated. For example, problems associated with plagiarism are clearly issues of fairness in receiving proper credit for work done. Determining the propriety of publications or the treatment of sensitive information is clearly an issue of authorship responsibility. However, determining the order of authorship or who counts as an author in collaborative work involves both attributing proper credit to each individual and assigning responsibility for the research reported. In what follows, we will treat issues of fairness and responsibility separately in order to address the main areas of contention in authorship disputes. We have also included a short section on authorship integrity that touches on a number of related, though infrequently discussed, authorship issues.

Fairness: Credit Where Credit Is Due

One of the chief reasons for publishing research is to receive appropriate credit for work. An author is one who receives the credit for work done in published manuscripts. Presumably this is why authorship is the currency of the academic marketplace; authorship is an indication of one's accomplishments. It is important, however, not only for the promotion and advancement of individual scientists' careers, but also for achieving the aims of science. Scientists may operate in a culture of competition for rights to first discovery, but that culture also highly values trust, openness, and the integrity of its practitioners. Giving proper credit to an individual's contribution to the advancement of science is crucial for that person receiving recognition for his or her work. It is also crucial for the smooth operation of science, by promoting openness and reproducible results. Not giving proper credit would be detrimental to the practice of science. If researchers believed that their ideas would be used without acknowledgment, then this would lead to distrust and inhibit the sharing of information. No doubt, competition among researchers generates some distrust and incomplete sharing of information, but on the whole receiving credit for contributions is seen as a valuable commodity. It is only fair that people get their due acknowledgment, and it produces good science.

Plagiarism

Plagiarism is a key area of dispute in accusations of scientific misconduct.[6] According to the federal Office of Research Integrity (ORI) definition, plagiarism is the appropriation of another person's ideas, processes, results, or words without giving appropriate credit. Plagiarism is a serious wrong for the obvious reason that it unfairly denies others the proper rewards of research and scholarship. It is also a form of theft and deception. Claiming another's work as one's own is, in principle, no different than stealing someone's property. It unfairly deprives the owner or originator of an idea and the fruits of that person's labor. It can also be argued that plagiarism violates certain principles of respect for others. Appropriating another person's ideas as one's own effectively treats that person as something to be used, as merely a means to some ends, not as a person of value in his or her own right. Clearly, it harms the victim of plagiarism, to say nothing of the integrity of the person who plagiarizes.

However, in academic and commercial research, the pressures to plagiarize are real, especially if the idea has marketable applications. How does one recognize plagiarism? Copying a published work word for word and passing it off as one's own is clearly a case of plagiarism, but not all cases are so obvious. For example, supervisors who rework the analysis of data done by graduate students in his or her lab, and then fail to credit the students in the resulting publication are misappropriating the work of the students as their own. Even if the reworking was substantial, the collection and analysis of data done by the graduate students should still be given full acknowledgement.[7] Other forms of plagiarism include paraphrasing without proper citation, claiming the spoken words (unpublished) of another without citation, and even summarizing the work of another without proper citation, sometimes called "citation amnesia." Even more subtle types of plagiarism exist.[8]

Ghost Authorship

A "ghost" author is someone who contributed substantially to the project, to a degree sufficient to be regarded as an author, but who is not listed as an author when the manuscript is published. This practice is improper, even if it takes place with the full consent of the "ghost." Ghost authors fail to receive the credit they deserve, instead allowing full credit to go to those who are listed on the manuscript. In addition, ghost authors also escape public responsibility for the published work (discussed below). Nonetheless, ghost authorship is surprisingly common. Flanagin et al. compared surveys of corresponding authors of articles in peer reviewed medical journals with published authorship information.[9] Their analysis indicated that 7% to 16% of the published articles contained evidence of ghost authorship. The prevalence of ghost authorship was higher in review articles in smaller-circulation journals.

Accidental Plagiarism

The most ethically problematic forms of plagiarism are when the plagiarist does it intentionally, as a way to promote themselves at the expense of others. Nevertheless, some plagiarism may occur accidentally. In the process of research, a great deal of information (published literature, discussions, experimentation, etc.) is reviewed and processed, so it is understandable that one might not remember a source when writing up information or ideas. In some cases, one might even think the plagiarized ideas are actually one's own. Although not usually considered as serious a form of plagiarism (once the error is recognized and corrected), accidental occurrences are still ethically troubling. In short, they demonstrate poor research practices. Part of the researcher's responsibility is to be familiar with the relevant literature so the work can be placed in proper context. Failing to identify the original sources of information amounts to sloppy science, and should be considered a form of blameworthy negligence.[10] The degree of blameworthiness increases with the professional level of the scientist; higher standards of professionalism can be applied to a more advanced student or faculty member than to a beginning undergraduate; with the latter, education is the more appropriate response. Accidental plagiarism can be avoided by keeping accurate and up-to-date research notes. Good research notes can act as an intellectual mapping of the terrain covered by one's research. They can also act as a rich source of data for the interpretation of findings and conclusions in the drafting of a manuscript. Thus, good research conforms to ethical standards of fairness. Sloppy science is simply bad science.

Self-Plagiarism

There is another form of plagiarism, sometimes referred to as "self-plagiarism," that poses unique problems.[11] Self-plagiarism is the practice of recycling one's own previously published work so that it looks original. Because of the pressures to publish, some may argue that this is an innocent practice. Recycling one's ideas is not necessarily a bad thing, because it promotes one's ideas by distributing them across a variety of publications, and it is not unusual to publish one's own work by building on previous work. Some duplication is necessary and acceptable. Self-plagiarism, however, misleadingly inflates an author's curriculum vitae. It may use

scarce and expensive journal space unjustifiably. Self-plagiarism often shades into other ethically questionable practices, such as wasteful publications or dividing research into least publishable units (discussed later). The chief problem with self-plagiarism occurs when the author fails to disclose or obtain permission from the original publisher for the use of the previously published information.[12] Even if the author is duplicating his or her own work, proper citation is essential, not just for providing credit where credit is due, but also for aiding other scientists in researching the experimental evidence for their own work. Self-plagiarism often leads to sloppy science or confuses the research record. It possibly also violates copyright laws.

Avoiding Plagiarism

Plagiarism is a serious concern because it deprives researchers of the proper credit due to them. It is ethically unfair and violates the trust and collegiality of scientists. How, then, does one avoid plagiarism? Most important is the diligent use of citation. Citation is always the responsibility of the researcher, never of the readers, editors, or publishers. Style guides and professional societies have recommendations for proper citations, but the general rule to follow is "when in doubt, always cite the source." Citations are not usually required when the information comes from common knowledge or general reference materials. However, this exception only applies to the information gathered from these sources, not the particular wording or phrasing of the information. Again, when in doubt, citation is the best way to make sure proper credit is given. At the very least, proper citation demonstrates a research trail that can be retraced by any researcher, which is the hallmark of openness and good research. Giving credit where credit is due properly acknowledges the discoveries and efforts of the scientific community, and, in the end, makes for good science.

Honorary Authorship

Another area of concern that deals with improper allocation of credit in scientific research involves the practice of giving credit where credit is not properly due. This includes what is called "honorary authorship"—listing a person as author for personal or professional favors or as a sign of respect or gratitude. For example, some laboratory directors insist that they be listed as an author on every publication that is produced by their lab, whether or not they were active in the production of that work.[13] This practice places questionable emphasis on unequal power relationships that hold between colleagues or between supervisors and graduate students, rather than on according proper credit for work done. It also involves violations of authorship responsibility and accountability, which is discussed later. Similarly, problems arise with a form of honorary authorship called "prestige authorship," in which a person with a recognized position of prestige or notoriety is listed as an author solely in order to give the publication more visibility.[14] In extreme cases, for example, pharmaceutical companies have asked physicians to be listed as authors on papers for which they did no research, planning, or writing, in order to give the paper greater status.[15] In other cases, researchers may want to add the name of a well-known scientist, perhaps a former advisor, so that the paper may more easily get published or be more likely to receive funding for the research. In all of these cases, the "author" is author in name only. Clearly this violates fairness issues when attributing credit; the author is receiving credit for work he or she has not done. Honorary authorship also raises problems for accountability. For instance, who is responsible for the work when errors are found, or when other researchers request data or methodological materials in order to reproduce the results? The practice of honorary authorship may also tend to establish and reinforce a culture of fealty among scientists, which raises issues of scientific politics and the effects this may have on research results. In the end, credit should be attributed only to those who deserve the credit for the work done. Fairness is a hallmark of proper research practices and of authorship.

Credit and Collaborative Research

Authorship is a time-honored and critical part of the practice of science. Publications promote the expansion of knowledge as well as the career of the individual scientists recognized as the originators or discoverers of new knowledge. Plagiarism and honorary authorship most likely result either from the pressures of tenure, promotion, recruitment, and securing of funding or even from sloppy scientific practice. The natural question to ask, then, is how should authorship be attributed? For single-authored papers the answer is easy: the one who did all the work gets the credit. This is why the manuscript is published under a single author. The difficult question arises for multiple-

authored papers. Determining the criteria for authorship in multiple-authored papers is not an easy task.

Scientific journals have increasingly published instructions for authors that provide some statement of authorship policy, along with the usual details about manuscript preparation and other journal policies. A common convention for multiple-authored papers is to list the first author (who takes primary credit), then any co-authors or contributors (who contributed some work to the manuscript, but do not get primary credit), and then lastly the senior author (who may be the same as first author, but is typically the mentor, director, or head of the laboratory). Although this practice may provide some clarity, two basic problems remain. First, different journals, as well as different disciplines, have different conventions for assigning authorship, co-authorship, and senior authorship. Moreover, the category of senior author is reminiscent of honorary authorship. Second, those criteria provided by professional societies, editorial boards, and publishers are still problematically vague. First authors are typically identified as those persons who provide "a significant intellectual contribution" to the work; but what counts as "significant" is up for debate and varies across disciplines. Does proposing the original hypothesis, but not drafting the manuscript or analyzing data, count as authorship? Does simply writing the paper constitute authorship, even if one had little or nothing to do with collecting, analyzing, and interpreting data? And should graduate assistants and doctoral students get first authorship credit for work done, or does their mentor or lab director deserve primary credit?

In order to resolve some of these problems a uniform code for authorship credit has been proposed by the International Committee of Medical Journal Editors (ICMJE) that serves as the standard for biomedical publications.[16] Social and behavioral sciences often refer to the American Psychological Association (APA) for accepted ethics codes, but regarding authorship both the ICMJE and APA are in accord with one another.[17] Authorship credit, according to the ICMJE uniform requirements,

> should be based on 1) substantial contributions
> to conception and design, or acquisition of data,
> or analysis and interpretation of data; 2) drafting
> the article or revising it critically for important
> intellectual content; and 3) final approval of the
> version to be published. Authors should meet
> conditions 1, 2, and 3.[18]

Many editorial boards and institutions have adopted this or similar codes. One common departure from this uniform requirement is worth mentioning, however. According to some institutions, authorship credit may be given to those who offer not only significant intellectual contributions, but also significant "functional" or "practical" contributions.[19] These latter qualifications confer on those who contributed technical expertise or assistance the ability to be considered authors (or coauthors). In large research labs, this may provide a fairer distribution of credit, but it also opens the door to more questionable practices, such as giving authorship title to those who provide routine technical assistance, simply provide access to labs or materials, and so on. What counts as significant or routine is not entirely clear. In addition, institutional adoption of ICMJE uniform requirements or similar codes may conflict with journal editorial policies regarding authorship. Regardless, it seems that the best course of action is to be as explicit as possible about the credit each author in the byline of a paper is receiving. Those who may have contributed, but don't merit authorship status should be acknowledged in the footnotes or in an introductory note.

Other proposals have been offered. One proposal is to designate the particular contribution made by each person in the authorship category.[20] The research effort can be divided up into different elements. For example, research efforts often involve such activities as conceiving the project, reviewing background literature, generating data, analyzing and interpreting the data, designing experimental methodologies, providing technical support, and editing the manuscript. First authors are the ones who have completed the most essential of these elements, usually understood to be the conception, design, interpretation, and drafting of the manuscript. Other proposals are more radical, suggesting the complete dissolution of the concept of authorship in favor of other categories of credit allotment, such as contributors, guarantor, and sponsorship.[21] One problem with these proposals for dissolving authorship is that they are too cumbersome to be attractive to editors and publishers. Thus the entrenched practice of a list order of authors without designating particular roles to each is unlikely to be changed in the near future.[22] Nevertheless, what each of these proposals agrees upon is that taking credit for authorship involves more than receiving one's due acknowledgments. Credit for work done also entails taking responsibility for the work done.

Finally, when collaboration is between faculty members and students, inequalities in skills and power complicate the attribution of authorship. A recent proposal by Fine and Kurdek[23] suggests that different criteria for contribution should be applied depending on the professional level of those involved in creating the work. In their view, it is fair to expect less of students, more as they become more advanced, and more still of faculty, in order to claim credit for work. Inequalities in power, however, should not affect the attribution of authorship, nor should whether or not the student is being paid for the work. Rather, authorship attribution should depend on relative scholarly abilities and professional contributions of the authors.

The identification of the first author is a special concern because of the credit that status implies. Student projects such as undergraduate honors theses, master's theses, and doctoral dissertations may draw considerably on the expertise of supervising faculty members. When publishable papers are drawn from such projects, faculty members may be substantially involved in reworking or rewriting the projects to meet publication developing research design, writing parts of the manuscript, or interpreting data. Fine and Kurdek offer guidance on when students should receive first authorship credit. They contend that as students become more advanced professionals (doctoral students as against undergraduates, for example), they should be expected to play greater roles in projects to earn first authorship credit. Their argument is that on grounds of justice when students have less expertise in such matters as research design and data analysis, lesser relative contributions should be expected to gain authorship credit. Nevertheless, students should not earn authorship credit unless they have overall perspective on the project and their contributions are professional in nature. The initial recommendation of the Ethics Committee of the American Psychological Association was that first authorship of articles based on dissertations should be reserved for students, with supervisors credited with second authorship when they made substantial contributions to the study. The 2003 version of the APA Ethical Principles of Psychologists and Code of Conduct states that authorship should "accurately reflect the relative scientific or professional contributions of the individuals involved, regardless of their relative status."[24] Usually, the principles continue. This means that the student should be listed as principal author on articles based primarily on theses or dissertations.

Moreover, Fine and Kurdek recommend discussion and agreement on authorship early in the collaborative process, to guard against concerns about power imbalance and exploitation. Students should be fully informed about the meaning of authorship decisions and should have the opportunity to participate fully in decisions about responsibilities for the work in the project. Authorship attribution should then appropriately track performance. When student–faculty coauthors cannot agree, Fine and Kurdek recommend outside consultation or, in intransigent cases, neutral arbitration.

Responsibility and Accountability

Along with credit for authorship goes responsibility. In scientific fields especially, where progress builds upon earlier published work, it is important to be able to identify who stands behind published results. When errors come to their attention, authors may be required to make them known publicly. Conversely, people should not be identified as authors if they do not bear and should not be expected to bear responsibility for the full published work.

In fields such as the humanities, single authorship is common. Indeed, works such as paintings or operas generally bear only the name of a single creator despite multiple contributions of studio artists, librettists, or performers.[25] In the sciences and social sciences, multiple authors are the norm. As early as 1981, Broad identified field variations in multiple authorship and its "exponential" growth in some fields such as medicine.[26] Broad attributed multiple authorship to the structure of clinical trials and the growth of interdisciplinary research, as well as to the desire to claim credit to extensive lists of work. In 1986, Huth attacked abuses of authorship including the "salami" science described above and the growth of unjustified authorship. For Huth,[27] inclusion of someone as an author on a paper requires sufficient involvement in the work and writing to be able to take public responsibility for the work's contents. People who performed routine laboratory work, managed laboratories, made technical suggestions, or provided materials or research subjects should not be listed as authors, according to Huth, but should of course be given credit for their respective contributions.

This view that inclusion as an author demands responsibility reflects the current scientific consensus. Nonetheless, recent data indicate that rates of undeserved, "honorary" authorship may be as high as 25% in some journals. From a confidential survey of corresponding authors of original research and review articles in medical journals, Flanagin et al. report a range of 11% to 25% of articles with honorary authors, with higher rates in review articles and no statistically significant difference between larger-circulation and smaller-circulation journals.[28] This study used the International Conference of Medical Journal Editors criteria to identify authorship as honorary. Authorship was classified as honorary if the corresponding author indicated that he or she did not meet the ICMJE criteria for authorship of conceiving and designing the work or analyzing and interpreting the data, writing the manuscript or part of the manuscript or revising the manuscript to make important changes in content, and approving the final version of the manuscript. Other sufficient conditions for honorary authorship were if the corresponding author indicated he or she would not feel comfortable explaining the major conclusions of the article or reported that another author on the paper performed only one of a list of seventeen functions such as recruiting subjects or conducting a literature search.

Honorary authors pose the obvious problem for responsibility that they are listed as authors without sufficient knowledge or involvement in the project to be able to vouch for the project's scientific merit. Overinclusive authorship lists pose more subtle problems of responsibility. Listed authors on many multiple-authored papers may be in positions to take responsibility for some, but not all, aspects of the manuscript. It is this feature that has led to the most radical proposal, that of Rennie, Yank, and Emanuel, to replace authorship altogether for the ideas of "guarantor" and "contributor."[29] Their proposal is that every manuscript should list the respective contributions of everyone who would be listed as authors under current practice. Contributions may include research design, identification, and management of study subjects, data analysis, manuscript writing, or editing. "Guarantors" are those who are responsible for the entire manuscript; they may, of course, be contributors as well. This proposal has the advantage of identifying exact responsibilities. It provides as well the backstop of a guarantor or guarantors for the entire manuscript. As discussed above, it is unlikely to be adopted because of the sheer volume of information that might need to be included in an article with multiple contributors. It also brings the risk of fragmenting responsibility by dissipating it among many contributors. The response to this proposal might be that people should not be identified as authors unless they are prepared to be guarantors for the manuscript; other contributions should be credited in notes.

Ghost authors pose the opposite problem for responsibility: they escape public responsibility for the published work. For this reason, their presence is especially troubling. A ghost author may be the person who should be called upon to explain aspects of a manuscript, but his/her contribution is unknown. Manuscript readers may also wish to evaluate a manuscript by knowledge of the author and his/her skills, reputation, or potential conflicts of interest; ghost authorship prevents this assessment.

Authors are expected to disclose conflicts of interest, if any, when submitting manuscripts for review. Some journals include this information in the published form of the article. There is evidence that conflicts of interest may affect results or their presentation. Publication of information about conflicts may enable readers to scrutinize articles for possible bias.[30]

In most scientific publications, it is also standard to identify a corresponding author with information. The corresponding author is the person to whom inquiries or requests for reprints should be directed. In other fields such as the humanities, the author is identified by institutional affiliation, but other contact information typically is not provided. Those seeking further information about published work must either contact the journal editor or attempt to locate the author directly. The corresponding author is responsible for responding to appropriate inquiries about a study and may, as well, be responsible for notifying the editor of identified problems with the research brought to his/her attention.

Authorship Integrity

Authorship is thus constituted by fairness in the sense of proper allocation of credit for work done and by the responsibility taken for the published research. But authorship raises other, less commonly recognized issues of integrity. Authors are judged on their scientific reliability and research reputations—the integrity of their science. They may also be judged on practices that raise issues of integrity of character. A number of ethically ambiguous practices raise questions of authorship integrity.

Wasteful Publication

Given the career value of publication, authors may attempt to increase their publications by dividing a single research project into as many self-contained articles as possible. Also gaining popularity is the republishing of duplicate material in successive articles in different journals. Slightly less problematic is the padding of articles that may not be significant enough to stand on their own with content from an article published at an earlier date. Given the pressures to "publish or perish," these phenomena are far from surprising.

Whether such practices are strictly unethical is open to debate. Republishing older content within an "original" article could be construed as a form of self-plagiarism, discussed previously. Nevertheless, the practice of dividing publications into "least publishable units" still seems to be a kind of dishonest manipulation.[31] Although career pressures may seem to justify such dubious practices, it is unclear whether market pressures should remove responsibility from the authors that engage in them. "When five papers report findings that could have been reported in one, the editorial process, including peer review, is turned on five times instead of once."[32] Wasteful publication does not merely limit another author's publication success; such articles (and the author responsible for them), have squandered four times as many resources of science, as well as four times as much space within a publication. Such practices may not only be wasteful, they may even impede scientific progress. Four other articles with potentially new content were then not shared with the scientific community. Information or analyses that should have been published together are in different locations that may not be easily linked. Redundant publication not only cheats the scientific community out of original and valuable research, but it also saps valuable time of any responsible researcher who endeavors to keep up with as many developments as possible.

Inappropriate Publications

Issues involving "sensitive research" include, but are not limited to, the use and publication of data gathered through unethical methods, research programs dealing with "delicate" social issues, as well as research with potentially harmful applications. An extreme example of unethical methods is Nazi science. Once such research has occurred, one might argue that the publication and use of such data cannot harm anyone after the fact. Other factors, such as the permission of test subjects or the potential justification of further research programs may also determine what moral decency should require of an author of an article (or the journal publishing it) that utilizes such research data. Others argue, however, that the use of such tainted material is not permissible, no matter the benefit.

Various research programs may simply deal with subject matter that could be considered socially damaging or just in poor taste.[33] Any kind of research that tracks or connects trends within specific racial, social, or gender groups might, at the very least, be construed as inflammatory in various ways. This is not to say that a researcher should ignore scientific progress for the sake of sentimentality, merely that such considerations might be countenanced when dealing with such potentially socially volatile subject matter.

Various research programs produce "sensitive information" of a different kind, namely research with potentially harmful application. Programs in the area of human reproductive cloning or genetically engineered bioweapons are just two examples of types of research some believe should be deemed "forbidden science."[34] Unfortunately, even data that stems from research meant to combat infectious disease may contrarily be used to generate even more deadly diseases. The potential for the "dual application" of research raises questions as to what kind of responsibility researchers have with regard to the use and misuse of information they may or may not attempt to publish. Still, if members of the public are used as research subjects they may have a claim to the results of that research. If public funding or natural resources are used in a research program, the public may have a right to know whether such resources are used appropriately; assuming such research has public benefit, they have a right to know about it.[35] Additionally, some have argued that the restriction of such research, specifically in its publication, would significantly hinder valuable advances in the sciences. Restricting publication would only slow down the dissemination of the information while making it difficult, if not impossible, to replicate claimed results. This would only restrict the potential to develop countermeasures to those who might utilize the information for ill.[36]

Some "scientific research is already subject to numerous ethical guidelines," and policies have been put into effect to restrict the publication of articles with potentially dangerous content such as the "statement on scientific publication and security," to the effect that a significant number of the world's leading journal editors will screen and deny publication to articles that are viewed as potentially dangerous.[37] Although this may be, as one commentator remarked, "a tactical act of good citizenship," one may still question the effectiveness of such a policy as there is little guarantee that an editor of any specific journal is qualified to make such a judgment.[38] Moreover, this does not address concerns with regard to scientific progress. Perhaps a better policy would work at restricting certain access rather than the complete denial of publication.

Editorial Policy and Authors

Conflicts involving the funding of a research project may confuse the convention of giving credit or assigning blame for accidental or even purposely reported findings that may be either mistaken or possibly incomplete. A shift from academic investigators to private contract research organizations (CROs) allows corporate sponsors an increased capacity for manipulating clinical trial reviews.[39] A possible countermeasure is editors requiring that articles be submitted along with written guarantees that the sponsor of the project has "imposed no impediment, direct or indirect, on the publication of the study's full results, including data perceived to be detrimental to the product."[40] Such guarantees may also include the financial records of the authors for the purpose of discovering additional conflicts of interest with any sponsors or their affiliates.

Additional conflicts have arisen with the practice of peer review in the editorial process. Articles submitted for publication are sent out by the editor of the journal to selected readers for review of quality and content. As readers are generally experts in their fields, it is likely that the reviewer knows the author on a professional or perhaps even a personal level. If the reviewer publishes in the same field, which is highly likely, the potential for conflict of interest is multiplied. While at least one study indicated that there are not any significant differences in quality of reviews when the identity of the authors are hidden, this no way speaks to the threat of conflicts specific to the actual content of an article.[41] A reviewer intending to publish contrary or even similar content may "sit" on a competing article as an effective means to facilitate his or her own work being published first. Such concerns notwithstanding, reviewers only make suggestions; journal editors make final decisions. Nevertheless, this cannot guarantee that an editor is even aware of possible bias or conflict between author and reviewer.

Lastly, how much responsibility for guaranteeing integrity should be placed upon an author of an article as opposed to the editor of the scientific journal? If published, are inaccuracies now the responsibility of the journal that published the article? Given their role, it is seems fair to attribute some responsibility to editors for matters such as style requirements, accidental errors in citation, and perhaps even tracking reviewing practices and possible biases among peer reviewers. Journals may take various administrative steps for guaranteeing accountability and protecting from such problems as duplicate publication, citation of unpublished manuscripts, or perhaps contractual agreements with those that may have sponsored the research project.[42] They may also seek to protect the public from dangerous or unethical research, although these practices may be problematic from the point of view of academic freedom and should at a minimum be openly announced. The signing of such "honor codes" is perhaps a step in the right direction, yet it tends to put a responsibility upon editors to "police" those taking part in the publishing game while not going far enough in requiring authors to hold themselves responsible for their own work. An important question is whether a system that has forced such misconduct upon its subjects should concomitantly dissolve them from their responsibilities.

Conclusion

In this chapter, we have provided a principled account of authorship. Authorship is important since it gives credit where credit is due. But it also carries with it corresponding responsibilities. Paying attention to both issues of fairness and responsibility provides guidelines for decisions about proper attribution of authorship, order of authorship in jointly-authored papers, and other features of responsible authorship. Additional issues of authorship integrity warrant further discussion.

• • • References

1. Wilcox, L. "Authorship: The Coin of The Realm, the Source of Complaints." *JAMA* 280 (1998): 216–217.
2. Ibid.
3. LaFollette, M.C. *Stealing into Print—Fraud, Plagiarism, and Misconduct in Scientific Publishing.* Berkeley: University of California Press, 1992; McLellan, F. "Authorship in Biomedical Publications: How Many People Can Wield One Pen." *American Medical Writers Association* 10 (1995): 11.
4. Jones, A. "Changing Traditions of Authorship." In *Ethical Issues in Biomedical Publication,* edited by A. Jones and F. McLellan, 3–29. Baltimore, MD: Johns Hopkins University Press, 2000.
5. Huth, E.J. "Editors and the Problem of Authorship: Rulemakers or Gatekeepers?" *Ethics and Policy in Scientific Publications,* 175–180. Bethesda, MD: Council of Biology Editors, 1990.
6. Steneck, N. "Confronting Misconduct in Science in the 1980s and 1990s: What Has and Has Not Been Accomplished." *Science and Engineering Ethics* 5 (1999): 161–176.
7. Barnbaum, D.R., and M. Byron. *Research Ethics: A Text with Readings.* Englewood Cliffs, NJ: Prentice Hall, 2001.
8. LaFollette, 1992; Goode, S. "Trying to Declaw the Campus Copy Cats." *Insight Magazine* (April 18, 1993): 10–29.
9. Flanagin, A., L.A. Carey, P.B. Fontanarosa, S.G. Phillips, B.P. Pace, G.D. Lundberg, and D. Rennie. "Prevalence of Articles with Honorary and Ghost Authors in Peer-Reviewed Medical Journals." *JAMA* 280 (1998): 222–224.
10. Barnbaum and Byron, 2001.
11. Resnik, D. *The Ethics of Science.* New York: Routledge, 1998; LaFollette, 1992; De Solla Price, D.J. "Ethics of Scientific Publication." Science 144, 655–657.
12. Macrina, F.L. *Scientific Integrity: An Introductory Text with Cases.* 2nd ed. Washington, DC: ASM Press, 2000.
13. Jones, 2000.
14. LaFollette, 1992; McLellan, 1995.
15. Jones, 2000; Flanagin et al., 1998.
16. ICMJE. "Uniform Requirements for Manuscripts Submitted to Biomedical Journals." International Committee of Medical Journal Editors, 2004, http://www.icmje.org/index.html (accessed August 29, 2005).
17. American Psychological Association. "Ethical Principles of Phychologists and Code of Conduct," 2003, http://www.apa.org/ethics/code2002.html (accessed September 17, 2004).
18. ICMJE, 2004.
19. Jones, 2000.
20. Resnik, D. "A Proposal for a New System of Credit Allocation in Science." *Science and Engineering Ethics* 3 (1997): 237–243; Shamoo, A.E., and D.B. Resnik. *Responsible Conduct of Research.* New York: Oxford University Press, 2003.
21. Rennie, D., V. Yank, and L. Emanuel. "When Authorship Fails: A Proposal to Make Contrib-

utors Accountable." *JAMA* 278 (1997): 578–585; Davidoff, F., C.D. DeAngelis, J.M. Drazen, J. Hoey, L. Hojgaard, R. Horton, et al. "Sponsorship, Authorship, and Accountability." *JAMA* 286, no. 10 (2001): 1232–1234.

22. Shamoo and Resnik, 2003.

23. Fine, M.A., and L.A. Kurdek. "Reflections on Determining Authorship Credit and Authorship Order on Faculty–Student Collaborations." *American Psychologist* 48, no. 11 (1993): 1141–1147.

24. American Psychological Association, 2003, Section 8.12(b).

25. Griffith, E., and T.F. Babor. "Shakespeare and the Meaning of Authorship." *Editorial in Addiction* 95, no. 9, 2000, 1317–1318.

26. Broad, W.J. "The Publishing Game: Getting More for Less." *Science* 211 (1981): 1137–1139.

27. Huth, E. "Irresponsible Authorship and Wasteful Publication." *Annals of Internal Medicine* 104 (1986): 257–259.

28. Flanagin et al., 1998.

29. Rennie, D., V. Yank, and L. Emanuel, 1997.

30. Rochon, P.A., J.H. Gruwitz, M. Cheung, J.A. Hayes, and T.C. Chalmers. "Evaluating the Quality of Articles Published in Journal Supplements Compared with the Quality of Those Published in the Parent Journal." *JAMA* 272 (1994): 108–113.

31. Broad, 1981; Ibid.; Huth, 1986.

32. Huth, E., 1986.

33. Barnbaum and Byron, 2001.

34. American Association for the Advancement of Science. "Part 5, Forbidden Science: Should Some Research Be Outlawed?" In *Science and Technology Policy Yearbook*, 2003, www.aaas.org/spp/yearbook/2003/Part5.pdf (accessed September 22, 2004).

35. Barnbaum and Byron, 2001.

36. Zilinskas, R.A., and J.B. Tucker. "Limiting the Contribution of the Scientific Literature to the BW Threat." *Monterey Institute of International Studies*, 2004, http://cns.miis.edu/pubs/week/021216a.htm (accessed June 21, 2004).

37. Ibid; National Academy of Sciences. "Uncensored Exchange of Scientific Results." *Proceedings of the National Academy of Sciences* 100, no. 4 (2003): 1464.

38. Falkow, S. " 'Statement on Scientific Publication and Security' Fails to Provide Necessary Guidelines." Editorial in *Proceedings of the National Academy of Sciences* 100 (May 13, 2003): 5575; also available in serial online at www.pnas.org/cgi/doi/10.1073/pnas.1232277100 (accessed June 29, 2004).

39. Davidoff et al., 2001.

40. Ibid.

41. Bressler, N.M. "Reviewers, Authors, and Editors." *Archives of Ophthalmology* 117 (1999): 524–526.

42. Davidoff et al., 2001.

49

Conflict of Interest in Research

John Chinn, MBA, and Elliott C. Kulakowski, PhD, FAHA

Introduction

If, after reading this chapter, you expect to finish off your institution's conflict of interest obligations after your first one hundred days, take a note from our late President Kennedy. Conflict of interest issues are not likely to be solved that easily.

The matter of *conflict of interest* has developed alongside the development of standards, rules, and laws that govern how a civilized society or group should conduct itself. Pronouncements of these rules can and often have been biased toward those making them or those who were in power. Not all those who made these pronouncements or rules had conflicts of interest: for example, the Ten Commandments are generally accepted as being made for the good of all, without conflict of interest.

The US Constitution was drafted by a group of men, the "founding fathers." We are taught that the rules and laws stemming from the Constitution were developed by individuals who had only the good of the new nation in mind. Still, the framers of the Constitution had the foresight to draft the Constitution to allow for changes as needed by the governing body so as to protect the integrity of its laws from issues, including conflicts of interest. Despite the foresight of the framers, there is continued need to legislate protections to battle against conflict of interest that exists in our government.

A most recent example of conflict of interest or perceived conflict of interest in government is the case a duck-hunting trip taken by US Supreme Court Justice Antonin Scalia and US Vice President Dick Cheney. At the time, the Supreme Court had a case before it that involved the Vice President. Was the trip appropriate? Did it represent conflict of interest? Should the Justice recuse himself, given his recent personal excursion with the Vice President? Given these questions and in his refusal to recuse himself from hearing the case, was Justice Scalia in violation of federal policy?

The requirement of conflict of interest policies as related to research is a fairly recent development. The concern of conflict of interest in academia was not as pronounced in the past as it is today. Two major changes came from the federal government that increased the potential for a conflict of interest among research faculty. The first was the 1980 Bayh Dole Act, which allowed colleges, universities, and nonprofit research institutions to retain title to inventions developed with federal funds. The institutions were to seek patent protection and to share any royalty with the research faculty inventors. (1)

The second was the 1982 establishment of the Small Business Innovation Research Program, which was designed to capitalize on federally funded research projects, in part by requiring 2.5% of extramural research budgets of federal research agencies be used to fund the engagement of small US businesses in research and development. As a result of this program, many researchers became entrepreneurs, establishing small businesses to commercialize their research activities and institutions began to license their inventions to these spin-off companies. (2)

As faculty began to take advantage of these programs, there was also an explosion in the sciences, in biotechnology, molecular biology, genetic engineering, and computer and robotic sciences. These new areas of research in science are largely funded by federal and private agencies. Boosted by newly available funds, many new areas in science (for example, biotechnology, including genetic bioengineering) have experienced unprecedented growth. As a result of these successes, investors have continued to fund expertise in these areas. Pioneer researchers in biotechnology have sought out university colleagues. Growth of the biotechnology market also caught the attention of the health care industry, which formed its own biotechnology divisions to get a share of the market. However there have also been issues of divided loyalties among those in the field; those caught between the lure of biotechnology and the scientist's commitments and potential conflict between scientists' work and their institutional commitments.

Major political developments have also drastically shifted some funding areas of science. The recent passage of the Homeland Security Act shifted many funding sources and foci of research including in the areas of computer science and robotics (e.g., unmanned vehicle technology development, recognition software and data mining).

Prior to the technology boom of the late 1980s and 1990s, federal research funding had not grown significantly. Researchers sought other sources of funding, often through collaborations with industry. These partnerships also led to concerns about potential conflict of interest. In response, the federal government promulgated regulations at the National Science Foundation (NSF) and the National Institutes of Health (NIH) to deal with issues of financial conflict of interest.

The NSF issued its "Financial Disclosure Policy" on June 30, 1994 (3,4) and revised its policy requiring institutions to disclose to NSF any financial ties between their principle investigators with any private interests who could potentially profit from NSF-funded projects. The policy also required that institutions describe the measures taken to minimize risk of conflicts of interest.

Subsequently, the Public Health Service (PHS) of the Department of Health and Human Services (HHS) released its regulation, "Objectivity in Research." (5) This policy requires disclosure of all "significant financial interests" of an institution and that institutional official(s) review these disclosures in accordance with an administrative process to be established by each institution. According to the policy, following this review, the institutional official(s) are to determine the acceptability of the reported financial interests and act to protect PHS-

funded research from any bias that is reasonably expected to arise from those interests. This regulation requires that each institution applying for PHS funds has written and enforced polices on conflicts of interest that:

1. Comply with the PHS regulations;
2. Inform faculty applicants of such policies;
3. Inform faculty applicants of their roles and responsibilities; and,
4. Inform each faculty applicant of PHS regulations.

In 2002, the NIH reported its study of the top 300 funded institutions to determine how their Objectivity in Research Policy was implemented. (6) Surprisingly, they found significant similarities among the respondents:

- 87% of the institutions did not disclose in each public presentation, the result of clinical research where the investigator had a disclosed or managed conflict of interest.
- 86% of these institutions did not define "research."
- 76% of the institutions did not require reporting of identified conflict of interest to the awarding component of PHS.
- 68% of the institutions did not report the corrective actions taken.
- 54% of the institutions did not address the flow-down requirements to their subcontractors.
- 52% of the institutions did not identify the PHS regulation on objectivity in research.
- 45% of the institutions did not require the reporting of the conflict to the PHS prior to grant fund expenditures.

It appears from these findings that many institutions had yet to develop adequate policies and procedures to address the federal requirements. These results were somewhat surprising based on the fact that organizations such as the National Council of University Research Administrators and the Society of Research Administrators International had continually addressed these regulatory issues in numerous workshops and sessions at their annual and regional meetings since 1994. (7–9)

The intent of the federal conflict of interest regulations is to ensure that research is not biased by and the public's trust in the integrity is not reduced by any financial conflict of those conducting research on the public's behalf.

Conflict of interest will continue to be an issue for institutions and researchers as long as conditions exists that lead institutions and researchers to stray from their missions and objectivity. Conflict of interest should not necessitate avoidance of the research; instead, conflict must be identified and diffused so that the research can continue and the mission of the institution is not compromised.

The intent of this chapter is to provide the information necessary to understand the issues of conflict of interest, to provide guidance to develop and implement policies, and to suggest ways to educate employees about conflict of interest. There are no immediate solutions, however, there are ways to manage conflicts that can work for the good of the institution, for the advancement of knowledge, and for the good of society on the whole.

Activities That May Result in Conflicts of Interest

There are several activities that can result in a conflict of interest. These can be consulting relationships with industry, relationships that involve technology licensing, clinical research, mentoring relationships, procurement, and institutional conflicts. (10)

Consulting

Consulting relationships hold the most potential for conflict of interest—for example, a faculty member who receives research support from a company and, at the same time, the company hires the faculty member as a scientific consultant or to serve on their scientific advisory board. With such appointments often comes an agreement that requires that faculty members assign their rights to any intellectual property to the company. However, in fact, there may be questions over the faculty member's right to sign over intellectual property developed under the sponsorship of the institution.

Licensing and Procurement

In today's entrepreneurial academic culture, faculty may establish their own company and license a technology from their institution for further development. However, unless appropriately managed, such relations can also raise questions about future or other technology developments by the faculty member. Some of these issues can involve procurement conflict, for example, if a faculty member seeks institutional funds to purchase a product from his or her own company. In this example, the faculty member may have developed a technology such as a particular reagent, media, or antibody

that the institution owns and licenses to the faculty member's company. In another case, a project might require a key product for a project produced by only one company owned solely by the investigator(s) or immediate family.

Clinical Trials

Clinical trials also present concern because of the potential for harm and even death to research participants. (11) Clinical trials are conducted to determine safety and efficacy of new therapeutic agents, diagnostic procedures, or medical devices. Physician–researchers may have been instrumental in development of the therapeutic agent. They also may own considerable stock or stock options in the company conducting the experimental agent. In addition, pharmaceutical companies often hire those clinicians who enrolled the largest numbers of subjects in a study and compensate them as authors for the major published articles and to speak at national meetings. The financial rewards from such endeavors can be very lucrative and have the potential to influence the actions of the physician–researcher. The conflicts of interest can extend to members who sit on the institutional review board (IRB) where their decisions can potentially be influenced unless appropriate precautions are taken.

Financial Relationships in Research

A 2000 report in the Journal of the American Medical Association assessed the financial relationships that faculty at the University of California, San Francisco, had with industry. (12) The report found that 7.6% of the faculty had financial ties with research sponsors. Of this group, slightly over one-third participated in speaking engagements that ranged in compensation from $250 to $20,000. A similar number had consulting relationships with companies that ranged from less than $1,000 to $120,000 per year (about a third held positions as members of scientific boards or boards of directors), and, in addition, multiple relationships among these interests existed among 12% of the study group.

Recognizing the serious potential for conflicts of interest, the federal government issued a number of reports on the issue of clinical research. These included reports from the Government Accounting Office, the Food and Drug Administration (FDA), the NIH, and the Office of Human Research Protections. (13,14,15,16) The Association of American Medical Colleges (AAMC) has also established task forces to develop guidelines for clinical investigators and on how institutions should deal with issues of conflict of interest. (17,18,19,20)

Development of a Conflict of Interest Policy

Policies, like laws, are designed to prevent unwanted outcomes. Developing a strong and effective conflict of interest policy will do your institution as much good as finding the cause of a dreaded disease or a technological breakthrough. It may not be of interest to the media, but then do you want your conflict of interest problems to be exposed in the media?

An effective policy includes the following essential elements:

- Definition of terms such as conflict of interest and significant financial interest.
- Steps taken to collect and review disclosures.
- Appropriate policy management plans, including methods to monitor the implementation of the plans.

The policy and procedures must be developed to fit the institution's environment, mission, and organizational structure. The following is adapted from the NIH, NSF policies, and other references from other institutional policies (listed in Appendix 1).

Definition of Terms

Conflict, according to Webster's dictionary, is a "fight, battle, struggle, emotional disturbances resulting from a clash of impulses in a person, a choice you do not want to make." (21) In high school, we learn about conflicts "man versus man," "man versus nature," and "man versus self." When we think of conflict of interest we are dealing with "man versus self." It may be the teacher versus the researcher, the physician versus researcher or the researcher versus the entrepreneur. It may be the desire to advance knowledge, help mankind, or provide the best care to your patients, which is pitted against a desire for recognition through new grants and publications, promotion and tenure, or fortune.

Interest is defined as "a right or claim to something . . . a share or participation in something . . . anything in which one participates or has a share . . . profit, benefits."(22)

Conflict of interest occurs when there is a conflict between an individual's private interests and his or her professional obligations to another entity such that an independent observer might reasonably question whether the individual's professional actions or decisions are affected by his or her private interest.

Institutional research consists of sponsored projects funded by an external funding source. PHS defines research as, "any systematic investigation designed to develop or contribute to generalizable knowledge relating broadly to public health, including behavioral and social-sciences research." (5) The term encompasses basic and applied research and product development, and includes any such activity for which research funding is available from a PHS awarding component through grant or cooperative agreement, whether authorized under the PHS Act or other statutory authority.

Technology transfer refers to all intellectual property and licensing activities, including those in which an institution may acquire equity or ownership.

Investigator or principle investigator refers to the project director, a co-principal investigator, research staff member, manager, and any other person at an institution who is responsible for the design, conduct, or reporting of research, educational or service activities funded, or proposed for funding, by an external sponsor. In this context, the definition of *investigator* also includes the investigator's spouse and dependent children or other family members whose involvement in a project matter may constitute conflict of interest.

Small Business Innovation Research (SBIR) is the PHS' extramural research program for small business that was established by the Awarding Components of the PHS and certain other Federal agencies under Public Law 97-219, the Small Business Innovation Development Act, as reauthorized in 2000. For purposes of these guidelines, the term SBIR Program includes the Small Business Technology Transfer ("STTR") Program. (2)

Significant Financial Interest refers to any means of monetary value, including, but not limited to:

- Salary or other payments for services (e.g., consulting fees or honoraria).
- Equity interests (e.g., stocks, stock options, or other ownership interests).
- Intellectual property rights (e.g., patents, copyrights, and royalties from such rights).
- Holding a management position or playing an advisory or consultative role (whether compensated or not) with a company or on the board of a for-profit company.

Significant financial interest does not include:

- Salary, royalties, or other remuneration from the university.
- Income from seminars, lectures, or teaching engagements sponsored by public or nonprofit entities.

- Income from service on advisory committees or review panels for public or nonprofit entities.
- An equity interest that, when aggregated for the investigator and the investigator's spouse and dependent children, does not exceed $10,000 in value as determined through reference to public prices or other reasonable measures of fair market value, and does not represent more than a five percent ownership interest in any single entity; or salary, royalties or other payments that, when aggregated for the investigator and the investigator's spouse and dependent children over the next twelve months, are not expected to exceed $10,000. (5)

Identifying Conflict of Interest

Some might describe conflict of interest using the same description as that for describing pornography: "I'll know it when I see it." Unlike pornography, however, *conflict of interest* can be defined.

As discussed earlier, there are many types of conflicts of interest, most often involving financial gain. The PHS's Policy on Objectivity in Research states that "a conflict of interest occurs when the financial or personal considerations of an individual may compromise or has the appearance of compromising an employee's judgment or performance of one's obligation to the institution." (5) The Association of American Medical Colleges defines the term *conflict of interest* in science as "situations in which the financial or other personal considerations may compromise, or have the appearance of compromising, an investigator's professional judgment in conducting or reporting research." (20)

Significant Financial Interest

The NIH and NSF policies are, on the whole, similar with only minor differences. The policies require that investigators conducting or proposing research using NIH or NSF funds disclose to their institution all significant financial interest of the investigator, his/her spouses, and dependent children. Significant financial conflict of interest is defined as anything that has financial value such as noninstitutional salaries or payments, consulting fees, equity interest, and revenues from patents or licenses, not including:

- Salaries, royalties, or other remunerations from the institution or ownership in the institution if the institution is an SBIR.

- Income from lectures or speaking engagements from public or other nonprofit entities.
- Financial interest in a for-profit entity of less than $10,000 or 5% ownership.

If an institution receives federal funding, the policy can be stricter than the agencies policy, but not less restrictive.

Covered Person

The institution's policy should name all those at the institution covered by the policy. The NIH and NSF policies identify those as the principal investigator, coinvestigators, or other persons responsible for the design conduct or reporting of the research or educational activities funded or proposed for funding. This may also include faculty, researchers, postdoctoral fellows, graduate or undergraduate students, technical support staff, nurses, biostatisticians, and data managers. The policy should also include research administrators, technology transfer managers, institutional procurement staff, and committee members such as members of the institutional review board.

In addition to those directly affiliated with the institute, the policy should include family members of principle persons, including spouses, life partners, unemancipated or stepchildren, and may also include parents, siblings and their children, business partners, and any dependents (as defined by the Internal Revenue Service). The scope of individuals covered must meet federal regulations but the breadth of disclosure beyond the regulations depends on the culture of the institution.

Disclosing Conflict of Interest

When reviewing disclosures of conflict of interest, it is good to keep in mind this proverb. To properly manage conflicts of interest, the institution must be informed of the truth, the whole truth, and nothing but the truth.

Both the NSF and PHS policies place the burden of collecting disclosures on the institution. Based on the institution's definitions of conflict of interest and significant financial interest, the policy should describe the form in which disclosure is to be made and when disclosure is to be made (some of the policies identified at the end of the chapter include copies of disclosure forms). The disclosure form should be in sufficient detail for a determination to be made as to whether a conflict of interest exists.

The filing of disclosures of conflict of interest can vary among institutions, but such reporting must be done before a proposal is submitted. Some institutions in their policy require annual disclosures of all faculty and staff at certain levels of responsibility. Others may require disclosures only of researchers and those responsible for the design conduct and reporting of the research activities. Still others, such as at the University of Utah, require disclosures with each proposal being submitted (22) or a certification that there has been no change in the previous disclosure form before a proposal is submitted to the funding agency. Policies generally call for updates in the disclosure form when changes occur.

Review of Disclosure and Resolution

We know that conflict of interest is not in and of itself bad, but *knowing* what to do about it is difficult.

Policies need to describe who is responsible for review of disclosure forms. The review can be by a senior administrator in the sponsored projects office, someone at the level of the vice president for research, by institutional council, or a designated conflict of interest manager, sometimes referred to as a designated official (DO).

The policy may also call for a triaging of disclosures where by those with identified conflicts are separated from those with no conflict. As someone once said, if there is not conflict, there is no interest. For those that report some conflicts, the DO should examine if the reported conflict exceeds the level of significance. If not, then a note should be made in the grant file. When the DO reasonably determines that a conflict of interest could directly and significantly affect the design, conduct, or reporting of the grant funded research activity, then the case needs to be brought to the attention of the conflict of interest committee for review and management.

The institute's conflict of interest committee should be defined within the conflict of interest policy. The committee may be composed of faculty and administrators. Administrators on the committee may include representatives from the sponsored programs office, the grants accounting office, the technology transfer office, IRB, and legal counsel. It

is advisable to have multiple faculty members on the committee to give credence to the committee's recommendations on determination and management of conflict of interest. The committee might also include ad hoc members with expertise in addressing issues of conflict of interest.

Appointment to the committee should come from senior administration (provost office, president, senior vice president). The committee generally reports to senior administration at the institution such as the vice president for research or general council as defined in the policy. Their charge is to review those disclosure forms where a conflict of interest or potential conflict of interest has been disclosed and to determine an appropriate resolution plan. The committee should be given the authority by senior administration to investigate fully the reported conflict of interest. This includes being able to request additional written information and have discussions with the employee. The committee should meet when a conflict of interest case has been identified, and then as needed until the case is resolved. Committee members can be assigned tasks to perform and report back at the next scheduled meeting. In this era of electronic communication, it is possible to hold committee meetings in cyberspace to confer with or determine the management of simple cases. For the more politically sensitive cases, a formal meeting could save a lot of time and effort.

In a presentation at the 2003 Society of Research Administrators International annual meeting, Barbara Winger of the University of Florida discussed review committee criteria. (10) Among them were the use of the individual's position; time commitments; continuing obligations; use of institutional resources such as equipment, facilities, personnel, inventions, and institutional name; employment of students; ability to influence decisions concerning the entity; and financial interests from an entity supporting or affected by the faculty member's research or educational program.

Essentially, the committee may recommend three basic resolutions from any review. They can accept it, manage it, or prohibit it.

Development of Management Plan

The policy should designate responsibility of development of a conflict management plan to the committee, the office of the vice president for research, institutional council, internal review board, or some other administrative body of the institution.

A management plan allows the activity to proceed. Just because a conflict of interest exists, it does not mean that it can not be allowed. There may be instances where the conflict is known and is allowed to occur. For example, an allowable conflict of interest may occur when a faculty member is involved with a company that is the only producer of a specific reagent needed for the faculty member's research, and, therefore, the faculty member must purchase the reagent from this company.

The management plan may include a variety of requirements. These requirements may include required disclosure in publications and at presentations; disclosure to sponsors, collaborators, staff, and students; disclosure in informed consent form and during the process of consenting a patient for a clinical trial; modification of the research plan; change in or restriction of the principle investigator's role; and/or appointment of an oversight committee or a data safety and monitoring board for clinical trials. There may also be other sanctions imposed. It is also not uncommon for there to be more than one requirement placed on a faculty member. The degree of requirements should be proportional to the level and the risk of the conflict as determined by the committee. Finally, the management plan may call for prohibition of an activity. The prohibition may include discontinuation of the external activity, divestiture of ownership or equity, or termination of the sponsored activity.

The outcome of the management plan should result in a memorandum of understanding between the employee and the institution that describes the requirements. However, if the employee is unwilling to enter into such an agreement the policy should provide for the institution to take appropriate personnel actions as is necessary.

Notifying External Sponsors

The NSF and HHS currently require institutions to report conflict of interest to the funding agency prior to grant fund expenditures. It also requires disclosure of the conflict in each public presentation of the result of clinical research when the investigator has had a disclosed or managed conflict of interest. Other nonfederal funding agencies will have their own policies on the reporting of activities. The policy should describe that sponsor guidelines will be followed in resolving any conflicts of interest, and that reports of conflict of interest determinations and actions are kept with the project files and typically in the sponsored programs office. These records are required to be kept for three years.

Periodic Review

Conflict of interest policies should be reviewed periodically (every one to three years) to determine if the policy needs to be modified or updated. Changes in institutional environment and position would necessitate updates; changes in external environments (economy, market forces, and political control) also may require modification to conflict of interest policy. Finally, it is important to keep abreast of changes in federal regulations (found in federal publications) and to participate in the various professional organizations identified elsewhere.

Educating Individuals About the Conflict of Interest Policy

After the policy has been developed and the appropriate signatures are affixed, the next step is to educate the research community about the policy. This should begin at the highest levels of administration.

The policies should be made available to affected employees. This can be through internal correspondence in the form of memoranda or e-mails. In today's electronic environment, most policies are placed on the institution's Web site. Typically there is a policy site or it may be placed in the institution's research administration's site.

Beyond publication of a policy, the institution must undertake an effective education program. The education program should precede the implementation of the policy. It may include presentations at the level of the faculty senate, discussions at the college level and at the department level, or at medial staff meetings. The policy should not be presented as a dictum, but rather how it benefits the institution and protects the individual. One method of education is the use of case studies (some are presented in Appendix 2). Others are available from the Council on Government Relations (COGR). (23)

An effective program to manage conflict of interest has many advantages. If both industry and other sponsors of research know that the institution takes such activities seriously and effectively manages conflicts of interests, there may be increased support for research from industry, a feeling of trust among researchers and the ability to build more interdisciplinary programs; it may enhance educational programs, earlier translation of basic to applied research with industry, and better opportunities to prepare students for careers in industry.

Institutional Conflicts of Interest

Currently, NSF and HHS do not require disclosure of conflict of interest from the institution. This is an issue that currently is receiving considerable attention and discussion. (10, 23) In the future there will be guidelines developed by the federal government and academic associations; in the meantime, institutional conflict of interest typically involves the governing or administrative bodies (trustees, senior management, procurement officers, legal counsel, contracting officers, and institutional officers) of the institution. Relationships with investors or with entities involving licensing of institutional patents and technologies are other potential sources of institutional conflicts of interest. Incidents of institutional conflict of interest can include:

- Gifts from commercial sponsors through the institutional development office.
- Revenues from licensing of institutional technologies.
- Master agreements with corporate sponsors.
- Research involving human participants of institutional technologies.
- Purchasing department activities.
- Participation with local venture capitalists to grow institutional technologies.
- Activities of board of trustee members.

The development of institutional policies are sure to become more frequent in the future. (24)

In Conclusion

You have read a lot about conflict of interest in this chapter, but we realize that there is far more to learn about the various issues and that new issues are bound to develop and will need to be understood and managed. The management of conflict of interest is one of many things of which research administrators must be cognizant. While Catherine Deangelis, editor of the Journal of the American Medical Association, commented in an editorial that "without trust medical research is doomed," (25) the truth of the matter is that without trust, the entire research enterprise is in jeopardy. It may not be the most glamorous nor the most important, but the reliability and integrity of research is very heavily dependent upon its proper oversight and the careful and principled management of conflict of interest.

This chapter contains the basic information necessary for research administrators to keep their institutions in compliance with federal grant regulations with respect to conflict of interest. The case studies (Appendix 2) present scenarios and situations of conflicts (fictitious) for the reader to consider.

We all know the answer to the question of what makes real estate sell: location, location, location. The answer to what the key to management of conflict of interest is disclosure, disclosure, disclosure. With full disclosure, the reasonable research administrator is able to manage the intriguing and complex subject of resolving conflict of interest issues.

Appendix 1. Sample Conflict of Interest Policies

East Carolina University. "ECU Policy in Conflicts of Interest and Commitment," (Appendix I of East Carolina University Faculty Manual) http://www.ecu.edu/data-fsonline/facultymanual/ appendixi/appendixi.htm (accessed August 28, 2005).

Emory University. Designing a Process for "Identifying and Controlling Institutional Conflicts of Interest (2002)," http://www.or.emory.edu/share/policies/institutional_conflict.pdf (accessed September 15, 2004).

Harvard University. "Principles Governing Commercial Activities (2001)," http://www.provost.harvard.edu/policies_guidelines/commercial_activities_summary.php (accessed September 15, 2004).

Johns Hopkins University. "School of Medicine Policy on Conflict of Commitment and Conflict of Interest," http://www.hopkinsmedicine.org/faculty_staff/policies/facultypolicies/conflict_commitment (accessed September 15, 2004).

Stanford University. "Policy on Conflict of Commitment and Interest," http://www.stanford.edu/dept/DoR/rph/4-1. html (accessed September 15, 2004).

Tulane University. "Conflict of Interest Policy," http://www.tmc.tulane.edu/researchadmin/coiPolicy.html#Institutional (accessed September 15, 2004).

University of Florida. "Guidelines, Policies and Procedures on Conflict of Interest and Outside Activities, Including Financial Interest," http://www.generalcounsel.ufl.edu/Conflict/COI. pdf (accessed August 28, 2005).

University of Kansas Medical Center. "Institutional Conflict of Interest Policy," http://www. kumc.edu/Pulse/policy/icoi.html (accessed September 15, 2004).

University of Pennsylvania School of Medicine. "Guidelines on Institutional Conflicts of Interest," http://www.med.upenn.edu/facaffrs/Policies/ Conflict_of_Interest_Guidelines.pdf (accessed September 15, 2004).

Appendix 2. Case Studies

Clearing your mind of preconceived notions will help you get the most out of these case studies. Just as determining the disposition of conflict of interest does not have clear cut answers, these case studies do not necessarily have right or wrong answers. These cases are to stimulate thought and allow the reader to practice thinking of the details involved in looking at conflicts of interest.

A Case of Conflicts of Interest in Mentoring

A graduate student is attending a professional national meeting where he learns about a project that is related to his current research. As he listens with great interest, he realizes that his work could have a positive impact to the presenter's work. He returns to his advisor to discuss this news. His advisor informs him that he is consulting for a firm that is competing with the presenter's company.

1. What is the graduate student to do about his research in light of what he has learned? Should the graduate student keep quiet about his research? If he does, how does this impact the advancement of science for the good of science?
2. What are the responsibilities of the advisor? Does informing his graduate student of his consulting with a competing firm satisfy the requirements for disclosure? What should the advisor do about his consulting arrangements since his graduate student's research could result in the company he is consulting with to gain by the research?
3. What happens to scientific advancement when there is conflict of interest?

A Case of Conflict in Commitment

There are faculty members who will believe and are confident that they are doing what is right. Be prepared to deal with that angry faculty.

Professor Jones, a full time faculty and researcher at ABC University has been in conversa-

tion with nearby XYZ Research Center to conduct his research at XYZ. XYZ is a modern, state-of-the-art research center and has excess resources that it wants to utilize so that it can be more efficient in the use of its resources. XYZ Research Center is nonacademic and has no ties or connections to ABC University. ABC University and XYZ Research Center do compete for research funding from the same funding sources. ABC University has grown large, cumbersome, inefficient, and bureaucratic. Thus Professor Jones is very interested in the discussion with XYZ. XYZ would make available its excess research resources to Professor Jones provided that Professor Jones would submit all future grants related to XYZ's research mission through XYZ. The relationship between XYZ and Professor Jones would be that of an employer/employee with Professor Jones' time commitment based upon the time and effort proposed on grants awarded to XYZ submitted by Professor Jones.

1. What should Professor Jones consider when deciding if he should or should not accept XYZ's offer?
2. If Professor Jones accepts XYZ's offer, should Professor Jones disclose his relationship with XYZ to ABC University? What should he disclose of the possible relationship and how much disclosure is necessary?
3. Professor Jones has disclosed the relationship with XYZ to ABC and ABC permitted the relationship. What impact does this arrangement have on Professor Jones' time and effort reporting for ABC and XYZ to the grantor? What restrictions would need to be in place for subcontracting arrangements between ABC University and XYZ Research Center?
4. What should ABC require of Professor Jones and/or XYZ so that ABC University's commitment policies and expectations of its faculty and the rights of ABC's students are not lost?
5. Is there another solution for ABC University that would create a win-win situation for Dr. Jones and ABC University?

A Case of Conflict of Interest in Clinical Research

Some conflict of interest that you may encounter may make you feel very, very disillusioned of your institution and faculty. The situation should not make you feel worst than it is.

Dr. Smith is well known in his specialty and the DrugsRus drug company representatives have good relationships with him because he often gives out their samples to his patients and prescribes their drugs. As such he has access to the marketing and senior management of DrugsRus. He has conducted many clinical trials for DrugsRus, as well as clinical research for other drug companies. DrugsRus and drug companies often award him educational grants. Dr. Smith uses these grants to send his nurses or interns or residents to national meetings.

When taking on a clinical trial, he tries to not conduct studies that compete for the same patient population but he views that having access to the latest and best drugs is best for his patients. He always has his patients' best interest in mind.

Dr. Smith also has a consulting relationship with DrugsRus. He serves on their medical board. Dr. Smith attends various meetings to present his research and is often the lead author on publications from DrugsRus. In exchange for his service to DrugsRus, Dr. Smith is able to exercise an option to purchase company stock at discounted prices. To avoid any perception of financial conflict of interest, Dr. Smith has not chosen to exercise his option to purchase and thus does not own any stock in DrugsRus.

At ABC Medical Center, Dr. Smith is able to use any residual funds from his research studies for other research or educational purposes. To gain access and the attention of pharmaceutical companies, Dr. Smith would often use these residual funds to conduct pilot studies for the drug companies. He hopes to get access to more lucrative studies by conducting these smaller pilot studies.

1. What should Dr. Smith report to ABC Medical Center when completing his conflict of interest form?
2. What action should ABC Medical Center take after reviewing Dr. Smith's form?
3. What should the IRB require on Dr. Smith's clinical research applications?
4. What should Dr. Smith's patients do or ask if they are considering participating in Dr. Smith's studies?

A Case of Conflict of Interest for Institutions and Inventors

Upholding your conflict of interest policies may be more difficult than one expects.

Professor Pat Pending at Intell Prop University (IPU) is the most prolific inventor at his institution. Through his patents, IPU is the envy of similar institutions in its class. Pat Pending has a new cell line that he believes can replace animals in the laboratory. IPU owns the license to the cell line and is looking for investors. An IPU board member contacts some of his business associates who contacts

Pat Pending in his laboratory. The investors are very interested in Pat Pending's cell line and make an offer to IPU for licensing rights. In addition, the investors convince Pat Pending to join the investor group in investing and marketing the cell line. Pat Pending would share in any royalty that the investing group gets from their investments.

Pat Pending takes the summer off from teaching to work full time to generate data for proving his cell lines could substitute for animals in testing labs and to market the cell lines to potential buyers.

IPU technology transfer in the meantime is consulting its patent attorneys to finalize the licensing agreement with the investing group.

1. What should the buyer ask?
2. What should Pat Pending disclose to IPU?
3. What should IPU include in the licensing agreement?
4. What needs to be done to manage any conflicts of interest?

● ● ● References

1. Bremer, H.W. "University Technology Transfer Evolution and Revolution." In *Research Administration and Management*, edited by E.C. Kulakowski and L.U. Chronister, 627–639. Sudbury, MA: Jones and Bartlett Publishers, 2006.
2. Nixon, R.A., R. Shindell, and J. Goodnight. "SBIR/STTR Programs." In *Research Administration and Management*, edited by E.C. Kulakowski and L.U. Chronister, 865–872. Sudbury, MA: Jones and Bartlett Publishers, 2006.
3. National Science Foundation. "Investigator Financial Disclosure Policy," http://www.nsf.gov/pubs/stis1996/iin117/iin117.txt (accessed on August 17, 2005).
4. National Science Foundation. "Investigator Financial Disclosure Policy," http://www.nsf.gov/pubs/stis1996/iin118/iin118.txt (accessed on August 17, 2005).
5. Public Health Service. "Policy: Objectivity in Research," www.grants.nih.gov/grants/guide/notice-files/not95-179.html (accesssed October 16, 2004).
6. National Institutes of Health. "Financial Conflict of Interest: Objectivity in Research," www.grants.nih.gov/grants/policy/coi/nih_review.htm (accessed on October 16, 2004).
7. Killoren, R., E. Kulakowski, and S. Smith. "Conflict of Interest in Sponsored Research." NCURA Workshop, Washington, DC 1994.

8. Mizzell, S. "Financial Conflict of Interest," grants.nih.gov/grants/compliance/coi_2003_regional_seminar.ppt (accessed September 12, 2005).

9. Wingo, B. "Conflict of Interest: Individual and Institutional." Presentation at Society of Research Administrators International annual meeting, Pittsburgh, PA 2003.

10. Association of American Universities. "Report on Individual and Institutional Conflict of Interest," http://www.aau.edu/research/COI.01.pdf (accessed October 16, 2004).

11. Lemmens, T. and P.A. Singer. "Bioethics for Clinicians: 17. Conflict of Interest in Research, Education and Patient Care." *Can. Med. Assoc. J.* 159 (October 1998): 960–965.

12. Boyd, E.A., and L.A. Bero. "Assessing Faculty Financial Relationships with Industry: A Case Study." *JAMA* 284, no. 17 (November 1, 2000): 2209–2214.

13. GAO. "Biomedical Research: HHS Direction Needed to Address Financial Conflicts of Interest," November 2001, http://www.aau.edu/research/gao.pdf (accessed September 15, 2004).

14. US Food and Drug Administration. "Guidance: Financial Disclosure by Clinical Investigators," March 20, 2001, http://www.fda.gov/oc/guidance/financialdis.html (accessed September 15, 2004).

15. National Institutes of Health. "Financial Conflicts of Interest and Research Objectivity: Issues for Investigators and Institutional Review Boards," June 5, 2000, http://grants.nih.gov/grants/guide/notice-files/NOT-OD-00-040.html (accessed September 15, 2004).

16. Department of Health and Human Services, Final Guidance Document Financial Relationships and Interests in Research Involving Human Subjects: Guidance for Human Subjects Protections (2004) http://www.hhs.gov/ohrp/humansubjects/finreltn/fguid.pdf (accessed August 28, 2005).

17. AAMC, Financial Conflicts of Interest in Clinical Research http://www.aamc.org/members/coitf/ (accessed August 28, 2005).

18. AAMC, Protecting Subjects, Preserving Trust, Promoting Progress: Policy and Guidelines for the Oversight of Individual Financial Interests in Human Subjects Research http://www.aamc.org/members/coitf/firstreport.pdf (accessed September 12, 2005).

19. AAMC, "Protecting Subjects, Preserving Trust, Promoting Progress II: Principles and Recommendations for Oversight of an Institution's Financial Interests in Human Subjects Research," http://www.aamc.org/members/coitf/2002coireport.pdf (accessed August 28, 2005).

20. AAMC. "Guidelines for Dealing with Faculty Conflicts of Commitment and Conflicts of Interest in Research," http://www.aamc.org/research/dbr/coi.htm (accessed September 15, 2004).

21. *Webster's Third New International Dictionary.* Springfield, MA: Merrian Company Publishers, 1966.

22. University of Utah, "Conflict of Interest Policy," March 8, 2004, http://www.admin.utah.edu/ppmanual/2/2-30.html (accessed September 15, 2004).

23. Council on Governmental Relations (COGR) Web site, www.cogr.edu (accessed September 15, 2004).

24. Emanuel, E.J. and D. Steiner. "Institutional Conflict of Interest." *NEJM* 332, no. 4 (January 26, 1995): 262–267, http://www.med.utah.edu/ethics/RCREthics/emanuel.html (accessed September 15, 2004).

25. Deangelis, C.D. "Editorial." *JAMA* 284, no. 17 (November 12, 2000): 27.

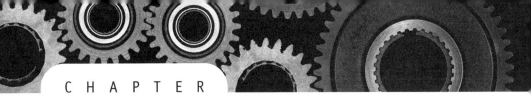

50

Beyond the Federal Definition: Other Forms of Misconduct

Chris B. Pascal, JD

Introduction

The federal definition of research misconduct adopted by the Office of Science and Technology (OSTP) in 2000 means fabrication, falsification, or plagiarism in proposing, performing, or reviewing research, or in reporting research results. This definition of misconduct is narrow and applies to all federally funded research. It was adopted to conform to the research community's own view of the most serious research infractions that that warrant federal response. However, there are many other forms of research or academic misconduct that are subject to institutional policy only. Some institutions rely solely on the federal definition of misconduct, while others augment the federal definition to allow for additional internal institutional standards that can be applied; these include research infractions defined as "inappropriate," but which do not fall under the more serious federally-defined infractions, described as "egregious and unacceptable."

The Office of Research Integrity (ORI) has long recognized the principle that research institutions have inherent authority in their role as employers, teachers, and managers of research funds to establish their own internal standards for misconduct and integrity that supplement any federal wide or federal agency specific standard. Consistent with this position, OSTP stated in announcing its definition of research misconduct that "this federal policy does not limit the authority of research institutions,

or other entities, to promulgate additional research misconduct policies or guidelines or more specific ethical guidance."[1]

This chapter addresses three main issues relevant to the role of the research administrator in providing guidance to the research institution in managing research integrity issues:

1. What other types of misconduct are relevant to the research institution?
2. How have these types of misconduct been described in institutional policies and applied in practice?
3. What are the pros and cons for the institution of supplementing federal definitions of misconduct with additional institutional standards?

Background and History: Other Types of Misconduct

In 1992, the National Academy of Sciences (NAS) issued a report, "Responsible Science: Ensuring the Integrity of the Research Process,"[2] which made a number of important recommendations on research misconduct and integrity issues to federal agencies and the scientific community. The report discusses three types of behaviors:

- Misconduct in science, which it defines as fabrication, falsification, and plagiarism;
- Questionable research practices that deviate from traditional norms of acceptable research

practice but are not considered serious enough to constitute formal misconduct, and;

• Other forms of misconduct.

The report makes a number of recommendations for how to deal with these various behaviors.

First, it recommends that research institutions and government agencies adopt a common framework for distinguishing among types of research misconduct, questionable research practices, and other misconduct. Secondly, it encourages scientists and institutions to take actions, "to discourage questionable research practices through a broad range of formal and informal methods,"[3] but with processes distinct from those for handling research or other misconduct. It also encourages institutions to establish policies and procedures for handling other forms of misconduct (discussed later in this chapter).

The report details a wide variety of other issues of misconduct, including sexual and other forms of harassment; misuse of funds; gross negligence in professional responsibilities; vandalism, including tampering with research experiments and instrumentation; and violation of research regulations, including regulations on radioactive materials, recombinant DNA research, and the use of human or animal subjects. Other forms of misconduct include issues related to the research misconduct process itself, including: coverup of misconduct; retaliation against whistleblowers; dishonest allegations of research misconduct; and violations of due process protections for accused scientists.

Although the NAS report uses a separate category to discuss questionable research practices and does not group them under the term "other misconduct," for our purposes it is useful to include questionable research practices in this chapter because they, like other misconduct, warrant institutional scrutiny and discipline in appropriate circumstances. In this regard, the report specifically notes that institutions "should also accept responsibility for determining which questionable research practices are serious enough to warrant institutional penalties."[4] The NAS report lists seven specific examples of questionable practices:

• Failure to retain significant research data for a reasonable period;

• Inadequate research records to support conclusions or published results;

• Improper authorship practices;

• Refusal of reasonable access to unique research materials or data that support published papers;

• Use of inappropriate statistical or other methods to enhance findings;

• Inadequate supervision of research staff or exploitation; and,

• Misrepresentation of speculation as fact or release of preliminary results without sufficient data to allow objective review.

However, there are certainly a number of other practices not listed in the NAS report which meet the report's criteria that questionable research practices erode "confidence in the integrity of research process, violate traditions associated with science, affect scientific conclusions, waste time and resources, and weaken the education of new scientists." These could include, for example, failure to disclose or manage a substantial conflict of interest, improperly dropping data points without adequate scientific justification, and use of a poor research design that leads to uninterpretable results in human or animal studies.

Another significant report on research and other misconduct was issued in 1995 by the statutory Commission on Research Integrity (CRI). That report, "Integrity and Misconduct in Research,"[5] also discusses research misconduct and other forms of professional misconduct. The report proposed a definition of research misconduct that included "misappropriation, interference, and misrepresentation." We will only discuss interference since misappropriation and misrepresentation are similar to the definitions of plagiarism and falsification or fabrication, respectively. Interference is defined to cover action, intentional or without authorization, to "take or sequester or materially damage any research-related property of another, including without limitation the apparatus, reagents, biological materials, writing, data, hardware, software, or any other substance or device used or produced in the conduct of research."[6] The very broad scope of this definition would certainly cover sabotage of another scientist's experiment, as well as theft of property. In this regard, it overlaps with the NAS report's coverage of other misconduct that includes vandalism and tampering with research experiments and instrumentation.

The CRI report also covers other forms of professional misconduct that includes "obstruction of investigations of misconduct" and "noncompliance with research regulations." Obstruction of investigations includes intentional destroying or withholding of evidence, falsifying evidence, soliciting or giving false testimony, and attempting to intimidate or retaliate against witnesses, potential witnesses, or potential leads. The "noncompliance" definition covers all applicable federal research regulations, including regulations on biohazardous materials and human and animal research. Serious noncompliance with such regulations by an investigator who had advance notice of the regulation would constitute professional misconduct.

Although the CRI report's proposed definitions of research misconduct and other forms of professional misconduct were not adopted, the CRI recommendation that a federal government-wide definition of research misconduct be adopted was accepted by the OSTP and ultimately led to the federal government-wide definition discussed previously. Though not implemented, the commission definitions remain as useful guidance for those institutions which choose to adopt institutional specific standards for research staff on misconduct and integrity issues.

ORI Study on Institutional Misconduct Policies

In 2000, ORI published under contract a study on a nonrandom sample of 156 institutional policies on research misconduct. One goal of the study was to determine how many institutions had definitions of research misconduct that were broader than the current Public Health Service (PHS) definition of misconduct, "research misconduct means fabrication, falsification, plagiarism, or other practices that seriously deviate from those that are commonly accepted in the scientific community for proposing, conduct, or reporting research. It does not include honest error or honest differences in interpretations or judgments of data."*,[7]

The report, which is available on the ORI website found that slightly over 50 percent of the institutions reviewed had adopted a misconduct

definition that exceeded the PHS definition. The major category of additional misconduct covered was "material failure to comply with governmental regulations," which was included in 33% of the reviewed policies.[8] The author believes that this category would cover a wide variety of investigator activity that did not comply with regulatory requirements, such as substantial failure to follow human subject protections, animal welfare requirements, or conflict of interest regulations. Thus, an investigator who fails to report a substantial conflict of interest covered by the regulations or to follow institutional directives to manage, reduce, or eliminate the conflict might be subject to institutional discipline, depending on the severity of the infraction and any specific institutional policies or guidance on the subject. Table 50-1 summarizes the main categories of behavior covered by institutional definitions that go beyond fabrication, falsification, and plagiarism.

Several institutional policies are discussed below to demonstrate how institutions have handled their plenary authority to set standards for research integrity by defining ethical conduct beyond fabrication, falsification, and plagiarism.

The institutional policies in Tables 50-2, 50-3, and 50-4, although using variable terminology, cover the basic categories of research misconduct, questionable research practices, and other misconduct we discussed in the background section. The

---

*The original PHS regulation uses the term "misconduct" or "misconduct in science." However, chapter uses the term "research misconduct" to be consistent with the terminology of the federal definition and the revised PHS regulation which was published on May 17, 2005; 42 CFR 93.103.

TABLE 50-1 Institutional policies exceeding the federal definition of research misconduct.[9]	Number of Policies	Percent of Policies
Number of policies containing a definition of research misconduct that includes types of misconduct other than fabrication, falsification, and plagiarism	82	53%
Other types of behavior most often defined as research misconduct:		
Material failure to comply with governmental regulations	52	33%
Unauthorized use of confidential information	39	25%
Retaliation or threat of retaliation against persons involved in the allegation or investigation of misconduct	25	15%
Improprieties of authorship	24	15%
Material failure to comply with nongovernmental regulations applicable to research	16	10%

TABLE 50-2	Excerpts from Michigan State University Misconduct Policy.[10]

The Research Integrity Policy of the University of Pittsburgh (Jan. 1, 2002) defines "research Misconduct" to include "misrepresentation of credentials, in proposing, performing, or reviewing research, or in reporting research results."

***

Questionable research practices as practices that do not constitute Misconduct or Unacceptable Research Practices but that require attention because they could erode confidence in the integrity of Research or Creative Activities.

***

"Unacceptable Research Practices" are defined as "practices that do not constitute Misconduct but that violate applicable laws, regulations, or other governmental requirements, or University rules or policies, of which the Respondent had received notice or of which the Respondent reasonably should have been aware."

***

The policy goes on to explain how MSU handles these practices:

Referral from Proceedings. An inquiry Panel or an Investigative Committee may find that, while a Respondent's conduct does not warrant an Investigation or constitute Misconduct, it nevertheless may constitute an Unacceptable Research Practice or a Questionable Research Practice. Any such finding shall be referred to the Responsible Administrator for review and further appropriate action.

Discovery and Report. Unacceptable Research Practices or Questionable Research Practices may also be discovered in other circumstances. When that happens, the alleged Unacceptable Research Practice or Questionable Research Practice should be reported to the Responsible Administrator for such review and further action, if any, as may be appropriate under unit guidelines.

Discipline. The University views Unacceptable Research Practices as grounds for appropriate action pursuant to existing University policies, procedures, and contracts.

A separate provision provides for grieving disciplinary decisions.

In addition to research misconduct, the Michigan State University (MSU) policy on "Procedures Concerning Allegations of Misconduct in Research and Creative Activities" (June 27, 2002), explicitly addresses "questionable research practices" and "unacceptable research practices." Selective provisions of the policy are set forth [later in the policy].

Michigan State University policy (Table 50-2) addresses questionable research practices, using the nomenclature and principles of the NAS, and "unacceptable research practices" that overlap with the "other misconduct" as defined in the NAS Report. The policy also provides for imposition of sanctions where the investigator's conduct falls under the proscribed activities.

The University of Pittsburgh policy (Table 50-3) uses different terminology, "research improprieties" to describe other practices considered not acceptable, that seems broad enough to cover both questionable research practices and other misconduct. This policy also provides for discipline where research improprieties are committed.

The University of Maryland-Baltimore policy broadly defines "academic misconduct" to include "fabrication, falsification, and plagiarism" (the core of the new federal definition of research misconduct) and other practices that would fall under the questionable research practices category or other misconduct. In particular, the examples of academic misconduct provided are broad enough to encompass the NAS Report's description of miscon-

duct in the research misconduct process (see Table 50-4, number 7, "inappropriate behavior in relation to academic misconduct").

By adopting approaches similar to the institutional policies described previously, a research institution can put in place a system to respond to behaviors outside of the formal federal definition of research misconduct when those behaviors constitute questionable research practices, other forms of misconduct, or breach specific standards set by the institution. Under this type of system, the types of behaviors subject to review and discipline by the institution could include:

- Substantial violation of research regulations, such as failure to obtain informed consent in a study involving high risk to the subject;
- Failure to disclose a significant conflict of interest when the conflict has the potential to bias the study; assuming improper authorship by not giving credit to other major contributors;
- Misusing privileged communications to obtain an unfair advantage in publishing or getting funded; deceptive analysis and reporting of research results; and,

TABLE 50-3	Excerpts from University of Pittsburgh Misconduct Policy[11]

"The Research Integrity Policy" of the University of Pittsburgh (Jan. 1, 2002) defines

"Research Misconduct" to include "misrepresentation of credentials, in proposing, performing, or reviewing research, or in reporting research results."

***

It also addresses **"research improprieties"** as follows: "If the research activities of the Respondent are found to involve research impropriety although not a nature or to a degree that might constitute Misconduct or that warrant additional investigation, the dean may take corrective or disciplinary measures."

***

The policy further describes "possible sanctions for research improprieties" as follows:

***

If the research activities of the Respondent are found to constitute research impropriety, although not of a nature or to a degree that might result in a finding of Research Misconduct, the dean may impose sanctions, such as:

   a. a reprimand;

   b. notification of the IRB or IACUC for possible actions in matters relevant to clinical or animal research, respectively;

   c. requirement to withdraw or correct abstracts, manuscripts, publications, and/or grant proposals;

   d. limitations on the Respondent's responsibility in research;

   e. requirements for participation in training programs;

   f. notification to sponsoring agencies, co-authors, editors, and other institutions involved in the research.

- Deliberate dropping of data points to improve study outcomes, short of outright fraud.

These issues cover some of the types of high profile lapses in research integrity that have occurred in the past few years that have brought criticism, or in some cases litigation, against the institutions involved.

Examples of Applying Other Misconduct in Practice

In this section, we will discuss several cases where institutions have applied policies going beyond the federal definition in specific circumstances. The first case involves a finding of misconduct by the University of Medicine and Dentistry of New Jersey. The institution found that the accused scientist published the same material twice without notifying the publisher or the readers of that fact. This practice has been variously described as "duplicate publication" or "self-plagiarism." The institution reported the matter to ORI for oversight review and ORI did not find misconduct on the grounds that it did not consider duplicate publication to be plagiarism under the PHS definition of research misconduct. Although journal editors consider the practice unacceptable and often instruct submitting authors

that they must certify that manuscripts are original work, ORI concluded that because the author had not taken the work of another and used it as his own, it would not find misconduct. However, ORI did notify the institution that it could find the author's practice unacceptable under its institutional policy. The institution did so and took administrative actions against the accused scientist. He then took the case to court. In *Shovlin v. University of Medicine and Dentistry of New Jersey*, the court upheld the institution's finding and stated that:

> [E]ven though the federal agency [ORI] to which the university reported may not have considered duplicate publication to constitute 'misconduct in science,' it recognized the university's right to hold such practice unacceptable.[12]

In *United States v. Arora*, the National Institutes of Health (NIH) filed a civil suit against an NIH scientist for sabotaging another's research project (wrongfully destroying cells).[13] Although the amount of damages awarded to NIH was small, the court upheld the principle that the conduct involved was unacceptable behavior. In its ruling, the court stated that the scientist's actions "undermined the honor system that exists among the community of scientists, a system which is ultimately

TABLE 50-4	Excerpts from University of Maryland, Baltimore Misconduct Policy.[14]

The University of Maryland-Baltimore "Policy and Procedures Concerning Misconduct" (revised Dec. 1998) define "**academic misconduct**" to include, in addition to fabrication, falsification, and plagiarism, "any form of behavior, including the making of allegations that involve frivolous, mischievous, or malicious misrepresentation, whereby one's work or the work of others is seriously misrepresented. Academic Misconduct may take numerous forms including, but not limited to, those listed in Section X, below. Academic misconduct does not include honest error or honest differences in interpretations or judgments of data."

***

Section X lists the following examples of academic misconduct, in addition to fabrication, falsification, and plagiarism:

***

3. **IMPROPRIETIES OF AUTHORSHIP:** Improper assignment of credit, such as excluding others by knowingly not citing their work; misrepresentation of the same material as original in more than one publication.

4. **MISAPPROPRIATION OF THE IDEAS OF OTHERS:** An important aspect of the scholarly activity is the exchange of ideas among colleagues. Improper or nonattributive use of information acquired in this process constitutes Academic Misconduct. New ideas gleaned from such exchanges can lead to important discoveries. Scholars can acquire novel ideas during the process of reviewing grant applications and manuscripts. However, improper use of such information or wholesale appropriation of such material constitutes Academic Misconduct.

5. **VIOLATION OF GENERALLY ACCEPTED RESEARCH PRACTICES:** Serious deviation from accepted practices in proposing or carrying out of research, improper manipulation of experiments to obtain biased results, deceptive statistical or analytical manipulations, or improper reporting of results.

6. **DELIBERATE VIOLATION OF REGULATIONS:** For example, failure to comply with regulations concerning the use of human subjects, the care of animals, health and safety of individuals and the environment, new devices, investigational drugs, recombinant products, or radioactive, biologic, or chemical materials.

7. **INAPPROPRIATE BEHAVIOR IN RELATION TO ACADEMIC MISCONDUCT:** Including bad faith accusation of Misconduct; failure to report known or suspected Academic Misconduct; withholding or destruction of information relevant to a claim of Academic Misconduct: and retaliation against persons involved in the allegation or investigation of Academic Misconduct.

8. **MISAPPROPRIATION OF FUNDS OR RESOURCES:** For example, the misuse of funds for personal gain.

9. **ABUSE OF CONFIDENTIALITY:** For example, improper use of information gained by privileged access, such as information obtained through service on peer review panels and editorial boards.

based on truthfulness, both as moral imperative and as a fundamental operational principle in the scientific research process."

A third case involved a major West Coast institution[*] where a scientist was alleged to have committed plagiarism by taking material from a former collaborator to use as his own in a grant application. The accused scientist argued that it did not constitute misconduct because ORI does not consider disputes between former collaborators to fall under its definition of plagiarism. ORI notified the institution of the ORI position, but also advised that the institution could establish different standards under its own policy. The institution found plagiarism in the case and this decision was upheld in an administrative hearing.

---

[*]The institution is not named here because the matter did not involve ORI jurisdiction and the details were not reported in public decision).

Another case does not involve an institutional finding of "other misconduct" per se, but is illustrative because it upholds damages against a whistleblower, who made public statements against an accused scientist when there was no institutional finding of misconduct. In *Arroyo v. Rosen*, the Maryland Court of Appeals upheld a jury verdict against Dr. Arroyo, the whistleblower, when she made disclosures to the Baltimore *Sun* about the allegation after the institution did not find misconduct and the paper then published a story on the matter.[15] Although not mentioned in the court's decision, Arroyo may also have violated the expectation of confidentiality provided in the PHS misconduct regulations, 42 CFR 50.103 (d) (3), "affording the affected individuals confidential treatment to the maximum extent possible." Similar provisions are also included in most institutional policies, providing a potential basis for institutions to find "other misconduct" in similar circumstances.

Although the number of published cases in the area of "other misconduct" is small, the cases demonstrate the institution's authority to fashion and enforce remedies in cases of "other misconduct."

Issues to Consider in Adopting Institutional Policies That Cover Questionable Research Practices or Other Forms of Academic or Research Misconduct

If the institution has adopted "other misconduct" policies, questions about other forms of misconduct or breaches of research integrity have already been asked. Regardless, it is still important to ask:

- What has the institution's experience been?
- Has the policy been applied in practice?
- Do the faculty and other research staff support the policies?
- Have there been specific cases where the policy applied but the institution chose not to enforce it? If so, this may undermine the principles enunciated and create cynicism among those affected.

If the policy has not been applied fairly, cynicism and morale problems can arise. Further, if the institution's policies have never been used or been used in an inconsistent or questionable matter, it may be time to consider updating or revising the policy.

For institutions that wish to consider adding new policies in this area, there are several issues that should be considered.

First, consider where problems have occurred. Have substantial difficulties occurred in human studies, animal welfare, conflict of interest, or other research areas? If so, it may be advisable to establish a committee or use an existing mechanism (e.g., faculty senate) to study the problem and make recommendations on how to proceed. There is advantage to involving the research community in these matters: their participation helps to substantiate the importance of the institute's policy and helps to identify issues and approaches that are unique to a particular institutional culture. Institutions that have had significant problems in other areas of research conduct but cannot redress them because of the lack of established policies may have the biggest incentive to modify or add to existing institutional policy. On the other hand, an institution with a superior culture of integrity and which has a history of few or minor issues of misconduct may conclude that additional policies are unnecessary and not worth the staff time and commitment of institutional resources. Of course, even when problems seem to be few and minor in nature, institutions can use institutional policies to set expectations for staff and encourage

positive behavior. In this regard, even where no sanctions are imposed for other types of misconduct, institutions may want to consider adding research guidelines that promote responsible research conduct in specific areas, such as responsible authorship and recording, retaining, and reporting data.

There are also potential negatives when adding new policies on "other misconduct." As demonstrated in the "other misconduct" case studies, there can be the threat of litigation if the institution plans to enforce the policy in a specific instance. Litigation can require substantial resources and may cost the institution in a number of ways, including negative publicity. In other cases, however, an institution may find publicity a positive in that it demonstrates the institution's commitment to a high level of research integrity.

Perhaps the single most important factor to consider is the culture of the individual research institution. If the institution's research standards are lax, and research infractions are common or serious, new policies that exceed the bare minimum of discouraging fabrication, falsification, and plagiarism may be exactly what is needed to set the institution on a new course. If the existing culture of integrity is strong, adding new policies may be a waste of institutional resources and could create new problems, such as faculty or research staff resistance. Each institution must answer this basic question for itself.

Conclusion

This chapter has discussed the types of "other misconduct" issues: those that exceed the federal definition of research misconduct and that have been identified by the research community; by existing institutional policies; and by case law. Research administrators considering supplementation of existing institutional policies on misconduct can choose from a variety of approaches and models, which include questionable research practices; and other forms of research, academic or other misconduct and research infractions. These policies are tools that institutions can use to provide new standards or guidance to institutional staff. Each institution must decide whether additional policies are worthwhile to promote the institution's research mission.

Author's Note

The opinions expressed herein are those of the author and do not necessarily represent the views of the Office of Research Integrity, the U.S. Department of Health and Human Services, or any other federal agency.

• • • References

1. Office of Science and Technology Policy. "Federal Policy on Research Misconduct." *65 Federal Register* 76260, December 6, 2000.

2. National Academy of Sciences. *Responsible Science: Ensuring the Integrity of the Research Process.* Volume I. Washington, DC: National Academy Press, 1992, http://www.nap.edu/books/0309047315/html/index.html (accessed September 15, 2005).

3. National Academy of Sciences, 1992.

4. National Academy of Sciences, 1992.

5. U.S. Department of Health and Human Services. "Integrity and Misconduct in Research." *Report of the Commission on Research Integrity*, 1995, http://ori.hhs.gov/documents/report_commission.pdf (accessed October 20, 2005).

6. U.S. Department of Health and Human Services, 1995, at 13.

7. 42 *Code of Federal Regulations* 50.102.

8. Office of Research Integrity, Analysis of Institutional Policies for Responding to Allegations of Scientific Misconduct, http://ori.dhhs.gov/documents/institutional_policies.pdf (accessed October 20, 2005).

9. Office of Research Integrity.

10. Michigan State University. "Procedures Concerning Allegations of Misconduct in Research and Creative Activities," June 27, 2002, http://www.hr.msu.edu/HRsite/Documents/Faculty/Handbooks/Faculty/ResearchCreativeEndeavor/vi-miscon-toc (accessed October 20, 2005).

11. University of Pittsburgh. *Policy on Research Integrity*, revised January 1, 2002, http://www.pitt.edu/HOME/PP/policies/11/11-01-01.html (accessed October 20, 2005).

12. State of New Jersey, 50 F. Supp. 2d 297, 314 (D. N.J. 1998), aff'd per curiam, 3rd, Cir. May 28, 1999.

13. *United States v. Arora*, 860 F. Supp. 1091 (D. Md. 1994), aff'd per curiam, 56 F. 3d 62 (4th, Cir. 1995), this is the U.S.

14. University of Maryland, Baltimore. *Policy and Procedures Concerning Misconduct*, http://www.umbc.edu/newsevents/Student/scholar.html (accessed October 20, 2005).

15. State of Maryland, Court of Appeals, 102 Md., App. 101, 648 A. 2d 1074, Md. Ct. App., 1994.

Human Research Management: Building a Program for Responsible Conduct and Oversight of Human Studies in a Brave New World

Greg Koski, PhD, MD, CPI, DSc (Honorary)

In a world of almost unimaginable beauty and complexity, mankind has developed remarkable capability to probe the workings of nature and its creatures, including how they behave and interact. Driven by insatiable curiosity and an apparently growing entrepreneurial spirit, scientists continue to push the limits of technology and creativity in their efforts to know even more about our world and ourselves; why we behave as we do; and to develop new products for diagnosis, prevention, and treatment of disease. As science searches for signs of intelligent life elsewhere in our universe, science also seems to be inching closer to creation of life here at home, unraveling and applying the coded messages of our genetic bible. The mysteries of mind seem less mysterious when the chemical and physical bases of thought and emotion can be probed with positron emission scanning and other sophisticated tools. Even the fusion of man and machine is no longer the stuff of science fiction.

Advances in science and technology are rightfully a source of wonder and awe for all of us. For some, this progress is also a source of pride and profit. For a growing number, it is becoming a source of concern and even fear. Discovery-related anxiety is hardly a new phenomenon. Through the ages, dramatic discoveries that challenge our beliefs or encroach upon things our cultures and societies hold sacred have given rise to a backlash of resistance. Some minds are simply not well prepared or disposed to accept "the truth" as disclosed by science. In the words of Bob Seger, a popular singer of the 1980s, in his classic song, "Against the Wind," there are some of us who may, "wish I didn't know now what I didn't know then." It is not that they are opposed to progress; they may just not be ready to deal with its consequences.

Many, even in the scientific community, are concerned that society may not be properly equipped to deal with the social, ethical, and legal issues that emerge when science opens a new black box. Experience teaches us that these concerns are often justified. Knowledge is power, and power can be used and abused. Abuses are most likely to occur when society has not yet established acceptable norms of conduct or developed effective mechanisms to prevent them. When abuses do occur, even when committed by only a few, society, in turn, reacts by implementing rules and regulations that impact everyone. Even though well intentioned, the consequences of regulation are far reaching and are not always beneficial or predictable. Such seems to be the case in human research.

Human Research Oversight: "Born of Abuse and Reared in Protectionism"

Carol Levine's often quoted line aptly and succinctly describes the evolution of the ethical and legal environment in which scientists have conducted human research for the past century. Whether in the biological, behavioral, or social sciences, a relatively small number of studies, by well intentioned investigators, have at times violated the sensibilities of society. The natural history of societal reaction to such abuses is a recurring cycle of disclosure and outrage followed by regulation and later reflection.

In modern day human research, the initial cycle of regulation began with revelations of atrocities perpetrated in the name of science in wartime concentration camps during the 1930s and 1940s. We know of atrocities that occurred in Europe and Asia and which may also have occurred elsewhere. War too easily allows individuals to engage in activities that they otherwise would abhor. Twenty years after the Nuremberg tribunal, the work of Beecher and Katz set the stage for disclosure in 1972 of the US Public Health Service Syphilis Study, commonly, but unfortunately, called the Tuskegee Study. In response to these events, the US Congress enacted the National Research Act in 1974 and established the National Commission for Protection of Human Subjects in Biomedical and Behavioral Research, generally referred to as the National Commission.

The commission's Belmont Report [1], issued in 1979, established an ethical foundation for regulations that established requirements for review boards and consent processes to prevent future abuses. Accordingly, our national system for institutionally based human research oversight was born. It was not something that institutions and scientists had asked for: the system of oversight was imposed upon them through the law.

With inadequate funding and an ineffective implementation strategy, it is not surprising that this system failed to realize its potential. By 1982, just one year after federal regulations for protection of human subjects were promulgated, the first of what is now a long series of federal advisory commission reports on this subject was issued. Disclosure of unethical human radiation experiments during the Cold War initiated yet another cycle of concern and reaction, and another report calling for reform. [2]

The situation in the United States reached a flash point with the death of Jesse Gelsinger in 1999. Gelsinger's death from multiple organ failure after infusion of an adenoviral vector in a failed gene-transfer study prompted congressional hearings to which the Department of Health and Human Services (HHS) reacted by creating the Office for Human Research Protections (OHRP) as part of an initiative to remodel and enhance the effectiveness of the national system for protection of human subjects. [3]

Recognizing that investigations after the fact do little to protect human subjects or the integrity of science, OHRP has been instrumental in initial efforts to move from a reactive, compliance-focused approach to oversight of human research toward a proactive, prevention-focused paradigm designed to enhance performance and effectiveness of the review, approval, and oversight process, while improving efficiency and reducing administrative and regulatory burdens that do little in and of themselves to protect research participants. [4]

During the initial stages of the current cycle of reform, the research community itself has displayed a new willingness to accept responsibility for ensuring the safety and well-being of research participants. In keeping with the philosophy that it is better to prevent the tragedy than to investigate and sanction after the fact, the research community has not only endorsed this approach, but has actually taken the lead in creating new, nongovernmental programs for enhancing protections for human subjects in research, including quality improvement initiatives, voluntary accreditation programs, and professional certification programs for research coordinators, investigators, and institutional review board (IRB) professionals. Notably, the Association of American Medical Colleges (AAMC) contributed substantially toward developing and launching the Association for Accreditation of Human Research Protection Programs (AAHRPP), an independent, not-for-profit organization supported by a host of major scientific and professional associations, which offers voluntary accreditation to human research protection programs that are able to meet its rigorous standards that actually exceed the requirements of federal regulations. AAHRPP, like OHRP, has promoted the philosophy that compliance with regulations alone is not an adequate or appropriate goal.

In human research, science has been granted the privilege to violate a fundamental principle of human rights: to use human beings as a means to an end. With that privilege comes responsibility. Research is not without risk. Indeed, risks attendant to research may threaten life, livelihood, and privacy. More often than not, individual research subjects are unlikely to benefit directly from their participation in research or to even know they are exposed to all of the attendant risks. Science and society are able to rationalize and justify this practice on utilitarian grounds. The benefits to science and society flowing from research are considered to be worth allowing some to be exposed to the risks provided the risks are reasonable in relation to the anticipated benefits, that the risks are minimized, and that participation is voluntary and with the informed consent of the subject. Along with the privilege of conducting research on fellow human beings comes the moral and legal responsibility to protect their safety and well-being, to protect their interests, and to ensure that their participation is fully informed and voluntary. Any failure to fill these responsibilities is an affront to the integrity of science and the dignity of our fellow man. The goal of this chapter is to help research managers who bear responsibility for human research administration and protection of human subjects to foster a values-based institutional culture that supports a programmatic approach to protection of human subjects that promotes and facilitates responsible conduct of human research at every level of the institution. While this article targets academic centers, the principles and practices described here are easily adaptable to other settings in which human studies are performed, including independent research performance sites.

The Importance of Institutional Culture

For too long, the research community has failed to appreciate and internalize the values that underlie responsible conduct of human research and accept its responsibilities. Compliance with regulations in human research is a necessary, but insufficient goal. When efforts to protect human subjects are viewed as little more than costly, inefficient administrative impediments to research productivity, it is not surprising that they do not receive the respect and resources necessary for effectiveness. When such attitudes emanate from the leadership of an organization or are tolerated by its leaders, the result can be disastrous.

The 2001 death of Ellen Roche in a physiological study of airway responsiveness at Johns Hopkins University Medical Center in Baltimore prompted an investigation by the Food and Drug Administration (FDA) and OHRP that revealed an institutional culture that was described by an independent advisory committee, chaired by Dr. Sam Hellman, Dean Emeritus of the University of Chicago's Pritzker School of Medicine, as "an adversarial relationship with federal regulators." [5] The committee found that "many people at Hopkins believe that oversight and regulatory processes are a barrier to research and are to be reduced to a minimum rather than their serving as an important safeguard." It is not unreasonable to assume that this view has been prevalent throughout the academic community for many years, not only at Hopkins, but this may be changing.

This painful chapter in the history of human research had far-reaching impact throughout the research community, as well as in Baltimore. The commitment of the leadership of Johns Hopkins to have the best program for human research in the world has been echoed by other institutions, including the University of Iowa, Washington University of St. Louis, and Duke University. These commitments have been met with resources and action. While some institutions are still in a reactive mode, responding in fear of "being shut down" by government regulators, others have begun to move beyond this reactive culture of compliance toward a culture of conscience and responsibility. This cultural evolution can have dramatic salutary results for an institution, as evidenced by the resurgence of Duke's clinical research programs in the wake of what has there come to be known as "the unhappiness," the 1999 assurance suspension by OHRP's predecessor, the Office for Protection from Research Risks (OPRR), when it found that the institution had failed to comply with federal regulations for protection of human subjects.

Building a Culture of Conscience: Taking It to the Top

The first step in creation of an effective management program for responsible human research is to secure a commitment from the very top leaders of the organization that all human research will be done right or not at all. Getting this commitment is not always easy, but it is both necessary and worthwhile. The several high-profile examples of what can (and does!) happen when this commitment is unfulfilled may provide a useful catalyst when there seems to be the reluctance at the top. Enlightened university presidents or deans of research, such as Dr. David Skorton at the University of Iowa, have realized that if a research institution is going to be in the headlines, it is better to do so for being the first academic medical center to receive accreditation of its human research protection program than for the death of a research participant!

When necessary, even if the goal is to establish a "culture conscience," applying the compliance enforcement card may be helpful and effective. Fear of enforcement actions and the adverse publicity that inevitably follows can provide the activation energy necessary to get the process moving. For the mid-level research manager, a forthright expression of concern to senior leaders regarding perceived deficiencies in human subjects protection program can be remarkably powerful, particularly when it is in writing, realizing that in some cases, the action may impact one's career pathway for better or for worse. Any responsible institutional leader should want to know if situations exist within an organization that renders it vulnerable to failure. One should establish an expectation that anyone, at any level, who sees a situation that could result in harm, injury, or failure to achieve the institutional mission will bring that situation immediately to the attention of the leadership, and should be rewarded for doing so. If the institutional culture discourages such behavior, the conscientious observer is likely to become a whistle-blower, reporting a situation to an outside authority, the press, or a regulatory agency. If so, the outcome is not likely to be flattering to the institution.

A useful step in bringing cultural change to an institution is to participate in a comprehensive program evaluation, either a directed self-evaluation or an independent external evaluation. Many institutions hired external consultants after federal regulators suspended research activities at major research sites in the late 1990s; as a result, some likely avoided similar consequences. More recently, the introduction of OHRP's quality improvement program and the emergence of voluntary accreditation programs have offered alternative pathways to the same end. In these cases, institutions are afforded an opportunity to "safely" review their programs for possible deficiencies and receive expert feedback on steps that can be taken to improve their programs. Many institutions have participated in these programs and their experiences have mostly been overwhelmingly positive. Some institutions have been wary to ask OHRP to examine their programs, but these fears are unwarranted. The OHRP quality improvement program was designed with just this concern in mind—to create an operational firewall between compliance oversight and quality improvement activities while strengthening programs for protection for research participants. Upon completion of the OHRP program or a pre-accreditation assessment, institutional leadership is given an objective analysis of their program's strengths and weaknesses. As both consultations consider "institutional culture" within their analytical framework, this feedback can be the needed catalyst for cultural change.

This kind of "managing upward" serves the institution very well, but is only a start of the process of cultural evolution at an institution. Nevertheless, these programs are essential if broader reform initiatives are to succeed. The most desirable outcome from these upwardly directed initiatives is an unequivocal, widely disseminated personal statement from the highest institution of commitment to "doing it right" as the institution's highest priority. Tangible actions to support that statement should be taken (including elevation of the oversight process within institutional management hierarchy; establishment and provision of necessary resources; and recognition of the contributions of those who fulfill their responsibilities) to lend credibility and foster acceptance of the normative values.

When President Clinton officially apologized to the survivors of the US Public Health Service–Tuskegee study, he acknowledged the immorality of what had been done by our government to some of its own people and, further, voiced a commitment to ensure that steps would be taken to prevent future research atrocities. [6] The creation of OHRP in June 2000 by then Secretary Donna Shalala and the agency's elevation with the Office of the Secretary, and a tripling of the agency's resources signified that the government was willing to take a step in the right direction to ensure and enforce protective measures. One can only hope that this sense of commitment and direction will continue within the government and that institutions operating under federal regulations for protection of human subjects will similarly demonstrate the strength of their commitments.

Finding oneself trapped in an institution that neither is willing nor able to make the necessary commitments is a no-win situation. Sooner or later, an unfortunate event will occur, and when it does, a small solo voice wailing, "I told you so," will likely be drowned out by much louder and more powerful voices. There will be a need for a scapegoat. One should make every effort to avoid being the recipient of this dubious distinction. Leaving because conditions prevent the job from being done is better for one's career than leaving because the system failed, no matter who is ultimately implicated as the responsible party. Whether one should go even further by actually bringing the situation to the attention of higher authorities beyond the institution is a matter for personal reflection. The decision to take action or not is both difficult and important, and one that can have far-reaching consequences for the institution and many individuals. It is never a decision made lightly.

Building an Effective Program: The Partnership Paradigm

Over the past thirty years, the "system for human research oversight," as it has euphemistically[1] been dubbed, has rested, somewhat precariously, upon the "twin pillars" of human subjects' protection, institutional review boards (IRBs), and the informed consent process. These concepts emerged directly from the discussions of the National Commission in the late 1970s. They were operationally implemented through regulations for protection of human subjects in biomedical and behavioral research promulgated by the US Public Health Service (PHS) and the Department of Health, Education and Welfare (HEW) in 1981. [7] The presumption that review and approval by an independent review board composed of both scientists and nonscientists, coupled with a signed consent document, would afford adequate protections for human research subjects were not unreasonable in and of themselves at the time, but in practice, they fell short of expectations.

The problem was less conceptual than operational. Implementation was inadequate. To illustrate this point, consider our national air transportation safety system. Prior to September 11, 2001, virtually anyone could buy a ticket, get on an airplane, take on board just about anything, and fly off to wherever, whenever they chose. Once the planes were in the air, an elaborate tracking system employing the most sophisticated radar communications and navigation systems insured that most collisions were avoided and planes landed safely because people were watching them and there were flight rules intended to keep pilots and planes on course and out of harm's way. The pilots followed the rules or they were not allowed to fly. All of these systems were in place to enhance safety with the general understanding that people would not fly if they did not perceive air travel as safe. For the most part, the air transportation safety system,

a network of well-functioning operational units governed by an agreed upon set of rules and standards, worked.

However, the situation on the ground was rather different. Yes, there were X-ray machines and security guards for screening passengers, but frequently the X-ray machines did not work and most screeners had little or no training, insufficient time, and inadequate experience to be able to recognize suspicious objects. The screeners did not check to see whether passengers were who they purported to be and bags were rarely subject to serious searches. The security guards, too, had minimal, if any, training and were sometimes disparagingly referred to as "bottom feeders" in the job market. Funding for airport security came directly from the airlines, many of whom viewed the entire process as an unfunded federal mandate that made their passengers unhappy, ground operations less efficient, and air travel more costly. The airlines and airports had incentives to keep the process as simple and unobtrusive as possible, using the lowest possible level of trained personnel and the least expensive equipment.

Neither the public nor the air travel industry placed much value in the process because they did not believe that a serious threat existed. The goal of their efforts was to be in compliance with regulations, even if that meant nothing more than going through the motions of a security process, whether or not in fact they made any real difference to the safety and security of air transportation.

Analogies to the so-called human subjects protection "system" established by the 1981 regulations are fairly obvious. In practice, it was not a system at all, but a collection of autonomous local review boards operating with little oversight or coordination. The review and approval of complex and potentially risky protocols by a group of well-intended but untrained and sometimes reluctant "volunteers," supported by overburdened administrative personnel, lacking adequate support from institutional officials who viewed the process as an administrative sticky wicket through which their investigators had to pass in order to get federal research dollars, were unlikely to provide effective protections for human subjects. The failure of the government to provide sufficient resources to enable grantee institutions to fulfill the mandatory requirements for space, personnel, and expertise compounded the burden on research institutions facing increasing costs from this and other federally

---

[1]A *system* as generally defined involves a group of interacting, interrelated, or interdependent elements or parts that function together as a whole to accomplish a goal. To refer to the highly independent and often idiosyncratic collection of institutional review boards as a *system* implies a degree of coordination, oversight, and interrelatedness that has not yet been achieved in practice.

mandated compliance programs. In both research and air travel, the cost of failure of these safety systems is enormous, not only in terms of the innocent people harmed or killed, but also in terms of the public's loss of confidence in the systems themselves. Trust betrayed is lost, and once lost, is very difficult to restore.

One can no more expect human subjects to be protected by passing a protocol through in ineffective IRB than to expect a broken metal detector to find a concealed weapon on an airline passenger. In both cases, the risks are very real, and yet, it is no surprise that investigators complain that the process is needlessly cumbersome and inefficient, just as disgruntled air travelers complain as they wait to take off their jackets, shoes, and belts before going through the arches of the metal detectors. Ultimately, these situations become confrontational and when they do, they can escalate. Some people can become enraged and unprofessional; others will try to evade the process entirely. Is there a reasonable alternative?

As can be seen in the business world, even the fiercest competitors can become partners when it is in their common interests to do so. This is the partnership paradigm, recognizing that to achieve a common goal, both parties must share responsibilities. In human research, IRBs and investigators share common goals to ensure that human studies are done in a responsible, scientifically, and ethically sound manner without anyone being harmed. No responsible investigator wants to intentionally hurt a research subject nor do IRBs want to arbitrarily establish roadblocks to research progress, even if it may sometimes seem that way to investigators at the time of review.

When IRBs and investigators recognize and accept their shared goals and responsibilities, a different paradigm emerges. If an investigator is as concerned about the safety of the subjects and ethics of the study design as the IRB is, the investigator will take the time to identify the specific safety and ethical issues inherent in the study designs and address them openly and in detail before sending a protocol for review. In turn, the IRB should not require idiosyncratic changes in study design or procedure when issues of subjects' safety are not involved. When legitimate differences in opinion are cause for concern, the parties should engage in a collegial discussion to explore the basis for the concern and possible resolution. With some concerted effort, experience, and goodwill, rarely is it impossible to find a safe and ethical way to answer an important research question, although some compromise may be necessary.

In the very rare instances in which a properly constituted, well-informed IRB must disapprove a study on ethical grounds, the investigator should be more grateful than resentful, for more likely than not, a potential tragedy has been avoided. In such cases, however, the action taken by the IRB must be based on sound information and principles that warrant respect for its judgment and decision. An effective human research program exists within a prevailing culture of conscience and an environment of collegiality. As with any partnership, its strength is only as great as the strength of each partner's commitment to making it work, and these commitments must be founded on mutual respect, trust, and a demonstrated willingness to work together.

Walking the Talk of Responsibility

Talking about changing institutional culture and establishing a collegial environment that recognizes shared goals and responsibilities is easy; actually doing it is harder, but not impossible. The key to success is not found with the leaders themselves; the key to success is held by the followers. When programs are developed to target shared goals, all parties that have a stake in the outcome must participate in their development. Doing so is only possible when the leaders clearly demonstrate through their actions a willingness to seek balance and fairness, and the process must be open. The policies and practices that emerge from these encounters must be true to the principles on which they are founded. If they are not, the credibility and the viability of the venture are lost. Hard decisions may be necessary, but when those decisions are based on sound principles, developed and endorsed by the stakeholders, they will be justifiable and fair.

Another general principle is familiar to all: put your money where your mouth is! Failure to invest in the development of an effective human research protection program (HRPP) as part of the critical infrastructure for a responsible human research initiative sends a very loud and clear message, however an unfortunate one. Dr. Rob Califf, Director of Clinical Research at Duke University Medical Center, once remarked during a conference on clinical research sponsored by the Association of American Medical Colleges that "it cost Duke more to have its assurance suspended for four days that it would have cost to run the entire human research protection program for a year." In such cases, hindsight is always crystal clear. Dr. Califf went on to say that "a decision to build a few less isolation cages" in the research animal housing facility "would have paid for the best human subjects protection program in the country." Had this message been clear to the senior leadership at Duke prior to the suspension in 1998 of its assurance and closing of its research programs by OPRR for noncompliance with regulations for human subjects protection, their priorities may have been different. Had this message been clear to the National Institutes of Health (NIH) and Congress when funds were appropriated for the human subjects protection programs in 1981, the 1998 report from the Office of the Inspector General declaring that IRBs "review too much, too quickly, with too little expertise . . . with limited personnel and resources" [8] might have read very differently. To a very large extent, how the government and grantee institutions choose to apply funds available for research support is a simple matter of priorities; building an effective infrastructure for protection of human subjects has never been placed highly enough on the list to ensure sufficient resources to do the job properly, largely because this has not been considered to be part of the science itself.

Still, simply throwing money at the challenge of building an effective human subjects protection program is obviously not the answer. The effective human research manager must insure that available resources are invested wisely in programs and activities that actually work. And of course, the greatest challenge of all is developing methods to evaluate the effectiveness of human subjects protection programs. In this regard, audits demonstrating that minutes have been kept, consent forms signed, protocols followed, and adverse events reported are all helpful in demonstrating that procedures have been followed, but insufficient to demonstrate that the safety, rights, and welfare of subjects are actually being protected. Such evaluations do little to demonstrate that an IRB exercises well reasoned analysis and judgment, and speak even less to whether subjects are actually protected.

The federal government failed in the implementation of our national system of IRBs by not incorporating specific plans for ongoing evaluation of program effectiveness and accountability as part of the process. Instead the government opted for an approach of pseudo-accountability, one that relied almost entirely upon negotiated written assurances of compliance without much follow-through to see that the system actually worked. When the government actually did look, it found that these assurances were in many cases no more than paper promises, even at some of the country's most prestigious and well-funded research institutions.

The hallmark of any program that is truly striving for excellence is a willingness to seek external validation of the program's quality, such as independent accreditation. Like an Olympic athletic team, a human subjects protection program must be willing to seek constructive external evaluation and criticism in order to improve its performance and be willing to be held accountable as part of a continuing effort to improve. Rarely is the institution anxious to open its programs to outside scrutiny when it is practicing only the bare minimum requirements to avoid an enforcement action. In contrast is the institution that actively participates in education programs and quality improvement initiatives; requires certification for its personnel and formal accreditation of its programs; and otherwise demonstrates through its actions its commitment to excellence and willingness to accept responsibility for its actions.

All of these options are now readily available to institutions and investigators, and the effective research manager can insist that his or her institution and staff participate. As these initiatives become more widely adopted, government regulators will soon find that only a few institutions will need the legal hammer to build their programs. It is toward these institutions that the regulators' compliance oversight attention, enforcement activities, and sanctions will be focused.

The benefits to the institution of "walking the walk" include a higher degree of confidence and comfort that the institution will not become the next focus of unflattering public attention. Even more importantly, the chances that anyone will be harmed in research are greatly reduced, and all at the institution can take pride in the excellence of a research program conducted responsibly and with full respect for those upon whom its continued success depends, the research subjects.

A Systems Approach to Responsible Conduct and Oversight

Several times in this chapter I have referred to our national system for protection of human subjects in research. As mentioned earlier, this reflects very loose usage of the term "system." It is true that when compared with the situation that existed 30 years ago, we are far better off today, at least as far as avoiding unethical and reckless human research is concerned, though questions about the cost-effectiveness of these efforts remain unanswered and hotly debated.

Today we have IRBs, statutes, regulations, policies, guidance documents, and lists of best practices. We have educational programs and an assurance process, a uniform registration process for IRBs and a federal policy for protection of human subjects that has been adopted by most of the federal agencies that support or conduct human subjects research. Collectively, don't these measures qualify as a system?

A system involves a specifically designed and selected set of interrelated components that work together to produce a desired result. Returning to our earlier analogy, consider what would happen in air transportation in every air traffic control center operated independently with its own interpretation of Federal Aviation Agency (FAA) rules for separation zones and made no effort to insure that an aircraft leaving one zone was not appropriately tracked and transferred in a systematic way to the next air traffic control zone as a flight progressed. The simple answer is that there would be no air traffic control system, just a collection of air traffic control centers and air traffic controllers operating independently and idiosyncratically. This does not mean that they would not be trying in good faith to do a good job. But in the absence of an effectively coordinated system, planes would run into each other daily and chaos would rule the skies. Death and metal would rain from above. The picture is not hard to imagine.

The prevailing institution-based model for human research oversight is fraught with conflicts of interest and mixed messages, as noted by the National Bioethics Advisory Commission and others.[2] One could reasonably have predicted that imposing requirements for human subjects protection programs on grantee institutions without sufficient funding to support them and without having an effective oversight process in place to ensure accountability would have limited effectiveness. Had the federal government been more serious about developing a true system for protection of human subjects three decades ago, it might have considered more effective alternatives to the chosen approach. The government oversight process itself, prior to the recent creation of OHRP, was conflicted by placement of its human research oversight office

in a position subordinate to the government agencies that support and conduct research. [9] Even the current placement of OHRP within the Office of the Secretary of the Department of Health and Human Services does not fully alleviate concerns that the autonomy of OHRP could be compromised by the huge research agencies within the department. A separate office outside of the existing agencies may be needed to ensure needed autonomy.

For institutional officials and research managers, the message is that effective human research protection programs must be positioned within the organization in such a way that they are visible, respected, and authoritative, and operate with the autonomy necessary to effectively carry out responsibilities. [5] In turn, the program must conduct its activities in a manner consistent with its position and importance so as to warrant the respect and trust of those within the institution who depend upon it.

Selecting the Components

Development of an effective system for responsible conduct of human research is similar to building an effective computer network. No single model is best; the basic principle is to ensure that each component has appropriate capability, capacity, and interconnectivity and that the network is sufficiently robust and efficient to reliably serve the clients. Network architectures range from mainframe models to completely distributed models, and several hybrid approaches are enabled by platform independent communication protocols. Extending this analogy to human research, each individual research protection program might be considered as a domain, and each domain will have several components that must be interconnected to provide critical functionality (see Figure 51-1). Linking the functionality of these operating units through a robust network to form a safety net creates a system.

[2]The National Bioethics Advisory Commission (NBAC) was established by Executive Order 12975, signed by President Clinton on October 3, 1995. NBAC's functions were defined as follows: a) NBAC shall provide advice and make recommendations to the National Science and Technology Council and to other appropriate government entities regarding the following matters: 1) the appropriateness of departmental, agency, or other governmental programs, policies, assignments, missions, guidelines, and regulations as they relate to bioethical

issues arising from research on human biology and behavior; and 2) applications, including the clinical applications, of that research. The Commission issued several reports during its lifespan, including a detailed assessment of the status of oversight and review of human subjects research. All NBAC reports are available through: U.S. Department of Commerce, Technology Administration, National Technical Information Service, Springfield, Virginia 22161 and at http://www.georgetown.edu/research/nrcbl/nbac/pubs.html.

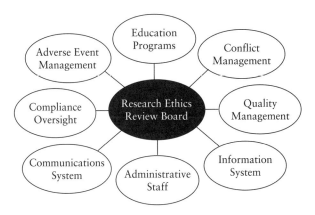

FIGURE 51-1 Components of an Effective Human Research Protection Program

The components of a good program include the research ethics review board or RERB,[3] which is the "motherboard" of the program, but the RERB cannot function properly without multiple support components as discussed later.

The RERB or IRB must be composed according to the federal regulations, which set a minimum of five members, at least one of which is unaffiliated with the founding institution, and one whose primary interests are not scientific in nature. The members are to be chosen to engender respect for its decisions by the institution's scientific community, and it should be appropriately balanced with respect to gender and ethnicity. In practice, the typical RERB at an academic medical center today generally includes about two dozen members, predominantly physician–scientists drawn from their group of peers, along with a sprinkling of lay members (clergy, ethicists, retired businessmen, lawyers, etc.). The membership frequently includes primary and alternate members in hopes of ensuring a necessary quorum.

Most members volunteer or are appointed to serve, generally without compensation, and with little or no formal training in the ethics, science, or regulatory requirements of human investigation. Although their review activities often focus on biomedical studies, most academic centers also engage in social and behavioral research involving human subjects, and this research is also subject to IRB review and approval whenever federal support is involved. This situation has been problematic at many centers. The willingness of some boards to review social and behavioral research even though they lack the expertise to do so has caused considerable distress among members of the social and behavioral science community who believe that a "clinical research model" has inappropriately and unfairly been applied to their nonmedical research protocols. These complaints are not without merit, and they highlight an important point: an IRB must have the expertise to review the science before it, and if not, to seek competent expert consultation as part of the comprehensive review process.

There are some, mostly in scientific circles, who believe that RERBs (and OHRP) should not be involved in review of the science of human research, but should focus only on the ethical aspects and regulatory compliance of proposals. [10] This view is too narrow. In human research, ethics and science are inseparable; they cannot and must not be considered in isolation from each other. Often, a study design that yields the fastest and cleanest data involves risks or other factors that are not ethically acceptable. Some degree of compromise and balance is likely to be needed. Investigators will find that their interests and those of their research subjects are well served, and communications with the IRB are more easily facilitated (i.e., more rapidly approved) when time and effort are devoted to careful consideration and justification of a chosen study design on the grounds of ethical and safety considerations. All investigators should be expected, indeed, directed by institutional requirement, to formally discuss in detail why a given design was chosen and others rejected, from the perspective of the interests of the human subjects. This single action would go very far toward clearing up the unfortunately all too common disagreements and misunderstandings between investigators and IRBs that may unnecessarily delay meritorious research and contribute to a confrontational relationship that may undermine the process.

The importance of selecting members carefully and wisely cannot be overstated. In the best of circumstances, members would all be highly qualified and committed individuals who fully understand the ethical, legal, and scientific dimensions of their responsibilities, and of course, are willing to work long hours to the effort for nothing. Officials at the Department of Health, Education, and Welfare must have thought that such individuals were in ready supply when the regulations were promulgated; but, as we have learned, sometimes painfully, that this is not so. Members are generally well-intentioned individuals who do want to responsibly exercise their duties, usually out of a sense of obligation or altruism, but they need training, support,

---

[3]RERB is the term recommended by the Institute of Medicine in its recent report, "Responsible Human Research: A Systems Approach," published in October 2002. The full report is available at http://www.iom.edu/report.asp?id=4459.

and time to do their best. When faculty members are asked to serve as RERB members, this service should be recognized for the special expertise it requires and its contribution to the academic mission of the institution. This can be accomplished through appropriate consideration during the academic promotions process, special recognition, and appropriate rewards. Good RERB members are extremely valuable to any institution, and their value should be acknowledged appropriately.

Everything stated here about general members applies several times over to the chairperson(s). An RERB chair should be recognized and respected throughout the institution as one of the most important contributors to its academic research mission. The individual's time commitments, financial support, and academic promotion should reflect this view. An institutional investment in a superb RERB chairperson is one of the two most important that can be made toward creating an effective program of responsible human research, the other being the program manager.

The program should be under the direction of a certified IRB professional. Certification is presently offered by national organizations such as the Boston-based Applied Research Ethics National Association (http://www.primr.org/membership/overview.html). The administrative support components and the communications and data-storage/processing infrastructures are also essential to an effective program. Software packages that facilitate, and may even automate every aspect of the oversight process are available. These can do much to strengthen the management, documentation, and record-keeping required by federal regulations, and in doing so, greatly enhance regulatory compliance.

Other important components may include an adverse event reporting process that may be linked to other institutional safety systems, such as incident reporting systems in hospitals and peer review programs. An independent quality improvement program that works with investigators and their research teams to implement best practices for recordkeeping, subject recruitment, and reporting can be extremely valuable. Some institutions have developed and implemented their own programs, while others have relied upon outside contractors to provide such services. Many investigators have noted dramatic improvements in enrollment and conduct of their studies after participating in such quality improvement efforts, and these programs may be more attractive to research sponsors and granting agencies. The importance of ongoing, quality education is widely recognized, and its value

amply demonstrated. An investment in education for all members of the research team and for potential participants yields high returns.

It is important to note that the many activities that are critical to an effective program are not the responsibility of the IRB or RERB. Certain activities, such as biosafety, radiation safety, and certain pharmacy activities, for example, are the primary responsibility of ancillary committees or processes that complement, but should not duplicate the IRB review and approval process. The same ought to be said for the process of evaluating conflicts of interest. Recent guidelines issued by national organizations and the US Department of Health and Human Services recommend that potential conflicts of interest be evaluated by a separate organizational entity or individual specifically dedicated to this task but appropriately interfaced with the RERB review process to ensure that conflicts are properly managed or eliminated without having this burden fall primarily upon the RERB. [11]

Not every program will be constructed in precisely the same way, but the selected components must be capable of efficiently performing all mission critical functions. As put so well by the Office of Inspector General of the Department of Health and Human Services, emphasis should be placed on performance, not process alone. [8] Current approaches to accreditation of HRPPs incorporate this principle, allowing flexibility with accountability, as recommended in the Inspector General's report. The federalwide assurance process developed and implemented by OHRP and its quality improvement program also support this approach. Participation in this program is a safe and effective way to insure that all critical functions are built into your program.

Putting the Pieces Together

Although every program must be tailored to meet specific organizational needs, there are general considerations that impact decisions regarding what a specific program will look like. The first consideration for the manager is whether to establish an institutionally based program at all. The "buy or build" decision has become increasingly important as the complexity and costs of maintaining an effective program increase, and consequences of maintaining an ineffective program are so readily apparent.

The flexibilities afforded by the new federalwide assurance process make consideration of outsourcing human subjects protections responsibilities a viable, practical, and in many cases preferable, alternative to establishing and/or maintaining an individual program, particularly at smaller institutions and sites that may not have all of the resources, expertise, and research volume necessary to justify and sustain an "accreditable" program of its own. This emphasis on accreditation is appropriate in light of the growing reliance upon accreditation both in United States and internationally to insure effectiveness of ethical review and oversight of human studies.

Recognizing the current realities of the US federal budget deficit, one can hardly imagine that OHRP, FDA, or any other human research oversight office or agency that might emerge from ongoing legislative activity will receive significant increases in funding for expanding oversight activities. Accordingly, federal regulators are likely to look toward voluntary private accreditation, either formally or informally, as an index of a program's quality and regulatory compliance. Because standards for accreditation exceed minimal requirements of the existing federal regulations for protection of human subjects, the likelihood that a duly accredited program will ever face serious enforcement action, especially the dreaded assurance suspension, is practically nonexistent.

Since the cost of operating an effective program is dramatically reduced by economies of scale, and since necessary technical expertise is more likely to be available at larger institutions, a small program can drastically reduce its costs and potential liability, while ensuring the strongest possible protection for its research participants by outsourcing these activities under a well-turned contract to a well-established and accredited human research protection program (HRPP). Such a program may be independent or institutionally based. The key is that a nationally or internationally recognized objective body accredits it.

Many institutions have been reluctant to outsource human research protection functions or even to participate in emerging collaborative review processes (e.g., as launched by the National Cancer Institute) because of concerns over liability and autonomy. [12] The question of liability is largely addressed by appropriate due diligence in selection of an accredited HRPP, and a good contract, along with continuing quality assurance activities on site. Any organization contemplating participation in off-site review programs must make certain that appropriate precautions, policies, and procedures are in place to insure necessary sensitivity to local factors and sensibilities. Even a research study that

has been approved by an accredited RERB and judged both scientifically and ethically sound may still not be appropriate for performance at a particular local site. This is not an ethical issue: it is an operational decision. If a site does not have an appropriate environment, facilities, personnel, or expertise, it should not participate in a study even if it has been thoroughly reviewed and approved by the finest RERB in the world.

In some cases an organization's HRPP may rely upon an external independent review board while retaining other functions in-house. This is not unlike a small organization using a hosting service provider to post and maintain its Web site. A good example in the human research world is the central RERB tandem models sponsored by the National Cancer Institute and developing cooperation with OHRP. Ultimately, whatever approach or model is chosen, the goal remains the same: to ensure that the research is done responsibly and well, in compliance with all regulations, and that all human subjects are treated with respect, justice, and a sense of beneficence. In this regard, a utilitarian approach is fully justified and acceptable; the end does indeed justify the means.

The Bottom Line: The Bottom Line?

It goes without saying that almost every one of the recommendations discussed above costs money, with the exception of marshalling the good will and conscience of well-intentioned individuals to do the right thing and to conduct their activities in a responsible, professional manner. Competition for resources in today's world of academia is intense. This competition has driven some institutions to look for alternative sources and arrangements for funding, sometimes in places that have yielded less than desirable results. Concerns that academia has sold its soul to industry are rampant and growing.

Much has been made of the public's loss of trust in the research enterprise. This loss of trust seems driven in part by increasing evidence that life sciences industries have engaged in questionable practices, including biased publication of results, concealing potential harmful information, price manipulation, unethical research practices in developing countries, and other activities that call into question our confidence in their motivations and conduct. The several high-profile tragedies in human research that have come to light recently at major academic research institutions, some of which were associated with financial relationships of the institutions and their investigators with industry that posed clear conflicts of interests have allowed the public's concern to rightfully extend to the academic research community.

In the final analysis, the costs of building, operating, and maintaining robust programs for responsible conduct of human research must be weighed against the costs of failing to do so. When an institution is receiving hundreds of millions of dollars in research grants and contracts, while concurrently investing trivial sums in programs to ensure that the work is done well and that subjects are not put at undue risk, the makings of yet another scandal are at hand. A friend in Tanzania once told me that one does not need to be mauled by a lion to know that it is an unpleasant experience. This lesson should be obvious to everyone in the academic scientific community, and such system failures should be preventable. Yes, the costs of doing it right may be steep, but the costs of not doing it right are immeasurable.

Resolution of this dilemma will come only with a realignment of priorities. We must look at the costs of the critical infrastructure for responsible human studies as an investment in responsible science rather than as an administrative liability. We must also strive to have government, industry, and academia work together to develop new and more effective models for funding these critical activities at a more realistic level, one that properly values these activities as the foundation upon which responsible research is conducted, both in the United States and around the world—a brave new world, indeed.

• • • References

1. National Commission for the Protection of Human Subjects in Biomedical and Behavioral Research. *The Belmont Report: Ethical Principles and Guidelines for the Protection of Human Subjects of Research*. Washington, DC: Government Printing Office, 1979, http://www.hhs.gov/ohrp/belmontArchive.html (accessed June 6, 2005).

2. Advisory Committee on Human Radiation Experiments. *Final Report: Advisory Committee on Human Radiation Experiments*. Washington, DC: Government Printing Office, 1995, http://www.eh.doe.gov/ohre/roadmap/achre/report.html (accessed June 6, 2005).

3. U.S. Department of Health and Human Services. Press release, June 6, 2000, http://www.hhs.gov/news/press/2000pres/20000606.html (accessed June 6, 2005).

4. U.S. Congress. House of Representatives. Committee on Veterans Affairs. *Human Subjects Protections: Hearing before the Subcommittee on Oversight and Investigations*, 108th Cong., 1st sess., June 18, 2003, http://veterans.house.gov/hearings/schedule108/jun03/6-18-03/gkoski.html (accessed June 21, 2003).

5. Hellman, S., et al. *Report of Johns Hopkins External Review Committee*. August 8, 2001, http://www.hopkinsmedicine.org/external.pdf (accessed June 6, 2005).

6. The White House. *Remarks by the President in Apology for Study Done in Tuskegee*. Press release, May 16, 1997, http://www.cdc.gov/nchstp/od/tuskegee/clintonp.htm (accessed June 6, 2005).

7. U.S. Department of Health and Human Services. *Code of Federal Regulations, Title 45: Public Welfare, Part 46, Protection of Human Subjects*. November 13, 2001, http://www.hhs.gov/ohrp/humansubjects/guidance/45cfr46.htm (accessed June 6, 2005).

8. Office of Inspector General, U.S. Department of Health and Human Services. *Institutional Review Boards: A Time for Reform*. Report No. OEI-01-97-0193. Washington, DC: Government Printing Office, 1998, http://oig.hhs.gov/oei/reports/oei-01-97-00193.pdf (accessed June 6, 2005).

9. National Institute of Health, Office for Protection from Research Risks Review Panel. *Report to the Advisory Committee to the Director, NIH*. June 3, 1999, http://www.nih.gov/about/director/060399b.htm (accessed June 6, 2005).

10. Drazen, J.M. "Controlling Research Trials," *New England Journal of Medicine* 348 (2003): 1377–80.

11. U.S. Department of Health and Human Services. *Final Guidance Document, Financial Relationships and Interests in Research Involving Human Subjects: Guidance for Human Subject Protection*. May 5, 2004, http://www.hhs.gov/ohrp/humansubjects/finreltn/fguid.pdf (accessed June 6, 2005).

12. Koski, G., et al. "Cooperative Research Ethics Review Boards: A Win-Win Solution?" *The Institutional Review Board: Ethics & Human Research*, 27 (2005): 1–7.

52

Ethical Review of Social and Behavioral Science Research

Michael Owen, PhD

Introduction

Critics of the ethical review of social and behavioral science research in the United States and Canada argue that Institutional Review Boards (IRBs)[1] are stifling social and behavioral science research by applying biomedical/clinical considerations of risks and harms on research protocols in the social and behavioral sciences. Further, many argue that IRBs do not understand the nature of social and behavioral (and humanities) research and impose unreasonable restrictions on research emerging from these disciplines.[2] Since "a major tenet in the protection of human subjects is that persons can be wronged even if they are not harmed,"[3] IRBs seek to ensure that participants in social and behavioral science research are not wronged nor harmed.

In this chapter, we discuss some of the issues related to human research in the social and behavioral sciences about which research administrators (pre-award grant specialists, post-award administrators and compliance officers) need to be aware and to manage. Research with human subjects drawing on social and behavioral science methodologies permeate the world in which we live. Many clinical trials have quality-of-life arms that employ survey and other techniques to assess the impact of new treatments on the lives of subjects and their families. Social and behavioral research with individuals on the "margins" of society (the homeless, gang members, sex workers, refugees, runaway children) as well as studies in schools, universities, and work and community settings contribute significantly to our understanding of the economic, polit-ical, and social environment in which we live and underpin a wide range of policies and legislation. These studies are not insignificant and the number and the potential impact on our lives may be as significant as clinical or other biomedical studies. It is therefore important for research administrators to develop their knowledge of the potential benefits, risks, and harms to the individuals and communities asked to participate in these studies.

Definition of Research

The definition of research employed by Institutional Review Boards (IRBs) is embedded in the Common Rule and ethical guidelines from other jurisdictions[4] and undervalues much research and scholarship in the human, social, and behavioral sciences.[5] HHS regulations define 45 CFR 46.102(d) research as, "a systematic investigation, including research development, testing and evaluation, designed to develop or contribute to generalizable knowledge." This definition of research suggests to IRBs, which are responsible for the review and approval of research involving humans, and investigators, that scholarship in the social and behavioral sciences and the humanities does not contribute generalizable knowledge and, perhaps, is of no value. Yet, the scholarship and research of social and behavioral scientists and humanists contribute to a body of knowledge within disciplines or professional practices and more directly and perhaps more often than clinic research to our understanding of the social, economic, and political systems in which we live.[6]

Definition of Human Subjects

The Common Rule (45 CFR 46, Section 102) defines research with human subjects. A "human subject" is a living individual or collectivity about whom an investigator conducting research obtains information or data through intervention or interaction with the individual or collectivity, or identifiable private information. Human subjects are often children in educational settings; individuals incarcerated in a prison or other facility; patients in a clinical setting; university and college students in classrooms or laboratories; prostitutes; individuals in immigrant, refugee, or alien communities; workers in a factory; or "the man on the street." It is the breadth of social and behavioral science research, the permeability of boundaries that shape such research, and the ill-defined and undocumented nature of potential risks and harms associated with such research that creates ethical issues for researchers and IRBs.

While oral history has been determined not to constitute research (therefore, the methodology employed by oral historians is excluded from US federal regulations), the American Anthropological Associations specifically identify ethnography as fitting the definition of research.[7]

Risks and harms to human subjects in social and behavioral science research are real. These risks and harms include: emotional distress, psychological trauma, invasion or loss of privacy, social embarrassment, loss of social status, loss of employment, or loss of political and other rights, among others. In addition, risks and harms associated with social and behavioral research are time and situation specific, are often very subjective, and there is little or no empirical data or research on the likelihood, permanence, or impact of risks and harms in social and behavioral research.[8]

Potential risks and harms are normally associated with individual subjects. Harms to communities arising from research in those communities should not be discounted or underestimated. Yet, IRBs are uncomfortable with the notion that they need to assess harm to a community as well as to individuals. It is not unusual, for example, for aboriginal communities in North America and Australia to resist the entreaties of or impose restriction on social science research conducted by scholars from universities and health centers. This resistance has grown from nearly three centuries of exploitation and disregard for the community, including the interests of the community to learn directly from researchers and to benefit from the outcomes of the research conducted within the community—either socially or economically.[9]

Issues for Research Administrators

IRB administrators in the United States[10] adhere to the Common Rule definition of research and of human subjects and many institutions voluntarily apply the Common Rule and related US federal regulations to both federally and nonfederally funded research involving human subjects.[11] Many institutions in the United States and elsewhere charge the IRB with broad responsibilities for the protection of human subjects who participate in research under the auspices of the institution and as the entity responsible for ensuring adherence to federal regulations.

While scholars and researchers in the social and behavioral sciences are aware of these federal regulations, institutional policies or professional codes of conduct for the ethical review of research involving human subjects. Moreover, humanists and behavioral and social scientists view IRBs, initially created to review research protocols emerging from the biomedical and clinical fields, as unable to effectively assess the breadth of research methodologies and practices common in the humanities and social and behavioral sciences, emerging or qualitative research designs, or the communities in and with which the research is conducted. As a result, humanists, social scientists, and behavioral scientists engage in research involving human subjects without understanding or recognizing their responsibilities for submission of protocols to IRBs or, while complying, are resistant to the application of institutional review procedures to their studies.

Most social and behavioral science researchers recognize the Common Rule and institutional guidelines as the "gold standard" and also adhere to codes of conduct of professional scholarly associations that guide research with human subjects (e.g., American Psychological Association, American Anthropological Association,[12] American Educational Research Association,[13] and the Oral History Association). However, association codes of conduct are not binding on members of a discipline and there may not be sanctions that the professional association is able to levy that prevent the researcher from carrying out her/his craft. Moreover, in spite of Sieber's admonition that "ethics of social research is not about etiquette,"[14] some social and behavioral scientists continue to ignore or resist the need to have their research protocols reviewed by IRBs, even where such research does not fall within exempt categories.[15] Categories of research studies for which an investigator may request a waiver or exemption from IRB review include:

- Research conducted in educational settings, involving normal educational practices;
- Research involving the use of educational tests, survey procedures, interview procedures, or observation of public behavior;
- Research involving the collection or study of existing data, documents, and records, if these sources are publicly available or if the information is recorded in such a manner that subjects cannot be identified, directly or through identifiers linked to the subjects; and,
- Research and demonstration projects, which are designed to study, evaluate, or otherwise examine public benefit or service programs.[16]

For IRB administrators, the dissonance between institutional expectations, the possible sanctions that may be imposed on research institutions that do not adhere to federal regulations, and academic prerogatives create tensions that need to be resolved.

The key elements within social and behavioral science research with human subjects for the research administrator are:

- The research protocol.
- Informed consent.
- Confidentiality and anonymity.
- Expedited review and exempt research, including balancing risks and harms with benefits primarily to knowledge enhancement.
- Educating the community of researchers.
- Educating the community of research subjects.
- Managing workloads as more social and behavioral science protocols enter the review process.

Research Protocol

Sieber describes the research protocol as a "planning tool" that is intended to define what is to be done, to whom, how, and why.[17] Research administrators recognize the parallels between the study protocol and a grant application. The protocol details:

- The purpose of the research, proposed research methods and procedures (what, how); Criteria for selection of subjects/participants (to whom)

and why (including some or all of demographic details such as age, ethnicity, religious traits, language, geographic, socioeconomic status and occupation);
- How risks and harms are identified and minimized, the manner with which the researcher will respect the autonomy of individual participants and collectivities, any benefits associated with participation in the research;
- How informed consent is to be obtained and maintained, and other related information.

If deception (also referred to as partial/delayed disclosure) is employed, the justification for deception is to be detailed in the research protocol. Where deception is involved, the administrator needs to be aware if subjects will be debriefed on the purpose of the study (if not, why not) and if there may need to be any special steps put in place to deal with sensitive issues arising from the study.

Informed Consent in Behavioral and Social Science Research

A key issue in all research involving human subjects is informed consent. Informed consent is not a form to be signed or a single event at which an individual or community agrees to participate in a research study. Rather, it is an educational process that takes place between the researcher(s) and the prospective subject(s) or participant(s) in which the subject and/or the community is informed of:

- The nature of the research study;
- The obligations which the subject or community may be accepting (e.g., time commitment, participation in a series of activities, etc.);
- The potential risks and harms associated with these activities;
- The potential benefits, if any, arising from their decision to participate; their rights as research subjects; and,
- The obligations of the researcher.

Researchers must recognize that their assessment of what is a potential risk or harm may not be viewed in the same way from the subjects' perspective. Thus, researchers, administrators at pre- and post-award stages, and IRB must be cognizant of the ways in which potential or actual research subjects may interpret the risks and harms of participating in any study. While pre-award administrators are somewhat distant from the actual research, their insights might assist researchers in the planning of a research proposal. At the post-award and IRB stages, administrators in their review of all research protocols must ensure that subjects are given sufficient information regarding the study to determine for themselves what the risks are and whether they want to assume those risks. They also need to ensure that subjects are provided with the opportunity and time to assess whether they wish to participate and that the researcher is able to assess whether subjects have the capacity to comprehend the nature of the research in which they are to participate.

Privacy, Confidentiality, and Anonymity

In behavioral and social science research there is often confusion about assurances of *confidentiality* and *anonymity*. Anonymity is an individual's right to privacy. Privacy refers to persons and to their interest in controlling the access of others to themselves. Confidentiality is an extension of the right of privacy and refers to data and how data are to be handled in keeping with the subjects' interest in controlling the access of others to information about themselves. Within the context of behavioral and social science research, anonymity means that names and other unique identifiers of subjects are not known, even to the researcher. Assurances of confidentiality, however, allow the researcher and perhaps others to know who the subjects are but does not allow for personal and private information or an individual's response to questions on a questionnaire, for example, to be linked to that individual.

Researchers need to understand the differences between anonymity and confidentiality and, at the same time, the limitations to assurances of confidentiality. Moreover, it is important to remember that not all research subjects wish to have their participation in research remain anonymous and may actually be offended if not provided with the opportunity to be identified. Oral history is one example in which research participants may desire to have their identities known and associated with data.

In other cases, however, it may not be possible to guarantee anonymity, confidentiality, or both. Research with focus groups is one example in which there will necessarily be limitations on the researcher's ability to assure both anonymity and confidentiality. In ethnographic research within communities, outsiders may not be able to identify participants, but individuals within a geographic or ethnic community or a community of practice may be able to identify respondents and participants.

Balancing Risks and Harms with Benefits

For an individual or community to voluntarily agree to participate in a research study, they need to be able to make informed decisions and consent to participate. A core element of informed consent is being able to understand and balance the possible risks and harms that a research study might pose to one or to a community with the potential benefits, primarily to knowledge creation and dissemination.

Risks and harms are real in social and behavioral science research. Possible risks and harms include (but are not limited to) emotional trauma and distress, psychological trauma, physical harm, loss of privacy, embarrassment, loss of social status, economic risk such as loss of employment, and legal risk, including possible incarceration, or inconvenience such as taking time from one's daily activities to participate in a study.

Consider, for a moment, the nature of much of the research undertaken in the social and behavioral sciences and the questions that these researchers are attempting to answer and social processes they are attempting to understand. The research subjects are often students in schools and universities; youth at risk; individuals engaged in social and economic behavior that is or may be questionable ethically or legally such as prostitution, gangs, and criminal behavior; individuals working in corporations or in unionized environments; or individuals who have experienced loss or trauma (e.g., death of a friend or loved one in a tragic accident). In the case of communities,[18] researchers often focus on those that are at the margins of mainstream society, e.g., First Nations, minorities, and immigrant and refugee communities, or with minority populations or dissidents in other nations. Experiences of these communities and individuals in them with central and local governments, security forces, or representatives of the First World may not be positive. Some communities fear that their knowledge of local flora and fauna might lead to exploitation by central governments or pharmaceutical companies if their "ways of knowing" are revealed. Others fear expropriation of lands or political suppression if political authorities or economic elites know their social, economic, or political views. Research in schools and universities engage populations—students and parents—who, eager to please a teacher–researcher or professor, might not understand the consequences of participating or not participating. A research study with first-year women students exploring dating behaviors, for example, might provoke emotional distress and psychological trauma arising from earlier experiences. Yet, such research might yield knowledge and lead to procedural, policy, or programmatic advances that benefit the individual, the community, and the society.

Research administrators recognize that their role is not to place barriers in the way of social and behavioral research on sensitive issues, but to identify ways for the researcher(s) to recognize risk and harms in their research studies and to support research subjects to balance these risks, harms, and benefits arising from their participation in the research. Moreover, in social and behavioral science research, as in all other research, it is not possible to anticipate all potential risks, harms, and benefits. Researchers and research administrators must, prior to the implementation of the research study, assess the potential risks and benefits and assess how these will or may be viewed by the population(s) being studied or requested to participate in a study. Also, it is important to recognize that one individual's or community's assessment of risk and benefits may be different from another's. More specifically, it is important to recognize that a researcher's perceptions of potential risks and harms will differ greatly from the assessment of risk by potential subjects.[19] The research administrator, therefore, should ensure that researchers are aware of possible sources of risk and have sought ways to meliorate those risks, consulted with individuals or experts who can help them identify and reduce risks, and are aware of their own biases, the assumptions underlying their theories and methods and the limitations thereof, and how others might interpret their research findings differently.

The components of research projects that involve risks and harms include (a) the theory of the research idea, (b) the research, (c) the research setting, and (d) the dissemination or uses of the results. That is, harms and risks may be imposed prior to the research beginning (e.g., the study design creates unnecessary risks for the population of participants), during the study, in the location that the study occurs (e.g., creating limitations on expectations of privacy and anonymity), and during the dissemination of the results of the research (e.g., reporting sample sizes that allow for the identification of individuals).[20]

Harms and risks are often inherent in the research process. These risks may be identified in designing of the research, recruitment of subjects, obtaining of informed consent, administering of research instruments (e.g., questionnaires, interviews), gathering of data, and analyzing and interpreting the results. Butz (2002) and Sieber (1992) identify risks and harms as emerging during:

Data Gathering. In research with individuals, groups or communities, the way in which data are collected can lead to unintended harms or risks to individuals. Data gathered through videotaping in social environments (e.g., classrooms) expose individuals to risks that would not otherwise occur.

Data Analysis. Sample size may allow for individuals and their personal/private information to be ascertained by a knowledgeable outsider. As a result, possible social, economic, or psychological harms may be inadvertently extended to individual subjects.

Data Sharing. Researchers are increasingly encouraged to share data, decreasing the likelihood of over-studying specific populations (e.g., aboriginal populations, school children), increasing the power of the analysis, and ensuring that the findings can be replicated or tested. If such data are not anonymized to remove unique identifiers, personal data or the identity of community-based informants may be revealed, thereby leading to unintended social, economic, or personal harms.[21]

The institutional setting of the research might create risks for participants. Research settings such as schools, hospitals, prisons, clinics, and churches may pose unintended risks/harms to potential participants, depending on the nature of the research. The research administrator will need to inform the investigator that institutional settings may have requirements for the administrative and/or ethical review and approval of the research prior to the initiation of the research. While these "institutional gatekeepers" (e.g., school principals or clinical directors) may facilitate the research process, they may place additional obligations on the researcher or barriers to access potential subjects.

An anticipated outcome of research with human subjects is its publication in the academic, scientific, and professional literature. More frequently, researchers are being required to take on obligations that may limit or place additional steps between the gathering and analysis of research data and its publication in a thesis, an article, or scholarly work. Communities such as aboriginal populations or ethnic/minority groups more often require, as a condition of being able to collect data using their members, that the researcher reports outcomes and policy issues to them prior to any other form of dissemination. In some cases, communities may demand the right to control the release of data and the findings. The research administrator will need to work closely with the researcher to assess what is the best strategy for the researcher when working with communities.

Maximizing Benefits

In the same way as risks and harms are situation-specific and vary depending on the individuals and communities engaged as the subjects of research, so too do benefits depend on the nature of the research process and the perspectives of the participants. Researchers typically identify the potential contributions to knowledge, science, and social advancement as the primary benefits of the research, rarely identifying any benefits to individual participants or to communities. It is not unusual, however, for individuals or their community to receive some benefit from a research study and for researchers to identify benefits, whether it be improvements to pedagogical processes in the classroom and improved learning outcomes, changes to social services, or an advocacy role on behalf of an aboriginal community or an indigent population. Moreover, the outcomes of social science research rarely provide short term benefits to society and the impact may, in fact, be ten to twenty years later, once the findings have worked their way through academic and professional publications and into public policy or program development.

Researchers and research administrators need to work through the risk/benefit analysis to ensure, wherever possible, that the benefits to individuals, communities, and society and knowledge development outweigh the potential risks and harms. Yet, the benefits need to be tangible and not false promises.

Occasionally individuals participate in research for personal benefits, including access to food or payment for their time; extra credit in a course; or social, medical, or mental health services. These "benefits" ought not be so large as to be considered coercive for populations with minimal access to these goods and services.

The researcher and her/his institution also benefit from research. These benefits may be research funding, research equipment, ongoing access to valuable study populations (e.g., school children), new methodological insights, publication of research outcomes, and career advancement. Unlike some clinical research, much sociobehavioral research is unfunded and hence the benefits to the institution rarely include revenue streams from products of the research.

Expedited Review and Exempt Research

Much social and behavioral science research poses minimal risks to research subjects. As a result, in accordance with US federal regulations and other international codes and regulations governing research with humans, such research may qualify as exempt research or for expedited review. Under Canadian,[22] US (45 CFR §46.110), and other regulatory frameworks, research with human subjects that poses no more than minimal risk to an individual or community may qualify for expedited review. The expedited review procedure permits the review to be conducted by the IRB chair and/or by one or more members of the IRB who are so designated by the IRB chair. These reviewers exercise all of the authorities of the IRB but cannot disapprove the research. Research protocols that are not approved are redirected to full board review.

As noted previously, exempt research in the United States has technical meanings.[23] However, researchers often fail to recognize that the application of the term "exempt" to a research protocol is not the prerogative of the researcher.

In both instances, it is the IRB or another institutional official such as a dean or department chair, as determined by the institution, not the investigator, who determines, under institutional and/or appropriate national and state/provincial guidelines, whether the protocol qualifies for expedited review or is exempt from IRB oversight.

Waiver of Consent Requirements

Federal and other regulations permit IRBs to consider alternate modes of consent. If informed consent is a process and not a form, IRBs should consider ways in which individuals or communities might provide or rescind their consent and assent, in the case of some vulnerable populations, to their participation in a research study.

In the United States, federal regulations (45 CFR §46.116) permit either written or oral consent and also permit the modification or waiver of consent requirements under specific circumstances.[24] These regulations do suggest, however, that written consent is the "gold standard," requiring the documentation of consent but allowing for its waiver in specific instances. An IRB may waive the requirement for the investigator to obtain a signed consent form for some or all subjects if it finds either:

1. That the only record linking the subject and the research would be the consent document and the principal risk would be potential harm resulting from a breach of confidentiality. Each subject will be asked whether the subject wants documentation linking the subject with the research, and the subject's wishes will govern; or

2. That the research presents no more than minimal risk of harm to subjects and involves no procedures for which written consent is normally required outside of the research context.

For many behavioral and social science researchers, especially those employing ethnographic, collaborative, and emerging design methodologies, *written* informed consent may undermine the research and the informed consent processes. In his ethnographic study of Northern Pakistan villagers, Butz (2003)[25] argued persuasively that his research could not have occurred if written consent were required, and he demonstrated that the community-based consent process, which did not formally require individual informed consent, and the reciprocal expectations and obligations between the researcher and the researched (the community) ensured a richer set of data, a deeper analysis and understanding of community structure and land use, and contextualization of the study within a highly charged politico-economic and ethnic environment. Studies with ethnic, economic, religious, or health-challenged (e.g., HIV-positive) groups and other vulnerable populations in North America, Europe, and Africa might benefit from more judicious employment of alternatives to written informed consent.

The research administrator (pre-award, post-award or IRB manager) who is knowledgeable about the range of research methodologies and issues confronting populations being studied can advise researchers and IRBs of the flexibility that exists for ensuring informed consent and that it is obtained and retained while eliminating barriers to the research that are imposed by a strict adherence to the practice of written, individual consents.

Educating the Community of Researchers

Research administrators have a responsibility to provide ongoing education and training for and on behalf of researchers and to continuous learning related to the responsible conduct of research for themselves. This obligation is shared with the research community and is more than a mere acknowledgement of federal, international, local, and institutional regulations and guidelines. It is a commitment to ongoing education and professional development to ensure that the community of scholars and researchers is aware of the fundamental principles underlying the need for the ethical review of research protocols (funded or unfunded) involving human participants, the changing regulatory and practice environment in which research is conducted, and principles of reciprocity with the potential participants.

Over the last decade governmental and nongovernmental agencies and institutions have developed strategies for educating research administrators and researchers in the principles underlying and processes for the ethical conduct of research. In Canada, the Interagency Panel on Research Ethics developed an on-line tutorial on the Tri-Council Policy Statement on Ethics in Human Research (TCPS). In the United States, the Office of Human Research Protection created an online tutorial and certification for institutional officials, IRB administrators and members, and researchers. Completing this tutorial is a requirement for institutions wishing to obtain and retain a Federal Wide Assurance (FWA) for their IRB. Many universities and consortia, too, have developed educational tutorials and workshops for their administrative and research staff. In some instances, evidence of completion of such workshops or tutorials is required prior to the initiation of research with human subjects.

Research administrators need to work with researchers at the pre-award (grant development) stage to ensure that the research design is appropriate to the questions to which they are seeking answers. Not only does this strengthen the research proposal, but it ensures that the ethics protocols do not become unduly burdensome and that researchers will have considered the ethical issues at the outset and be able to address these in the protocol submission to the IRB. At the post-award stage, research administrators need to work closely with the research community to adjust research design, if necessary and as recommended by external peer reviewers and by the emerging nature of the research, to meet ethical requirements and put in place appropriate measures to protect the potential subjects from harm and to inform the research subjects, as well as the scholarly and public policy communities, of the outcomes of the research project.

Throughout the research process, research administrators have obligations to the research community to ensure that a series of on-going professional development, educational, and technical training programs is offered. Such educational and technical programs provide researchers with advice on hot topics such as deception, field research with minority populations, research with aboriginal groups, and research in international settings. Recently professional and scholarly organizations have developed tools for their members and consortia such as the Responsible Conduct of Research (RCR) Educational Consortium are bridging the divide between administration and researchers, are building the capacity of institutions to provide educational resources for RCR training, and are encouraging the integration of RCR education in the curricula of courses and programs at the undergraduate and graduate levels.

Educating the Community of Research Subjects

The education of the community of actual and potential research subjects is often an overlooked responsibility amongst researchers and research administrators, including IRB administrators. The challenge of educating the community of research subjects is extraordinary, and individual researchers, IRBs, and research administrators can only take small steps in this regard. The primary responsibility for educating the community of participants falls on the researchers in their efforts to (1) recruit research subjects and (2) to inform the research subjects and their communities (e.g., schools, communities of patients, ethnic or immigrant communities) of the outcomes of the research. Only through proactive education will negative effects attributed to research involving humans be overcome (e.g., research on diverse populations such as First Nations). Senior research administrators such as vice presidents of research and researchers themselves may also engage in outreach efforts to local communities to understand the importance of engaging in all aspects of social and behavioral research to identify the benefits of such research to the community: understanding of the ways in which children and youth engage with others or use the Internet; developing advice to regional planning boards on the social and economic impact of development of transportation systems; or devising interventions that affect the personal health of individuals within communities.

Communicating Outcomes

One of the major barriers to continued community- and institution-based (e.g., school) research is the inability of researchers to demonstrate benefit and/or to provide communications to the participants and communities of the research findings and outcomes. Many researchers do not provide feedback to the individuals and communities (e.g., schools, hospitals, ethnic organizations, aboriginal populations) on the outcomes of the research that they have conducted. Many aboriginal communities in the United States, Canada, Africa, and Asia have developed a mistrust of researchers and refuse to be the objects of research. School boards often decline invitations to have their classroom be the location of research because researchers often fail to provide timely or any information on the outcomes of the research to the teachers, students, and school board.

More recently, leading scientific journals have implemented codes of conduct for authors, some of which require attestation that the research study was completed in accordance with research ethics standards and a declaration of any conflicts of interest.

Research administrators, when working with investigators to design research studies and IRBs, have an obligation to identify mechanisms for communicating the outcomes of the research. Embedded in this obligation is a need to review any grant and contract agreements to ensure that publication of the results is permitted within institutional guidelines.

International Studies

There is considerable debate with regard to the ethical review of research in international settings. Some of the debate focuses on power relationships between the researcher and the researched, particularly when the researcher is from a developed country and the researched are individuals or communities in lesser-developed nations. Another aspect of the debate focuses on whose regulations, guidelines, or practices govern research with human subjects in an international setting. Are the regulations those of the sponsoring agency or nation or the regulations, guidelines, conventions, and/or community customs of the population in the subjects' nation? Whose regulations or conventions govern the research when, for example, the studies are being conducted by Canadian researchers, funded by Canadian agencies, with populations in the United States? Would the same reasoning apply when US researchers, funded by US federal agencies, in Canada, conduct the research? Would researchers require IRB approval in both nations?

Many countries have legislation, regulations, and conventions that govern research conducted within their boundaries, and with their citizens.[26] While research administrators cannot be informed on all international guidelines and legislation governing research that their investigators might conduct in foreign states (including, for some readers, the United States), it is the research administrator's responsibility to require that the investigator inform her/himself of local laws, statutes, regulations, or conventions. The documentation of these local requirements will allow the investigator, research administrator, and the IRB to assess the environment in which the investigator will be working, maintain the highest possible level of adherence to ethical principles, and be compliant with local as well the researcher's governing regulations and legislation.

Researchers need to be aware that when dealing in cross-cultural settings, what is practicable in a developed nation (Canada or the United States) might not be practicable in another environment. For example, the standard of written informed consent may not be acceptable as many individuals may not be literate or not be willing to sign consent forms, fearing that their identity may be revealed to authorities or that they are under other obligations.[27]

Managing Workloads

A common concern amongst research administrators and IRB administrators is the ever-increasing workload of IRBs, projects ranging from those related to the biomedical and clinical studies to those in the social and behavioral sciences. The sheer increase in the number of protocols places burdens on the research administrator and IRB administrator as well as on the IRB members and reviewers and the research community. With a renewed emphasis on the ethical review of research from the social and behavioral sciences, research managers and IRB administrators must ensure that their committees are familiar with the research methodologies used by behavioral and social scientists and the ethical issues that emerge from the use of those methodologies. The burden on IRB members can be reduced if IRBs are suitably knowledgeable of these issues and do not read into protocols concerns that are primarily those of clinical scientists. The burden of increased workload may be, in part, the result of overexamination of protocols rather than a proportionate review, including the assessment of research studies based on the level of risk and potential for harm.

A number of institutions have introduced social and behavioral science IRBs or subcommittees of full IRBs. These IRBs or subcommittees meet the standards required of any IRB. With a broader membership, these IRBs are able to review protocols more effectively and efficiently.

Strategies for managing the increased workload on IRBs arising from increased scrutiny of social and behavioral science research include the more judicious use of exempt categories, expedited reviews,[28] and information technologies (IT). For example, it

may be possible, where authority is provided by the institution to the IRB administrator to triage protocols based on the nature of the research, research methodologies, and the assessment of risk/harm to have minimal risk protocols reviewed in an expedited manner employing one or two, depending on the institutional requirements, IRB members. Should one or both of these members suggest that the protocol require full IRB review, it would be directed to the next meeting of the IRB. Should the reviewers assess the protocol favorably, meeting the requirements of applicable governing regulations, guidelines, and procedures, the IRB administrator or chair would issue an approval to the researchers and report to the IRB on the action of the review subcommittee. Thus, the effect would be the implementation of an effective review of all protocols, a reduction in the workload of the IRB, and, probably, a more rapid turnaround for the researcher.

In some institutions, increased workload of IRBs derives not solely from an increase in the number of graduate student and class-based studies. Institutions employ a variety of strategies to deal with this dramatic increase in reviews. Many institutions employ expedited review processes or departmental-based IRBs to manage the protocol review at a local level. A recent innovation at the University of Minnesota was the creation of an IRB devoted solely to student protocols, which reviews student protocols and provides ethical training for student members as well as student researchers. By removing student protocols to this IRB, it balanced the workload of the university's behavioral and social science IRB, provided more effective service to students, and met Association for the Accreditation of Human Research Protection Programs Inc.'s (AAHRPP) accreditation requirements.[29]

Research managers must consider how IT facilitates the management of increased workloads. Vendors offer IRB management tools that permit the electronic submission and review of protocols by IRB members in advance of face-to-face meetings. Such tools allow the research manager to log protocol submissions, respond to researcher inquiries, prepare IRB minutes, prepare and send letters to investigators, and maintain databases that alert the administrator to critical dates/required action. Moreover, these tools allow the IRB administrator to focus not on the paper workload but on providing high quality service to the researcher, the institution, and the sponsor; improving the educational role of the research administrator, and enhancing compliance with specific regulations and guidelines.

Useful Resources

While the environment in which we work changes constantly, there are online and professional resources that will assist the research administrator to become more knowledgeable of issues related to and concerns affecting social and behavioral research with human subjects. The IRB Listserv (http://www.irbforum.org/), while focusing primarily on issues related to clinical and biomedical research, addresses issues related to social and behavioral science research. The Hastings Center's periodical, *IRB: A Review of Human Subjects Research*, is an excellent resource on all aspects of human subject research. Many institutions and consortia provide online tutorials, as do federal oversight agencies in the United States and Canada, focusing not solely on regulations but on principles of ethical research involving humans and issues related to the social and behavioral sciences.[30]

Professional organizations' (Society of Research Administrators International, National Council of University Research Administrators, ARENA, PRIMR, and RCR Educational Consortium) and scholarly associations' annual meetings and Web sites and Listservs are outstanding resources and tools for the administrator to seek out best (or at least current) practices at other research institutions.

Concluding Comments

"Ethical research is research which not only 'does not harm,' but also has positive outcomes (in the short and long term) for the communities in which the research is conducted and often more broadly."[31] The research administrator needs to be aware of the nuances of the discourse on research ethics involving human subjects. The research administrator must be aware of the broad range of regulations, disciplinary practices and ethos, the contours of the ever changing methodological environment in which researchers operate and the ways in which different disciplines become aware of different research methodologies, the process of ethical review of research studies at her/his institution and, most importantly, the principles underlying the need for ethical research involving human subjects. This includes the pre-award administrator who is assisting the investigator in the development of a research study that may/will involve human subjects, the post-award (financial and non-financial) administrator who is required to know when/if funds might be released prior to an IRB approval, and the IRB officer who is responsible for administering the ethical review process. Research administrators are assets to investigators in their pursuit of

new knowledge for the benefit of the society in which we live—not hurdles to be overcome or barriers which researchers must contrive to avoid. In many postsecondary institutions the majority of researchers are in the humanities and social and behavioral sciences, and many of these conduct research with human subjects. Our IRBs have, until recently, focused nearly entirely on clinical research, and the US federal regulations and other nations' regulations and guidelines appear to be aimed primarily at research involving humans in a clinical environment. Thus, as research administrators we need to engage our community of investigators to become knowledgeable of the principles of ethical conduct of research involving human subjects and be sensitive to the constraints and practicalities of applying these principles and regulations to research from a range of nonclinical disciplines, employing a wide range of methodologies, and engaging a diversity of populations not considered when the codes of conduct, regulations, and review boards were first established.

Acknowledgment

The origins of this paper emerged from discussions and workshops with colleagues in the Society of Research Administrators International as well as debates at professional meetings of SRA, the Canadian Association of Research Ethics Boards, and the National Council for Ethics in Human Research (NCEHR). Among the colleagues whose advice was sought are J. Terrence Manns, Dr. Edward Gabriele, and Deborah van Oosten. The responsibility for interpretation, errors, or omission remains the author's.

• • • Endnotes

1. Institutional Review Boards are also known as Research Ethics Boards, Research Ethics Committees, and Ethics Research Committees.
2. See Nancy Janovicek, "Historians and the Tri-council Policy Statement on Research Involving Humans," *Canadian Historical Association Bulletin* 29, no. 2, (2003): 1–2; John H. Mueller and John L. Furedym, "Reviewing for Risk: What's the Evidence That It Works?" *American Psychological Society Observer* 14, no. 7 (2001), http://www.psychologicalscience.org/observer/0901/irb_reviewing.html (accessed December 6, 2003); Tim Lougheed, "A Ques-

tion of Ethics," *University Affairs,* June/July 2003, 10-13; Michael Owen, "Engaging the Humanities: Research Ethics in Canada," *The Journal of Research Administration* 33, no. 3 (2002): 5–12; Will van den Hoonaard, ed. *Walking the Tightrope: Ethical Issues for Qualitative Researchers* (Toronto: University of Toronto Press, 2002); Social Sciences and Humanities Research Ethics Special Working Committee to the Interagency Advisory Panel on Research Ethics, "Giving Voice to the Spectrum," June 2004, http://www.pre.ethics. gc.ca/english/workgroups/sshwc/SSHWC VoiceReportJune2004.pdf (accessed August 1, 2005); Constance F. Citro, Daniel R. Ilgen, and Cora B. Marrett, editors, *Protecting Participants and Facilitating Social and Behavioral Sciences Research* (Washington, DC: National Academies of Science, 2003); J. E. Sieber and R. M. Baluyot, "A Survey of IRB Concerns about Social and Behavioral Research," *IRB: A Review of Human Subjects Research* 14, no. 2 (1992): 9–10; American Association of University Professors, "Protecting Human Beings: Institutional Review Boards and Social Science Research," 2000, http://www.aaup.org/ statements/Redbook/repirb.htm (accessed February 1, 2004).

That such complaints are not limited to the social and behavioral sciences, see the consultation of the Natural Sciences and Engineering Research Council of Canada and the Interagency Advisory Panel on Research Ethics, "NSERC Community Whose Research Involves Human Subjects: Results of a Survey about Their Needs and Supports in Research Ethics," November 2003, http://www.pre. ethics.gc.ca/english/publicationsandreports/ publicationsandreports/nsercsr2003_a.cfm (accessed August 1, 2005), and "Response to the Recommendations in the Report of the Survey of the Natural Sciences and Engineering Community Whose Research Involves Human Subjects," November 2003, http://www.pre. ethics.gc.ca/english/publicationsandreports/ publicationsandreports/nsercsr2003_c.cfm (accessed August 1, 2005); Robert H. Gilman and Hector H. Garcia, "Ethics Review Procedures for Research in Developing Countries: A Basic Presumption of Guilt," *Canadian Medical Association Journal* 171, no. 3 (2004): 248–249; and Hester J.T. Ward et al., "Obstacles to Conducting Epidemiological Research in the UK General Population," *BMJ*, 329 (2004): 277–279.

3. Cynthia McGuire Dunn and Gary Chadwick, *Protecting Study Volunteers in Research* (Boston, MA: CenterWatch, Inc., 1999).

4. 45 CFR §46, "Basic DHHS Policy for Protection of Human Research Subjects," Originally adopted May 1974, revised January 13, 1981 and June 18, 1991. Additional protections for vulnerable populations are contained in Subparts B-D. The Federal Policy for the Protection of Human Subjects ("The Common Rule" June 18, 1991) was extended to Departments of Agriculture, Energy, Commerce, HUD, Justice, Defense, Education, Veterans Affairs, Transportation, the HHS, NSF, NASA, EPA, AID, Social Security Administration, the CIA, and the Consumer Product Safety Commission.

5. A number of disciplines, such as history, are viewed as both humanities and social sciences and often employ research participants to inform their scholarship.

6. For example, the Oral History Association (OHA) defines oral history as "a method of gathering and preserving historical information through recorded interviews with participants in past events and ways of life." The OHA argues:

> It is primarily on the grounds that oral history interviews, in general, are not designed to contribute to "generalizable knowledge" that they are not subject to the requirements of the HHS regulations at 45 CFR §46 and, therefore, can be excluded from IRB review. Although the HHS regulations do not define "generalizable knowledge," it is reasonable to assume that this term does not simply mean knowledge that lends itself to generalizations, which characterizes every form of scholarly inquiry and human communication. While historians reach for meaning that goes beyond the specific subject of their inquiry, unlike researchers in the biomedical and behavioral sciences, they do not reach for generalizable principles of historical or social development, nor do they seek underlying principles or laws of nature that have predictive value and can be applied to other circumstances for the purpose of controlling outcomes. Historians explain a particular past; they do not create general explanations about all that has happened in the past, nor do they predict the future.

See the Oral History Association Web site, http://dickinson.edu/organizations/oha/ (accessed August 1, 2005).

7. See American Anthropological Association Executive Board, "American Anthropological Association Statement on Ethnography and Institutional Review Boards," June 4, 2004, http://www.aaanet.org/stmts/irb.htm (accessed September 9, 2004).

8. See American Anthropological Association Executive Board, "American Anthropological Association Statement on Ethnography and Institutional Review Boards," Section 3, What are the risks and benefits of ethnographic research, and Section 4, Does ethnography exempt from IRB review? http://www.aaanet.org/stmts/irb.htm, (accessed August 1, 2005).

9. That this phenomenon is not limited to aboriginal or ethnic communities, see Carolyn Ellis, "Emotional and Ethical Quagmires in Returning to the Field," *Journal of Contemporary Ethnography* 24, no. 1 (1995): 68–69. See also Deborah Zion, "Restoring Lost Time: Indigenous Health and Research," *Monash Bioethics Review* 22, no. 4: 1–2; Joseph M. Kaufert and Josee G. Lavoie, "Comparative Canadian Aboriginal Perspectives on Draft Values and Ethics in Aboriginal and Torres Strait Islander Health Research," *Monash Bioethics Review* 22, no. 4:31–37; William Freeman, "Restoring Lost Time: Indigenous Health and Research: A View from the USA," *Monash Bioethics Review*, 22, no. 4:38–44.

10. While IRB administrators elsewhere employ different sets of guidelines and/or regulations, the ethical principles underpinning these guidelines and regulations have common origins, including but not limited to the Declaration of Helsinki and the Belmont Report. In Canada, for example, the Tri-Council Policy Statement (TCPS) asserts:

> The fundamental ethical issues and principles in research involving human subjects are common across the social sciences and humanities, the natural sciences and engineering, and the health sciences. They reflect shared fundamental values that are expressed in the duties, rights, and norms of those involved in research. Research subjects reasonably expect that their rights shall be equally recognized and respected, regardless of the researcher's discipline. . . .

Canadian society legitimately expects that the benefits and harms of research shall be fairly distributed. (TCPS, "Goals and Rationale of the Policy," in *Tri-Council Policy Statement: Ethical Conduct for Research Involving Humans*, 1998 (with 2000, 2002 updates) http://www.pre.ethics.gc.ca/english/policystatement/goals.cfm#A (accessed August 1, 2005).

The TCPS further states: "The cardinal principle of modern research ethics is respect for human dignity." Respect for human dignity in research with human subjects incorporates (1) respect for free and informed consent; (2) respect for privacy and confidentiality; (3) balancing harms and benefits, including minimiz-

ing harm: a principle directly related to harms—benefits analysis is nonmalfeasance, or the duty to avoid, prevent, or minimize harm to others, while maximizing benefit; (4) respect for vulnerable persons; and (5) respect for justice and inclusiveness (TCPS, "Context of an Ethics Framework," in *Tri-Council Policy Statement: Ethical Conduct for Research Involving Humans*, 1998 (with 2000, 2002 updates) http://www.pre.ethics.gc.ca/english/policystatement/context.cfm (accessed August 1, 2005).

11. 45 CFR §46.101 states:

> (a) Except as provided in paragraph (b) of this section, this policy applies to all research involving human subjects conducted, supported or otherwise subject to regulation by any Federal Department or Agency which takes appropriate administrative action to make the policy applicable to such research. This includes research conducted by Federal civilian employees or military personnel, except that each Department or Agency head may adopt such procedural modifications as may be appropriate from an administrative standpoint. It also includes research conducted, supported, or otherwise subject to regulation by the Federal Government outside the United States.

Other exceptions are noted in 45 CFR§46.101 (b).

12. See American Anthropological Association "Commission to Review the AAA Statements on Ethics," 1995, http://www.aaanet.org/committees/ethics/ethrpt.htm (accessed September 13, 2005).

13. See the American Educational Research Association Web site, www.aera.net (accessed February 1, 2004).

14. Sieber and Baluyot (1992): 3.

15. 45 CFR §46.101 identifies categories of research that may be exempt from IRB review. In most situations, it is the IRB, not the researcher, that determines what research meets the criteria for exemption.

16. See US Department of Health and Human Service regulations 45 CFR §46.101.

17. Joan E. Sieber, "Planning Ethically Responsible Research," *Applied Social Research Methods Series*. Newbury Park, CA: Sage Publications. 31 (1992): 14–15.

18. Not all researchers, IRB members, or commentators on research ethics agree that IRBs ought to consider the impact on communities. See Sieber and Baluyot (1992): 76.

19. TCPS, *Tri-Council Policy Statement: Ethical Conduct for Research Involving Humans*

(1998, with 2000, 2002 updates) http://www.pre.ethics.gc.ca/english/policystatement/policystatement.cfm (accessed August 1, 2002); Sieber and Baluyot (1992): 94–95.

20. David Butz, "Consent in Community-based Ethnographic Research," National Council on Ethics in Human Research (NCEHR) Conference on Informed Consent, Alymer, Quebec, March 2003. In this report on his ethnographic research on portering relationships and transcultural interaction in Northern Pakistan, Dr. Butz covered issues of consent by focusing on two core issues: (1) the type of research (ethnographic) and (2) focus of the research (community rather than individual). He argued that issues of language, literacy, and cultural difference between researcher and researched are important, but subsidiary to these two primary concerns. Paulina Onvomaha Tindana of the Navrongo Health Research Centre in northern Ghana demonstrated that to be effective and ongoing, informed consent is a consensual contract between the researchers, the community leadership, and individuals. Such robust processes that include substantial community engagement may place traditional first world principles of individuality and anonymity but do not jeopardize principles of confidentiality of personal data. See Paulina Onvomaha Tindana, "The Informed Consent Process in a Rural African Setting," paper presented at the National Council on Ethics in Human Research Annual Meeting, Ottawa, March 5, 2005.

21. For a discussion of issues related to sharing of data, consent for secondary use of data, most of which is gathered using social science methodologies, see *Guidelines for Protecting Privacy and Confidentiality in the Design, Conduct and Evaluation of Health Research: Best Practices* (Ottawa: Canadian Institutes of Health Research, 2004). The July 31, 2004 issue of the *British Medical Journal* (Vol. 329) identifies concerns of research on barriers placed on social and behavioral research as a result of "overregulation" of research protocols.

22. See TCPS, Section D1, "A Proportionate Approach to Ethics Assessment," in *Tri-Council Policy Statement: Ethical Conduct for Research Involving Humans,* 1998 (with 2000, 2002 updates), 1.7–1.8, http://www.pre.ethics.gc.ca/english/pdf/TCPS01e.pdf (accessed August 1, 2005).

23. See 45 CFR §46.101 (b). In addition, the Office for Protection from Research Risks (OPRR) has determined that the following criteria (see 48 FR 9266-9270, March 4, 1983) must be satisfied to invoke the exemption for research and demonstration projects examining "public benefit or service programs" as specified under Department of Health and Human Services (HHS) regulations at 45 CFR §46.101(b)(5):

(1) The program under study must deliver a public benefit (e.g., financial or medical benefits as provided under the Social Security Act) or service (e.g., social, supportive, or nutrition services as provided under the Older Americans Act).

(2) The research or demonstration project must be conducted pursuant to specific federal statutory authority.

(3) There must be no statutory requirement that an Institutional Review Board (IRB) review the project.

(4) The project must not involve significant physical invasions or intrusions upon the privacy of participants.

Institutions should consult with the HHS funding agency regarding the above conditions before invoking this exemption. In addition, it is extremely important that staff in all HHS agencies understand and respect the following principles, which are critical to the successful implementation of human subject protections under HHS regulations:

(1) Institutions conducting (nonexempt) HHS-supported human subjects research must provide OPRR with an acceptable Assurance of Compliance with the human subjects regulations [45 CFR §46.103(a)]. Under the terms of such Assurances, it is typically the responsibility of the Institutional Review Board (IRB) or other designated institutional official(s), **not the investigator,** to determine whether research activities qualify for exemption. Institutions holding OPRR-approved Assurances generally require that all research involving human intervention/interaction or **identifiable private information** [45 CFR §46.102(f)(2)] be subjected to independent verification of exempt status.

(2) Institutions may elect under their Assurance not to claim the exemptions provided in the regulations, choosing instead to require IRB review of all research involving human intervention/ interaction or identifiable private information.

(3) While HHS requires neither an Assurance nor a Certification of IRB Review [45 CFR §46.103(f)] for exempt research, institutional requirements regarding review of such research are, nevertheless, binding on investigators. It would be inappropriate for staff of any HHS agency to discourage potential awardees from submitting their activities for institutionally required IRB review.

24. 45 CFR §46.116 (c). An IRB may approve a consent procedure which does not include, or which alters some or all of the elements of informed consent set forth above, or waive the requirement to obtain informed consent provided the IRB finds and documents that:

(1) the research or demonstration project is to be conducted by or subject to the approval of state or local government officials and is designed to study, evaluate, or otherwise examine: (i) public benefit or service programs; (ii) procedures for obtaining benefits or services under those programs; (iii) possible changes in or alternatives to those programs or procedures; or (iv) possible changes in methods or levels of payment for benefits or services under those programs; and

(2) the research could not practically be carried out without the waiver or alteration.

It should be noted that the US Department of Defense (10 USC 980) cannot waive the process of informed consent unless a waiver is granted by higher authority such as the Secretary of Defense (or his or her delegate).

25. David Butz, "Consent in Community-based Ethnographic Research," National Council on Ethics in Human Research (NCEHR) Conference on Informed Consent, Alymer, Quebec, March 2003.

26. US research administrators need to be aware of the requirements of 45 CFR §46.101(h).

27. See, for example, Lauren Clark and Ann Kingsolver, "Briefing Paper on Informed Consent: AAA Committee on Ethics," http://www.aaanet.org/committees/ethics/bp5.htm (accessed September 13, 2005), and Joe Watkins for the AAA Committee on Ethics, "Briefing Paper on Consideration of the Potentially Negative Impact of the Publication of Factual Data about a Study Population on Such Population," http://www.aaanet.org/committees/ethics/bp4.htm (accessed September 13, 2005).

28. Secretary, US Department of Health and Human Services, "Categories of Research That May Be Reviewed by the Institutional Review Board (IRB) through an Expedited Review Procedure," identifies the following as eligible for expedited review:

Research activities that (1) present no more than minimal risk to human subjects, and (2) involve only procedures listed in one or more of the following categories, may be reviewed by the IRB through the expedited review procedure authorized by 45 CFR §46.110 and 21 CFR §56.110. The activities listed should not be deemed to be of minimal risk simply because they are included on this list. Inclusion on this list merely means that the activity is eligible for review through the expedited review procedure when the specific circumstances of the proposed research involve no more than minimal risk to human subjects. (See the list at http://www.hhs.gov/ohrp/humansubjects/guidance/expedited98.htm, accessed August 1, 2005).

29. "HRPP Innovations: University of Minnesota Student IRB," *AAHRPP Advance*, 4, 8, http://www.aahrpp.org/Documents/D000062.PDF (accessed August 1, 2005).

30. See the Interagency Advisory Panel on Research Ethics' (PRE) online Introductory Tutorial for the *Tri-Council Policy Statement: Ethical Conduct for Research Involving Humans* (TCPS), http://www.ethics.gc.ca/english/tutorial/ (accessed August 1, 2005) and The Office of Human Research Protection Program's "Human Subject Assurance Training," http://137.187.172.153/CBTs/Assurance/login.asp (accessed May 6, 2005).

31. Jane McKendrick and Pamela Aratukutuku Bennett, "The Ethics of Health Research and Indigenous Peoples," *Monash Bioethics Review*, October 2002. This issue of the *Monash Bioethics Review* has a number of articles on the issue of ethics or health research and indigenous peoples, focusing primarily on the National Health and Medical Research Council's recently released document entitled "Draft Values and Ethics in Aboriginal and Torres Strait Islander Health Research."

53

The Impact of Health Insurance Portability and Accountability Act (HIPAA) on Research

Ada Sue Selwitz, MA, Helene Lake-Bullock, PhD, JD, and Joe R. Brown, MHS

Introduction

Health Insurance Portability and Accountability Act (HIPAA) of 1996 is a complex statute that was designed to standardize transmission of electronic health information.[1] It authorized multiple new regulations, which focus on security of electronic transmission, transactions and code sets, and privacy.

Since it went into effect on April 14, 2003, the HIPAA Privacy Rule has had an impact on research administrators, Institutional Review Boards (IRBs), and researchers nationwide. The Privacy Rule regulates use and disclosure by entities covered by the rule of certain individually identifiable health information designated as protected health information (PHI). The regulations do not replace the existing human research protection regulations. Federal agencies have adopted the "Federal Policy for the Protection of Human Subjects," referred to as the Common Rule.[2] The HIPAA privacy requirements are in addition to the Common Rule and other existing federal protection of human subjects requirements.

The HIPAA Privacy regulations are intricate and were not written with research in mind. HIPAA was established "... to improve portability and continuity of health insurance coverage in the group and individual markets, to combat waste, fraud, and abuse in health insurance and health care delivery, to promote the use of medical savings accounts, to improve access to long-term care services and coverage, to simplify the administration of health insurance ..."[1] "... Congress recognized that advances in electronic technology could erode the privacy of health information. Consequently, Congress incorporated into HIPAA provisions that mandated the adoption of Federal privacy protections for individually identifiable health information."[3] The new federal regulation affects researchers who access, create, use, and/or disclose protected health information from HIPAA-covered entities. The regulation has made access to patient information for research more complex, making it more difficult to share a patient's PHI information with collaborators or sponsors who are not employed by the covered entity. HIPAA has added a considerable number of new concepts and requirements not included in the preexisting IRB regulations. These new requirements and concepts include covered entity status; protected health information; restricted options for accessing and sharing PHI; minimum necessary standards; business associate agreements; privacy notices; and designation of patient legal rights for privacy. Research administrators, IRBs, and researchers have struggled with the complexity of the rule and with the additional burden of being responsible for applying new concepts and complying with multiple sets of regulations simultaneously.

The HIPAA Privacy Rule includes a limited set of provisions that specifically focus on research. In those provisions, entities covered by the rule are given the option of delegating the responsibility for waiving selected HIPAA requirements to an existing IRB or to a privacy board. The requirements for membership and operation of a privacy board are included in the HIPAA privacy rule. Some entities covered by the regulations chose to establish privacy boards, but many others, especially higher education institutions, chose to delegate HIPAA research responsibilities to the IRB.

Key Provisions

The purpose of this chapter is to assist research administrators in understanding the HIPAA Privacy Rule requirements by providing an overview of key provisions that impact research and research administration. Some of the questions discussed in this chapter are:

- When does HIPAA apply to research?
- What penalties can be applied if a covered entity or individual conducting HIPAA regulated research fails to comply with HIPAA requirements?
- How do researchers access or share protected health information under the HIPAA Privacy Rule?
- What privacy rights has the HIPAA rule provided to patients who participate as subjects in research?
- What additional requirements impact research and research administration?

It is beyond the scope of this chapter to provide detailed information on the lengthy and complex HIPAA statute. For in-depth guidance on the HIPAA privacy rule requirements, research administrators should check with their own privacy officer, if one is available, or their legal counsel. This chapter does not address all of the HIPAA Privacy Rule provisions that impact research. It includes only those key provisions that impact research administration.

When Does HIPAA Apply to Research?

For research to be covered by the Privacy Rule, it must fall within a "covered entity" and meet the definition of protected health information (PHI). To determine whether a research project falls under HIPAA, research administrators, IRBs, and researchers must understand HIPAA requirements regarding who is covered by the rule (i.e., what type of entity employs the investigator and whether the investigator is in a covered component of the entity). Also, research administrators, IRBs, and researchers need to determine whether the data to be collected or created meet the definition of protected health information.

Who is covered by HIPAA?   HIPAA applies to covered entities that are defined as "a health plan, a health care clearinghouse or a health care provider who transmit[s] health information in electronic form."[4] If a researcher is employed by a covered entity, then his/her research that uses protected health information must comply with the Privacy Rule. If a researcher is not employed by a covered entity, then his/her research would not be covered by HIPAA unless the study design requires that protected health information be collected from a "covered entity."

There are several different types of covered entities including:

Free Standing, Single Entity. A single legal entity such as a freestanding hospital or private physician practice could be designated as a single covered entity. All research involving protected health information conducted by an employee would fall under the Privacy Rule.

Hybrid Entity. "The Privacy Rule permits a covered entity that is a single legal entity and that conducts both covered and non-covered functions to elect to be a 'hybrid entity'."[5] For example, a comprehensive university that included a hospital would have both covered health care components and noncovered components (e.g., college of education) and could be designated as a hybrid entity.

Affiliated Covered Entity. "Legally separate covered entities that are affiliated by common ownership or control may designate themselves (including their health care components) as a single covered entity for Privacy Rule compliance."[5] For example, a group of affiliated university hospitals which are legally separate could be designated as an affiliated covered entity.

Organized Health Care Arrangement. "The Privacy Rule identifies relationships in which participating covered entities share protected health information to manage and benefit their common enterprise as organized health care arrangements. Covered entities in an organized health care arrangement can share protected health information with each other for the arrangement's joint health care operations."[5]

Research administrators, IRBs, and investigators need to know whether the researchers or researchers' employer is covered by HIPAA (i.e., health care plan, clearinghouse, or provider). If so, research administrators need to know which type of covered entity has been designated. Also, researchers who want to create, use, and access protected health information must know whether the data are held by a HIPAA covered entity.

The type of covered entity in which an investigator is employed will impact how health information can be accessed or shared within that entity. For example, many universities are designated as "hybrid entities," which means that they perform both covered and noncovered functions as part of their business operations. A researcher who is employed in a noncovered department is not regulated by HIPAA unless he/she wants to access PHI from the covered component of the university. To access data from the covered component, the researcher must comply with the Privacy Rule, but once the researcher is in possession of the PHI it is no longer regulated by the Privacy Rule. There may be other federal and possibly state protections that cover the use of the data, but many of the HIPAA requirements such as patient rights, which are discussed below, would not apply.

HIPAA regulated entities will have a designated privacy officer. Research administrators that are unsure about their institution's HIPAA status should check with legal counsel or the designated privacy officer, if one is available.

What types of data are covered by HIPAA? HIPAA requirements apply to protected health information (PHI). A designated covered entity may not use or disclose PHI except as permitted or required under the Privacy Rule. PHI is defined as individually identifiable health information transmitted by electronic media, maintained in electronic media, or transmitted or maintained in any other form or medium.[6]

According to the Department of Health and Human Services Office of Civil Rights, which is responsible for HIPAA oversight, "individually identifiable health information" is information, including demographic data, which relates to:[7]

- The individual's past, present, or future physical or mental health or condition;
- The provision of health care to the individual; or,
- The past, present, or future payment for the provision of health care to the individual, and that identifies the individual for which there is a reasonable basis to believe it can be used to identify the individual.[7]

Individually identifiable health information includes eighteen types of identifiers. The types are as follows:

1. Names;
2. All geographic subdivisions smaller than a state, including street address, city, county, precinct, zip code, and their equivalent geocodes;
3. All elements of dates (except year) for dates directly related to an individual, including birth date, admission date, discharge date, date of death;
4. Telephone numbers;
5. Fax numbers;
6. Electronic mail addresses;
7. Social Security numbers;
8. Medical record numbers;
9. Health plan beneficiary numbers;
10. Account numbers;
11. Certificate/license numbers;
12. Vehicle identifiers and serial numbers, including license plate numbers;
13. Device identifiers and serial numbers;
14. Web Universal Resource Locators (URLs);
15. Internet Protocol (IP) address numbers;
16. Biometric identifiers, including finger and voice prints;
17. Full face photographic images and any comparable images; and
18. Any other unique identifying number, characteristic, or code.[8]

If a researcher is employed by a covered entity and uses any of the 18 identifiers, all of the provisions of the HIPAA Privacy Rule would apply.

If the researcher is not employed by the covered entity or works in a noncovered component of a hybrid entity, but is accessing any of the eighteen designated identifiers held by a covered entity, access is HIPAA regulated. What is confusing to the research community is that once the data are removed from the entity the data are no longer HIPAA regulated unless the covered entity has required the researcher to sign an agreement extending the HIPAA requirements.

How can data be de-identified so that the HIPAA Privacy Provisions no longer apply? The HIPAA Privacy Rule states that if protected health information is de-identified, HIPAA does not apply. This means that if a researcher who is employed by a covered entity or who is accessing data from a covered entity can conduct his/her research using de-identified data, the study does not fall under the HIPAA Privacy Rule requirements. PHI can be de-identified in one of two ways:

1. Remove all 18 identifiers from the data.
2. Use statistical methods to certify there is very small risk that the information released could identify the individual.

Utilizing the first option raises questions about whether the researchers can be the individuals to de-identify the data. Each covered entity sets up its own policies and procedures regarding who can de-identify and under what circumstances. The second statistical method option includes additional HIPAA requirements that must be met. Consequently, to apply either of the de-identification options, researchers need to check with the covered entity to determine what policies and procedures it has in place.

Can the covered entity extend the HIPAA requirements to noncovered entities that need to use or access PHI? The HIPAA Privacy Rule includes a mechanism for indirectly extending the applicability of the Privacy Rule to individuals or entities outside of the covered entity. HIPAA requires the covered entity to sign written business associates agreements with parties outside of the covered entity. Business associates are external entities that or individuals who perform a service on the covered entity's behalf and create or have access to identifiable health information.[9]

Generally, collaborating researchers outside of the covered entity (e.g., investigators at another university) are not considered to be business associates. Also, sponsors, funding agencies, and statistical centers are usually not considered to meet the HIPAA requirements for business associates. However, researchers conducting HIPAA regulated research and research administrators need to know that these requirements exist and ensure whenever HIPAA covered PHI is being shared outside of the covered entity that a business associate agreement is not needed. For example, if in a study, a Web hosting data storage company is hired to store the PHI collected for the research, a business associate agreement might be necessary either as a stand-alone agreement or part of a larger subcontract.

What penalties can be applied if a covered entity or individual conducting HIPAA regulated research fails to comply with HIPAA requirements? Covered entities that fail to comply with the Privacy Rule may be subject to a variety of penalties. HIPAA regulations could result in civil fines and criminal penalties imposed on the covered entity and/or the individual researcher. Civil fines range from $100 per violation to $25,000 per person per year for each violation. Criminal penalties range from $50,000 to $250,000 and up to ten years in prison for knowingly violating the HIPAA regulations. Oversight and civil enforcement responsibility for the Privacy Rule are under the auspices of the Office of Civil Rights (OCR), Department of Health and Human Services (HHS). Enforcement of the criminal penalties for violations of the Privacy Rule is under the auspices of the Department of Justice (DOJ).[10]

These penalties stand in sharp contrast to the IRB DHHS regulations and the Common Rule sanctions which, depending on the source of funding, include a variety of corrective actions from letters of reprimand to withdrawal of funding. The federal regulations that govern human subjects research, 45 CFR 46, provide for the termination or suspension of federal support for protocols that "materially failed to comply" with 45 CFR 46. They do not include civil or criminal penalties.

How do researchers access or share protected health information under the HIPAA Privacy Rule? Research administrators, IRBs, and researchers are often confused about how protected health information held in covered entities can be accessed or shared under the HIPAA Privacy Rule. To minimize the confusion, research administrators, IRBs, and researchers need to have a sophisticated understanding of the options for accessing and sharing that HIPAA regulations provide.

How do researchers access protected health information under the Privacy Rule? Frequently, research protocols will require that protected health information be accessed from existing medical records or existing research databases that are covered by HIPAA. For example, in clinical research to identify potential subjects, researchers need access to medical records. Or, during the implementation of the research, researchers need to collect data from medical records during the administration of the drug or device and during the follow-up phase of the trial. Another example would be when a researcher from covered entity "A" is collaborating with a researcher at another covered entity "B" and needs access to the protected health information owned by entity "B."

The HIPAA Privacy Rule does allow researchers to access protected health information maintained by a covered entity using any of the five options listed below:

1. The individual from whom the protected health information has been collected provides written authorization for access. The written authorization must include six mandated core elements, three required statements, and two additional requirements (see Table 53-1).[11,12] The authorization can be combined with the informed con-

TABLE 53-1	HIPAA Authorization

Required Elements

1. Specific description of information to be used/disclosed class of persons
2. Identification of person/authorized to make disclosure/use
3. Identification of person/class of persons to whom CE releases the information
4. Description of each purpose of the requested use or disclosure
5. Expiration date related to purpose of the use/disclosure
6. Signature of individual and date (if personal representative, description of authority to act for individual)

45 C.F.R. § 164.508(C)(1)

Required Statements

1. Individual's right to revoke authorization in writing
2. Ability or inability to condition treatment, payment, enrollment, or eligibility for benefits
3. Potential for information to be subject to redisclosure

45 C.F.R. § 164.508(C)(2)

Must be in plain language and subject must be given a copy of the signed authorization

sent in which case it must be reviewed and approved by an IRB. Or, it can be a separate document in which case HIPAA does not require IRB approval. The local covered entity may require IRB approval of the separate authorization form, but this is not a federal requirement.

2. An IRB or Privacy Board can waive the requirements for written authorization if the HIPAA dictated criteria for waiver are met (see Table 53-2).[13] The IRB or Privacy Board must document that the waiver criteria have been met and the approval letter must be signed by the IRB or Privacy Board chairperson or IRB designee if expedited procedures are used.

3. Researchers submit to the covered entity assurances that the use of the protected health information meets three criteria for preparatory work (see Table 53-3).[14] The preparatory work option is typically used by researchers to obtain access to PHI without authorization in order to collect aggregate data to determine of there are enough prospective subjects to justify conduct-

ing a study or to identify prospective subjects that meet the inclusion/exclusion study criteria.

4. Researchers who need to access decedent protected health information must submit assurances that meet three criteria for decedent PHI (see Table 53-4).[15]

5. Limited type of identifiers can be released to a researcher by a covered entity if the data set includes only the limited data set elements specified in the Privacy Rule (see Table 53-5).[16] In addition, the researcher and the covered entity must sign a data use agreement. The Privacy Rule includes specific requirements regarding what information must be included in the data use agreement. If the researcher who wants access to the limited data set wants to prepare the data set, then depending upon the covered entity's policy and procedures, there may be additional requirements. For example, if a researcher who is outside the covered entity wants to abstract from the records a limited data set, he/she might be allowed to do so if he/she signed both a data use agreement and

TABLE 53-2	Authorization Waiver Criteria

1. The use or disclosure involves no more than minimal risk because of an adequate plan/assurance:
   a. To protect PHI from improper use or disclosure
   b. To destroy identifiers at earliest opportunity
   c. That PHI will not be inappropriately reused or disclosed
2. The research could not practicably be conducted without the waiver
3. The research could not practicably be conducted without access to and use of PHI

45 C.F.R. § 164.512(i)

Waiver of authorization must be approved by IRB or privacy board. Decision making should be documented. Approval letter should include chair's signature.

TABLE 53-3	Preparatory Work

Researcher Must Submit to Covered Entity Assurances That:

1. Use of PHI solely to prepare protocol
2. No PHI removed from covered entity
3. PHI necessary for preparation of research

45 C.F.R. § 164.512(i)(1)(ii)

TABLE 53-4	To Access/Share PHI from Deceased Individuals

Researcher Must Assure the Covered Entity That:

1. Use or disclosure of PHI solely for research
2. PHI necessary for research
3. At request of covered entity, documentation of death may be requested

45 C.F.R. § 164.512(i)(1)(iii)

TABLE 53-5	Limited Data Set

Elements That Cannot Be Included

1. Name (including relatives, employers, and/or household members)
2. Street address
3. Telephone number
4. Fax number
5. E-mail address
6. Social Security number
7. Medical record number
8. Health plan beneficiary number
9. Account number
10. Certificate/license number
11. Vehicle identifiers/serial numbers
12. Device identifiers/serial numbers
13. Web URLs
14. IP address numbers
15. Biometric identifiers
16. Full face photographs and any comparable images

Elements That Can Be Included in Data Set

1. Zip codes
2. City and state
3. Dates of birth
4. Other date info
5. Any other code not specified above

45 C.F.R. § 164.514(e)

business associate agreement. Policies and procedures will vary from covered entity to covered entity.

Determining which of the five options or combination of options apply in a specific research study requires the researcher to have a sophisticated understanding of the complexities surrounding the HIPAA requirements for each of the five options. A single study may require use of several of the options. For example, in a clinical drug trial, researchers often need to review medical records to identify prospective subjects. If the researcher works in the covered entity, he/she may be able to use the preparatory work option to review medical records to identify prospective subjects, without prior authorization. After the individual has been contacted using IRB approved procedures, the researcher would use the authorization option to obtain access to medical record data throughout the life of the trial.

Most covered entities have established their own policies and procedures dictating how the five options are to be applied within their respective entity. At a minimum, a research administrator should know the HIPAA expert within his/her organization regarding the covered entity's procedures.

How does a researcher who is employed by a covered entity share the PHI? In many studies, the research design or funding source will require that the PHI be shared with a variety of different of groups such as the sponsor or sponsor subcontractors; collaborating researchers at other institutions; collaborating researchers that work in noncovered components of the covered entity; federal inspectors and the IRB. The HIPAA Privacy Rule provides the researcher with options that the researcher can use to share PHI. Five of the options are identical to those that the covered entity can use to share PHI with a researcher within the covered entity:

1. Authorization
2. IRB or privacy board waiver of authorization

3. Preparatory work assurances
4. Decedent data assurances
5. Limited data set

In addition, a researcher can de-identify the data before sharing it outside of the covered entity. HIPAA also allows researchers to share PHI without an authorization for public health activities and when required by law.

Typically, in clinical research, sharing of PHI is accomplished by using the authorization option. The authorization form or the combined informed consent/authorization form includes a detailed listing of the individuals or classes of individuals with whom the PHI will be shared. If, however, the researcher changes plans regarding with whom data will be shared, he/she cannot share the PHI with a class of individuals that was not listed in the original authorization without applying one of the HIPAA options.

What privacy rights does HIPAA provide to patients who become subjects in research? The HIPAA Privacy Rule provides patients in the clinical setting and research subjects participating in HIPAA regulated research with the following privacy rights:

1. Patients/subjects are given the legal right to receive an accounting of disclosure of their PHI provided certain HIPAA conditions are met.
2. Patients/subjects may access the PHI maintained by the covered entity or by the researcher in a HIPAA covered study. HIPAA Privacy Rule does allow researchers to include specific statements in the authorization that would restrict subject access until the end of the research. However, if the statement is not included in the authorization, subjects in HIPAA covered research may access PHI at any time.
3. Patients/subjects may amend their PHI in records if specific HIPAA conditions are met.
4. Patients/subjects may revoke their authorization, although researchers may continue to use the data collected prior to the date when the authorization was revoked unless the IRB objects to this use.
5. Patients/subjects can request restrictions on use and disclosures of their PHI.
6. Patients/subjects can request receipt of communication of PHI by alternative means.[17]

What is confusing in applying the HIPAA requirements is that these rights do not extend to subjects participating in studies where the researcher is not employed by the covered entity (i.e., is outside of the covered entity). The HIPAA patient privacy rights do not apply once the PHI is removed from the entity by a researcher who is not employed by a covered entity. In these cases, researchers are not required to set up systems to ensure that these patient/subject rights are upheld. Subjects cannot access PHI using these HIPAA rights if the research is not HIPAA covered.

These rights are provided to subjects participating in HIPAA covered research (i.e., researchers work in the covered entity or covered component of a hybrid entity and in the study PHI will be accessed, used, or created). These researchers must set up systems to ensure that privacy rights are observed. Researchers in covered entities should check with the privacy officer to determine if the covered entity has a system for handling subjects' requests pertaining to their rights.

The privacy right that researchers find most difficult to comply with is the requirement that a subject has a right to receive an accounting of all of the disclosures that have been made by the covered entity of the PHI. HIPAA defines disclosures as sharing the PHI outside of the entity. The HIPAA requirements are complicated and specify the circumstances under which an accounting is required and the circumstances under which an accounting is not required. Table 53-6 lists the conditions when researchers must be able to supply an accounting and the conditions under which they have no obligation to provide the subjects with a list of each incident when the PHI was shared outside of the covered entity.[16] At most covered entities, the HIPAA privacy officer is given the responsibility for assisting researchers in setting up systems of accounting or in responding to privacy rights requests.

What additional requirements impact research and research administration? The HIPAA Privacy Rule includes a number of additional requirements that directly or indirectly impact research and research administration. It is beyond the scope of this chapter to discuss these areas in detail. Some of the requirements that most directly impact research include:

State Law. The Privacy Rule does not preempt state privacy laws. When state laws give greater protections to subjects, state laws will apply. Researchers, IRBs, and research administrators need to be knowledgeable about any state laws that overrule the HIPAA Privacy Rule.

HIPAA "Minimum Necessary" Requirements. The Privacy Rule imposes a minimum necessary

TABLE 53-6	Accounting of Disclosure	
Researcher Must be Able to Provide Accounting if PHI Obtained or Disclosed through:	**Researcher Not Required to Maintain Accounting if PHI Created or Accessed with:**	
1. Waiver of authorization 2. Preparatory research 3. Decedent PHI 4. Disclosure to public health authorities 5. Disclosure to law enforcement officials 45 C.F.R. § 164.528 45 C.F.R. § 164.508 45 C.F.R. § 164.514(e) 45 C.F.R. § 164.502 45 C.F.R. § 164.506 45 C.F.R. § 164.512(K)(5)	1. Authorization 2. Limited data sets with agreement 3. Disclosure to individual 4. De-identified information	

requirement on covered entities for permitted uses and disclosures of PHI. This means that the covered entity or covered researcher must try to limit the PHI to be collected, used, or disclosed in the research to the minimum necessary to achieve the research purpose. The rule is complicated because it also specifies circumstances when this standard applies (i.e., when PHI is collected under the waiver, decedent, preparatory work, or limited data set options) and when it does not apply (i.e., collection of PHI with subject authorization, treatment disclosures or requests, disclosures for compliance, or uses or disclosures as required by law).

Privacy Notice. A covered entity must tell individuals how their PHI will be used and disclosed. The covered entity provides a privacy notice to each patient. Researchers may have an obligation to ensure that the patient/subject has received a copy of the privacy notice.

Documentation Retention Requirements. HIPAA Privacy Rule includes requirements for length of time that documents such as the authorization form, Data Use Agreement, statistical certification of de-identification, IRB/Privacy Board waiver of authorization, or accounting of disclosures must be maintained. The length of retention is usually six years from date of creation of the document or from the date when the document was last in effect, whichever is later. It is not clear who within the covered entity is responsible for maintaining which document. Further confusion is created because the six-year requirement differs from the IRB requirements that research records must be maintained three years after completion of the study.

Researchers, IRBs, and research administrators who need in-depth knowledge about HIPAA requirements and advice on how to apply the requirements in a research setting can find assistance by reviewing

documents and guidance that have been issued by the Department of Health and Human Services' Office of Civil Rights and the National Institutes of Health's Office of the Director, Office of Science Policy.[i]

Conclusion

The HIPAA Privacy Rule is a complex statute that has had a significant impact upon researchers' access, use, and sharing of protected health information within a covered entity. Whether a research administrator needs in-depth knowledge of the HIPAA requirements depends upon his/her role within the institution in which he/she is employed. At a minimum, all research administrators should know if their employer is a covered entity and if so, which components of the organization are covered by the HIPAA requirements. Research administrators at covered entities need to know the key HIPAA contact individuals within the organization. Usually, these individuals are designated a legal counsel, a privacy officer, or an IRB HIPAA specialist.

---

[i]Office of Civil Rights, U.S. Department of Health & Human Services, 200 Independence Avenue, S.W., Room 509F, HHH Building, Washington, D.C. 20201. HIPAA toll-free number—(866) 627-7748. Web site: http://www.hhs.gov/ocr/hipaa/.

National Institutes of Health (NIH), Office of Science Policy, Office of Science Policy and Planning, Building 1, Room 218, 9000 Rockville Pike, Bethesda, MD 20892-0152; Phone number: 301-496-1454. The NIH Web site states that "for formal guidance on interpretation of the Privacy Rule, contact the Office for Civil Rights, http://www.hhs.gov/ocr/hipaa.

Research administrators who negotiate clinical trial agreements, contracts, or subrecipient agreements need to be familiar enough with HIPAA requirements and the covered entities policies to identify clauses that may be in conflict with local or federal requirements. Whenever clauses raise concern, the research administrator should ensure that they are reviewed by the appropriate individual such as a legal counsel or a privacy officer. Also, research administrators should have enough understanding of the business associate provisions to advise researchers that they need to contact the designated business associate agreement expert. Depending upon the HIPAA Privacy Rule requirements that have been put in place in a covered entity, IRB or departmental research administrators may need an extensive knowledge of the Privacy Rule in order to effectively advise either the researcher, IRB, or privacy board.

• • • References

1. Public Law 104-191, Health Insurance Portability and Accountability Act of 1996, http://aspe.hhs.gov/admnsimp/pl104191.htm (accessed August 21, 2005).

2. Federal Policy for the Protection of Human Subjects, http://www.hhs.gov/ohrp/references/frcomrul.pdf (accessed August 21, 2005).

3. Department of Health and Human Services, Standards for Privacy of Individually Identifiable Health Information; Final Rule 45 CFR Parts 160 and 164 http://www.hhs.gov/ocr/hipaa/privruletxt.txt (accessed August 21, 2005).

4. National Institutes of Health. "Protecting Personal Health Information in Research: Understanding the HIPAA Privacy Rule," http://privacyruleandresearch.nih.gov/pr_02.asp (accessed August 21, 2005).

5. United States Department of Health and Human Services. "Summary of the HIPAA Privacy Rule," http://www.hhs.gov/ocr/privacysummary.rtf (accessed August 12, 2004).

6. National Institutes of Health. "Protecting Personal Health Information in Research: Understanding the Privacy Rule, HIPAA Privacy Rule," http://privacyruleandresearch.nih.gov (accessed August 12, 2004).

7. United States Department of Health & Human Services. "Standards for Privacy of Individually Identifiable Health Information; Final Rule," *45 Code of Federal Regulations Part 160 Section 103,* Washington, DC: US Government Printing Office, 2002.

8. United States Department of Health & Human Services. "Standards for Privacy of Individually Identifiable Health Information; Final Rule," *45 Code of Federal Regulations Part 164 Section 514(b),* Washington, DC: US Government Printing Office, 2002.

9. National Institutes of Health. "Protecting Personal Health Information in Research: Understanding the Privacy Rule," http://privacyruleandresearch.nih.gov (accessed August 12, 2004).

10. National Institutes of Health. "HIPAA Frequently Asked Questions," http://privacyruleandresearch.nih.gov/faq.asp#1 (accessed August 12, 2004).

11. United States Department of Health and Human Services. "Standards for Privacy of Individually Identifiable Health Information Final Rule," *45 Code of Federal Regulations Part 164 Section 508(c)(1),* Washington, DC: US Government Printing Office, 2002.

12. United States Department of Health and Human Services. "Standards for Privacy of Individually Identifiable Health Information; Final Rule," *45 Code of Federal Regulations Part 164 Section 508(c)(2),* Washington, DC: US Government Printing Office, 2002.

13. United States Department of Health and Human Services. "Standards for Privacy of Individually Identifiable Health Information; Final Rule," *45 Code of Federal Regulations Part 164 Section 512(i),* Washington, DC: US Government Printing Office, 2002.

14. United States Department of Health and Human Services. "Standards for Privacy of Individually Identifiable Health Information; Final Rule," *45 Code of Federal Regulations Part 164 Section 512(i)(1)(ii),* Washington, DC: US Government Printing Office, 2002.

15. United States Department of Health and Human Services. "Standards for Privacy of Individually Identifiable Health Information; Final Rule," *45 Code of Federal Regulations Part 164 Section 512(i)(1)(iii),* Washington, DC: US Government Printing Office, 2002.

16. United States Department of Health and Human Services. "Standards for Privacy of Individually Identifiable Health Information; Final Rule," *45 Code of Federal Regulations Part 164 Section 514(e),* Washington, DC: US Government Printing Office, 2002.

17. United States Department of Health and Human Services. "Standards for Privacy of Individually Identifiable Health Information; Final Rule," *45 Code of Federal Regulations Part 164 Section 528,* Washington, DC: US Government Printing Office, 2002.

54

Management of Human Tissue Resources for Research in Academic Medical Centers: Points to Consider

Jeffrey R. Botkin, MD, MPH, Mark A. Munger, Pharm D,
Patrick A. Shea, JD, PC, Cheryl Coffin, MD, Geraldine P. Mineau, PhD

Abstract

Human tissue specimens are increasingly valuable resources for research at academic and commercial institutions. In recent years, there has been active debate over appropriate human subject protections in the use of tissue specimens in research. However, discussion over broader institutional policies governing human tissues has been limited. In this article, we propose a set of governing principles and a series of points to consider in developing policies in academic institutions for the management of human tissue resources for research. The points cover issues arising from the protection of human subjects, sharing between investigators, academic institutions, and commercial collaborators and the protection of intellectual property rights.

Introduction

Contemporary medical research in a number of fields increasingly is utilizing large collections of human tissues. The National Bioethics Advisory Commission (NBAC) estimated in 1999 that there were 282 million biological specimens in the United States and that this number was growing by 20 million per year.[1] At academic medical centers, stored tissues are derived from residual samples from research projects, tissue repositories established for research, pathology specimens from clinical care, and residual blood or fluid specimens from clinical testing. These human tissues are recognized as an increasingly valuable resource in biomedical sci-

ence, and their management is an emerging challenge for academic research institutions.

In the past decade, there has been a vigorous national and international debate over the appropriate use of these specimens.[2-5] This debate has focused on informed consent issues and the protection of individuals providing tissue specimens.[6-9] Increasingly, academic institutions must focus on collaborations between clinicians, institutional investigators, and investigators at other academic institutions. This focus requires attention to issues beyond consent, including academic freedom, promotion of research, and fairness in the allocation of research resources. Collaboration with for-profit companies who conduct biomedical research requires attention to issues of conflicts of interest, academic freedom, and obtaining appropriate financial return for product development for academic institutions.

In the emerging literature on research with tissues, little has been published to guide institutional policies regarding tissue resources. In response to emerging issues at the University of Utah, an Ad Hoc Tissue Advisory Committee (TAC) was convened to provide recommendations to the university with respect to its management of human tissue resources. The TAC was composed of representatives from within and outside the institution. The TAC approached its task by reviewing relevant literature, developing a set of guiding principles, and then analyzing issues in three domains: human subject concerns, concerns arising in academic collaboration, and concerns arising in collaborations with for-profit companies. Subsequently, the university established a standing advisory committee on human tissue resources to assist in the implementation of policies and procedures.

We review here a subset of the TAC recommendations that may be relevant to policy development in other academic institutions. Given the diverse nature of academic institutions, we present these as points to consider in the development of institutional policy. This discussion does not address policy issues in clinical care, organs acquired for transplantation, or special tissues relevant to human reproduction such as sperm, eggs, or embryos.

The appropriate management of human tissues requires the balancing of competing values. The TAC identified four principles relevant to the use of tissue resources. In general order of priority, these principles are individual welfare, academic freedom, public welfare, and commercialization.

- The primary institutional obligation in the management of tissues, tissue data, and clinical data is the protection to the fullest extent possible of the welfare, confidentiality, and privacy of individuals who provide tissues to the institution.
- Second, institutions should encourage the exchange of ideas and resources to maximize the opportunities for investigators to pursue new knowledge.
- Third, management of tissues, tissue data, and clinical data should encourage collaboration with governmental agencies and nonprofit organizations involved in basic science and disease detection, prevention, and treatment.
- Finally, the institution should encourage collaboration with commercial companies to promote the conduct of science and the development of products for the welfare of patients, the general public, the research community, and industry.

Conflicts between these principles are anticipated and must be negotiated and resolved in individual cases and policy provisions.

Patient and Research Participant Issues

Tissues are acquired from patients through diagnostic and therapeutic clinical services, including blood and body fluid testing, surgical procedures, tissue sampling, and autopsy specimens. Research participants may provide tissues through projects designed to acquire tissue for specific research testing, or to establish tissue repositories as an ongoing resource

for research. The College of American Pathologists requires the maintenance of paraffin blocks and glass slides from surgical and autopsy specimens for at least ten years.[10] Blood and body fluid samples generally are only retained for several days and then discarded, unless they are stored for approved research purposes. There are three issues we raise for discussion in the retention of tissues for research: ownership of tissues, the definition of research subjects, and the context and process of informed consent.

Ownership

The TAC considered whether the appropriate model for management of human tissues is one of stewardship or ownership. The concept of stewardship over tissues acquired for research is consistent with the general model adopted by pathologists with respect to tissues acquired through clinical care. Stewardship is an attractive concept since it incorporates the sense that tissues are managed in order to protect and foster the welfare of patients and research participants.[11,12] As articulated in the above principles, the protection of patients and research participants is the highest priority in the management of tissue resources. Further, respect for the autonomy of patients and research participants requires that research conducted with tissues is consistent with the informed wishes of the patient or participant (or his or her surrogate). In these respects, academic institutions must be good stewards of all tissues obtained for clinical and research purposes.

However, the concept of stewardship is not sufficiently broad to encompass the other rights and responsibilities academic institutions hold with respect to tissues. In particular, negotiations with external research institutions or commercial companies with respect to use of tissues and the intellectual property that may derive from tissue-based research cannot be based on the concept of stewardship alone. Academic institutions have clear responsibilities to patients and research participants, but they also have broader responsibilities to enhance public welfare through research, education, and product development. In the judgment of the TAC, academic institutions must own tissues if they are to maintain control over these resources to promote medical science and health product development. However, the prerogatives of ownership of tissues provided for research are clearly limited by federal and state regulations governing the ethical conduct of research. Therefore, the concept of ownership does not eliminate the substantial responsibilities institutions owe to those who provide their tissues to health care or research institutions.[13]

The law on ownership of tissues acquired through clinical care or research remains unresolved.[14–16] To date, the limited case law on the issue does not support ownership of tissues by patients or research participants.[17] In most legal jurisdictions, there remains an element of uncertainty about how ownership would be assigned if directly contested in court and, of course, legal decisions would depend on the facts in individual cases.

Point 1 Academic institutions should proceed in their management of tissues on the assumption that tissues acquired through clinical care or research become the property of the academic institution, unless federal or state legislation or case law clarify this issue to the contrary.

When tissue is obtained primarily for clinical purposes, it is essential that sufficient tissue be available to clinical pathology for a complete evaluation. Research interests in tissues should never jeopardize the clinical care of patients.

Point 2 Quality of care considerations and guidelines from such organizations such as the Joint Commission on Accreditation of Healthcare Organizations and the College of American Pathologists recommend that all tissues removed from patients be routinely submitted for pathological examination unless specific exceptions are approved by the hospital medical staff. Therefore, permission and collaboration of the pathologist should be obtained before any portion of a clinical tissue specimen is taken for research purposes.

Defining Research Subjects

If clinical specimens are utilized in research, then a question arises over whether patients who were the sources of the specimens become subjects of the research. The Common Rule (45CFR46) is the body of federal regulations for human subject protections for seventeen federal agencies that sponsor human research. Many academic institutions have signed a Multiple Project Assurance or a Federal Wide Assurance that guarantees that all research conducted at the institution, or by faculty employed by the institution, will adhere to these standards, whether or not the research is funded by the federal government. It is the responsibility of the institution's institutional review board (IRB) to provide peer review for research covered by the MPA and to establish policies and procedures to assure the protection of human subjects in research at the institution.

The Common Rule is a federal minimal standard and the IRB may establish local policies and procedures that are more stringent than those articulated in the Common Rule. The regulations (45CFR 46.102(f)) stipulate that human subjects are living individuals. Research conducted with tissues of a deceased individual, whether obtained before or after death, obviously cannot harm that individual. However, such research may have important implications for the deceased individual's living family members or close associates. Particularly through genetic research and research on infectious diseases, information relevant to family members or close associates may be generated through the analysis of tissues from deceased individuals. Adequate protection of all individuals potentially affected by the conduct of research requires that the interests of living family members and other close associates of deceased individuals be considered in the peer review of research protocols by the IRB.[18,19]

Point 3 Research conducted with tissue specimens obtained from identifiable individuals whether living or deceased should be subject to IRB oversight. Whether human tissue or tissue data are individually identifiable is an essential criterion for determining whether the tissue source is considered a research subject. In some circumstances when there is no data linked with a specimen, then the specimen becomes truly anonymous and its source individual is not the subject of research. In other circumstances, the specimen may be linked with clinical data that could be sufficiently informative to identify the tissue source. The Health Insurance Portability and Accountability Act of 1996 (HIPAA) lists eighteen identifiers that cannot be associated with specimens or data if the sources are unidentifiable for the purposes of the privacy rules.[20] When extensive databases of genotype information are created in the future, specimens may be individually identifiable through genetic analysis and cross-linked databases. Therefore the removal of names, medical record numbers, or specimen numbers may not be sufficient to "unlink" specimens from their sources.

Point 4 Procedures used to unlink personal identifiers from human tissues should be subject to IRB oversight and approval.

Informed Consent Issues

At least three issues are relevant to the content and process of informed consent in this context:

1. Research with tissues obtained in autopsies or postmortem examinations;
2. Tissues obtained for clinical or research purposes and "banked" for future, unspecified research; and,
3. Consent for use of tissues in commercial product development.[1] Consent for autopsy specimens:
   (A) *Consent for Autopsy Specimens*: As noted in Point 3, IRB oversight of research conducted with tissues obtained from deceased individuals should be considered.[21] A simple autopsy consent process and content may be sufficient if specimens are unlinked.

Point 5 Language in the autopsy authorization form should address the retention of unlinked tissues for use in education or research, for example:

> I hereby authorize [the institution] to dispose of, or to use for educational or research purposes any tissues, parts or body fluids which may be removed as long as personal identifiers have been permanently removed from the tissues, parts or fluids.

If linked tissues from autopsies are to be used in research, then information relevant to the health of living family members may be generated. For example, analysis of tissues obtained at autopsy for disease-associated mutations, such as a BRCA1 mutation, may reveal that the deceased individual's children are at 50% risk of being mutation carriers and/or that a parent is an obligate mutation carrier.

Point 6 The IRB should consider a requirement for informed consent from one or more first-degree relatives for research with linked tissues obtained at autopsy or postmortem examination when the research poses greater than minimal risk to family members.

Consent for use of specimens in future, unspecified research: When tissues are linked, informed consent from the tissue source may be necessary.[22] If the linked tissues will be used for a single research project, then the consent can be tailored to that proposed use. A more complicated situation arises when tissues are to be "banked" in a repository for unspecified future use in research. The National Bioethics Advisory Commission (NBAC) recommends a check-box format to offer research participants a range of options for use of their specimens.

Their approach addresses three basic elements of choice for research participants: use of linked or unlinked tissues; research on a limited range of conditions or a broad range; and permission for recontact for new consent or no recontact. Additional elements of choice might include use of tissues in collaboration with commercial companies and permission to return results to family members if the patient/subject is dead or incompetent.

The number of potential choices can become quite complex, perhaps in excess of reasonable expectations of subjects, investigators, or IRBs.[23] In general, investigators should design their consent process and content to reflect the needs of the research project and they need not offer choices that are not essential for their work. The broadest range of choices will only be relevant to projects that seek to establish a large repository as a resource for a wide variety of future, unspecified research projects.

NBAC's determination that it can be appropriate for research participants to be asked their permission for unspecified future uses proved to be controversial within the commission and this option was controversial within the TAC and other professional groups.[24] Some commissioners and TAC members argue that participants should not be asked to approve future, unspecified research with their linked samples because participants cannot weigh the risks and benefits of the research without information about the specific project. Other commissioners and TAC members believe that participants who are not concerned about risks should have the authority to permit unrestricted and unspecified future research on their specimens. However, our institutional legal interpretation of the subsequent HIPAA regulations indicates that consent for unspecified future research cannot be requested of research participants (although reliance on such consent obtained prior to the HIPAA compliance date is permitted).[25] Therefore, our institutional policy no longer permits asking consent for unspecified future research on specimens, although requesting use within a domain like "cancer research" is permitted.

A check-box approach to consent requires that a system be in place to track the choices of the research participant with their tissues. For large tissue repositories with a consent process that offers a number of choices, this tracking system would be essential to effectively honor the restrictions posed by participants.

Point 7 The institution should support investigators and research participants through the evaluation and development of a tracking system that will facilitate the ability of investigators to honor research participant choices with respect to the use of their tissue specimens. If an investigator plans to offer choices to research participants about the management of their tissues, then investigators should document in the protocol how these choices will be recorded, stored, and accessed.

Consent for use of tissues in commercial product development: Collaboration between academic institutions and for-profit entities is increasingly common and important for translating research into beneficial health products.[26] With respect to informed consent, some research subjects may wish to know if their tissues will be used in commercial product development. Further, some subjects might expect to receive compensation or a share in the profits of a commercial product derived from the use of their tissues. As noted above, case law to date has not recognized ownership rights by research subjects in their tissues. The Moore case, which involved investigators who developed a commercial product from a cell line derived from an individual patient, is the primary case precedent in this arena.[27] Ultimately, the California Court of Appeals decided that Mr. Moore did not have property rights in the cell line, but that investigators had an obligation to inform him of the commercial implications of the research in the informed consent process. Based on this precedent, many IRBs require that investigators indicate to potential research subjects that commercial products may be developed from their tissues and whether participants will share any financial gains from product development (although typically they will not).

Point 8 IRBs should consider the requirement of a discussion in the consent process about commercial aspects of research with subjects if known commercial products are being developed wholly or in part from their tissue or tissue data. It is necessary to inform subjects whether they will share in financial gains from product development. When investigators collaborate with advocacy organizations or special populations, negotiations over intellectual property issues may be appropriate.[28,29]

Collaboration between Academic Investigators

Because tissues are a valuable resource for research, institutions should encourage management of tis-

sues to promote research within the institution and between research institutions. Tissues acquired by faculty through clinical care or through research grants or contracts provided through the institution are not owned by faculty members but are owned by the institution. Principal investigators typically are responsible for obtaining grant funding for tissue acquisition and storage, use the tissues in their research, have physical control over the tissues, and oversee the day-to-day management of the tissues. However, investigators may not recognize the substantial contribution made by the institution in developing and maintaining research resources. Further, grants to conduct research are awarded typically to the institution rather than to faculty members.

Nevertheless, a strong sense of ownership by the investigator is understandable. Investigators often expect, appropriately, to maintain substantial control over tissues acquired in their research in order to maximize their own productivity. At the same time, investigators may want to limit access to "their" tissues by other investigators, whether at the institution or elsewhere, in order to limit competition for research goals. While limiting competition for research goals may be in the interest of an investigator and his or her team, it is not always in the interests of the institution or the general public. Accordingly, the institutions must balance their support for investigators who develop tissue resources with their obligations to other faculty and to the pursuit of new knowledge.

Point 9 Academic institutions should foster the sharing of tissue resources within the institutional community in order to maximize the pursuit of new knowledge. Education of the research community should emphasize that tissues acquired in clinical care or research are owned by the institution and not by its individual faculty.

Sharing of tissues arises in three general contexts:

1. Sharing of tissues with other investigators at the same institution.
2. Sharing of tissues with investigators at other academic institutions.
3. Sharing of tissues with commercial companies

Sharing of Tissues within the Institution

Sharing of tissue specimens and/or tissue data must be conducted in a manner consistent with the informed consent obtained from the research participant. If the original informed consent was explicitly for use by only one investigator or project, then sharing of linked tissues within the institution may not be appropriate without new consent by the research participant. However, it is unlikely that most research participants understand the departmental and program divisions within academic institutions, nor is it likely that many subjects care whether tissues and/or tissue data are shared between investigators at the institution, as long as there are no additional risks or benefits involved. Therefore it may be beneficial for the institution to request consent from participants to use and share tissues and/or tissue data for specified research purposes, and not inadvertently restrict consent to one project or one set of investigators.

Point 10 The IRB should foster consent language that permits the sharing of tissues and/or tissue data between investigators at the institution without the need for recontacting subjects, whenever possible, for example:

> . . . I permit investigators at [the institution] to use my tissues . . .

The risk to research subjects can be minimized by limiting the degree to which tissues are linked with identifiable, private information. The ability to link tissues or tissue data with their source should be limited to those investigators who have a valid scientific need for this information. Whenever possible, tissues and/or tissue data should be shared with investigators without identifying information and with only the demographic or clinical information that is essential for the research.

Point 11 Personal identifiers should only be shared between investigators in conjunction with tissue specimens and/or tissue data when essential for the conduct of the research.

The sharing of tissues between investigators raises issues beyond human subject protections. Questions concerning the extent of use of the shared resource, subsequent redistribution to third parties, authorship rights for publications, and intellectual property rights should be the subject of discussion and written agreement between the investigators. Prior agreements on the nature of the collaboration between investigators will minimize conflicts and promote collegial collaboration. The academic institution should consider developing a mechanism to promote these agreements.

Point 12 Investigators who share tissue specimens or tissue data within the institution should prepare an informal, written agreement governing the use of the tissues and data by the recipient investigator. We have termed this agreement a Material Transfer Memorandum (MTM) to distinguish it from the formal legal agreement between institutions, termed a Material Transfer Agreement (MTA). These documents should include the items noted in Table 54-1.

Sharing of Tissues between Investigators at Different Academic Institutions

Due to the potential loss of control of tissues or data that is shared outside the institution, additional scrutiny for these transactions is necessary. As always, the protection of patients and research subjects is the primary concern.

Point 13 Transfer of tissues and tissue data from the academic institution and use of tissues and tissue data at the home institution from other research institutions is subject to IRB oversight. IRB approval at the donor and recipient institution(s) should be documented prior to the transfer of tis-

TABLE 54-1	Guidelines for Elements To Be Included in Material Transfer Memorandum between Investigators and Material Transfer Agreements between Institutions

- Detailed description of the resources to be shared
- Nature and extent of research conducted using shared resources
- Documentation of IRB approval for
  1) acquisition of tissues by donor-investigator
  2) transfer and use of tissues/data by recipient
- Permission for, or prohibition of, further distribution of tissue and/or tissue data by the recipient
- Intellectual property rights for discoveries made with shared tissues and/or tissue data
- Authorship on publications developed from use of shared tissues and/or tissue data
- Participation on future grant applications emerging from shared resources
- Disposition of residual tissues and/or tissue data (returned, retained, or destroyed)
- Termination date for the agreement

sues/data. An MTA must be completed through the institutional technology transfer office (or its equivalent) before tissues can be transferred from, or to, the home academic institution. Negotiations toward an MTA can be conducted in parallel with IRB application and approval; however, IRB approval should precede completion of the MTA because the IRB may limit the use of tissues in ways relevant to the MTA.

Point 14 Tissues with any personally identifying information acquired at the home institution should not be shared with other research institutions, unless there is past or present informed consent and HIPAA authorization by research subjects for the sharing of individually identifiable tissues or information.

Point 15 Certain tissue sets represent a limited and valuable resource. In rare circumstances when conflicts arise, transfer of tissues from the institution should be subject to review and approval by an oversight committee and/or by the research vice president (or officer with similar authority).

Point 16 Investigators should retain portions of tissues that are shared with other research institutions, when feasible, as insurance against loss of these resources.

Prior to the transfer of tissues, institutional investigators, in collaboration with a technology transfer office, typically must prepare an MTA to be signed by the sending investigator, the institutional technology transfer office, and by an authorized person at the receiving institution.

Point 17 Faculty who leave the home institution for employment at other academic or commercial institutions should not take tissues or tissue data with them without a formal, written agreement with the home academic institution.

Point 18 Faculty who gain employment at the home institution from other institutions should not be permitted to bring tissues and/or tissue data with them unless:

a) The new faculty member can document personal ownership of the tissues and/or tissue data, or,

b) A formal agreement has been entered between the home institution and the institution where the tissues and/or tissue data originated.

Collaborative Research with Commercial Companies

In the past decade, there has been a rapid expansion in biomedical research being conducted by commercial companies. Biotechnology companies often seek to collaborate with academic institutions as a source of clinical and research expertise, tissues, and data. Further, many biotechnology companies are emerging in close association with academic institutions as faculty work to translate their creative efforts into commercial products.[30,31] In general, this collaboration between academic institutions and commercial companies is valuable and often essential to the translation of basic research into useful products.

In this context, the key set of issues arising in the collaboration with commercial companies pertains to ownership and control over tissues and tissue data that are shared in the collaboration. Acquisition of tissues and associated clinical data often requires the extensive resources of the academic institution. Accordingly, the academic institution should expect and seek substantial control over, and rewards for, its contributions to collaborative research. In addition, academic institutions highly value academic freedom, education, the integrity of their faculties, and the pursuit of new knowledge. These values must be protected as the academic institutions pursue a fair balance of risk and reward for collaborative research and product development.

Point 19 When sharing tissues with commercial companies, academic institutions should retain ownership rights of tissues acquired at the institution. Transfer of tissues to a commercial company should not occur without an MTA signed by an authorized representative of the academic institution. [Note: In general, individual faculty members are not authorized representatives of the institution.]

Point 20 Whenever possible, the academic institution should, by appropriate agreement, acquire or maintain ownership or joint ownership rights over tissue data derived from tissues established, maintained, and/or acquired at the academic institution, including tissue data generated by a for-profit company.

Point 21 When the creation of a tissue resource at the academic institution is funded wholly or in part by a commercial company, only limited restrictions on additional uses of the resource by the academic institution should be negotiated. Agreements with commercial companies should permit the use of tissue resources by the academic institution for:

- Research that is not competitive with the research goals of the commercial company for which the tissue resource is being used in collaboration; and,
- Unrestricted research after a negotiated time period unless a new agreement is signed.

Collaboration with for-profit companies may entail an analysis of tissues by the company, with the return of data to the academic institution for further work toward a shared goal. Companies have a legitimate interest in restricting the use of tissue data they have generated to work toward the shared goal, and restricting use by academic institutions for other purposes, including work with other commercial collaborators. However, it is contrary to the interests and values of academic institutions to permit extensive restrictions on data derived from collaborative research.

Point 22 Negotiations concerning tissue data provided to an academic institution by a for-profit company (but derived from tissues owned by the academic institution) should stipulate a reasonable time period in which use of the tissue data by the academic institution will be restricted to a specific set of research goals and a specific set of additional collaborators, if any. Beyond that time period, the academic institution should be able to use the tissues and/or tissue data without restrictions.

Conclusions

The public has a strong tradition of supporting academic research. This tradition is based, in part, on the many benefits derived from such research conducted in the past. Further, the tradition is based on the trust that research universities will work to sustain the public's trust. Contemporary research has been highly productive in identifying acquired and hereditary genetic mutations associated with conditions that are relatively common and those associated with single gene mutations. Rare conditions and those with more subtle genetic factors involved have proven to be more challenging. In addition, the influences of many environmental exposures on human disease, growth, and development remain poorly understood. These research priorities increasingly require large populations and research efficiency requires the use of large tissue repositories with linked clinical data by investigators with a

range of expertise. In this emerging era of human research, careful management of tissue resources will be essential both for scientific quality control and to maintain the public's trust. Attention by academic institutions to these policy issues and consistency between institutions on policies enhance the quality and efficiency of research and promote equitable agreements with for-profit collaborators. This attention also can help to sustain the support and trust of the public in academic research institutions.

Acknowledgments

We would like to thank the following individuals for their valuable contributions to the Tissue Advisory Committee: Michele Ballantyne, JD, Lisa Cannon-Albright, PhD, William Carroll, MD, Lynne Chronister, Edward Clark, MD, Brent Brown, JD, Chris Jansen, PhD, Mark Leppert, PhD, Patricia MacCubbin, Karen McCreary, JD, Susan Poulter, JD, PhD, Jean Wylie, MS, Kurt Albertine, PhD.

• • • References

1. National Bioethics Advisory Commission. "Research Involving Human Biological Materials: Ethical Issues and Policy Guidance," 1 (1999) (accessed August 30, 2005).
2. Clayton, E.W., K.K. Steinberg, M.J. Khoury, E. Thomson, L. Andrews, M.J. Khan, L.M. Kopelman, and J.O. Weiss. "Informed Consent for Genetic Research on Stored Tissue Samples." *JAMA* 274 (1995): 1786–1792.
3. Knoppers, B.M., and C.M. Laberge. "Research and Stored Tissues: Persons as Sources, Samples as Persons?" *JAMA* 274 (1995): 1806–1807.
4. Wier, R., ed. *Stored Tissue Samples: Ethical, Legal, and Public Policy Implications.* Iowa City, IA: University of Iowa Press, 1998.
5. Botkin, J.R. "Informed Consent for the Collection of Biological Samples in Household Surveys." In *National Research Council Committee on Population, Cells and Surveys: Should Biological Measures Be Included in Social Science Research?* edited by C.E. Finch, J.W. Vaupel, and K. Kinsella, 276–302. Washington, DC: National Academy Press, 2001.
6. American Society of Human Genetics. "Statement on Informed Consent for Genetic Research." *Am J Hum Genet* 59 (1996): 471–474.
7. Merz, J.F., D.G.B. Leonard, and E.R. Miller. "IRB Review and Consent in Human Tissue Research." *Science* 283 (1999): 1647–1648.

8. American College of Medical Genetics. "Storage of Genetics Materials Committee: Statement on Storage and Use of Genetic Materials." *Am J Hum Genet* 57 (1995): 1499–1500.

9. Steinberg, K.K., E.J. Sampson, G.M. McQuillan, and M.J. Khoury. "Use of Stored Tissue Samples for Genetic Research in Epidemiologic Studies." In *Stored Tissue Samples: Ethical, Legal, and Public Policy Implications*, edited by R.F. Weir, 82–88. Iowa City, IA: University of Iowa Press, 1998.

10. College of American Pathologists, Commission on Laboratory Accreditation. "Laboratory Accreditation Program." *Anatomic Pathology Checklist*, March 2003, www.cap.org/apps/docs/laboratory_accreditation/checklists/anatomic_pathology_March2003.pdf (accessed August 30, 2005).

11. College of American Pathologists. "Stewardship of Pathologic Specimens," College of American Pathologists, 2000, http://www.cap.org/governance/policies/policy_appf.cfm (accessed April 28, 2004).

12. Jeffres, B.R. "Human Biological Materials in Research: Ethical Issues and the Role of Stewardship in Minimizing Research Risks." *Adv Nurs Sci* 24, no. 2 (2001): 32–46.

13. Skene, L. "Ownership of Human Tissue and the Law." *Nature Reviews Genetics* 3 (2002): 145–148.

14. Gottlieb, K. "Human Biological Samples and the Laws of Property: The Trust as a Model for Biological Repositories." In *Stored Tissue Samples: Ethical, Legal, and Public Policy Implications*, edited by R.Weir, 182–197. Iowa City, IA: University of Iowa Press, 1998.

15. Reymond, M.A., R. Steinert, J. Escourrou, and G. Fourtanier. "Ethical, Legal, and Economic Issues Raised by the Use of Human Tissue in Postgenomic Research." *Digestive Diseases* 20 (2002): 257–265.

16. McHale, J. "Waste, Ownership and Bodily Products." *Health Care Analysis* 8 (2000): 123–135.

17. Hakimian, R., and D. Korn. "Ownership and Use of Tissue Specimens for Research." *JAMA* 292 (2004): 2500–2505.

18. DeRenzo, E.G., L.G. Biesecker, and N. Meltzer. "Genetics and the Dead: Implications for Genetics Research with Samples from Deceased Persons." *Am J Med Genet* 69 (1997): 332–334.

19. Azarow, K.S., F.L. Olmstead, R.F. Hume, J. Myers, B.C. Calhoun, and L.S. Martin. "Ethical Use of Tissue Samples in Genetic Research." *Military Medicine* 168, no. 6 (2003): 437–441.

20. U.S. Department of Health and Human Services Office for Civil Rights. "Standards for Privacy of Individually Identifiable Health Information," as amended 2003, http://www.hhs.gov/ocr/combinedregtext.pdf (accessed August 30, 2005).

21. Roberts, L.W., K.B. Nolte, J.D. Warner, T. McCarty, L.S. Rosenbaum, and R. Zumwalt. "Perceptions of the Ethical Acceptability of Using Medical Examiner Autopsies for Research and Education: A Survey of Forensic Pathologists." *Arch Pathol Lab Med* 124 (2000): 1485–1495.

22. Merz, J.F., P. Sankar, S. Taube, and V. Livolski. "Use of Human Tissues in Research: Clarifying Clinician and Research Roles and Information Flows." *Journal of Investigative Medicine* 45 (1997): 252–257.

23. Wendler, D., and E. Emanuel. "The Debate over Research on Stored Biological Samples: What Do Sources Think?" *Arch Intern Med* 162 (2002): 1457–1462.

24. Deschenes, M., G. Cardinal, B.M. Knoppers, and K.C. Glass. "Human Genetic Research, DNA Banking and Consent: A Question of 'Form?'" *Clin Genet* 59 (2001): 221–239.

25. *Federal Register* 67, no. 157 (2002), 53226.

26. Gelijns, A.C., and S.O. Their. "Medical Innovation and Institutional Interdependence: Rethinking University–Industry Connections." *JAMA* 287 (2002): 72–77.

27. *Moore v. Regents of the University of California*, 793 P. 2d 479 (Calif. 1990).

28. Merz, J.F., D. Magnus, M.K. Cho, and A.L. Caplan. "Protecting Subjects' Interests in Genetics Research." *Am J Hum Genet* 72 (2002): 215.

29. Terry, S.F., and C.D. Boyd. "Researching the Biology of PXE: Partnering in the Process." *Am J Med Genet* 106, no. 3 (2001): 177–184.

30. Brown, J.R. "Privatizing the University: The New Tragedy of the Commons." *Science* 290 (2000): 1701–1702.

31. Martin, J.B., and D.L. Kasper. "In Whose Best Interest? Breaching the Academic–Industrial Wall." *New Engl J Med* 343 (2000): 1646–1649.

55

Welfare of Research Animals

Kathryn A. Bayne, MS, PhD, DVM, and John E. Harkness, DVM, MS, MEd

Introduction: Welfare and Rights

The use of vertebrate animals in research, teaching, and testing in institutions and corporations, public or private, affords great opportunities for the improvement of the lives of man and other animals. At the same time, these uses elicit in most people, in some more than others, considerable concern. The resulting discussions and debate, among segments of a continuum of views, have resulted in institutional animal care and use becoming one of the most emotive, contentious, and significant issues of our time and an endeavor molded by international, national, and local public opinion, financial interests, and regulation and policy, including regulations discussed in this chapter and the policies of professional organizations, funding agencies, and editorial boards. Few issues are as complex, as promising for the progress of mankind, or as strongly opposed by a highly vocal component of the population as is the use of animals in research, testing, and teaching.

Humans and animals have interacted for millennia, with humans using and caring for animals to obtain food, skins, bone and antler utensils, ritualistic icons, pleasure from sport, and, since ancient times, knowledge of the normal and abnormal aspects of mankind through observation and ultimately rigorous research and study. As a consequence of this interdependence, humans have developed a spectrum of feelings and concerns toward animals, especially toward those animals that have directly met human needs, have included those ranging from fear and recognition of utility of animals to feelings of empathy, urge to control, and interest in and desire to manage animals' welfare. In modern culture, these interests have led to the present-day controversy over the use of animals in testing, teaching, and research.

Fundamental to understanding human concerns about animal care and use is the term "animal welfare." Although there is no one standard definition of "welfare," considering that the species of man cannot know with certainty the optimal conditions for other animal species, the definition of the term promulgated by the American Veterinary Medical Association (AVMA) (1) includes the views of many:

> Animal welfare is a human responsibility that encompasses all aspects of animal well-being, including proper housing, management, nutrition, disease prevention and treatment, responsible care, humane handling, and, when necessary, humane euthanasia.
>
> Tannenbaum, while cautioning against a precise definition of welfare, lists as welfare attributes (paraphrased) absence of unpleasant sensations and availability and opportunity for pleasurable experiences. The state of welfare or "faring well" is evidenced by good health, absence of abnormal behavior, and fulfillment of basic biological drives. (2)

The term "animal rights" presents a greater challenge to wide acceptance and is often linked by the scientific community with opinions or movements inimical to biomedical and agricultural research, despite pragmatic advantages for removing this pejorative connotation. The AVMA (1) states that "Animal welfare and animal rights are not synonymous terms," and that "the AVMA cannot endorse the philosophical views and personal values of animal rights advocates when they are incompatible with the responsible use of animals for human purposes . . ."

This view of animal rights is shared by the Foundation for Biomedical Research (FBR). (3) An alternative view of "animal rights" is discussed by Tannenbaum, (2) who cites the World Veterinary Association's "certain provisions of care" as worthy examples of five basic rights that are accepted widely as basic, intrinsic "moral claims" or "rights" of sentient beings, including many animals. The association's list includes freedom from hunger and thirst, from physical discomfort and pain, from injury and disease, from fear and distress, and freedom to conform to essential behavioral patterns. These rights are said to exist apart from any human obligations (welfare concerns) due animals but are compatible with those obligations. This concept, that animals possess intrinsic rights to "faring well," does not abrogate human decisions or animal instincts to override those rights for their own purposes, but rather deepens human concern for animals.

As FBR notes, animal rights activists (now often referring to themselves as animal protectionists) believe that animals should have the same moral rights as do humans. Alex Pacheco, cofounder of the People for the Ethical Treatment of Animals (PETA), for example, states that "animals have the same rights as a retarded human child, because they are equal mentally in terms of dependence on others." (4) Beauchamp (5) makes an effective case for the recognition of animal rights when he notes that modern legal systems encounter little or no opposition (except in advocacy of rights for a fetus) when assigning rights to impaired human beings who may have fewer cognitive and emotional capacities than do many animals, whose cognitive and emotional capacities continue to be a source of public and scientific interest and research. Peter Singer, the philosopher who helped raise the issue of animal rights into an international movement, underscores this notion of equality between humans and nonhumans in his remarks that "An animal experiment cannot be justifiable unless the experiment is so important that the use of a brain-damaged human would be justifiable." (6) These concerns for welfare and rights and the evolving recognition of animal capacities underlie many of the regulatory and policy documents and positions described in this chapter.

Historical Perspective

Pet Theft, Dog Concentration Camps, and New Laws

Federal laws for the humane treatment of animals have been in place since 1873, when Congress passed a law governing the treatment of livestock during shipment for export. The law was called the "28 Hour Law" after the maximum length of time animals could be transported before receiving food, water, and rest. (7) This law was later repealed and a new version of the "28 Hour Law," passed in 1906, is still in effect today. However, the first federal law to protect nonfarm animals, called the Laboratory Animal Welfare Act, administered by the Animal and Plant Health Inspection Service (APHIS) of the US Department of Agriculture (USDA), was not passed until 1966. At first, this law was primarily concerned with dog and cat dealers, requiring that individuals or corporations that bought or sold dogs or cats for laboratory activities be licensed and adhere to certain minimum standards for the care of animals and that users of cats or dogs for research register with the USDA and also meet minimum standards for animal care. For animal users, the law applied only to animals held prior to or after the laboratory activity.

The impetus for the 1966 Laboratory Animal Welfare Act has its roots in two stories published in popular magazines that captured the public's interest and fueled the demand for increased Congressional attention to animal welfare. The first story was that of Pepper, a pet Dalmatian stolen from her owners in Pennsylvania. Pepper was eventually traced, but not before she had been sold to a New York state dog dealer and subsequently sold to a New York City hospital for use in research where she was used in an experiment and euthanized as part of a study. Pepper's story was told in a November 1965 *Sports Illustrated* article, "The Lost Pets That Stray to Labs." Within the year, *Life Magazine* published an article, "Dog Concentration Camps: Your Dog is in Cruel Danger," which included photographs taken during a raid at a dealer facility by Maryland state police and pictured a dog owner and pet, who wore an identification tag of the research facility clearly visible on the dog's collar.

The *Life Magazine* article engendered enormous public outcry regarding the possible future of pet dogs that were lost or stolen; the magazine received more feedback from readers about this article than on any it had published about the Vietnam War. Pet theft continues to be a rallying point for animal rights activists today, whereas the USDA's "trace-back" audits of research animals' dealerships do not support that animal theft occurs. (8)

The Laboratory Animal Welfare Act of 1966 (9) has been repeatedly amended (in 1970, 1976, 1985, 1990, and 2002) to modify the scope of the law. For example, the Animal Welfare Act (AWA) of 1970 (Public Law 91-579) included regulation addressing use of animals for teaching, exhibition, and the wholesale pet industry. Animals covered by the law included most warm-blooded animals. The law also required that research facilities register with and submit an annual report to the Secretary of Agriculture. (10) Animals specifically exempted from the law included horses (not used in research) and animals used in food and fiber research; animals distributed through retail pet stores; and animals used in state and county fairs, rodeos, purebred cat and dog shows, and agricultural exhibitions. The AWA Amendments of 1976 (Public Law 94-279), included common commercial carriers, such as airlines, under the law, which subsequently led to standards being developed for shipping containers (such as design and construction standards) and conditions of shipment.

Public and Congressional interest in animal research was recaptured in 1981 when an NIH-sponsored Maryland scientist, Dr. Edward Taub, was charged with cruelty to animals. Investigation into Dr. Taub's practice began after a volunteer worker called police to report cruelty to animals at the facility where Dr. Taub used nonhuman primates to study how the central nervous system adapts to the neurological trauma that may follow stroke or spinal cord injury. Over the course of the next decade, the media continued to cover the fate of Dr. Taub and the so-called "Silver Spring monkeys" (named after the location of the research facility). Dr. Taub was tried and convicted on six counts of animal cruelty and acquitted on eleven other charges. In an appeal, his conviction was reduced to one count involving one animal. Ultimately, in 1983, the Maryland Appeals court overturned Dr. Taub's conviction on the remaining count on the grounds that the state's anticruelty law did not apply to federally sponsored research. In a

separate decision, the NIH itself terminated the research grant based on noncompliance with the PHS policy requirement for adequate veterinary care. Due to the wide media attention, members of Congress held hearings in the Science Subcommittee to review practices of laboratory animal care, use, and treatment. (11) Testimony from these hearings laid the foundation for additional hearings on the same subject, and the subsequent legislation pertaining to laboratory animal welfare, including the 1985 Improved Standards for Laboratory Animals Act (Public Law 99-198). The act included many new provisions regarding animal welfare, including:

- Minimization of animal pain and distress and consideration of alternatives to painful procedures; consultation with a doctor of veterinary medicine for any practice that could cause pain to animals;
- Limitation of conducting more than one major survival surgery on an animal;
- Establishment of an Institutional Animal Care and Use Committee (IACUC) to provide oversight of the animal care and use program and facilities;
- Provision of specific training to personnel;
- Provision of exercise to dogs; and,
- Stipulation to promote the psychological well-being of nonhuman primates.

More recently, the Food, Agriculture, Conservation, and Trade Act of 1990 (Section 2503, Protection of Pets, Public Law 101-624) established that a holding period occur for dogs and cats at shelters and at other holding facilities prior to sale to dealers, and thus into the research stream. This law also requires dealers to provide written certification to the recipient regarding the background of each animal. The Animal Enterprise Protection Act of 1992 makes "physical disruption" of animal enterprises by property damage, theft, economic damage exceeding $10,000, serious bodily injury, or death a criminal offense. In 1998 the Alternatives Research and Development Foundation (ARDF) petitioned the USDA to amend the AWA to include rats, mice, and birds in the definition of "animal," and thus include them in the Animal Welfare Regulations and the resulting annual inspections of research institutions. A year later the USDA faced further pressure when it was sued by the ARDF regarding the same issue. In a settlement, the USDA agreed to regulate the handling of rats, mice, and birds. This agreement was partially preempted by Senator Jesse Helms' introduction of a section to the 2002 Farm Bill that amended the Animal Welfare Act by modifying the definition of "animal" to exclude rats of the genus *Rattus*, mice of the genus *Mus*, and birds bred for use in research.

Federal Oversight

In the United States, oversight of animal care and use for research, testing, and teaching is achieved by numerous laws, regulations, policies, and guidelines from two principle government organizations, the USDA and the PHS. (12) Other guidance may be derived from scientific panels and endorsed by the government as required standards. Federal laws are compiled and categorized annually into their respective subjects (e.g., agriculture) and published as the United States Code (USC). The USC includes a discussion of the intent of Congress for establishing the law and any interpretations from the courts. Regulations are promulgated to enforce the corresponding law. Proposed regulations are published in the Federal Register for public comment. After the responsible agency reviews and addresses the public comments, the regulations are again published in the Federal Register in final format and are then incorporated into the Code of Federal Regulations (e.g., 9 CFR[13]). (13–15) In general, laws address two specific areas: animal welfare and procurement and animal importation and shipment.

US Government Principles for the Utilization and Care of Vertebrate Animals Used in Testing, Research, and Training (US Government Principles) (16)

The activities of the Interagency Research Advisory Committee (IRAC) date back to 1983 when the Interagency Primate Steering Committee (IPSC), at the time the only federal interagency committee engaged in the review of issues involving research animals, was asked to represent the United States at a meeting of the Council of Europe. (14) It quickly became evident that representation on the committee needed to be expanded; this recognized need became the impetus to the IPSC to be broadened into the IRAC. The IRAC's primary concerns are the "conservation, use, care and welfare of research animals" and its main responsibilities are "information exchange, program coordination, and contribution to policy development." (16) In 1985, IRAC published the nine principles to be taken into consideration by federal agencies that develop requirements for testing, research, or training procedures involving vertebrate animals. Because the federal principles also appear in the PHS "Policy on Humane Care and Use of Animals" (17) (PHS Policy, see below) and the *Guide for the Care and Use of Laboratory Animals* (*Guide*) (18), institutions required to conform with either or both of those documents must also adhere to these principles.

US Department of Agriculture

The USDA has been vested by Congress with both promulgation and enforcement authority of the AWA through its Animal Welfare Regulations (AWRs). The USDA is required to conduct unannounced annual inspections of research facilities with follow-up inspections until any cited deficiencies have been corrected (exempt from this provision are federal research facilities). It is required that research facilities, intermediate handlers, and common carriers register with the USDA, whereas animal dealers and exhibitors must be licensed. Research facilities and federal government agencies are required to purchase animals only from licensed sources, unless the source is exempted from obtaining a license. In addition, the USDA publishes polices meant to clarify the AWRs and requires annual reporting from registered institutions. USDA policies have the force of interpretive rule, and thus must be strictly followed by the regulated community. Facilities that fail to comply with regulatory requirements can face fines, suspension of authority to operate, and even permanent revocation of the facility's license to operate. Penalties can be imposed on the facility such that some portion of the fine is mandated to be spent on the operation of the facility (e.g., physical plant repairs) to improve the program of animal care and use. Thus, the enforcement component of the USDA's oversight responsibility is strong, and has been used over the years to improve animal welfare at dealers, animal exhibits, and research facilities.

Public Health Service Policy

The other federal agency charged with oversight of research animal care and use is the PHS. First implemented in 1973, the PHS Policy was revised in 1979, 1986 and 2002. Today, the PHS authority is derived from the Health Research Extension Act of 1985, Section 495 (Public Law 99-158), Animals in Research. Under this act, institutions conducting animal research using PHS funding, (e.g., the NIH), must comply with the PHS Policy. (17) The policy requires submission by the funding recipient (referred to as an "awardee institution") of an Animal Welfare Assurance Statement, which must be approved by the PHS's Office of Laboratory Animal Welfare (OLAW), and NIH, which commits the filing institution to follow the federal principles, and the *Guide*. The PHS Policy covers all vertebrate animals used in research, testing, or teaching. In addition to stating a commitment to animal welfare, the Animal Welfare Assurance Statement must designate clear lines of authority and cite responsibility for the institution's oversight of the work, inclusive of a designated "Institutional Official," who is ultimately responsible for the animal care and use program. The statement must also identify a qualified veterinarian involved in the program and must provide a description of the occupational health and safety program for relevant personnel in the program; a description of mandated training; and a description of the facility. Assurances are renegotiated with OLAW every five years. OLAW can approve, disapprove, restrict, or withdraw approval of an assurance.

PHS awarding agencies, such as the NIH, may not make an award for an activity involving live, vertebrate animals unless the prospective awardee institution and all other institutions participating in the animal activity have an approved assurance with OLAW and provide verification that the IACUC has reviewed and approved those sections of the grant application that involve use of animals. applications from organizations with approved assurances must address five specific points pertaining to the use of animals:

1. A detailed description of the proposed work, including species, strain, sex, age, and number of animals to be used in the proposed work.
2. Justification of the use of animals, species, and number of animals.
3. Information on the veterinary care for the animals.
4. Description of the procedures for ensuring that discomfort, distress, pain, and injury will be minimized.
5. Description of the method of euthanasia and the reason for the selection of that method, including a justification for any method that does not conform with the AVMA's 2000 Report of the Panel on Euthanasia. (19)

Awardee institutions that do not comply with the standards of the *Guide*, the USDA's Animal Welfare Regulations, and other standards referenced in the PHS Policy (e.g., the AVMA's 2000 Report of the Panel on Euthanasia [19]), may have

their Assurance Statement restricted, which in turn can limit access to PHS funding for research. Sustained noncompliance with the PHS policy can result in withdrawing the approval of the assurance and cessation of all PHS funding for animal-based activities.

The awardee institution must also submit an annual report indicating any changes in the program or facilities, including changes in accreditation status. Institutions not accredited by an external review group (Category 2) must provide copies of their IACUC's latest semiannual program review and facility inspection with the initial assurance submission and subsequent renewals.

The role of the IACUC in providing local oversight of animal care and use is a key element of the PHS Policy. Although the required composition of the IACUC for the PHS differs slightly from USDA requirements, the "Memorandum of Understanding" concerning laboratory animal welfare sets forth procedures for cooperation among the three agencies (the APHIS/USDA, the Food and Drug Administration [FDA], and the NIH) in their oversight of animal care and use programs, and ensures that general functions and responsibilities of the IACUC are compatible among the federal agencies.

OLAW conducts site visits of awardee institutions both for cause and not for cause. In addition, an ongoing significant mission of OLAW is the educational outreach it performs in collaboration with awardee institutions. Jointly sponsored workshops focus on information of value to institutional officials and IACUC's to provide appropriate oversight of animal care and use. OLAW also provides guidance through articles in journals, commentary on other articles, NIH Guide Notices, and a Listserv.

Other Laws, Regulations, and Policies

The Department of Defense (DoD) developed a "Policy on Experimental Animals" in 1961 to ensure that all research at DoD facilities involving animals was conducted in accord with certain principles of animal care. (20) Later versions of this policy also included care in overseas sites. Subsequently, the DoD issued a 1995 Directive, "The Use of Laboratory Animals in DoD Programs," (21) that applies to the Office of the Secretary of Defense, the military departments, the Uniformed Services University of the Health Sciences and the Defense Agencies, which requires that all DoD facilities apply for accreditation by AAALAC International and establish local institutional animal care and use committees. The directive also assigns to the DoD oversight responsibility for DoD-sponsored, extramural animal-based research, testing, and training under DoD grants or contacts.

Office of Research Oversight (ORO), Department of Veterans Affairs

At the time of this writing, the ORO serves as the primary component of the Veterans Health Administration to advise the Under Secretary for Health on all matters affecting the integrity of research by ensuring the welfare of research animals through promoting conformance with relevant regulations and policies. Through VA Handbook 1200.7, the VA has adopted the standards of the PHS Policy for all animal research conducted under VA auspices, and further requires that VA medical centers conducting animal studies and accepting any PHS funds should have a PHS Animal Welfare Assurance (1200.7.7e). However, a bill before Congress would establish the Office of Research Compliance and Assurance within the Veterans Health Administration of the Department of Veterans Affairs. The mission of the office would be to promote the ethical conduct of research, to prevent the mistreatment of laboratory animals in research, to observe external accreditation site visits for animal welfare, and to negotiate and maintain a research assurance with each medical center of the department conducting animal research.

State Laws

State laws to protect animals have a long history: the first anticruelty law was passed in 1641 in the Massachusetts Bay Colony to prevent riding or driving farm animals beyond established limits. (22) Subsequently, all fifty states and the District of Columbia enacted anticruelty laws. (23) The overarching goals of these laws are to protect animals from cruel treatment; to require that animals have access to suitable food and water; and that animals are provided shelter from extreme weather. Some state laws define "animal" and some do not. State laws consist of a number of diverse approaches to providing protection to animals, however; for example, some states have additional provisions for animals used in research, while many states prohibit the sale of pound animals into the research stream. In general, criminal penalties are imposed for offenses. Historically, state anticruelty laws have been used against research facilities and in recent years, state and federal laws have even been used by private citizens or citizen groups claiming "standing to sue" on behalf of animals. The issue of "standing" has undergone a long litigation process and a synopsis of this issue has been compiled by the National Association of Biomedical Research. (24)

Other Relevant National and International Laws

Because animal research can involve a variety of different species, several other federal acts, laws, and treaties have bearing on animal use and their welfare, including:

- The US Endangered Species Act, restricting the research conducted on these animals to those that would directly benefit the species under investigation;
- The Marine Mammal Protection Act, which provides authority for scientific research on marine mammals by special permit;
- The Convention on International Trade in Endangered Species of Wild Fauna and Flora (CITES), requiring signator countries to obtain a permit for the import or export of certain species;
- The Lacey Act, which governs import, export and interstate commerce of foreign wildlife; and,
- The Migratory Bird Treaty Act, which makes it unlawful to take or possess any protected bird except by permit.

AAALAC International

The Association for Assessment and Accreditation of Laboratory Animal Care (AAALAC) International is a nonprofit organization incorporated in 1965. AAALAC's mission is to promote the humane treatment of animals in science through confidential, voluntary accreditation of animal care and use programs. The association is comprised of a board of trustees of more than 60 scientific organizations, patient advocacy groups, animal welfare organizations, and research lobby groups; a council on accreditation made up of veterinarians, animal researchers, research administrators, and facility managers who are experts in the field of laboratory animal science and medicine; and an office staff. The board of trustees sets the vision and general direction of the association, the Council on Accreditation is responsible for the conduct of site visits and for determining the accreditation status of institutions, and the office staff (United States and Europe) serves as a point of coordination of these activities and as an information resource to the laboratory animal using community.

AAALAC does not establish policies with which institutions must conform. Rather, AAALAC International relies principally on the *Guide*, as well as national laws, regulations, and policies, and numerous scientifically based standards, referred to as "reference resources," which address specific subject areas (e.g., recombinant DNA, surgery, euthanasia) for evaluation of animal care and use programs around the world. (25, 26) AAALAC International has developed a limited number of position statements pertaining to adequate veterinary care, occupational health and safety, multiple major survival surgical procedures, and *Cercopithecine herpesvirus*-1, to name a few, to provide clarification to the *Guide* and other resources. The accreditation process includes an extensive internal review conducted by the institution that is summarized in an animal care and use program description. On-site visits are announced and are conducted every three years. There is also an annual report requirement. The standards and process for accreditation are described in the association's Rules of Accreditation. Nonconformance with AAALAC International standards results in formal notification that full accreditation has not been granted and a provision of a timeline for correcting identified deficiencies. Revocation of accreditation can ultimately result from sustained nonconformance.

A Program Status Evaluation (PSE) service is also offered by AAALAC International. Former members of the Council on Accreditation and the associate director conduct these evaluations. The PSE is designed to assist institutions in determining if their animal care and use programs meet AAALAC International standards for accreditation. The PSE also familiarizes institutions around the world with the AAALAC accreditation process. It is more consultative than the accreditation site visit, and has occasionally been referred to as a "pre-AAALAC" visit.

Institute for Laboratory Animal Research

Founded in 1952, the Institute for Laboratory Animal Research (ILAR) is a component of the National Research Council, National Academy of Sciences. ILAR reports on subjects of importance to the animal care and use community through the use of expert committees, published in the quarterly *ILAR Journal*. In addition, the ILAR manages the Animal Models and Genetic Stocks Information Program, which includes the maintenance of an international database on Laboratory Registration Codes. In its role as a provider of information, ILAR reports have substantially shaped the standards of laboratory animal care and use. Foremost among these reports is the *Guide* currently in its seventh edition; it has been translated into six languages in addition to English. The *Guide* emphasizes performance standards, which define an outcome and provide criteria for assessing that outcome—standards less prescriptive than engineering standards (18).

The *Guide* provides direction on appropriation of institutional policies and responsibilities regarding general animal environment, housing, and management; veterinary care; and the physical plant. In addition, ILAR publications have addressed rodent management; dog management; the recognition and alleviation of pain and distress; the psychological well-being of nonhuman primates; monoclonal antibody production; cost containment methods for animal research facilities; and issues of occupational health and safety.

Good Laboratory Practice Regulations

The Food and Drug Administration (FDA) promulgates "Good Laboratory Practice Regulations" (21 CFR 58) for the conduct of animal experiments relating to existing pharmaceutical medicinal substances, food additives, or other chemicals. (27) Companion regulations for conducting studies relating to health effects, environmental effects, and chemical fate testing are found in GLP regulations administered by the Environmental Protection Agency (EPA). (28) Like the guidelines found within the AWRs and the *Guide*, both the FDA and EPA GLPs require that:

- Personnel using animals be appropriately trained and qualified to conduct the work.
- Animals be free of disease at the start of the study.
- Sanitation of animal cages and equipment occur at suitable intervals.
- Food and water be free of contaminants at levels higher than those specified in the protocol.

Adherence to the regulations is achieved primarily through voluntary compliance. Compliance is assessed through an active program of periodic inspections carried out by trained field inspectors. Serious noncompliance is dealt with by procedures ranging from study rejection to laboratory disqualification. (29)

Local and Institutional Oversight

Institutional oversight of an animal care and use program is influenced by the factors noted in the introduction, but the regulatory basis for institutional oversight is based on a mandated or voluntary adherence to the regulations and policies discussed in Section III (specifically, the AWRs, the PHS Policy, and the *Guide*). There are also many corollary policies, articles, and texts (see References) that facilitate understanding of pertinent issues (see References).

Lines of Responsibility/Authority

Unless otherwise indicated, the discussion below quotes or is derived from the AWRs and PHS Policy.

An institutional organization for managing and overseeing animal care and use must be compatible with institutional responsibilities under the regulations. The chief executive officer (CEO), the highest operating official of the organization, appoints or delegates specifically and in writing the responsibility to another to appoint, a minimum of three to five members to an Institutional Animal Care and Use Committee (IACUC). The institution must also designate an Institutional Official (IO) authorized (with the needed authority) to legally commit on behalf of the institution that regulatory requirements are met and that required reports, notifications, and assurances are accurate and submitted. The IACUC reports to the IO and through the IO to the regulatory agencies. The institution must also have a formal arrangement with an "attending veterinarian" (AV), who has appropriate training and credentials and direct or delegated authority and responsibility for activities involving animals at the institution. Most institutions do not combine for reasons of checks and balances the responsibilities of IO, AV, or IACUC chairperson in one or two persons, but such a combination may occur in some institutions. This basic administrative triumvirate is usually supported by animal care personnel, office staff, technicians, and offices of regulatory compliance; the latter are increasingly obtaining a prominent role in the coordination and support of institutional animal welfare compliance efforts. Effective organizations possess clear lines and definitions of authority, minimal potential for conflicts of interest, where neither the IO, the AV, the IACUC chairperson, nor the regulatory compliance officer(s) are more than one or two levels removed from the CEO in the chain of command.

The Institutional Animal Care and Use Committee

This critically important committee may have various names, but its considerable responsibilities and authority are clearly described in the AWRs, PHS Policy, and in the *Guide*. A comprehensive review of IACUC structure and function is found also in the *Institutional Animal Care and Use Committee Guidebook* (30) and *The IACUC Handbook*. Formally, the IACUC must include three (according to the AWRs) or five members (if covered by PHS Policy), including a veterinarian, practicing scientist, nonscientist, and person not affiliated in any way with the institution, except as an IACUC member.

Although there is no regulatory restriction on duration of IACUC service, most institutions' members serve one or two two- to three-year terms. There may be additional members and nonmember consultants to the committee. In any case, another institutional authority "may not approve an activity involving the care and use of animals if it has not been approved by the IACUC."

Primary responsibilities of the IACUC as effected by at least a majority of the members (i.e., a quorum) include:

- Review of the institution's animal care and use program and facilities (programmatic reviews have been traditionally a challenge for institutions).
- Submission of appropriate reports and recommendations to the IO; review and investigation of complaints regarding the programs.
- Review and approval, modification, or disapproval of proposed and ongoing activities related to animal care and use.
- Suspension of activities that do not comply with the AWRs, PHS Policy, the *Guide*, the assurance, or if so authorized, with state or local regulations or public relations imperatives.

Ultimately, the institution, not solely its IACUC, is responsible also for ensuring that the animal care and use procedures described in proposals to funding agencies are congruent with those in the corresponding institutional animal use protocols.

Program of Veterinary Care

If the institution uses species defined as "animals" in the AWRs, receives PHS support, is accredited by AAALAC International, or receives support from an entity requiring compliance with the AWRs or PHS Policy, both an IACUC and an AV position must be established.

A qualified veterinarian must be an IACUC member, but an appropriate program of "adequate veterinary care" may require two or more veterinarians, a support staff, supplies and equipment, and facilities. The veterinarian(s) must:

- Have appropriate programmatic authority and ready access to animals to observe animals;
- Possess the ability to prevent, control, diagnose, and treat diseases and injuries at all times;
- Have the ability to receive and communicate timely information about animal health;
- Provide guidance regarding handling, immobilization, management of pain relief and distress, euthanasia, disease recognition; and,

- Provide guidance regarding management of occupational health and safety, periprocedural recognition, and record keeping.

In situations requiring measures to ensure animal well-being, veterinarians may intervene in the conduct of an approved study, including the decision to stop a study to treat or even euthanize animals, assuming timely concurrence of the IACUC. This prerogative, however, should be described in institutional policy and noted in the program for veterinary care submitted to APHIS/AC.

Training Programs

The US Government Principles (16) mentioned in Section III include the requirement that "Investigators and other personnel shall be appropriately qualified and experienced for conducting procedures on living animals." The AWRs, PHS Policy, and the *Guide* amplify this mandate. Almost everyone associated with an animal care and use program must be trained (or closely supervised by one who is) when working with and around animals. Groups and individuals to receive appropriate training are IACUC members; investigators, instructors, and their assistants; animal care personnel; veterinarians; all persons at risk from hazards in the animal and work environment; and institutional officials with animal program responsibilities. Many training modalities may be used, but ultimately the institution and the IACUC must determine that "Personnel conducting procedures on the species being maintained or studied will be appropriately qualified and trained in those procedures" (18) and that "Personnel at risk should be provided with clearly defined procedures for conducting their duties, should understand the hazards involved, and should be proficient in implementing the required standards." Required or suggested content for training courses are provided in the AWRs and in other publications.

Reporting Deficiencies

PHS Policy states that the IACUC, through the IO, shall promptly report to OLAW with an explanation of circumstances, a plan and schedule for correction of serious or continuing noncompliance (with PHS Policy), serious deviations from provisions of the *Guide*, or suspension of an activity by the IACUC. The AWRs require that noncompliant circumstances that threaten the health or safety of animals that are not corrected according to an IACUC plan and schedule be reported to APHIS/AC within fifteen business days of the determination of noncompliance.

In addition, the AWRs [Section 2.32 (c) (4)] include instruction regarding, "Methods whereby deficiencies in animal care and treatment are reported" that underscores the point that "No facility employee, Committee [IACUC] member, or laboratory personnel shall be discriminated against or be subject to any reprisal for reporting violations." The institution must provide for the promulgation of this requirement and for careful processing of complaints received as a result. This process, as with many other processes mentioned in this chapter, may require a supporting institutional policy compatible with relevant regulations.

Open Meeting and Freedom of Information Laws

All states, the District of Columbia, and the federal government have open meeting or "sunshine" laws that allow public access to certain group meetings to discuss public business. (31) Similarly, IACUC meetings in public institutions may be subject to such a law. Laws differ among the states, and some laws allow closed meetings for specified purposes, such as discussions of proprietary information, personnel and certain legal matters, and other topics (e.g., visitors may be allowed to attend meetings, but not be permitted to take part in discussions or to address the IACUC members).

In addition, Freedom of Information laws allow public access to documents of state agencies (and in some states, entities receiving state funds) and of the federal government (but not necessarily to entities receiving federal funds). Request procedures for documents (animal use protocols, IACUC meeting minutes, animal acquisition records, and records of semiannual reviews) vary among states and targeted state agencies may argue that release of requested information is not in the public's interest or that state-mandated exemptions to release of certain categories of information apply. There is usually a charge for preparing documents for release (31).

Conclusions

Quality science demands quality animal care. Because the goal of biomedical research is that of good science, it is within the best interest of all research institutions to have a high quality animal care and use program. There are ethical, legal, and public relations reasons for ensuring that programs using animals in research, testing, and teaching meet contemporary standards and guidelines for animal use.

No animal care program can be successful unless personnel using or caring for animals are well-qualified by training or through experience. Lines of authority, policies, and procedures for animal care and use programs should be set forth in writing, be well understood, and must be adhered to by all personnel. Administration must remain fully aware of the status of the animal care and use program. A quality animal care and use program requires the integrated support of many persons that make up the research team, including institutional officials, program investigators and their research technicians, veterinarians, and the animal care staff. Sustained and visible support from institutional officials and other research administrators is essential to establishing and maintaining a high quality program as they are in positions to influence institutional priorities and ensure that appropriate and adequate resources are allocated to the program. (32)

• • • References

1. American Veterinary Medical Association. "Policy on Animal Welfare and Animal Rights." In *AVMA Directory*, 71. Schaumburg, IL: The Association, 2003.

2. Tannenbaum, J. *Veterinary Ethics—Animal Welfare, Client Relations, Competition and Collegiality*. 2nd ed. New York: Mosby, 1995.

3. Foundation for Biomedical Research. "Animal Welfare vs. Animal Rights," 2003, http://www.fbresearch.org/animal-activism/welfare-vs-rights.htm (accessed August 16, 2005).

4. Bishop, K. "From Shop to Lab to Farm, Animal Rights Battle Is Felt," *New York Times*, January 14, 1989.

5. Beauchamp, T.L. "Philosophical Foundations." In *Bioethics and the Use of Laboratory Animals: Ethics in Theory and Practice*, edited by A.L. Kraus and D. Renquist, 1–13. Dubuque, IA: Gregory C. Benoit Publishing, 2000.

6. Singer, P. *Animal Liberation: A New Ethic for Our Treatment of Animals*. 2nd ed. New York: New York Review of Books, 1990.

7. McPherson, C.W. "Laws, Regulations, and Policies Affecting the Use of Laboratory Animals." In *Laboratory Animal Medicine*, edited by J.G. Fox, B.J. Cohen, and F.M. Loew, 19–30. New York: Academic Press, Inc., 1984.

8. Foundation for Biomedical Research. "The Pet Theft Myth," 2003, http://www.fbresearch.org/education/pet-theft-myth.htm (accessed August 16, 2005).

9. *Animal Welfare Act of 1966*, Public Law 89-544 and its amendments, U.S. Code, 7 (1966) § 2131–2157 et seq.

10. Anderson, L.C. "Laws, Regulations, and Policies Affecting the use of Laboratory Animals." In *Laboratory Animal Medicine*, edited by J.G. Fox, L.C. Anderson, et al., 19–33. New York: Academic Press, 2002.

11. Brown, G.E. "Thirty Years of the Animal Welfare Act." In *Animal Welfare Act 1966-1996: Historical Perspectives and Future Directions*, edited by M. Kreger, D. Jensen, and T. Allen, 11–15. Washington, DC: WARDS; 1996.

12. Bayne, K. and P. deGreeve. "An Overview of Global Legislation, Regulation, and Policies on the Use of Animals for Scientific Research, Testing, or Education." In *Handbook of Laboratory Animal Science*, Vol. 1, Essential Principles and Practices, 2nd ed., edited by J. Hau and G.L. Van Hoosier Jr., 31–50. New York: CRC Press, 2003.

13. Animal Welfare Act. *Code of Federal Regulations*. Title 9 (Animals and Animal Products), Subchapter A (Animal Welfare) (1985).

14. Johnson, D.K., M.L. Martin, K.A.L. Bayne, and T.L. Wolfle. "Laws, Regulations, and Policies." In *Nonhuman Primates in Biomedical Research: Biology and Management*, edited by B.T. Bennett, C.R. Abee, and R. Henrickson. 15–31. New York: Academic Press, Inc., 1995.

15. Johnson, D.K. and M.L. Morin. "U.S. Laws, Regulations, and Policies Important to Managers of Nonhuman Primate Colonies." *J. Med. Primatol* 12 (1983): 223–238.

16. Interagency Research Animal Committee. "U.S. Government Principles for the Utilization and Care of Vertebrate Animals Used in Testing, Research, and Training," *Federal Register* 50, no. 97, May 20, 1985, Washington, DC: Office of Science and Technology Policy.

17. Office of Laboratory Animal Welfare, National Institutes of Health. *Public Health Service Policy on Humane Care and Use of Laboratory Animals*. Bethesda, MD, 1986 (revised 2002), http://grants.nih.gov/grants/olaw/references/phspol.htm (accessed August 31, 2005).

18. National Research Council. *Guide for the Care and Use of Laboratory Animals*. Washington, DC: National Academy Press, 1996.

19. American Veterinary Medical Association. "2000 Report of the AVMA Panel on Euthanasia." *J. Amer. Vet. Med. Assoc.* 218 (2001): 669–696.

20. Rozmiarek, H. "Origins of the IACUC." In *The IACUC Handbook*, edited by J. Silverman, M.A. Suckow, and S. Murthy, 1–9. New York: CRC Press LLC, 2000.

21. Department of Defense. "Use of Laboratory Animals in DoD Programs," Directive Number 3216.1, 1995.

22. U.S. Congress, Office of Technology Assessment. "State Regulation of Animal Use." In: *Alternatives to Animal Use in Research, Testing, and Education*, 305–331. Washington, DC: Government Printing Office, OTA-BA-273; 1986.

23. Bayne, K. "Developing Guidelines on the Care and Use of Animals." *Annals of the New York Academy of Sciences* 862 (1998): 105–110.

24. National Association for Biomedical Research. "Private Right of Action and Standing Under the Animal Welfare Act," 2005, http://www.nabr.org/AnimalLaw/Proposals/ (accessed August 16, 2005).

25. Bayne, K. and J.G. Miller. "Assessing Animal Care and Use Programs Internationally." *Lab Animal* 29, no. 6 (2000): 27–29.

26. Bayne, K. and D.P. Martin. "AAALAC International: Using Performance Standards to Evaluate an Animal Care and Use Program." *Lab Animal* 27, no. 4 (1998): 32–35.

27. *Code of Federal Regulations*. Title 21: Food and Drugs; Chapter 1: Food and Drug Administration, Department of Health and Human Services; Subchapter A: General; Part 58: Good Laboratory Practice for Nonclinical Laboratory Studies (rev. 1998) http://www.access.gpo.gov/nara/cfr/waisidx_01/21cfr58_01.html (accessed August 31, 2005).

28. *Code of Federal Regulations*. Title 40: Protection of the Environment; Chapter 1: Environmental Protection Agency; Subchapter E: Pesticide Programs; Part 160: Good Laboratory Practice Standards (rev. 1997) http://ecfr.gpoaccess.gov/cgi/t/text/text-idx?c=ecfr&sid=b9b607af1eab55c20d813ffe4a146ee7&rgn=div5&view=text&node=40:23.0.1.1.10&idno=40 (accessed August 31, 2005).

29. Office of Laboratory Animal Welfare, National Institutes of Health. "Memorandum of Understanding Among the Animal and Plant Health Inspection Service, U.S. Department of Agriculture and the Food and Drug Administration, U.S. Department of Health and Human Services and the National Institutes of Health, U.S. Department of Health and Human Services Concerning Laboratory Animal Welfare," 2001, http://grants1.nih.gov/grants/olaw/references/finalmou.htm (accessed August 16, 2005).

30. ARENA/OLAW. *Institutional Animal Care and Use Committee Guidebook*. 2nd ed. Washington, DC: US Government Printing Office, 2002.

31. The Reporters Committee for Freedom of the Press. "Freedom of Information Acts." In *The First Amendment Handbook*. The Reporters Committee for Freedom of the Press: Arlington, VA, 2003, http://www.rcfp.org/handbook/viewpage.cgi (accessed August 16, 2005).

32. National Institutes of Health. *Institutional Administrator's Manual for Laboratory Animal Care and Use*. NIH Publication No. 88-2959, 1988.

56

Environmental Health and Safety

Matthew D. Finucane, MS, CIH

Introduction

Environmental health and safety issues are integral to the satisfactory management of sponsored programs. Increasingly, sponsors require that institutions provide written assurances that they are in compliance with a myriad of federal, state, and local laws and regulations, and that they meet granting agency and sponsor guidelines. Sponsored program directors must also establish procedures to consult with environmental health and safety professionals to provide the expertise needed to protect the institution from misrepresenting the institution's compliance status. The health and safety assurances must often be integrated into other regulatory requirements; for example, assurances needed to obtain both institutional biological safety committee (IBC) approval of human gene transfer experiments, as well as approval of the institutional review board (IRB).

Mandated compliance requirements in the environmental health areas have developed over time, as have compliance requirements in other areas. For example, the US Army Medical Research and Materiel Command (USAMRMC) now mandates the submission of a certificate of environmental compliance for each proposal; NIH requires the submission of an animal welfare assurance for:

all research, research training, experimentation, biological testing, and related activities, hereinafter referred to as activities, involving live, vertebrate animals supported by the Public Health Service (PHS) and conducted at this institution, or

at another institution as a consequence of the subgranting or subcontracting of a PHS-conducted or supported activity by this institution.[1]

Such assurances provide a convenient model to describe a comprehensive safety program to effectively support sponsored programs.

Environmental Protection

The receipt of federal support, whether through grants, cooperative agreements, or contacts, may trigger the National Environmental Policy Act of 1969 (NEPA).[2] Under NEPA, the federal agency providing funds may conduct an environmental assessment (EA) to determine if an environmental impact statement (EIS) is warranted, based on the activities associated with the funding. Should an EIS be required, the institution receiving the funding is required to devote significant resources in order to provide answers to complete the EIS. The EIS is conducted by the funding agency, usually through its own and/or contractor resources. However, much of the information needed must be supplied by the institution receiving funding. A partial list of the major laws reviewed in an EIS includes:

- Endangered Species Act
- The Clean Air Act (CAA); 42 U.S.C. s/s 7401 et seq. (1970)
- The Clean Water Act (CWA); 33 U.S.C. ss/1251 et seq. (1977)

- Comprehensive Environmental Response, Compensation, and Liability Act (CERCLA or Superfund) 42 U.S.C. s/s 9601 et seq. (1980)
- The Superfund Amendments and Reauthorization Act (SARA); 42 U.S.C.9601 et seq. (1986)

Each of these laws has proscriptive requirements that institutions must meet. If any of the activities to be funded has the potential of violating environmental impact laws, the institution must develop measures to mitigate any impact on the environment.

Fortunately, most funding decisions do not require funding agencies to conduct EAs; however, grantees must still comply with many federal, state, and local laws and regulations, and in many instances must comply with guidelines that are, for all intents and purposes, regulations. An overview of the salient laws, regulations, and guidelines that affect an institution's compliance status is provided in the following section.

Workplace Safety and Health

The Occupational Health and Safety Act of 1970[3] created the Occupational Safety and Health Administration (OSHA), and the standards and regulations promulgated by OSHA govern workplace safety and health for private employers. Many states have chosen to assume the responsibility for enforcement of safety and health standards in place of OSHA through state plans. A state may choose to cover state workers as well as private employers under its OSHA state plan. Some states and territories (Connecticut, New Jersey, New York, and the Virgin Islands) have state or territorial plans that cover only public employees, whereas federal government employees are covered by Executive Order 12196.[4] Wherever they are located, grantees are obliged to comply with the health and safety regulations that are relevant in the locale where the research is conducted (e.g., research conducted in mines or quarries would be governed by regulations promulgated by the US Mine Safety and Health Administration [MSHA],[5] which are different than OSHA regulations). State plan regulations may also be more stringent than federal regulations; for example, local codes and regulations such as fire and building codes may place additional requirements on the use, storage, and disposal of hazardous materials. The safe conduct of research often has regulatory and guideline requirements that are different than those of commercial or industrial activities. Each proposal should be evaluated to assure that all safety and compliance issues are addressed for each location where research will be conducted.

The safety evaluation of research proposals requires the participation of individuals with expertise in the many different areas. Safety and health committees with representation from across the institution are a mechanism to conduct the comprehensive reviews that may be needed. Depending on the types of research materials used, there are specific requirements for types of safety committees and the composition of those committees. The requirements for each committee will be discussed in the general categories of research below. Given the dynamic nature of regulations and guidelines and research itself, institutions must continually review safety requirements to assure they understand sponsor expectations. Safety and health programs must have stated objectives and defined responsibilities through program administration.

Safety and Health Program Policy

Institutions should develop an overarching policy statement, signed by senior management, which clearly states the goals, objectives, and responsibilities of the institution's safety and health program(s). Ideally, such a statement is no more than one page and commits the institution only to goals that are achievable.

The policy statement should succinctly state management's commitment to the policy and that all personnel associated with the institution must adhere to goals, objectives, and responsibilities as outlined within the policy. A single entity, for example, as the institution's safety and health office, should be identified as responsible for coordination of the policy under the direction of a safety and health committee(s) that, in turn, advises and reports to senior management. The purpose of the policy must be clearly stated as should the scope of the policy.

There are many safety and health programs that generally fall beyond the scope of sponsored research programs, such as underground storage tanks and air permits for stationary sources, that need not be part of sponsored program reviews, except in those cases where the federal government sponsor requires an environmental impact statement. There are, however, several programs that should be considered at a minimum in sponsored research. They are:

Biological Safety:

- Pathogenic agents
- rDNA
- Human gene transfer
- Bloodborne pathogens
- Select agents

Chemical Safety:

- Chemical hygiene plan
- Hazard communications

Radiation Safety:

- Radioactive materials (RAM)
- Machine produced ionizing radiation
- Non-ionizing radiation
- Radioactive waste

Environmental Management:

- Hazardous waste disposal
- Biohazardous/medical waste
- Chemical waste

No list can be all-inclusive because research by its very nature entails working at the frontier of knowledge (in uncharted territory) and, therefore, may create unanticipated hazards. A thoughtful review process with appropriate risk assessments minimizes unpleasant surprises.

Biological Safety

Pathogens The purpose of biological safety is to establish safe laboratory practices, procedures, and the proper use of containment equipment and facilities by laboratory workers in a biological/biomedical environment to prevent occupationally-acquired infections or release of organisms to the environment. Biological safety is the responsibility of everyone who manipulates pathogenic microorganisms and recombinant DNA molecules.

Risk assessment is a fundamental principal of biological safety. The principal investigator or laboratory director must conduct a risk assessment to determine the proper work practices and containment requirements for work with biological materials. The risk assessment process must identify the

inherent ability of microorganism to cause disease as well as the host range and environmental factors that influence the potential for health effects in humans, animals, and plants.

The National Institutes of Health (NIH) Office of Biotechnology Activities provides criteria to be used in risk assessment in the "NIH Recombinant DNA Guidelines":[6]

Basis for the Classification of Biohazardous Agents by Risk Group (RG)

Risk Group 1 (RG1) - Agents that are not associated with disease in healthy adult humans

Risk Group 2 (RG2) - Agents that are associated with human disease which is rarely serious and for which preventive or therapeutic interventions are often available

Risk Group 3 (RG3) - Agents that are associated with serious or lethal human disease for which preventive or therapeutic interventions may be available (high individual risk but low community risk)

Risk Group 4 (RG4) - Agents that are likely to cause serious or lethal human disease for which preventive or therapeutic interventions are not usually available (high individual risk and high community risk).

The American Biological Safety Association (ABSA) also provides guidance on conducting risk assessment that includes references to international standards.[7] Factors to consider when evaluating risk include the following:

Pathogenicity. The more severe the potentially acquired disease, the higher the risk.

Route of transmission. Agents capable of transmission by the aerosol route are known to cause the most laboratory-acquired infections. Therefore, the greater the aerosol potential, the higher the risk of infection.

Agent stability. The greater the potential for an agent to survive in the general environment, the higher the risk. Factors including desiccation, exposure to sunlight or ultraviolet light, or exposure to chemical disinfections must be considered when looking at the stability of an agent.

Infectious dose. The amount of an agent needed to cause infection in a normal person must be considered. An infectious dose can vary from one to hundreds of thousands of organisms or infectious units. An individual's immune status can also influence the infectious dose.

Concentration. Consider whether the organisms are in solid tissue, viscous blood, sputum, etc.; the volume of the material; and the laboratory work planned (amplification of the material, sonication, centrifugation, etc.). In most instances, the risk increases as the concentration of microorganisms increases.

Origin. This may refer to the geographic location (domestic or foreign), host (infected or uninfected human or animal), or nature of the source (potential zoonotic or associated with a disease outbreak).

Availability of data from animal studies. If human data is not available, information on the pathogenicity, infectivity, and route of exposure from animal studies may be valuable. Use caution when translating infectivity data from one species to another.

Availability of an effective prophylaxis or therapeutic intervention. Effective vaccines, if available, must be offered to laboratory and animal care and maintenance personnel in advance of their potential exposure to putative infectious material. However, immunization does not replace engineering controls, proper practices and procedures, and the use of personal protective equipment (PPE). The availability of post-exposure prophylaxis should also be considered.

Medical surveillance. Medical surveillance programs may include monitoring employee health status, participating in post-exposure management, employee counseling prior to offering vaccination, and annual physicals.

Experience and skill level of at-risk personnel. Laboratory workers must become proficient in specific tasks prior to working with microorganisms. Laboratory workers may have to train with noninfectious materials in trial runs to ensure they have or develop the appropriate skill level prior to working with hazardous materials. Laboratory and animal care workers may have to go through additional training (e.g., Biological Safety Level-3 training, etc.) before they are permitted to work with certain materials or in a designated facility.

Inherent in risk assessment is the concept of containment of hazardous agents. The Centers for Disease Control (CDC) describes four biological safety levels (BSLs), which consist of combinations of laboratory practices and techniques, safety equipment, and laboratory facilities. Each combination is specifically appropriate for the operations performed; for the documented or suspected routes of transmission of the infectious agents; and for the laboratory function or activity. The recommended biological safety level for an organism represents the conditions under which the agent ordinarily can be handled safely. When specific information is available to suggest that virulence, pathogenicity, antibiotic resistance patterns, vaccine and treatment availability, or other factors are significantly altered, more (or less) stringent practices may be specified.

- *Biological Safety Level 1* (BSL-1) is appropriate for work done with defined and characterized strains of viable microorganisms not known to cause disease in healthy adult humans. It represents a basic level of containment that relies on standard microbiological practices with no special primary or secondary barriers recommended, other than a sink for hand washing.

- *Biological Safety Level 2* (BSL-2) is applicable to work done with a broad spectrum of indigenous moderate-risk agents present in the community and associated with human disease of varying severity. Agents can be used safely on the open bench, provided the potential for producing splashes or aerosols is low. Primary hazards to personnel working with these agents relate to accidental percutaneous or mucous membrane exposures or ingestion of infectious materials. Procedures with high aerosol or splash potential must be conducted in primary containment equipment such as biological safety cabinets. Primary barriers such as splash shields, face protection, gowns, and gloves should be used as appropriate. Secondary barriers such as hand washing and waste decontamination facilities must be available.

- *Biological Safety Level 3* (BSL-3) is applicable to work done with indigenous or exotic agents with a potential for respiratory transmission and which may cause serious and potentially lethal infection. Primary hazards to personnel working with these agents (i.e., *Mycobacterium tuberculosis*, *St. Louis encephalitis virus*, and *Coxiella burnetii*) include auto-inoculation, ingestion, and exposure to infectious aerosols. Greater emphasis is placed on primary and secondary barriers to protect personnel in adjoining areas, the community, and the environment from exposure to infectious aerosols. For example, all laboratory manipulations should be performed in a biological safety cabinet or other enclosed equipment. Secondary barriers include controlled access to the laboratory and a specialized ventilation system that minimizes the release of infectious aerosols from the laboratory.

- *Biological Safety Level 4* (BSL-4) is applicable for work with dangerous and exotic agents that pose a high individual risk of life-threatening disease, which may be transmitted via the aerosol route and for which there is no available vaccine or therapy. Agents with close or identical antigenic relationship to BSL-4 agents should also be handled at this level. Primary hazards to workers include respiratory exposure to infectious aerosols, mucous membrane exposure to infectious droplets, and auto-inoculation. All manipulations of potentially infected materials and isolates pose a high risk of exposure and infection to personnel, the community, and the environment. Isolation of aerosolized infectious materials is accomplished primarily by working in a Class III biological safety cabinet or a full-body, air-supplied positive pressure personnel suit. The facility is generally a separate building or a completely isolated zone within a complex with specialized ventilation and waste management systems to prevent release of viable agents to the environment. Few institutions have facilities that can support work at BSL-4.

Vertebrate Animal Biological Safety Levels (ABSLs) There are four animal biological safety levels for work with infectious agents in mammals. The levels are combinations of practices, safety equipment, and facilities for experiments on animals infected with agents that produce or may produce human infection. In general, the biological safety level recommended for working with an infectious agent *in vivo* and *in vitro* is comparable.

- *Animal Biological Safety Level 1* (ABSL-1) is suitable for work involving well characterized agents that are not known to cause disease in healthy adult humans, and that are of minimal potential hazard to laboratory personnel and the environment.
- *Animal Biological Safety Level 2* (ABSL-2) is suitable for work with those agents associated with human disease. It addresses hazards from ingestion as well as from percutaneous and mucous membrane exposure.
- *Animal Biological Safety Level 3* (ABSL-3) is suitable for work with animals infected with indigenous or exotic agents that present the potential of aerosol transmission and of causing serious or potentially lethal disease.
- *Animal Biological Safety Level 4* (ABSL-4) is suitable for addressing dangerous and exotic agents that pose high risk of life-threatening disease, aerosol transmission, or related agents with unknown risk of transmission. Few institutions have facilities that can support work at ABSL-4.

Complete descriptions of all biological safety Levels and Animal Biological Safety Levels are outlined in the 4th edition of *Biological Safety in Microbiological and Biomedical Laboratories* published by the US Department of Health and Human Services.[8]

Recombinant DNA Molecules Institutions receiving any federal funding for research that plan to use or construct recombinant DNA (rDNA) molecules must comply with the NIH Guidelines for Research Involving Recombinant DNA Molecules (NIH Guidelines).[9] The Recombinant DNA Advisory Committee is the public advisory committee that advises the Department of Health and Human Services (DHHS) Secretary, the DHHS Assistant Secretary for Health, and the NIH Director concerning recombinant DNA research.[10] The guidelines, while not regulations, have the force of regulations in that an institution could lose all or part of its federal funding for not adhering to them. Many of the risks governed by the guidelines are similar to those for work with pathogens and require similar risk assessments. Compliance with the guidelines requires the appointment of an institutional biosafety committee and adhering to a delineated approval process. There are:

> ...six categories of experiments involving recombinant DNA: (i) those that require Institutional Biosafety Committee (IBC) approval, RAC review, and NIH Director approval before initiation, (ii) those that require NIH/OBA and Institutional Biosafety Committee approval before initiation, (iii) those that require Institutional Biosafety Committee and Institutional Review Board approvals and RAC review before research participant enrollment, (iv) those that require Institutional Biosafety Committee approval before initiation, (v) those that require Institutional Biosafety Committee notification simultaneous with initiation, and (vi) those that are exempt from the NIH Guidelines.[11]

Human Gene Transfer (Human Gene Therapy) Particular care must be taken in the case of human gene transfer protocols experiments. These experiments require an extraordinary amount of coordination between the IRB and the IBC. Changes made by the principal investigator at the behest of either IBC or IRB may have to be rereviewed and reapproved by each committee. Adverse event reporting must also be coordinated with all relevant administrative committees. Failure to do so may put the institution afoul of the NIH or the Food and Drug Administration (FDA) or both.

Bloodborne Pathogens OSHA has a specific standard to deal with occupational exposure to bloodborne pathogens (BBP) for employees, including faculty.[12] Bloodborne pathogens are pathogenic microorganisms that are present in human blood and can cause disease in humans including but not limited to hepatitis B virus (HBV), hepatitis C virus (HCV), and human immunodeficiency virus (HIV). The standard requires training, a written "Exposure Control Plan," offering hepatitis B vaccination, among other requirements.

Select Agents and Toxins The Public Health Security and Bioterrorism Preparedness and Response Act of 2002 (Public Law 107-188)[13] placed restriction on the possession, use, and transfer of certain materials designated as "select agents" and "toxins." This law and a previous federal law, the US Patriot Act,[14] imposed criminal and civil penalties for unregistered possession of select agents and toxins and restricted access to select agents and toxins. The Department of Agriculture[15] and the Department of Health and Human Services[16] have published final rules about select agents and toxins.

It is important to be aware that a section of the US Patriot Act[17] requires the possession of biological agents be restricted to use for *bona fide* purposes. Therefore, researchers must be told that the storage of biological agents without specific plans for their use is unlawful and can lead to arrest.

Chemical Safety in the Laboratory/Research Area

Chemical Hygiene Plan

The use of chemicals in laboratories is regulated by the OSHA standard (29 CFR1910.1450), "Occupational exposure to hazardous chemicals in laboratories (Lab Standard),"[18] whereby institutions must develop and implement a written institution-specific set of safety requirements called a chemical hygiene plan (CHP). The CHP must protect lab workers from the health hazards associated with chemicals used in the institution's labs. When institutions choose not to develop and implement a chemical hygiene plan they must comply with standards specific to each substance used in labs. In general, substance-specific standards are more burdensome than instituting a CHP. The CHP

must be capable of protecting employees from health hazards associated with all hazardous chemicals in laboratories; must maintain employee exposures to chemicals below the permissible exposure limits (PELs), as specified in the Subpart Z of the OSHA standards;[19] and must be readily available to employees, employee representatives, and OSHA inspectors. The CHP must also include:

- Standard operating procedures relevant to hazardous chemicals in the lab.
- Designation of a chemical hygiene officer (CHO), who is an employee of the institution (consultants may not be retained to serve as the CHO) and who is qualified by training or experience to provide technical guidance in the development and implementation of the provisions of the Chemical Hygiene Plan. If appropriate, a chemical hygiene committee should also be established.
- Stipulation of control measures that the employer will use to reduce exposures to hazardous chemicals to keep lab worker exposures below the limits specified in the OSHA standards, include:
  - Fume hoods and other containment or protective equipment used in labs;
  - Training and information about hazardous chemicals and the content of the chemical hygiene plan;
  - Provisions for additional protective measures for employees working with particular hazardous substances such as select carcinogens, reproductive toxins, and acutely toxic materials;
  - Medical exams and consultations for employees using hazardous chemicals; and,
  - Appropriate and proper employee protective measures for particularly hazardous chemicals.

All employers, including colleges and universities, are subject to OSHA regulation except public employers in states without federal-state OSHA agreement plans. However, prudent safety practices dictate similar procedures and practices for all laboratories. Employers must understand that OSHA enforcement actions can be based on the employer's written CHP. Therefore, the CHP should be simple, easy to understand, and easy to implement. OSHA provides a fact sheet about hazardous chemicals in labs on its Web site.[20] The CHP should be considered a part of a hazard communication program.

Worker Right-to-Know (Hazard Communications)

There are state and local worker right-to-know programs that predate OSHA's Hazard Communication Standard[21] and the Lab Standard. Worker right-to-know (RTK) laws and regulations were adopted to assure that information concerning chemical hazards employers and employees. Localities may not have adopted OSHA's Lab Standard for public employees, therefore, RTK regulations may govern the use of hazardous chemicals in sponsored research. RTK regulations require that hazardous materials be labeled, that Material Safety Data Sheets (MSDSs) be available, and that training be provided to employees in the hazards of the chemicals used and how to use MSDSs. Initial training and training whenever new chemicals are introduced are required. There may also be requirements for periodic training in some locales.

RTK regulations require chemical suppliers to provide hazard information through MSDSs and labels for chemical purchasers. RTKs require a written hazards communication program similar to the CHPs. RTK laws may require reporting hazard information and chemical inventories to fire and/or police departments. There may also be provisions for public assess to hazard information. Additionally, providing hazard information and inventories are often mandated by local fire and building codes independent of RTK laws.

Radiation Safety

Ionizing radiation produced by radioactive materials (RAM) and radiation-producing devices is potentially hazardous and as a consequence their use is stringently controlled through federal and state laws and regulations. Despite the strict requirements for its use, ionizing radiation is a common tool in research and medicine. Institutions using radioactive materials or radiation-producing devices develop and implement controls such that their use does not create health hazards. A written program describing mandated administrative and operational controls constitutes the radiation safety program. The basic elements of a radiation safety program are discussed below.

Licensing and Registration Requirements

The use of radioactive materials (RAM) requires licensing with the appropriate regulatory agency before RAM may be received. Both the type of ionizing radiation and the state in which the institution is located determine which agency issues the license. In most states, the Nuclear Regulatory Commission

(NRC) regulates special nuclear material (plutonium, uranium, and by-product material, which is chemically or physically separated fission product material). Machine source radioactive materials (such as those produced by cyclotrons or linear accelerators) are regulated by state departments of health or environmental protection. The NRC has a number of guides available on its Web site to assist in developing programs for compliance.[24] States may also have information available at their Web sites.

In order to obtain appropriate licensing, institutions must determine the types of RAM needed. Institutions that require limited amounts of RAM for specific uses generally receive licenses that prescribe in detail how the RAM will be used and who may use it. Larger institutions that have greater diversity in RAM use and that have more procedures in place may apply for and receive broad scope licensure.

As mentioned previously, a written radiation safety program governing the use of all radioactive materials must be developed. A radiation safety officer (RSO) must be designated. The RSO need not be an employee of the institution. A radiation safety committee (RSC) must be established for broad scope license activities. This committee is composed of the RSO, a management representative, and members of the personnel who have experience or training in the use of RAM. The RSC has the authority and responsibility to review and approve all uses of radioactive material at the institution. In addition, the RSC establishes institutional policies and oversees the operation of the radiation safety program.

Machine source ionizing radiation (e.g., X-rays) is found in science and engineering research laboratories, as well as in medical and dental facilities. State departments of health or environmental protection generally regulate machine source ionizing radiation. States may require that each X-ray producing device be registered.

Personnel Training

Current federal regulations mandate training for individuals likely to receive, within a year, an occupational radiation dose in excess of 1 mSv (100 mrem).[25] States have adopted similar regulations regarding the training of those working with or near radiation sources. The types of personnel requiring training may include such diverse groups as laboratory personnel, custodians, maintenance personnel, and construction workers, as well as various emergency personnel. Stipulations in individual institution licenses may obligate the institution to meet more stringent training requirements.

Accountability for Materials and Devices

Institutions authorized to use RAM must maintain an accurate account of the types and quantities of these radiation sources in their possession at any given time. Large institutions possessing a variety of radiation sources may require complex systems for tracking the possession, use, and disposal of RAM.

Radiation Surveys

Institutions using RAM are required by state and federal regulations to perform periodic surveys of all areas where RAM is used or stored. The frequency of surveys is determined by risk posed by RAM in an area. The frequency may also be stipulated in the institution's license.

Personnel Monitoring

Personnel dosimeters are devices worn to measure external radiation doses. Federal and state regulations require the use of monitoring devices for workers who are likely to receive 10% of the regulatory dose limit. All personnel monitoring results must be maintained by the institution and available to individuals upon request. In addition, personnel monitoring results are routinely distributed to the licensee and should be posted in the areas where RAM is used. When using radioactive material, accidental intakes may occur. These exposures can occur as a result of a spill or surface contamination, or as a result of using volatile radioactive materials such iodine and tritium. If volatile radioactive materials are used, the institution's license may require a bioassay program to assess internal radiation dose assessment in people.[26] Bioassay determines the kinds, quantities or concentrations, and, in some cases, the locations of radioactive material in the human body, whether by direct measurement or by analysis materials excreted from the humans. At research institutions a common method of bioassay is thyroid counting for radioactive iodine.

Radioactive Waste Management

Radioactive materials waste management is a demanding and expensive element of a radiation safety program. There are high per unit volume costs for commercially disposing of radioactive wastes costs. Considerable effort should be directed at minimizing RAM waste generation and maximizing the use of local treatment and disposal options to reduce the total volumes requiring commercial disposal. The options such as compaction and decaying short-lived materials in storage, and methods involving small releases to the environment, such as incineration and disposal by way of the sanitary sewer, are labor and capital intensive. Disposal methods involving radioactive releases to the environment, however, are strictly controlled by federal and state regulations and must often be specifically approved in the institution's license.

Nonionizing Radiation

The control of potential hazards related to the use of sources of nonionizing radiation such as lasers, microwave ovens, microwave antennae, radiofrequency (RF) induction furnaces, ultraviolet radiation sources, magnetic resonance devices, and sputtering devices must be integrated in health and safety programs. In many cases no state or federal regulations mandate the control of nonionizing radiation. However, consensus standards such as those of the American National Standards Institute standard on the safe use of lasers and the American Conference of Government Industrial Hygienist Threshold Limit Value (TLV) magnetic fields have been established.[27,28] Many guidelines have been adopted by institutions to control hazards to a recognized acceptable level.

Environmental Management

Hazardous Waste Management

Hazardous Waste Defined   Hazardous materials have hazardous characteristics such as: flammable, corrosive, reactive, toxic, radioactive, poisonous, carcinogenic, or infectious. In a general sense, these materials are considered hazardous because they present a potential risk to humans and/or the environment. A waste is basically any discarded material. By law, a hazardous waste is defined as a waste, or combination of wastes, that, because of quantity, concentration, or physical, chemical, or infectious characteristics, may cause or significantly contribute to an increase in serious irreversible, or incapacitating reversible illness or pose a substantial present or potential hazard to human health, safety, or welfare, or to the environment when improperly treated, stored, transported, used, or disposed of or otherwise managed. Hazardous waste management plans generally separate waste into three broad groups: radioactive, chemical, and biological. This section addresses only chemical waste.

Hazardous waste includes a wide range of material, including discarded commercial chemical products, process wastes, and wastewater. Some chemicals and chemical mixtures are hazardous wastes because they are specifically listed as such by the EPA. Most of the common laboratory solvents are listed wastes. A chemical waste that is not listed by the EPA is still a hazardous waste if it has one or more of EPA's four hazardous characteristics: ignitability, corrosivity, reactivity, or toxicity.

Institutions must establish policies to manage all hazardous wastes in a safe and environmentally sound manner that complies with all applicable federal, state, and local regulations. Biological and chemical wastes are also discussed in this section. Radioactive waste is discussed in the later section on radiation safety.

Biological/Medical Waste Management

The institution must assign the generators of potentially infectious waste with the responsibility to properly sort and dispose of all infectious waste following the policies and procedures established by the institution. Infectious waste management varies from state to state. For specific information on infectious waste disposal procedures, institutions should contact their state departments of environmental protection or health departments.

Categories of materials that are generally considered potentially infectious waste:[22]

- Cultures and stocks
- Pathological wastes
- Human blood, blood products, and body fluid waste
- Animal wastes
- Isolation wastes
- Used sharps

Handling The primary responsibility for identifying and disposing of infectious material rests with principal investigators or laboratory supervisors. This responsibility must not be shifted to inexperienced or untrained personnel.

Generally, potentially infectious and biohazardous waste must be separated from general waste at the point of generation (i.e., the point at which the material becomes a waste) by the generator into the following three classes as follows:

- Used sharps
- Fluids
- Other

Other infectious waste must be discarded directly into containers or plastic (polypropylene) autoclave bags that are clearly identifiable and distinguishable from general waste. Containers must be marked with the universal biohazard symbol. Autoclave bags must be distinctly colored red or orange and be marked with the universal biohazard symbol. These bags must not be used for any other materials or purpose. Materials designated as infectious waste generally must be treated before final disposal. Treatment may be by disinfection such as autoclaving, dry heat, or destruction such as incineration. These treatments may take place at the institution or the materials may be transported off-site for treatment. Requirements for the final deposition of wastes vary by locale and transportation of these materials is governed by federal and state regulations.

Chemical Wastes

The institution must establish policies and procedures to assure that potentially hazardous chemicals are disposed of in accordance with state and/or federal regulations. Each unit within the institution may wish to develop procedures to best manage the wastes generated in its area, but this may lead to regulatory violations. It is generally best to establish one overarching hazardous waste policy and supporting procedures to effectively and efficiently manage chemical wastes.

Because states often have primacy in hazardous waste regulation, it is important to assure that the institution is complying with the regulations in the locale in which the waste is generated.

Classification of Chemical Waste A chemical waste is considered to be a hazardous waste if it is specifically listed by the EPA or state environmental protection agency as a hazardous waste or if it meets at least one of the four hazardous characteristics (ignitability, corrosivity, reactivity, and toxicity). If a chemical waste is not on the EPA list of hazardous wastes and does not meet any of the hazardous waste characteristics, it is a nonhazardous waste. For complete definitions of hazardous characteristics of waste, see the EPA regulation 40 CFR 261, "Identification and Listing of Hazardous Waste." [23]

The regulatory burden associated with the management of hazardous waste is very high. It is important to ensure that waste generated from a process at the institution has a bona fide affordable disposal option. A procedure may generate a hazardous waste with disposal costs so high as to be prohibitive as the waste is unique and no commercial facility is permitted to dispose of the material.

Wastes composed of multiple hazards are considered "mixed wastes." Mixed wastes may be mixtures of hazardous chemical wastes and radioactive wastes, or mixtures of biological wastes and chemical wastes, or a combination of these wastes. Special handling and disposal procedures that are required for mixed waste and the procedures may vary depending on the governing regulations in the locale where the wastes are generated.

Large scale projects that use large volumes of chemicals may have substantial disposal costs associated with terminating the project. For large scale projects decommissioning plans should be incorporated into the original grant proposal to assure funds are available to close out the project.

Record Keeping

As with all formal health and safety programs, a radiation safety program must maintain comprehensive records. Regulations or license conditions often explicitly state what types of records must be kept and for what period they must be maintained. The institution may be required to devote significant effort and resources to the record keeping area of the program.

Summary

Sponsored research programs should encourage the participation of safety and health personnel in the proposal review process to assure regulatory compliance and more importantly to assure that the research can be conducted safely with the available institutional resources. Every proposal need not undergo review by health and safety personnel but the institution should develop procedures to identify protocols/proposals that may require review and perhaps approval by the safety office. By developing partnerships among animal husbandry staff, the animal care committee, the institution review board, the institutional biosafety committee, and the safety office, sponsored program offices can act as a conduit to provide researchers the information needed to submit proposals that meet the ever growing compliance burden.

References

1. National Institutes of Health, Office of Extramural Research, "Public Health Service Policy on Humane Care and Use of Laboratory Animals," 2002, http://grants2.nih.gov/grants/ olaw/references/phspol.htm (accessed August 21, 2005).
2. *The National Environmental Policy Act of 1969*, as amended, Public Law 91-190, 42 U.S.C. 4321-4347 (January 1, 1970), as amended by Public Law 94-52 (July 3, 1975), Public Law 94-83 (August 9, 1975), and Public Law 97-258, § 4(b) (Sept. 13, 1982), http:// ceq.eh.doe.gov/nepa/regs/nepa/nepaeqia.htm (accessed February 8, 2004).
3. *The Occupational Health and Safety Act of 1970* (amended 1998), http://www.osha.gov/ pls/oshaweb/owasrch.search_form?p_doc_type =OSHACT&p_toc_level=0&p_keyvalue= (accessed August 21, 2005).
4. Executive Order No. 12196 (1980), http://tis. eh.doe.gov/feosh/resource/eo12196.htm (accessed February 9, 2004).
5. U.S. Department of Labor Mine Safety and Health Administration, "Title 30 Code of Federal Regulations Parts 1–199," http://www. msha.gov/30cfr/0.0.HTM (accessed August 21, 2005).
6. National Institutes of Health, "Guidelines for Research Involving Recombinant DNA Molecules," 2002, http://www4.od.nih.gov/oba/rac/ guidelines_02/NIH_Guidelines_Apr_02.htm#_ Toc7261553 (accessed February 15, 2004).
7. American Biological Safety Association, "Risk Group Classification for Infectious Agents," http://www.absa.org/resriskgroup.html (accessed August 30, 2004).
8. Centers for Disease Control, *Biological Safety in Microbiological and Biomedical Laboratories* (BMBL) 4th ed., http://www.cdc.gov/od/ ohs/biosfty/bmbl4/bmbl4toc.htm (accessed August 30, 2004).
9. Ibid.
10. Ibid.
11. Ibid.
12. US Department of Labor, Occupational Health and Safety Administration, *Bloodborne Pathogens*, 29CFR 1910.1030, http://www.osha.gov/ pls/oshaweb/owadisp.showdocument?p_table= STANDARDS&p_id=10051 (accessed August 30, 2004).
13. *Public Health Security and Bioterrorism Preparedness and Response Act of 2002*, http:// thomas.loc.gov/cgi-bin/query/z?c107:H.R. 3448.ENR (accessed February 15, 2004).
14. United and Strengthening America by Providing Appropriate Tools Required to Intercept and Obstruct Terrorism (USA Patriot Act) Act of 2001, http://frwebgate.access.gpo.gov/ cgibingetdoc. cgi?dbname=107_cong_public_ laws&docid=f:publ056.107.pdf (accessed August 21, 2005).

15. Department of Agriculture, Animal and Plant Health Inspection Service, Agricultural Bioterrorism Protection Act of 2002; Possession, Use and Transfer of Biological Agents and Toxins; Final Rule, http://a257.g.akamaitech.net/7/257 /2422/01jan20051800/edocket.access.gpo.gov/ 2005/pdf/05-5063.pdf (accessed August 21, 2005).

16. Department of Health and Human Services, Possession, Use and Transfer of Select Agents, and Toxins, Final Rule, 42 C.F.R. Parts 72 and 73 CFR Part 1003, http://www.cdc.gov/ od/sap/pdfs/42_cfr_73_final_rule.pdf (accessed August 21, 2005).

17. *US Patriot Act*, 18 USC § 175, http:// uscode.house.gov/uscode-cgi/fastweb.exe? getdoc+uscview+t17t20+222+0++%28USA%2 0PATRIOT%20act%29%20%20AND%20% 28%2818%29%20ADJ%20USC%29%3ACI TE%20AND%20%28USC%20w%2F10%20 %28175%29%29%3ACITE%20%20AND% 20%28CHAPTER%20ADJ%20%2810%29 %29%3AEXPCITE%20%20%20%2 (accessed August 30, 2004).

18. US Department of Labor, Occupational Health and Safety Administration, *Occupational Exposure to Chemicals in Laboratories*, 29 CFR, 1910.1450, http://www.osha.gov/pls/oshaweb/ owadisp.show_document?p_table= STANDARDS&p_id=10106 (accessed August 2, 2005).

19. US Department of Labor, Occupational Health and Safety Administration, *Authority for 29 CFR, 1910 Subpart Z*, http://www.osha.gov/ pls/oshaweb/owadisp.show_document?p_table =STANDARDS&p_id=10147 (accessed August 2, 2005).

20. US Department of Labor, Occupational Health and Safety Administration, OSHA *Fact Sheet, Hazardous Chemicals in Labs*, 2002, http:// www.osha.gov/OshDoc/data_General_Facts/ hazardouschemicalsinlabs-factsheet.html (accessed August 30, 2004).

21. US Department of Labor, Occupational Health and Safety Administration, *Hazard Communication*, 29 CFR 1910.1200, http://www.osha. gov/pls/oshaweb/owadisp.show_document? p_table=STANDARDS&p_id=10099 (accessed August 2, 2005).

22. Adapted from 25 Pennsylvania Code Subsection 271.1, http://www.pacode.com/secure/ data/025/chapter271/s271.1.html (accessed August 30, 2004).

23. Title 40: Protection of Environment Part 261— Identification and Listing of Hazardous Waste, http://ecfr.gpoaccess.gov/cgi/t/text/text-idx? c=ecfr&sid=46744c91555f9baeadebf5bce6e60 da4&rgn=div5&view=text&node=40:25.0.1.1. 2&idno=40 (accessed August 21, 2005).

24. US Nuclear Regulatory Commission, "NRC Regulatory Guides—General (Division 10)," http://www.nrc.gov/reading-rm/doc-collections/ reg-guides/general/active/ (accessed August 2, 2005).

25. U.S. Nuclear Regulatory Commission 10 CFR part 19.12 Instruction to Workers, http://www. nrc.gov/reading-rm/doc-collections/cfr/part019/ part019-0012.html (accessed August 21, 2005).

26. US Nuclear Regulatory Commission, "Conditions Requiring Individual Monitoring of External and Internal Occupational Dose," *10 CFR 20.1502*, http://www.nrc.gov/reading-rm/ doc-collections/cfr/part020/part020-1502.html (accessed August 2, 2005).

27. Laser Institute of America, *American National Standard for Safe Use of Lasers ANSI Z136.1, 1-2000.* Orlando, FL: 2000.

28. ACGIH. "TLVs and BEIs, Threshold Limit Values for Chemical Substances and Physical Agents, Biological Exposure Indices," presented at the 2003 American Conference of Government Industrial Hygienists in Cincinnati, OH.

57

Bioterrorism: Policy Considerations for Research Institutions

Bryan Benham, PhD

Introduction

The attacks of September 11, 2001 raised critical awareness of the threat of terrorism on US soil. The subsequent mailings of anthrax spores to government and media offices further heightened awareness of the existing vulnerabilities to biological attacks by terrorists, enough so that it is widely believed that bioterrorism "represents a serious threat to our nation and the world."[1] The immediate governmental response, understandably enough, has been to severely increase security measures and divert funds to defend against bioterrorist threats.

The most notable changes in national security have occurred through the 2001 passage of the Patriot Act, which granted increased surveillance powers to governmental agencies, largely through the creation of the Department of Homeland Security (DHS), a new regulatory agency with oversight power of the government. Other significant post-September 11th legislation has included passage of the 2002 Bioterrorism Preparedness and Response Act, mandating close monitoring of sensitive research and materials in the life sciences. The act has inadvertently posed issues of censorship of information in the academic world: for example, reclassification of some types of information as "sensitive" has restricted publication of information that was formerly widely available. In addition, the act has tightened visa requirements for foreign students and scholars. The government has also dramatically increased funding for counterbioterrorism efforts, spurring research on biological

pathogens and vaccines, development of biodefense technology (e.g., detection systems), and the construction of laboratories and programs focusing specifically on counterbioterrorism efforts.

Each of these legislative and governmental actions—increased security and funding—has had serious consequences for research institutions. For one, research institutions are now expected to produce research and technology that responds to bioterrorism threats, while at the same time, institutions are expected to forbear increased security to protect this technology. Increased expectations to produce counterterrorism solutions and increased security measures conflict with the ideals of scientific freedom and civil liberties, which many see as essential to the practice of effective science and critical to a democratic society and the preservation of human rights. The increased funding opportunities also pose a challenge for research institutions: institutions must decide whether they are going to take advantage of new funding opportunities and how new funding areas will affect current and future missions. Of great concern is that new emphasis on "missiles and medicine" research will divert resources away from other critical areas, such as public health problems and other areas already considered underfunded. There is also concern that increased research for biodefense violates present international treaties on biological weapons research and that such violation could initiate a new biological arms race. The central challenge facing research institutions is to balance these competing issues; in other words, research institutions must balance the needs of increased security along with the needs of scientific freedom and openness, while also continuing to define their proper roles in the war on terrorism.

The purpose of this chapter is to examine some of the central questions that research institutions face as a result of current policies and practices initiated in response to the threat of bioterrorism. A comprehensive review of current policy and policy recommendations since the 9/11 attacks would be too difficult to attempt here, because of the rapidly changing legislative and regulatory landscape of bioterrorism policy. Nevertheless, this chapter attempts to identify the major trends in response to the threat of bioterrorism that most directly affect research institutions. The goal is to provide a rough sketch of the issues and implications of this changing landscape. The issues discussed in this chapter focus primarily on public institutions, such as research universities, but much of what is discussed can also be applied to private institutions, and, to a lesser degree, to private industry involved in biotechnology and related fields.

There are three emerging areas of concern for research institutions as a result of increased security and funding for counterbioterrorism efforts. First among these are the proposed restrictions and regulatory oversight concerning biological research and the publication of research findings, which includes the increased scrutiny directed at foreign students and scholars doing research in the United States. Second, there are issues relating to public safety and preparedness against bioterrorist attacks. Much of the research for biodefense will be conducted at public universities, which raises concerns over the measures in place to protect facilities, faculty, and public health in those areas. Third, though not entirely separable from the above concerns, the threat of bioterrorism itself raises questions regarding the changing role of the university and other research institutions associated with the biodefense effort. The impact that federal regulations and increased funding will have on the mission and continued existence of research institutions is yet to be fully evaluated.

Regulating Research

Government regulations are not new to the scientific community, but the heightened security measures that have been implemented since the attacks of 9/11 and the subsequent mailings of anthrax spores to government offices have brought to the forefront questions about the proper balance between scientific freedom and civil liberties, on the one hand, and national security on the other. Research institutions are at the center of this debate because they have historically and currently provide the scientific know-how and instrumentation to carry out biodefense research.

The threat of bioterrorism, in particular, poses special problems. Although terrorists will likely continue to use conventional weapons, many think that biological or chemical weapons may become the weapon of choice by terrorists for a number of reasons.[2] The materials and techniques needed for developing and deploying biological weapons are readily available, relatively easy to disguise, and have the devastating potential to cause large scale death, disease, and panic. What is perhaps most troubling, for national security purposes, is that much of the technology and techniques associated with biological weapons are dual-use. Dual-use technologies are those that have the beneficial use of saving lives, curing disease, and improving the human condition, but which can also be used for less benevolent purposes. The same technology that can produce vaccines can also make biological agents more virulent. The same technology that increases the effectiveness of certain drugs can also be used to weaponize those drugs. National security strategy has been to regulate those dual-use technologies so that they cannot be used against the United States. The challenge facing national security biodefense measures, then, is to adequately regulate dual-use technologies in the life sciences without hindering the potential benefits of those same technologies. But it has been argued that regulation of scientific research fundamentally restricts the exchange of ideas and limits access to essential materials, which thus inhibits progress in biodefense exactly at the time we need it most.

At least since World War II and the subsequent Cold War, the government has employed regulation that restricts certain sensitive research. The central mechanism of regulation was classification of research. Research that was potentially dangerous was classified and funded under government contract. The government maintained direct control over the research, and where necessary, could limit access to research by locating it at national laboratories under close security. Unclassified research remained under the control of individual researchers and institutions. Funding for that research was provided by private or federal grants and had no restrictions on the publication of research findings. The system of classified/not-classified research provided a clear mechanism for restricting certain information while not hindering scientific progress in other areas.[3] In 1985, President Reagan reaffirmed the importance of this mechanism in his National Security Directive 189 (NSDD-189), which states:

> ... to the maximum extent possible, the products of fundamental research remain unrestricted ... [and] where the national security requires control, the mechanism for control of information generated during federally-funded fundamental research in science, technology and engineering at colleges, universities and laboratories is classification. ... No restrictions may be placed upon the conduct or reporting of federally-funded fundamental research that has not received national security classification, except as provided in applicable U.S. Statutes.

Accordingly, NSDD-189 remains in effect today with the support of universities, the scientific community, and each Presidential administration to date.[4] However, recent legislation points to problematic extensions of governmental regulations that introduce a new category of "sensitive but unclassified" research.[5] The designation of research as "sensitive but unclassified" (SBU) is a new regulatory category created in the November 2002 Homeland Security Act. According to the Department of Health and Human Services (DHHS), the SBU category refers to any research that involves a Select Agent, as defined by the US Centers for Disease Control, *and* can achieve one or more of the following bioweapons related goals:

1. Make human or animal vaccines ineffective;
2. Grant resistance to therapeutically useful antibiotics or antiviral agents for humans, animals, or crops;
3. Increase the virulence of human, animal, or plant pathogens, or make nonpathogens virulent;
4. Make pathogens more easily transmissible or alter their host range;
5. Help evade diagnostic or detection methods; or,
6. Enable weaponization of biological agents or toxins.[6]

The use of this new category of "sensitive but unclassified" research has implications for the funding, publication, and oversight of scientific research

as well as on the monitoring of foreign students and scholars in these sensitive research areas.

Research Funding and Publication

One of the most significant regulatory measures taken in response to the threat of bioterrorism is the recent creation of the National Science Advisory Board for Biosecurity (NSABB) announced in March 2004. The NSABB will be managed by the National Institutes of Health (NIH), and "will advise on and recommend specific strategies for the efficient and effective oversight of federally conducted or supported potential dual-use biological research taking into consideration both national security concerns and the needs of the research community."[7] The NSABB is designed to work in a similar fashion as the Recombinant DNA Advisory Committee (RAC) that has developed national guidelines and principles since the mid-1970s for the safe and ethical conduct of recombinant DNA research. But unlike the RAC, the NSABB will set policy and assess the efficacy of such policy across all federal agencies.[8] Aside from its main functions as a public forum for discussion of dual-use technologies and as a liaison for federal agencies that support research in the life sciences, two other mandates stand out as having a significant impact on how research institutions address biodefense research. According to its mandate, the NSABB will "advise on strategies for local and federal biosecurity oversight for all federally funded or supported life sciences research," and it will "advise on strategies to work with journal editors and other stakeholders to ensure the development of guidelines for the publication, public presentation and public communication of potentially sensitive life sciences research."[9] In these two capacities the NSABB is concerned to advise only on "sensitive but unclassified" research, namely, the type of research that may inadvertently aid bioterrorists.

The creation of NSABB and its particular mandate to provide oversight for funding and publication of "sensitive but unclassified" research raises a number of issues for research institutions. First, there are concerns over the effect this type of oversight might have on current and future research in the biological sciences. As it is designed, the NSABB will not directly review or control research. Decisions about the appropriateness of certain SBU research will be made at the level of the research institutions, by institutional biosafety committees or other bodies that review research at the institutional level. The NSABB is meant to act only on those cases in which institutional biosafety committees request assistance. The purpose of the NSABB is only as an advisory board. Compliance with NSABB guidelines is completely voluntary at this time. Nevertheless, there is a concern that "in the future, federal grant agencies could potentially withhold or rescind funding to an institution or grantee who doesn't comply with the board's guidelines."[10] The worry is that NSABB oversight will eventually be a mechanism whereby funding and funding decisions are limited to certain research areas. Eventually this oversight will either scare away qualified researchers because certain areas have become highly regulated and restrictive, or NSABB oversight will channel funding in ways that might be detrimental to the biodefense effort and basic scientific research in other areas. What is needed, according to critics, is a way to motivate qualified researchers to actively pursue relevant research without overregulating dual-use research. The NSABB potentially has detrimental effects on the flow of dollars to biodefense research efforts.

Second, there are serious concerns raised about the NSABB advisory role in publication of SBU research. Most scientists and professional organizations prefer the classification system employed previously for national security measures (NDD-189), and the former Secretary of Homeland Security, Tom Ridge, reaffirmed that the SBU label will "not apply to federally funded grants to universities and other private sector entities."[11] Yet a number of universities have raised issues regarding grant and contract clauses that request prepublication review for disclosure of sensitive information.[12] Several schools, including MIT and Stanford, have refused federal research grants and contracts because, they argue, prepublication review undermines academic freedom and professional obligations of the university and scientific communities.[13] According to the American Association for the Advancement of Science (AAAS), universities worry that the removal of SBU documents from the public domain could negatively impact existing research and undermine biodefense efforts.[14] University officials, such as James Siedow, the Vice Provost for Research at Duke University, have expressed reservations over the SBU category, saying that "if the government decides to tighten up, a lifetime of research can become, essentially, classified, overnight."[15]

The central criticism raised against federal oversight by the NSABB and the category of SBU research, is that it will unduly hinder much needed scientific research by limiting access to critical information. The scientific process depends on maintaining open and uncensored exchange of scientific results in publication.[16] In addition, according to Nicholas Cozzarelli, editor-in-chief of the *Proceedings of the National Academy of Sciences*, editors and researchers alike already monitor for inappropriate material.[17] External governmental control over the process is likely to impede timely scientific publication. Moreover, it is unclear how the NSABB will provide advice to journal editors and publishers about problematic areas of research when the board will meet only quarterly. Additional oversight on SBU research in the biological sciences will do little to help the already existing practices.

Other criticisms raised against the NSABB question the effectiveness of the oversight provided by the NSABB. There are, for instance, no mechanisms of punishment for failure to comply with NSABB guidelines. As mentioned previously, compliance is currently entirely voluntary. Moreover, any future punitive measures may only have an impact on those researchers who are already acting conscientiously. Scientists who want to research in SBU areas or use select agents will not be touched by these regulations, if they have nonfederal funding or are working internationally. Even though private industry (e.g., pharmaceutical companies) often complies with federal regulations and recommendations, the NSABB has no power to monitor or control commercial research institutions.[18] Likewise, the NSABB has no authority over international research which is increasingly focused on biotechnology. Biotechnology is "not a technology that is restricted to a few nations like using nuclear missiles is," so the effectiveness of NSABB advisory power is severely limited.[19] In addition, critics argue that the percentage of researchers actually affected by NSABB guidelines is extremely small because the NSABB is only concerned with research that is categorized as SBU.[20] Such a narrow focus misses the mark. Nearly all biological research (SBU or otherwise) has the potential to be used for malicious purposes. This is the dilemma of dual-use technologies. Regulation of SBU biodefense research only marginally delays the dissemination of sensitive information and, in the process, will delay the development of legitimate countermeasures to the threat of bioterrorism. Thus, most scientists call for open and uncensored access to this critical research.

Alternatively, some argue that the creation of the NSABB, like the creation of the RAC, is essential for security purposes, and has not unduly prevented scientific progress in the past.[21] Moreover, critics of the NSABB have not provided any detailed alternatives that would adequately protect against, for example, the publication of sensitive information.[22] The balance between security needs and scientific freedom is still an area open for debate. One example that attracted international attention and is illustrative of the divisiveness of this issue occurred in February 2001, before the 9/11 attacks, when Australian researchers published a paper in the *Journal of Virology* that raised serious concerns regarding the effectiveness of self-regulating practices of scientific journals. While trying to develop pest population control mechanisms, researchers inserted a gene for an immune-system molecule for the mousepox virus. Rather than producing infertile mice, the experiment produced a far more deadly engineered virus that killed even the mice already vaccinated against mousepox.[23] Critics argued that the paper "shouldn't have been published. You don't want to publish how to make an organism more virulent." However, proponents of scientific freedom point to the Australian researchers' own statement that "The best protection against any misuse of this technique was to issue a worldwide warning . . . We also want researchers to use this knowledge to help design better vaccines."[24] It is clear that proponents and critics alike have legitimate concerns.

Even though a number of reservations have been raised about the formation of the NSABB and SBU categories, most scientists appear to be in agreement that some oversight would be helpful in directing decisions regarding sensitive or dangerous information. It is only that the announced program for the NSABB is currently too vague to be of much help. It is in need of development. Research institutions will have to address the appropriate balance between the demands of national security, especially under the NSABB, and the openness requisite for productive scientific research.

Foreign Students and Scholars

Another key issue in the regulation of scientific research is the monitoring of foreign students and scholars working at US research institutions. At least since the Cold War, US immigration policy has been concerned about access to educational and technological information by foreign students and scholars, especially in physics and nuclear science.[25] With the 1993 bombing of the World Trade Center, which was perpetrated by foreign nationals in the United States with student visas, increased measures were taken to screen and monitor international students. The 1994 amendment to the Immigration and Nationality Act (8 U.S.C. 212(a)(3)(i)(II))

required consular officials to deny visas for international students who wanted to study in sensitive fields identified by the State Department's "Technology Alert List." The Alert List includes sixteen categories of study that students from countries identified as "state sponsors of terrorism" should not be admitted to the United States to study. But perhaps most importantly, the Illegal Immigration Reform and Responsibility Act of 1996 authorized an electronic foreign student tracking system, the Student Exchange Visa Information System (SEVIS), which was designed to make the names, residences and educational status of foreign students more accessible to immigration officials. However, because of lack of funding and concerns over the financial cost to foreign students, the system was not fully implemented before the attacks of September 11, 2001.

Increased security measures since September 11, 2001 have continued the monitoring and restrictions of foreign students and scholars. Shortly after the 9/11 attacks, the White House proposed the Interagency Panel on Advanced Science and Security (IPASS) that would review the visa applications of foreign students and faculty whose research touched on sensitive areas. The US Patriot Act of 2001 and the Enhanced Border Security and Visa Entry Reform Act of 2002 (P.L. 107-173) strengthened and expanded SEVIS by increasing foreign student monitoring, restricting access to hazardous biological agents, provided the government with access to some information about students and their Internet usage, and provided for the Immigration and Naturalization Service (INS) to periodically review compliance efforts of educational institutions enrolling foreign students. In addition, these acts authorized $36 million to fully implement the SEVIS and required that it be fully operational by January, 30, 2003.

The aim of this legislation is to "assure that foreigners cannot enter the U.S. on student visas in order to cause harm to the U.S. and that foreign students cannot receive education in sensitive areas that they could then turn against the U.S."[26] Yet, many have raised objections to the specifics of increased monitoring of foreign students and scholars visiting the United States. The complaints are threefold: the laws are too restrictive, overreach proper security needs, and may, in fact, threaten the defense efforts and the US leadership role in science and technology that relies on major research institutions.

First, the increased surveillance capabilities granted to the US government with regard to foreign students raise a number of questions about the preservation of individual civil liberties. SEVIS requirements place a special burden on research institutions that enroll foreign students, because the institutions are primarily responsible for entering students into the SEVIS database. In addition, universities are required to act as police, rooting out suspected terrorist activity by monitoring student activity to a degree not previously required. This raises questions about the proper mission of universities in their dual role as educational and research institutions (and is further discussed in the last section of this chapter). Nevertheless, increased access to student information and Internet usage by the federal government has prompted the academic community to respond to civil liberty concerns. As a result, several institutions have refused to implement the system or release data on students.

Second, the balance between civil liberties and security is made more complex by the categories of surveillance proposed by recent legislation. The State Department's "Technology Alert List" originally identified areas such as nuclear technology and information security as sensitive areas of study. Proposed expansions of the list have included areas in microbiology and biotechnology. As sensible as these additions may appear, it will be difficult to implement these measures. For example, it will be difficult to differentiate which courses in microbiology and biotechnology might be properly considered sensitive and which are not, because the techniques taught in even the most basic courses can be used to create biological or chemical weapons. Dual-use technology in the biological sciences is not like dual-use technology in nuclear sciences. The techniques, materials, and equipment required to build a nuclear weapon are not readily available, and so are relatively easy to regulate. Biotechnology builds on very basic and widely accessible techniques, materials, and equipment. Identifying which information should be made available to foreign students and scholars becomes extremely difficult to define and even more difficult to enforce. Other proposed expansions of the technology alert list include such areas as architecture, city planning, and civil engineering. In each of these cases institutions argue that the government has overstepped its proper role as guardian of national security, imposing requirements that are impossible to define.

Third, and the most problematic feature of legislation concerning foreign students and faculty, is the effect visa and reentry restrictions will have on the US position as a leader in science and technology. The overall worry is that these restrictions will discourage students from applying to and continuing to study in the United States, thus draining the United States of valuable scientific, economic, and social resources needed to fight bioterrorism, disease, and other technological problems.[27] In 2000, approximately 36% of graduate students in science and engineering were foreign students and about a third of US science and engineering PhD recipients were foreign students (of these 52% in engineering, 49% in mathematics and computer sciences, and 40% in physical sciences).[28] Although many of these students return to their country of origin after receiving degrees to contribute to the scientific and technological efforts in those nations, a large number remain in the United States, providing important contributions to scientific and technological success.

Continued restrictions on foreign students and faculty in sensitive security areas may hinder scientific progress as well as hurt the US economic future. Surveys conducted in early 2004 by several national educational organizations documented a substantial drop in applications by international graduate students to leading US research institutions for the 2004-05 academic year.[29] Continued declines in foreign student applications are indicators of negative economic and social impacts. It is estimated that during the 2001–02 academic school year, approximately 583,000 international students were expected to add almost $12 billion to the American economy in terms of scientific discovery and contribution.[30]

The main problem with the new policies, according to the American Association for the Advancement of Science (AAAS), is "the amount of time it takes for a visa to be issued to a foreign student, and the process seems especially difficult for foreign students studying science and technology."[31] One year after the 9/11 attacks, at least 10,000 men from 26 predominantly Muslim countries experienced delays of two months or more, if they were not rejected outright.[32] According to statements issued by the National Academies, there have been many delays in research collaborations, scientists have not been able to reenter the United States to continue their research, and many scientists and students have not been issued visas in time to attend scientific conferences or start their program of study at US universities.[33] The increased restrictions have created a backlogged system of visa review. In 2000, nearly 1,000 nonimmigrant visa applications were marked for review under US screening systems. By 2002, that number had increased to 14,000. According to John Marburger, the US President's science advisor, by the spring of

2003 approximately 1,000 cases were under review at any point in time.[34] The delays that result from such an increased number of cases prevents scholars from participation in research and conferences, and prohibits many students from attending school. The visa delays compound problems with cooperation in international research and education that promise to aid efforts against bioterrorism as well as public health, medicine, and other areas of technology.

While recognizing the need for increased national security, the AAAS and other organizations argue for a more streamlined process for issuing visas and for those reentering the United States who already have a visa.[35] In May 2004, the AAAS and more than twenty other science, higher-education, and engineering groups, which represent approximately 95% of the US research community, issued a statement and recommendations that they urged the US government to adopt in order to solve current visa-processing problems.[36] On the whole, the recommendations attempted to remove unnecessary barriers to international cooperation in research. In addition, other concerns about visa restrictions focus on the trend that increased security measures point to for international relations. Visa restrictions promote the idea that the United States does not welcome international students, scholars, and scientists, and leads to xenophobic tendencies within the United States.[37]

How research institutions, professional organizations, and researchers respond to these new policies will determine the course of action of government officials and policy. The need for national security appears to require some regulation of research practices, including the monitoring of foreign students and scholars. However, a balance must be struck between security issues and the fundamental need of science to operate in an open environment. As the above discussion indicates, the criticism of recent policy from the scientific community has been largely negative. While researchers, institutions, and professional organizations all realize the need for sound security measures to face the threat of bioterrorism, they also see the trend of current policy as too heavy-handed. Refinements are needed to streamline the policies and open scientific dialogue and international exchange, both essential for the war on terrorism.

Public Safety and Preparedness

In addition to federal policies regulating research and monitoring foreign students and faculty,

research institutions face further challenges in their effort to defend against bioterrorism. Research institutions must secure their facilities against potential terrorist exploitation, and, for those institutions that conduct biological research, they must insure the health and safety of the population in their vicinity. Security, public health, and preparedness are essential components of any research institution's response to the threat of bioterrorism. Recent federal policies regarding each of these issues pose additional challenges for research institutions. Two pieces of recent legislation are of particular interest.

Bioterrorism Act of 2002

In response to the October 2001 attack of anthrax-laden letters mailed to government officials in Washington, DC, and several media agencies in New York and Florida, the US government adopted the Public Health Security and Bioterrorism Preparedness Act of 2002 (P. L 107-188). It is a measure intended to control biological agents that might be used as biological weapons. Under its provisions the Center for Disease Control (CDC) was directed to issue a "select agents" list "of each biological agent and each toxin that has a potential to pose a severe threat to public health and safety" (P. L. 107-188, 202(a)). Facilities or individuals who possess, use, or transfer any of the agents or toxins on the list are required to register with the CDC or the Animal and Plant Health Inspection Service (APHIS). The CDC is responsible for monitoring and regulating the use of select agents. In addition, the Bioterrorism Act specifies that only institutions or individuals with "lawful purpose" are allowed to posses these select agents, and facilities that use any of these agents are required to have secure facilities.

The control of these potentially dangerous select agents is an important step in securing materials that may be used by bioterrorists. However, each requirement of the Bioterrorism Act has raised a number of worries. First, the implementation of this act as a legal tool to pursue potential terrorists has already been placed under scrutiny. A number of academics, students and faculty, have been charged under the Bioterrorism Act. The first to be charged was Tomas Foral, in July 2002. A student at the University of Connecticut, Foral was charged with possessing anthrax in a university freezer. Reportedly, he failed to destroy several anthrax-infected animal tissue samples after being told to do so. Another incident involved Thomas Butler, a Texas Tech University researcher, who was arrested in January 2003 for "smuggling bacteria into the

U. S. from Tanzania and lying to FBI agents about the disappearance of 30 vials of CDC-listed bubonic plague bacteria."[38] The most recent incident was the arrest of Steven Kurtz, an art professor from State University of New York, Buffalo and Robert Ferrell, head of the human genetics department at the University of Pittsburgh Graduate School of Public Health. Kurtz was accused of illegally possessing suspected bacteria, and Ferrell was accused of illegally shipping the bacteria. The case is pending, but circumstances of the incident are troubling. Paramedics arrived at Kurtz's house, responding to a call that his wife had died of a heart attack overnight; they noticed an array of lab equipment and notified Buffalo police. FBI agents confiscated the material, including two species of bacteria that Kurtz planned to use in an exhibit. It turned out that neither bacterium was on the select agents list and that both are considered harmless. Nevertheless, prosecutors pursued both Kurtz and Ferrell, who supplied Kurtz with the bacteria, for illegal shipping of the bacteria. According to interviewed colleagues, both "fall on no one's radar screen as a potential terrorist."[39] This immediately raised worries about the potential for overreaching application of these laws in academic settings that use or potentially use biological materials and equipment that are otherwise innocuous, but can be interpreted as posing a threat.[40] The effect this and future cases will have on the research interests of faculty and private industry is yet to be seen. Research institutions are subsequently faced with the legal enforcement of these ill-defined laws on campus and in the laboratory.

Second, the security and registration requirements of the Bioterrorism Act have been criticized for instituting "requirements for implementation without necessarily providing resources to accomplish governmental security mandates."[41] Compliance with the Bioterrorism Act raises questions about the financial capacities of research universities, especially smaller universities, and the budget priorities of these research institutions. The cost of upgrading existing laboratories to meet security requirements is not trivial. Louisiana State University reported $130,000 in expenditures to upgrade their laboratories. The design of new science buildings at the University of Louisville, Kentucky was altered to separate secure labs from faculty offices, so that students without clearance could meet with their professors. A number of other universities are considering remodeling their laboratories to meet security requirements of the Bioterrorism Act.[42] The cost of security upgrades, coupled with a downward trend in higher education budgets, has placed additional financial burdens on research institutions to either reallocate resources, potentially at the cost of other departments, or to drop research efforts effected by the select agents list. The latter course of action would effectively lock out certain institutions from such research and potentially restrict the number of institutions doing biodefense research on select agents. Some universities without enough funding have instituted policies that focus "attention and resources on existing areas of expertise that fit well with the funding priorities that have evolved since September 11."[43]

The financial cost of research under the Bioterrorism Act is not the only deterrent. Increased paperwork to register select agents with the CDC or APHIS and increased tightening of regulation for research on biological agents incline universities and individual researchers to avoid these problems by "disposing of potentially problematic research materials."[44] Moreover, the practice of disposing of undesired materials may weaken the biodefense effort because the specimens may be irreplaceable. "Many of the specimens being discarded are key to understanding the workings of biological weapons and biodefense." They are also "essential to understanding the evolution of pathogens in nature," thus providing key information to combat naturally occurring diseases.[45] In an effort to address some of these concerns the federal government has established a temporary repository to help preserve unwanted select agents.[46] In the end, the requirements of the Bioterrorism Act appear to restrict access to certain biological agents, but perhaps not in the ways intended. The mandates of the act attempt to restrict unwanted access to potential terrorists, but also place financial restrictions and additional responsibilities on the very institutions that should be doing research on these select agents. The net effect of the Bioterrorism Act could end up being a complete restructuring of the research landscape in the biosciences—a restructuring that may have unintended but dire consequences by unduly limiting scientific research.

The third worry that is associated with the mandates of the Bioterrorism Act includes doubts about its actual effectiveness in protecting against the potential use of biological agents as weapons of bioterrorism. CDC-listed select agents are readily accessible in areas experiencing outbreaks of infectious disease and the equipment and material for weaponizing agents is publicly available.[47] Additional concerns were raised in July 2002, when the publication of a synthetic poliovirus was made public. It demonstrates that "infectious diseases can be built from off-the-shelf smidgens of DNA that are individually benign."[48] Control of the "DNA synthesis industry" (nationally and internationally) and tighter control over exports of genetic material may provide some measure of security, but would also severely hamper legitimate research and business activities.

There is wide concern that the restrictions placed on research institutions as a result of the Bioterrorism Act appear to affect only the very individuals and institutions that are not a threat, while terrorists intent on using biological agents on the CDC select list will not be effectively restricted from access. Careful consideration of the effectiveness and consequences of legislation such as the Bioterrorism Act of 2002 is called for. Regulation may be necessary, but not at the cost of eliminating institutions from effectively responding to the threat of bioterrorism. Some have suggested as an alternative to the Bioterrorism Act a reconsideration of the 1975 Biological and Toxin Weapons Convention (BWC) occur. The BWC prohibits "the development, production, or stockpiling of biological or toxic agents and of devices to deliver such agents," but it does not prohibit research.[49] However, the BWC does not have an enforcement mechanism to deter nations, institutions, or individuals from developing biological weapons. The US government did recognize this potential and proposed a draft protocol to address this problem, which included national criminal legislation against convention violators; however, this effort was rejected. It faces the same challenges for research as the Bioterrorism Act. In addition, since BWC provides a blanket prohibition against developing, producing, or stockpiling biological or toxic agents, it might also effectively eliminate current US efforts to develop and stockpile these agents for purposes of vaccination and other treatments.

Project Bioshield, 2004

In his 2003 state of the union address, President Bush announced Project Bioshield, in which nearly $6 billion will be made available to researchers over the next ten years and which provides incentives for the biotech industry to develop bioterrorism countermeasures. In May 2004 the Project Bioshield bill received final approval by Congress with a nearly unanimous vote. Among its mandates, the bill provides for purchase of vaccines and other medicines as part of a national bioterrorism protection plan. It also streamlines the peer-review process for FDA approval for new drugs, and, in case of national emergency, allows the government to distribute treatments that may not have received final approval by the FDA. The project promises to increase financial incentives so that much needed drugs and vaccines can be developed in the fight against possible terrorist attacks with biological weapons. This is an opportunity for research institutions, including public universities, where much of the proposed biodefense research will be conducted. This marks an expansion of high-security biocontainment laboratories from a small number of classified government facilities, such as the Centers for Disease Control (CDC) and the US Army Medical Research Institute of Infectious Diseases (USAMRIID), to a larger number of Biological Safety Level (BSL) 2, 3, and 4 laboratories in academic settings around the nation. BSL indicates the potential risk associated with biological agents studies as well as the level of containment and safety measures required to handle these agents; the higher the number, the greater the containment measures required. Although such a move is seen as warranted, several have raised concerns about public health and preparedness of local communities in these areas because of the secrecy surrounding biodefense research. Those research institutions that undertake this research are called upon to address these issues.

The Bioterrorism Act of 2002 establishes a national database that tracks the identities of researchers working with select agents, as well as the locations and nature of those agents. However, access to this database is restricted so that local authorities, public health officials, and those who act as first response units for outbreaks of infectious disease do not have information regarding the type of research being performed at local laboratories. Laura Kahn (2004) argues that this is a serious issue that needs to be addressed. This situation raises a number of serious problems, including the fact that "secrecy can invite misinterpretation of intentions, not only by a nation's citizens but also by its international allies."[50] There is no indication that research under Project Bioshield will be classified, but activities of other government agencies may be pushing the limits of BWC and other restrictions on biodefense research.

Another problem, according to Kahn, is that there are a number of high security laboratories being built at highly classified sites designed for nuclear weapons design (Lawrence Livermore National Laboratory and Los Alamos National Laboratories). These facilities have a history of security lapses and environmental contamination.

There are additional concerns whether a nuclear weapons design facility is properly designed to contain biocontamination that may result from biodefense research. For many research institutions, this level of security and decontamination may not be necessary, but it stresses the importance of having proper safeguards in place.

But the more pressing problem that faces research institutions undertaking biodefense research is the issue of public health and preparedness. Although the public health risk of exposure to dangerous pathogens varies with the type of research being conducted, and the likelihood of such a public outbreak as a direct result of failed laboratory security is low, the risks of laboratory-acquired infections for laboratory workers is considerable. Workers may have contact with the local community and possibly to the international community. A recent example illustrates this problem:

> The Severe Acute Respiratory Syndrome (SARS) virus infected 2 medical researchers in Taiwan and Singapore, who were working in BSL-4 and BSL-3 laboratories respectively. In the BSL-4 laboratory, liquid waste had spilled into a transporting chamber, and the researcher likely became infected after opening the chamber to clean it. After being exposed, the Taiwanese researcher traveled to a conference in Singapore before becoming ill; this event resulted in the quarantining of 90 people in both countries. In the second case, the BSL-3 laboratory in Singapore was faulted for poor safety practices after a researcher, working with West Nile virus, became infected with a SARS-contaminated specimen. The need to quarantine contacts was not reported in this case.[51]

Although neither of these incidents resulted in secondary cases of infection, they did require public health responses: vaccination, surveillance, and quarantine. If the local authorities were not aware of these agents, the response would have been much slower, resulting in more severe consequences. Because of the secrecy involved in biodefense research, public health officials are unable to alert emergency room physicians of possible infectious agents, plan a proper response to possible outbreaks, and mobilize the necessary detection systems and treatment equipment. The need for proper safety procedures, as well as the proper information channels is obvious. Guidelines are published by the CDC and NIH and most research universities have a biosafety board that oversees that these procedures are followed. To overcome some of these difficulties, Kahn reports that some states might adopt further measures. As of the date of this chapter, Maryland is the only state that has passed legislation establishing its own biological agents registry, which effectively duplicates the federal Bioterrorism Act and requires all individuals in possession of select agents in Maryland to register with the state database, as well as the federal one. Secure access to the Maryland database by state public health officials can help to avoid a potential epidemic outbreak. Although many research institutions may not have the power to enact such legislation, they can, however, exert influence on local government or implement similar public health measures.

The danger of naturally occurring infectious diseases poses a far greater risk than the possibility of a bioterrorist threat. However, public health programs designed to detect and respond to infectious disease outbreaks, let alone bioterrorist attacks, are woefully inadequate.[52] According to the TFAH, in July 2004, only thirteen states had a plan or a draft of a plan to confront infectious disease outbreaks such as an influenza pandemic,[53] while the CDC itself, as of this writing, has not yet released a federal plan for such an outbreak. The worry is that little has been done to plan for infectious disease outbreaks, even though significant federal money has been made available to counter bioterrorist threats. The rapid global response to the 2003 SARS outbreak demonstrates that planning, surveillance, and decisive action by public health organizations can prevent epidemics.[54] Given the secrecy involved in registering select agents under the Bioterrrorism Act of 2002 and the increased funding for research on select agents at institutions around the nation, increased planning would be wise policy. It is up to research institutions to take the lead in formulating plans, organizing resources with public health organizations, and even lobbying for public health policies that meet security requirements for biodefense but also adequately protect public health.

The burden placed on research institutions as a result of federal policy meant to combat the threat of bioterrorism is increasingly restrictive of research practices, stresses the budgets of these institutions, and potentially places the public health at risk. Efforts to negotiate these hazards and, at the same time, effect a productive biodefense research program are under development. How research institutions respond will depend in large part on how these institutions define or redefine their mission in the face of the threat of bioterrorism.

The Role of the Research Institution

The threat of bioterrorism poses serious challenges for the mission of research institutions. The primary role of public universities has been education and research. Intimately associated with this mission is a commitment to the open and free exchange of ideas, both across campus and across national borders. The pursuit of knowledge requires it. Yet, this openness, which is the strength of any research institution, is also one of the greatest vulnerabilities we have against terrorism. The very same technology that results from the exchange of ideas and designed to aid society can also be used against that society. Thus, the immediate governmental response to protect against terrorism was to limit, restrict and control the flow of information and technology that might be used against it. It is an understandable reaction to a terrible threat. But it is also one that places research institutions and national security needs in a difficult and uncomfortable tension. Eugene Skolnikoff remarks on this state of affairs:

> . . . universities are moving in one direction, toward greater internationalization while jealously guarding the essential openness of the campus. At the same time our national concerns about proliferation, movement of information, and access of foreign students are intensifying in the opposite direction.[55]

The critical challenge facing research institutions is how to address this essential tension so that both national security needs can be met and the prospect of scientific research is not unduly hindered. It is clear that a balance must be struck between these two competing aims. The central question is how are research institutions going to respond? Other questions are also pressing. What responsibilities do research institutions have in the biodefense effort? How will this affect the mission of research universities? There are no easy answers.

The connection between universities and national interest is not unfamiliar. In the midst of World War II, researchers in physics and engineering provided essential contributions to the war effort. They also had to balance the needs of national security with the open exchange of ideas. Funding opportunities for research institutions were increased, and with the formation of the GI Bill increased enrollment also increased the educational and research training demands of universities. The onset of the Cold War brought with it new funding and research agendas from the federal government, as well as security issues of its own. The fall of the Soviet Union marked a post-Cold War environment of increased economic development, and the creation of the World Wide Web also impacted the research agendas of universities.[56] The new War on Terrorism will likely have similar effects. However, the War on Terrorism has a couple of unique features.[57] Unlike World War II and the Cold War, the enemy is not easily identifiable. The terrorist threat is diffuse and crosses traditional national boundaries. There is no geographically recognizable war front, and though no war is constrained by clearly defined time limits, we are reminded that the War on Terrorism will be of indefinite duration and fought using a diverse arsenal of military, legal, and diplomatic strategies.

These are troubling features, especially when we consider that short-term answers to these problems may have detrimental long-term consequences for research institutions. For example, many worry that excluding many international students from US research institutions or limiting the topics of study available to them may secure the short-term goal of restricting access to sensitive material and methods to potential enemies, but will, in fact, have long-term consequences. Limiting foreign enrollment may limit the pool expertise at research institutions, also limiting industrial and governmental development of new technologies, and may set the United States on a path to isolationism that would be disastrous for international relations.[58] "The nebulous, diffuse nature of terrorism makes a simple prescription for the responsibilities of academic institutions impossible."[59]

In order to chart a more sensible course of action, research universities and their partners must seriously consider their role in the defense against bioterrorism and more generally in the War on Terrorism. A large number of things should be considered, but three central concerns all research institutions should and must address follow.

Perhaps most importantly, research institutions should develop or strengthen their partnership with government and policy-making bodies. According to Eugene Skolnikoff (2002), "It is imperative that the universities understand what the issues are, how they believe they should respond to them, how far they should go in accepting certain restrictions, and how they should work with government on these matters," crucial because "the climate in the government on these issues is such that, outside science agencies, the concern of universities are not well respected."[60] Research universities should take the lead in advising and molding policy, lest they find themselves under mandatory legislation that goes counter to the mission of the university. But it is more than mere self-protection that should motivate universities to take an active role in policy formation. Universities, by their very nature, offer much needed resources for the War on Terrorism. Obviously, research institutions have the facilities and know-how in their faculty and students to address a wide range of technical problems. However, as Lewis Branscomb (2002) observes, the current War on Terrorism poses unique problems that need to be addressed because the enemy is ill-defined, diffuse, and the war is of indefinite duration; it requires cross-disciplinary approaches in counterterrorism efforts.[61] However, the government is traditionally inept at coordinating and drawing together the efforts of multiple departments, not originally defined to deal with problems that call for crossdepartmental solutions. Universities, on the other hand, have a great deal of experience and the facilities to handle cross-disciplinary problems. In the last couple of decades, research has become increasingly interdisciplinary and international. The success of these projects speaks volumes for the types of resources that universities can offer governmental agencies in terms of organizational capacities and interdisciplinary work. Regardless of how universities decide to employ this capability, most every researcher and research institution have called for continued openness in the exchange of ideas and development of technologies. Thus the role of the research institution should be in large part as an active advisory partner for government at the federal, state, and local levels.

The mission of universities is to be a repository of new knowledge and research that advances science, hopefully for the betterment of society. This is usually translated into a focus on science and technology. The threat of bioterrorism requires a scientific and technological response. However, this is not the sole benefit of universities. In determining what role to play in the War on Terrorism, research universities should consider the whole university. M. R. C. Greenwood (2002) reminds us:

> . . . the word 'university' is derived from the Lain root *universitas*, meaning 'whole' or 'body,' yet we often forget the whole and work in departmentalized, segmented units. We must keep in mind the whole university, as we will need the full complement of intellectual tools within those institutions to ensure our national security and well being.[62]

Greenwood's point is relevant in several ways.

First, the resources needed to address bioterrorism and terrorism, in general, require more than simply technological achievement. The social sciences and humanities play a critical role, as well. Understanding the roots of terrorist ideology, understanding and remedying the conditions under which terrorism is viewed as a legitimate means to some end, calculating and evaluating risk to cultural structures, assessing responses to terrorist threats, and any number of other problems faced by the threat of terrorism can and must be addressed by the social sciences and humanities. Their contribution is often overlooked in times of war, where emphasis is quickly placed on immediate technological solutions to security issues.

Second, research institutions should consider the whole university because policy and funding decisions effect the operation of the whole university. In responding to current regulations, many universities will undoubtedly want to avoid increased governmental control over research, and the accompanying limits it poses on research. Such decision may limit the funding opportunities for that university, especially in the life sciences and engineering. In an era of already decreasing budgets, this is likely to affect programs across the curriculum. Likewise, a decrease in foreign students and faculty because of visa restrictions may have a negative impact on the functioning of the research institution. Even if universities adopt the strategy of tailoring programs to take advantage of biodefense funding, a risk of drawing other necessary resources from across the campus still exists. This may disadvantage nonscience and nontechnology components of the university.

Lastly, research institutions should consider the whole university because the mission of research institutions is not only research, but also education. The education of scientists and other students is crucial in a time of threat. The problems that face us today are not ones that are easily compartmentalized. The current and next generations of scientists, engineers, and citizens will require a variety of tools and background knowledge to deal with the challenge. This includes broad-ranging education across disciplines. The mission of the university may change in response to national interests and global priorities, but the basic tenet of the research university is still to educate its students, and to continue to educate the public.

The final concern that should be addressed by research institutions has to do with identifying the responsibilities the university has to the wider public. Most universities, public universities especially, are funded and maintained by public money and public interest. Thus it is said that universities must uphold public trust by contributing to the public good. Part of this involves securing public safety and public health. Many research institutions are associated with hospital or other medical facilities. Institutions deciding to pursue counterbioterrorism research have the additional responsibility to secure the health and safety of the facilities, personnel, and local community. Defining the mission or research agenda of a university incorporates internal needs and goals, as well as external needs. These external needs should include those who most have a stake in the outcome. In so far as research risks the health and safety of a community in order to fulfill its mission, the research institution has a responsibility to adequately address that risk. Doing so will involve cooperation and coordination with local officials, but it will also involve educating the public at-large.

Incorporating the mission of research universities with the needs of national security is a difficult and demanding challenge, but one that must be approached thoughtfully and with the full compliment of abilities at hand to the research institutions.

Conclusion

This chapter has identified three main trends in the response to the threat of bioterrorism that affect research institutions:

1. Current policies restricting and regulating research pose an especially worrisome challenge for research universities.
2. Public health and preparedness issues pose another challenge not often discussed.
3. The response to bioterrorism also raises questions about the proper role of research universities.

Each of these issues deserves serious and thoughtful action on the part of research institutions. As the major receptacle for the nation's scientific research and technical knowledge, research universities will play a critical role in the War on Terrorism. In addressing the very real threat of bioterrorism, the role of research universities and other research institutions is no less critical. Nevertheless, a balance between the needs of national security and scientific freedom must be carefully achieved. The importance of this is best summarized by MIT President, Charles Vest, in his 2002–03 state of the university address:

> As we respond to the reality of terrorism, we must not unintentionally disable the quality and

rapid evolution of American science and technology, or of advanced education, by closing their various boundaries. For if we did, the irony is that over time this would achieve in substantial measure the objectives of those who disdain our society and would do us harm by disrupting our economy and quality of life.[63]

Acknowledgments

I would like to acknowledge the assistance of Jonathan Mareno, Nils Hasselmo, Mark Frankel, Alice Gast, and of the research assistance of Dale Clark.

• • • Endnotes

1. Field, K. "Residents fight Boston U.'s 'biosafety' laboratory," *Chronicle of Higher Education* [serial online] 50, no. 42, June 25, 2004, A28, http://chronicle.com/weekly/v50/i42/42a02801.htm (accessed July 7, 2004); See also Bowers, S.R., and Keys, K.R. "Technology and terrorism: The new threat for the millennium," *Conflict Studies*, May 1998; Alcabes, P., letter to the editor, *The Chronicle of Higher Education* 50, no. 31, April 9, 2004, B17.

2. Clark, B. *Technological Terrorism*. Old Greenwich, CT: Devin-Adair, 1980; Cole, L. "The specter of biological weapons," *Scientific American* [serial online], 1996, http://www.sciamdigital.com/browse.cfm?ITEMIDCHAR=41096E69-3C0C-4AEF-80263FA4A990642&methodnameCHAR=&interfacenameCHAR=browse.cfm&ISSUEID_HAR=F3512189-9123-4A3AB7553602FE08C78&ArticleTypeSubInclude_BIT=1&sequencenameCHAR=itemP (accessed September 1, 2005).

3. Chamberlain, A., American Association for the Advancement of Science. "Science and national security in the post-9/11 environment: Federal grants and contracts," August 2004, www.aaas.org/spp/post911/grants/ (accessed August 29, 2005).

4. Gast, A.P. "The impact of restricting information access on science and technology," in *A Little Knowledge: Privacy, Security, and Public Information after September 11*. Edited by J. Podesta, P.M. Shane, and R.C. Leone. 1–13. New York and Washington, DC: The Century Foundation, 2004.

5. Ricks, R., American Association for the Advancement of Science. "Science and national security in the post-9/11 environment: 'Sensitive but unclassified' information," July 2004, www.aaas.org/spp/post911/sbu/ (accessed August 29, 2005).

614 Part V Responsible Conduct of Research

6. See also The National Academies, news release. "Balanced approach needed to mitigate threats from bioterrorism without hindering progress in biotechnology," October 8, 2003, http://www4.nationalacademies.org/news.nsf/isbn/0309089778?OpenDocument (accessed August 29, 2005).

7. Department of Health and Human Services, news release. "HHS will lead government-wide effort to enhance biosecurity in 'dual use' research," March 4, 2004, www.fas.org/sgp/news/2004/03/hhs030404.html (accessed June 29, 2004).

8. Miller, J.D. "New US board for biosecurity," The Scientist [serial online], March 5, 2004, www.biomedcentral.com/news/20040305/04 (accessed June 29, 2004).

9. Department of Health and Human Services, 2004.

10. Miller, 2004.

11. Chamberlain, August 2004, "Federal grants and contracts."

12. Norris, J.T. "Restrictions on research awards: Troublesome clauses, a report of the AAU/COGR task force," http://www.aau.edu/research/Rpt4.8.04.pdf (accessed September 1, 2005); Tucker, J.B. "Research on biodefense can get generous funding, but with strings attached," The Chronicle of Higher Education 50, no. 26, March 5, 2004, B10.

13. Chamberlain, August 2004, "Federal grants and contracts."

14. Ibid.

15. Brickley, P. "Contract conflicts," The Scientist [serial online], January 7, 2003, http://www.the-scientist.com/news/20030107/02 (accessed August 29, 2005).

16. Journal Editors and Authors Group. "Uncensored exchange of scientific results," Proceedings of the National Academy of Sciences [serial online] 100, February 18, 2003, 1464, www.pnas.org/cgi/doi/10.1073/pnas.0630491100 (accessed June 29, 2004).

17. Cozzarellie, N.R. "PNAS policy on publication of sensitive material in the life sciences," Proceedings of the National Academy of Sciences [serial online] 100, February 18, 2003, 1463, www.pnas.org/cgi/doi/10.1073/pnas.0630514100 (accessed June 29, 2004); see also, Zilinskas, R.A, and Tucker, J.B. "Limiting the contribution of the scientific literature to the BW threat," Monterey Institute of International Studies, December 16, 2002, http://www.cns.miis.edu/iiop/cnsdata?Action=1&Concept=0&Mime=1&collection=CNS+Web+Site&Key

=pubs%2Fweek%2F021216a%2Ehtm&QueryText=Zilinskas+Tucker+Limiting+contribution&QueryMode=FreeText (accessed August 29, 2005).

18. Marburger, J. "Science and technology in a vulnerable world: Rethinking our roles," Keynote address for 27th annual AAAS colloquium on science and technology policy, Washington, DC, April 11, 2002, ostp.gov/html/02_4_15.html (accessed June 24, 2004).

19. Miller, J.D. "US biosecurity board reviewed," The Scientist [serial online], March 8, 2004, www.biomedcentral.com/news/20040308/01 (accessed June 29, 2004).

20. Cozzarellie, 2003.

21. Perpich, J.G. "The recombinant-DNA debate and bioterrorism," The Chronicle of Higher Education [serial online] 48, no. 27, March 15, 2002, B20, http://chronicle.com/weekly/v48/i27/27b02001.htm (accessed July 12, 2004).

22. Falkow, S. "Statement on scientific publication and security fails to provide necessary guidelines," Proceedings of the National Academy of Sciences [serial online] 100, May 13, 2003, 5575, www.pnas.org/cgi/doi/10.1073/pnas.1232277100 (accessed June 29, 2004).

23. Monastersky, R. "Publish and perish? As the nation fights terrorists, scientists weigh the risks of releasing sensitive information," The Chronicle of Higher Education 49, no. 7, October 11, 2002, A16.

24. Ibid.

25. Gast, 2004.

26. House Committee on Science, US House of Representatives. "Conducting research during the war on terrorism: Balancing openness and security," October 10, 2002, www.house.gov/science/hearings/full02/oct10/charter.htm (accessed September 14, 2005).

27. This is a debatable claim. See, for example, Monastersky, R. "Is there a science crisis? Maybe not," The Chronicle of Higher Education. 44, July 9, 2004, A10–A14.

28. House Committee on Science, US House of Representatives, 2002; Gast, 2004.

29. AAAS. Joint statement. "Leading science, higher-education and engineering groups urge six improvements to U.S. visa-processing quagmire," AAAS news archives Web site, May 12, 2004, www.aaas.org/news/releases/2004/0512visa.shtml (accessed June 24, 2004).

30. House Committee on Science, US House of Representatives, 2002.

31. Chamberlain, A., American Association for the Advancement of Science. "Science and national

security in the post-9/11 environment: Foreign students and scholars," July 2004, www.aaas. org/spp/post911/visas/ (accessed August 29, 2005).

32. Nakashima, E., and Sipress, A. "Tighter U.S. policy leaves foreign students in limbo," *Washington Post*, September 24, 2002, A17.

33. National Academies. "Current visa restrictions interfere with U. S. science and engineering contributions to important national needs," December 13, 2002 (Revised June 13, 2003), http://www4.nationalacademies.org/news.nsf/isbn/s12132002?OpenDocument (accessed September 1, 2005).

34. Marburger, J., 2002.

35. Ibid.

36. American Association for the Advancement of Science. "Leading science, higher-education and engineering groups urge six improvements to U.S. visa-processing quagmire," AAAS news [serial online], May 12, 2004, www.aaas.org/news/releases/2004/0512visa.shtml (accessed June 24, 2004).

37. Ibid.; House Committee on Science, US House of Representatives, 2002.

38. Malakoff, D. "Plague of lies lands Texas scientist in jail," *Science* 299, 2003, 489–490; Malakoff, D. and Enserink, M. "A recap of the events in the Butler case"; Malakoff, D. and Enserink, M. "Scientist on trial," *Science Now* [serial online], www.sciencenow.sciencemag.org/feature/data/butlertrial.shtml.

39. Couzin, J. "Indictment of academics raises worries," *Science Now* [serial online], July 2, 2004, http://sciencenow.sciencemag.org/cgi/content/full/2004/702/4 (accessed July 5, 2004).

40. Matthews, A. "SUNY Buffalo art: It's not bioterror, but is it illegal anyway?" *CNN Headline News* [serial online], July 13, 2004, http://www.cnn.com/2004/SHOWBIZ/07/12/buffalo.art/ (accessed August 29, 2005).

41. Bloedel, J.R. "Impact of September 11 on funding priorities and campus programs. Science at a time of national security," Merrill Advanced Studies Center, June 2003, 106, http://merrill.ku.edu/publications/2002whitepaper/bloedel.html (accessed September 14, 2005).

42. Chamberlain, A. American Association for the Advancement of Science. "Science and national security in the post-9/11 environment: Select agent rules," August 2004, www.aaas.org/spp/post911/agents/ (accessed August 29, 2005).

43. Bloedel, J.R., 2003.

44. Malakoff, 2003.

45. Chamberlain, August 2004, "Select agent rules."

46. Ibid.

47. Ibid.

48. Weiss, R. "Mail-order molecules brew a terrorism debate," *The Washington Post*, July 17, 2002, A1.

49. Chamberlain, 2004, "Select agent rules."

50. Kahn, L.H. "Biodefense research: Can secrecy and safety coexist?" *Biosecurity and Bioterrorism: Biodefense Strategy, Practice, and Science* 13, no. 2, 2004, 1–5; See also, Field, 2004; Brainard, J. "World's most dangerous germs, coming to a campus near you?" *The Chronicle of Higher Education*, April 25, 2003, www.chronicle.com/weekly/v49/i33/33a02101.htm (accessed July 7, 2004).

51. Ibid.

52. Henderson, D.A. "Public health preparedness," in *Science and Technology in a Vulnerable World*. Edited by A.H. Teich, S.D. Nelson, and S.J. Lita, 33–40. Washington, DC. Committee on Science, Engineering, and Public Policy, American Association for the Advancement of Science, 2002.

53. Glasser, R.J. "We are not immune: Influenza, SARS, and the collapse of public health," *Harper's Magazine*, July 2004, 35–42.

54. Gast, 2004.

55. Skolnikoff, E.P. "Research universities and national security: Can traditional values survive?" in *Science and Technology in a Vulnerable World*. Edited by A.H. Teich, S.D. Nelson, and S.J. Lita, 65–73. Washington, DC. Committee on Science, Engineering, and Public Policy, American Association for the Advancement of Science, 2002.

56. Greenwood, M.R.C. "Risky business: Research universities in the post-September 11 era," in *Science and Technology in a Vulnerable World*. Edited by A.H. Teich, S.D. Nelson, and S.J. Lita, 1–20. Washington, DC. Committee on Science, Engineering, and Public Policy, American Association for the Advancement of Science, 2002; Gast, 2004.

57. Greenwood, 2002; Skolnikoff, 2002.

58. Gast, 2004.

59. Vest, C.M. "Response and responsibility: Balancing security and openness in research and education," Report of the President [of Massachusetts Institute of Technology] for the academic year 2001–2002, 2002, http://web.mit.edu/president/communications/rpt01-02.html (accessed July 7, 2004).

60. Skolnikoff, 2002.

61. Branscomb, L.M. "The Changing Relationship between Science and Government Post September 11" in *Science and Technology in a Vulnerable World*. Edited by A.H. Teich, S.D. Nelson, and S.J. Lita, 21–32. Washington, DC. Committee on Science, Engineering, and Public Policy, American Association for the Advancement of Science, 2002.

62. Greenwood, 2002.

63. Vest, 2002.

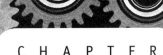

58

Dealing with Allegations of Research Misconduct: The Other Side of Responsible Conduct of Research

Elliott C. Kulakowski, PhD, FAHA

Introduction

The number of people involved in research pursuits has increased significantly within the past decade, including an increasing number of faculty, researchers, physicians, postdoctoral fellows, graduate trainees, as well as undergraduate students. They also include those who support the research enterprise, including research technicians and research nurses, who work in colleges and universities, hospitals, independent research institutes, government laboratories, and in industry. Despite the large number of individuals involved in the whole of research enterprise, the number of individuals who engage in research misconduct is miniscule.

We have heard the expression that "one bad apple spoils the whole bunch." Truer words have never been spoken, especially when it comes to the area of science. While the public appreciates the advances that science has made in our lives (e.g., the transistor, computers, and new treatments for diseases), some people have distrust for science and scientists, alike. Much of this distrust stems from images promulgated by Hollywood depictions of scientists (e.g., Frankenstein and in other stories of science fiction). It can be considered that, overall, recent scientific advances have outpaced ethical discussions about the meanings and repercussions of advances in science. It is very appropriate to question and debate certain advances and it is no wonder that within the general public there is concern about electromagnetic waves from cell phones and genetic engineering of our food supply.

Similarly and unfortunately, the general public does not consider one scientist's implication in research misconduct as an isolated event; instead, general public opinion interprets such misconduct as representative of scientists' collective conduct. In the lay press, stories of research misconduct sell airtime and newspapers. At times Congress has held hearings into allegations of research misconduct and Congressmen have been reelected based on public support for their vigilance over the expenditures of public funds for research. Overall, the impact of such scrutiny and, at times, sensationalism regarding research misconduct is felt not only by the scientists in general, but also by their institutions.

This chapter addresses the responsible conduct of research, for which there is an unfortunate need. When allegations are made that someone has engaged in actions not consistent with responsible conduct of research, research institutions and the scientific community are obligated to verify the allegations and to take appropriate action accordingly. For the sake of the reputation of the institution and research community, the response must be considered both fair and unbiased. Response to an allegation must protect the rights of the complainant (the person making an allegation) and respondent (the person alleged to have engaged in the misconduct).

Definition of Research Misconduct

There is no one uniformly accepted definition of research, previously referred to as scientific, misconduct. The basic definition of research misconduct was established by the federal government in policies of the National Institutes of Health (NIH) and the National Science Foundation (NSF). However, many institutions have gone beyond these basic definitions, adding to them. There are also some distinctions between the definitions of research misconduct versus other types of misconduct.

The NIH regulations were published in 1989:

> Misconduct or Misconduct in Science means fabrication, falsification, plagiarism, or other practices that seriously deviate from those that are commonly accepted within the scientific community for proposing, conducting, or reporting research. It does not include honest error or honest differences in interpretations or judgments of data.(1)

The NIH definition had come under some criticism for the ambiguity of the phrase "other practices that seriously deviate from those commonly accepted by the scientific community..."(1) In 1991 the NSF promulgated its final policy of scientific misconduct in which it defined misconduct:

> Misconduct means fabrication, falsification, plagiarism, or other serious deviation from accepted practices in proposing, carrying out, or reporting results from activities funded by NSF; or retaliation of any kind against a person who reported or provided information about suspected or alleged misconduct and who has not acted in bad faith.(2)

The White House Office of Science and Technology Policy (OSTP) released a government-wide publication "Federal Policy on Research Misconduct," in December 2000, which defined research misconduct as:

> ... fabrication, falsification, or plagiarism in proposing, performing, or reviewing research, or in reporting research results. Fabrication is making up data or results and recording or reporting them. Falsification is manipulating research materials, equipment, or processes, or changing or omitting data or results such that the research is not accurately represented in the research record. Plagiarism is the appropriation of another person's ideas, processes, results, or words without giving appropriate credit. Research misconduct does not include honest error or differences of opinion.(3)

Shortly after the release of "Federal Policy on Research Misconduct," agencies began to revise their policies to be consistent with the new policy, including the NSF in 2002.(4) The National Aeronautics and Space Administration and a number of other agencies have followed suit.(5) In April 2004, the Office of Research Integrity (ORI) of the Department of Health and Human Services (DHHS) announced a proposal to update the Public Health Service (PHS) Policy on research misconduct to make it comply with the new federal policy.(6) The PHS *Policy on Research Misconduct; Final Rule* was published May 17, 2005 and took effect June 16, 2005.(7) This new policy conforms to the OSTP Policy.

In developing their policies, some institutions extended the federal definition of research misconduct. In an analysis of institutional policies, the ORI found that over half of the institutions surveyed went beyond the federal definition of research misconduct, and included other categories in their policy.(8) The largest category among these included the category of "material failure to comply with federal regulations," entailing "serious or substantial, repeated, or willful violations involving use of funds, care of animals, human subjects, investigational drugs, recombinant products, new devices, or radioactive, biologic or chemical materials." Other categories identified by the ORI report included unauthorized use of confidential information; improprieties of authorship; material failure to comply with nongovernmental regulations applicable to research; inappropriate behavior in relation to misconduct, including failure to report allegations, withholding or destruction of relevant information, and retaliation.

An effective research misconduct policy also should define what is not research misconduct. In 1992, the Panel on Scientific Responsibility and the Conduct of Research, under the auspices of the National Academy of Sciences, National Academy of Engineering, and Institute of Medicine, released a report, *Responsible Science Ensuring the Integrity of the Research Process Volume I*,(9) which went beyond the NSF and NIH definitions of what did not constitute research misconduct and further addressed issues of questionable research practices and other types of misconduct. The panel's definition of questionable research practices include:

> failure to retain significant research data...; maintaining inadequate research records...; conferring or requesting authorship on the basis of a specialized service or contribution...; refusing to give peers access to unique research materials or data...; using inappropriate statistical methods...; inadequate supervision...; and misrepresenting speculations as facts...(8)

Other types of misconduct identified by the panel include:

> ...sexual ... harassment...; misuse of funds; gross negligence by persons in their professional activities..., vandalism..., and violations of government research regulations.(8)

It should be noted that some institutional policies surveyed by ORI classified one or more of these areas as research misconduct.

The federal policies on research misconduct have also set the baseline for institutions that qualify to receive federal funding. The extent that the institution expands on the definition of research misconduct also depends on state regulations and on the culture of the institution.

Developing a Policy for Dealing with Research Misconduct

Institutions receiving federal funds must establish research misconduct policies that meet standards set within the federal regulations. A research misconduct policy should include:

1. A definition of research misconduct.
2. A description of whom a complainant can contact when there is a question about research misconduct.
3. The rights of the complainant and the respondent.
4. The process that the institution will undertake to assess allegations that includes an inquiry, investigation, and adjudication process.

   * The outcomes that may result from an investigation.
   * The educational process to inform research personnel about the policy.

The cornerstone for any policy of research misconduct is the definition of what an institution considers to be research misconduct. While the federal definition of research misconduct has been modified, it is clear from the ORI analysis that over half the institutions they surveyed have a more stringent definition of research misconduct.

Following the 1989 augmentation of the federal regulations, the Council on Government Relations (COGR), the Association of American Medical Colleges (AAMC), the American Association for the Advancement of Science (AAAS), and many other organizations developed booklets discussing the issue of science misconduct. Despite the

involvement of these and other organizations, the research community did not yet know how to adequately respond when faced with allegations of research misconduct. Two workshops were organized to address this issue. The first, "Responding to Allegations of Research Misconduct: A Practicum," sponsored by the AAMC and AAAS, was held in 1992. A second, "Investigating Allegations of Research Misconduct: A Practicum," was held in 1994 and was sponsored by AAAS/ABA National Conference of Lawyers and Scientists, AAMC, Association of American Universities, and the National Association of State Universities and Land Grant Colleges. The workshops provided detailed step-by-step instructions on how to appropriately conduct an inquiry and an investigation, respectively. Subsequently, the Office of Scientific Integrity released "Model Policy for Responding to Allegations of Scientific Misconduct" and "Model Procedures for Responding to Allegations of Scientific Misconduct" in 1995 (revised in 1997).(10, 11)

The process described in this chapter is based on the ORI model and federal-wide policy.(3,11)

Disclosure of an Allegation of Research Misconduct

Every member of the research community must report allegations of research misconduct. Some institutional policies cite failure to report research misconduct as a violation of policy.

Because there can be uncertainty about what is research misconduct, some institutions allow informal discussions between the complainant and someone they trust or the research integrity officer (RIO) without a formal allegation. Some polices may allow a complainant, if he or she is willing, to informally discuss the issue with a potential respondent to try to resolve a misunderstanding before it reaches a formal allegation. While this may resolve a misunderstanding at the institutional level, the ORI has indicated that its policy does not support an informal process.

Institutional policies may include various definitions regarding types of disclosure and to whom allegations are reported (e.g., the dean, the vice president for research, the chief medical officer, institutional office of council, president, or a designated research integrity officer). Some institutions do not accept anonymous allegations, while others treat anonymous allegations formally in cases where the complainant may be uncertain about career repercussions (e.g., students or other persons who report to the potential respondent). Still other institutions require a more formal, open process, whereby allegations are submitted in writing and the complainant is known. In some cases, the institution's research integrity officer (RIO) may put the allegation in writing following a discussion with the complainant. Overall, it is advisable that the institution make reasonable efforts to protect the identity of the complainant.

Inquiry

Once an allegation has been lodged, the institution is to follow its policy and implement its procedures. The RIO has certain responsibilities that include:

- Informing the respondent in writing that an allegation has been made.
- Disclosing the nature of the allegation(s).
- Providing the respondent with a copy of the institutional policy.
- Informing the respondent of the procedures that will be followed.
- Securing data or samples as necessary.
- Establishing an inquiry committee to conduct a preliminary assessment into the allegations.
- Informing the complainant and respondent that they will have an opportunity to address the inquiry committee.

The respondent should be informed that the institution will make reasonable efforts to prevent the allegation from becoming public, but that confidentiality cannot be guaranteed.

Depending on institutional policy, the RIO may need to inform other administrative officials of an allegation. Officials may include institutional council, human resources, and other senior institutional executives. In special circumstances, the institution must report the allegations to the federal sponsor.

The inquiry committee may be either standing or *ad hoc*. The committee structure may differ depending on whether the respondent is faculty or staff or if there is a union contract; for example, the University of Pennsylvania has separate procedures for faculty and staff.(12,13) The committee may consist of only the RIO or be composed of several members, faculty and/or nonfaculty or can include members who are not affiliated with the institution. The members of the inquiry committee must not have any relationship with the respondent, complainant, or issue that would present any conflict of interest; however, members of the committee should have sufficient knowledge to make a comprehensive

assessment to evaluate the case. Once an inquiry committee has been established to review an allegation, both the complainant and respondent should be given written notice that also identifies the committee members.

The inquiry committee is responsible for first assessing the allegations and then determining whether there is cause to warrant an investigation. Once the inquiry committee members can make a determination whether or not the issue warrants an investigation, their job is done.

The inquiry committee may conduct interviews and reviews supporting documentation and ultimately produces a report, submitted to the RIO, that describes the allegations, the evidence reviewed, the results of any relevant interviews, and the results of the deliberations. If the committee has found evidence to substantiate the allegations, the committee recommends an investigation; otherwise, the committee recommends that no further action is required. The committee report is shared with the respondent and the complainant, and, often, each is permitted to present comments, which are included in the final report. The final inquiry report is forwarded to the deciding official (DO), the president, CEO, provost or other cognizant vice president. The report should be presented to the DO within a reasonable period of time. As described by OSTP, should be completed within sixty days from the first meeting of the inquiry committee.(3)

If the recommendation of the inquiry committee is that there does not appear to be substance to the allegations, the DO can accept the recommendation of the inquiry committee and take no further action. However, the DO can overrule the recommendation of the committee and decide to proceed with an investigation. At times, the inquiry committee may determine that no research misconduct has occurred, but that other types of misconduct have occurred. In this instance, the DO may not pursue research misconduct but refer the issue to others, for example, to human resources if other forms of misconduct are identified.

If the inquiry committee determines that there is substance to the allegation(s) and they recommend an investigation, it is unlikely that the DO overrules the inquiry committee. Once the DO has made a determination, responsibility falls to the RIO to implement the subsequent decisions and related activities. If no further action is necessary, the RIO should undertake efforts to restore the reputation of the respondent, especially if the issue has become known within the institutional community. The institution also has a responsibility to protect the complainant from any reprisals if, indeed, their allegations have been made in good faith.(14,15) The RIO is also responsible for maintenance of information obtained during the course of the inquiry in the event that the action of the inquiry committee comes into question or if other issues arise. Such information should be held in a secure place.

If the DO determines that an investigation is to be conducted, typically the issue is referred back to the RIO for handling. The RIO is responsible for notifying the respondent and complainant of the decision of the DO. If the allegations are related to a federally funded project, and if the allegations meet the federal definition of research misconduct, the federal agencies are also to be notified that an investigation of research misconduct is being undertaken. Some institutions may require that other individuals or offices be notified (e.g., human resources or faculty senate).

Investigation

The OSTP criteria for determining that research misconduct has occurred include whether:

- There is departure from the standard practice of the research discipline.
- The act was committed willfully and knowingly.
- There is a preponderance of evidence that research misconduct has occurred.(3)

If determined that there may be merit to the allegation of misconduct, the RIO then convenes an investigation committee consisting of members with area-related expertise to make an assessment of the allegations. Ex-officio members may include representatives from the research administration office, institutional council, or other offices as appropriate. The investigation committee is to be free from any conflict of interest.

The investigation committee is to conduct a thorough, fair, and detailed analysis of the allegation(s) and investigate any new allegations identified during the inquiry phase. The committee accomplishes such through interviews, and review of research data, notebooks, data tapes, samples, abstracts, publications, grant applications, and relevant communications (including e-mails). Interviews may include the complainant, respondent, and other witnesses who may have something material to contribute. Interview summaries are prepared and the witnesses are allowed to make comments to their summary, which becomes part of the investigation report.

Both the complainant and respondent may have legal council present in an advisory capacity,

but such counsel may not participate directly in the proceedings.(11) In addition, the complainant, respondent, and each of the witnesses must be interviewed separately in order to maintain confidentially.

At the conclusion of its investigation, the investigation committee provides a written report summarizing its activities and conclusions. The report is presented to the RIO; it includes reference to the institutional policy and the allegations being investigated; a summary of each of the interviews conducted and information reviewed; and a recommendation for action based on a preponderance of the evidence. The complainant and respondent are generally permitted within a reasonable period of time to review and comment on the report. Their written comments, if any, become part of the final report.

The recommendations of the investigation committee may determine that:

1. There is insufficient evidence to conclude that research misconduct has occurred and recommend that the allegations be dismissed.
2. The respondent conducted misconduct, but not of the type that falls under the institutional definition of research misconduct; therefore, the committee recommends that the issues be referred to other institutional offices for appropriate action.
3. The criteria set forth at the beginning of this section are met, and the committee concludes that research misconduct has occurred.
4. Issue may involve a combination of the second and third factors, as above.

Investigations should take place within a reasonable period of time as determined by institutional policy, federal regulations, or other sponsor. For example, the ORI requires that cases involving Public Health Service support be completed and submitted to the DO within 120 days of initiation of the investigation. This period may be extended if necessary, upon notification and consent of the ORI.(7)

Adjudication

The OSTP policy separates the inquiry and investigation phases from the adjudication phase.(3) For example, in the adjudication phase, the DO makes the determination based on the recommendations of the investigation committee and takes appropriate action in the following cases:

- If the DO agrees with the recommendation of the IC that—based on a preponderance of the evidence that no research misconduct has occurred—the institution has responsibility to see that the reputation of the respondent is restored.

- If it is agreed that other types of misconduct have occurred, the DO refers the issue to other appropriate offices for action.

- If, based on a deviation from normal practices, on evidence that the act was committed willfully and knowingly, on a preponderance of the evidence and recommendation of the investigation committee, the DO concurs that research misconduct has occurred, appropriate disciplinary measures are to be recommended and/or implemented depending of the severity of the misconduct. Among potential actions there can be a letter of reprimand in the personnel file, required retraction of publications, termination or restrictions on research activities, and termination of employment.

- Because of both research misconduct and other misconduct, the DO may take appropriate disciplinary in conjunction with other offices, such as human resources, according to institutional policy.

Institutional policies as to whom internally is notified of the final actions of the DO vary greatly. The respondent and complainant are notified. The outcome of the investigation also may be conveyed to the institution's dean, department chair, the academic senate, board of trustees, human resources, or other institutional body, as outlined in the institutional policy or as deemed appropriate.

Sponsor Actions

It is also incumbent upon the institution to notify any project sponsors of any inquiry of research misconduct. The sponsor, in turn, may impose its own sanctions against the respondent. If the sponsor is an industrial or a nonprofit organization, it may terminate support for the investigator, request retractions of any publications, and/or prohibit the investigator from receiving future funding.

In the case of a federal award, the institution must provide the federal agency or the lead agency (if more than one agency is involved) with a copy of the investigation report and the evidence reviewed, and must inform the agency of any proposed actions or of any implemented by the institution against the respondent. The agency then reviews the materials presented and may itself undertake an independent investigation and, potentially, if criminal violations are identified, the agency may also undertake disciplinary action in the form of reprimand, termination of research support, debarment, and/or case referral to the Department of Justice. (Lists of individuals debarred by the federal government can be found on the general federal government Web site.)(16) The respondent, however, can appeal federal government sanctions.

Research misconduct that occurs over the course of conducting federally funded research is considered tantamount to fraud. The Department of Justice (or individual citizens who have appropriate knowledge of fraud) may file a *qui tam* suit on behalf of the federal government to recover such funds. An individual bringing suit is entitled to a portion of any funds recovered by the federal government under the False Claims Act (31U.S.C. section 3729 – 3733). The act basically states that if an individual or group of individuals knowingly submits a false claim for payment of government funds, they are liable for three times the government's damages plus civil penalties. The False Claims Act and a discussion of its importance can be found on the Taxpayers Against Fraud Web site.(17,18)

Relatively few cases of research misconduct, however, have been filed under the False Claims Act. One of the few cases of such action involved Dr. Berge and the University of Alabama (UAB). Dr. Berge originally made allegations of scientific misconduct against a former student at the UAB for plagiarism of Dr. Berge's work. Two investigations found the allegations baseless. However, Dr. Berge subsequently filed under the False Claims Act stating that UAB provided false statements to the NIH in various progress reports. A jury originally found against UAB and awarded the United States $1.66 million, of which $500 thousand would go to Dr. Berge. The appellate court subsequently overturned the lower court ruling because of a "lack of materiality to the government's funding decisions of the alleged false statements; the insufficiency of the evidence that UAB made false statements to the government…and the preemption, by federal copyright law, of the state law conversion of intellectual property claim."(19)

Despite the few cases involving federally sponsored research that have been prosecuted under the False Claims Act, the US Sentencing Commission announced in April 1994 new sentencing guidelines that relate to research compliance and ethics programs.(20) It is uncertain whether in the future there will be an increase in the filings of such cases brought on behalf of the US government.

Protection of the Complainant and the Respondent

Institutions are responsible for protecting the rights and reputation of the complainant and the respondent in any allegations of research misconduct, throughout the inquiry and investigation phases, and afterward.

A complainant (sometimes referred to as a whistleblower) who make allegations in good faith needs to be reassured that his or her rights will be protected from any form of retaliation. Complainants may have concerns about their careers and their reputations, and they may fear or face harassment and physical harm. Institutions need to take appropriate measures to ensure confidentiality and to protect complainants from retaliation. To help understand what sort of measures can be taken, ORI has published guidelines for protection of whistleblowers and has issued rule-making standards.(14,15)

The rights of the respondent also need to be protected. It is a terrible experience for a respondent to go through the scientific misconduct process, especially if the allegations are unfounded. Regardless, the institution needs to reassure the respondent that throughout the investigation, the institution will strive to maintain confidentiality. Ultimately, if the respondent is found not to have engaged in research misconduct, the institution must make effort to restore the reputation of the respondent.

Special Issues That Require Contacting the Agency

In certain instances when the federal government is the sponsor, the institution can contact the funding agency any time it has a question about an inquiry or an investigation. OSTP policy requires that, during any stage of investigation into allegations, institutions notify the federal agency:

- If public health or safety is at risk;
- If agency resources or interests are threatened;
- If research activities should be suspended;
- If there is reasonable indication of possible violations of civil or criminal law;
- If federal action is required to protect the interests of those involved in the investigation;

- If the research institution believes the inquiry or investigation may be made public prematurely so that appropriate steps can be taken to safeguard evidence and protect the rights of those involved; or,
- If the research community or public should be informed.(3)

Conclusion

This chapter discusses the policy about research misconduct that any institution receiving federal funds must have in place; and the one policy that institutions hope is never to be invoked. The best way to prevent the need to invoke the policy is through the offering of educational programs that fully address the risks and consequences of research misconduct. It is through formal education and example where students, faculty, and staff learn the ethics of appropriate responsible conduct of research. These courses are being offered at most institutions today with a good deal of success. The Responsible Conduct of Research Educational Consortium is one program that offers institutions educational materials on responsible conduct of research. Other organizations offer compliance certificate programs for administrators and special interest groups, present workshops or satellite or teleconferences, and have available reading materials and videotapes. The actual benefits of education of responsible conduct of research to prevent cases of scientific misconduct may never be known. However, cases of scientific misconduct hurt the reputation of all scientists and their institutions, can do physical harm to research participants of clinical trials, increase public distrust for science, jeopardize future research support from our legislators, and as a result can slow the progress of development of new cures for diseases and new technologies to make our lives easier. Conversely, the positive benefits of conducting research responsibly can be overwhelming for each of us.

• • • References

1. U.S. Department of Health and Human Services, National Institutes of Health. "Responsibilities of Awardee and Applicant Institutions for dealing with and reporting possible misconduct in Science," *NIH Guide for Grants and Contracts* 18 no. 30 (1989): 1–10, http://

grants2.nih.gov/grants/guide/historical/1989_ 09_01_Vol_18_No_30.pdf, (accessed June 6, 2005).

2. National Science Foundation. "Misconduct in Science and Engineering Research: Final Rule." *Federal Register* 56, no. 93 (1991): 22287–22290.

3. Office of Science and Technology Policy. "Federal Policy on Research Misconduct," December 6, 2000, http://www.ostp.gov/html/ 001207_3. html (accessed September 15, 2004).

4. National Science Foundation. "Research Misconduct: Final Rule." 45 CFR Part 689 2002, http:// www.washingtonwatchdog.org/documents/fr/ 02/mr/18/fr18mr02-19.html (accessed September 1, 2005).

5. National Aeronautics and Space Administration. "NASA Grant and Cooperative Agreement Handbook—Research Misconduct; Final Rule." 514 CFR Parts 1260, 1273, and 1274 2005, http://a257.g.akamaitech.net/7/257/2422/01jan 20051800/edocket.access.gpo.gov/2005/05 9952.htm (accessed September 1, 2005).

6. Department of Health and Human Services. "Public Health Services Policies on Research Misconduct, Proposed Rule," 42 CFR parts 50 and 93. *Federal Register,* Part V, April 16, 2004, http://a257.g.akamaitech.net/7/257/2422/14mar 20010800/edocket.access.gpo.gov/2004/pdf/04-8647.pdf (accessed September 15, 2004).

7. Department of Health and Human Services. "Public Health Service Policies on Research Misconduct; Final Rule," 42 CFR parts 50 and 93, *Federal Register,* May 17, 2005, http://ori. hhs.gov/documents/FR_Doc_05-9643.shtml (accessed June 5, 2005).

8. Office of Research Integrity. "Analysis of Institutional Policies for Responding to Allegations of Scientific Misconduct," http://ori.hhs.gov/ documents/institutional_policies.pdf (accessed August 29, 2005).

9. National Academy of Sciences. Panel on the Responsible Conduct of Science. *Responsible Science: Ensuring the Integrity of the Research Process.* Vol. 1. Washington, DC: National Academy Press, 1992.

10. Office of Research Integrity. "Model Policy for Responding to Allegations of Scientific Misconduct," http://ori.hhs.gov/documents/model_ policy_responding_allegations.pdf (accessed August 29, 2005).

11. Office of Research Integrity. "Model Procedures for Responding to Allegations of Scientific Misconduct," http://ori.hhs.gov/ documents/ model_procedures_responding_allegations.pdf (accessed August 29, 2005).

12. University of Pennsylvania. "Procedures Regarding Misconduct in Research," http://www. upenn.edu/assoc-provost/handbook/iii_c.html (accessed September 15, 2004).

13. University of Pennsylvania. "Procedures Regarding Misconduct in Research for Nonfaculty Members of the Research Community," University of Pennsylvania Almanac, September 13, 2004, http://www.upenn.edu/almanac/ volumes/v51/n01/OR-research.html (accessed September 15, 2004).

14. Office of Research Integrity. "ORI Guidelines for Institutions and Whistleblowers: Responding to Possible Retaliation Against Whistleblowers in Extramural Research," November 20, 1995, http://ori.hhs.gov/misconduct/Guidelines_ Whistleblower.shtml (accessed August 29, 2005).

15. Office of Research Integrity. Handling Misconduct—Whistleblowers, http://ori.dhhs.gov/ misconduct/whistleblowers.shtml (accessed September 1, 2005).

16. Excluded Parties List System Web site, http:// epls.arnet.gov/ (accessed September 15, 2004).

17. Taxpayers Against Fraud Education Fund. "Title 31. Money and Finance Subtitle III. Financial Management Chapter 37. Claims Subchapter III. Claims against the United States Government," Section 3729, http://www.taf. org/federalfca.htm (accessed September 15, 2004).

18. Taxpayers Against Fraud Education Fund. "What Is the False Claims Act & Why Is It Important?" http://www.taf.org/whyfca.htm (accessed September 3, 2004).

19. *United States of America ex rel. Pamela A. Berge, v. The Board of Trustees of the University of Alabama, et al.* United States Court of Appeals for the Fourth Circuit. No. 95-2811 (CA-93-158-N) (1997), http://www.law.emory. edu/4circuit/feb97/952811.p.html (accessed September 15, 2004).

20. U.S. Sentencing Commission, news release. "Sentencing Commission Toughens Requirements for Corporate Compliance and Ethics Programs," U.S. Sentencing Guidelines, Revised, April 13, 2004, www.ussc.gov/PRESS/ rel0404.htm (accessed September 15, 2004).

VI

Technology Transfer

59

University Technology Transfer: Evolution and Revolution on the 50th Anniversary of the Council on Governmental Relations

Howard W. Bremer, JD

"Upon this gifted age, In its dark hour
Rains from the sky a meteoric shower
Of Facts-; They lie unquestioned, uncombined—
Wisdom enough to leech us of our ill
Is daily spun, but there exists no loom
To weave it into fabric.

—*from a poem by Edna St. Vincent Millay*

Prologue

Apropos to the basic research function at universities, it is suggested that the loom for weaving into a substantive fabric the wisdom derived from the conduct of research lies in the enlightened cooperation between the universities, industry, and the government that, through voluntary acts and legislative initiatives, has permitted and continues to permit the transfer of that wisdom to the public for its use and benefit.

Technology Transfer Defined

The concept of technology transfer—the transfer of the results of research from universities to the commercial sector—is said to have had its origins in a report made to the President in 1945 by Vannevar Bush[1] entitled *Science: The Endless Frontier*. Having witnessed the importance of university research to the national defense for its role in the successful Manhattan Project, Bush projected that experience to recognition of the value of university research as a vehicle for enhancing the economy by increasing the pool of knowledge for use by industry through the support of basic science by the federal government. The report stimulated substantial and increasing funding of research by the federal government leading to the establishment of several research-oriented governmental agencies, e.g., the National Institutes of Health (NIH), the National Science Foundation (NSF), the Office of Naval Research, and, ultimately, to the acceptance of the funding of basic research as a vital activity of the federal government.

Long before Vannevar Bush's report, but absent federal support in their research endeavors, the universities had been engaged in the "technology transfer," although that specific term may not have been applied to their activities.

Universities' greatest technology transfer efforts have probably been expended in preparing papers on research results for publication in scientific journals. Another area in which universities have been active in this effort has involved the activities of the extension services, particularly the agricultural extension services, which communicate a great variety of useful information, largely technical, but also in social and economic fields to many users, both rural and urban. Continuing education programs, e.g., in law, medicine, pharmacy, and engineering, have also served in the communication of information, keeping professionals in those fields abreast of the latest developments. Technical consultants provide technology transfer in both directions—the consultant imparts information to the engaging party while the consultant, in turn, can expect some professional enrichment from that activity. Another means for transferring technology is by making tangible products of research available to others with or without a view toward commercialization, for example, seedling plants for propagation by others, appropriate fragments of tissue for tissue culture, cell lines, hybridomas, and seeds, as well as mechanical or electronic prototypes and computer programs.

Thus, technology transfer occurs in many ways—through the simple spoken word, through the physical transfer of a tangible product of research, or through the relative complexity of an intellectual property licensing program.

Although all of these forms of technology transfer have been and are being practiced today, the focus of this chapter is upon the transfer of technology as represented by the transfer of a property right as the result of ownership of the intellectual property generated during the conduct of research. Such ownership may be manifested by patents, copyrights, trademarks, trade secrets, or a proprietary right in the tangible products of research.

Intellectual Property

Constitutional Basis

As we all know, the Constitution was drafted in the context of a struggle with a government that had abused its obligations to defend the rights of its citizens. It was no accident, therefore, that the salient portion of the Constitution drafted for the purpose of protecting liberties, the Fifth Amendment, made the government the servant and protector and not the master of individual rights. The Fifth Amendment of the Bill of Rights provides that:

> No person shall—be deprived of life, liberty, or property, without due process of law; nor shall private property be taken for public use without just compensation.

Thus, the Fifth Amendment provides generic protection for individual property. Since there is little doubt that the term "property" as used in the Fifth Amendment includes intellectual property, it would seem that the protection afforded the individual by that amendment would be adequate. Yet, the framers of the Constitution felt compelled to be even more explicit about intellectual property and provided the following language in Article 1, Section 8:

> The Congress shall have Power–To promote the Progress of Science and useful arts, by securing for limited Times to Authors and Inventors the exclusive Right to their respective Writings and Discoveries.

Why this special handling of intellectual property?

There was no recorded debate in the Constitutional Convention on September 5, 1787, when Article I, Section 8, was presented and was unanimously approved. That intellectual property, the products of the mind, should prospectively receive legal protection, even from a centralized government yet to be formed, was a principle upon which no one disagreed.

The power given under this clause is not general. Hence, it expressly appears that Congress is not empowered by the Constitution to pass laws for the benefit of the protection of authors and inventors except as a means to "promote the Progress of Science and useful arts."

Under this specific power the present patent statute, Title 35 of the United States Code (35 U.S.C.) was enacted. It is significant that the face of the patent document contains the following statement:

> —these Letters Patent are to grant unto the said claimant(s)—the right to exclude others from making, using, or selling the said invention throughout the United States.

Title 35 U.S.C. 261 characterizes this right to exclude as a property right. The technology transfer function is in great part based upon the recognition of and the specific provision for that very special property right.

Nature of University Research

During the prevalence of the "ivory tower" concept of universities and the research that was carried out in them, little thought or impetus was given to the transfer of the results of that research to the public other than through the accepted and acceptable route of scientific publication. In fact, under that "ivory tower" concept, a researcher who accepted a corporate subsidy aroused the suspicion among his colleagues that he had been diverted from his basic research and had become a tool of vested interests. He had accepted "tainted money."

In 1924, it was suggested at the University of Wisconsin that a plan be developed to make use of patentable inventions generated by faculty members, which would:

1. Protect the individual taking out the patent;
2. Insure proper use of the patent;
3. Bring financial help to the university to further its research effort.

The purists, then, quickly applied the "tainted money" theory to the plan. It was feared that any such arrangement would divert the scientist from basic research to work only on those ideas which appeared to have commercial potential. In other words, the research function would no longer be driven by the seeking of new knowledge, but by the dollar-driven need to solve current problems in the real world, even to the development of products and processes to market-ready condition.

However, the fears then propounded by the purists, fears still embraced in academia by some, did not materialize. There was no great rush toward patenting. There was no evident movement among university researchers toward applied research tied directly to actual product development. Nor was there any observable change in the research scientists' attitude. In fact, university research then, even as now, remained essentially basic in character.

The generation of inventions is almost never the main objective of basic research. If inventions do flow from that research activity, it is a largely fortuitous happening that takes place because the researcher, or perhaps an associate, had the ability to see some special relationship between the scholarly work product and the public need. It is from the recognition of this connection, which can convert a discovery or invention into patentable invention, that innovation arises.

Not too many years ago there was little appreciation of the value of that intellectual property generated during the course of research being conducted on the university campus or of the value of that intellectual property to the university, if properly transferred to the private sector for development and marketing through appropriate arrangements. In fact, on numbers of campuses, those activities would have even been considered unwelcome as an incursion into academic pursuits, as was the early experience at Wisconsin. Nevertheless, prior to the legislative initiatives under which, today, most universities engage in the protection and licensing of intellectual property, several universities and organizations carried out such practices with the attendant opportunity to generate funds to aid in supporting research efforts. Prominent among such institutions were the University of California, Iowa Sate University, Battelle Development Corporation, Research Corporation, which represented a number of universities, and the University of Wisconsin through its patent management organization, the Wisconsin Alumni Research Foundation.

The Government Vector

During the early history of the United States very little technical development work was done by the government and, therefore, as a practical matter, the question of the government owning a patent never arose. Gradually, federal agencies began to undertake the practical kind of development work which led to inventions. Since prior to World War II most government-financed research and development work was conducted in federal laboratories by full-time government employees, there was a small but recurring problem of what to do with inventions resulting from such work—inventions that, if made by private parties, would have become the subject of patent applications.

This situation changed rapidly during and after World War II, when the technological demands imposed by more and more sophisticated military requirements, as well as the increasing complexity of support services, made it quickly evident that there were not sufficient resources within the government to undertake all the scientific projects necessary to a war-winning effort. The absolute necessity to utilize the best technical ability available, regardless of its locus, spawned a rapid proliferation of government-sponsored and government-funded research and development contracts.

The proper disposition of rights to patents resulting from this work was theoretically as important then as now, but was never seriously addressed as a major problem because of the exigencies of wartime needs.

The basic issue was whether the government should always take the commercial rights to patentable inventions generated under a government-sponsored contract or from government-funded research, or whether such rights would be better left with the contractor or grant recipient to permit utilizing the patent system for transferring the technology developed to the public sector for its use and benefit.

After World War II, the rapid technological strides made under the impetus of a wartime footing and the obvious necessity for continuing technological superiority, at least in defense-oriented efforts, made it imperative to continue to provide public support for science. This support was not limited to the military. For example, in 1950

Congress finally provided an annual budget of $15 million for the National Science Foundation to conduct university-based basic scientific research. During this same period, hundreds of millions of dollars were appropriated by the government in the area of medical research in the beginning of an all-out attack on disease.

With the rapid expansion of scientific projects undertaken and supported by the government, the same shortage of technical ability and facilities continued to prevail as had been experienced under the pressures of World War II. Since the government could not do all the necessary work in its own facilities, the government sought out qualified private companies, universities, and nonprofit organizations to perform many of the programs through contractual arrangements. In each arrangement, the same old problem of ownership of patent rights existed, but was seldom, if ever, directly addressed. In the case of universities and other nonprofit organizations, few were engaged at the time in patenting the results of research and in technology transfer activities. Since one of the prime objectives of such an institution was to support its respective research efforts and since the government was a ready source of funds for supporting such efforts, the prevailing attitude was simply to "take the money and run," with little thought given to the underlying property rights and the value of those rights in the long term.

The government itself had not developed a uniform patent policy for all of its agencies regarding the disposition of rights in intellectual property generated during the course of research and supported by those agencies. In fact, there was no existing statutory authority giving agencies the right to hold patents or license technology. Such acts were viewed as objectives of the agency mission. Consequently, each governmental agency that supported a research and/or development effort through either contractual or grant arrangements developed its own policy. The ultimate result was that many and varied policies evolved to the point that the university sector was faced with the prospect of having to deal with some twenty-six different agency policies. Also, to support a given research pursuit, funds from different agencies were often comingled, and more than a single agency policy had to be considered with the most restrictive policy becoming the controlling policy.

Operating under the various agency policies, the government had accumulated in its portfolio about 30,000 patents of which only about 5% had been licensed and an even smaller percentage of the patented inventions had found their way into commercial use. Thus, with the government, as represented by its agencies, espousing, in the main, a nonexclusive licensing policy, the experience of licensing a government-owned patent had been irrefutably one of nonuse. For example, in 1978 NASA reported that up until 1978 it had had 31,357 contractor inventions reported to the agency. Of those, title had been waived to the contractor in 1,254 cases or fewer than 4%. The results of NASA's own licensing program were said to have been disappointing, representing a commercialization rate of less than 1%. In contrast, the rate of commercialization of the waived inventions was consistently in the 18% to 20% range. Therefore, the intended benefits, which were to flow to the public in the form of new products and processes as a result of federal support of research (both intramurally and in the university sector and stimulated through use of the patent system) were left unrealized.

An interesting comparison along these lines was made by Harbridge House[2] in its 1968 study of government-funded patents put into use in 1957 and 1962. The study found that contractor-held inventions were 10.7 times as likely as government-held inventions to be utilized in products or processes employed in the private sector for the benefit of the public.

Moreover, under the agency policies then in place, government ownership of a patent was in a sense an anomaly. The patent system had been created as an incentive to invent, develop, and exploit new technology to promote science and useful arts for the benefit of the public. When the government held title to those many inventions under the aegis that the inventions should be freely available to all—much the same as if the invention had been disclosed in a publication, the patent system could not operate in the manner in which it was intended. The incentive inherent in the right-to-exclude conferred upon the private owner of the patent (the inducement to development efforts necessary to the marketing of new products or the use of new processes) was simply not available. The ineffectiveness and inadvisability of such agency policies and their adverse effect on the public benefit should have been apparent.[3]

Government Policy—Move Toward Uniformity

In 1963, Jerome Weisner, President Kennedy's Science Advisor, recognized the need for guidelines to effect a more uniform government policy toward inventions and patents on a government-wide basis. The results of Dr. Weisner's study culminated in the policy statement issued on October 10, 1963 by President Kennedy[4] to establish government-wide objectives and criteria, subject to existing statutory requirements, for the allocation of rights to inventions between the government and its contractors, which would best serve the overall public interest while encouraging development and utilization of the inventions.

Since the policy, as promulgated, would most likely have to be revised after experience had been gained in operating under it, a Patent Advisory Panel was established under the Federal Council for Science and Technology to assist the agencies in implementing the policy, acquiring data on the agencies' operations under the policy, and making recommendations regarding the utilization of government-owned patents. In December 1965, the Federal Council established the Committee on Government Patent Policy to assess how the policy was working.

The studies and experience of the committee and the panel culminated in the issuance of a revised Statement of Government Patent Policy by President Nixon on August 23, 1971.[5] The changes effected in the Nixon policy statement were made as a result of analysis of the effects of the policy on the public interest over the seven years from the Kennedy policy statement. The fundamental thrust of that statement was:

> A single presumption of ownership of patent rights to government-sponsored inventions either in the government or its contractors is not a satisfactory basis for government patent policy and, that a flexible, government-wide policy best serves the public interest.

The considerations basic to the Statement of Government Patent Policy included:

(a) The government expends large sums for the conduct of research and development that results in a considerable number of inventions and discoveries.

(b) The inventions in scientific and technological fields resulting from work performed under government contracts constitute a valuable national resource.

(c) The use and practice of these inventions and discoveries should stimulate inventors, meet the needs of the government, recognize the equities of the contractor, and serve the public interest.

(d) The public interest in a dynamic and efficient economy requires that efforts be made to encourage the expeditious development and civilian use of these inventions. Both the need for incentives to draw forth private initiatives to this end, and the need to promote healthy competition in industry must be weighed in the disposition of patent rights under government contracts. Where the contractor acquires exclusive rights, the contractor remains subject to the provisions of the antitrust laws.

(e) The public interest is also served by sharing of benefits of government-financed research and development with foreign countries to a degree consistent with international programs and with the objectives of US foreign policy.

(f) There is growing importance attaching to the acquisition of foreign patent rights in furtherance of the interest of US industry and the government.

(g) The prudent administration of government research and development calls for a government-wide policy on the disposition of inventions made under government contracts reflecting common principles and objectives, to the extent consistent with the missions of the respective agencies. The policy must recognize the need for flexibility to accommodate special situations.

Although there is evidence that the guidelines did bring the patent practices of the agencies into greater harmony, divergent policies still existed, and there was a strong presumption, if not evidence, in terms of the transfer of technology to the public sector, that the more restrictive the policy of the agency, i.e., the more title-oriented the agency was toward inventions and patents generated under its funding (the agency generally took title to most if not all inventions made with the use of the funds), the less was the likelihood that the technology would be transferred for the public benefit.

Institutional Patent Agreements

During the period from 1963 to 1971, while experience with the Weisner-Kennedy effort was being gained, further efforts were made to persuade several federal agencies, specifically the Department of Health, Education and Welfare (now Health and Human Services [HHS]) and the NSF, to enter into Institutional Patent Agreements (IPAs) with universities. The policies of both of these agencies permitted a waiver of rights to the inventions made with their funds (referred to as an 8.2[b] grant of greater rights). However, on the very few occasions where such a waiver was granted, it was so fraught with restrictive provisions that it presented an unworkable basis for transferring technology to the private sector. No commercial firm was willing, under the conditions imposed under many of the waivers, to risk the expenditure of the necessary development funds.

Subsequently, after five years of negotiation, the then Department of Health, Education and Welfare issued its first new IPA to the University of Wisconsin in 1968. This was followed in 1973, after another five years of effort, by an IPA[6] between the NSF and the University of Wisconsin, the first such agreement with that agency.

That evidence of not only the availability of an IPA, but that those two agencies would actually grant them, appeared to provide some impetus to universities to engage in the technology transfer business. Nevertheless, some of the provisions of the IPAs available from those two agencies were unacceptable under some university policies, while many other governmental agencies still clung tenaciously to the policy of taking title to all inventions made with funds they had supplied.

Fundamental to the success of technology transfer under the IPAs was the vestment of certainty of title to inventions held by the universities under those agreements. That factor and, in addition, the ability of universities to grant exclusive licenses were instrumental in the subsequent willingness of private sector industry to engage in licensing arrangements with universities that had IPAs.

Although limited to two agencies, the IPAs were not only important as manifesting a change in the attitude of those agencies and potential licensees but, more importantly, as establishing, through negotiation, terms and provisions that were carried into and set the tone for the legislative effort that culminated in the 1980 passage of Public Law 96-517, the Patent and Trademark Law Amendments Act (the Bayh-Dole Act). In fact, the law is often looked upon as a codification of the terms and provisions of the IPAs.

The Bayh-Dole Act[7]

The passage of the Bayh-Dole Act was the reward for almost 20 years of effort by the nonprofit sector to stimulate the transfer of technology through the vehicle of the patent system. It was the culmination of the many pieces of legislation introduced over many years that had sought to establish a uniform patent policy within the government. It should be considered a landmark piece of legislation in that, after many false starts and unsuccessful efforts, it was, finally, a recognition by Congress that:

1. Imagination and creativity are truly a national resource;

2. The patent system is the vehicle that permits us to deliver that resource to the public;

3. Placing the stewardship of the results of basic research in the hands of universities and small business is in the public interest;

4. The existing federal patent policy was placing the nation on peril during a time when intellectual property rights and innovation were becoming the preferred currency in foreign affairs.

The most significant feature of the act was that it changed the presumption of title to any invention made by small business, universities, and other nonprofit entities through the use, in whole or in part, of government funds from the government to the contractor-grantee. Another factor, often overlooked, is that the act did away with the distinction between grants and contracts that agencies had often made when dealing with universities; a distinction that a number of agencies rigorously applied in their zeal to retain rights to intellectual property as a contractual obligation.

It is not universally recognized that the act provided, for the very first time, statutory authority for the government to apply for, obtain, and maintain patents on inventions in both the United States and abroad and to license those inventions on a nonexclusive, partially exclusive, or exclusive basis. The passage of the law was not, however, the end of the battle. It took over a year to settle the controversy that arose over the drafting of the regulations under the law. During the course of the legislative effort, an almost adversarial relationship had developed between the university sector on the one hand and the Department of Energy, Department of Defense, and NASA on the other hand. The nature of that relationship became very clear when those agencies combined to voluntarily draft regulations that actually controverted the law and its intention. As a consequence, much greater attention was given to the regulations by a university group that promulgated regulations that afforded protection against both arbitrary exemptions to the law at agency discretion and to the exercise of march-in rights by the government.

The Bayh-Dole Act represented the first cautious step into a new relationship between the government, as represented by its agencies, and universities. It also presaged a new and closer relationship with industry. The certainty of title in the universities to inventions made with government funds afforded by the Bayh-Dole Act, which was the stimulus to successful technology transfer under the IPAs, provided the major impetus to new and expanding university-industry relationships. Inasmuch as the government always receives an irrevocable royalty-free license under any such invention, and because of other provisions of the Bayh-Dole Act and the ensuing regulations under that act, the relationship is, in reality, a university-industry-government relationship.

The Economic Climate

To more fully appreciate what has evolved through the sequence of events that has been enumerated, it must be kept in mind that through this period, the economy of the country as a whole, as well as the economy of each state, was and still is in transition. Today, universities operate in an economic climate that:

1. Is knowledge-based, not capital-based (although, without question, availability of capital is a necessity);
2. Is entrepreneurially based; witness the large numbers of new companies created in recent years;
3. Involves world markets; the international aspect of protection for intellectual property generated through the research function must be a consideration;
4. Reflects continuous and often radical technology changes;
5. Is becoming more decentralized, making state and local options and initiatives more significant;
6. Is an economy of appropriateness, not one of scale, i.e., merely increasing the size of a production plant will not necessarily reduce the cost of product or increase its quality;
7. Is increasingly competitive on a global scale; witness the advent of the European economic community and other geographic economic blocks.

In view of this continually evolving economic climate, and since new products arise from new fundamental ideas as well as from new applications of existing technology, the necessity for supporting research is evident. However, support of research is not enough. That support must be coupled with a creative technology transfer capability. Invention without innovation has little economic value.

With the passage of the Bayh-Dole Act and, in the same year, the decision of the Supreme Court in the Chakrabarty Case,[8] which stood for the proposition that merely because something was alive (in that case a bacterium) it was *not* precluded from being patentable, along with the evolution of genetic engineering concepts, the universities were literally propelled into an awareness of the potential economic value of the technology that was being generated in their research programs. That fact made it self-evident that steps had to be taken to make innovation follow invention since invention alone holds little hope for generating needed revenues to support an expanding research effort. Because the government has been and still is the primary source of the funds supporting the research effort at universities, the passage of the Bayh-Dole Act permitted the universities to position themselves, through the establishment or expansion of technology transfer capabilities, to better insure that innovation would, indeed, follow invention.

Government Patent Policy Reshaped

At the outset, it must be presumed that government research dollars are made available with the expectation of not only developing basic knowledge, but also with the expectation that the funded research will lead to products, processes, and techniques that will be useful and acceptable in all or part of our society to improve the well-being of society in general.

In the face of this presumption it is apparent that inventions, whether made through the expenditure of private or governmental funds, are of little value to society unless and until they are utilized by society. In order to achieve such utilization it is essential that the invention be placed in a form or condition that will be acceptable and beneficial to the public. In other words, the technology must somehow be transferred to the public sector. To quote Thomas Edison, "The value of an idea lies in the using of it."

In a free enterprise system, such transfer is normally accomplished as the result of pertinent and appropriate activities of private enterprise. Since such activities obviously entail the commitment and expenditure of substantial monies—many times the amount needed to make the invention—adequate and appropriate incentives to such commitment and expenditures must be afforded. Consequently, and since the patent system provides such incentives and is the most viable vehicle for accomplishing the transfer of technology, full and careful consideration must be given to the making of any policy that will affect the transfer of technology that has been generated in whole or in part by government-funded research. In addition, careful consideration must also be given to proposed changes in the patent laws, including proposed treaty accommodations, that could adversely affect the technology transfer capabilities.

One would not disagree that the primary objectives of a government patent policy should be to:

1. Promote further development and utilization of inventions made in whole or in part with government funds;
2. Ensure that the government's interest in practicing inventions resulting from its support is protected;
3. Ensure that the intellectual property rights in government-sponsored inventions are not used for unfair, anticompetitive or suppressive purposes;
4. Minimize the cost of administering patent policies through uniform principles;
5. Attract the best qualified contractors.

However, of all the considerations attendant upon the establishment of a governmental patent policy, only one consideration should be paramount:

In whose hands will the vestiture of primary rights to inventions serve to transfer the inventive technology most quickly to the public for its use and benefit?

The passage of the Bayh-Dole Act was the beginning of the reshaping of Federal Patent Policy. Subsequent events between 1981 and 1985 further shaped that policy. The Bayh-Dole Act, the first event, became effective on July 1, 1981. The Congressional intent in its passage is abundantly clear from the recitation of the Policy and Objectives portion of the Act 35 U.S.C. 200.[9]

The second event was the issuance in 1982 by the Office of Management and Budget (OMB) policy guidance to federal agencies for implementing the Bayh-Dole Act in the form of OMB Circular A-124.[10] This circular clarified provisions in the Bayh-Dole Act regarding:

1. Standard patent rights clauses for use in federal funding agreements;
2. Reporting requirements for universities electing title;
3. Special federal rights in inventions.

A third event was the issuance of a Presidential Memorandum on Government Policy,[11] under which federal agencies were directed to extend the terms and provisions of the Bayh-Dole Act to *all*

government contractors with a follow-on amendment to the Federal Acquisition Regulations (FAR) to assure that all federal R&D agencies would implement the Bayh-Dole Act and the Presidential Memorandum.

The fourth event was the amendment of the Bayh-Dole Act by Public Law 98-620[12] to remove some politically motivated restrictions on exclusive licensing placed in the original Bayh-Dole Act. That law, in essence, made the Department of Commerce the lead Agency in administration of the Bayh-Dole Act as amended.

The fifth event, which did not occur until 1987, comprised publication of rule-making[13] by the Department of Commerce that finalized the provisions of the Bayh-Dole Act, P.L. 98-620, the OMB Circular A-124, and the Presidential Memorandum.

Also, in this same period, the establishment of the Court of Appeals for the Federal Circuit, under the able leadership of Chief Judge Howard Markey, gave further impetus to the value of patents and uniformity to their interpretation that put to rest the disparities that existed among the Judicial Circuits and had led to forum shopping in patent litigation. To paraphrase Chief Judge Markey, no institution has done so much for so many with so little understanding as the United States Patent System.

The government patent policy, as reshaped by the events noted, presented a charge and a challenge: a charge to show, through performance, that the confidence that was placed in the hands of the universities by Congress to transfer technology for the public benefit was not misplaced; and a challenge to maximize the benefits that can be derived from the opportunity offered through that patent policy to aid in maintaining the United States as the world leader in innovation.

These events, led by the passage of the Bayh-Dole Act, created the revolution in university technology transfer.

The Impact of the Bayh-Dole Act

How can we measure the practical impact on universities of the Bayh-Dole Act and the reshaped government patent policy? Since we are dealing for the most part with the transfer of technology from a protected base, i.e., patents and other forms of intellectual property protection, an obvious answer is to look at the change in the number of patents issued to universities and other nonprofit entities,

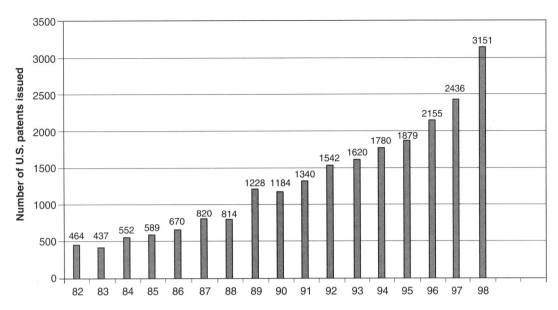
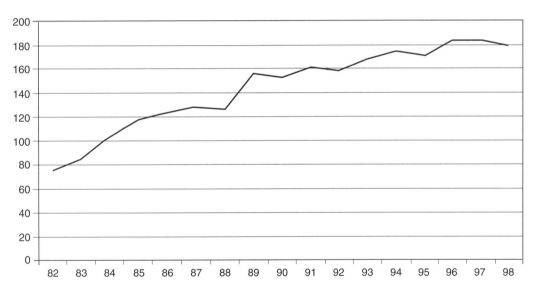

FIGURE 59-1 Patents Awarded to Academic Institutions 1982–1998

FIGURE 59-2 Academic Institutions Receiving Patents 1982–1998

e.g., teaching hospitals, since the effective date of the Bayh-Dole Act in 1981. The increase in numbers of patents issued can be readily seen from Figure 59-1. The growth and trend lines are evident. The figure is also significant in that it evidences that in the period from 1982 to 1985, the university sector was gearing up to either engage in or expand technology transfer efforts and that the fruits of those efforts became abundantly clear in the large increase in patents in the post-1986 period. That

trend continues today. In the last few years universities have received approximately 3% of all US origin patents issued, up from about 1% in 1980.

It is tempting to view patents issued on a year-to-year basis as evidence of current activity, particularly for those who are not familiar with the patenting process. Because of the varying periods of time patent applications are in prosecution in the United States Patent and Trademark Office, over the short term that kind of assessment can be very misleading. Over the longer term, however, since the passage of the Bayh-Dole Act in 1980, the number of patents issued to the university sector is a more meaningful measure.

Perhaps even more significant is the increase in the number of US universities receiving patents. This is strongly indicative of more universities engaging in technology transfer activities. It can be seen from Figure 59-2 that the number of universities receiving patents doubled from 1982 to 1989. It is reasonable to assume that this was in great measure due to the Bayh-Dole Act.

The real measure of technology transfer is not, of course, the number of patents that the university sector holds, but the amount of technology represented in and by those patents that has been transferred to the private sector for further development into products and processes useful to mankind.

What has been the licensing experience? The most recent licensing survey by the Association of University Technology Managers (AUTM)[14] shows a continuing growth in patenting and licensing activities by the university sector. The data presented in the AUTM survey was utilized by the General Accounting Office in part in formulating its required periodic review of the administration of the Bayh-Dole Act.[15]

Licenses and options executed have increased steadily since the passage of the Bayh-Dole Act, representing both an increase in the number of universities engaging in patenting and technology transfer activities and in the increasing activities of those universities already engaged in those functions. In accordance with the GAO report for fiscal 1996, the percent increase from the previous year was 8.4% for recurring correspondents in the AUTM survey. About 10.9% of the licenses or options granted were to start-up companies, 54.7% to small businesses. At the end of fiscal 2002, the university sector (based on response to the 2002 AUTM survey) reported 26,086 active licenses or options. The number of such licensees and options producing income was 10,866, generating a net license income of $1.267 billion.

Although the foregoing figures represent the effect of all licensing activities and not only those attributable directly to operation under the Bayh-Dole Act, it is submitted that because of the overwhelming support of research and development in the university sector by government funding, being 58% of the funding for R&D performed in academic institutions in 2000 (Science and Engineering Indicators 2002) and 62.5% in 2002 (from responding institutions of the 2002 AUTM survey)

with the recognized and traditional comingling of funding by the universities in funding research, it is legitimate to conclude that the bulk of patenting and licensing activity in the university sector is government-fund-driven and falls within the ambit of the Bayh-Dole Act.

Without question, the economic impact of university licensing activities is substantial—adding billions of dollars to the US economy.

Significant as this is, it should not be overlooked that university inventions, arising as most of them do from basic research, have led to many products which have or exhibit the capability of saving lives or of improving the lives, safety, and health of the citizens of the United States and around the world. In that context their contribution to society is immeasurable.

Another measure of the effect of the Bayh-Dole Act is the growth of membership in the AUTM and its predecessor, the Society of University Patent Administrators. That growth, which is demonstrated in Figure 59-3, is perhaps the most direct measure of the interest in and growth of the technology transfer functions in the university sector. It also evidences the creation and growth of technology transfer as a professional calling.

The Heritage of the Bayh-Dole Act

The Bayh-Dole Act can be given credit for focusing congressional interest on intellectual property-oriented legislation. With that focus established, the years since have seen many pieces of such legislation introduced. Some have become law; most have not. One piece of legislation, which could be considered to have been almost directly spawned because of or as the result of the Bayh-Dole Act, is the Federal Technology Transfer Act of 1986 (FTTA). That act was introduced as an amendment to the Stevenson-Wydler Act of 1980, which had been intended to promote the utilization of technology generated in government laboratories, but was singularly unsuccessful in accomplishing that goal.

The FTTA was largely a response to the increasingly tough international competition facing the United States and the prevalent complaint that "the United States wins Nobel Prizes, while other countries walk off with the market." The designers of the FTTA built the act under certain fundamental principles:

1. The federal government will continue to underwrite the cost of much important basic research in scientifically promising areas that takes place in the United States.

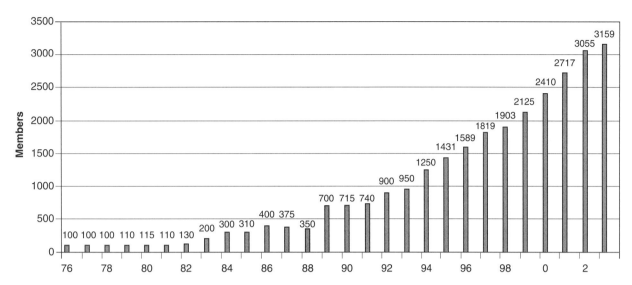

FIGURE 59-3 AUTM Membership by Year 1976–2003

2. Transferring this research from the laboratory to the marketplace is primarily the job of the private sector, with which the federal government should not compete.

3. The federal government can encourage the private sector to undertake this by judicious reliance on market-oriented incentives and protection of proprietary interests.

The principles enumerated were first tested through experience with the Bayh-Dole Act and the FTTA responded to the lessons learned from that law, perhaps the most important of which was its success in promoting university–industry cooperation.

The FTTA is clearly a direct, highly beneficial legacy of the Bayh-Dole Act, as has been additional legislation designed to expand the use of the results of research carried out within government-owned, government-operated laboratories by expanding the licensing opportunities for those laboratories.

Commentary

The growth of technology transfer has taken place over the last 30 years in an environment that slowly progressed from hostile to favorable. That progression was given major impetus by the passage of the Bayh-Dole Act. During that period we have seen a dramatic change in the attitude of the justice department and the interpretation of the antitrust laws where patents and antitrust are no longer

viewed as antithetical. We have seen a move toward a favorable statutory basis under which we have much greater freedom to operate. We have had an active effort by various administrations to obtain equitable treatment for US citizens in foreign venues, both in trade and intellectual property pursuits. We have had numerous and far-reaching changes in the patent laws of those foreign venues that have provided greater opportunities for technology transfer in and to these venues. We have also experienced extensive changes in our own patent laws and practices that have further expanded the opportunities to engage in technology transfer. We have had the benefit of a knowledgeable court in the Court of Appeals for the Federal Circuit that has slain many of the mythical dragons attached to intellectual property laws to provide uniformity of interpretation of those laws and before which we can expect equitable treatment. We have obtained the attention of Congress and, particularly, the attention in that body to the university sector's perspective on intellectual property law issues. We have seen the introduction and passage of legislation favorable to the universities and their technology transfer efforts. We have also seen developed, not only in the university sector, but in university–industry relationships and university–industry–government relationships, a greater awareness of technology transfer and a growing recognition of the possibilities that can be made available through creative technology transfer efforts and a much greater sophistication in handling those possibilities. Today, we operate in a climate that recognizes the value of intellectual property and the technology transfer function. We would like to think that much of this has come about because the universities, as a source of fundamental discoveries and inventions, have been the source of enlightenment for recognition of the value of innovation.

A word of caution, however. We work in a very uncertain business where, on the average, it takes in excess of ten years and hundreds of thousands, even millions, of dollars to bring an invention to the marketplace. We must also remember that, as a licensor, we have very little actual control over the process by which an invention is brought to the market or how, ultimately, it is marketed. We are always vulnerable to the attacks of special interest groups, whether inside or outside government, that are based not on fact but on emotion or that may be waged for psychological reasons. As long as envy and jealously are part of the human condition, such attacks are inevitable—only the intensity will rise and fall.

The emphasis today, as well as the "buzzword" in Washington is "competitiveness." That the university sector has made a tangible contribution to the competitiveness of the United States in a global market through the technology transfer function cannot be denied. The seminal piece of legislation that made that contribution possible was the Bayh-Dole Act. Without doubt, the objectives[16] of the act have been realized. Through operation under the Bayh-Dole Act:

1. Small business, which is frequently the test bed for embryonic university technologies, has benefited to a very large extent;
2. The government is comforted in knowing that taxpayer dollars, which support the bulk of basic research in the university sector, have led to the development of products and the use of processes that have advanced the quality of life for its citizens.
3. Industry can rely on a source of technology, data and information, and a pipeline of manpower that fulfills its needs and feeds the production processes.

In sum, all sections of society enjoy both the protection and benefits afforded under the Bayh-Dole Act and its progeny.

In recent years we have been experiencing an increasing incidence of efforts to restrict or curtail the technology transfer capabilities of the university sector under the Bayh-Dole Act through government agency actions, agency programs and legislative activities and through agency–industry consortiums. For example, pending legislation would disenfranchise the universities, as well as other nonmanufacturing entities utilizing the patent system, from exercising the constitutional-based right vested in the patentee to exclude others from practicing the invention patented.

We must understand that no matter how much money we spend on research and development the findings are not going to benefit the public unless there are suitable incentives to invest in commercialization. And because no one knows which venture will succeed, we must strive for a society and an environment ruled by the faith that the guarantee of reasonable profits from risk-taking will call forth the endless stream of inventions, enterprise, and art necessary to resolve society's problems. The words of the poet Edna St. Vincent Millay quoted at the beginning of this chapter seem most apropos to this situation.

We have already passed through an era where science was being made subservient to politics. In today's technologically intense atmosphere, where the maximum protection for intellectual property is more than ever necessary to provide protection for the heavy investment necessary to technology development, we must remain alert.

Even in the current favorable climate for university technology transfer as the heritage of the Bayh-Dole Act, views on the control of intellectual property, whether by government or special interests, can lend themselves to emotional molding. Outspoken claims to the guardianship of the public interest or welfare is a rich field in which to cultivate political power. We must never forget that freedom demands a constant price and that vigilance is essential. To quote Pogo, "We have met the enemy and he is us."

In the struggle to obtain the passage of the Bayh-Dole Act, as well as on other pieces of proposed legislation that impinged on the university sector, universities collectively spoke with a loud and single voice. We must continue to do so in all circumstances that threaten the rights and opportunities that we have earned over many years by dint of perseverance, patience, and hard work. This will require a unified, active, and continuing participation by all members of the university sector.

THE HERITAGE OF THE PAST IS THE SEED THAT BRINGS FORTH THE HARVEST OF THE FUTURE.[17]

Author's Note

This chapter is a slightly updated version of the article published by the Council on Governmental Relations on behalf of its 50th anniversary.

• • • **Endnotes**

1. Vannevar Bush held the following positions in government: Chairman—National Defense Research Committee, 1940; Director—Office of Scientific Research and Development, 1941; Chairman—Joint Research and Development Board, 1946–47; Member—Research and Development Board of National Military Establishment, 1944–48.

2. Harbridge House, Inc., *Government Patent Policy Study for the FCST Committee on Government Patent Policy*, Vol. II, Parts II and III, Washington, DC. (May 15, 1968).

3. See Betsy Ancker-Johnson-Les Nouvelles, "Resume of U.S. Technology Policies," *Journal of the Licensing Executives Society* 11, No. 4 (1976): 186.

4. "Presidential Memorandum and Statement of Government Patent Policy," *Federal Register* 28, no. 200 (October 12, 1963).

5. "Presidential Memorandum and Statement of Government Patent Policy," *Federal Register* 66, no. 166 (August 26, 1971).

6. For historical interest regarding institutional patent agreements and early DHEW practice, see Comptroller General of the United States, "Report to the Congress on Problem Areas Affecting Usefulness of Results of Government-Sponsored Research in Medicinal Chemistry," Washington, DC. August 12, 1968.

7. *Patent and Trademark Amendments Act of 1980*, Public Law 96-517, *U.S. Code* 18 §§ 200–212. This law amended Title 35 United States Code by adding Chapter 18, Sections 200–212.

8. *Diamond, Commissioner of Patents v. Chakrabarty*, 206 USPO 193, U.S. Supreme Court 1980.

9. *Bayh-Dole Act, U.S. Code* 35 (1981) § 200, "Policy and Objective": It is the policy and objective of the congress to use the patent system to promote the utilization of inventions arising from federally supported research or development; to encourage maximum participation of small business firms in federally supported research and development efforts; to promote collaboration between commercial concerns and nonprofit organizations, including universities; to ensure that inventions made by nonprofit organizations and small business firms are used in a manner to promote free competition and enterprise; to promote commercialization and public availability of inventions made in the Unites States by United States industry and labor; to ensure that Government obtains sufficient rights in federally supported inventions to meet the needs of the Government and protect the public against nonuse or unreasonable use of inventions; and to minimize the costs of administering policies in this area.

10. OMB Circular A-124 was subsequently codified at 37 *Code of Federal Regulations* Part 401.

11. "The Presidential Memorandum on Government Policy" was incorporated into the text of OMB Circular A-124 on March 24, 1984.

12. *The Trademark Clarification Act*, Public Law 98-620, amended Chapter 18 of Title 25 U.S. Code.

13. Final rules were published on March 18, 1987 (52FR8552) and subsequently codified at 37 *Code of Federal Regulations* Part 401.1–401.16.

14. "Survey Summary," AUTM Licensing Survey 2002, Washington, DC. FY 2002.

15. General Accounting Office, "Technology Transfer—Administration of the Bayh-Dole Act by Research Universities," *Report to Congressional Committees*. Washington, DC. May 7, 1998.

16. See note 9.

17. From a tablet affixed to the front of the National Archives in Washington, DC.

60

How to Organize a Technology Transfer Office

Patricia Harsche Weeks, MS

Why Establish the Technology Transfer Office? An Understanding of the Public Mandate

How have we arrived to where we are today? Until the mid-twentieth century, the academic institution existed to produce knowledge for knowledge's sake. Technology transfer existed in the form of the educated student, the production of scholarly works, in particular in scientific journals, and in the sharing of materials with colleagues. Vannevar Bush first articulated the idea of the academic institution as the reservoir of the nation's innovation. He is generally given credit for advancing the idea of governmental support of research in order to enhance the public good. In his 1945 report, *Science: The Endless Frontier*, submitted to President Roosevelt, Bush argued:

> Advances in science will bring higher standards of living, will lead to the prevention or cure of diseases, will promote conservation of our limited national resources, and will assure means of defense against aggression. But to achieve these objectives—to secure a high level of employment, to maintain a position of world leadership—the flow of scientific knowledge must be both continuous and substantial. . . The publicly and privately supported colleges, universities, and research institutes are the centers of basic research. They are the wellsprings of knowledge and understanding. As long as they are vigorous and healthy and their scientists are free to pursue the truth wherever it may lead, there will be a

flow of new scientific knowledge to those who can apply it to practical problems in Government, in industry, or elsewhere.[1]

Following this remarkably prescient report, which was instrumental in the formation of the National Institutes of Health (NIH) and the National Science Foundation (NSF), a public mandate began to emerge that academia had the obligation to move knowledge into the marketplace for the public good. Today, in addition to the traditional mechanisms for transferring technology, there is broad understanding that the technology transfer function is needed:

- To commercialize research for public good.
- To reward, retain, and recruit faculty.
- To forge closer ties to industry.
- To promote economic growth.
- To generate income for research and education.

As the 1970s arrived, however, so did the realization that less than 5% of the 30,000 patents issued by the US government had been licensed to industry with a corollary lack of products or services developed. After many false starts, the 1980 passage of the Bayh-Dole Act finally assured that academic institutions that had developed inventions with government funding were entitled to benefit from the fruits of that research. The Bayh-Dole Act recognized the value of academic innovation, the need for a uniform method of handling inventions, and the conviction that development of technology is best accomplished on a local basis. Technology Transfer Offices (TTOs) were first established at the nation's premier research universities and today there are more than 400 at universities nationwide.

Establishing the Mission: Aligning the TTO Mission with the Mission and Core Values of the Institution

The first and essential task of every technology transfer director is to ensure that the technology transfer office (TTO) is aligned with the goals and missions of the academic institution. Technology transfer is now a recognized profession both within and outside the university community. However, misunderstanding of the purpose, goals, and outcomes of academic technology transfer persists. As one of the deans of the profession, Howard Bremer, remarked in his 2001 address to the National Association of State Universities and Land-Grant Colleges:

> Of all the controversial subjects which have been addressed by members of Congress and discussed by newspaper editors and columnists over the years none appears to be less understood than the allocation and disposition of rights to inventions arising from government-funded research and development. In addition, the US patent system has always seemed to be mysterious to the lay public as well as its duly elected representatives. In the words of Howard Markey, Chief Judge of the Court of Appeals for the Federal Circuit, 'No institution has done so much for so many with so little public and judicial understanding as has the American patent system.' That dichotomy on disposition of rights to inventions and the lack of understanding of the operation and contribution of the patent system to the benefit of the public persists today.[2]

In establishing the technology transfer office, the prudent professional is careful to maintain complementary and related foci:

- The public mandate, as first articulated by Vannevar Bush and later codified in Public Health Service regulations, related to the award of extramural grants;
- The mission of the academic institution within which the office operates; and,
- The expectations of the different stakeholders within the institution that may include faculty and researchers, administration, deans and department heads, legal and finance, university relations, alumni affairs and the development

department, as well as members of the board of trustees.

Who Are the Customers? What Do They Want?

TTOs operate within private and public universities, large land-grant universities, and small, single mission institutes—all of which hold dearly the core values of the creation of knowledge within an atmosphere of free inquiry. However, each institution strikes a balance of teaching, research, service, and economic development activities that is unique to each. Interviews with the key stakeholders, noted previously, to understand how each of them interpret these functions is essential. Asking the question of each stakeholder, "How will you know the tech transfer operation is successful?" can be used to lead discussion, to measure expectations, and to set metrics for success.

Ultimately the successful technology transfer (TT) director must arrive at an understanding of the mix of functions (service, production of income, and economic development) that suits the institution. The exercise of keen political acumen is essential. While it is doubtless true that the diversity of stakeholders assures that not all of them will be satisfied, the astute TT director will leave as many stakeholders understanding and supporting, if not agreeing completely, with the focus of the office.

Strengths, Weaknesses, Opportunities, and Threats (SWOT): The Strategic Analysis

Whether establishing an office where none has ever existed or assuming responsibility for an established office, the TT director is well served to perform an analysis of the strengths, weaknesses, opportunities, and threats of the office. To the extent possible, this analysis should be done with the participation of as many of the stakeholders as possible. In obtaining participation for this analysis, the TT director ultimately can obtain substantial agreement with office goals and the operating model. This agreement is critical when difficult future decisions that may demand trade-offs among the stakeholders must be made.

Strengths may include an experienced and well-seasoned staff; a long, positive history of interaction between the university and industry; an administration with reasonable expectations of the office as measured by national standards; good office systems; and sufficient funds to invest in a robust patent portfolio systems and people. Weaknesses frequently include opposite factors: inexperienced or poorly trained staff; an administration with unrealistic expectations; a divisive or negative history of interactions with industry; bad or nonexistent office systems and procedures; and insufficient funding. Opportunities may include close proximity and access to venture capital and entrepreneurial management and a supportive local business community with local assistance programs. A unique capability or program within the university may be in place with key potential partners as a basis for doing business. Star faculty can serve as the magnet for attracting important funding for research projects through research consortia and the creation of intellectual property. Board members may offer both connections and expertise. Threats to the TTO can include a risk-averse university or local environment and/or absence of an economic development infrastructure and/or business assistance programs.

Broad goals can be established for the office when working with understanding of the institute's mission, of the interests of key stakeholders, and of the environment within which the TTO operates. As noted above, maintaining strategic relevance to the mission of the larger institution requires that the director continue to check back with key stakeholders to ensure that the primary activities of the office match the expectations of the stakeholders. Regular meetings and reports also ensure an opportunity to educate stakeholders to the technology transfer process, engage them in the challenges facing the office, and arrive at mutually agreed upon solutions for challenges.

Creating the Strategic Plan

The key to accomplishing this level of concurrence is the environmental assessment, a careful analysis of the strengths, weaknesses, opportunities, or threats (SWOT) to the successful operation of the office.

It is important to emphasize here that these analyses and discussions are not one time events. Any environment continues to change. At minimum, the TT director surveys customers informally or perhaps formally at least once a year to ensure that expectations are being met. As internal customers begin to interact with a TTO, their perceptions and demands may change. As an example, the office may become trusted to review consulting agreements to ensure that both faculty and institutional needs are

being met. This nonrevenue-producing activity is a valuable service that can encourage disclosure and discussion of key inventions. The external environment may change as well; as an example, the larger community may put in place financing structures that can enable start-ups in a way that would never have been feasible before.

The Working Models

In the majority of offices in the United States versions of three operating models predominate: service, income, and economic development.

In the *service* model, the emphasis is on service to faculty, not on the generation of income. In this model, each disclosure or case receives the same attention. While customer satisfaction is generally high, one drawback of this model, which should be discussed with stakeholders during the environmental assessment period, is that significant income earning opportunities can be lost because all disclosures are treated with equal urgency. Therefore, this office can require higher institutional subsidy to compensate for lost income.

The *income* model emphasizes the generation of income over service. This demands an experienced staff with good understanding of the markets and industries to which technologies might be licensed. It requires a vigorous triage process to separate the potential hits from the losers. It has the potential to generate significant income, which will satisfy administration and those inventors whose technologies are successful. However, it is likely to result in a generally overall lower level of satisfaction from faculty, most of whose technology is not a blockbuster income producer.

The *economic development* model emphasizes the formation of companies, especially local companies around university technologies. It has the potential for significant long-term income through shares of equity. It tends to downplay straightforward licensing to established companies and requires significant skill sets in company start-ups. It is a long-term, higher risk investment in the time and resources of the university. If successful, it permits the university to enjoy substantial public recognition for the creation of jobs and enhancement of the local economy. Because so few technologies can serve as the platforms upon which companies may be formed, measures of general faculty satisfaction are likely to be low.

In reality, no office can afford not to have some combination of the models above. At all times, the TT director must balance conflicting expectations and priorities. Thus, the director must have significant communication skills and be proficient in using them in order to stay attuned to the various constituencies within the university community.

Resources and Organization of the Office

Typically, university TTOs operate as departments within the university, reporting to the provost, vice president of research, or vice president for finance. On occasion, as in the cases at Cornell University, the Wisconsin Alumni Research Foundation (WARF), or Florida State University, offices are established as freestanding corporations with obligations to commercialize technologies arising out of the parent university. This discussion, however, does not address the benefits and drawbacks of these models.

The TTO is a complex operation with many skill sets required. To be successful, the TTO must have the capacity to encourage and receive invention disclosures from faculty and staff; to manage the flow of paperwork and income through the office; to understand the opportunity presented by each disclosure; to perform appropriate reporting functions to the government and funding agencies; to evaluate and make a decision regarding protection of potential inventions, manage patent prosecution, market and license technologies; and to report regularly to all stakeholders appropriate to their interests.

Every office, regardless of size should have the skill set to understand disclosures, evaluate them according to a set of criteria, establish a general business plan in cooperation with the inventor, and then manage that plan to conclusion. For example, the goal that Wake Forest University has set for itself of "faster, better, cheaper,"[3] is both stimulating to staff and responsive to customers.

People

Depending upon the size of the research operations of the university, TTOs average one licensing professional or case manager per twenty-five disclosures. Data from the Association of University Technology Managers (AUTM) indicates that an institution with a fully mature office may expect one disclosure per every $2.3 million in research funding.[4] Similarly, as patent filings increase, so does the need for people managing the significant paperwork associated with these legal documents. The following describes the functions and experience required in the office. Clearly, in the small office, some of these functions may be performed by the same person. In larger offices, several people may perform the same function.[5]

Director   This is the individual primarily responsible for relationship management, inside and outside the institution. This individual ensures a regular and ongoing dialog with faculty and administration. This may be informal, or, as is the case in some large institutions, may include a regular monthly luncheon meeting with the vice president of research and university counsel. On an ongoing basis, this individual ensures that a plan is in place to stay in touch with customers and stakeholders. This individual may be responsible for or participate in the establishment of policy, but certainly is responsible for interpretation of policy, in some cases working with university counsel. He or she supervises the case managers or licensing associates. This individual is the face of the university to the business community and manages the relationships with the various law firms who are engaged to carry out the legal needs of the office.

Office Manager   This person performs the human resources functions for the office, ensuring that appropriate records are kept in accordance with university policy. He or she manages the support staff, including the accounting function. Working with the director, he or she establishes office procedures; manages the files and maintains the office docketing and record system, often a computer-based system for tracking disclosures, maintaining information on inventors, managing reporting functions to funding agencies, keeping track of patent applications, income, and expenses.

Accountant   In some institutions, this function may reside in the financial office. In larger TTOs, there may be sufficient volume to justify having this skill set reside within the office. In any case, this function maintains a ledger for general office expenses, as well as legal expenses, tracks royalties and royalty distribution to inventors, and legal fee reimbursement by licensees. A computer-based system now in place in many offices is a critical and useful tool in accurate accounting for the TTO. These systems, whether paper- or computer-based, are the source of information to produce the reports measuring office accomplishments.

Docket Clerk   This individual (in a small office, often the office manager) logs disclosures into the office database, sends acknowledgements of receipt, sends reminders of funding sources, maintains the database, and is responsible for government and foundation reporting. Under Public Health Service (PHS) rules in the United States, this latter function includes entering data into the government iEdison database and sending the necessary election of title and confirmatory license required under Bayh-Dole legislation.

Case Manager This individual has the critical role of evaluation according to whatever scheme is set up in the office. He or she makes recommendations for patenting. In some offices, this decision is made by a team of case managers working with the director, using a set of triage criteria. After a patenting decision is made, this individual manages patent prosecution performed by counsel, usually outside counsel, markets and licenses the technology, manages existing licenses and, on occasion, manages material transfer agreements (MTAs).

Finances

MTAs are license agreements used by universities and industry to protect their rights in materials while permitting experimental use of those materials. They create an interesting dilemma for the TTO since they usually produce no income, but consume time and effort within the office. Certainly, the efficient management of these agreements is regarded as a valuable function of the office by faculty. Some larger offices put the management of MTAs into the hands of a single person to ensure consistent management of terms. Others place income-producing MTAs in the hands of case managers, since MTAs may serve as option agreements leading to a license. Whatever model is used, it is important that an office handle these agreements in a professional and timely manner in order to maintain faculty satisfaction. Details of MTAs are handled elsewhere in this volume.

While TTOs vary significantly in their budget structure, most include salaries and benefits, supplies and office systems, outside legal costs, rent, telephone, travel, software, and professional memberships and education in their budgets. Some offices may enjoy the support of accounting services through the university financial office; others must staff in order to maintain financial accounts, invoice licensees, monitor and pay attorney invoices. Space and furnishings may be part of overhead or a direct expense.

Based on the number of expected disclosures coming into the office, provision should be made to fund patent filings. This is an institutional commitment that recognizes that few companies will be interested in technologies that do not have some level of protection. The cost to file patents in the United States ranges from about $25,000 to $30,000. Assuming a rigorous triage system that will identify and assign effort to the most promising disclosures, efforts should be made to locate a licensee in the first year after filing in order to shift foreign filing costs to the exclusive licensee when applicable or to create sufficient revenue from nonexclusive licensees to support further patent costs. Patent costs must be rigorously managed. Larger offices should consider a patent professional, such as a registered patent agent or lawyer, along with the appropriate financial professional, to manage patent costs and outside firms. These costs can easily run away if not actively managed as part of an ongoing evaluation scheme. Too often, patent costs that have no business rationale are incurred. Regular review of the patent portfolio to ensure that the technology is moving along according to the original plan is essential.

In his 2003 presentation to the First Globelics Conference on Innovation Systems and Development Strategies for the Third Millennium, Tony Heher noted that "the cost of operating a technology transfer office varies from 0.5% of research expenditure in a large university to around 1% in smaller institutions."[6]

The rare blockbuster technology notwithstanding, experience tells us that sufficiently self-sustaining funds may not be generated by an office for at least ten years; according to Tornatzky, 50% of offices in the year 2000 operate at a net loss.[7] This data undoubtedly reflects the range of time that offices around the world have been established, with those established ten years or longer, now self- supporting. Nevertheless, the prudent institution should be prepared to sustain the costs of operating the office for at least that long or longer, if the office emphasizes service over income. Heher offers the following to illustrate the typical phasing of the value chain.[8]

Space

As is true of any function within the university, the space allotted for the TTO should be sufficient and of a quality to permit the functions of the office to be performed efficiently and effectively. These offices are ideally located central to research operations at the university to enhance interaction. In very large universities, consideration should be given to some degree of decentralization in order to enhance service. As an example, the medical school may benefit from having a licensing professional present even when the main TTO may be located elsewhere. This decision to physically decentralize must be balanced against the very real threat of isolating that professional and the inevitable inefficiencies of operations that will result.

Since this office frequently hosts meetings with industry licensees, entrepreneurs, investors, local government and economic development professionals, consideration must be given to appropriate meeting space to conduct operations.

Tools

Mention has been made of the need to establish a system to handle the volumes of paperwork and funds flowing through the TTO. In the past, universities were frequently forced to create their own systems. Today, there are several software systems on the market that may be selected to manage office operations. Careful attention should be paid to the trade-offs of each system. It is prudent to include university information system professionals in the final selection of a system in order to ensure that they will be able to support the system once installed. Clearly, the office manager and docket clerk should have a role in the selection of a system since these individuals will be working most closely with it. Time and funds should be set aside to provide sufficient training for all members of the office to ensure its most effective use. The office manager may be the person designated to set up protocols for use of the system to ensure consistent data input and set-up and to manage system reports.

Another critical management tool for the office is a triage system that weighs generally recognized criteria in order to come up with a total score for a disclosure. This score is then used to help make a decision regarding the effort and resources dedicated to a particular technology. An example of a form commonly used is included in Appendix 60-A.

Advisors and Other Resources

Good business decisions cannot be made in isolation. Just as the TT director has assessed the environment and the strengths, weaknesses, opportunities, and threats confronting the organization, so should that individual reach out to understand what is happening in other offices and what is evolving as best practice in the larger community.

Some of these resources are close to home: professionals within the office, selected members of the board of trustees, faculty. Business faculty and the inventors themselves can assist in provid-

ing perspective, market assessment, and a sense of the environment for any particular technology. Colleagues who manage similar offices are key resources in improving the operations of the office as well as specific deal construction. Some offices conduct the very useful practice of having colleagues from other offices visit and consult in overall office operations or specific skill sets, such as how to triage disclosures. This continuing quality improvement ensures that the office is continually reenergized with the best ideas and that stakeholders remain satisfied with the office work product.

Consideration should be given to exposing office staff to a broad range of related training. General sales and marketing techniques, as well as principles of customer service are widely applicable. One- or two-day courses are available in most major cities around the country. Thought should be given to establishing a regular education process for all members of the office to introduce new skills and refresh old ones. Getting out of the office and meeting individuals from other industries is useful, energizing, and good for morale.

The Internet provides resources in the form of Listserves such as techno-L that provides a forum for technology transfer professionals to exchange questions and information, and, newsletters from a broad range of industry sources. General business newsletters, such as from McKinsey or Recombinant Capital, as well as from specific industry Web sites (those found on Genomeweb or other information technology Web sites) can be helpful in monitoring the general environment and understanding the practice of deal making and technology transfer at all stages of the innovation process.

Professional Associations

The Association of University Technology Managers (www.autm.net) is generally regarded as the premier organization for academic technology transfer managers. AUTM offers profession-specific courses, publishes a newsletter and journal, and conducts national and regional meetings that offer the academic technology transfer manager courses at all levels of experience and aspects of the profession.

Other academic professional organizations, such as the Society of Research Administrators (www.srainternational.org), the National Council of University Administrators (www.ncura.edu), and the National Association of State and Land Grant

Colleges (www.nasulgc.org) serve as resources for technology transfer professionals. The Licensing Executive Society (www.usa-canada.les.org) is another useful organization. AUTM and LES membership includes those from both academia and industry.

The Council on Governmental Relations (www.cogr.edu) and the Association of American Universities (www.aau.edu), and the American Association of Medical Colleges (www.aamc.org) are other professional organizations that provide thoughtful material and suggestions for policy as they relate to the practice of technology transfer in academic institutions.

Each member of the TTO should be encouraged to join any one of these organizations and to participate actively in their education programs.

Marketing and Communications

The TTO has a number of audiences, both internally and externally, and it must develop a capacity to speak to each one in a way that is important to that audience. (Think "customers" here.)

University administrators, senior management, and the board of trustees have invested resources in the TTO. Regular communication with this group to inform them of the office's successes, in the context of the larger environment, and to inform them of important policy and legislative issues is critical. Managing the expectation of this group is essential. Typically, it takes ten to fifteen years for university technology to produce income, if it ever does. At Stanford, one of the "granddaddies" of university technology licensing, only 31 cases have generated more than $1 million or more in cumulative royalties. Overall, only one in 4,850 university technologies becomes a big income producer for its institution.[9]

In fact, experience tells us that on average it takes up to ten years for an institution to obtain a positive rate of return. Around the world, the cost of an effective technology transfer system is about 1% of R&D. An invention disclosure rate of $2 to $2.3 million of research per invention disclosure is remarkably consistent across the United States and around the world.[10]

Faculty, especially those who are inventors, need to know about the progress of the office, in general, and about the progress of their invention,

in particular. Getting out to departmental meetings, holding seminars, sending newsletters or placing articles in institution newsletters are all good general mechanisms that help maintain interest, encourage disclosures, and provide reporting. Meeting with inventors, copying them on correspondence, and including them in meetings ensures their greater cooperation and continued disclosure.

It is important as well that TTOs relate effectively with offices of public and legislative affairs in the institution, as well. Public affairs offices can be very helpful in getting attention for successful deals. This media exposure elevates the profile of the office, smoothing the way for interactions with potential licensees and investors. The legislative affairs officer in the institution is a key member of the team in ensuring that local, state, and federal policies continue to support the technology transfer agenda of the institution.

Outside the institution, the offices must cultivate a presence in their cities and regions as well as with their potential licensees. Academic technology transfer is widely seen as the engine of economic development. The challenge for most TTOs is balancing the large numbers of meetings and events held any year to promote new business and start-ups with the routine tasks of the office. A careful selection needs to be made to ensure that the TTO obtains the optimal value for its participation to support its goals. Technology transfer officers should attend and participate whenever possible in meetings dedicated to bringing together sellers and buyers of technology.

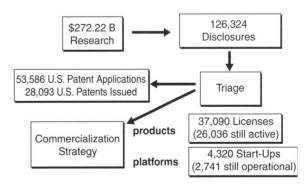

FIGURE 60-1 Academic Technology Transfer Productivity. Source: AUTM Licensing Surveys, FY 91–FY 02.

Measuring Success

For eleven years, the Association of University Technology Managers (AUTM) has performed an annual survey of academic technology transfer. Figure 60-1 illustrates the results obtained from FY 1991 through FY 2002. As noted, the TTO must, at minimum, be able to measure the amount of research dollars coming into the institution; the disclosures received; patents filed for and issues and licenses; and options and start-ups formed. These national standards can then become the norm against which the office is measured. Some offices, especially in their early years with deals yet to come to fruition, measure the number of contacts with faculty members to signify that they are reaching out, as well as to reassure themselves that they are seeking the very first fruits of research: disclosures. Disclosures are important because they are the first step toward identifying and protecting intellectual property.

Other measurements include research support negotiated that is related to a licensing or option deal; numbers of confidentiality; material transfer agreements; and consulting agreements reviewed. Other metrics may be established in concert with faculty and administration, which may include a satisfaction survey. In the discussion of what metrics to be used is an opportunity to set expectations and market the office. The office may want to consider publishing a yearly report; this provides an opportunity to present results, set them in a national and international context, honor inventors, and create a public image.

Every TTO exists in a continuously changing environment requiring flexibility and continuous learning and improvement. New technologies and new approaches to solving scientific problems are constantly appearing. Local, state, and federal governments continue to seek new ways to make use of intellectual assets to improve the economy and create jobs. Faculty members come and go. Professional development, as noted earlier, should be a central and ongoing component of the operation of each office. Each member of the office, according to the duties of the job, should be budgeted to attend at least one annual meeting to enhance job skills. Much can be learned from consulting with others from more established offices during one-day seminars and/or operations audits. It is also essential to retain ongoing formal and informal dialogue with customers of the office to assure that their needs are being met.

When it is well run, it is difficult to imagine a more exciting business than academic technology transfer, which exists at the nexus of scientific discovery, business, and law.

••• Bibliography

Heher, Anthony D. "Return on Investment in Innovation: Implications for Institutions and National Agencies." Presentation to the First Globelics Conference on Innovation Systems and Development Strategies for the Third Millennium, Rio de Janeiro, Brazil, November 2003.

Severson, James A. "Structure and Function of Technology Transfer Offices." Presentation to the Association of University Technology Managers, Atlanta, GA, 2000.

Watanabe, Mary. "Stanford Office of Technology Licensing." Presentation to the Association of University Technology Managers, Atlanta, GA, 2000.

••• References

1. Bush, Vannevar. "Science: The Endless Frontier," 1945, http://www1.umn.edu/scitech/assign/vb/Vbush1945.html (accessed December 2, 2003).

2. Bremer, Howard. "First Two Decades of the Bayh-Dole Act as Public Policy." Speech given to the National Association of State Universities and Land Grant Colleges (NASULGC), Washington, DC, November 11, 2001, http://www.autm.net/index_ie.html (accessed January 10, 2004).

3. Lemons, Spencer, and David Winwood. "Technology Transfer Offices: Structure, Goals and Evaluation," Presentation to Association of University Technology Managers, Atlanta, GA, 2000.

4. Association of University Technology Managers, "2002 Survey," www.autm.net.

5. Severson, James A. "Structure and Function of Technology Transfer Offices," Presentation to the Association of University Technology Managers, Atlanta, GA, 2000.

6. Heher, Tony. "Return on Investment in Innovation," Presentation to the First Globelics Conference on Innovation Systems and Development Strategies for the Third Millennium,

Rio de Janeiro, Brazil, November 2003. From an unpublished paper with permission of the author.

7. Tornatzky, Louis G. Building state economies by promoting University-Industry technology transfer prepared for the National Governor's Association. April 2000, http://nga.org/cda/ files/UNIVERSITY.PDF (accessed September 6, 2005).

8. Ibid.

9. Watanabe, Mary. "Stanford Office of Technology Transfer," Presentation to AUTM, Atlanta, GA, 2003.

10. Heher, 2003.

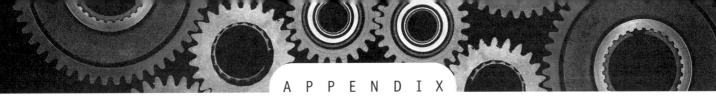

60-A

Sample Assessment Form

Initial Technology Assessment
Score 1-5 (5=highest)
Date: Docket #:   Score: Inventor: Tech. Mgr.:

Technology:

Patent/Science Issues   Yes   No

                               Rating (1-5)

1. Literature search completed and clear.
2. Patent search completed and clear.
3. No prior claims to the technology.
4. Pending publications/presentations?
5. Technology is patentable?

Technology Issues
1. Major breakthrough? Basis of new industry/company?
2. Stage of development.
3. Animal data?
4. Human data?
5. Technology state of the art.
6. Functioning prototype?
7. Time to market?
8. Long product life cycle?
9. Addition to FCCC patents?

Marketing Issues
1. Fills identifiable need.
2. Market sizable and growing?

3. Definable market niche?

4. Advantages over existing technologies?

5. Market accessible (no dominant competing technology).

6. Sustainable competitive advantage?

7. Conforms to relevant standards?

Management Issues

1. Inventor is technology champion.

2. Inventor has realistic expectations.

3. Inventor is cooperative.

4. Inventor is team player.

What is of the greatest concern?

What is the opportunity?

Critical information needed/data that need to be gathered for commercial viability

Estimated patent costs: Domestic $

                             Foreign $

Estimated return $ Time span (yrs):

Recommendation:

☐ Return for research

☐ Not patentable

☐ Patent application

☐ Commercialize without patent

☐ Return to inventor

61

Elements of an Intellectual Property Policy

Elliott C. Kulakowski, PhD, FAHA

Introduction

Institutions should develop a policy about how to manage the intellectual property that is developed by their faculty and researchers. Many larger or established institutions already have such policies, but new research institutes and independent hospitals that engage in research may not have such policies. This chapter presents an overview of what may be included within an intellectual property policy.

A policy should define the obligations of the inventor and institution to protect intellectual property rights. The policy must meet federal regulations related to the Patent and Trademark Law Amendment Act, commonly referred to as the Bayh-Dole Act (Public Law 96-517 and 98-620, as amended), if the institution receives federal funds.[1,2] Refer to the discussion of the Bayh-Dole Act in this section.[3] States may also have statutes that govern intellectual property developed by state academic institutions. An institution's intellectual property policy also serves as the cornerstone to help define an institution's position in conducting research with for-profit companies and ownership of any intellectual property that may develop.

There is no standard format for an intellectual property policy. This chapter references several different policies from nonprofit institutions, including universities (public and private), academic medical centers, and nonprofit research institutes. The policies range from being very short and general, to very long and specific with several appendices. The different policies also represent the culture of the institution from being very conservative to very entrepreneurial.

Despite the differences, several segments of a policy are generally universal. The three basic parts of an intellectual property policy are:

1. Ownership of the intellectual property.
2. Obligations and responsibilities of the parties.
3. Accounting for income, expenses and royalty distribution.

Some policies include an introduction or preamble and definition of terms that may be codified in patent law or may be unique to a given institution. A policy may also discuss copyrights or creative works of art. These areas are not discussed in this chapter, but examples are presented in the references.

Readers are encouraged to look at the various institutional policies that are referenced to note the diversity among policies from different institutions.

Preamble

While not universal, many policies have a preamble that may describe the institution's mission and purpose and objective of the intellectual property policy. The preamble also may reference the responsibilities of the parties that are described elsewhere in the policy. Finally, the preamble may discuss the relationship to federal laws and state law, if applicable.

The mission of the institution is a clear and concise statement. Academic institutions typically describe their mission as teaching, research, and service, while academic medical centers and hospitals focus on patient care, teaching, and research. The overall mission of independent research institutions is primarily the discovery of new knowledge. For example, the University of Florida states in its policy "Central to the purpose of the University of Florida are teaching, research and service."[4] Its policy then elaborates on its mission statement.

This is in contrast to the preamble of the intellectual property policy of the University of Pennsylvania that focuses primarily on the research aspect of their mission. Their policy states "The mission of the University includes the stimulation of basic and applied research activities of faculty, employees and students of the University, and the dissemination of the results of their research for the purpose of adding to the body of knowledge and serving the public interest."[5]

Another segment of the preamble may be to describe the objectives of a policy. Cincinnati Children's Hospital, for example, states that its "responsibility is to encourage creativity and innovation, promote the use of novel discoveries and inventions for the good of the public, and provide equitable distribution between CCMC (Children's Hospital Medical Center) CCRF (Cincinnati Children's Research Foundation) and the inventor/investigator(s) of licensing revenues resulting from the commercialization of novel discoveries and inventions."[6]

The intellectual property policy of the Albert Einstein Healthcare Network (AEHN) in Philadelphia expands on this to discuss that its purpose also is "to facilitate the transfer of AEHN-developed research results to industry, to provide AEHN Inventors with assistance in assessing patentability and marketability of inventions and to facilitate the processes of patenting and licensing such inventions, and to define the obligations of AEHN, Inventors, and Sponsors regarding inventions and to safeguard the property rights and obligations of AEHN and its Inventors."[7]

State universities may add a reference to or description of their state policy to their preamble. For example, the policy of the University of Colorado states "The purpose of this Administrative Policy Statement is to implement Regent policy, 'Intellectual Property on Discoveries and Patents for Their Protection and Commercialization.' "[8,9]

Definitions

Many policies have a section where terms used in their policy are defined. Some of the definitions may be codified in law; others are used to define

terms used in a particular policy. The United States Patent and Trademark Office has a rather extensive glossary of terms and provides good definitions of patent and patent rights, copyrights, trade and service marks, mask works and tangible research property, and trade secrets.[10] Similar terms are found in the Massachusetts Institute of Technology policy[11] and in the two from Colorado.[8,9] In this chapter, we do not identify all the terms that can be included in a policy. However, when we use a specific term, we will provide a defnition.

Ownership

Ownership, as defined in a policy, describes what types of intellectual property are covered by the policy, what is excluded from the policy, and who is entitled to such ownership.

While the wording of ownership may differ from institution to institution, the basic premise remains the same. The institution claims ownership of the intellectual property rights to any invention developed in whole or in part by a covered person under the institution's intellectual property policy, unless the institution elects to waive its ownership rights (see discussion of covered person below), including any patents resulting from the invention. Covered persons are required to assign their rights and interests to the institution. Some institutions limit applicability of their ownership to only those inventions that effectively utilize in whole or in part the institution's personnel, resources, facilities, or funds. However, when an institution's personnel are involved in the origination or development of the concept, the institution may also claim ownership. In instances where the external funds are provided by the federal government, nonprofit associations, or industry, the institution may claim rights to the intellectual property unless there are specific restrictions as to who owns the intellectual property that is agreed upon between the sponsor and the institution, in advance.

It should be noted that it is not unusual in industrial or clinical trial agreements that institutions seek to protect any intellectual property of their faculty, staff, and students. It is not unrealistic to expect institutions to have wording in their agreements stating that what the institution develops belongs to the institution. Conversely, what the company develops through the conduct of its own activities and personnel belongs to the company, and in instances where both contribute to the development of an invention, both own the technology, but the institution is required to offer the technology to the corporate sponsor.

Ownership of intellectual property covers not just the embodiment of the invention, but includes the underlying materials needed to support the preparation, submission, prosecution, and protection of an institution's intellectual property. Notebooks or other documentation in written or electronic form such as computer tapes, video or audio tapes, photographs, drawings, radiographs, disks, source codes, biological samples, chemical structures, samples, or models are the property of the institution and should be described in the policy. Many institutions already claim ownership rights to these materials developed by their faculty and supported by their institution and any other external sponsor, especially the federal government, through specific policies such as a data ownership policy or scientific misconduct policy. However, it also may be mentioned again in the intellectual property policy. The institution needs to have ownership of these materials to be able to protect its intellectual property. While an institution rarely takes physical control of the data and underlying materials, it retains the ownership rights to them for its own purposes.

When an institution accepts an assignment of intellectual property, it is also implied that it assumes control and responsibility for costs of protecting such intellectual property.

Some institutional policies specifically exclude certain ownership rights in their policy that they may otherwise claim. Institutions may specifically exclude from their policies pure works of art, musical compositions, literature, theatrical productions, and copyrighted works such as lectures, presentations, journal articles, chapters for books, books or monographs which may be developed during the course of their employment at the institution. The University of Colorado does not apply this exclusion if it commissions the work for its own purposes, if it supports the specific work, or if it is subject to contractual obligations.[8] Other institutional policies may be silent on these issues.

While some institutions claim ownership to the entire embodiment of intellectual property developed by a person covered by their policy (covered person), others are somewhat less constraining. In today's entrepreneurial environment, covered persons may have their own companies or be involved in other external activities. For example, Temple University's policy states that "an inventor shall be entitled to all right, title, and interest to any discovery or invention which is developed wholly on the inventor's own time and with the inventor's own facilities and which does not involve use of any Uni-

versity funds, equipment, facilities, or personnel. Where such right, title and interest are claimed and agreed upon, the University shall not assume any responsibility for costs or liability of patent prosecution, maintenance or enforcement, or licensing."[12]

The University of Pennsylvania requires that an inventor disclose inventions that the inventor believes to be outside of the scope of the institution's policy. The inventor must provide the technology transfer office with "a written statement of the circumstances leading to the making of the INVENTION." If it is determined that the invention is not covered by their policy, the institution "shall confirm in writing that the university has no right, title and interest to the INVENTION."[5] However, if it is determined that the university believes that it should claim ownership or that it can not make a determination about who should have intellectual property rights, the issue is referred to their Intellectual Property Committee for resolution.

Some intellectual property policies also state that a covered person cannot hide the fact that he or she has made an invention, and that if a covered person fails to disclose an invention to the institution, the institution retains its rights to the invention unless it relinquishes its rights in writing. The institution alternately may seek to exercise its rights and regain any lost revenues from the inventor. In addition, the institution also may take appropriate disciplinary action against the covered person. This is especially true regarding any invention derived from federal funds and where the institution is required to notify the federal government and in industrial agreements where the institution is required to disclose such inventions.

Parties: Roles and Responsibilities

Institutional policies invariably define who is covered under their intellectual property policy. The main players are the covered person and the institution. While not a party to the ownership of intellectual property, many policies also define the roles and responsibility of an intellectual property committee.

Covered Persons

The use of the term *covered person(s)* is not universal and is used in this chapter to define those individuals at an institution who may be covered under the institution's intellectual property policy. It also is used in defining their roles and responsibilities. In the simplest definition, a covered person(s) may be limited to full- or part-time employees, when some institutions may describe more specifically to include faculty, physicians, and staff.

In an expanded definition, a covered person may include trainees in postdoctoral fellows, residents, graduate students, and undergraduate students. An intellectual property policy should clearly define the role and responsibilities of trainees, when at certain institutions they may not be considered employees. Many institutions include them in their policy because their research is conducted at the institution and uses institutional resources; may or may not be supported by a grant or contract from the federal government or other external sponsor; and as such should be covered under the policy. This should include work toward a dissertation.

Activities by an undergraduate student may be a little more complicated when they are part of a cooperative educational program as described in the University of Pennsylvania policy. In this instance, their academic institution is receiving tuition from the student, and the student is involved in a training experience at a company. Since the institution provides neither space nor resources directly for this activity, an institution should decide whether the student should be covered under the institution's policy. In addition, the company may require, as a condition of the work experience, that the student be covered under the intellectual property policy of the company. An institution should resolve the issue of intellectual property ownership with the company and the trainee before the work/training experience begins. A good description of undergraduate students is in the policy from the University of Pennsylvania.[5]

Others who may be considered covered persons can be agents for the institution and nonemployees who use the institution's resources. Issues can arise when the individual, possibly a visiting scientist or a faculty member on sabbatical, who is covered under their home institution's intellectual property policy and who is supported in whole or in part by their home institution or a grant at their home institution from a sponsor, is required to abide by the intellectual property policy of the host institution. In this instance, the policy may describe that a resolution should be determined between the two institutions in advance of the activity.

An institution may require that all covered persons be informed of the policy and refer the covered person to the policy's location on the institution's Web site or give them a paper copy of the policy. This can happen at the time of employment or when changes are made to the policy. The University of Pennsylvania includes in its intellectual property policy a requirement that covered persons sign a participation agreement, which is an addendum to its policy that spells out the responsibilities of a covered person.[5] The required signing of the participation agreement ensures that the covered person is aware of the institution's policy and agrees to comply with it.

Inventor

For purposes of this chapter, once a covered person invents something he is referred to as an *inventor*. The United States Patent and Trademark Office defines an inventor as one who contributes to the conception of an invention.[10] The patent law of the United States of America requires that the applicant in a patent application must be the inventor.

Inventors have specific responsibilities to their institution that should be described in the policy. First and foremost, the inventor must disclose any and all inventions, whether the inventor believes that such an invention belongs to the institution or not. It is only through the disclosure of intellectual property and who was involved in its development that the true inventor(s) can be determined, and whether the invention is covered under the institution's intellectual property policy.

The intellectual property policy should require the inventor to disclose any invention as soon as feasible to allow the institution the opportunity to take appropriate action to protect the intellectual property. Unfortunately, it is not unusual for an inventor to contact the technology transfer office about a possible invention just before there is to be public disclosure in the form of an article or abstract for publication, or the inventor is to make a presentation at a scientific session or in a meeting with industry sponsors. While patent protection may be obtained in the United States, failure of a covered person to disclose an invention in a timely manner may result in loss of international patent protection, and thus reduce the potential commercial value of the invention.

The inventor is required to assist in patent prosecution. This means that the inventor may be required to meet with staff of the technology transfer office to refine the scope of the invention, with the institution's internal and/or external counsel responsible for patent filing and prosecution, and marketing individuals to develop appropriate materials to advertise the invention.

An inventor also would be required to assign any intellectual property that the institution is entitled to own. This includes an assignment initially required by the institution, and assignment for US patent filing purposes, and an assignment for any international patents that may be required.

The inventor has a responsibility to assist, where applicable, in marketing the technology to potential licensees. Inventors know best the technology and its applications; the state of the science; and leaders in the area and possibly colleagues in related fields in industry who may be interested in the technology or who can provide contacts in the company. For these reasons, they can be very useful in marketing the technology. The inventor also can be the best salesperson for a technology, because an inventor can make appropriate presentations to company technology transfer staff and to industry scientists about the technology. The inventor can describe the technology, its potential applications and the benefits of the technology over other current technologies. In addition, inventors may be useful in developing of marketing materials.

Another role of the inventor is to assist in further development of the technology. It is not unusual for an inventor to be retained by a licensee to further develop the technology through a research agreement that supports further related research of the inventor. In addition the inventor may be retained by the company through a consulting agreement, which should be disclosed and monitored by the institution.

The responsibility of the inventor remains throughout the life of the patent. This exists even if the inventor should leave the institution that holds the patent. This responsibility exists because the inventor in essence is in partner with the institution and the inventor shares in any financial gain that the institution obtains.

Institution Responsibilities

Every institution wishes to benefit from the results of its research. The outcomes of the research may be to further general knowledge through the publication of journal articles by its faculty, their presentation of research results at international meetings, and/or the prizes that their faculty may receive from the research. Other benefits may be the translation of fundamental research to practical application through applied and developmental research. The intellectual property of faculty also may lead to inventions and potentially to commercial products. To this end, when an institution assumes ownership of intellectual property, it assumes a fiduciary responsibility to attempt to bring the technology to market.

A policy should state who is the responsible party at the institution for managing issues of intellectual property. Depending on organizational size and structure, the institution's technology manager

may be the research director, medical director, or institutional counsel, or he or she reside in a dedicated technology transfer office.

As a party to the intellectual property of its faculty, an institution assumes certain responsibilities to protect and manage its intellectual property while maintaining academic freedom. These obligations may be mandated by federal regulations, sponsor agreements, or by convention of the institution itself. Regardless of the source, in the interest of openness and collegiality, the duties and responsibilities of the institution should be articulated clearly in the intellectual property policy.

Institutions may identify what services they provide to inventors in developing an invention disclosure. There may be informal discussions about an invention, or formal discussions with assistance from institution staff and external consultants, such as patent counsel. The assistance in developing the invention disclosure also may depend on the complexity of the invention, the potential scope of the application, and the expertise of institutional staff managing technology transfer.

Invention disclosure forms may be provided on specific forms of the institution that may be an attachment to the institution's policy such as in the Massachusetts Institute of Technology policy.[11] The disclosure should include a description of the technology, what the novel features are, what its utility is, who the inventors are, and what input they had into the invention. Disclosures by the inventor should be in sufficient detail that the institution could adequately assess its interest in the technology.

Once an invention disclosure is made to the institution, the institution's policy should state what is to be done with the disclosure; namely, what action the institution will take to determine whether to retain ownership of the technology or release it back to the inventor. The description may involve consultation with internal staff, review of funding source and agreements, external market analysis, and determination about patent ability. An institutional technology manager, intellectual property committee, or senior executive may make the final decision. Some policies set a time limit for the institution to make a decision about whether it will retain its ownership rights or not.

A policy should state that if an institution determines that it does not wish to retain ownership of an invention to which it otherwise would be entitled, the invention would be released back to the inventor. In this instance the inventor would be free to purchase patent protection, to market it, and to license it or otherwise develop it further without institutional support. The institution would not be responsible for any costs or liabilities related to the invention and it would not be eligible to any royalties. However, the institution may retain rights to a royalty free use of the invention.

The responsibilities of an institution are greater if it elects to retain rights to an invention. If the institution elects to retain ownership in an invention, the policy should state in the broadest terms what the institution will do with the IP or tangible property, such as, it will administer the invention consistent with its objectives. These may vary among institutions but would include patenting, marketing, licensing, commercialization agreements, establishing a spin-off company, or taking equity in a company that is to develop the technology. The uniqueness of each technology requires different approaches. The policy may describe that the institution assumes all the costs associated with its activities unless it relinquishes its rights to the invention.

The institution has several other responsibilities that it must fulfill and that can be described in the intellectual property policy. This can be the establishment and periodic review of the policy; development of procedures for management of the technology transfer operations; ways in which it makes covered persons aware of the intellectual property policy; and a description of its accounting of costs, income, and distribution of income.

It is not unusual for an institution, at some time after electing to retain rights, to waive its rights to the invention. The policy may describe what procedures the institution will undertake to relinquish its rights and if any rights will be retained by the institution. First and foremost, the institution should determine whether any sponsors of the research have any rights to the invention before the inventor. If they have rights, they are to be contacted first. If none exists or they waive their rights, the rights, title, and interest in the intellectual property may be returned with or without limitations placed on the inventor depending on the circumstances. For example, the institution may elect to retain a non-exclusive, royalty-free license to use the invention for its own educational or research purposes. If improvements to IP are made and are covered by the policy, the inventor must disclose these to the institution, which must review these improvements and its interest in them. If there was more than one inventor, the institution should release the rights in the same percentage as directed by patent law. Such

a procedure should be with the knowledge and concurrence from the intellectual property committee if one exists.

Intellectual Property Committee

A third party who can be involved in the technology transfer process and who is often described in the intellectual property policy is the intellectual property committee. This body can be viewed as a semi-autonomous committee overseeing the technology transfer operations of the institution and can serve as a useful buffer between the covered person/inventor and the institution on issues that may arise.

Depending on the level of detail desired, the intellectual property policy can define who appoints the committee, the composition of the committee, term of appointments, the reporting line, and the committee's charge. The intellectual property committee can be appointed by and report to the institution's board of trustees, president, chief operating officer, executive vice president, provost or other similar executive leader depending on the institutional organization. The composition of the committee may be described in general terms or describe particular individuals who may be on the committee or serve in an ex-officio capacity. The committee appointment can be described to include faculty and nonfaculty, and areas of expertise. Members may include faculty from specific areas such as biomedical research and engineering, who produce a large number of invention disclosures, from the school of business, or school of law. Other representation in an ex-officio capacity may include deans, legal counsel, finance officer or treasurer, and members of the technology transfer office and the sponsored projects office. External members may also be appointed to the committee such as from business, venture capital companies, and local or state economic leadership. Terms of appointment for committee membership may be defined, for example, for three-year appointments.

The responsibilities of the intellectual property committee should be clearly delineated in the policy. These roles may vary from institution to institution and examples are taken from the policies reviewed. The responsibilities may include the following:

- Development of the intellectual property policy with the institution, and its periodic review;
- Monitoring policy implementation by the institution;
- Working with technology transfer office staff to development of means to encourage discovery

at the institution and to educate faculty about the technology transfer program;

- Together with institutional staff development of appropriate procedures and guidelines for the use, marketing, licensing, financing, and manufacturing of inventions, as appropriate;
- Reviewing the actions of the institution to ensure that services are provided fairly to all inventors, and that the quality of the services is maintained and continuously improved;
- Reviewing invention disclosures and reports about patentability and potential markets and to make recommendations about whether the institution should retain a particular invention or return it to the inventor;
- Recommending resolutions to disputes between the inventor and the institution regarding whether a particular invention is covered by the IPP;
- Reviewing any disagreements about expenses charged against gross income from a license or other agreements about an invention;
- Reviewing any institutional or individual conflicts of interest that may arise because of a financial or fiduciary relationship between a party covered by the policy including members of the institution involved in representing the institution and a potential or actual licensee;
- Developing a management plan for issues arising between the inventor and institution;
- Resolving any disputes that may be develop between inventors; and
- Attending to any other such matters that may be referred to them and covered under the IPP.

Royalty and/or Equity Distribution

An institutional policy should define what it considers revenues, expenses, and net royalty or equity income. The policy should define the accounting practices and procedures for distribution of net royalties or net equity.

Revenues

Revenues for the purpose of a policy can be revenues received from the signing of a license agreement licensee fees, license maintenance fees, milestone payments, minimum royalties, sublicense fees, royalties on the sale of products, and settlements from any legal actions. It should not include any money received from a research agreement that supports ongoing research of the inven-

tor, because of the potential future benefit to the inventor and institution if there are new inventions or advancements. It also refers to the proceeds received from equity in a company in terms of dividends or the sale of equity.

Expenses

Institutions, in accepting an assignment of intellectual property rights to seek patent protection, license a technology or enter into other agreements that hopefully will result in financial benefits to the institution and the inventor and agree to pay upfront expenses related to these activities. It is the institution that incurs the financial loss should a technology prove to be unpatentable, a licensee cannot be identified, or there is no market for the product. Institutions should be entitled to recover these costs if financial gain is realized.

Expenses incurred by an institution may be defined in an intellectual property policy broadly or in detail. The largest expense categories generally are legal fees associated with patent application, copyrights and trademark protections, and any marketing costs, especially if an external company is used to market the technology. Other related costs may be legal fees associated with licensing, development costs related to start-up companies, money due another institution if inventors are from more than one institution, legal fees associated with protection against patent infringement or other disputes, and applicable taxes. Some institutions may also invest further in the technology with the understanding that they will recoup these costs as opposed to changing the royalty distribution. These may be expenses directly related to the research that led to the intellectual property, such as special research personnel or equipment.

What is generally excluded in a policy from being considered an expense are the salary and benefits of the inventor, and any usual and ordinary expenses that the institution may incur. This can include technical support, secretarial support, supplies, lab space, overhead, and any internal institutional costs.

Net Royalty or Net Equity

Simply put, *net royalty* or *equity income* is revenue received less any expense that the institution incurs. While there is no set method for net royalty distribution, the intellectual property policy should clearly describe the distribution between inventor and institution. Distributions can be very simple or very complex. The simplest forms can be a straight percentage distribution, and the most complex are those with sliding scales.

The simplest description is a policy where the inventor and the institution receive a fixed distribution of royalties. The policy for the Albert Einstein Healthcare Network in Philadelphia provides for a 50/50 distribution between the institution and the inventor. The institutional share is not subdivided in the policy.[7]

A slightly more complex example of a royalty distribution described in a policy is a fixed percentage given to the inventor and a subdivided share to the institution. An example is in the Temple University policy, which describes internal allocations of the institution's share. The institution's share is distributed 35% to the department or research unit responsible for the invention, 15% to the school or college responsible for the invention, and 50% to the university.[12]

A more complex model is a simple sliding scale. In this instance the royalties are shared between the inventor and the institution, but the percentage of royalties to the inventor decreases as more and more royalties are endeared. There are various models that have three or more levels to the sliding scale, and the dollar ranges in each are also variable. The intellectual property policy adapted by the Arizona board of regents provides the employee inventor with "a minimum of fifty percent (50%) of the first net ten thousand dollars ($10,000) received by the university and a minimum of twenty-five (25%) of the net amount received by the university in excess of the first net ten thousand dollars ($10,000)."[13]

The most complex case of royalty distribution has a sliding scale between the inventor and the institution as described above, however, the institution also maintains a sliding scale within and among the internal groups eligible for royalty income. "For net adjusted income up to $500,000" at the University of Florida, the inventor receives 40% and the institution 60%, which is divided among the program(s) (10%), inventor's department (7.5%), inventor's college (7.5%) and the Office of Research, Technology, and Graduate Education (ORTGE) or the University of Florida Research Foundation (UFRF) (35%). For net adjusted income over $500,000 the inventor's share is reduced to 25%, and the institutional distribution is 10% to the program, 10% to the inventor's department, 10% to the inventor's college, and 45% to ORTGE or UFRF.[4]

Some institutions, such as the University of Utah, may allow an inventor to participate with the institution in furthering the technology. In this instance, the university may allow the inventor to assume certain expenses. As a result, the inventor is provided a higher than normal royalty or other revenue percentage after the inventor is reimbursed for any approved expenses.[14]

Consistent with the net income, there should be a requirement in the policy that, at least annually, the institution conducts an audit of each of its patent accounts. In the interest of openness, a copy of the yearly revenues received and expenses incurred and any royalty distribution should be made to each inventor.

Some policies describe how an inventor can donate his or her share of royalties back to the institution, if so desired. This may be the entire amount or a portion thereof. The donation could be to the institution itself, or the inventor's school, department, or clinical entity.

Conclusion

Intellectual property policies are as varied as the institutions that exist. The right policy must be developed and adapted for the institution and be reviewed in terms of organization's culture and the regulations. This chapter has shared with you some of the issues common to most policies and where major differences occur. Many differences relate to the degree of detail in some of the policies.

• • • References

1. U.S. Congress. "To Amend the Patent and Trademark Laws," http://thomas.loc.gov/cgi-bin/bdquery/z?d096:HR06933:@@@L%7CTOM:/bss/d096query.html%7C (accessed August 29, 2004).

2. U.S. Congress. "A Bill To Amend Title 28, United States Code, with Respect to the Places Where Court Shall Be Held in Certain Judicial Districts, and for Other Purposes," http:// thomas. loc.gov/cgi-bin/bdquery/z?d098:HR06163: @@@L&summ2=m&|TOM:/bss/d098query. html (accessed August 29, 2004).

3. Bremer, Howard. "University Technology Transfer Evolution and Revolution." In *Research Administration and Management*, edited by Elliott C. Kulakowski and Lynne U. Chronister,

627–639. Sudbury, MA: Jones and Bartlett Publishers, 2006.

4. University of Florida. "University of Florida Intellectual Property Policy," http://rgp.ufl.edu/otl/pdf/ipp.pdf (accessed August 29, 2004).

5. University of Pennsylvania. "Patent and Tangible Research Property Policies and Procedures of the University of Pennsylvania," http://www.med.upenn.edu/postdoc/patent.policy.02.22.05.pdf (accessed September 16, 2005).

6. Cincinnati Children's Hospital Medical Center. "Intellectual Property and Venture Development: Policy on Inventions, Patents and Intellectual Property," http://www.cincinnatichildrens.org/research/administration/ipvd/invention-policy.htm (accessed August 29, 2004).

7. "Intellectual Property Policy," *Albert Einstein Healthcare Network*, 2002.

8. University of Colorado System, Office of the Vice President for Academic Affairs and Research. "Intellectual Property Policy on Discoveries and Patents for Their Protection and Commercialization," http://www.cusys.edu/policies/Academic/IP_discoveries.html (accessed August 29, 2004).

9. University of Colorado, 5-J. "Intellectual Property Policy on Discoveries and Patents for their Protection and Commercialization," http://www.cusys.edu/regents/Policies/Policy5J.htm (accessed September 1, 2005).

10. United States Patent and Trademark Office glossary, http://www.uspto.gov/main/glossary/index.html (accessed August 29, 2004).

11. Massachusetts Institute of Technology. "Guide to the Ownership, Distribution and Commercial Development of MIT Technology," June 1999, http://web.mit.edu/tlo/www/guide.pdf (accessed August 29, 2004).

12. Temple University. "Temple University Invention and Patent Policy," http://www.patents.temple.edu/ip_policy.html (accessed August 29, 2004).

13. Arizona Board of Regent's Intellectual Property Policy http://www.abor.asu.edu/1_the_regents/policymanual/chap6/6-908.pdf (accessed September 1, 2005).

14. University of Utah. "Patents and Inventions," March 8, 1999, http://www.admin.utah.edu/ppmanual/6/6-4.html (accessed August 29, 2004).

62

Industrial Research Collaborations before a Product Is Developed

Colin Cooper

Introduction

One of the fundamental activities of a contemporary university is to engage in collaboration with external bodies where both parties can use the generation of new knowledge to further their own core activities. In this chapter we review how universities collaborate with industry and what makes a successful partnership. With technological advances happening on a daily basis, it has never been more important for universities to develop long-term relationships with industry. The current level of knowledge being generated globally in areas such as genetics, proteomics, environmental science, and others means that industry can use that knowledge to create new products and services that benefit mankind, while, at the same time, achieve the economic growth and profits demanded by their stakeholders. Globally this has become known as the knowledge-based economy.

The major problem in establishing partnerships between industry and academia is that realms of academia and industry operate in totally different environments; their basic aims and interests are different (Table 62-1). It is important, therefore, that the value of the proposed collaboration (partnership) and the potential areas for conflict should be explicitly understood and addressed at the outset in order to foster valuable relationships.

Most national governments recognize the knowledge-based economy as the main driver for economic growth at the regional and national level; to this end governments have been proactive in facilitating links between industry and academia. Research-led univer-

TABLE 62-1	Comparison between Academia and Industry	
	University	**Industry**
Purpose	Knowledge	Profit
Accountability	Public	Shareholders
Operational Area	Freedom	Competition
Time Lines	No specific time or limits	Short time scope
Scientific Results	Publish	Concealment

sities have established offices responsible for generating these forms of partnerships that are responsible to ensure that the universities' knowledge, ideas, and products are transferred to the external markets. These offices are now regarded as mainstream in the university's operations and, further, in research-led universities, these offices are responsible for a significant share of the university's total income stream. Major industrial sponsors, in turn, have offices and staff responsible for interactions with academia. The offices within each organization are acutely aware of the need for collaboration (see Table 62-2). At the national level, industries have formed groupings such as the Inter-Company Academic Relations Group (ICARG) in the United Kingdom and Business Higher Education Forum (BHEF) in the United States. More recently in the United Kingdom, as a result of the government's review of funding for research, there has been the formation of a Funders' Forum. Those industries that have had significant collaborations now include them in their business and development plans.

TABLE 62-2	Main Drivers for Collaboration
University	**Industry**
Potential income source	Gearing of funds
Access to specialized equipment	Access to latest technologies
Supply of raw materials	Recruitment of graduates
Publications	Prestige
Government funding	Regional presence
Increased research ratings	Product development
Personal income	Public relations
Establishment of research centers	Potential for multi-disciplinary teams
Student placements	Access to expertise
Increased skills base	Increased skills/knowledge base
Improved teaching base	Outsourcing

There are many obvious benefits to both academia and industry, but there are also other intangible benefits that can be reached when collaboration is managed professionally, for example, increased experience and expertise of staff within each organization.

There are different stages in the course of establishing a partnership. Further discussed in this chapter are the various elements that make up a successful partnership and the key elements from a research administration perspective.

Stage 1. Identifying the Need

Most universities would like to engage with industrial partners for carrying out funded research projects. Before trying to attract industrial funding, however, it is important that to be completely aware of the skills index of the academic staff to ensure that the university has the "critical mass" of expertise that can support the relationship. It is also recommended that the current industrial funding base be assessed and resources benchmarked against those of the competition. It is no use trying to attract a particular company if they are already engaged at significant level of activity with another university. To start in a partnership, the university must agree on and understand the main drivers for the collaboration, including the potential benefits and the risks (Table 62-2). Once this criteria has been agreed upon within the university and there is awareness about the specific areas in which collaboration can be achieved, then an appropriate industrial partner can be found.

Stage 2. Finding the Partner

One would be surprised at the level of contacts that the university has with industry. First, there is a requirement to gather as much information as possible on the current relationships that exist within the university. Senior personnel must be made aware of relationships with industry that already exist. Industry performs a significant amount of due diligence in the selection of the academic partners they want to have a relationship with, it is important that universities similarly take this approach before selecting potential industrial partners. Once this information has been collated, combined with the selection of the particular scientific areas in which the university wants to foster relationships, the institution is then in a position to select the industrial sector in which to operate and be able to target within that sector and to market the university. Generally, the university and industry contacts and points of interaction are spread across a wide operating area and include:

- Current research collaborations
- Suppliers
- Careers office
- Continuing professional development
- Industrial representatives on governing bodies
- Sponsored chairs
- Endowments
- Industrial board
- Alumni
- Personal relationships
- Industrial student placements
- Visiting staff
- Technology transfer offices
- Donations
- International office

After having selected the target, it is then important to find the appropriate person within the target area to whom the initial approach can made. This person should be as senior as possible and any initial contact should be made at vice principal or vice chancellor level. It is critical that before making this initial approach that the university has completed a significant amount of detailed analysis on the sectors needs and in particular the problems that the selected target currently faces and how the university can address their requirements. This information is now freely available, as most companies place their mission statements, research plans, and key issues on their corporate Web sites. Other good sources for gathering this type of information include conference proceedings, trade associations, local development agencies, professional interest groups, and industry marketing reports (e.g., Keynote, Reuters and Snapshot, although these reports are costly).

Stage 3. The Research Proposal

When the partner has been found and has agreed to the benefits and outcomes of the planned collaboration, the next stage is to develop a potential research plan. The research plan forms the basis for any eventual formal binding agreement. In a potential research plan, the following areas should be explicitly addressed:

- Participants
- Scope of the project
- Overview
- Background
- Aims and objectives
- Description of the research
- Duration
- Budget requirements
- Management/reporting requirements
- Dissemination and exploitation
- Success criteria

Extensive discussions between the academic staff at the university and the technical staff from industry are required before the research plan can be drafted. A good reason for having a comprehensive project plan is that this document can be used as a reference by the academic staff at the university when carrying out the work (instead of using the actual contract put in place for carrying out the project). A research administrator can facilitate these preliminary discussions by providing direct input into the nontechnical areas of the project such as budget requirements, management, dissemination, exploitation, and the drafting and issuing of any required agreements. The level of involvement and the requirements for each element depend on the scope of the planned relationship. At this early stage, ensuring that documents are dated and marked as confidential, where appropriate, demonstrate to the potential partner the university's intention to act in a professional manner. It is, however, important that these inputs are also performed in a timely manner with both the research administrator and the academic realizing that industrial sponsors tend to work with different timelines than do gov-

ernment sponsors and that delays can destroy a potential relationship before it has even begun.

Stage 4. Costing and Pricing a Partnership

A university must be aware of all the costs involved in carrying out sponsored research and must have a clear and precise costing and pricing policy that enables administrators to estimate accurately both the direct and indirect costs of any sponsored research partnership. The cost of the partnership and each party's respective contributions will help influence the terms and conditions of the contractual instrument put into place to help manage the partnership (Figure 62-1). Actual recovery rates can vary significantly between sponsor types and on industrial projects; there is always a requirement to be aware of the income-achieved set against the academic rewards.

The full cost of participation by both parties should be as accurate as possible; and both parties should be able to view each other's estimates. In the long run, inaccurate cost estimates can lead to problems in the relationship if projects are under-resourced and greater commitments are required over and above anticipated levels of participation. The funds needed for protection and exploitation of arising intellectual property and dissemination of the results are important and must be addressed during preparation of costings. It is always important to remember that in its commitment to university research, the industrial partner will have to budget beyond its current fiscal year: in essence, this means that approval may have to be sought at a senior level for signing off the required financing.

Stage 5. Forms of Engagement

It is still the case that most university–industry collaborations are performed on a single project or a one-time consultancy basis. As further discussed, these research partnerships can take many forms.

Specific Goal-Orientated Research Partnerships Addressing a Particular Problem

This is a standard model for most university–industry relations and one of the more frequently used models. In these cases, the funds supplied by industry are for a one-time research project to address a problem specific to the industry or to produce incremental developments to an existing product

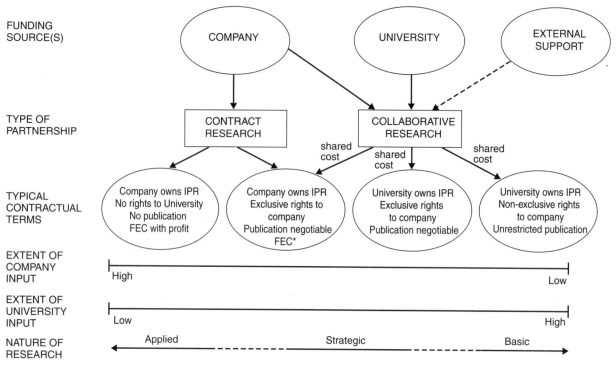

FUNDING SOURCE(S)

TYPE OF PARTNERSHIP

TYPICAL CONTRACTUAL TERMS

EXTENT OF COMPANY INPUT

EXTENT OF UNIVERSITY INPUT

NATURE OF RESEARCH

*FEC: Full Economic Cost

FIGURE 62-1 Research Partnerships: Possibilities for Ownership and Use of Results

that is already on or near the marketplace. The research plan therefore is usually set by the industrial partner based on its own background knowledge and intellectual property (IP) and the results are commercially confidential and hence the ownership of arising IP would normally rest with the industrial partner. In these cases, the university can expect, depending on the level of industrial funding, to have a negotiated right to publish and a share in any future commercial exploitation of the results (Figure 62-1).

Collaborative Research Partnerships

In a collaborative project the research plan is generally set by both parties and is based on background IP of both parties, the results of the research will be of benefit to both. Each party contributes to the funding of the project, either in cash or in kind, and both can expect to share in the results with joint ownership of inventions.

Project Partners on Government-Funded Research Programs

Increasingly in the knowledge-based economy, governments are providing third-party funding to foster the development of partnerships between industry and academia. There are many schemes that

encourage partnerships between small-to-medium-size enterprises (SMEs) and universities. With these programs, the research plan and the formal agreement are based on the particular scheme chosen, and proposals are normally peer reviewed. In these cases, it is good practice to designate a head of agreement at the proposal stage so that funding agencies and their reviewers are aware that consideration has been given to the outputs of the collaboration.

Consultancy/Subcontracts

Consultancy agreements are for smaller one-time goal-orientated services; for example, the use of a specific piece of equipment or for academic specialist knowledge. In these cases, there is no research plan, as there is no expectation for the generation of new knowledge. Instead, industry normally expects to own all the results and there are no publication rights. These projects normally have short time spans. A consultancy agreement is a good tool for marketing the university's skills to business and these should be encouraged as a first stepping-stone to develop longer term relations with industry.

Sponsored Research Studentships

A sponsored studentship is a most effective tool for fostering relationships with industry, providing students with an opportunity to spend some time in industry, and even the potential of employment at the end of the project. In these agreements, the research plan is first drawn up between both parties, usually based on a specific industrial theme. A sponsored studentship is an affordable alternative to a sponsored research project for industry. The contractual terms for this form of partnership are particularly important, as there must be a right to publish allowed so that students can be awarded their higher qualifications through the production of a thesis. This can be a stumbling block for projects that are commercially sensitive and industrial partners have to consider this when accessing the appropriate form of engagement with the university. Studentships can take many forms, depending on whether the student is studying at undergraduate or postgraduate level; the length of the project; and placement time of the student with the industrial partner. For postgraduate students, the industrial partner must commit to funding the project for the length of time it will take the students to complete their studies (up to three years).

Networks

There are some industrial sectors that fund research at universities through a consortia arrangement. This allows the consortia to fund projects that address generic problems across a particular area. An arrangement that addresses generic issues lessens the problems that can arise with IP; however, IP background and IP generated during the partnership can be problematic within consortia. The main area of concern in relation to IP is the retention of ownership of background IP, this can be resolved in the consortium agreement with a clause that stipulates background IP remains the property of the party that brings it to the project, is only available during the course of the project, and can only be used under license by other members for the exploitation of IP generated during the project (foreground IP).The memberships to these consortia are normally based on an annual fees, as well as on research projects. It is also typical for consortia to run workshops and symposia for their staff.

Long-Term Partnerships in Training and Research

If a university is to be truly successful in achieving a long-term relationship, it is preferable to have a corporate relationship with the industrial partner (Figure 62-2).

The benefit of a corporate relationship is in its longevity, as it means that there can be a mutual and beneficial input into the association over an extended and predicted period. Other benefits include the opportunity to develop joint interdisciplinary and multidisciplinary teams to address industry's applied problems, while still looking to address the university's fundamental motivation in producing new knowledge through basic research programs. In a one-to-one relationship built around only a small number of individuals, if a member of the party leaves his or her employment, then the relationship is often ended, and, thus, the organization's time and resources spent on supporting the relationship have been wasted. A long-term corporate relationship, instead, allows the university to plan a research strategy rather than an *ad hoc* one, as there is a guaranteed funding stream with which to plan. From industry's perspective, such an arrangement allows for product development planning and, of course, the potential to hire experienced university graduates. In Figure 62-2, it is suggested that there is a single point of contact from both sides to ensure that initial enquiries are dealt with effectively and that any conflicts that might arise in the event of establishing a corporate relationship can also be dealt with expeditiously.

Each of the models described requires a legal agreement so that potential areas for dispute can be resolved at the earliest stage. In each case, specifics (e.g., ownership, confidentiality, and publication rights) must be addressed. Before any formal agreement is reached, there has to be extensive discussion on the focus and research area of the project. To enable free discussion, it is always advisable that both parties sign a confidentiality agreement. This enables both parties to discuss the objectives of the project and to supply background knowledge and any new ideas they may have. The agreement also ensures that the information exchanged will not be used beyond the fledgling partnership and that, in commercial terms, no information will be made available to third parties without the prior and mutual permission of both interests (Appendix 62–A). When seeking third party support, for example from government schemes, it is also a good idea to have a heads of agreement (HAO) signed between the partners. An HOA reaffirms the partner's intention to work together in the event that the proposal is selected for funding and outlines the planned ownership and dissemination of the results of the work. This shows to potential reviewers of the work that the project and the relationship have been thought out and mutually developed by the participants. (An example of an HOA is given at the end of this chapter.)

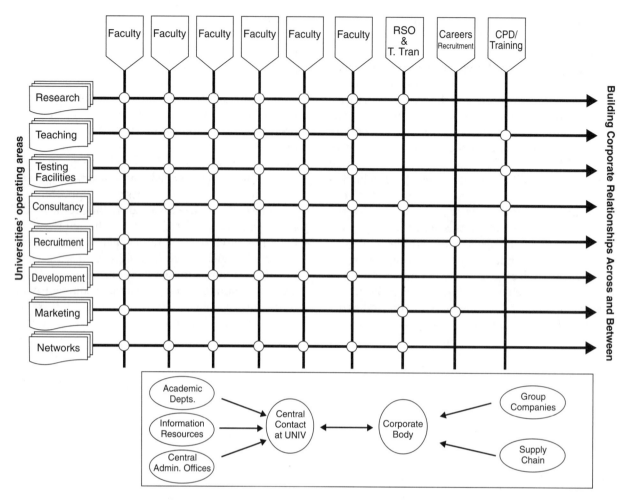

FIGURE 62-2   Corporate Relationship

Stage 6. Negotiating an Agreement

The negotiation of an agreement to cover the planned partnership is one of the key areas. The agreement governs how the project and the relationship are run and each agreement varies because each partnership is unique. The areas within a well-structured research plan are duplicated in any formal agreement (Table 62-3). When negotiating, it is important for both parties that the negotiation process is not prolonged. From the academic side, delays can result in missed opportunity to appoint suitable research staff or students to work on the project. From the industrial side, delays can mean a loss of potential market advantage. There is no advantage in getting drawn into lengthy negotiations with a resultant detailed and expensive legal agreement when the project is a one-time arrangement or of limited value. Conversely, there are advantages for negotiating a master or corporate

agreement where there is a significant level of activity between the parties.

Most companies that invest in research at universities have their own standard (model) agreements; research-led universities have theirs, too. These standard agreements are a good starting point for the negotiation, but rarely do they become the final signed document (Appendix 62-B, 62-C, and 62-D.)

The main stumbling block in any contract negotiation is the ownership of IP generated through the research work. Each industrial partner and each university will have its own policy in relation to IP rights and, indeed, the rules and regulations vary worldwide. There are no standards, and each case has to take account of a number of factors in the decision-making process that can include the contributions from each party, the particular industrial sector, the cost of protecting the IP, and academic pressure to publish. Figure 62-1 explores

TABLE 62-3 Mirroring the Research Plan and the Research Agreement

Research Plan	Research Agreement
Participants	Parties
Scope of the project	Work program (normally an annex)
Overview	Recitals
Background	Recitals/IPR ownership
Aims and objectives	Consideration
Description of the research	Title
Duration	Start and date
Budget requirements	Price and payment
Management	Reports, confidentiality, warranties, liability, termination
Dissemination and exploitation	Publication, IPR ownership
Success criteria	Exploitation rights, papers, thesis, journals, products, patents, trained staff

TABLE 62-4 University–Industry Partnership

Marriage	Research Administration
Flirting	Marketing
Finding the right one	Partner searches, due diligence
Opposites attract	University/industry
Engagement	Heads of agreement, MOU
Prenuptial agreement	Feasibility study, background IP
Marriage license	Corporate agreement, master agreement
Honeymoon	!*!+$!*
Anniversary	Annual reports
Children	Outputs
Any marriage has its problems...	
In-laws	Lawyers
Rows	Disputes
Affairs	Loose sponsors or academic staff
Trial separation	Fixed contract
Divorce	End of contract
But all problems can be resolved..	
Marriage guidance counselor	Research administrator

some of the potential routes for ownership and exploitation.

Just for Fun

The most important partnership that most research administrators enter into is a marriage partnership, and the elements of that relationship bear an unnerving similarity to a university–industry partnership (Table 62-4).

• • • Suggested Resources

1. The University–Industry Research Collaboration Initiative. "Working Together Creating Knowledge," Business Higher Education Forum, http://www.acenet.edu/bookstore/pdf/working-together.pdf (accessed September 29, 2005).
2. Laidler, D. A. *Research Partnerships between Industry and Universities Partnerships for Research and Innovation*. Runcorn, UK: CBI Publications, 1988.
3. Duncan, D. "Partnerships between Industry and Academia in Information Technology," *Journal of Business Education* 1, Proceedings 2002. http://www.abe.villanova.edu/proc2000/n086.pdf (accessed October 20, 2005).
4. Lambert, R. "Lambert Review of Business-University Collaboration (UK Government)," 2003, http://www.hm-treasury.gov.uk/media/DDE/65/lambert_review_final_450.pdf (accessed October 20, 2005).
5. United Kingdom Government. "Research and Development Scorecard," London, UK 2002.
6. Kurfess, T. R. and Nagurka, M. L. "Fostering Strong Interactions between Industry and Academia." Proceedings of ASEE Annual Conference & Exposition, Milwaukee, WI, June 1997.
7. Conn, R. W., Jacobs, I., and Jacobs, J. *The University of California's Relationships with Industry*. San Diego University of California, 1999.
8. Princeton University, *Research Relationships with Industry*, http://www.princeton.edu/patents/forms/resrel.html (accessed October 20, 2005).
9. Paone, J. "When Big Pharma Courts Academia." *The Scientist* 16, no. 2 (January 21, 2002): 48.
10. Farrell, J. A. *University and Corporate Research Partnerships: Developing Effective Guidelines to Promote Change and Transformation*. Ann Arbor, Michigan, University of Michigan, 2000, http://www-personal.umich.edu/~marvp/facultynetwork/whitepapers/farrell.html (accessed October 20, 2005).

11. Eickmann, K. "Leveraging Learnings: Industry and Academia." Presentation at Construction Industry Institute 2002 ASEE Annual Conference, Montréal, Canada, June 15–19, 2002.

12. *Corporations, Colleges and Universities: What Makes Great Relationships So Great?* The Consulting Network, in Network vol. 2, 1–8, 1998, http://www.theconsultingnetwork.com/pdfs/nl_fall98.pdf (accessed October 20, 2005).

13. R.W. Johnson Research Triangle Institute, *Working with the Private Sector and Foundations*, Manchester, UK, 2000.

14. Tornatzky, L. G., Waugaman, P. G., and Gray, D. O. "New University Roles in a Knowledge Economy," Southern Growth Policies Board, 2002, http://ip.research.sc.edu/PDF/Innovation UniversityBook.pdf (accessed September 29, 2005).

15. Higher Education Funding Council of England, *HE Business Interaction Survey*. January 2004, http://www.hefce.ac.uk/pubs/hefce/2004/04_07/ (accessed October 20, 2005).

16. Leigh, B. *Research Partnerships*. Vancouver, Canada Society of Research Administrators International annual meeting, 2001.

All model agreements are used by the author's research administration and therefore certain terms and conditions that may not be applicable to universities outside of the United Kingdom.

62-A

Confidentiality Agreement

Part A

DATED   2005*
(1) THE UNIVERSITY OF
(2) [ ] LIMITED/PLC
        CONFIDENTIALITY AGREEMENT
DATE: 200*
PARTIES:

(1) THE U* address ("U*") acting on behalf of itself and its employees, students and persons otherwise engaged at U* in a research or teaching capacity involved with the Development (defined below) ("U* Staff");

(2) _____ LIMITED/PLC (registered in _____ number _____) whose registered office is at _____ acting on behalf of itself and each and everyone of its subsidiaries, holding companies, and any subsidiary of such holding companies (together referred to as "the Company")

(Hereinafter referred to collectively as "the Parties")

BACKGROUND:

(A) U* acting on behalf of itself and its employees owns intellectual property and other rights in and to _____ ("the Development").

(B) U* and/or U* Staff has/have disclosed and/or will be disclosing to the Company information designated by U* and/or the U* Staff to be confidential, whether expressly or not relating to the Development which may include, without limit, drawings, samples, know-how and/or data in any form ("the Confidential Information").

(C) The Company may also disclose secret and confidential information relating to its business (to be included within "the Confidential Information").

OPERATIVE PROVISIONS:

In consideration of U* and/or any of the U* Staff agreeing to disclose the Confidential Information to the Company, and vice versa, the Parties agree that:

1. they will:

  1.1 only use the Confidential Information for the express purpose of evaluation of the Development [in order to decide whether or not they wish to be involved with its commercial exploitation] ("the Purpose") and for no other purpose, whether commercial or otherwise whatsoever;

  1.2 keep the Confidential Information confidential and exercise at least the same degree of care with it as they exercise with their own confidential information which they do not wish to be disclosed;

  1.3 not disclose or divulge the Confidential Information or any part of it or extracts from it to any third party without the prior written consent of U* or the Company, as appropriate, except as required by law;

  1.4 divulge Confidential Information only to those of its employees, agents or representatives ("the Parties' Staff") who need to have access to it for the performance of their duties, and then only to the extent actually needed for the Purpose;

  1.5 ensure that each member of the Parties' Staff is fully aware of and complies with the restrictions placed on the Parties in this Agreement [and the Parties shall obtain a written undertaking to do so from each such member of the Parties' Staff];

1.6 conspicuously label, where possible, all Confidential Information received by the Parties or any of the Parties' Staff as being Confidential Information and the property of U* or the Company, as appropriate;

1.7 not copy or reproduce in any manner or form, without the prior written consent of U* or the Company as appropriate, the Confidential Information or any part of it or of any notes in any form which they or any of the Parties' Staff make of the Confidential Information;

1.8 not store the Confidential Information in a computer or electronic retrieval system accessible from outside their usual place of business and not transmit it in any form by any means outside their usual place of business without the consent of U* or the Company as appropriate; and

1.9 return all copies in any form of the Confidential Information to U* or the Company if so requested at any time by U* or the Company within [30] days from the date of such request and delete the Confidential Information and any notes of it which have been made by the Parties or any of the Parties' Staff from any computer or electronic retrieval system where it is stored;

2. for the purpose of this Agreement any disclosure of any Confidential Information by any member of the Parties' Staff will be deemed to be disclosure by the Parties and the Parties will be responsible to each other for such disclosure;

3. the restrictions contained in Clause 1 do not apply to any of the Confidential Information which:-

3.1 was already known by the Parties prior to the disclosure by U* or the Company, if either of the Parties informs the other that it was so known as soon as the Company or U* is aware of the fact;

3.2 at the time of disclosure by or on behalf of the Parties is public knowledge or subsequently becomes public knowledge other than through a breach of this Agreement on the part of the Company or U*;

3.3 is lawfully received by the Parties from a third party without any breach of a confidentiality relationship with U* or the Company; or

3.4 is generated independently by the Company or U* without use of any of the Confidential Information;

4. the Parties understand and acknowledge that whilst the Parties believe the Confidential Information to be accurate and sufficient for the Purpose, neither U* nor the Company give any warranty or representation to this effect;

5. this Agreement does not grant the Company any rights in the Development or U*'s contribution to the Confidential Information and vice versa; it does not oblige either of the Parties to enter into any negotiations or other agreement relating to the Development;

6. this Agreement shall continue in force notwithstanding the return of all the Confidential Information belonging to U* and the Company as appropriate;

7. any waiver or forbearance in relation to this Agreement shall operate only if in writing and shall apply only to the specified instance and not affect the existence of or continued applicability of the terms of this Agreement; and

8. this Agreement shall be construed and governed in accordance with English Law and the Parties agree to submit to the exclusive jurisdiction of the English Courts.

SIGNED by _____
For and on behalf of _____
THE UNIVERSITY OF _____
and each of the U* STAFF _____
SIGNED by _____
For and on behalf of _____
[COMPANY] LIMITED/PLC _____

Part B

CONFIDENTIALITY AGREEMENT

DATE: _____ 200*

During discussions and/or demonstrations relating to _____ to be held today or subsequently between _____ ("U* Staff Member") and the other signatories of this Agreement ("the Participants"), information may be disclosed to the Participants, which must remain confidential to U*.

In consideration of the U* Staff Member disclosing such information to the Participants, each of the Participants agrees to keep such information confidential at all times and not disclose such information to any third party without prior written consent from U*. Information obtained by the U* Staff Member from any of the Participants in the course of such discussions and/or demonstrations will also be subject to the same confidentiality obligations.

The obligations of confidence and non-disclosure will be without limit in time, unless approval to publish is given by U* in writing in relation to its confidential information and by the relevant Participant in relation to that Participant's confidential information.

The restrictions contained in this Agreement do not apply to any of U*'s confidential information which:-

1. was already known by the Participants prior to the disclosure by the U* Staff Member, if the Participants inform U* that it was so known as soon as the Participants become aware of the fact;

2. at the time of disclosure by or on behalf of the U* Staff Member is public knowledge or subsequently becomes public knowledge other than through a breach of this Agreement on the part of any of the Participants;

3. is lawfully received by the Participants from a third party without any breach of a confidentiality relationship with U*; or

4. is generated independently by the Participants without use of any of U*'s confidential information.

The obligations of confidentiality in relation to the information obtained by the U* Staff Member from the Participants will be subject to the equivalent exceptions as set out above.

SIGNED by [U* STAFF MEMBER] _____
SIGNED by [PARTICIPANT] _____
SIGNED by [PARTICIPANT] _____

62-B

Research Collaboration Agreement

HEADS OF TERMS

1. PURPOSE

Subject to the obtaining of mutually acceptable [EPSRC] Funding U* and the Company wish to collaborate on a programme of research relating to the Project (defined in paragraph 4) on the terms below.

2. PARTIES

The University of Manchester Institute of Science and Technology of PO Box 88, Manchester M60 1QD ("U*"); and _____ [Limited/PLC] (registered number _____) of [REGISTERED OFFICE] ("the Company").

3. INTENTION

This document is intended neither to create a legally binding contract between U* and the Company (except for paragraph 9 which is intended to be legally binding on U* and the Company) nor set out an exhaustive list of matters to be incorporated into a legally binding contract in relation to the Project.

4. PROJECT

[INSERT DETAILS OF PROJECT] ("the Project").

5. CONDUCT OF RESEARCH

5.1 U* will use all reasonable endeavours to carry out the Project in accordance with the details outlined below:-[INSERT DETAILS OF THE PROJECT PLAN].

5.2 The Company will provide the following resources for use in the Project:
[INSERT DETAILS OF SUPPORTING RESOURCES].

5.3 If financial support is not approved by [the EPSRC] on terms mutually acceptable to the parties, then any work which has already been undertaken pursuant to these Heads of Terms shall cease.

6. USE OF INTELLECTUAL PROPERTY

6.1 U* and the Company will each contribute, to the extent possible, for the purpose of and duration of the Project any background intellectual property rights necessary to undertake the Project.

6.2 Any background intellectual property will remain the property of the contributing party, but the other party will, on terms negotiated between the parties, have continuing access to it to the extent necessary to exploit the Project results.

6.3 Prior to the commencement of the Project, the parties will negotiate arrangements to enable the other party to access any intellectual property rights generated under the Project for the purpose of in-house research and commercial exploitation. The arrangements will include financial provisions related to the respective inputs of the staff of each party to any exploitable intellectual property arising out of the Project and the respective contributions made by U*, [the EPSRC] and the Company.

7. PUBLICATION OF RESULTS

7.1 Publication of the results of the Project are to be in accordance with academic and scientific practice, and shall not be published by one party without the consent of the other party, consent not to be unreasonably withheld.

7.2 Any support by the Company will be acknowledged in the publication.

7.3 If the results of the Project are patentable, no publication shall be made until an application for such patents has been filed.

8. COSTS

Each party shall bear its own costs which may arise pursuant to these Heads of Terms.

9. CONFIDENTIALITY

The Company undertakes to keep confidential all information (except for that which is already in the public domain) in relation to the Project which is disclosed to it or its advisors by U* or their advisors and will not without U*'s consent divulge such information save to its professional advisors and employees for the sole purpose of entering into a binding contract in respect of the Project. The Company will ensure that its employees and professional advisors are made fully aware of these obligations of confidence to U*.

10. GOVERNING LAW

These Heads of Terms shall be construed and governed in accordance with English law and are subject to the [non-]exclusive jurisdiction of the English Courts.

SIGNED by [NAME] _____
for and on behalf of _____
THE UNIVERSITY OF _____
SIGNED by [NAME] _____
for and on behalf of _____
_____ [LIMITED/PLC] _____

62-C

Research Contract Agreement

RESEARCH CONTRACT AGREEMENT
DATE: 200*
PARTIES:

(1) THE U* (insert full name and address) ("U*")
(2) _____ LIMITED/PLC (registered in _____ number _____) whose registered office is at _____ ("the Company")

BACKGROUND:

(A) U* has the research capability and experience to carry out research relating to _____.
(B) The Company wishes to appoint U* to carry out such research.

OPERATIVE PROVISIONS:

INTERPRETATION
In this Agreement the following expressions have the following meanings unless inconsistent with the context:-

"Background Intellectual Property" any Intellectual Property made available by either party for use in the Project or necessary to exploit the Project Intellectual Property, but not generated under the Project and belonging to such party or any of the Research Staff or to which U* has rights which permits its use in the Project [all such Intellectual Property being listed in Schedule 2 or subsequently notified in writing by one party to the other before it is used in the Project];

"Company's Research Staff" all scientific and technical staff who are employees of the Company and are to

participate in the Project and/or any third parties appointed by the Company to participate in the Project;

"Designated Officer" the officer of U* designated by U* as responsible for the Project;

"Intellectual Property" all intellectual and industrial property rights including without limitation patents, know-how, trade marks, registered designs, applications for and rights to apply for any of the foregoing, unregistered design rights, unregistered trade marks and copyright (including, without limitation, copyright in drawings, plans, specifications, designs and computer software), database rights, topography rights, any rights in any invention, discovery or process, in each case in the United Kingdom and all other countries in the world;

"Milestone Dates" the dates set out in the Project Plan by which various stages are projected to be completed;

"Project" the research and development work to be undertaken by U* in accordance with the Project Plan in relation to [SHORT DESCRIPTION];

"Project Plan" the plan setting out the scope and objectives of the Project, the stages of the Project, the payments due and key dates as set out in Schedule 1;

"Project Intellectual Property" any and all Intellectual Property generated directly under the Project;

"U* Research Staff" all scientific and technical staff, who are under contract (whether as employees or independent consultants) to U* who are to participate in the Project.

Insert Name U*'s wholly owned intellectual property management and exploitation company, U* (insert name).

1 The headings in this Agreement are for convenience only and are not intended to have any legal effect.

2 APPOINTMENT OF U* TO CONDUCT RESEARCH WORK

   a. In consideration of the payments to be made under clause 4 U* agrees to use its best endeavours to undertake the Project in accordance with the terms and conditions of this Agreement and the Project Plan.

3 DURATION OF AGREEMENT

   a. This Agreement shall operate for [NUMBER] months commencing on the [INSERT START DATE].

   b. This Agreement may be extended, beyond its original term, for successive further periods by written agreement between the parties, to be agreed and entered into before the expiry of the original term or, in the case of a second or subsequent extension, before the expiry of the prior extended term.

   c. U* may at any time during the term of this Agreement, by notice in writing to the Company, be released from all its obligations, save for those of confidentiality, if any department of U* to which the performance of this Agreement is for the time being delegated is closed for a period exceeding 30 days or is amalgamated with another department [or if any member of the U* Research Staff whom U* deems to be key to the Project ceases to be employed by U* and a suitable replacement cannot be found].

4 PAYMENT FOR RESEARCH

   a. In consideration of U* undertaking the Project, the Company agrees to make payments to U* in accordance with the Project Plan.

   b. In the event of U* invoking clause 3.c above all payments accrued and owing to U* at the date of occurrence of the event relied upon by U* in invoking the clause shall remain payable and shall be paid to U* immediately, including any costs incurred by U* in carrying out its obligations under this Agreement but all subsequent payments shall cease to be payable.

   c. If U* terminates this Agreement due to any breach by the Company of its obligations under this Agreement, the Company shall pay U*'s costs in relation to its employment of any PhD student required to take part in the Project.

   d. All payments under this Agreement are quoted exclusive of VAT which shall be chargeable and payable in addition where applicable.

   e. If the Company fails to make a payment within 30 days of the date of the receipt by the Company of an invoice setting out the payment due in accordance with clause 4.a, interest shall be payable at the rate of 4% (four per cent) per annum above the base rate from time to time of Barclays Bank PLC on the amount due calculated from the date payment became due until the date of actual payment. The date of payment shall be the date such amounts are received by U*.

5 CONDUCT OF THE RESEARCH STAFF

   a. The U* Research Staff and the Company Research Staff will while engaged on the Project and on premises under the control or in the possession of U* act at all times in accordance with the rules and regulations of U* governing such research work and with the instructions of the Designated Officer.

   b. The Company accepts sole responsibility for the health and safety of the U* Research Staff and the Company Research Staff on premises other than premises under the control or in the possession of U* and will indemnify U* in respect of any claims made against U* by or on behalf of any such persons in respect of personal injuries or other loss and damage suffered by such persons in the course of the Project.

   c. The Company and U* will promptly notify each other in writing of any information which comes into its possession which may affect the health and safety of persons engaged on the Project arising from the nature of or location of the research work being undertaken in the course of the Project.

   d. The Company and U* will ensure that all the Company's Research Staff and the U* Research Staff shall execute:-

     i. acknowledgements of confidentiality concerning any confidential information relating to and coming into their possession in the course of the Project;

     ii. undertakings to act at all times in accordance with the rules and regulations of U* governing such research work and to follow the instructions of the Designated Officer whilst on premises under the control or in the possession of U*;

iii. [appropriate documents of acknowledgement of title or assignment in favour of [U* TT COMPANY][the Company] [any third party] of the Project Intellectual Property and each member of the U* Research Staff and the Company Research Staff is obliged to waive (to the extent that such rights are waiveable) all moral rights and rights of a like nature in the Project Intellectual Property.]

6 REPORTING RESULTS OF RESEARCH

a. Subject to clause 6.b below, U* will:-

i. report [in writing] to the Company all and any results of the Project on a confidential basis at the intervals and in the form set out in the Project Plan; and

ii. present a final written report to the Company on a confidential basis not later than [INSERT NUMBER] months after the conclusion of the Project, including a full and comprehensive statement of the work done and the results accomplished and an evaluation of them; and

iii. without prejudice to the above, not disclose such information as is contained in the reports made under clauses 6.a.i and 6.a.ii to third parties for so long as it remains confidential without the prior consent in writing of the Company, which consent shall not be unreasonably withheld or delayed.

b. The obligations undertaken by U* in clause 6.a above do not extend to any information concerning the progress of the Project or its results which is already publicly available at the time of such information or results being discovered.

c. Notwithstanding clause 6.a:

i. the Company shall not withhold its consent under clause 6.a.iii to disclose such information to the extent that it shall effect or delay submission of an examination of a thesis or other examination in relation to the Project or the Project Results;

ii. U* reserves the right to disclose to third parties the fact that U* is conducting the Project for the Company and may announce, if any, the fact that it has received any grant in relation to the Project.

7 INTELLECTUAL PROPERTY RIGHTS

a. [All Project Intellectual Property shall from the time it arises vest in the Company. U* assigns to the Company all Project Intellectual Property and all statutory or common law rights attaching to it including the right to sue for past infringement and to retain damages obtained as a result of any such action. [CONSIDER EXPLOITATION BY U* TT COMPANY IN NON-COMPETITIVE FIELD].]

N.B. Ensure Research Staff have agreed to vest their rights where necessary.

[OR]

[All Project Intellectual Property shall from the time it arises vest in U*. Pursuant to an agreement between U* and U* TT COMPANY, all such intellectual property rights and improvements are exploited through U* TT COMPANY. Accordingly, the Company agrees to execute all such documents at the cost of U* TT COMPANY as may be necessary to vest all such rights in U* TT COMPANY and all statutory or common law rights attaching to it including the right to sue for past infringement and to retain damages obtained as a result of any such actions.]

b. U* and the Company will promptly notify each other on a confidential basis of any actual or potential Project Intellectual Property of which either party becomes aware.

c. Notwithstanding clause 7.a U* may publish articles relating to the results of the Project, with the prior consent of the Company, not to be unreasonably withheld. U* acknowledges that it will not publish such results prior to any applications for a patent in respect of the Project Intellectual Property being made provided that such application is made as soon as reasonably practicable.

d. The Project Intellectual Property shall be exploited in accordance with the terms set out in Schedule 3.

e. To the extent that there is Background Intellectual Property which is necessary or useful in the manufacture, sale or maintenance of any product or service arising out of the results of the Project, U* grants the Company a non-exclusive, [worldwide,] [irrevocable] [royalty-free] [perpetual] licence to use the Background Intellectual Property to the extent necessary to manufacture, sell or maintain such product or service and for no other purpose whatsoever. [The licence in this clause shall be royalty-bearing in accordance with the terms set out in Schedule 3.]

[Only include 7.f and 7.g if assigned to Company under 7.a]

f. [The Company shall be free, at its own expense, to apply for a patent or other similar protection in respect of the Project Intellectual Property. Such application shall be filed in the name of the Company and where appropriate members of the Research Staff and Company Research Staff will be named as inventors or co-inventors in any patent application. The costs of filing and maintaining such applications for patents and other registered intellectual property shall be borne by the Company.]

g. [U* undertakes that it will and procures that U* TT COMPANY will, where appropriate, at the Company's cost (such cost to include fees for the time spent by U* and/or U* TT COMPANY in carrying out the work in accordance with this clause 7.g), execute such further documents and do such acts as may be necessary for securing, confirming or vesting absolutely the Company's full rights, title and interest in the Project Intellectual Property in the Company and to confer on the Company all rights of action in respect of any claim of infringement by third parties.] U*'s and/or U* TT COMPANY's fees for the purposes of this clause 7.g shall be [ ] per hour plus VAT.

8 INFRINGEMENT

a. Each party shall give notice to the other if it or the U* Research Staff or the Company's Research Staff becomes aware of:-

   i. any infringement of the Background Intellectual Property or the Project Intellectual Property; and

   ii. any claim by a third party that an action carried out under the Project infringes the Intellectual Property or other rights of any third party.

b. Where any infringement or suspected infringement arises or a claim by a third party alleging infringement of that third party's Intellectual Property or other rights arises in respect of any [Project Intellectual Property or] Background Intellectual Property, U* and/or U* TT COMPANY shall promptly consult with the Company and take such action to bring or defend such action (as appropriate, if any) as is agreed between the parties. The Company shall give such assistance as is reasonably requested by U* and/or U* TT COMPANY to assist U* and/or U* TT COMPANY, at U* and/or U* TT COMPANY expense, in the prevention of any infringe-

ment. U* and/or U* TT COMPANY shall meet the costs of any legal proceedings instituted by U* and/or U* TT COMPANY, but shall be entitled to keep any awards of damages made in its favour. [The Company shall not have any rights itself to take action.]

c. [If U* and/or U* TT COMPANY fails to agree what action shall be taken to bring or defend an action then the Company may take all such action as it shall consider to be necessary or appropriate, at its own expense, to bring or defend an action and shall be entitled and subject to all damages and other sums which may be recovered or awarded against it as a result of such action. In such event U* and/or U* TT COMPANY shall provide all reasonable assistance to the Company, at the Company's expense.]

d. [Where any infringement or suspected infringement of the Project Intellectual Property arises or a claim by a third party alleging infringement of that third party's Intellectual Property or other rights arises in respect of the Project Intellectual Property the Company shall in its absolute discretion determine what action, if any, shall be taken in respect of such matter and shall have sole control over and shall conduct such action as it shall deem necessary at its own cost. U* and/or U* TT COMPANY shall at the request of the Company, at the Company's cost promptly provide all reasonable assistance to the Company in respect of any such claim.]

[Only insert clause 8.d if Project Intellectual Property assigned under clause 7.a]

9 TERMINATION

a. Either party may terminate the Project with immediate effect by notice in writing to the other and shall be released from all its obligations under this Agreement for a material breach by the other party of any of the terms of this Agreement which in the case of a breach capable of being remedied, is not remedied within 30 days of receipt by the party in default from the aggrieved party of a notice specifying the breach and requiring its remedy.

b. U* may terminate this Agreement by notice in writing to the Company if:

   i. an encumbrancer takes possession or a receiver is appointed over any of the property or assets of the Company; or

   ii. the Company makes a voluntary arrangement with its creditors or becomes subject to an administration order; or

iii. the Company goes into liquidation (except for the purposes of an amalgamation, reconstruction or other reorganisation and in such manner that the company resulting from the reorganisation effectively agrees to be bound by or to assume the obligations imposed on the Company under this Agreement); or

iv. any distrait execution or other process is levied or enforced on any property of the Company and is not paid out withdrawn or discharged within 21 days; or

v. the Company ceases or threatens to cease to carry on business.

c. Any termination of this Agreement shall operate without prejudice to the rights of the parties already accrued at the time of termination.

d. Any waiver or forbearance in regard to the performance of this Agreement shall operate only if in writing and shall apply only to the specified instance and not affect the existence of and continued applicability of the terms of this Agreement.

10 FORCE MAJEURE

Neither party to this Agreement shall be liable to the other party in any manner whatsoever for any delay or non-performance or for the consequences of any delay in performing or non-performance of any of its obligations under this Agreement if such delay or non-performance is due to cause beyond that party's reasonable control including, without limitation, acts of God, acts of any governmental or supranational authority, war or national emergency, riots, civil commotion, fire, explosion, flood, epidemic, lock-outs (whether or not by that party), strikes and other industrial disputes (in each case, whether or not relating to that party's workforce), restraints or delays affecting carriers, inability or delay in obtaining supplies or adequate or suitable materials and currency restrictions and the party so delayed or non-performing shall be entitled to a reasonable extension of time for performing such obligations.

11 RELATIONSHIP BETWEEN THE PARTIES

Nothing in this Agreement shall constitute the parties as parties to a legal relationship of partnership, employer-employee, principal-agent or otherwise render one party liable for the acts of the other save insofar as expressly provided under the terms of this Agreement.

12 GENERAL

a. This Agreement represents the whole agreement between the parties and supersedes any previous agreement or representations written or verbal relating to the subject matter of this Agreement and may be amended only by writing signed by both parties.

b. No employee or agent of the parties has any authority to bind either party to terms in any way inconsistent or warrant or give any advice in respect of the Agreement or its interpretation save when such term representation or warranty is made in writing by an authorised director of the Company or designated responsible officer of U* (as the case may be).

c. The failure of either party to enforce or to exercise, at any time or for any period of time, any term of or any right arising pursuant to this Agreement does not constitute, and shall not be construed as a waiver of such term or right and shall in no way affect that party's right later to enforce or to exercise it.

d. The invalidity or unenforceability of any provision of this Agreement shall not prejudice or affect the validity or enforceability of any other provision of this Agreement.

e. Each party acknowledges that on entering into this Agreement it does not do so on the basis of and does not rely on any representation, warranty or other provision except as expressly provided in this Agreement and all conditions, warranties or other terms implied by statute at common law are excluded to the fullest extent permitted by law. Nothing shall exclude the liability of either party for fraudulent misrepresentation.

13 LAW AND JURISDICTION

a. [All disputes and questions whatsoever which arise either during the subsistence of this Agreement or afterwards between the parties touching this Agreement or the construction or application thereof or as to any other matter in any way relating to this Agreement shall be referred to a single arbitrator in accordance with and subject to the provisions of the Arbitration Acts 1950-1979 (or any statutory modification or re-enactment thereof for the time being in force). Either party may serve notice upon the other party to agree upon an arbitrator and in default of such agreement within [seven] days of the date of such notice the arbitrator shall be appointed at the request of either party by the President for the time being of the Institute of Arbitrators. The costs of any such arbitration shall be paid by one of more parties as determined by the Arbitrator.

b. The arbitration proceedings will be conducted in the English language and will be held in London, England. The decision of the arbitrator will be final and binding on the parties.

c. Notwithstanding the provision of clause 13.a above, either party shall have the right to seek appropriate injunctive relief against the other party in an English court.]

d. This Agreement shall be construed and governed in accordance with English Law [and the Company agrees to submit to the exclusive jurisdiction of the English Courts].

SCHEDULE 1

Project Plan

1. PROJECT TITLE:
   [insert]

2. PROJECT OBJECTIVES:
   [outline main objectives of the Project]
   The Project will be split into [number] stages:
   [outline stages of Project]

3. MILESTONE DATES:
   U* undertakes to complete each of the above stages of the Project by the following dates:
   Stage: Completion Date:
   [   ]   _____

4. PROJECT DELIVERABLES:
   [insert details of work to be delivered as a result of the Project]

5. LOCATION OF PROJECT WORK:
   [insert details of location for research]

6. FINANCE:
   [insert details of staff costs etc.]
   U* will invoice the Company for quarterly payments, in advance, for the contracted total.

SCHEDULE 2

Background Intellectual Property
(This to be inserted here)

SCHEDULE 3

Intellectual Property/Commercial Explanation
[It would be better to try to fix a royalty rate, include specific dates for payment, and detailed definition of net sales value etc., upon signature of this agreement]

1 All Background Intellectual Property which both parties agree to make available for the effective undertaking of the Project shall remain the sole property of that party.

2 [If U* makes any invention or discovery arising from the Project the Company shall have the exclusive benefit of the Project Intellectual Property. U* TT COMPANY shall take all steps requested by the Company, at the expense of the Company, in order to enable the Company to file and prosecute and defend any Project Intellectual Property. If any commercial benefit accrues to the Company through its entitlement to the Project Intellectual Property the Company shall make payments to U* TT COMPANY in respect of the contributions made by U* as are, in all circumstances, reasonable. Such payments shall recognise the commercial value of the invention to the Company, the inventive contribution of U* and the financial risks and efforts of the Company in developing the invention or discovery. Any such payments shall not exceed 7% of the gross sales value of any products sold or otherwise disposed of or services supplied by the Company arising out of the Project Intellectual Property. The Company shall grant U* TT COMPANY a [non-]exclusive, [non-]transferable licence free of charge, for all countries concerning all results for the purposes of teaching and research [and to exploit the Project Intellectual Property in any field, provided always that U* TT COMPANY shall not exploit the Project Intellectual Property in such a way as to compete with the activities of the Company carried out in the course of the Company's business].]

[If U* makes any invention or discovery arising from the Project, it shall have the exclusive benefit of the Project Intellectual Property. If any commercial benefit accrues to U* through its entitlement to the Project International Property, U* TT COMPANY shall make payments to the Company in respect of the contributions made by the Company as are, in all circumstances, reasonable. Such payments shall recognise the commercial value of the invention to U*, the inventive contribution of the Company and the financial roles and efforts of U* and/or U* TT COMPANY in developing the invention or discovery. Any payments shall not exceed 7% of the net sales value of any products sold or otherwise disposed of or services supplied by U* TT COMPANY arising out of the Project Intellectual Property. U* TT COMPANY shall grant the Company a [non-]exclusive, [non-transferable] licence free of charge, for all countries concerning all results [for the purposes of {INSERT PURPOSE}).]

3 [The Company/U* TT COMPANY] agrees that [U* TT COMPANY's/the Company's] rights to receive payments from [the Company/U* TT

COMPANY] in accordance with clause 2 of this Schedule in respect of the Project Intellectual Property will not be prejudiced by any sale of such Project Intellectual Property by [the Company/U* TT COMPANY] to any third party. [The Company/U* TT COMPANY] agrees to ensure that any purchaser of any of the Project Intellectual Property will continue to make payments to [U* TT COMPANY/the Company] at a rate at least as high and for a period at least as long as under this Agreement or any subsidiary agreement reached between the Company and U* TT COMPANY.

4 [The Company/U* TT COMPANY] shall be obliged to keep [U* TT COMPANY/the COMPANY] informed on an annual basis from the date of this Agreement of any income due to [U* TT COMPANY/the Company] under the above clauses and shall send to [U* TT COMPANY/the Company] at the same time as each royalty payment is made a statement setting out [in respect of each country/region in which products are sold] the quantity of products sold and the total gross sales value of the products sold expressed both in local currency and pounds sterling and the conversion rates used if applicable.

5 Should [the Company/U* and/or U* TT COMPANY] not wish to exploit any invention or discovery arising from the Project, whether or not patents have been filed, it shall discuss with [U* and/or U* TT COMPANY/the Company] the option of assigning some or all rights to [U* TT COMPANY/the Company]. Under these circumstances [the Company/U* TT COM-PANY] agrees not to disclose any such inventions or discoveries to third parties before it is informed by [U* TT COMPANY/the Company] that [U* and/or U* TT COMPANY /the Company] has no interest in exploiting the inventions or discoveries.

6 If a member of U* Research Staff makes a contribution to any Project Intellectual Property which becomes the subject of any patents, then the member of U* Research Staff shall be named as inventor or co-inventor in such patents.

SIGNED by _____

for and on behalf of _____

THE UNIVERSITY OF _____

_____

Date _____

SIGNED by _____

for and on behalf of _____

U* TT COMPANY _____

Date _____

SIGNED by _____

for and on behalf of _____

_____ LIMITED/PLC _____

Date _____

I have read the terms and conditions of this Contract, agree with them and agree to abide by them.

SIGNED by _____

Date _____

Print Name _____

_____ Designated Officer

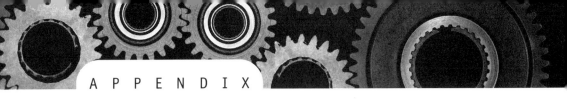

62-D

Research Studentship Agreement

DATE: 200*

PARTIES:

(1) THE U* INSERT FULL NAME AND ADDRESS ("U*"); and

(2) _____ LIMITED/PLC (registered in _____ number _____) whose registered office is at _____ ("the Company").

BACKGROUND

(A) U* has identified a suitable student, [name] ("the Student") who will work under the supervision of [name] of the department of [name] ("the Academic Supervisor").

(B) The Company has identified a suitable supervisor [name] ("the Industrial Supervisor") who will liaise with the Academic Supervisor in the supervision of the Student.

(C) The Student will undertake a programme of research training in the field of [description] that will normally culminate in the Student submitting a thesis for examination for the award of a postgraduate degree ("the Research Training Programme"), the Research Training Programme has been devised by the Academic Supervisor and the Industrial Supervisor and details are provided in Schedule 1.

(D) [The Student will be co-funded by the Company and [sponsor name], details of these funding arrangements are given in Schedule 2.]

(E) [The undertaking of the Research Training Programme by the Student will be carried out in accordance with the [sponsor] rules, available at [website] that apply to [sponsor] funded studentships, where there is any conflict between this agreement and the rules that apply to [sponsor] studentship, the latter will take precedence.]

(F) U* and the Academic Supervisor are in possession of certain know-how, techniques and expertise in the field of [describe] ("U*'s Existing Intellectual Property") that will be used in the undertaking of the Research Training Programme.

OPERATIVE PROVISIONS

1. CONFIDENTIALITY AND PUBLICATION OF RESULTS

   a. The Company shall be given reasonable and prompt access to all results and information directly arising from the Research Training Programme. It is the understanding of the Company, U*, the Student and the Academic Supervisor that wherever possible the results of the Research Training Programme will be published in accordance with normal academic practice subject to the following confidentiality provisions of this clause 1.

   b. Subject to clauses 1.c and 1.d below, the Student and the Academic Supervisor shall keep secret all results and conclusions arising from the Research Training Programme and shall not disclose the same to any person other than employees of the Company directly concerned with the Research Training Programme without the express written permission of the Company.

   c. The Student and/or the Academic Supervisor shall give the Company a written draft of any thesis, publication, presentation or other form of proposed disclosure relating to the Research Training Programme which either or both of them wishes to release. The Company shall examine the draft and shall inform the Student and/or the Academic Supervisor within one month of receipt whether it consents to the proposed disclosure or intends to enforce the secrecy obligation expressed in clause 1.b in order to obtain patent protection or for other good reason, and;

i. if the Company does not provide a response to the submission of a draft disclosure within one month of the submission of the draft by the Student and/or Academic Supervisor then it will be assumed that the proposed disclosure will not be subject to the secrecy obligation expressed in clause 1.b; or

ii. if the Company does intend to enforce the secrecy obligation expressed in clause 1.b it will identify precisely those results and conclusions that are to be subject to the secrecy obligation and will assist the Student and/or the Academic Supervisor in amending the proposed disclosure in such a way that it will not prejudice the obtaining of patent protection by the Company. The Company will also earnestly endeavour to minimise the period of any such enforcement of the secrecy obligation that in no case shall exceed 3 months from the receipt of the original draft by the Company.

d. In the case of a thesis or other internal report the Company shall not object to examination by any examiner or committee appointed by U* to adjudicate on the award of any degree provided that the Academic Supervisor makes it clear to the examiner(s) or committee(s) that the contents of the thesis are disclosed in confidence. Upon the successful outcome of a final examination of the Student's thesis, the thesis will be stored in U*'s main library. If the Company makes a specific request that the contents of the thesis are to be subject to the secrecy obligations expressed in clause 1.b, U*'s main library will restrict access to the thesis for a period of 5 years.

e. The Student and the Academic Supervisor shall keep secret all other information relating to the business or research activities of the Company that they may learn as a result of collaboration with the Company in conducting the Research Training Programme.

f. The restrictions contained in clauses 1.b and 1.e do not apply to information which:-

i. was already known to the Student or the Academic Supervisor prior to disclosure by the Company, if the Student or Academic Supervisor informs the Company that it was so known as soon as the Student or Academic Supervisor is aware of the fact;

ii. at the time of disclosure by or on behalf of the Company is public knowledge or subsequently becomes public knowledge other than through a breach of this Agreement on the part of the Student or the Academic Supervisor;

iii. is lawfully received by the Student or the Academic Supervisor from a third party, without any breach of a confidentiality relationship with the Company.

g. Notwithstanding the termination of this Agreement and the return of any confidential information the obligations of this clause 1 shall continue in full force for 5 years following the date of submission of the thesis for final examination.

2. INTELLECTUAL PROPERTY RIGHTS

a. U*'s Existing Intellectual Property will be made available to the Student and the Company solely for the purpose of undertaking the Research Training Programme and shall remain in the ownership of U*. If the Company wishes to use U*'s Existing Intellectual Property [and/or any Intellectual Property arising from the Research Training Programme] *(if this insertion is left in, clauses 2.2 to 2.7 and schedule 3 should be deleted)* for commercial purposes, U* will consider a request from the Company for a licence to be negotiated on fair and reasonable terms.

b. [All Project Intellectual Property shall from the time it arises ("Arising IPR") vest in U*.] [U* shall assign to the Company [IDENTIFY RIGHTS TO BE ASSIGNED] and all statutory or common law rights attaching to it including the right to sue for past infringement and to retain damages obtained as a result of any such actions.

c. In respect of any Arising IPR owned by U*, U* will offer to the Company the option to take either a non-exclusive or exclusive licence, which may or may not be restricted by field.

d. The terms of any licence agreement provided for in Clause 2.3 above shall be negotiated in good faith by the Company and U*'s wholly owned intellectual property management and exploitation company, U* Ventures Limited ("U* TT COMPANY") and shall contain all such terms and conditions which are usual and customary in a licence agreement, including but not limited to liability, audit provisions, termination, governing law provisions. The financial terms of any licence will be fair and reasonable in the circumstances and will be negotiated on a case-by-case basis taking into account the scientific and financial contributions of the Parties to the Arising IPR being licensed and the subsequent scientific and financial contribution of the Parties that will be necessary to commercially exploit such Arising IPR.]

[OR]

2.2 [If the Student and/or the Academic Supervisor shall make any invention or discovery during the Research Training Programme ("the Invention"), any intellectual property rights arising shall vest in the Company. The Student will assign his/her intellectual property rights in relation to the Research Training Programme to U*'s wholly owned intellectual property management and exploitation company, U* Ventures Limited ("U* TT COMPANY") by signing the deed provided in Schedule 3. The Academic Supervisor will assign his/her intellectual property rights in relation to the Research Training Programme to U* TT COMPANY by signing the declaration provided in Schedule 4. The Student and the Academic Supervisor shall execute such further documents and take all steps as may be necessary, at the expense of the Company, to secure the vesting in the Company of such intellectual property rights, in order to enable the Company to file, prosecute and defend any intellectual property rights in the Invention.

2.3 If any commercial benefit accrues to the Company through its entitlement to such intellectual property rights the Company will make payments to U* TT COMPANY at an appropriate percentage of relevant gross sales that reflects the contributions made by the Student and/or the Academic Supervisor as are in all the circumstances reasonable.

2.4 The Company grants U* and/or U* TT COMPANY an irrevocable, non-exclusive, non-transferable, royalty-free licence throughout the world to use all results obtained from the Research Training Programme for the purposes of teaching and research.

e. [The Company also grants U* TT COMPANY an irrevocable, exclusive licence throughout the world to commercially exploit all results obtained from the Research Training Programme providing that such commercial exploitation does not compete in any way with the commercial activities of the Company. If any commercial benefit accrues to U* TT COMPANY though its entitlement to such a licence U* TT COMPANY will make payments to the Company that reflect the contribution made by the Company as are in all circumstances reasonable.]

f. The Company agrees that U* TT COMPANY's rights to receive payments from the Company in accordance with the provisions of clause 2.3 above in respect of intellectual property rights and payments will not be prejudiced by any sale of such intellectual property rights by the Company. The Company agrees to ensure that any purchaser of any such intellectual property rights will make payments to U* TT COMPANY at a rate at least as high and for a period at least as long as under this Agreement or any subsidiary agreement reached between the Company and U* TT COMPANY.

g. Should the Company not wish to exploit the Invention, whether or not patents have been filed, it shall discuss with U* the option of assigning all rights to U* TT COMPANY. Under these circumstances the Company agrees not to disclose the Invention to third parties before it is told by U* and/or U* TT COMPANY that U* and/or U* TT COMPANY has no commercial interest in the Inventions.]

3. SUBSTITUTION OF SUPERVISOR AND/OR STUDENT

a. Unless U* and the Company otherwise agree, if the Academic Supervisor ceases to hold his present academic appointment he shall cease to be the Academic Supervisor but shall continue to be bound by the obligations of confidentiality in clause 1. U* shall obtain the Company's agreement in writing before any substitute Academic Supervisor becomes involved with the Research Training Programme, such agreement not to be unreasonably withheld.

b. If absolutely necessary at any time during the Research Training Programme U* and the Company will consider the substitution of the Student and/or the Academic Supervisor by suitable replacement to be agreed by U* and the Company. Any Student or Academic Supervisor replaced under the provisions of this clause shall continue to be bound by the obligations of confidentiality in clause 1.

4. TERM AND TERMINATION

a. This Agreement shall commence on [start date] of the Research Training Programme and may be terminated by either party on giving a minimum of 6 months prior written notice to the other. In the event of such termination the Company will pay U* a sum sufficient to cover all outstanding and unavoidable commitments in connection with the Research Training Programme that would normally be payable by the Company. [For the avoidance of doubt such unavoidable commitments will include the Student's stipend and tuition fees.]

b. U* shall be entitled to terminate this Agreement on giving the Company 14 days written notice if the Company fails to make the payments as required by clause 5.b below.

c. Unless otherwise terminated in accordance with clauses 4.a or 4.b, this Agreement shall terminate on completion of the Research Training Programme.

5. PAYMENT

a. In consideration of the research carried out under the Research Training Programme, the Company shall pay U* on the basis of the costs set out in Schedule 2.

b. U* shall invoice the Company on a quarterly in advance basis for the fees due for the following 3-month period beginning on the date of this Agreement. All payments due under this Agreement shall be paid to U* within 30 days of the date of receipt by the Company of such invoice.

6. Value Added Tax or similar tax shall be paid by the Company in addition to the payments made to U* under this Agreement.

7. ENTIRE AGREEMENT

This represents the whole agreement between the parties and supersedes any previous agreement or representations written or verbal relating to the subject matter of this Agreement and may be amended only by writing signed by both parties.

8. GOVERNING LAW

This Agreement is construed and governed in accordance with English Law and the Company agrees to submit to the exclusive jurisdiction of the English Courts.

SCHEDULE ONE

THE RESEARCH TRAINING PROGRAMME
[To be devised by the supervisors]

SCHEDULE TWO

U* COSTS (FULLY FUNDED STUDENTSHIP)
Based on the 3-Year Research Training Programme

Student stipend
Technical Support
Equipment Access
Consumables
Travel*
Overheads (50% of above costs)
Student Fees**
Total

*This budget is for travel to relevant conferences and meetings during the Research Training Programme. In addition to this, the Company will directly pay the travel and accommodation expenses incurred by the Student and Academic Supervisor as a result of undertaking visits and secondments at the Company's premises, providing that approval for such expenses is obtained in advance from the Company.

**This figure is based on rates applicable to UK/EC students for the academic year 200*/200*, and will therefore be increased as appropriate to take into account agreed increases determined by the UK Research Councils.

SCHEDULE TWO

U* COSTS (CO-FUNDED STUDENTSHIP)
Based on the 3-Year Research Training Programme

Cost Item	[sponsor]	the Company
Student stipend	*	
Consumables		
Travel**		
Student Fees*		
Total		

These figures are based on rates applicable to UK/EC students for the academic year 200/200*, and will therefore be increased as appropriate to take into account agreed increases determined by the [sponsor].

**This budget is for travel to relevant conferences and meetings during the Research Training Programme. In addition to this, the Company will directly pay the travel and accommodation expenses incurred by the Student and Academic Supervisor as a result of undertaking visits and secondments at the Company's premises, providing that approval for such expenses is obtained in advance from the Company.

SCHEDULE THREE

ASSIGNMENT OF INTELLECTUAL PROPERTY RIGHTS

(STUDENTS WORKING ON SPECIFIC PROJECTS)

To: U* TT COMPANY

("Outside Body") [LEGAL NAME OF OUTSIDE BODY]

("Project") [DESCRIPTION OF PROJECT]

1. ACKNOWLEDGEMENT

   I wish to carry out work in connection with the Project as part of the study I am undertaking at The University of ("U*"). As a condition of being allowed to do so I understand that it is necessary to ensure that:-

   1.1 confidential information received or generated in connection with or arising out of the Project is protected ("Confidential Information"); and

   1.2 ownership of any intellectual property rights created by myself and others in the course of undertaking work for the Project belongs to U*'s wholly owned intellectual property management and exploitation company, U* TT COMPANY ("U* TT COMPANY") (and/or the Outside Body).

2. CONFIDENTIALITY

   2.1 I confirm that I shall keep all Confidential Information, which I receive or generate, secret and confidential and not disclose it to anyone else, except to another person who is involved in the Project and has given an equivalent undertaking of confidentiality or who is aware of the obligations of confidentiality under this Agreement.

   2.2 My obligation of confidentiality does not apply to Confidential Information which is public knowledge unless it has become public because I have disclosed it.

   2.3 I may disclose Confidential Information if I have to do so by law, but only to the extent I am required to do so.

   2.4 Upon completion of the Project I shall return all documents or other materials incorporating any of the Confidential Information to U* and/or U* TT COMPANY as directed.

3. ASSIGNMENT

   3.1 I assign to U* TT COMPANY, with full title guarantee, all copyright, design rights and related rights and in relation to future copyright, design rights and related rights, by way of present assignment of future rights, and agree to assign upon request by U* TT COMPANY, with full title guarantee all other intellectual property rights in existence existing in any part of the world which have been created or invented or are in the future created or invented by me in the course of my undertaking work on the Project ("IPR").

   3.2 I acknowledge that IPR includes copyright, design right, patents, inventions and applications or rights to apply for such rights.

   3.3 I waive my moral rights arising from the IPR, so far as I can, including any rights I may have to be identified as the author of the IPR or to object to derogatory treatment of them.

   3.4 I shall do all things and sign all documents which U* TT COMPANY reasonably requires me to do or sign to confirm U* TT COMPANY's (or the Outside Body's) ownership of the IPR. This will be at U* TT COMPANY's cost and expense. I appoint U* TT COMPANY as my attorney to execute any such documents, including assignments of IPR.

   3.5 U* TT COMPANY will try to ensure that I am given attribution for the work which I carry out under the Project and that I receive an equitable share of any benefits arising from the IPR (which could include a share of any royalties).

Dated   200*

SIGNED AND DELIVERED AS A DEED _____

By _____

Name of Student _____

of (Address) _____   Signature

_____

_____

Witness signature:

Witness address:

Witness occupation:

SIGNED by _____

for and on behalf of _____

THE UNIVERSITY OF _____

_____   Signature

U* TT COMPANY _____

Witness signature:

Witness address:

Witness occupation:

SCHEDULE FOUR

STAFF DECLARATION FOR CONTRACT RESEARCH WORK

NAME OF STAFF MEMBER [EMPLOYEE'S FULL NAME] ("the Employee") of [HOME ADDRESS]

[RESEARCH CONTRACT/NUMBER] ("the Project")

[COMPANY PARTY TO RESEARCH CONTRACT WITH U*] ("the Company")

DATE: 200*

In consideration of:-

[(i) the rewards stipulated under U*'s Intellectual Property policy [as detailed in Addendum 1]/U* allowing the Employee to take part in the Project; and]

(ii) U* and/or the Company disclosing Confidential Information to the Employee, including but not limited to intellectual property, drawings, samples, know-how and/or data in any form, and/or other proprietary information of or information relating to the business activities of U* or the Company or any third party in relation to and/or arising out of the Project ("Confidential Information");

the Employee agrees that [he/she] shall not either during or after the completion of the Project, without the prior written consent of U*:-

(i) disclose the existence of the Project nor any of the Confidential Information nor the Company's involvement to any third party not directly involved in the Project;

(ii) publish or otherwise disclose to any third party outside U* or its wholly owned intellectual property management and exploitation company, U* Ventures Limited ("U* TT COMPANY") any of the Confidential Information;

(iii) use any of the Confidential Information for any purpose other than the Project whether or not such use is in connection with his/her employment with U*; nor

(iv) copy or reproduce in any manner or form any of the Confidential Information except as is reasonably required to carry out the Project.

The Employee's obligations in respect of Confidential Information shall apply whether or not such Confidential Information is labelled as such.

The restrictions contained in this Agreement do not apply to Confidential Information which:-

(i) was already known to the Employee prior to the disclosure by U* or the Company, if the Employee informs U* that it was so known as soon as the Employee becomes aware of the fact;

(ii) at the time of disclosure by or on behalf of U* or the Company is public knowledge or subsequently becomes public knowledge other than through a breach of this Agreement on the part of the Employee;

(iii) is lawfully received by the Employee from a third party without any breach of a confidentiality relationship with U*; or

(iv) is generated independently by the Employee without use of any of the Confidential Information.

The Employee agrees that by operation of law, all intellectual property rights and improvements of any kind, recorded in any manner, created or invented by [him/her] in the course of the Project shall belong to and vest in U* exclusively. Pursuant to an agreement between U* and U* TT COMPANY, all such intellectual property rights and improvements are exploited through U* TT COMPANY. Accordingly, subject to any agreement between U* and/or U* TT COMPANY and the Company, the Employee agrees to execute all such documents at the cost of U* TT COMPANY as may be necessary to vest all such rights in U* TT COMPANY or the Company (as U* directs) [and assist in the resolution of any question in relation to any patent application which may arise out of the Project]. Nothing in this Agreement shall affect the Employee's rights under the Patents Act 1977.

The Employee agrees to conduct [him/her]self in a manner consistent with the obligations undertaken by U* in any agreement entered into by U* and/or U* TT COMPANY in relation to the Project to the extent that such obligations have been brought to the Employee's attention.

The obligations undertaken by the Employee in this Agreement will survive the termination of [his/her] employment with U*.

On termination of the Employee's employment with U* or at any time, if requested by U*, the Employee undertakes to return all Confidential Information in [his/her] possession (including any copies of it or notes made in relation to it) to U* within seven (7) days of such termination or request.

The confidentiality obligations in this Agreement shall continue in force notwithstanding the return of all Confidential Information or the completion of the Project.

This Agreement shall be construed and governed in accordance with English Law and the Employee agrees to submit to the exclusive jurisdiction of the English Courts.

SIGNED by _____

for and on behalf of _____

THE UNIVERSITY OF _____

SIGNED by [EMPLOYEE] _____

ADDENDUM 1

Where no other party claims any intellectual property rights arising from the Project U* agrees to pay to the Employee a share of the payment made to U* by the Company as compensation for U*'s assignment of all IPR arising from the Project. This represents full and final payment to the Employee.

Payment will be allocated as follows:-

Payment by the Company as Compensation for Arising IPR Assignment	*Percentage payable to the Employee*
The first £5,000	75% of net revenue
The next £15,000	60% of net revenue
Thereafter	50% of net revenue

SIGNED by

for and on behalf of _____

THE UNIVERSITY OF _____

Date _____

SIGNED by _____

for and on behalf of _____

U* TT COMPANY _____

Date _____

SIGNED by _____

for and on behalf of _____

[THE COMPANY] LIMITED/PLC

_____

Date _____

SIGNED by _____

THE ACADEMIC SUPERVISOR

_____

To confirm that I have read and will abide

_____

by this Agreement _____

SIGNED by _____

THE STUDENT _____

To confirm that I have read and will abide

_____

by this Agreement _____

Identifying and Triaging Technologies

Joseph Fondacaro, PhD

Introduction

There are many documents that one might consider essential to an active, robust academic technology transfer program. Perhaps the most important of these is the invention disclosure. For without inventions being disclosed to the technology licensing office, there are no technologies to patent, to market, or indeed, to transfer. The very existence of an academic technology transfer program depends almost exclusively on having technologies to license to for-profit entities as a basis of products for the benefit of the public. Thus, the invention disclosure is truly the "cornerstone" of a technology transfer program.

This chapter provides an in-depth analysis of the invention disclosure as to its form, its meaning, and, utmost, its evaluation and utility. A stepwise process of evaluation is discussed and a decision-tree format is presented to assist in the understanding of the critical steps in this evaluation process. After reading this chapter, one should be equipped to begin, in earnest, the process of managing more effectively the technologies described within the invention disclosure.

Formatting the Invention Disclosure

As with any form document, the invention disclosure is only as valuable as the information that it contains. Therefore, asking for the right information (i.e., within the format of the disclosure) is of utmost importance. The questions asked should be straightforward and easy to understand. This effort is not to minimize the intelligence of academic research faculty. It is intended to point out that, rather, even after more than twenty years of active academic involvement, technology transfer and licensing is still not an integral part of the culture in many institutions. The most difficult task facing the academic technology transfer professional is to maintain a "business" presence within an academic environment. It is true that many faculty (indeed many centers) are now well-tuned to these processes; however, there remain many that are not facilitating the process of evaluating invention disclosures with a well-planned, coherent and understood form document. Many of the problems encountered by academic technology transfer professionals can be lessened or eliminated altogether by meeting with potential inventors prior to submission of the disclosure. Thus, in the "education process," technology transfer managers should encourage academic faculty to schedule a predisclosure meeting.[1] A sample guide to a predisclosure meeting is included as Appendix A at the end of this chapter.

The main objective behind the questions included in an invention disclosure form is straightforward. The completed document should represent a sharing of information that allows someone with reasonable skill to completely duplicate the invention. While it may take some time for a licensing professional to attain sufficient knowledge to truly comprehend the art of such a process, having the appropriate set of questions can facilitate the needed level of understanding and confidence. It should be kept in mind that this document represents the first step in the patenting or copyright process. Thus, the information requested should also be familiar to patent and/or copyright attorneys. The invention disclosure must identify the inventor(s); clarify information about prior art; and include the inventor's signature on an "assignment of rights" form that assigns property rights to the academic center.

The information collected within an invention disclosure is not only important as the cornerstone of a technology licensing or transfer program, but also documents and validates the invention for patent application and, ultimately, its issued patent. In the United States, patent law recognizes the party who is "first to invent," unlike most other countries that grant "first to file" patents. Thus, if two separate patent applications claim the same invention, the United States Patent and Trademark Office (USPTO) would seek, in the form of documented evidence, proof of the first to conceive of the patentable invention from the two entities applying for the patent. Failure to provide such proof (because of lack of evidence or incomplete documentation) may result in loss of patent rights by one of the parties. The invention disclosure, with key accompanying documents, may be the only complete record of the invention available to determine these discrepancies. Thus, accurate and thorough collection and documentation of invention-related data is critical to a successful technology patenting and licensing initiative (M. Mark Crowell's chapter in the *Technology Transfer Practice Manual* also provides extensive, detailed coverage of this topic).[2]

The invention disclosure form generally begins with the title of the invention, as described by the inventor(s). This is usually followed in the disclosure by a request for the date of original conception and the first date of reduction to practice (or proof of concept), followed by a section requesting the full name(s), home address, and contact information of each named inventor. Each inventor's academic title and affiliation is also important information to collect. Each inventor should sign the disclosure in full name, along with the date of the signature.

The matter of inventorship vs. authorship is difficult, yet, one of the critical issues encountered by many, if not most, licensing and technology transfer managers. Faculty, customarily and typically, are encouraged to publish the results and interpretations of their research, at least to satisfy requirements for reappointment, promotion, and

tenure. It goes without saying that academic faculty/inventors are eager to publish. Academic research faculty often recognize the contributions of other members of their research team and seek acknowledgement for their contributions, and often, these contributors are included as co-authors. For example, in the biomedical research field, senior investigators often include the name of a graduate student or senior technician as co-author on a publication. However, patent law requires that only inventors (those contributing to the creation and/or reduction to practice of an invention) be listed as inventors on a patent application. Since the logical sequence of events leads from an invention disclosure to a patent application (later discussed), only those persons directly contributing creative or inventive steps should be listed in or should sign the invention disclosure form. Inappropriate listing of inventors, either by addition or omission, may jeopardize the validity of a patent. Therefore, the technology transfer manager in an academic research environment often times must ask the difficult questions regarding inventorship. It is often advisable, and perhaps necessary, to defer this task to a neutral third party, i.e., the patent attorney selected to prepare, submit, and to prosecute the patent application generated from an invention disclosure.

The Invention

There are several key elements of the invention that should be requested within the invention disclosure form. First, the inventor(s) must provide a clear, concise, but all-inclusive written description of the invention. This text should contain two critical characteristics: a) it should be understandable to someone who is not skilled in the art and, b) it should be complete to a point where someone who is skilled in the art can reproduce the invention. Therefore, questions should be clear to all involved parties, principally the inventor. Answers to the questions within the form of the disclosure will not only be important to the initial evaluation by the technology transfer professional, but will and can be the basis of any or many, if not most, of the claims of a patent application ultimately derived from this disclosure.

In order to enhance understanding of the invention and assist in the evaluation of the invention and its utility, the inventor(s) should be asked to provide documented evidence of reduction to practice of the invention. This may take the form of drawings, charts, graphs, tables or any other illustration of data to support the invention.

The inventor(s) should also be asked to envision the invention's use as or in a product, if a product is not obvious within the invention or, in the case of a device, a prototype has not yet been assembled. This information can aid in the overall evaluation of the invention disclosure and can provide key information on utility for preparation and prosecution of a patent application.

Prior Art

Essential to the evaluation of a newly disclosed invention is the collection and assessment of prior art. There are generally three categories of prior art that are important to have: publications by the inventor(s), publications that the inventor(s) is (are) aware of from other laboratories', and issued patents and published patent applications. It is necessary, therefore, that the invention disclosure form requests the inventor(s) to submit a copy of all known publications that fall within the scope of the invention. Additionally, it is advisable to request a list of all recent publications and presentations of the inventor(s) as, again, it may be helpful in completing a thorough review of the invention disclosure. Likewise, the inventor(s) should submit, and the form should request a copy of any manuscripts either in press or in preparation that may be relevant to the invention.

Most academic researchers are not aware of patent literature, however, some may very well be able to provide such information. Thus, it is not unusual to request this on the disclosure form in such a way as to be collegial, such as, "If the inventor(s) is (are) aware of any patents or published patent applications that may be relevant to the described invention, please provide the identification numbers of such patents or patent applications." It will, however, generally be the task of the technology transfer professional or the selected patent attorney to gather such patent-prior art.

Other Information

The invention disclosure form should ask the inventor(s) to provide any knowledge they may have regarding companies working in the same area of technology as their invention. The names of these companies themselves may be sufficient. This will provide some level of confidence to the technology transfer professional that this technology has poten-

tial value in the marketplace in terms of the evaluation of the invention. It will also suggest whether the invention (or better still, the envisaged product) is novel and potentially competitive with current marketed technologies. In addition, having some initial information on companies marketing similar products or even working in the area of the invention provides a potential starting point for building a licensing strategy when the time comes to begin marketing efforts for the technology. The invention disclosure form should include a statement of "assignment of rights." This statement should be worded such that all rights relating to the described invention are assigned to the academic center. The assignment should be signed and dated by each listed inventor.

Invention Disclosure "Triage"

Once the basic information described above is received, the technology transfer manager is ready to begin the evaluation of the invention disclosure. This process is often referred to as a *triage*. Webster's New Collegiate Dictionary defines triage as: "The sorting and allocation of treatment to patients...according to a system of priorities designed to maximize the number of survivors."[3] The application of this definition to the evaluation of invention disclosures is well-founded, not in the sense of medical treatment, but certainly as a system of priorities used in the evaluation so as to increase the likelihood of building a successful portfolio of technologies to market and license. It is a thoughtful, stepwise, and thorough evaluation process. This requires dedicated time and often several conversations with inventors, office colleagues, and perhaps patent attorneys. The process should be applied similarly to all disclosures received so that each disclosure has an equal opportunity to enter the patent and licensing portfolio of technologies available for licensure by the academic technology transfer office.

Each invention disclosure received should be stamped with the date of submission and assigned a case number. The case numbering system is totally arbitrary but should be consistent throughout the life of the program. The case number will follow the invention disclosure and the invention throughout the process of evaluation, decision to retain ownership rights, and patent application. Next, details, including title, case number, inventors, date of submission, and other information to follow should be entered into a database of all invention disclosures in order to facilitate tracking of the time and events applied to the invention disclosure. This provides an excellent opportunity to make sure that all sections of the disclosure form are complete (especially regarding the dates requested) and to ensure that all the supporting documents are attached. If portions of the invention disclosure are incomplete, it is recommended that a phone call be placed to the inventor(s) to request the missing information or documentation.

In the academic setting, it is important to remember that one is generally working against the clock of a date of publication or other types of disclosures. Thus, the initial review for completeness of the invention disclosure form should occur within one to two days of receiving the disclosure.

An often overlooked piece of information is the listing of grant support. While most technology transfer managers are aware of the need to inform a governmental research granting agency of the submission of an invention disclosure, it is now becoming the norm with several private research funding agencies to request the same information. Private foundations that provide research grants to academic centers now request information on inventions resulting from research funded by these agencies. Having the information on grant funding, therefore, is critical to this responsibility and one should make sure that, if this section of the disclosure form is blank, the inventor is asked directly if a grant provided by any agency supported the research out of which came the described invention.

Description of the Invention

Following the initial cursory review for content, it is now time to delve into the invention itself. The written description of the invention, with all the supporting documents handy, is reviewed carefully. In the biological, chemical, or engineering sciences, these supporting documents usually consist of graphs, charts, tables, and drawings and are necessary to present a complete understanding of the invention. Recalling also that an invention consists of two parts—a conception and a reduction to practice—the reviewer should focus on identifying these two components. This may require reading and studying the written description and the supporting documents several times. However, as one gains experience in this field, one does become more proficient at identifying these two elements of an invention.

As one is moving through this process of review, it is inevitable that one contemplates the patenting process. In this, it is essential that the three basic requirements of a patentable invention—novelty, utility, and nonobviousness—be considered. A comparison of the described invention to the prior art documents that accompany the disclosure should provide the first clues on novelty. While often times it is not possible to initially determine novelty, as the technology manager matures to the task (which includes frequent conversations with patent attorneys), he or she becomes somewhat facile in assessing the novelty of an invention. The final deliberation usually rests with the experienced intellectual property attorney. However, as technology managers themselves become experienced in this process, they are able to address novelty with the attorney and, more importantly perhaps, with the inventor(s). If novelty is clearly not gleaned from the description of the invention, a conversation with the inventor(s) is most definitely in order.

Utility is somewhat more easily assessed. How an invention would be used is something an inventor should be asked to describe and should be readily visualized by the technology transfer professional. Again, as experience is gained, utility becomes easier to determine. It is also recommended that during some later meeting with the inventor(s), other uses of an invention be explored.

The discussion of utility would not be complete without addressing technology validation.

Technology Validation and the Demonstration of Utility

In the opinion of most, the validation of any technology is essential to satisfying the utility requirement. Validation is the very demonstration of utility. A mechanical or surgical device takes life when such a device is shown to perform the task for which it is designed. A biological target becomes real when studies demonstrate that manipulation of the target results in a desired effect. A new chemical entity likewise becomes a meaningful creation when it performs the contemplated chemical or pharmacological interaction. Technology validation not only demonstrates usefulness, it adds value to a technology and, in the eyes of a licensee, reduces the risk of accepting the technology. Therefore, academic technology transfer programs should strive to establish some means of technology validation not only to demonstrate the utility of an invention but also to enhance its licensing opportunities.

Patentability and Commercial Potential

An integral component of evaluating an invention disclosure is assessment of the patentability and commercial potential or marketability of the described invention. This is particularly critical in the academic research setting since these commercially oriented matters are not typically part of the culture. Thus, unlike the for-profit environment where an invention disclosure addresses a targeted market and usually includes some level of patent prior art, academic research-derived inventions are not always afforded this level of initial thought by the academic inventor. Furthermore, academic technology transfer offices usually do not have budgets that allow for anything less than a conservative approach to filing patent applications. Thus, it becomes the responsibility of the academic technology transfer manager to gather and assess as much patentability and marketability information as possible.

Approaching the patentability question is somewhat routine. The faculty inventor, as discussed above, should provide a fairly comprehensive review of the scientific literature and perhaps even some patent information. Although somewhat time consuming, a search of the USPTO Web site[4] using a few key words can provide the technology manager some initial impressions of the patent prior art. Some offices subscribe to search engines (e.g., NERAC® or Delphion®) that provide a more in-depth search. The safe route at this point is a discussion with the inventor and a patent attorney or agent that will result in the most efficient, yet economical approach to answer the question of whether an invention might be patentable. Regardless of the mechanism chosen to gather this information, it is important for academic technology transfer offices to engage in this process and to have the information at hand to help in the evaluation of a disclosure.

Addressing the question of commercial viability may be somewhat more difficult and intensive. Again, search engines (e.g., NERAC®), as well as Web sites for nonprofit agencies can be used. For example, some information on the market size for (or prevalence of) specific heart diseases can be gathered from the Web site of the American Heart Association.[5] This may require conversion of incidence or prevalence data into dollars and thus will often require the opinion or assistance of someone in the field. General online searches are also helpful. Ultimately, a licensee of the technology will conduct a much more in-depth search than can be performed by an academic licensing office. However, having such information beforehand will greatly assist in determining how to negotiate financial terms of a license. The more immediate question is, "Does this technology have enough commercial attraction for us to decide to move forward with the patent process?" Adding to the difficulty of market assessment is the fact that academic technology is most often at a very early stage. As such, it is in a very practical sense, several years from being a marketed product. Thus, the additional burden of projecting the market needs, competitive environment, and overall economic landscape several years out is a daunting task. The final answer may rest with information obtained from a professional market search firm. While this approach may seem expensive, especially for the beginning technology transfer program, the potential savings on patent expenses or the potential long-term financial return of a license may warrant the expense. Excellent coverage of the commercial evaluation of an invention disclosure is provided by Nelson.[6]

Meeting with the Inventor

As we continue through the "triage" of the invention disclosure, and if it has not already occurred, a face-to-face meeting with the inventor(s) is the next logical step in the process. In this discussion, the invention disclosure is reviewed with the inventor(s) with particular emphasis on some key points.

While a full written description of the invention is part of the disclosure, the inventor(s) should be asked to describe the invention and how it is envisaged to be a product if it is eventually patented and licensed. Often times a somewhat different perspective on the invention is gained and is usually helpful in understanding more fully the reported technology. It also allows for an opportunity to ask questions of clarification and detail about the invention. One of these questions should be, "At what stage toward product development do you see the technology now?" This may give the technology transfer manager an opportunity to ask about target validation, prototype development, or proof of concept testing.

The inventor(s) may also be asked to describe the uniqueness of the invention over current technologies and how it is seen as nonobvious from similar technologies already disclosed in either the scientific or patent literature. Recalling the three criteria for patentability defined as novelty, utility, and nonobviousness to one skilled in the art, this discussion may provide some guidance for the technology manager and the patent attorney in understanding and describing the uniqueness of the invention.

A more important discussion point that needs to be raised with the inventor(s) is the question of inventorship. Recall that only the true inventor(s), the one(s) who provided inventive concepts that later are created in a claim, should be named as the inventor(s). A person who merely follows directions, regardless of the volume of work performed, is not and should not be named as a co-inventor. A person whose inventive contribution is recited in at least one claim of a patent is a legal co-inventor.[7] As stated earlier, this can be one of the uncomfortable topics to discuss with academic inventors. Thus, the technology transfer professional should have a good grasp of the topic of inventorship and be prepared to explain the details of this issue. It is, however, important to remember that preserving the relationship with faculty is critical to the success of an academic technology transfer program. Likewise having patents on which inventorship cannot be challenged is also a critical success factor for the office. Therefore, it may be wise to bring a patent attorney into this discussion early in the disclosure review process.

One topic that academic inventors should be and usually are willing to discuss is publications, both their own and those belonging to others. Even though a technology manager may have copies of the inventor's publications relating to the invention, it is a wise practice to ask inventors to elaborate on recent publications, if for anything, just to get a better appreciation for what generated the concept for the invention. More importantly, what may be revealed during this discussion is a realization that previous publications by the inventor(s) disclose the invention or somehow would bar the allowance of a patent. If one senses that a disclosure of the invention has been made previously, then an assessment as to whether that disclosure is enabling, that is, describes how to make the invention, and should be initiated. The same holds true for the inventor's interpretation of publications of other scientists or professionals in the field. If this is suspected, a patent attorney should be brought into the process so that a professional opinion and perhaps a patenting decision can be rendered. It is important to stress that the technology man-

ager should have copies of all relevant publications, including abstracts, and of manuscripts either in press or in preparation. A rapidly approaching publication date will raise the priority of the disclosure review and may hasten the course of filing a patent application.

In continuation of the technical discussion, the inventor(s) should be asked where the current research is leading relative to the disclosed invention. Experiments or studies that support the invention, validate a target, prove a concept or principle, or otherwise enhance the novelty and/or utility of the invention may be ongoing or planned. Improvements are also a likely outcome of these studies and thus the technology manager should be aware and be kept informed of the progress of these studies.

At this point it is also useful to explore the inventor's ideas regarding the potential commercial aspects of the invention. To begin, the technology manager might ask the inventor to discuss his/her vision of how the technology will be used in the commercial setting or to simply ask, "How do you envision a product being made and sold using your invention?" This may be one of the questions on the actual invention disclosure form. While the objective is to keep the form as short and simple as possible, this is important information to gather. One must then assess the ease of filling out the form, while not sacrificing helpful information. This is why a meeting with inventors is essential to the overall process of disclosure evaluation.

Other commercial questions should address the inventor's thoughts on the market for such a product, whether there is such a product available currently, what the competitive landscape is, where they see this market going in the future, and whether they have any leads on companies working in or have a franchise in the area of the technology. This last point may be somewhat easy for the inventor to comment on since many company scientists are publishing regularly in broadly distributed scientific and technical journals.

This section has stressed the importance of meeting with the inventor(s) in the evaluation of the invention disclosure. Such a meeting provides the technology transfer manager a greater understanding of the inventor's thoughts on the commercial potential of the technology and affords the technology manager a first-hand opportunity to clarify and confirm statements contained in the disclosure form. In this respect, taking notes during the meeting and preparating a summary immediately following the meeting are critical elements of the total evaluation package. As the technology transfer professional becomes more experienced in extracting verbal information from academic inventors, the process becomes easier and more meaningful for both parties. The opportunity to build a relationship with a faculty member during this process is of the utmost importance. Faculty, in turn, can appreciate this meeting as a vehicle for learning more about the technology transfer process and about the people and workings of the technology transfer office, in general. The establishment of mutual trust and understanding between faculty and the technology transfer office are a desired intangible outcome of this meeting; and, in the academic environment, word of such a positive reputation will spread rapidly throughout the ranks of the faculty. This relationship is important later in the patenting and licensing processes and it is important that the relationship be cultivated and nourished from the very outset.

The Decision to Patent

At this point in the invention disclosure "triage," the key pieces of information have been gathered: the technology transfer manager now has the needed information on the "patentability" and prior art relevant to the invention and on the market and commercial applicability of the technology; the manager has the answers to key questions from the invention disclosure form and has verbal descriptions of the invention along with a vision from the inventor as to how the invention could be utilized as or within a commercial product. At this point, too, the technology transfer official has likely had at least one conversation with a patent attorney or patent agent about the invention. Critical questions focusing on novelty, utility, nonobviousness, and inventorship have been addressed and satisfactorily answered. Having these elements in place, the technology transfer manager can now address the question of whether or not to move forward with the filing of a patent application.

In most, if not all cases, encouraging reports of patentability and marketability and all of the accompanying information on the technical and commercial aspects of the invention should direct the technology manager to proceed with a patent application. In the academic setting, a "yes" to the question of whether or not to file brings into play other important questions on the type and timing of the application. With a pressing publication or other public disclosure date looming (not uncommon in this environment), the provisional applica-

tion process may be the wise choice. However, caution is advised as to the content and elements of this type of application, as well as to the one-year requirement for nonprovisional filing. These points are covered in greater detail in other chapters of this book. A more critical look at the decision not to file a patent application is warranted here.

The Decision Not to Patent

The question is often asked, "What percent of academic invention disclosures result in a patent application?" The answer to this question is somewhat variable but, on average, about 30% to 35% of academic invention disclosures lead to the filing of a patent application (according to this author's survey). There are several reasons why only about one third of submitted disclosures result in patent applications, the most important being mission and budget. The mission of academic research is not the achievement of an invention but the discovery and dissemination of new knowledge. And, in the opinion of most persons in this field, creation of new inventions should not be the objective of academic research. Inventions, innovations, and commercial discoveries, however, are a natural outcome or "fallout" of academic research. Any other approach would seriously compromise the academic culture. Likewise, filing, prosecuting, and maintaining patents is expensive and often a budgetary challenge. Thus, academic technology transfer offices are selective as to what technologies are taken forward to the patenting process. As stated above, only those inventions that are supported by positive patent and research prior art and market data should be considered for patenting.

How does the technology transfer manager handle the majority (about two thirds) of technologies reported in invention disclosures in academic research centers? The answer to this question is dependent upon the results obtained from patent and market searches. If market data is not supportive of a commercial opportunity and patentability is questionable or barred altogether, the property rights to these inventions should be assigned back to the inventor(s) with an appropriate explanation, including the results of the respective searches. Likewise, if patentability is achievable but the market is unfavorable, these disclosures are generally not worth the expense of taking forward to patenting since the risk (i.e., the expense) is not commensurate with the potential return.

Often, what one finds in an invention disclosure is that there is no invention. For example, in the biomedical sciences, academic invention disclosures often define a novel therapeutic target. This usually takes the form of a new receptor, a novel intermediate in a regulatory pathway, or perhaps a newly identified gene or series of genes. Many of these targets are reported to be involved in the etiology of diseases. The rapid technological advances of molecular genetics, namely the ability to create "knockout" mice has brought many of these concepts forward. However, what is often lacking is evidence of functional involvement of these new targets in a disease state and, more importantly, that the inhibition of such a target (e.g., receptor or pathway intermediary) defines a new therapy. This is often referred to as *proof of concept* or *proof of principle*. Academic research, by definition, is geared toward cutting-edge discovery, while proof of concept is often thought of as a development step that should be the focus of a commercial enterprise. In most situations where proof of concept or proof of principle is not demonstrated, patentability is questionable, and it is recommended that these disclosures be returned to the inventor(s) with an explanation that further proof of invention, with supportive data, needs to be provided.

Often times, an invention disclosure will describe an unpatentable technology or a technology with a very narrow claim profile, but one for which market data suggests a potential return. These inventions often become licensable as research tools. For example, in the biomedical arena, certain areas (e.g., monoclonal antibodies, genetically-engineered mice, specific cell lines, genetic constructs, and other such inventions) have value in the research laboratory or perhaps within the drug discovery sector. Research tools can provide a company with a much needed shortcut to discovering or screening new drugs. Licensing of research tools licensing is a widely practiced form of technology licensing in the academic technology transfer field. While not the much sought-after home run, a tools license can provide a steady income stream to the technology transfer program and is well accepted by industry.

Conclusion

This chapter focuses on the evaluation or "triage" of the academic invention disclosure for the purpose of obtaining licensable technologies. As with all evaluative processes, having accurate, timely, and complete information about the invention and information about its potential use and commercial market is essential. Some suggestions relative to timing and other considerations regarding the decision to file a patent application are also provided. More importantly, selecting the right options on those inventions on which the decision is made not to file may be critical to the success of the academic technology transfer program and to future academic relationships as well.

It is stressed that the suggestions provided in this chapter are those of the author and that there are undoubtedly other ways of "triaging" the disclosure and managing others that are not taken forward to the patenting process. The belief that the invention disclosure is indeed the cornerstone of the academic technology transfer process is universally understood. Without it, there are no technologies to transfer—in short, there is no need for an office or a program. Thoughtful and thorough attention to information gathering, support of faculty relationships, and the evaluation of invention disclosures will lead to growth of a successful academic licensing program and also to a fulfilling career for the technology transfer professional.

• • • References

1. Hoffman, D.C. "Invention Disclosure," in *Technology Transfer Practice Manual*. 2nd ed. Edited by Marjorie Forster. Washington, DC: Association of University Technology Managers, 2001.

2. Crowell, M.C. "Documentation of Inventions," in *Technology Transfer Practice Manual*. 2nd ed. Edited by Marjorie Forster. Washington, DC: Association of University Technology Managers, 2001.

3. Merriam-Webster online dictionary, 2005, http://www.merriam-webster.com (accessed June 10, 2005).

4. United States Patent and Trademark Office Web site, http://www.USPTO.gov (accessed June 10, 2005).

5. American Heart Association Web site, http://www.americanheart.org (accessed June 10, 2005).

6. Nelson, L. "Evaluation of Inventions," in *Technology Transfer Practice Manual*, 2nd ed. Edited by Marjorie Forster. Washington, DC: Association of Univesity Technology Managers, 2002.

7. Pressman, D. *Patent It Yourself*. Berkeley, CA: Nolo Press, 1999, 3.

63-A

Confidential

INVENTION, TECHNOLOGY, AND DISCOVERY DISCLOSURE

It is the responsibility of the (academic center) to facilitate the application of the results of research to the benefit of society in partnership with other organizations, both for-profit and nonprofit. This Invention and Technology Disclosure is designed to record an invention and related circumstances and to serve as the basis for an evaluation by the (academic center) and the Office of Technology Transfer of its protectability and potential for commercial application.

Thus, this disclosure form should be filled out as accurately and with as much attention to detail as possible. Do not hesitate to contact the Office of Technology Transfer at (phone number) if you need assistance or have questions.

As defined by Title 35 of the United States Code, a patentable invention may be any process, machine, or material that is new and useful and may result when research yields unusual or unexpected results. To be patentable, an invention should not be obvious to others in the field, not be used by others previously, and not be described in a publication or other public disclosure.

This form is available on paper or electronically through the (academic center) intranet site. Please return the completed form to the **Office of Technology Transfer, (address), (fax number).**

For your reference, an updated copy of the (academic center) Intellectual Property Policy on Inventions is available.

1. **Title:** Please provide a brief title that is descriptive of the invention and its potential application.

_____

_____

_____

_____

_____

_____

_____

_____

_____

_____

2. Inventor(s): Include the names, addresses, and affiliations of all likely inventors. An inventor is an individual who has conceived an essential part of the invention, either independently or jointly. Please note if any named individual has an appointment at an institution other than (academic center). Also, please designate one of the Inventors as the primary contact for the Office of Technology Transfer.

If more space is needed, photocopy this page, attach, and check here [ ]

Inventor who will serve as primary contact regarding the disclosure:

_____

| Name 1 | Institution(s) | Department | Email | Extension/Fax |

Describe the contribution made by individual 1:

_____

_____

_____

Additional Inventors:

_____

| Name 2 | Institution(s) | Department | Email | Extension/Fax |

Describe the contribution made by individual 2:

_____

_____

_____

_____

_____

_____

_____

| Name 3 | Institution(s) | Department | Email | Extension/Fax |

Describe the contribution made by individual 3:

_____

_____

_____

_____

3. **Sponsors:** Please give the name of the organization and grant numbers that provided any funding for yourself and/or other Inventors that led to the invention (at other institutions if applicable).

_____   _____

Organization   Grant No.   P.I.   Organization   Grant No.   P.I.

Was any of the funding from another institution? If so, name:

_____

Were biological materials from another institution used? If so, what materials and from where:

_____

4. **Assignment Statement and Signatures:** <u>All</u> inventors **MUST** read and sign this section.

I/We agree to assign all right, title, and interest to this invention and any subsequent patent applications to (academic center) in accordance with the terms of my appointment and/or employment at the (academic center) and with its policies:

Inventor Signature/Date: _____

Inventor Signature/Date: _____

Inventor Signature/Date: _____

5. **Description:** Please describe what the invention is and what it does, e.g., its general purpose, technical details, advantages or improvements over existing methods or materials, patents or publications by others that may be similar. You may attach or insert an abstract from a manuscript, presentation, manuscript, or abstract for publication, or grant application. Also, attach any supporting materials, for example, drawings, tables, and figures.

If additional materials are attached, check here [ ].

_____

_____

_____

_____

_____

_____

_____

Please identify several key words that may be used to describe your invention. This will assist in the patent availability search.

_____

_____

_____

_____

What or who is a source of information on existing technology (e.g., reference books, colleagues, contacts within companies) to help us evaluate the advantages of your invention?

_____

_____

6. **Commercial Interest:** Has anyone from a company expressed an interest in the invention or research related to the invention, or do you know of a company that may be interested in the invention or the research related to the invention? Please give the names (if possible) of individuals or companies who have been or may be interested.

_____

_____

_____

7. **Conception and Disclosure to Others:** Accurate dates are important and may affect the likelihood of obtaining a patent. When was the invention conceived? Has or will the invention be described (disclosed) outside the (academic center) (e.g., in a poster session, publication, thesis, or grant application) or was any material associated with it transferred to others outside the (academic center)?

_____

Date of Conception. Is this date documented? _____ Yes _____ No. If so, where?

_____

Date and name of first publication containing sufficient description to enable someone to make or use the invention. Attach publication and check here: [ ].

_____

Date and location of first public oral disclosure containing a sufficiently enabling description. Abstract attached: [ ].

_____

If undisclosed as of now, please provide the date of the anticipated publication or oral disclosure and the name of the periodical or conference to which the description was or will be submitted. Publication or abstract attached: [ ].

Patent Law

Steve Highlander, PhD, JD

Introduction to Patents

A United States patent is an official document issued by the United States Patent and Trademark Office (USPTO), a division of the Department of Commerce. It defines, in technical and legal terms, the intellectual property claimed by the patent owner. The legal terms or claims describe the metes and bounds of the invention. The remaining portion of the patent is used to provide support for the claims, such as defining terms, equivalent alternatives, and methodology by which the invention may be made and used.

A patent is, in effect, the grant of a property right to the inventor. The term of a patent is twenty years from the date the patent application was first filed in the United States or from the filing date of an earlier related application, subject to the payment of maintenance fees after the patent issues. A United States patent grant is effective only within the United States, United States territories, and United States possessions.

A patent conveys "the right to exclude others from making, using, offering for sale, or selling" the invention in the United States or importing the invention into the United States. However, it does not give any affirmative right to the inventor to practice his or her own invention. Some refer to a patent as a "monopoly," limited by time and geography, but it really is more like an ownership right in a piece of land—one may keep others off owned property, but the land owner may nonetheless be limited in how he or she can exploit the land.[1]

Utility Patents

Patent law (set forth in Title 35 of the US Code) specifies the general field of subject matter that can be patented and the conditions under which a patent may be obtained. There are, in fact, three different kinds of patents: utility, design, and plant. The most familiar is the utility patent, which is named for the requirement that the subject matter claimed must be useful.[2] The term "useful" in this context refers to the requirement that the subject matter have a useful purpose and also is operable; that is, an invention that is inoperable to perform its intended purpose would not be useful, and therefore could not be the subject of a patent grant.

For an invention to be patentable, it must also survive an evaluation of statutory requirements known as novelty and nonobviousness (requirements that give rise to prior art rejections).[3] Novelty is defined literally in this context as the invention must be "new." This simply means that no one may have previously practiced a method or made a machine, manufacture, or composition that falls within the scope of the patent claims. Nonobviousness is a more daunting hurdle. Even if an invention is novel, it may nonetheless be unpatentable if the advance is trivial (more on this concept latter). These statutes, along with the one setting forth the utility requirement, are further discussed in greater detail.

Once an inventor has established the right to patent protection, he or she becomes a patentee and may file suit against those who infringe the claims of the issued patent. Remedies in a legal action under a patent include: (a) injunctions, where the

[1]See the United States Patent and Trademark Web site at http://www.uspto.gov/web/offices/pac/doc/general/whatis.htm.

[2]See 35 USC §101.
[3]See 35 USC §102 and §103.

infringer is instructed by the court to cease and desist the infringing activity; and (b) damages, which are often measured by reasonable royalty, though other factors, such as lost profits, can come into play. Damages are by far the more frequent outcome in a successful infringement action. Treble damages are available in a case of willful infringement, which means that the infringer knew of the patent and did not have a good faith belief of either noninfringement or invalidity of the patent. A potential infringer will often seek an opinion of counsel that establishes the basis for noninfringement, invalidity, or both, thereby avoiding trebling of damages.

Design Patents

As mentioned previously, there are three different kinds of patents governed by Title 35 of the US Code (USC). So far, we have discussed utility patents. Design patents, not surprisingly, cover designs. While the designs may be part of a useful thing, the design itself cannot be utilitarian. The design patent protects only the appearance of an article, but not its structural or functional features. (Examples include water fountain patterns, silverware patterns, car bumpers, shoes, etc.)

The general process relating to granting of design patents is the same as that relating to utility patents, including the requirements of novelty and nonobviousness, with a few minor differences. The major differences are that the specification of a design application is usually short and ordinarily follows a set form. Only one claim is permitted, and it often simply refers to a drawing in the patent (e.g. piece of silverware having the specific design). Also, the term of a design patent is 14 years, but no maintenance fees are required.

Plant Patents

A third patent type is the plant patent.[4] Plant patents cover only plants propagated by nonsexual means.[5] Thus, the law provides specifically for the granting of a patent to anyone who has invented or discovered any distinct and new variety of asexually reproduced plant, including cultivated sports, mutants, hybrids, and newly found seedlings, other than a tuber-propagated plant or a plant found in

an uncultivated state. Asexually propagated plants are those that are reproduced by means other than from seeds, such as by the rooting of cuttings, by layering, budding, grafting, inarching, and such. Again, the process for obtaining a plant patent is generally the same as for a utility patent. The primary difference is the heavy reliance of drawings, which are often in color. The term of a plant patent is 20 years from filing or the earliest claimed priority.

The specification of a plant patent should include a complete detailed description of the plant and the characteristics that distinguish the same over related known varieties, and its antecedents, expressed in botanical terms. The description should be in the form followed by standard botanical textbooks or publications, rather than a broad nonbotanical characterization commonly found in nursery or seed catalogs. The specification should also include the origin or parentage of the plant variety sought to be patented and must particularly point out where and in what manner the variety of plant has been asexually reproduced. Where color is a distinctive feature of the plant, the color should be positively identified in the specification by reference to a designated color as given by a recognized color dictionary. Where the plant variety was originated as a newly found seedling, the specification must fully describe the conditions (cultivation, environment, etc.) under which the seedling was found growing to establish that it was not found in an uncultivated state.

Because of the criticality of plant patent drawings, they should be artistically and competently executed. The drawings must disclose all the distinctive characteristics of the plant capable of visual representation. When color is a distinguishing characteristic of the new variety, the drawing must be in color. Two duplicate copies of color drawings must be submitted. Specimens (the plant, its flower or fruit) need not be submitted unless called for by the examiner.

---

[4]See 35 USC §161.

[5]In contrast, the Plant Variety Protection Act (PVPA), provides for a system of protection for sexually reproduced varieties, under the administration of a Plant Variety Protection Office within the Department of Agriculture. See Public Law 91577, approved December 24, 1970. Requests for information should be addressed to Commissioner, Plant Variety Protection Office, Agricultural Marketing Service, National Agricultural Library Bldg., Room 0, 10301 Baltimore Blvd., Beltsville, MD 20705-2351.

Defining an Invention

Each invention has two parts: a conception and a reduction to practice. These terms are key to understanding a number of different areas of patent law.

Conception is the formation in the mind of the inventor of a complete and permanent idea of the invention in the form in which it will ultimately be practiced. The critical point to understanding conception is that the invention need not actually have been made: no method need be practiced, no article need be produced, and no composition need be obtained. However, in order for the conception to be considered complete, only routine skill must be required to actually practice the invention. In addition, one must be able to describe the invention with sufficient detail such that it can be distinguished from the prior art.

Reduction to practice, on the other hand, is the actual making of a machine, the obtaining or synthesis of a composition of matter, or the performance of a process. This is what is called an *actual* reduction to practice. Filing of a patent also constitutes reduction to practice, although this form is termed *constructive* reduction to practice.

Some inventions cannot be conceived until they are reduced to practice. These inventions are subject to the doctrine of "simultaneous conception and reduction to practice." An example of such inventions is DNA sequences. The Federal Circuit, the USPTO's reviewing court, has held that one cannot have a legal conception of a DNA molecule until the sequence is known. However, to obtain the sequence, the DNA must be isolated, and thus reduced to practice.

Patentability Under 35 USC §101

The patent statutes define what subject matter can be patented. According to the law, any person who "invents or discovers any new and useful process, machine, manufacture, or composition of matter, or any new and useful improvement thereof, may obtain a patent,"[6] subject to the conditions and requirements of the law. The following describes the patentable categories:

- Process: A process, act, or method.
- Machine: A mechanical device that serves to create other types of articles or accomplish a given task.
- Manufacture: Articles that are made either by humans or machines.

- Composition of Matter: Chemical compositions including mixtures of known ingredients (such as multivitamins), as well as wholly new chemical compounds (such as Prozac) and purified forms of natural compounds (such as Taxol).

Courts have interpreted these four categories to mean that just about anything under the sun made by man is patentable. However, this case law has set some limits on patentable subject matter. For example, under these decisions, it has been held that printed matter, laws of nature, physical phenomena, pure algorithms, products of nature (in unmodified forms), and abstract ideas are not patentable. Similarly, patents will not be issued on inventions that are contrary to public policy.[7] It also should be noted that a patent cannot be obtained upon a mere "idea" or "suggestion." Rather, the patent is granted for invention of a new process, machine, manufacture, or composition of matter. Thus, a reasonably complete description of the subject matter for which a patent is sought is required.

In addition to falling within one of the statutory criteria above, the invention must also achieve at least one useful objective or goal. The invention need not achieve all objectives stated in the specification, but must achieve at least one objective, normally one that is stated in the patent application as filed. This requirement is generally an easy one to satisfy as "[t]o violate [the requirement for utility] the claimed device must be totally incapable of achieving a useful result. . . ."[8] One of the seminal cases on utility dealt with the "one-armed bandit"— the slot machine. There, the US Supreme Court held that entertainment of the player (and presumably monetary gain for the owner) was a useful undertaking sufficient to satisfy the utility requirement. Thus, in general, the utility requirement is not difficult to satisfy, especially in established arts. It can, however, present significant issues in emerging technologies.

---

[6]35 USC §101.

[7]The Atomic Energy Act of 1954 prohibits the patenting of inventions that are used solely in atomic energy or atomic weapons.

[8]*Brooktree Corp. v. Advanced Micro Devices Inc.*, 977 F.2d 1555, 1571 (Fed. Cir. 1992).

Prior Art Rejections

As indicated above, in order for an invention to be patentable, it must be novel and nonobvious. These determinations are made by comparing the claimed invention to the existing body of knowledge at the time of invention: the *prior art*. Put another way, prior art is the collective sum of existing technologic information against which an invention is judged to determine if it is patentable. The statute that defines what is and is not prior art is 35 USC 102. This statute has seven subsections, each defining a different type of prior art. If a particular prior disclosure qualifies as prior art under one of these seven subsections, then it is available as prior art. If the prior art contains each limitation of a patent claim, then that claim is said to lack novelty over, or be anticipated by, that prior art. However, even a trivial difference between the cited art and the claimed invention will preclude a rejection for lack of novelty.

35 USC §102(a)

The first subsection of §102, §102(a), identifies that which "was known or used by others in this country, or patented or described in a printed publication in this or a foreign country, before the invention thereof by the applicant for patent" as prior art. The key aspects of this statute are the types of disclosure (knowledge, use, patented, or published), source of the disclosure (by others) and the relevant time frame (before the invention). Thus, even if a particular disclosure by another occurred prior to a patent's filing date, and thus is *prima facie* prior art under §102(a), the inventor can still establish patentability over that reference by showing invention prior to the effective date of the reference. This is accomplished by filing an affidavit, filed under 37 C.F.R. 1.131, "swearing behind" the date of the disclosure. However, there is a critical limitation on the swearing behind approach—the one-year bar of 102(b) (discussed below).

So, if A is the inventor on a patent application filed on January 1, 2001, the disclosure of the same subject matter on July 1, 2000 would not be prior art against the application as this disclosure was not "by another." In contrast, the disclosure by B on October 1, 2000 of the claimed subject *would* be prior art. However, we know that A had possession of the invention on at least July 1, 2000. That is earlier than B's disclosure, and thus A can "swear behind" B's disclosure, effectively removing it as prior art.

35 USC §102(b)

The second subsection of §102, §102(b), defines a disclosure that is not removable as prior art, the so-called "statutory bar." The content of a reference qualifies as §102(b) art if it was "patented or described in a printed publication in this or a foreign country or in public use or on sale in this country more than one year prior to the application for patent in the United States." Also, the relevant time frame is measured by the patent application's filing date, thus emphasizing why early filing is desirable. Notably, this subsection is not limited to the actions of others, and thus can include the disclosures of the inventor. This part of the statute, taken with §102(a), is said to define a one-year "grace period" in which the inventor can still file for a patent after he or she makes a disclosure. In other words, if a disclosure by the inventor is less than one year prior to filing, it does not qualify as art under 102(a) ("by another"), but if it is more than one year prior to filing, it becomes §102(b) art.

For example, if A filed a patent application on July 1, 2001, a disclosure on July 1st or later of 2000 would not constitute a "statutory bar" under §102(b) (although it might be relevant under §102(a) if made by "another"). However, a disclosure on June 30, 2000 or earlier would be prior art regardless of when A made his or her invention, and regardless of who made the disclosure.

35 USC §102(c)

Section 102(c) addresses "abandonment" of invention. This statute, along with §102(d), is one of the more rarely invoked statutes, and when it is invoked, it is by infringers in the context of litigation, not by examiners. The standards for establishing that an inventor has abandoned his or her invention are fairly stringent—clearly even long periods of delay are not enough. Rather, there must be some affirmative evidence that the inventor had intended to dedicate the invention to the public. This may take the shape of such acts as destroying materials, data, prototypes, or it may take the form of verbal or written indication that the inventor had dismissed the value or promise of the invention.

35 USC §102(d)

Like §102(c), §102(d) is rarely invoked. The basis of the statute is activity by the applicant in foreign patent offices prior to activity in the United States. Thus, if an invention was first patented (or was the subject of an inventor's certificate) in a foreign country prior to the date of application for a patent in this country, and the application for the patent or inventor's certificate was filed more than twelve months before the filing of the application in the United States, the activity is a bar.

35 USC §102(e)

A significant amount of prior art is established through the publication of patents and patent applications. As we have seen previously in the discussion of §102(a) and (b), patents or application may constitute a public description of an invention. However, patents, and more recently patent applications, can constitute a far more dangerous kind of prior art, sometimes referred to "secret prior art." The "secret" aspect arises from the fact that some art may be given an effective publication date prior to it actually becoming publicly known. Section 102(e) art is just that type.

Section 102(e) states as follows:

> A person shall be entitled to a patent unless ...
> (e) the invention was described in a patent granted on an application for patent by another filed in the United States before the invention thereof by the applicant for patent, or on an international application by another who has fulfilled the requirements of paragraphs (1), (2), and (4) of section 371(c) of this title before the invention thereof by the applicant for patent. . . .

What this means is that when a patent issues or a patent application becomes published, the relevant date for determining whether it is prior art to the invention is not the patent or application's publication date but, rather, the date upon which the application was filed. Thus, since the art was unknown to anyone but the inventors, the assignee, and the attorneys filing the application, it was effectively secret to the general public.

This is a very dangerous type of art that cannot be accurately assessed at the time the application is filed. This is true since most patents do not issue for 1.5 to 2.5 years from filing, and all countries that publish applications do so 18 months after the earliest claimed priority date. There is some good news about §102(e) art. First, one can swear behind this kind of art so long as it does not *claim* the same subject matter as the application. Second, if the §102(e) art was commonly owned at the time of filing, it is excluded as prior art.

So, assume A filed a patent application on January 1, 2001. A thorough prior art search made at the time revealed no significant prior art. On September 1, 2001, a patent to B issued that was based on an application filed on June 1, 2000. The patent, when issued, becomes prior art against A's application. If B's patent only discloses but does not claim what A's application claims, and A can show an invention date prior to June 1, 2000, swearing behind is an option. However, if B also claims the same invention, the only option is to invoke an interference (see §102(g), below). [Note: The same result arises if B did not yet obtain a patent but, instead, had the patent publish December 1, 2001, eighteen months after filing. This applies to the publication of US applications filed after November 29, 2000.]

35 USC §102(f)

Another form of prior art is that communicated from one individual to another in such a way that it cannot be said to be "published," i.e., private communications. If the information communicated is sufficiently detailed to constitute a conception of an invention (more on this later), the person receiving this information cannot obtain a patent independent of the person giving the information. If one attempts to take a complete conception and obtain a patent on the relevant subject matter, that person is said to have derived the invention from another. This is not permitted under the statutes.

Presume A and B are colleagues who once worked together at company X. At a trade convention, the two have dinner, during which A tells B about a new idea A has for converting donuts into rocket fuel. The series of chemical reactions are all defined by A and communicated to B. Intrigued, B returns home and tests A's method. Much to B's delight, the method works. He then applies for a patent naming only himself as an inventor. Under 102(f), B is barred from the patent as he derived the invention from A. [Note: If B had named A as a "joint" inventor, he might have been able to secure a patent for both A & B, if A's conception was not "complete," thereby necessitating B's inventive contribution.]

35 USC §102(g)

The last form of secret prior art arises under §102(g). As stated in the statute:

> A person shall be entitled to a patent unless ...
> (g) before the applicant's invention thereof the invention was made in this country by another who had not abandoned, suppressed, or concealed it. In determining priority of invention there shall be considered not only the respective dates of conception and reduction to practice of

the invention, but also the reasonable diligence of one who was first to conceive and last to reduce to practice, from a time prior to conception by the other. . . .

What happens when two people have filed patent applications claiming the same subject matter? In that case, the USPTO will declare the two applications (or one patent and one application) to be "interfering," and an interference proceeding is initiated. In the interference, the USPTO will determine which party was the first to invent. A discussion of the proceeding, including how the determination of priority is made, follows later.

Nonobviousness

Nonobviousness is one of the more fuzzy concepts of US patent law. Put as simply as possible, the issue of nonobviousness may be framed as whether the differences between the invention and the most closely related work that took place prior to the invention in question are trivial. There are many facets to nonobviousness, and even those inventions that at first blush appear obvious may still be patentable.

While nonobviousness ultimately is considered a question of law, one must first ascertain the following facts:

- The most relevant prior art.
- The differences between the prior art and the claims at issue.
- The scope and content of the prior art.
- The level of ordinary skill in the art.

As stated previously, the *prior art* is the existing body of technological information against which an invention is judged. Thus, one must first establish if a given piece of art is, in fact, prior art as defined by one of the §102 categories. Once one or more references are determined to be valid prior art, one must then ascertain exactly what is disclosed and how it relates to the claimed invention. Finally, what skill is ordinary depends on the field in question. In some cases, it may be the average consumer (low skill), while in others, a doctoral degree followed by some additional expertise may be required (high skill). Making each of these factual inquiries is a prerequisite to undertaking an obviousness analysis.

Once the underlying facts have been obtained, one asks the following questions, from the perspective of those with ordinary skill in the art:

- Is there a teaching of each claimed element in the prior art?
- Does the art itself provide sufficient motivation to modify the prior art device, composition, or method so as to arrive at the claimed invention?
- Is there a likelihood of success in making and using the claimed invention?

If the examiner believes the answer to each of these questions is "yes," then a rejection will be made. Applicants can attempt to defeat the rejection by arguing that it is improper for one or more reasons. This is done by attacking the factual bases of the rejection or the legal conclusions drawn therefrom. For example, one may argue that the prior art lacks one or more of the claimed elements. Alternatively, one may argue that there is a lack of motivation in the cited art to make the necessary modification(s), or that even if there is such motivation, the outcome of making such changes is uncertain. If any of these arguments are successful, the rejection should be withdrawn.

In examining the propriety of a rejection, one must be wary of the examiner asserting a lesser standard for a finding of obviousness, such as obvious to try, flash of genius or lack of synergism in combining known elements. None of these standards is proper, yet some examiners have a tendency to fall back on such arguments despite a clear instruction in the case law to the contrary. In addition, examiners tend to perform an impermissible hindsight reconstruction of the invention (i.e., using the applicant's disclosure as a road map with which to connect otherwise unrelated prior art).

It also is important to note that the burden is initially on the examiner to demonstrate each of the specified elements. If each of these elements is demonstrated, then the invention is said to be "*prima facie* obvious" over the cited art. At this point, the burden shifts to the applicant to rebut the examiner's position. However, even if the examiner has made out a valid *prima facie* case, all is not lost. In some cases, objective evidence of nonobviousness, also known as secondary considerations, may save the invention. Such secondary indicia include:

- Long-felt need: The field has recognized the need for an improvement like that offered by the invention but has yet to achieve it.
- Commercial success: The public has found value in the invention (must show a nexus with the invention and not an unrelated phenomenon like strong marketing), demonstrated by sales of the product or licensing.

- Failure by others: The art has attempted to make an improvement like that now claimed and failed.
- Copying: Others find value in practicing the invention.
- Initial disbelief by experts: Indicates that, at the time of invention, there is doubt as to the ability to achieve the invention, undercutting predictability.
- Acclaim by experts: Another indicator of value.
- Unexpected advantages or surprising results: The invention is actually better than could have been predicted, extending the value beyond what might have been obvious.
- Difficulty in achieving: Perhaps the results were not as simple as they initially seemed.

The idea behind these secondary indicia is that despite the facial appearance of obviousness, the facts argue that the invention is nonetheless worthy of patenting.

A key to rebutting an obviousness rejection, be it in the form of a valid *prima facie* case or not, is a *factual* showing. Examiners are, as a practical matter, limited in the kind of evidence they may rely on. Applicants, on the other hand, may have ready access to other kinds of information, such as unpublished data and the opinions of experts. When this sort of evidence is available, it puts the examiner in a difficult position if the rejection is to be maintained. Of course, the evidence must be relevant and support the applicant's position. But where such evidence is provided, examiners are much less likely to maintain a rejection than if facing argument alone.

In sum, obviousness is a difficult thing to define with any particularity, both due to the subjective nature of the analysis and to the fact that there are varying standards depending on the complexity of the field. It is sufficient to say that obviousness rejections are probably the most common of all rejections made, with each one presenting important factual nuances that make predicting the best approach for response (and the eventual outcome) with absolute certainty all but impossible.

Enablement, Written Description, and Definiteness (§112)

The narrative portion of a patent application, which includes descriptions of the purpose, structure and operation of the invention, is called the specification. It also may include a description of the prior art, figures, and a brief description thereof, and must include an abstract and sum-

mary of the invention. The legal requirements of the specification are set forth in 35 USC §112, first paragraph, which states that the specification must contain a written description of the invention in such full, clear, concise, and exact terms as to enable any person skilled in that art, or with which it is most nearly connected, to make and use the invention. This means that the specification must provide enough information that a person of ordinary skill would understand what the inventor has invented and how one goes about exploiting that invention. The second paragraph of §112 sets out the requirement that the invention be defined by one or more claims that describe the invention with sufficient clarity that one of skill in the art can determine the metes and bounds of the invention. In other words, the claims must sufficiently notify the relevant public of what the applicant considers the invention to encompass.

While enablement and written description are technically requirements of the patent specification, they also give rise to rejections of the claims as allegedly being based upon an insufficient specification. This is why one often sees voluminous applications for inventions in new or rapidly developing fields. In the more established arts, it is more likely that enablement will be provided by the general knowledge of those skilled in the art, and thus need not be repeated in the specification. Nonetheless, patent attorneys and agents tend to err on the side over-inclusion. Too much information is rarely a problem, although it certainly can add to the cost of the application. As with anything, however, there is a point of diminishing returns, and finding the balance between description and cost only comes with experience.

Enablement

Enablement is a far-ranging requirement that takes many different forms during prosecution. At its most fundamental, enablement challenges will arise when the specification simply fails to provide key information for practicing the invention. Generally, a good patent attorney or agent will be able to predict what the critical issues are and avoid them by including the necessary information.

Another version of the enablement rejection is the scope rejection. This is a way of saying that while some aspects of the invention are enabled, the breadth of the claims is such that they encompass far more than the specification supports. Sometimes this rejection can be dealt with quite easily by amending the claims to be commensurate in scope with what the examiner considers to be enabled. However, where the examiner identifies a scope that applicants have not anticipated, there may be no support in the application for the claim that would be of the right scope. In this case, the applicant may be forced to adopt a much narrower claim for which there is support, or possibly to cancel the claim altogether.

Perhaps the most difficult kind of enablement rejection is one based on a perceived lack of operability. While this could also be cast as a utility rejection (see above), examiners have found it much easier to defend this position as a matter of enablement given the historically high threshold for showing lack of utility. For example, in the case of human therapies, examiners often argue that the absence of clinical data on human subjects, while not giving rise to utility concerns, leaves open a significant question as to whether one of ordinary skill could in fact practice the claimed therapy on a human subject.

There are two ways to address this kind of rejection. First, one can simply show that the invention is operable as described in the specification. For many applicants, this is simply not feasible due to costs and/or time constraints. Second, one may provide an expert affidavit in support of the specification. Such affidavits are best obtained from third parties (i.e., not the inventors) so that they cannot be attacked for bias. They also should not express a legal conclusion, such as that the application is enabling, but instead provide the factual basis upon which an attorney can formulate an argument in favor of enablement.

Written Description

Written description had, for decades, been of relatively limited value to the examining corps. The test for written description appeared to be quite simple, asking whether the application literally described the claim descriptions. Even in rare instances where the specification did not contain literal support for a claim, the specification itself could be amended to include such a description, so long as the claim was an original claim (i.e., it had not been added or amended during prosecution). Only rarely, in cases when the applicant's claims were so wildly exaggerated, would written description become a challengeable issue. For example, a chemical compound claim where the substituents were defined so broadly that they would encompass unheard of compounds of extremely diverse structure was rejected. Written description was also an issue when applicants attempted to claim subject matter

beyond that which was included in the original filing. This was often accompanied by a rejection under 35 USC §132, a so-called "new matter" rejection.

These circumstances changed, however, in the mid-1990s, when certain judges at the Federal Circuit Court sought to invigorate the written description requirement. The seminal case was *Regents of the Univ. of Calif. v. Eli Lilly Co.*[9] This case dealt with the University of California's patent on various forms of growth hormone and the DNAs that encode these proteins. The issue of written description developed from the fact that, at the time the application was filed, the inventors had only isolated the rat growth hormone gene. With this gene, they arguably provided a way to obtain the human gene, and hence arguably enabled this subject matter. On the basis of this presumption, they prosecuted claims to not only a rat growth hormone gene, but to human and mammalian growth hormone genes, as well.

In finding that these latter claims were invalid due to lack of an adequate written description, the Federal Circuit Court noted that with respect to the mammalian claim, this encompassed a genus of dozens of growth hormone genes that were not described in the application by a particular structure that would allow one of skill in the art to identify them as distinct members of the genus to which they belonged. In other words, a single species could not provide the basis for claiming a genus. With regard to the human gene claim, the Federal Circuit Court stated that an important function of the written description requirement was to prevent inventors from claiming that which they did not possess at the time of filing. Since they had not actually obtained the human gene at the time of filing, and thus could not describe it in the application in a way that distinguished it from, say, the rat gene, this claim too failed to find an adequate written description in the specification. While the first holding was of little surprise or controversy among the patent bar, the latter holding caused quite a stir. Since the *Eli Lilly* decision, a series of cases have issued on the written description requirement, several of which have expanded upon the possession test promulgated in that case.

It is not possible to provide evidence obtained after one's filing date to substantiate written description. It also is somewhat more difficult, though still possible, to address such rejections by

---

[9] 119 F.3d 1559 (Fed. Cir. 1997).

expert affidavits. Thus, the critical time for establishing written description is as of its filing. This makes the written description a particularly critical issue for many applicants whose claims cannot live up to these new more stringent standards. It also seems as if some examiners in particular arts have unique types of rejections based on written description. For example, in the plant biology area, examiners may object to the use of open-ended claim language that permits the inclusion of unspecified (though noncritical) elements.

Best Mode

The specification of a patent application must also set forth the best mode contemplated by the inventor at the time of filing the application. The unique US requirement of best mode stems from the basic notion of patent protection, where the inventor is given a limited period of exclusivity in return for full disclosure of the invention to the public. The notion is that when the term of the patent expires, the public will be on equal footing with the inventor. However, if the inventor keeps secret the best way of practicing the invention, the inventor still has advantage after the patent has expired. This is not formally permitted, as it avoids the essential *quid pro quo* of the patent system, but it is this requirement that explains why trade secrets and patent protection are normally incompatible with each other.

Definiteness

Generally considered to be one of the more straightforward requirements, rejections for lack of definiteness are rarely fatal. In many cases, they arise from errors of a very routine nature (misspellings, improper claim dependency, failure to provide proper antecedent basis). Thus, correcting these kinds of errors is quite easy. Occasionally, if a key term is not adequately defined in the specification, and it does not have an accepted definition in the field, significant problems may ensue.

Beginning the Patent Process

The first step in the patent process is to obtain a disclosure. If you are lucky, the inventor will be familiar with the patent process and provide all the information necessary to perform an evaluation of patentability and marketability. More likely, the inventor will have little or no idea of how to go about preparing a disclosure. Here is a list of information that is helpful to gather at the beginning the patent process:

- Name, mailing address, phone and fax number, and email address for all inventors.
- Brief synopsis of the novel features of the invention and its intended use.
- Listing of any funding source or relevant agreements (SRA, CDA, MTA, etc.).
- Listing of potential companies that might be interested in licensing.
- Listing of the most relevant prior art.
- Listing of the inventor's relevant publication record and future publication plans.
- Detailed description of the invention including experimental data (ideally a manuscript).
- Federal grant information.

The next step is often a prior art search. Some institutions conduct a search in house, at least in a preliminary form. If the invention makes it past this first stage, an outside attorney may be contacted. Searches usually rely on key words that define the key aspects of the invention. Clearly, this may be more or less difficult depending on the technology. Another type of search seeks to identify the publications of the inventor(s), which often constitute the most damaging prior art. Regardless, these searches are only about 80% successful in identifying the most relevant prior disclosures. The alternative is to hire a professional search firm to conduct a prior art analysis. These firms tend to focus more on prior patents and, for certain types of inventions, this may be the most efficient way to proceed.

It is also important to examine whether there are any utility, enablement, or written description issues. The process involves a thorough review of the invention record that may include preliminary data produced by the inventor that tends to prove or disprove the operability of the invention. It also may involve a review of relevant literature to determine if there are general problems in the field that would lead an examiner to apply a higher standard for demonstrating enablement.

At various points during this process, it may prove useful to discuss the invention with the inventor. Many times a discussion can reveal previously unknown issues. At one level, this may simply involve clarifying what the inventor believes is the essential advance represented by the invention. It also may help illustrate embodiments of the invention that would have been evident merely by reviewing the invention disclosure and supporting documents.

There are other advantages to sponsoring a discussion between outside counsel and the inventor; for example, by explaining to the inventor the various kinds of disclosures that can result in a loss of rights, prior and upcoming disclosures may be uncovered. Collaborations that may impact inventorship and/or ownership also may be discovered. Finally, the inventor's future research plans, which may be relevant to the ability to strengthen or defend enablement, can be explored.

Once the most relevant information on all of these topics is obtained, one then makes an assessment of how this information would be viewed by an examiner. While it is impossible to predict with certainty how an examiner will treat any given case, an experienced patent attorney can give a reasonably good guess as to what the first office action will entail. Thus, the overall patentability assessment can range from a situation where the prospects for patentability are very high, to those where the chances are extremely low. This analysis alone may provide sufficient information for making a decision on whether to proceed with patenting of the invention.

However, it is more common that various other factors will bear upon the decision to proceed. For example, the following are all relevant considerations:

- The invention's stage of development.
- The time needed to bring a product to market.
- The potential duration of value for the technology.
- The level of cooperation expected from the inventor.
- The likely costs associated with patenting.
- The existence of dominant patents.
- Impending deadlines.
- Third party encumbrances through MTAs or SRAs.
- Potential ownership/inventorship disputes.
- The accessibility (or lack thereof) of enabling technology, i.e., will you infringe other patents in practicing the claimed invention?

While the last issue can be addressed by the outside counsel, the remaining factors are normally best addressed by the technology transfer professional.

One question is whether to reduce the results of a patentability assessment to writing, and if so, when to do so. Generally, the conventional wisdom is to avoid written records that might indicate perceived weaknesses in the patenting prospects. Although there are some cases that hold such infor-

mation governed by the attorney–client privilege, the more conservative approach is to assume that every document in your possession will be discovered in litigation, and the less you end up having to explain away, the better. However, there may be reasons to have the patentability opinion put in writing that are sufficient to override potential litigation concerns. If so, a good patent attorney will know how to phrase the opinion to create the minimal exposure to later attack.

Duty of Candor

Closely related to an applicant's review of patent prospects is the so-called "duty of candor," for example, when the inventor asks whether the examiner is likely to find the same references as were discovered in the patentability search. The answer is a resounding "yes" since the applicant is obligated to provide the references to the examiner. After all, a patent is, by its very nature, affected with a public interest. The public interest is best served, and the most effective patent examination occurs when, at the time an application is being examined, the USPTO is aware of and evaluates the teachings of all information material to patentability.

Each individual associated with the filing and prosecution of a patent application has a duty of openness and good faith in dealing with the USPTO. Included is a duty to make known to the office all information known to that individual that is relevant to patentability. The duty to relate information exists with respect to each pending claim until the claim is canceled or withdrawn from consideration, or the application becomes abandoned. On the other hand, there is no obligation to submit information that is not material to the patentability of any existing claim, nor is there an obligation to seek out information which is not known.

However, the consequence of failing to fulfill this duty is that the entire patent may be declared invalid. This is true even if the applicant's failure relates only to a single claim. In fact, some cases have established what is called "infectious unenforceability," where the applicant's failure is so pervasive that an entire family of patents may be held invalid by a single act during the prosecution of one patent. A violation of the duty is known as "inequitable conduct."

As stated above, there is no affirmative obligation to seek out the most relevant information regarding patentability. However, it is a good idea to take extra care to identify the following information for submission to the USPTO:

- Each piece of prior art cited in search reports of a foreign patent office in a counterpart application.
- Prior art authored by any of the inventors.
- Prior art from related US applications.

Recent decisions have also identified other areas of concern; for example, in a case where a declarant failed to disclose a potential bias (he had previously worked with the inventors), the courts held that failing to cite this information (which might have caused reason to question the declarant on the grounds of bias) constituted inequitable conduct. Another case held that, where inventors made false statements regarding inventorship, the patents arising therefrom were unenforceable even though innocent third parties (the excluded inventors) could seek to correct the inventorship of the patents.[10] Interestingly, the facts in this case were highly debatable, enough to cause one judge's dissent. The judge had argued that not only was the inventorship correct, but also that no false statements had been made to the USPTO.

Parts of the Application

There are two primary parts to a patent application: the specification and the drawings. The specification describes the invention in writing. As discussed previously, it must be clear and complete enough to allow any person skilled in the field to make and use the invention. The application must include the following: a title, a detailed description of the invention, an abstract, and at least one claim (unless the application is provisional). Drawings are often included, though they are optional. The application must also be filed in the name of at least one real person who is an inventor. The following is a breakdown of the different sections typically found within a patent specification, as set out in 37 CFR 1.71-79.

Title Page

The title should be brief, but also technically accurate and descriptive. On occasion, examiners will request a change in the title if the claims have been amended or canceled to the point that the title no longer tracks what is being claimed.

Background of the Invention

In general, the background of the invention provides a discussion of relevant art. However, the effective presentation of previous work focuses on its shortcomings, creating a clear need in the field for further advances. In so doing, one sets the stage for the improvement represented by the present invention.

Summary of the Invention

Typically, the summary of the invention provides literal support for the claims. This may be accomplished by rephrasing the claims in more prose-like fashion. One may also choose to provide additional embodiments that, while not being claimed at present, may prove useful as fall-back positions during prosecution. Generally speaking, this is not the place to include detailed information about how to make and use the invention.

Brief Description of the Invention

This essentially constitutes the figure legend(s) for the accompanying drawing(s). Obviously, if there are no drawings, there is no need for a description.

Detailed Description

The bulk of most applications results from the detailed description. There are three goals one has in mind in drafting this portion of the application. First, one needs to provide enablement for the full scope of the claimed invention. Enablement simply means that the patent must provide sufficient information that would permit one of ordinary skill to make and use the invention as defined by the claims. Thus, information, including various techniques that support the invention, is included. For example, a pharmaceutical case might include information on how one formulates a drug for human administration. An application for a new hammer might describe various methods for making hammers (casting, forging, etc.). While it is generally accepted that what is well-known in the art need not be included, there is little downside to including such information. Thus, particularly in newly emerging technologies, it is not unusual to see applications that read like textbooks. It also is typical to include examples, which provide experimental details of work done by the inventor. These serve the important purpose of demonstrating to

---

[10]*PerSeptive Biosystems, Inc. v. Pharmacia Biotech, Inc.*, 225 F.3d 1315 (Fed. Cir. 2000).

the examiner that the invention is real, and not just a paper patent of theoretical origin. Many times the examples also encompass the best mode at the time of filing. Of course, there are problems associated with applications that are excessive in length, so it is important to use good common sense in deciding what to include. Each case is different, and the wise practitioner will examine this each issue afresh for each case.

The second goal of the detailed description is to broaden the invention beyond that aspect for which the invention may have actually been made. Again, taking our pharmaceutical example, the inventor may have administered the drug by injection in testing, but oral formulations are likely to be more practical. In this case, incorporating a "canned" disclosure on oral drug formulations can go a long way toward ensuring that the examiner will not insist that the claims be limited to injectable embodiments. Of course, this sort of broadening is, in one sense, at odds with the new written description trend. However, it remains clear that applicants are entitled claim beyond that which they have exemplified: the question simply is to what extent. By adding information about the broader aspects of the invention, the wise practitioner is increasing the likelihood that these broader aspects will be accepted.

The third goal of the detailed description is to provide a variety of fall-back positions for prosecution. Let's return to our pharmaceutical example: even if a drug has been tested for its ability to limit the growth of lung cancer cells, there may be good reason to believe that it will treat other cancers. Such reasons might include action upon a target common to multiple cancers, or a structural similarity to drugs shown to be effective at treating different types of cancer. Thus, the practitioner may seek a claim such as, "a method limiting the growth of cancer cells comprising administering drug 123 to a subject." In all likelihood, the application will contain data relating to the lung cancer studies. In prosecution, an examiner may well find that the applicant's rationale for extrapolating to all cancers is insufficient. If no other disclosure regarding the *type* of cancer to be treated is included in the specification, the only fallback would be "lung cancer." However, if a section had been added to the application that included a discussion of various types of cancers, for example those treated with the structurally related compound, a more acceptable subgeneric claim could be presented. Even a laundry list of different cancers might prove sufficient if data were provided by affidavit showing that at least some of these cancers were, in fact, inhibited by the new drug.

Thus, one of the key decisions made during the patent drafting process relates to what should be included in the specification, and how much detail is appropriate. It is worth mentioning that one easy way to beef up a patent specification is to incorporate by reference. Strictly speaking, incorporation by reference is permitted only for issued US patents. When referenced this way, the entire text of the issued patent is deemed to be part of your application, and may be relied upon for enablement and written description just as the text of the specification. It is also possible to incorporate other public disclosures by reference (patent applications, journal articles, etc.). Though technically this is an improper incorporation, this can be cured (if necessary) at any time prior to issue by physically importing relevant portions of the references into the specification. This is usually done only in extreme cases where, for some reason that could not have been predicted beforehand, the reference contains information *not literally found in the specification*, yet essential for enablement and/or written description.

Claims

The claims of a patent define the scope of protection. Therefore, a valid, broad claim will cover infringing devices or processes that a narrower one may not. The inclusion of narrower claims is important, however, since it is possible that an infringer may be successful in proving that a claim is not valid due to prior art that was not considered during prosecution of the application. Similarly, narrower claims provide the basis for fall-back positions (as earlier discussed) should the examiner find reason (prior art, enablement, etc.) to reject the broader claims. The presence of additional elements or further delineation of broadly defined elements in narrower claims may further define the invention so as to distinguish over the prior art, or move the invention into the realm of enablement.

Structurally speaking, patent claims are detailed statements of exactly what the invention is intended to encompass. An apt analogy might be the deed to the property on which your house sits—it refers to a particular parcel of property with clearly identified boundaries. Because the scope of patent rights is based on the boundary of its claims, they constitute the most important section of the application. Therefore, they deserve a great deal of attention and care. And while many inventors profess not to understand patent claims, it is of critical importance that they carefully review and comment on their content and scope.

A patent claim is a single sentence describing the elements required to distinguish an invention over the prior art. A claim generally has a preamble, a transition, and a body. The preamble is a short introductory phrase that summarizes the general type of invention. For example, the preamble may begin: "A composition. . . ." or "A method. . . ." In short, the preamble sets the stage for the elements that define the invention. There is an interesting series of cases that deal with whether the terms presented in the preamble are actually affirmative limitations on the scope of the claims. The general rule emanating from these cases is that if the body of the claim refers back to the preamble, or "breathes life" into one or more aspects of the preamble, the terms included therein *can* be construed as meaningful limitations.

The transition should be one of the following three words or phrases: "comprising," "consisting of," or "consisting essentially of." The transition is used to express the degree of breadth of the scope of the claim. "Comprising" is considered open language, indicating that all the recited elements must be present, but that any other element also may be present. "Consisting" is at the other end of the spectrum (closed language) and the effect is that *only the recited elements, and no others, are included.* Obviously, this is a very narrow claim, and for that reason, it is very unusual to find this language used appropriately. Finally, "consisting essentially of" is considered partially open (or partially closed). What this means precisely in any given situation varies, but the general rule is that these claims encompass the recited elements, and other things that do not materially affect the nature or function of the recited elements. Again, this is fairly uncommon language in patent claims, but it does have its time and place.

Finally, the body of the claim is where the limitations or recitations are placed: this information indicates how the invention is distinguishable over the prior art. For a method claim, the elements usually take the form of steps, but obviously these may be further characterized by compositions or objectives as they relate to the steps. For a composition of matter, the elements may be physical characteristics, such as size and weight. For machines, the different parts of the machine, and how they relate to each other, are typical elements. One may also use functional limitations, where a thing is defined not by any particular structure or characteristic, but instead by what it does. This can be a powerful

claiming tool, but it also is dangerous given the potentially large scope of prior art encompassed, and the large scope of protection that must be enabled. As such, it is not particularly favored by examiners, and may in some cases be seen as overreaching on the part of the applicant.

Abstract

The abstract is a brief description of the invention. It should be 150 words or less, and it should contain key words that would be used by someone looking for information relevant to the invention's field of interest. Since many databases do not have full text searching capabilities, the abstract may very well be the best opportunity to identify your patent to the public.

Sequence Listing

For biotech applications dealing with nucleic acid or protein sequences, it is necessary to provide a sequence listing that sets relevant sequences in a particular format suitable for searching by the USPTO. Applicants must also submit a separate paper copy and disk copy of the listing, in addition to identifying each nucleic acid of "greater than 10 bases and each protein of greater than 4 residues by a 'SEQ ID NO'." While this requirement is eminently reasonable where the sequence is part of the claimed invention, the USPTO rules are, unfortunately, overly broad in requiring that *any* sequence, regardless of its remoteness to patentability, must be included.

The Application Process

Attorneys approach the application process in slightly different ways. There is consensus, however, regarding the general approach. The most critical issue to resolve prior to drafting is to precisely identify what the applicant wants to claim. Presumably, through searches and review of the prior art, the decision to proceed with preparation and filing of an application has also established what can be claimed. Sometimes, the client decides to limit the scope of what *is* to be claimed for financial or political reasons. Thus, simply knowing what *can* be claimed is insufficient. Regardless, it is important to have a game plan before starting the application.

Almost every attorney begins the drafting process with the claims. There are a number of reasons why this is the ideal place to start. First, starting with the drafting of claims provides the attorney with an opportunity to identify any misapprehension with regard to what is being claimed. Thus, it is important to distribute the draft claims to the inventor and the client (assuming they are different). Claims also provide an outline for the application: one approach is to highlight key terms in the claims and later check to see if these terms are adequately defined. Upon receipt of comments on the claims, one can begin drafting the application in earnest (preliminary drafting can proceed earlier).

When the application is ready, applicants have two choices for filing. If the application is mailed through the US Postal Services' Express Mail, the filing date is the date on which the application is mailed. Through other mail services (First Class, Priority Mail, private courier service or via hand delivery), the filing date is the date the application is received by the USPTO mail room. Thus, with the exception of Washington, DC area law firms, Express Mail is the preferred choice.

In order to be accorded a filing date, the application must contain at least one claim and name at least one inventor. The following are items that must be submitted to obtain a valid filing, but may be submitted after the application is filed:

(a) **Oath/declaration:** Identifies the inventor(s), attests to the truthfulness of the claims and specifications, and identifies other patents that disclose the invention.

(b) **Power of attorney:** Gives either an attorney or patent agent the power of attorney to submit the patent application, unless the inventor chooses to prosecute the application.

(c) **Fees:** Dependent upon the number of claims and the ability of an applicant to claim small entity status.

Other items that may be submitted include:

(a) **Assignment:** Establishes a formal legal transfer of ownership rights from the inventor(s) to the real owner, usually the employer.

(b) **Fee calculation and transmittal:** Assists with and identifies the calculation that is the basis of the filing fees submitted.

(c) **Information disclosure statement (IDS):** Satisfies the duty of candor listing US and foreign patents, published patent applications, and literature references.

Prosecution

Once all the requirements for a completed filing have been met, the application is assigned to a particular art unit based on the kind of technology involved. Then, it is assigned to a particular examiner. Depending on the workload that examiner is subject to, the application may simply sit for a period of time up to two years. However, a more common period of time before examination commences is 6 to 12 months.

Restriction Practice

The first significant correspondence from the USPTO is likely to be a restriction requirement. This type of action will issue where the examiner determines that there are multiple, patentably distinct inventions being claimed. In addition, there must be an undue burden upon the examiner to conduct the search. The rules for restriction requirement are arcane and complicated, the result being that the examining corps has plenary power to issue and maintain restrictions.

A response must be made either with or without disagreement or traverse. In responding, the applicant must be careful in choosing a strategy. Acquiescence means that the applicant may be forced to file one or more divisional applications to prosecute the different inventions. While this does not affect the effective filing or priority date of the respective divisional applications, it means that the applicant must pay to prosecute multiple applications at once or give up the post-issuance patent term, if the filing of divisional applications is delayed. It also means payment of multiple maintenance fees once the applications issue as patents.

The other area of concern is that in order to effectively traverse a restriction, it is almost always necessary to argue that the claims are not distinct. This can be dangerous, as such an admission, if made, permits the examiner to reject a wide variety of distinct claims over art that would otherwise have been insufficient to establish their unpatentability. Thus, before an applicant makes such an argument, it is wise to carefully consider whether doing so is even advisable.

Office Action(s)

The applicant (or the applicant's attorney) next receives an official action, more commonly referred to as an office action. Applicants should not be dismayed to find that the USPTO, on its initial review, has found most (if not all) of the claims to be unpatentable. There are numerous reasons that most first office actions are considered unfavorable. First, an aggressive attorney will attempt to claim up to or beyond that which truly is patentable in order to not leave anything on the table, and to provide an opportunity to meet the examiner halfway.

It should also be understood that the USPTO is very big on building the record, i.e., forcing the applicant to explain in more detail than presented in the application (e.g., why the invention is novel, nonobvious, and enabled). Through such record building, the USPTO believes stronger patents with clearer boundaries can be generated. Third, it must be realized that USPTO examiners are given little time to examine each case and, thus, it is not surprising when they misconstrue either the claims of the application or the prior art (or both).

Once an office action that rejects one or more claims is received, a response must be prepared. The deadline for responding is normally three months, with three additional one-month extensions available for a fee. A response or answer to an office action need not follow any particular format, however, the response should help to place the application in a position for allowance or, at a minimum, the response should reduce the number of issues to be appealed. Most responses include one or more of the following:

1. Amendments to the claims and/or specification; care must be taken not to introduce new matter in the application.
2. Scientific or technical argument as to how the invention is patentably distinguishable from the cited references, or why it is enabled.
3. Legal arguments as to why the amended claims are in condition for allowance, or a combination of these items; in some cases, argument alone will be needed to overcome the references, and amendments to the claims will not be necessary.
4. Evidence supporting (2) and/or (3) above, including journal articles, data, affidavits of experts, and case law.

With regard to prior art rejections, the response may argue that the prior art is not, in fact, prior art. Such an argument may arise from an inaccuracy in determining the art's effective disclosure date, by swearing behind the reference with an earlier invention date by the applicant (only good for §102(a) and §102(e) art) or by establishing a claim for benefit of priority under 35 USC §119 (foreign priority filing or provisional filing) or 35 USC §120 (domestic priority filing). One can also submit evidence arguing against lack of novelty or obviousness, including expert affidavits, unpublished data and peer-reviewed publications. Enablement rejections may be addressed in a similar fashion, although unpublished data from the inventors is often more useful in this context.

The examiner normally issues only one office action before making the rejections final, although the examiner can issue as many nonfinal actions as he or she deems appropriate. Similarly, an applicant may respond to as many nonfinal actions as desired, but once a claim has been twice rejected, an appeal may be sought. When a final office action is issued, applicants have only one more response of right, after which the examiner can effectively shut down the prosecution process. When a response to final office action is submitted, the examiner either allows the application or issues what is called an "advisory action." An advisory action is very brief and often contains only conclusory statements regarding the nonallowability of the claims. At this point, the applicant's ability to submit new evidence or to amend the claims is severely restricted. This is one reason why applicants must be careful to make their first response as complete as possible.

In the unfortunate event that claims are not allowed after a response to final office action has been filed, and an advisory action issues, the applicant has a choice to make. The case may be abandoned (clearly not a favorable outcome). The case may be refiled as a continuation, where by paying fees the applicant is given a "second bite of the apple," so to speak. This permits one to amend the claims and adduce new evidence. Finally, the applicant may appeal the examiner's rejection of the claims to the Board of Patent Appeals and Interferences.

Appeal

An appeal is initiated by filing a notice of appeal, and the payment of fees. This often is done at the time the response to final office action is filed, especially where the chances of securing allowance are low. Within two months of filing the notice of appeal, a brief from the applicant arguing the remaining rejections must be filed. This deadline is extendable as well; a total of five one-month extensions are available. Unlike the response, the brief must have a very particular structure and will be "bounced" if it does not. The brief must be filed in triplicate and, not surprisingly, with additional fees. Briefs tend to be a bit more focused on legal issues, though some may not. The examiner will then issue an answer to the brief, usually within 2 to 6 months after the brief is filed. [Note: No new grounds of rejection are permitted in the examiner's answer.] This rule often gives rise to reopening of prosecution; where the examiner realizes that the appeal cannot be won, but nonetheless believes the claims are not patentable. In this case, a new office action with new and more troubling rejections is often issued.

Upon receipt of the answer, the applicant may file a reply brief with additional arguments. If applicants wish to have the opportunity to argue the appeal in person in front of the three-member board (which does not include the examiner), a notice of oral argument (including fees) is required. The applicant must then wait, sometimes for several years. At some juncture, the board issues the notice of oral hearing that is either confirmed or waived. If waived, the board decides the appeal based on the brief, answer, and reply (if filed). If confirmed, applicant and/or applicant's representative travels to the USPTO in Crystal City, Virginia, for the argument to be heard. Examiners are also entitled to be heard at these hearings; rarely do they attend. After the hearing, a decision on the appeal, in writing, will issue within two to six months. Any unfavorable results can be appealed to the Court of Appeals for the Federal Circuit.

Allowance, Issue, and Continuing Applications

After all of rejections have been overcome and withdrawn, the notice of allowance is mailed. The notice sets forth a period of three months in which the issue fee must be paid and may also indicate the need to submit formal drawings, if the drawings previously filed were sufficient only for examination, but were otherwise found too informal for publication purposes. It is important to review the notice of allowance for the examiner's reasons for allowance. Occasionally, examiners make disparaging remarks about the claims or the applicant's alleged acquiescence on certain points. Failure of the applicant to rebut these statements is deemed as an admission that the statements are true—an unfortunate event should the patent ever be litigated. Patents normally issue within 3 to 6 months after payment of the issue fees and usually (though not always) are preceded by 7 to 10 days by an issue notification, setting the issue date and patent number.

The payment of the issue fees marks the final step the applicant must take to secure issuance of the patent. As such, it is an important time to reflect upon the need to file additional applications (claiming benefit of the issuing patent's priority date) to secure additional coverage. Reasons for such filings include: (a) a prior restriction requirement resulting in cancellation of restricted claims; (b) amendments to secure allowance that narrowed the claims beyond which applicants feel are truly necessary; or (c) to advance claims to previously unclaimed, though adequately disclosed, subject matter. Such applications must be filed no later than the day the patent issues, or else the priority claim will not be valid.[11]

---

[11]Note that patents only issue once a week, on Tuesdays.

This period is also the last opportunity to consider issues of inventorship, duty of candor, claim scope (in terms of operability and enablement), and benefit of priority. Sending a copy of the allowed claims to the inventor and client following payment of the issue fee is always a good idea.

Kinds of Applications

As mentioned earlier, there are several kinds of applications (described below) based upon their relationship to each other. Related applications have the following three features in common: (a) common subject matter (such that claims of the latter find support in the specification of the former); (b) common inventor(s) (at least one); and (c) copendency (a latter application is filed before a former issues). Cases of copendency must also contain a reference in the specification to the earlier application(s).

Provisional Application

A provisional application is not examined, but remains pending for 12 months after filing. It cannot claim priority to any other application, but serves as a source for priority claims to other kinds of applications. One of the biggest misconceptions is that a provisional can be filed with less effort than nonprovisional applications. This misunderstanding arises from the fact that a provisional patent application has fewer formalities than nonprovisionals, need not have claims, and never issues as a patent. However, as with a nonprovisional application, a provisional must fulfill the 35 USC §112 requirements for enablement, written description, and description of best mode. In other words, the law does not distinguish between a provisional and nonprovisional application on the grounds that it must contain full, clear, concise, and exact disclosure of the invention so as to enable any person-skilled in the art to make and use the invention, including the best mode contemplated by the inventor.

There are two ways that a provisional application can serve as the basis for a priority claim. First, the provisional application can be converted by petition to a nonprovisional claim. This is only appropriate where there is no need to add new information to the application at the time of conversion. While inexpensive, this approach has the downside of allowing up to a year of patent term (a claim for benefit of priority to a provisional application does not count against the twenty-year patent term), since the petition retroactively makes the provisional a nonprovisional as of its initial filing date. The other, and much more common way to claim priority to a provisional, is to simply file a nonprovisional application and make a claim under 35 USC §119 for benefit of the provisional's filing date. New data may be included in the nonprovisional or it may merely be a copy of the provisional.

No amendment, other than to make the provisional application comply with the patent statute and all applicable regulations, may be made to the provisional application after its filing date. Instead, should an update of the provisional claim be required, a second provisional can be filed including the new and/or corrected information. At one year from the original provisional claim's filing date, a nonprovisional claim would be filed claiming benefit from both earlier filed provisionals.

[Note: Failure to convert or file a nonprovisional claiming priority within one year of the provisional application's filing date means loss of the right to claim priority. The provisional application cannot be revived and thus the loss of this right is unrecoverable.]

Nonprovisional

The main distinguishing feature of the nonprovisional, as compared to a provisional application, is that it is examined and may issue as a patent. It also may claim priority to other applications and must have claims. The other aspects of nonprovisional applications have been discussed elsewhere in this document.

Divisional

A divisional application contains claims to restricted inventions that were canceled in response to a restriction requirement. It has the same specification as the parent application from whence the restricted claims were canceled. A divisional application may be filed after receiving a restriction requirement and canceling of restricted claims, or applicants may delay until just shortly before the parent application issues. More than one divisional claim may be filed claiming priority of a parent application, and a divisional application may thereafter also have divisional applications claiming priority of it. A patent derived from the parent application (or one of the divisionals) cannot be used as prior art against a divisional (or its parent), if the applications were pending simultaneously.

Continuation

A continuation uses the same specification as its predecessor "parent." Normally, the claims are different in some way from those pending in the parent application, for example, narrower or broader than claims currently in prosecution or filed with the original application. The determination of continuation really depends on why the continuation was filed in the first place. If the continuation purpose is to claim previously unclaimed, but disclosed subject matter, then no claim like those of the continuation will have been prosecuted in the parent. If the continuation is filed to pursue subject matter lost in the parent through amendment, then the claims may be broader than those currently pending in the parent. Finally, if the continuation is filed to secure entry of amendments that would place the claims in condition for allowance, then they likely are narrower than those currently pending.

An example of the latter approach involves the filing of a continuing prosecution application (CPA) or the simpler request for continued examination (RCE). Both applications rely on the same disclosure as the parent application, without the addition of any new matter. Unlike the CPA, however, the RCE is not a new application; it simply reopens the prosecution for the application; normally for the purpose of submitting amendments and/or new evidence of patentability. For applications filed prior to May 29, 2000, both the CPA and RCE are available for continuing prosecution. Only the RCE is available for applications filed after May 29, 2000.

Continuation-in-Part

A continuation-in-part (or C-I-P) is just that: it continues with some material found the parent, yet also contains some new material. By definition, this application will have the possibility of having claims with distinct priority dates. For example, if application A is filed on June 1, 2002 disclosing subject matter A, and application AB is filed on December 1, 2002 disclosing subject matter A + B, claims drawn to A take priority over the June 1st filing; where claims drawn to B will have priority only to the December 1st filing. C-I-Ps are rarely a good idea, however. Reverting to the example, if subject matter A is adequately disclosed in application A, why confuse the matter by filing a new application with new information? Further, if subject matter B is not adequately disclosed in application A, why claim benefit to application A, when it will do no good (and can result in a reduced patent term)? Overall, one must think carefully before filing a C-I-P.

Reissue

Reissue applications are one of two postissuance actions that an applicant may institute. Reissues are designed to deal with defects such that:

> The applicant believes the original patent to be wholly or partly inoperative or invalid by reason of a defective specification or drawing, or by reason of the patentee claiming more or less than the patentee had the right to claim in the patent, stating at least one error being relied upon as the basis for reissue.[12]

The applicant may make such a statement in an oath, and further swear that the defects arose without deceptive intent. Once taken up by the USPTO, the application will be examined as a normal application, with exception that division of the claims is not permitted. If filed within two years, the reissue may broaden or narrow the claims; if filed after two years, only narrowing the claims is permitted.

Reexamination

Reexamination is the other postissuance procedure. However, in contrast to reissues, it deals with prior art. Reexaminations may be requested by the applicant, by a third party, or instituted *sua sponte* by the USPTO. There are two different third party procedures, one permitting more involvement by the third party than the other (i.e., the opportunity to comment upon the patentee's submissions). Reexaminations are often the result of a patent infringement lawsuit, where the alleged infringer produces art that was not considered by the examiner during prosecution. Thus, the patent owner can request reexamination over the art, possibly while staying the lawsuit, as a way of defeating the alleged infringer's challenge. While the alleged infringer may still argue unpatentability in the lawsuit, an outcome favorable to the patentee during reexamination can make it very difficult for the alleged infringer to prevail.

Legal Interests in Patents

Employees who have signed an agreement with an employer to assign patent rights to that employer

are still inventors, but they are not considered the owners of the patent. Similarly, if an employee was initially hired or later directed to solve a specific problem or to exercise inventive skill, in most cases, the employer is the owner of the patent rights. Though the agreements on face value establish the ownership rights, it is wise to also obtain a written transfer of rights and to record this instrument with the USPTO.

Today a fairly rare situation can arise from what are known as "shop rights." A shop right gives the employer the right to make and use the invention if the employee used the employer's resources (tools, materials, or facilities) to conceive or reduce the invention to practice. The shop right is a nonexclusive, royalty-free, and nontransferable license.

Another important concern arises regarding federally sponsored projects (e.g., projects funded by the National Institutes of Health, the Departments of Defense, Agriculture, Education, etc.). These rights must be noted in the application itself, and most often subject the applicant to certain rules and regulations.

Finally, one of the most difficult interests to track arises under sponsored research agreements (SRAs) and materials transfer agreements (MTAs). These agreements may give rights of third parties, based solely on the specific terms set out therein. Thus, it is essential to have control over who makes such deals, as they can result in development of technology with preexisting (and often inconsistent) obligations to multiple third parties. Moreover, even when proper steps have been taken initially, any prior comingling of materials or of funds can create problems.

Inventorship

In the United States, a patent application must be made or authorized to be made by an inventor, even if the patent rights are owned by someone else (e.g., the inventor's employer), as is often the case. Even employees who have signed away rights to their invention must still be named as the inventors, and their names must appear on the patent. Any person or entity that finances an invention (e.g., a relative helping to pay for material and supplies) or an employer is not considered an inventor and cannot be named on the application. However, by obtaining an assignment of the inventor's rights, the owner can step in to control the prosecution.

There are only a few circumstances when people other than the inventor can apply for a patent, when:

---

[12]U.S. Department of Commerce, United States Patent and Trademark Office, 1414 Content of Reissue Oath/Declaration [R-3] in "Manual of Patent Examining Procedure, Original Eighth Edition, August 2001, latest revision August 2005 available at http://www.uspto.gov/web/offices/pac/mpep/documents/1400_1414.htm (accessed November 22, 2005)

i. The inventor has died (then a member of the inventor's estate may apply for the patent);

ii. The inventor is insane (then a guardian may apply); or

iii. The inventor refuses to apply for a patent or cannot be found (then a coinventor or interested party may apply).

An invention may have single, joint or coinventors. If two or more people invent together, they must both apply for the patent. Joint inventors jointly contribute to the same claim; coinventors contribute to different claims. An inventor may be a sole inventor if he or she conceives of the novel and nonobvious features of the invention. This is true, even in the case where others have first identified the problem that the invention solves; have made nonessential suggestions; have provided money or starting materials; or have contributed to the reduction to practice. However, an inventor may be a joint inventor if he or she has made some unique contribution to the conception, even if the contributions of the respective inventors are not equal. Furthermore, there is no requirement that joint inventors work together in the same place or at the same time, though some sharing of information is required.

Inventorship law is case made, i.e., there is no statutory definition of an inventor. Some of the more important conception/inventorship rules are:

- The threshold question in determining inventorship is who conceived the invention. Unless a person contributes to the conception of the invention, he is not an inventor . . . [and] reduction to practice, *per se*, is irrelevant.[13]

- For conception, we look not to whether one skilled in the art could have thought of the invention, but whether the alleged inventors actually had in their minds the required permanent and definite idea.[14]

- A conception is not complete if the subsequent course of experimentation, especially experimental failures, reveals uncertainty that so undermines the specificity of the inventor's idea that it is not yet a definite and permanent reflection of the complete invention as it will be used in practice.[15]

- The question is not whether [the inventors] reasonably believed that the inventions would

work for their intended purpose ..., but whether the inventors had formed the idea of their use for that purpose in sufficiently final form that only the exercise of ordinary skill remained to reduce it to practice.[16]

- An inventor may use the services, ideas, and aid of others in the process of perfecting his invention without losing right to a patent.[17]

- A person is not precluded from being a joint inventor simply because his or her contribution to a collaborative effort is experimental.[18]

Only through a thorough understanding of the subtleties of these rules and how they are applied in practice may one accurately determine inventorship. Here are some good rules of thumb:

i. Conception may be the key, but reduction to practice may be very instructive in determining who the inventors are.

ii. Look at the claims to determine inventorship; also worth paying some attention to what is a patentable invention.

iii. Determine first what the invention is, and then examine both the conception and reduction to practice to determine whether the conception was complete.

iv. Ask, who did what, under whose instruction, and at what time? Is there evidence of these facts?

One must remember that changes to the claims during prosecution, as are commonly made, can have an impact on inventorship. When this happens, the inventorship then must be amended. For example, if the claims are amended to include additional aspects of the invention that were not previously included in the claim (but were mentioned in the patent application), those aspects may be the result of an inventive contribution by someone not earlier considered an inventor because those aspects were not originally included in the claims. Deletion of claims also might eliminate an inventor whose contribution is no longer reflected in the remaining claims.

If the inventorship is not correctly named on a patent application, even if it has issued as a patent, one can change the inventorship so long as there was no deceptive intent. If the application has been filed recently and no inventor's oath/declaration has been submitted, it is a simple act to modify the inventorship. If an oath/declaration has been filed,

[13]*Fiers v. Revel*, 25 USPQ2d 1601, 1604-05 (Fed. Cir. 1993)

[14]*Burroughs Wellcome Co. v. Barr Laboratories*, 32 USPQ2d 1915, 1923 (Fed. Cir. 1994)

[15]*Burroughs Wellcome Co. v. Barr Laboratories*, 32 USPQ2d 1915, 1920 (Fed. Cir. 1994)

[16]*Burroughs Wellcome Co. v. Barr Laboratories*, 32 USPQ2d 1915, 1922 (Fed. Cir. 1994)

[17]*Hobbs v. Atomic Energy Comm'n*, 171 USPQ 713, 724 (5th Cir. 1971)

[18]*Burroughs Wellcome Co. v. Barr Laboratories*, 32 USPQ2d 1915, 1921 (Fed. Cir. 1994)

or if the patent has issued, it is slightly more complicated, requiring a petition and statements from the inventors.

[Note: A key practice point relating to inventorship (as with the following section on interferences) is the need to keep good records that can defend from fraudulent allegations of sole or co-inventorship by others (colleagues working elsewhere, transient faculty or students, etc.).]

Interference Practice

One of the unique aspects of US patent law is the rule that the patent is awarded to the person or persons first to invent, as opposed to the rest of the world where the patentee is determined based on the first to file. The basis for this rule is 35 USC §102(g) (discussed earlier), which gives rise to US interference practice, a pseudo-litigation proceeding within the USPTO that determines who was, in fact, the first to invent.

Recalling our earlier discussion of invention—which is comprised of conception and reduction to practice—priority of invention in an interference is determined based upon who was: (a) first to reduce to practice; or (b) the first to conceive followed by continuous diligence through to reduction to practice. What is most important to remember about these requirements is that each must be supported by sufficient corroborative evidence, which means evidence that goes beyond the inventors' own testimony. This corroboration may take the form of notebooks, although unattested notebooks are of questionable value on their own. Normally, the best corroboration is the testimony of third parties who were aware of what the inventors were doing during the key times at which the invention was being made.

Generally, an interference is broken into two parts: preliminary motions and proofs. The preliminary motions stage allows the parties to change the playing field by adding or deleting claims; substituting applications; arguing the unpatentability of claims to the other party; substituting the count (the count is like a claim, and it defines the contested subject matter); or allowing argument that no interference should exist. If both parties survive the motions phase, the junior party (that party with the later effective priority date) will put on its proofs (i.e., the evidence showing earlier invention). The senior party may then put on its proofs or rely on its earlier filing date, if the proofs offered by the junior party are, for one reason or another, deemed

defective. A board panel, comprised of three administrative patent judges, then conducts a hearing and renders a decision. An appeal from this decision may be taken to either the Federal Circuit Court (restricted to the record already established), or to a competent federal district court (trial *de novo*, meaning new evidence may be adduced).

A detailed review of interference practice is beyond the scope of this presentation. However, suffice it to say that interferences are one of the most complicated procedures conducted by the USPTO; they can be very expensive (approaching that of smaller patent litigations); and they are fraught with pitfalls for the unwary client and practitioner.

International Patents

Before technology can be exported to a foreign country, a foreign filing license is required from the US government. This usually appears on the filing receipt of a patent application, which is received between three and six months after the filing date. If there is a need to file in a foreign jurisdiction prior to receipt of the license, one may petition an expedited foreign filing license, which can be obtained in as little as forty-eight hours. Also, if an error occurs and a foreign application is filed prior to obtaining of a foreign filing license, a petition for a retroactive foreign filing license may be made.

The major difference between US practice and most foreign jurisdictions is regarding the first to file and who, subsequently, receives the patent. As we know from the preceding section, the United States determines who is first to invent, whereas, in other countries, inventorship is awarded on a first-to-file basis. However, in the United States, in a post-issuance process known as an opposition, the validity of a patent may be challenged based upon prior invention by another. The other major difference in foreign practice is the absence of the one-year grace period for the inventor's own publications, which arises from the different provisions of 35 USC §102(a) and §102(b). In almost every foreign jurisdiction (with the exception of Canada and Japan), *any* disclosure of the invention prior to filing will bar patenting—with no ability to swear behind. This strict application of a prior disclosure bar is also referred to as "absolute novelty."

The foundation of international patent law is the Paris Convention Treaty, which gives an applicant one year following his or her home country filing to file abroad in all signatory countries, while maintaining the effective priority date of the home country filing. However, after one year, only a non-convention application may be filed, which gains a priority date only of the date on which is it filed. [Note: This is one of the few deadlines that cannot be recovered through the payment of extra fees.]

The Patent Cooperation Treaty (PCT) is a vehicle to maintain foreign rights for relatively minimal cost. By most measures, it is a patent application as would be filed in the United States or any other country. It has inventors, claims, a description of the invention, and it is searched and examined by an appropriate searching and examining authority. However, no patent will issue from a PCT—it is merely a way to: (a) get an idea of how the invention will fare, in terms of patentability, in foreign jurisdictions; and (b) delay the date at which applications must be filed in individual foreign countries or foreign patent communities (such as the European Patent Community). Almost every industrialized country in the world is a member of the PCT, though a very few exceptions exist, such as Taiwan and Malaysia.

Also, certain types of claims may not be available in foreign countries. For example, claims to diagnostics and therapies on the human body are precluded in most countries outside the United States. However, this can be partially circumvented by the use of "Swiss-type" claims, which follow the format of preparation of a medicament for use in treating a disease ..... Also, the ability to patent engineered plants and animals varies widely from country to country, largely based upon morality and/or safety concerns.

Infringement

The USPTO has no jurisdiction over questions relating to the infringement of patents. In examining applications for patent, no determination is made as to whether the invention sought to be patented infringes any existing patent. An improvement invention may be patentable, but it may nonetheless infringe one or more prior unexpired patents for the invention improved upon.

Infringement of a patent consists of the unauthorized making, using, offering for sale, or selling any patented invention within the United States or United States Territories, or importing into the United States of any patented invention during the term of the patent. If a patent is infringed, the patentee may sue for relief in the appropriate federal court; state courts are not a proper venue for patent cases. The patentee may ask the court for an injunc-

tion to prevent continuing infringement, and may also ask the court for an award of damages because of past infringement. In an infringement suit, the defendant may raise the question of the validity or enforceability of the patent, which is then decided by the court. The defendant may also aver that what is being done does not constitute infringement. Primarily, the language of the claims of the patent determines infringement, and if what the defendant is making or doing does not fall within the language of any of the claims of the patent, there is no literal infringement. There are several types of literal infringement:

- Direct infringement: Making, using, selling, importing, or offering for sale an invention patented in the United States (35 USC §271(a)).
- Inducement to infringe: "Actively induces" the infringement of a patent (35 USC §271(b)); good where the "deep pocket" is not the actual infringer.
- Contributory infringement: Offers for sale or sells a component that is known to be especially adapted to be used in infringement of a patent (35 USC §271(c)); key issue is whether the component has a substantial noninfringing use.
- Product by process: A product made anywhere in the world by a process patented in the United States (35 USC §271(g)) and targeted at offshore infringers (though few cases have interpreted this statute since its inception).

Clearly, one of the key questions in litigation is, therefore, whether the accused device or method falls within the scope of the claims. In coming to this determination, a two-step approach is taken. First, the scope of the claims must be determined. This task has evolved into a minitrial of its own, called a Markman hearing.[19]

Whereby each side presents its evidence, including reliance upon claim terms (as defined in the specification), common usage of undefined terms, the prosecution history, and even expert witnesses. The judge then decides the proper scope of the claims. The second step involves determining what the infringing device/method includes. At this point, a straightforward comparison should lead to the proper result. However, anyone experienced with patent litigation knows that getting it right is far from an easy task.

Even if no literal infringement exists, one may still argue for infringement under an equitable doc-

---

[19]The hearing gets its name from *Markman et al. v. Westview Instruments, Inc.* et al., 517 U.S. 370 (1996).

trine called the "doctrine of equivalents." The basic concept is that the patentee will still be granted relief against an infringer who has avoided literal infringement by narrowly skirting the specific language of a patent claim, while can still benefit from the essence of the patentee's advance. Though thousands of pages have been written on this topic in recent years, and dozens of high profile cases decided such as *Warner Jenkinson Co., Inc. v. Hilton Davis Chemical Co.,* and *Festo Corp. v. Shoketsu Kinzoku Kogyo Kabushiki Co., Ltd.,*[20] it is difficult to state precisely where we are in the evolution of the doctrine. Clearly, the lower courts and the Federal Circuit Court find the malleable character of this remedy objectionable, but the Supreme Court has repeatedly stated that it exists as a refuge for patentees whose claims are not literally infringed. Thus, for the time being, one can expect that such claims will continue.

Suits for infringement of patents follow the rules of procedure of the federal courts. From the decision of the federal district court, an appeal may be taken to the Court of Appeals for the Federal Circuit. The Supreme Court may thereafter take a case by *writ of certiorari.* If the United States Government infringes a patent, the patentee has a remedy for damages in the United States Court of Federal Claims. The United States Government may use any patented invention without permission of the patentee, but the patentee is entitled to obtain compensation for the use by or for the government. Patent cases are also sometimes brought in conjunction with actions in front of the International Trade Commission (ITC).

What Is Not Infringement?

Now that we have discussed infringement, we need to look at the other side of the coin—that which is not infringement. This is important from a patentee's standpoint (i.e., knowing what they cannot prevent) and from the public's standpoint (i.e., knowing what they can do without fear of infringement).

Outside the Scope of the Claims

So long as infringement is avoided, the patent system itself is created to permit others to design around a patent's claims. To determine what is per-

mitted, that is, to determine what actions will fall outside of the patent claims, requires a similar analysis to that of infringement. First, the scope of the claims needs to be ascertained. Next, the infringing device or method is reviewed and is compared to the claims, as analyzed. From this, the need to license or modify the infringing device or method is determined. Although designing around a patent is legitimate, it should be approached with caution, since it is not absolutely certain that a given court or jury will agree, or that a doctrine of equivalents issue will not arise.

11th Amendment Issues

Under the 11th Amendment to the US Constitution, citizens of another state or country may not sue a state in federal court. Though cast in narrower terms, the 11th Amendment has long been recognized as a reformulation of state sovereign immunity. Thus, where a state or state-owned entity is accused of patent infringement, one cannot resort to the federal court system due to 11th Amendment constraints, thus giving rise to an exception to the normal patent infringement law. It is very significant for state-owned universities, since they are considered branches of the state itself, and hence are exempt (at least in theory) from patent infringement. The only exception is where the state has waived it immunity to suit: however the suit still cannot be brought under the federal patent statute, as there is exclusive federal jurisdiction.

Patenting or Licensing

A common assumption is that the filing of a patent application constitutes infringement: careful review of 35 USC §271 reveals that this is false. While the actions of the inventors in reducing the invention to practice may constitute infringement, those acts are separate and distinct from the preparation and filing of a patent application.

Similarly, the licensing of a technology to a third party does not constitute inducement to infringe. A license simply gives a third party the ability (should they choose to proceed) to practice an invention without risk of infringing its patent. In many cases, licenses to patents covering distinct, dominant, and/or subservient technologies may be needed. It is not the licensor's obligation to inform the third party of these technologies nor is the licensor subject to liability merely because the licensee chose to move forward with a particular commercial endeavor that turns out to infringe other patents. There can be exception where the

[20]*Warner Jenkinson Co., Inc. v. Hilton Davis Chemical Co.,* 520 U.S. 17 (1997) and *Festo Corp. v. Shoketsu Kinzoku Kogyo Kabushiki Co., Ltd.,* 56 U.S.P.Q. 2nd 1865 (Fed. Cir. 2000).

licensor warrants that no other licenses are needed to practice a particular invention or where the licensor agrees to indemnify the third party for patent infringement. Rare as such clauses may be, they still do not constitute patent infringement per se, but rather reflect remedies under the license.

Performance of a Government Contract

Where the federal government, through the issuance of a contract, has induced a third party contractee to infringe a patent, that third party is immune from suit, due to the federal government's sovereign immunity. Thus, the patentee's only resort would be a claim against the government for damages. Though the contractee would be immune, it can be party to the damages suit.

Used Solely for Regulatory Submissions

Under the Hatch-Waxman Act, 35 USC §271 was amended as follows:

> It shall not be an act of infringement to make, use, offer to sell, or sell within the United States or import into the United States a patented invention . . . solely for uses reasonably related to the development and submission of information under a Federal law which regulates the manufacture, use, or sale of drugs or veterinary biological products.

The original intent of this statute was to create patent term extension to patentees who faced delays in the regulatory approval process before they could practice their patented inventions (e.g., drugs). Since extension for regulatory delays was restored to patentees, Congress believed it only fair to give future competitors an equal opportunity to accomplish their regulatory testing prior to the expiration of existing patent rights. Thus, this statute creates a limited exemption for generic drug manufacturers to complete the necessary approval process *prior* to the expiration of the original patent. However, recent cases have made it clear that "solely" means just that. Thus, if there are other benefits to the potentially infringing act, then the exception will not apply.

Research Exemption

Historically, the courts have recognized an exemption to patent infringement where the alleged infringer is engaging solely in basic research, i.e.,

research that is conducted without commercial purpose. However, in recent years the courts have done much to abrogate the exception, and recent cases have all but done away with it. Suffice it to say that *any* university should consider the research exemption null and that it likely applies only to individuals working for their amusement and self-edification.

How to Know If You Are Getting Effective Representation

It is very easy to become complacent when dealing with outside patent counsel and simply rely on the status quo. Are you really getting good service though? On the other hand, outside counsel may fail to live up to your expectations. Are you expectations reasonable? Here are a few tips to apply when reviewing outside counsel's performance.

The number one complaint against attorneys in the United States is nonresponsiveness: if your calls are not returned promptly, and/or work product is not completed on time, you are probably not getting quality representation. All good attorneys are busy—that's because people want their time. However, good attorneys budget their time appropriately, decline new representation if they are at capacity, and offer to pay for extensions taken solely because their workload did not permit an earlier response.

A second frequent complaint against attorneys is that they do not explain issues so that the client fully understands what is going on. After you speak with the attorney, you should understand the strategy and why it has been chosen. An attorney's primary job, other than to get results, is to make his or her client feel at ease with the decisions and execution of the strategy. For many of you, your actions will be reviewed and even second-guessed by supervisors and inventors, so you should feel confident that you are doing the right thing. It is the attorney's job to guide you through this process. It is your job, though, to take thorough notes and not ask the attorney to recreate the strategy for you every time you return to the file.

Making inventors happy is a good thing, but sometimes you cannot do that while fulfilling your primary obligation to your employer. Sometimes the attorney needs to play the "bad cop," i.e., take the brunt of the inventors' unhappiness. However, a good attorney usually communicates the message without alienating the inventor. This is important, for example, where the invention simply is not ready for patenting, but when you want to encourage the inventor to return with new data down the road. On the other hand, don't set the attorney up as a sacrificial lamb; make outside counsel aware (if possible) of strong personalities and political undercurrents.

It is also important to be careful how you measure the success of your outside counsel. Simply getting an application allowed quickly can be a hollow victory if the claims do not cover commercially relevant aspects of the invention and/or are easily circumvented. Similarly, an up-front cost-savings can end up costing more money down the road. Still, attorneys should be flexible in dealing with cost constraints. Not every application needs to be the best application ever written, but it is also not fair to pin down your attorney to produce the cheapest application.

If costs are a concern, however, ask for an estimate. An experienced attorney should know an approximate application cost. However, there may be valid reasons why a cost estimate will not hold: you still need to take responsibility for inventors whose inventions evolve during the drafting process or for those who reveal prior art only after the decision to go forward. Cost overruns do occur, but you should hear about these long before the project is finished.

Know, too, that when comparing the prices of various law firms, different firms make their practices profitable in different ways, and, thus, a task-by-task cost comparison may be misleading. In the end, the best assessment is through a start-to-finish cost comparison for comparable technologies.

Finally, even though the attorney and inventor have the most frequent contact during prosecution, the outside counsel must keep you apprised on actions, deadlines, costs and with, just as importantly, the requests of the inventor. More than once, an attorney has lost of sight of the fact that the inventor is *not* the client, incurring unauthorized expenses based purely on the inventor's word. You need to stay involved and to take responsibility for the file, and it is critical that you have some professional quality review of the work product other than of the inventor.

What You Can Do to Make Your Attorney's Life Easier (and to Lower Your Bills)

Finally, some practical advice is offered to help make your job easier:

- First, respond to requests for authorization from outside counsel in a timely fashion, even if it is only to say, "We don't know yet." You must remember that your attorney is watching hundreds of deadlines, and keeping his or her mind on your particular matter is in everyone's interest.

- Second, take responsibility for your inventors. You may have little leverage over your researchers, but your attorney has even less. Thus, when information is needed, and the attorney has tried but failed to get such information, step in and take an active role.

- Third, keep copies of relevant documents and keep your patent files current. Doing so facilitates prompt decision making and avoids the added expense of having counsel retrieve, copy, and resend the information.

- Fourth, be reasonable in your expectation of success. It is not always possible to turn a sow's ear into a silk purse. This becomes particularly important where the inventor's and/or licensee's expectations diverge from those of the institution.

- Fifth, be reasonable in your time constraints. Emergencies come up in life, and your outside counsel will go to extreme lengths to avoid loss of rights. However, don't make waiting to the last minute a habit, as this will eventually lead to serious problems.

- Sixth, once the application is filed, you still need to be involved enough to move the process along. Keep on top of deadlines, request input from your inventors, update outside counsel on the licensing status, and keep everyone apprised of changes in the strategic objectives.

- Seventh, be clear in your instructions and, when asked for information, answer completely (preferably in writing so that the attorney has a written record). Many law firms use forms for securing information on various task. If requested, follow the law firm's procedures to a letter.

- Eighth, a kind word regarding a job well done goes a long way. Knowing that a client appreciates the efforts their attorneys make is likely to motivate an attorney to go the extra yard for that client.

Applying for United States Patent Protection

John S. Child, Jr., JD, B. Litt, and Kathleen D. Rigaut, PhD, JD

Introduction

Affording clever inventors a limited monopoly on their inventive contributions is not a new legal concept. An early patent statute enacted in Venice, Italy in March of 1474 reads:

WE HAVE among us men of great genius, apt to invent and discover ingenious devices; and in view of the grandeur and virtue of our City, more such men come to us every day from diverse parts. Now if provision were made for the works and devices discovered by such persons, so that others who may see them could not build them and take the inventor's honor away, more men would then apply their genius, would discover and would build devises of great utility and benefit to our common wealth. Therefore:

BE IT ENACTED: that, by the authority of this Council, every person who shall build any new and ingenious device in this City, not previously made in our Commonwealth, shall give notice of it to the office of our General Welfare Board when it has been reduced to perfection so that it can be used and operated. It being forbidden to every other person in any of our territories and town to make any further device conforming with and similar to said one, without the consent and license of the author, for the term of 10 years. And if anybody builds it in violation hereof, the aforesaid author and inventor shall be entitled to have him summoned before any magistrate of this City, by which magistrate the said infringer shall be constrained to pay him hundred ducats: and the device

shall be destroyed at once. It being, however, within the power and discretion of the Government, in its activities, to take and use any such device and instrument, with this condition that no one but the author shall operate it.[1]

The framers of the United States Constitution, like the Council in Venice, believed that providing patent protection to inventive Americans was highly desirable to encourage dissemination of new technological developments to the public. Accordingly, Clause 8 of Section 8, Article I of the United States Constitution provides that Congress has power:

To promote the progress of science and the useful arts, by securing for limited times to authors and inventors the exclusive right to their respective writings and discoveries.[2]

In 2003, about 170,000 US patents were issued for an enormous variety of inventions—from toys to computers to food supplements to new drugs. US

---

[1]Mandich, *"Venetian Patents (1450–1550),"* 30 *J. Patient Office Society.* 166 (1948) 172–174.

[2]*The United States Constitution*, Section 8, Article I. Article I led to the creation of the United States patent system. Under Section 271(a) of the United States Patent Law, Title 35 USC 271(a), a patent provides its owner with the right to exclude others from making, using, offering to sell or selling any patented invention within the United States, or to import into the United States any patented invention during the term of the patent.

patents are obtained each year by individuals developing inventions as a hobby and researchers in high tech facilities. Although inventions and inventors may differ, the process for obtaining US patent protection is the same for everyone.

The process for obtaining a US patent begins with filing a patent application with the United States Patent and Trademark Office (hereby referred to in this chapter as "Patent Office" or "Office"). In order for a patent application to issue as a patent, the invention must be new and nonobvious over subject matter already in the public domain or described in the prior art. The invention must also have utility, i.e., it must be useful for its designated purpose. Finally, the application for a patent must describe the invention in such clear and concise terms such that "undue experimentation" is not required to practice the invention as claimed. The patented invention is set forth in one or more claims that follow the description portion of the application.

Types of US Patent Applications

A patent application falls into one of three types, depending on the subject matter for which patent protection is being sought: a design patent application, a plant patent application, or a utility patent application.

Design Patent Application

A design patent application is filed to obtain patent protection for any new, original, and ornamental design for an article of manufacture such as a new lamp or bottle shape. A design patent has a term of 14 years from the date of grant of the patent. If the design of the invention is new, has commercial value, and the inventor would not be entitled to file a utility patent application on the article, design patent protection may provide the only available coverage for the invention. A design patent contains a single claim and a clear and concise description of the design including drawings of the article of manufacture.

Plant Patent Application

To obtain patent protection for a new plant variety, a plant patent application is filed. Although a rose may be a rose by any other name, there have been many plant patents directed to different varieties of roses. A plant patent application consists of a description and drawing or picture of the new variety of plant, a declaration averring that the plant has been asexually reproduced or newly located in a cultivated area, and a single claim to the plant as described and shown. Plant patents and utility patents have terms of 20 years from the earliest filing date of an application that issues into the patent.

Utility Patent Application

Subject Matter of Application The most common type of patent application is the utility or nonprovisional patent application. As indicated in 35 USC § 101, patentable subject matter includes any new and useful process, machine, manufacture, or composition of matter or any new and useful improvement thereof. George Washington's patent for a plow and the Wright Brothers' patent for the airplane are examples respectively of a manufacture and machine.

Patents covering new uses of a composition are also patentable under 35 USC § 101, provided that other conditions for patentability are satisfied. Patented inventions directed to a new use are described in terms of a method for accomplishing the use. A famous example is the patent concerning the use of DDT as an insecticide. At the time of that invention, DDT was a known composition. Accordingly, the patented invention was a method of killing flies by contacting the flies with DDT.

Contents of Application A utility application consists of the following parts: title of the invention; background of the invention; summary of the invention; brief description of the drawings; detailed description of the invention, claims; and drawings and abstract of the disclosure. Also required to be filed with the application is a small entity statement (if appropriate) and an oath or declaration of the inventors stating that they are the true inventors of the subject matter.

The *background of the invention* sets out the problem that the invention solves. The *summary of the invention* should directly track the claim language, providing a "legal fence" around the inventive subject matter: i.e., the definition of the patented invention from which the patent owner can exclude others from making, using and selling, offering to sell, or importing into the United States. The *detailed description of the invention* must be written in such explicit terms that one of ordinary skill in the art to which the invention pertains can make and use the invention as claimed. Importantly, the patent statutes require that the inventor provide the best mode for practicing the invention in order to ensure the invention is truly placed in the hands of the public upon expiration of the patent.

Initial Filing of an Application by Means of a Provisional Application In some circumstances, it is necessary to file a patent application as promptly as possible. This objective is accomplished through filing a provisional application for patent (provisional application), which provides the means to establish an early effective filing date in a design, plant or utility patent application filed under 35 USC 111(a) without a formal patent claim, oath or declaration. It also allows the term "Patent Pending" to be applied to the invention.

The provisional application was designed by the Office to provide a lower-cost first patent filing in the United States and to give the US applicant parity with a foreign applicant under the General Agreement on Tariffs and Trade (GATT) Uruguay Round Agreements.

A provisional application cannot issue as a patent. It has an unextendable pendency of 12 months from the filing date of the provisional application. Therefore, an applicant who files a provisional application must file a corresponding nonprovisional application for patent during the twelve-month pendency period of the provisional application in order to benefit from the earlier filing of the provisional application. In accordance with 35 USC 119(e), the corresponding nonprovisional application must contain or be amended to contain a specific reference to the provisional application.

Preliminary Steps for Preparation of a Patent Application

In order to facilitate preparation of a patent application, many institutions request that their inventors provide a record of invention. A typical question form for inventors appears below. These forms are useful for performing an initial evaluation of the invention as to its commercial value and patentability, identifying the inventor(s), fixing relevant dates of invention, identifying references that may be relevant to the patentability of the invention, as well as honing the inventive concept underlying the technology.

Development of a Record of the Invention

1. Provide a short, descriptive title of the invention.
2. Give a brief summary of the invention, particularly including its novel features and advantages.

3. State when the invention was conceived.
4. Provide the date of the first written record of the invention (e.g., notebook, letter, proposal, or drawing).
5. State when the invention was first successfully tested.
6. State when, under what circumstances, and to whom the invention has been disclosed:
   (a) Orally.
   (b) In writing.
   (c) In actual use or demonstration.
7. Identify any references about the invention, including any patents, patent applications, or other publications of which the inventors are aware and believe to be pertinent to this invention. A copy of such references should be attached.
8. Companies which might be interested in marketing the invention should be suggested.
9. Identify any inventors of the invention's general subjects area.
10. Present a sample claim.

Patentability Search

As the preparation of a patent application is time-consuming and expensive, a prudent, cost-effective step before authorizing the preparation of the application is to request a search for prior art pertinent to the invention. If the subject matter of the invention is already described in the prior art, the invention cannot be patented and there is no benefit obtained from filing a patent application on the invention.

Preservation of Evidence of Conception and Reduction to Practice

Dates of conception and reduction to practice become important in interference proceedings that occur when two or more inventors claim the same invention. In such proceedings, the Patent Office will determine, based on evidence provided by each party (e.g., notebooks, sketches, oral and written communications), which inventor was the first to invent and further, that the invention was not abandoned, suppressed, or concealed. Only the first qualified inventor is granted the right to a patent, as in the celebrated case in which Alexander Graham Bell was determined to become the first inventor granted a patent for the telephone.

Determination of Inventorship

Under 35 USC § 111(a), an application for patent is made or authorized to be made by the inventor or inventors. Such inventors own the subject matter claimed in the patent application unless the inventor has made an assignment of his rights. Accordingly, a determination of who is an inventor is a prerequisite to the filing of an application. Inventorship is a legal determination. A sole invention is the conception by one person of the solution to a problem, i.e., the means to the desired end, which constitutes the subject matter of the invention set forth in the claims. A joint invention occurs when more than one person contributes to the conception of the solution to a problem. According to a 1984 amendment to the US patent statutes, inventors may apply for a patent jointly even though: (i) they did not physically work together or at the same time; (ii) each did not make the same type or amount of contribution, or (iii) each did not make a contribution to the subject matter of every claim of the patent.

One becomes an inventor neither by merely suggesting a desired end or result, with no suggestion of the means for accomplishing it, nor by merely following the instructions of the person or persons who actually did conceive the solution. By the same token, one who merely contributes an obvious element to an invention is not considered a joint inventor. Moreover, including someone as a coauthor on a journal article does not necessarily imply that such a person is a coinventor.

It is possible to correct the inventive entity by petition and an averment that the error in determining inventorship occurred without deceptive intent on the part of the true inventors of the subject matter. Notably, a patent listing an incorrect inventive entity may be invalidated if it can be shown that the error in inventorship determination was made with deceptive intent.

Preparation of the Application

In order to provide the best possible coverage of the commercial value of the invention, a patent application should be drafted by a competent patent attorney. The time required by the attorney to draft the application may be reduced by having the inventor involved in the drafting process. The inventor can help by drafting a paper describing the features of the invention and by providing detail of any laboratory work related to the invention, including the best mode for practicing the invention. The inventor should keep the patent attorney apprised of all prior art and distinguish the art from the invention.

As noted, the invention record should include claims that declare the subject matter as patented. Ideally, the inventor assists the patent attorney in drafting these claims that are respectively broad, intermediate, and narrow in scope.

Broad claims have few words because each word can potentially limit the terms of a claim. For example, compare the following two claims:

1. A chair.
2. A blue chair with three legs.

Each additional word in Claim 2 limits the scope of protection afforded by the "legal fence." Accordingly, Claim 1 encompasses chairs of all colors and leg number, while Claim 2 is limited to blue chairs with three legs only.

Claims may be independent or dependent. Claims 1 and 2 above are independent. An example of a dependent claim is provided as Claim 3:

3. The chair as claimed in Claim 1, which is three-legged and blue.

Dependent claims provide further limitations that do not exist in the broader independent claims. The breadth of the claims decreases as further features are added.

For utility patent applications, claims are generally directed to the subject matter of the invention, i.e., a machine, manufacture, or composition of matter and a process of making the machine, manufacture, or composition of matter. Claims to the machine, manufacture, or composition of matter are usually more valuable than process claims. Potential licensees of the patented invention are most interested in having an exclusive right to manufacture, use and/or sell a product. In addition, many products can be made by a process other than the patented process so that claims to a process for making a product may not prevent others from making the product.

In summary, a patent application should be prepared and prosecuted in order to obtain a patent having claims that cover the invention in a manner that would enable the owner of the patent to prevent others from freely adopting the commercially valuable features of the invention.

Filing the Patent Application

Once the specification and claims sections of the application have been completed, and the correct inventive entity determined, a patent application may be filed with the Office. An application filed with the Oath or Declaration and the filing fee comprises a complete application. As noted above, the applicant is either the inventor absent an assignment of title to the application, or the assignee of such an assignment. The application may be filed without the fee or declaration. The applicant then receives a notice to file missing parts. Upon filing the declaration, fee, and surcharge for filing an incomplete application, the application will be deemed completed and given the filing date of initial receipt in the Patent Office. In connection with filing the application, the applicant should inform the Patent Office whether or not the applicant is entitled to claim small entity status. If the applicant is entitled to claim small entity status, all patent fees are reduced by half. Small entity status is afforded to individual inventors, small businesses with not more than 500 employees, and nonprofit organizations such as universities, provided the application has not been licensed by the university to a business which is not entitled to claim small entity status.

Prosecution of a Patent Application before the United States Patent and Trademark Office

The decision of whether to allow a patent application to issue as a patent is made by an official of the Office known as an examiner. This decision generally results following an exchange of papers concerning the patentability of the claimed subject matter between the examiner in the form of official actions and responses to the actions by the attorney representing the applicant. This process is customarily referred to as the prosecution of the application.

Duty of Disclosure

During the prosecution of the application, the applicant and other interested persons have certain responsibilities. An applicant seeking patent protection before the Office has a duty of candor. According to 37 CFR 1.56:

> Each individual associated with the filing and prosecution of a patent application has a duty of candor and good faith in dealing with the Office, which includes a duty to disclose to the Office, all information known to that individual to be material to patentability. . . . The duty to disclose information exists with respect to each pending claim until the claim is cancelled or withdrawn

from consideration, or the application becomes abandoned.

Accordingly, the inventor and any other individual associated with the filing and prosecution of the application has a duty to supply the patent examiner with prior art of which they are aware that is known to be material to the patentability of each of the pending claims. A failure to satisfy this duty constitutes a fraud on the Office and, if discovered, may invalidate the patent.

Relevant information is submitted to the Patent Office accompanied by an information disclosure statement (IDS) and a PTO 1449 form listing the references to be considered. At this time, the examiner performs a prior art search to identify relevant prior art and lists any references or patents identified on a PTO 892 form. It is important to submit the IDS and PTO 1449 form prior to receipt of a first official action on the merits as submission of prior art after a first action, but before a second and generally final action, requires payment of a fee. [See 37 CFR §1.97(c).]

Restriction Requirements

The claims of a patent application may often encompass more than one patentably distinct invention. For example, a patent application directed to a new gene that encodes a protein involved in the progression of cancer will often contain claims to the nucleic acid encoding the protein, the protein itself, an antibody having binding affinity for the protein, and a method for detection of the protein or nucleic acid for determining cancer progression. After approximately 14 months of pendency before the Office, the applicant often receives a restriction requirement, wherein an examiner divides the claims into groups of distinct inventions. In the example above, the nucleic acid encoding the protein would comprise one invention; the protein and fragments thereof would comprise a second invention; and claims directed to antibodies against the protein would fall into yet a third group. Whether or not the method claims would be included in any of the foregoing groups is at the discretion of the examiner. Normally, the examiner only examines one group of claims per application.

The applicant may, however, traverse the restriction and present arguments that the different groups are not directed to separate and distinct inventions. Traversing the requirement preserves the right to petition the commissioner as to whether or not the restriction is proper. However, in order to be fully responsive to the requirement, the applicant must elect one of the groups for further prosecution. Since patent term is calculated as of the filing date, the applicant may consider filing one or more divisional applications on the other groups of inventions. A divisional application is a later application for a distinct or independent invention carved out of a pending application and disclosing and claiming only subject matter disclosed in the earlier or parent applications. Delay in filing such divisional applications results in a loss of patent term which, as noted above, is 20 years from the initial filing date of the utility and plant parent patent applications.

Examiner's Action on the Patentability of the Claims

Rejections of Claims Based on Prior Art and Applicant's Response to the Rejection   Once a group is elected for further prosecution, the applicant receives a first official action on the patentable merits of the claims. In the first action, the examiner will typically reject the claims over prior art and may also raise enablement issues. Prior art rejections can take two forms. In a rejection made under 35 USC 102, the examiner relies on a single prior art reference to make a rejection based on a lack of novelty. In other words, the examiner contends the prior art reference discloses each and every element of the claim and therefore anticipates the invention. In a rejection made under 35 USC §103, the examiner relies on one or a combination of references asserting that the reference(s) renders the invention, as claimed, obvious to one of ordinary skill in the art.

In refuting rejections based on prior art, the applicant has several options. The applicant can argue that the examiner has not considered an essential element of the claims, which confers patentability over the prior art cited. The applicant may wish to amend the claims in such a way that they no longer read on the prior art. By means of a declaration, the applicant can provide further evidence of patentability, or evidence that the claimed invention was conceived of and reduced to practice before the effective filing date of the reference in order to remove the reference as prior art. It is often necessary both to argue against the merits of the rejection and amend the claims.

Rejection of Claims Based on the Specification or as Indefinite and Applicant's Response   The examiner may also reject the claims and/or specification under 35 USC §112, first paragraph, for inadequate enablement and/or inadequate written description. The examiner may reject claims under 35 USC §112, second paragraph, as indefinite for failing to particularly point out and distinctly claim the subject matter regarded as the invention. In response to these types of rejections, the applicant can direct the examiner's attention to the enabling sections of the disclosure or prior art that enables the invention. It is well-settled that a patent application need not disclose, and preferably omits, that which is well known to those of skill in the art. An examiner may assert that certain terms in the claims lack clear meaning. These types of rejections may be overcome by providing evidence that the term is readily understood by those of skill in the art. Such evidence may include definitions from the dictionary or technical manuals.

A complete response to the first official action must address all of the issues raised by the examiner. A failure to overcome all rejections of the claims will result in the issuance of a final official action. A statutory period of six months is given to respond to the first official action. If the response is filed within the first three months of receipt, no fee is required. Extensions of time are available for the fourth, fifth, and sixth months with payment of extension fees that increase with the passage of time from approximately $110 to $420 to $950, respectively. If the applicant qualifies for small entity status and licenses the application only to a licensee that qualifies for small entity status, the rates are reduced by half.

Further Prosecution of the Application

After the applicant's response to a first official action on the merits, the applicant can anticipate receipt of either a second official action, a final official action or, if the examiner is convinced by the arguments presented, a notice of allowance. A second nonfinal official action is received if the examiner raises new issues, such as art not of record in the first official action. Upon receipt of a notice of allowance, the applicant has up to three months to attend to payment of the issue fee.

Receipt of a final official action indicates that the examiner was not convinced that the arguments and claim amendments, if any, place the application in condition for allowance. The applicant's options to provide further evidence of patentability in the form of the declarations and present claim amendments after a final rejection are limited as such evidence and amendments are entered only at the discretion of the examiner. Generally, an examiner will refuse to enter such evidence and amendments after a final action if they introduce new matter for search and consideration. In such cases, the examiner will forward an advisory action to the applicant explaining why the amendment was not entered, or if it was entered, why it does not place the claims in condition for allowance.

After the issuance of a final action, the applicant has six months to take one of the following steps: obtain allowance of the application by further communicating with the examiner, file a request for continued examination (RCE), file a continuation application (i.e., a second application that contains the same disclosure as the original application), or appeal the decision.

If the applicant has obtained further compelling data regarding enablement and nonobviousness of the claims, the RCE or a continuation application may be filed. As mentioned above, it is extremely difficult to have such data entered during prosecution after a final official action. If the RCE is filed, the examiner must consider such evidence that can result in the issuance of a notice of allowance.

Appeal of Examiner's Final Action Rejecting the Claims

If the applicant disagrees with the examiner's position, a notice of appeal to the board of patent appeals and interferences is filed. Within the appropriate time period, the applicant must file an appeal brief and fee and must set forth the authorities and arguments on which the appellant will rely to maintain the appeal. The brief shall contain the following items under appropriate headings:

1. A statement identifying the real party in interest;
2. A statement identifying by number and filing date all other appeals or interferences known to appellant that will directly affect or be directly affected by the board's decision;
3. A statement of the status of all the claims, pending or canceled and identifying the claims appealed;
4. A statement of the status of any amendment filed subsequent to a final rejection;
5. A concise explanation of the invention defined in the claims involved in the appeal;
6. A concise statement of the issues presented for review;
7. A grouping of the claims; and
8. A statement of the appellant's position on the issues which refute the assertions made by the examiner in support of the final rejection of the claims.

The primary examiner may furnish a written statement in answer to the appellant's brief including such explanation of the invention claimed and of the

references and grounds of rejection as may be necessary. The examiner may not introduce a new ground of rejection at this time. If the appellant desires an oral hearing to better present the issues to the board, such a request must be made within two months of the examiner's answer. The appellant may also file a reply brief to the examiner's answer. If the appellant's arguments are compelling, an examiner may withdraw the final rejection and reopen prosecution. In cases where the examiner is still not convinced that the claims are patentable, the receipt of the reply brief will be acknowledged and the reply brief entered into the prosecution history. The appellant then awaits the decision of the board, which may affirm or reverse the decision of the examiner in whole or in part. In cases where the rejection is upheld, the applicant may file an appeal of the board's decision to the US Court of Appeals for the Federal Circuit or file a civil action. Currently, it takes approximately three years to conduct the appeal process.

Action After Notice of Allowance

Upon receipt of the notice of allowance, the claims in the allowed application should be reviewed with the inventor to determine whether the claims cover the patented invention. As noted, consideration should be given to filing a divisional or continuation application if the allowed claims do not cover all the commercial features of the invention. Also as noted, if, during prosecution of the allowed application, the inventor developed improvements to the invention, such improvements may be incorporated in a continuation-in-part application claiming priority from the allowed application. A continuation-in-part application is a second application repeating some substantial portion or all of the earlier application and adding matter not disclosed in the allowed application. In order to properly claim priority to the allowed parent patent application, such divisional, continuation, or continuation-in-part applications must be filed when the parent application is pending, i.e., before its issuance as a patent.

Commercialization of the Patented Invention

One theme of this chapter has been to suggest ways of applying for US patent protection that protects the most valuable features of the invention. This objective is important in order for the applicant to license the patent or otherwise commercialize the patented invention. As the applicant's success may, in fact, be measured by the ability to obtain revenue from licensing the patent, the following suggestions may be helpful toward accomplishing that goal.

Identifying Potential Licensees

As noted above, the invention record should include an identification of companies interested in licensing the invention. Efficient licensing of patented inventions must start with identifying and contacting companies that are likely to be interested in the patented invention. An initial step in any contract is to determine whether the company has any history of licensing patented inventions.

Obtaining License Initiation Fee

Most licenses provide for a royalty based on a percentage of licensee's sales of products coming within the patented invention. As most patented inventions are not successfully commercialized, the applicant should try to obtain a license initiation fee upon execution of the license to ensure receipt of some revenue from the license.

Shifting Burden of Costs of Patent Program to Licensor

In any license agreement, the applicant should try to have the licensor bear costs relating to the maintenance and prosecution of the licensed patent applications. This objective is particularly desirable if the applicant is trying to obtain foreign patents based on US patent application.

Conclusion

The foregoing provides a brief overview of the process of obtaining US patent protection. As the preparation and prosecution of a patent application is a complex process, it is highly recommended that the applicant enlist the aid of a patent attorney. In the case of university clients, it is often necessary to retain the services of patent attorneys of several firms to find patent attorneys who have the requisite technical expertise in the various technologically diverse areas of academic research.

66

Marketing University Technology: Selling the Promise

Richard Kordal, PhD

Introduction

In some respects the marketing of university technology or intellectual property is not unlike the marketing of consumer products. You must know your customers and target your advertisements to their market sector. Since all products have a limited lifecycle, you should perform your marketing and selling (or more accurately, "licensing") while the window of opportunity is still open. Unlike fine wine, the value of technology declines with age as new and improved technologies are developed. In the extreme case, older technologies become obsolete.

There are also many differences that make the marketing of university technology and associated intellectual property uniquely challenging. For example, unlike a consumer product that people can actually touch, feel, see, and easily compare against the competition, most often what we are "selling" is something intangible, at most an issued patent but often just a pending patent application that represents a promise of a product. Given the basic nature of university research, rarely do you have a prototype to show. It takes vision to get your hands around the potential products and all the uncertainties and risks that come with such early stage technology. Not only are there product development risks to contend with, but with pending patent applications there is also the uncertainty over what, if any, claims may ultimately be allowed. Until the patent actually issues, the issue of claims remains an unknown. At best all one can do is to assess the probability that commercially important claims will issue. Perversely, this sometimes works

to one's advantage. Typically a patent application is drafted with a broad set of claims that is narrowed (or eliminated) during the examination process. Therefore, a potential licensee must at least give some weight to the chance that these broadly written claims may issue; and because of this, many companies only license issued patents, and/or apply such a discount to the royalty rate of pending patent applications as to not be worth the effort of negotiating a license.

Another significant difference between marketing actual products and university intellectual property is that university technology has a "pedigree"; universities do not simply market a product, but also market the reputation and track record of its inventor. A Howard Hughes Fellow or Nobel Laureate inventor adds significant creditability (and thus value) to the technology. Other inventor factors that nudge up the value of university technology include whether the inventor is a strong proponent of the technology; has a reputation as being cooperative; is still active in the area (i.e., doesn't have a new research focus); and expresses a willingness to work with industry (e.g., accepts industrial-sponsored research to further a product's development).

Universities have not escaped the shortened product cycle phenomenon that has faced most industries. Once the decision is made to risk money on a new, unlicensed technology and to file a US patent application, the clock starts ticking as to when foreign applications must be filed, prosecuted, and ultimately nationalized. Generally the cost of preparing and filing a US and Patent Cooperation Treaty (PCT) (for certain foreign countries) application is small compared to the prosecution costs and costs of nationalizing foreign counterparts and because of the large expense, most universities cannot afford to nationalize the original PCT application in a wide number of member countries (beyond maybe one or two major countries) without first having a licensee willing to foot the bill. With PCT applications, a common strategy is to delay the nationalization through the filing of a Chapter II demand for preliminary examination. In this way, the decision to nationalize to thirty months after the filing of the original US application can be put off. This strategy, though helpful, still only gives the institution a two-and-half-year window during which to find a licensee before incurring large patent expenses.

If the researcher has no immediate plans to publish the discovery, then the filing of the patent application and marketing of the technology nonconfidentially can be delayed at least until which time the decision has been made to publish the findings. The risk of this strategy is that another inventor might make the same invention and then file foreign applications. Most foreign countries, unlike the United States, which grants a patent to the first to invent (and diligently reduce to practice), grant the patent to the first party to file.

Development of Marketing Strategy

In developing the technology marketing plan, it is important to ask, "What problem does the technology solve and who stands to directly benefit from it?" The answer to these questions help to clarify how best to market the technology. For example, if the technology helps to cure a particular disease like diabetes, the beneficiaries of the technology (aside from diabetics themselves) are the firms already marketing therapeutic products to diabetics. These firms should be the first targets for licensing this technology. It should be noted that the preferred market targets are the companies that are already involved in the target market. A company with only a fringe connection to the target market can be as bad as a company with no connection to the market at all (for example, a therapeutic technology to a firm only supplying syringes or lancets to diabetics).

If the technology has broader application, then it is important to identify all industries and industry segments that might have an interest in the technology. This is a thorough approach that helps to ensure that no licensing opportunities are overlooked and increases the likelihood that the same

technology can be licensed to multiple parties for separate and distinct applications or "fields of use" (discussed later in greater detail). The biomedical industry contains many segments (pharmaceutical or therapeutic, diagnostic and medical device) and some industry segments are further subdivided; the pharmaceutical industry, for example, includes firms that concentrate exclusively on the development of biotherapeutics (e.g., recombinant proteins like insulin) and firms that specialize on the development of small molecule drugs.

To successfully identify the profiles of all the possible licensing candidates in all the possible industry segments/subcategories, the university licensing professional must take pains to create a plate of spaghetti out of the technology (i.e., brainstorm all possible applications of the technology), build a "wall" from all known relevant industry segments/subcategories, then throw this spaghetti plate against the wall. What "sticks" on the wall as a result tells what you can license and to whom. While the spaghetti plate analogy is literally wasteful and messy, the following illustration may make the concept more appetizing.

To make the "spaghetti," assume that a researcher discovers a new gene that controls the expression of protein regulating cardiac function through the modulation of a cardiac receptor. Further assume that he or she has discovered a mutation in the gene that leads to the overproduction of the protein modulator; left unchecked, the condition can lead to cardiac disease. Fortunately, the researcher has identified a family of compounds that can bind to the protein modulator and inhibit its effect on the receptor. At this point, the university technology officer steps in to take the "dough" of the researchers' discovery and make the plate of spaghetti. As the research officer cooks, he should ask: What uses might these compounds have? Are they useful in their own right, useful as research tools, or both? After recognizing the significance of these discoveries, the technology transfer office files comprehensive patents on the inventions.

Next, the research officer builds the wall, which involves the natural industry segments/subcategories, including diagnostics firms, pharmaceutical firms, and RNA interference firms.

Finally, it is time to throw the spaghetti against the wall. What has stuck? Diagnostic firms that develop genetic tests may be interested in licensing the technology for the in vitro diagnostic or pharmacogenomics field of use in order to screen people for the presence of the mutation. More traditional diagnostic firms that develop routine antibody-based tests may have an interest in licensing the technology to develop immunoassays for measuring the level of the protein modulator to determine if it is abnormally high. Additionally, pharmaceutical firms may be interested in the protein modulator as a drug screening target to identify new compounds that may be more efficacious or safe. Alternatively, they may wish to license the class of compounds already discovered. New RNA interference firms may also find the technology interesting from the standpoint of developing drugs that provide a therapeutic benefit by interfering with the gene expression of the protein modulator.

Performing the "spaghetti exercise" not only helps identify potential licensees, but also helps to identify how the technology can be licensed exclusively to more than one licensee by granting each a license to one particular industry segment. To do so, the licenses should include "fields of use" restrictions tailored to the particular industry segments. Since the licensees will not be developing products in the same industry areas, competition among them should not be an issue.

Conduct Market Research

Once a marketing strategy that identifies a profile of licensing candidates in industry segments has been developed, typically the next step is to find actual companies that fit the profile and to identify the companies' key contacts. The aim here is to use a rifle rather than a shotgun approach by identifying companies with a realistic interest in the technology. To find companies that fit the strategy profile, a number of sources of information should be consulted, including business databases such as BioScan and CorpTech.

BioScan, published by American Health Consultants (a division of The Thomson Corporation), contains information on over 1,800 international companies involved in biotech product R&D. The directory service also contains detailed company profiles, including information on new products in development. Their service is available online, on CD-ROM, or in print form.

CorpTech, produced by OneSource Information Services, Inc., contains company profiles on over 50,000 public and private US technology companies. Companies in the CorpTech database are categorized within 17 high-tech industries and by 250 major technology codes and 3,000 product codes (SIC and NAICS codes are also included). The high-tech industries covered in the CorpTech database include:

1) advanced materials, 2) biotechnology, 3) chemicals, 4) computer hardware, 5) computer software, 6) defense, 7) energy, 8) environmental, 9) factory automation, 10) holding companies, 11) manufacturing equipment, 12) medical, 13) pharmaceuticals, 14) photonics, 15) subassemblies and components, 16) test and measurement, and 17) transportation. The CorpTech database is available as a tiered subscription service online, via CD-ROM, or in print. Individual company reports can also be accessed on a pay-per-view basis. There are several types of subscriptions: a high-end gold subscription for unlimited access and downloading of the CorpTech database, which can be downloaded into MS-Excel or comma-delimited formats, a silver subscription service that does not include download services but offers unlimited viewing of the database, and a special library service to public and university libraries. On CorpTech's database, companies can be searched by name, geography (state, MSA, or zip code) or by product (industry, SIC, NAICS, or CorpTech Codes).

Knowledge Express offers a convenient, one-stop way to search several key business databases from one portal. The firm provides unlimited use of over 25 different proprietary databases (including BioScan and CorpTech).

Organizations (both companies and universities) issue press releases and news stories to the major news wire services (e.g., PR Newswire, BusinessWire) each day about major events in technology licensing (pending mergers and technical breakthroughs). Often these press releases and new stories appear in newspapers around the country. In addition, regional and national business papers or journals (e.g., *Wall Street Journal, Cincinnati Business Courier,* and *Indianapolis Business Journal*) continually report on the business activities of companies around the globe. Daily news releases can be accessed by visiting the news wire service Web sites directly. Individual.com, for example, classifies the day's news stories into categories (e.g., health care) and subcategories (AIDS, Alzheimer's, etc.) to facilitate searching for relevant news releases. The site allows registered users to create individual profiles where fields or areas of interest can be specified. When a breaking news story matches one of the fields, the service emails the story to the user. These stories often provide valuable information about a company's business strategy and future product development plans.

While convenient for monitoring or tracking new developments, such Web sites do not serve as sources to conduct market research because they usually only list current stories (older stories are typically deleted). To research a complete history of a company's business news stories and other public information, one generally has to turn to a service like Lexis-Nexis that collects and archives such information. The academic version of Lexis-Nexis is available at most university libraries.

While all of the databases described here require the user to perform the searches personally, service provided by Nerac, Inc. does not. The firm has a large staff of information specialists with expertise in a variety of disciplines—many staff have had careers in science or engineering and are proficient at searching the firm's proprietary databases. Information requests are submitted to Nerac staff and the results are returned by e-mail, usually within a couple of days. Fees for the service are based on a usage structure and annual subscription rates.

Though often overlooked, the most valuable resources in conducting market research are inventors themselves. A recent study found that inventors were responsible for leading approximately 50% of academic technology transfer licensing deals.[1] This finding is not surprising given that many academic researchers have consultant and/or collaborative relationships with members of industry and frequently rub shoulders with leading industrial scientists at conferences and scientific meetings. As a result of this interaction, inventors come to know the industrial landscape well, and understand the areas in which different companies operate. One of the advantages of using inventors as lead sources is that generally they can put you into direct contact with the scientist of the company who is able to champion the technology from the technical, rather than business, standpoint.

Often licensing leads are found by reviewing job advertisements in weekly scientific periodicals, for example, *Science* and *Chemical and Engineering News*, published by the American Association for the Advancement for Science and American Chemical Society, respectively—organizations with large memberships. These publications with significant readership are widely used by industry to advertise job openings. In addition to listing job qualifications, job advertisements can include great detail about the company's research focus, products, and other key information about the company and, as a result, these advertisements can often provide information about potential licensees.

Some specialty companies organize conferences on the hot topics du jour (e.g., angiogenesis, stem cells, etc.), including companies like Strategic Research Institute.[2] Often these conferences are packed with speakers from industry who are recruited specifically for being active and well-known in their fields. Often included in the conference brochures or flyers are speakers' affiliations, which can provide contact information. Similarly, International Business Forum Conferences[3] are directed primarily toward business executives on research-related business topics (e.g., venture investing in biopharmaceuticals). These conferences are excellent sources for business contacts and are typically attended by venture capitalists, chief executive officers, new business development executives, and corporate decision makers.

Many companies have a long tradition of leveraging their internal R&D capabilities through partnerships, alliances, collaborations and in-licensing of new technology. A recent article in *Businessweek* indicates a growing trend among companies to look for technology externally and to be open to "forging ties with university labs even if this means sharing prized intellectual property rights."[4] At a recent Licensing Executives Society meeting,[5] Scott Foraker, Vice President of Licensing at Amgen, Inc. remarked that they expect that only 30% to 50% of their new products will be the result of in-licensing activity. Lately, Amgen has been receiving more than 2,000 in-licensing opportunities annually. Firms like AstraZeneca post detailed information about their licensing process on their Web sites[6] and include areas of interest, company wish lists, and contact information of the licensing managers. It is not uncommon for large companies like AstraZeneca to list technology licensing responsibilities by business focus (e.g., therapeutic areas like infectious diseases or cardiovascular diseases) and/or by territory (e.g., North America, Asia, Europe). Thus very often information about a company's licensing interests can be found on a company's Web site.

Other useful sources of information to consult regarding company interests and business activities are business newsletters like *BioWorld Today*[7] (published by BioWorld Publishing Group, a division of Thomson BioWorld) and *BioCentury*®[8] (published by BioCentury Publications Inc). The publications provide business intelligence on the biotech industry. Many industry organizations (e.g., Biotechnology Industry Organization or Bio)[9] maintain alphabetized lists of their membership on their Web sites; lists, which commonly include links to the member company's Web site address. In addition there are industry specific directories to consult: some are online (e.g., *Genetic Engineering News Biotechnology Database*)[10] and others are available in print (e.g., *Peak Publishing, Inc. Regional Life Science*

Directory[11] that conveniently organizes companies by geographical region.)

If others have been busy patenting technology similar to that you are attempting to license, you may be able to take advantage of "patent mining" software tools that can help identify potential licensees through analysis of patent citation linkages. Firms like Wisdomain[12] and Metrics Groups[13] offer services to identify patents (held by others) that cite or reference your patent in their specification. This information can be a good indication of who might have an interest in your technology. In addition, most of versions of the software have capabilities that can determine how frequently your patent is cited in other publications or patents. This metric is generally a good measure of the value of the technology because there is a strong and positive correlation between the value of a patent and frequency of its citation; the more frequent the citation, the greater its value.

Typically, the type of information one gathers from searching the business databases and the other sources is of high level staff, for example, about the upper management (e.g., chief executive officer, president, etc.). It is, after all, important to get information into the right hands, as it is to get to know the names of the people within the company who assess new technologies and/or negotiate license agreements (i.e., the licensing or business development manager). One way to ascertain this information is to cross-reference the target company information against the Association for Technology Managers[14] and/or Licensing Executives Society[15] membership directories, which include companies' technology scouts (it is necessary to update this information on an ongoing basis).

Types of Marketing

There are many different ways to get the word out or to market technology. In general it is best to reach out to potential licensees in different ways. The most commonly employed method of marketing technology today is through direct mail, where typically a packet of information is sent for review containing as much nonconfidential information about the technology as possible (e.g., an executive summary, copies of published journal articles, copies of issue patents, etc.).

Although cost-effective, direct mail has some notable drawbacks: information sent to most large companies needs to be in an easily disseminated form that can be captured electronically for storage in their databases. The main reason for this is that most reviews are conducted by a team or group composed of technical, business, and legal personnel and, therefore, it is easier for companies to distribute information to all team members electronically. Hardcopy form requires photocopying and/or scanning, which can invariably lead to review delay.

For this reason e-mail is overtaking regular mail as the preferred means to market technology. Another big advantage of e-mail is that by sending the information electronically, one can get some immediate indication as to whether or not the contact person is still employed at the company: for example, a bounced e-mail reply can quickly indicate that new contact information is needed, not so readily understood via regular mail service.

Difficulties associated with receiving information by regular mail have led some companies, for example, Abbott Laboratories,[16] to only accept information electronically, which requires that before an electronic submission can be made, one must agree to the company's policy regarding electronic submissions.

In addition to e-mail and regular mail, most universities market technology passively via the Internet by listing all available technologies and issued patents on their technology transfer offices' Web sites (see, for example, the University of Cincinnati's Intellectual Property Office Web site).[17] To make searching convenient, institutional Web sites often list the technologies in groups or according to field area (e.g., life sciences or physical sciences). Some regional and affiliated institutions have attempted to post all technology developments within a single site, notably Harvard University and its affiliated hospitals, via Harvard Biomedical Community Gateway.[18] For the most part, however, institutions prefer to maintain individual Web sites because of the need to ensure the accuracy of the information. Therefore, most often, it is necessary to search institutional Web sites individually.

A recent development in the marketing of university technology has been the advent of online technology transfer brokering forms. The pioneer and leading online network for technology transfer in the life sciences is TechEx™,[19] originally created by Jon Garen, a former Yale University technology transfer professional, and operated by Yale University (the company was recently acquired by UTEK Corporation).

The TechEx system works as follows: at one end, companies register their contact information (i.e., name and address) along with a list of technologies they are seeking to acquire. These "wish lists" are kept confidential. On the other end, universities (technology owners) post descriptions about their available technologies. If keywords are matched in these listings, TechEx sends an email to the company with a description of the university technology and notes to the university contact, to whom the information has been sent. The list of recipients is continually updated as additional companies whose profiles match the search criteria become subscribers to the service. After reviewing the technology description, if the company desires additional information, it then is able to contact the university representative directly. At present, TechEx provides this match-making service free of charge to universities and other nonprofits, but charges potential licensees (for-profit companies) a subscription fee for the service.

Since the establishment of TechEx, several companies have sprung up trying to duplicate the TechEx business model, but with unique variation. Some of these companies include University Ventures,[20] Pharma-Transfer,[21] Yet2.com,[22] and Pharmalicensing.[23] Some older, more established firms like Knowledge Express and Micropatent are also upgrading their traditional methods of promoting or advertising university technologies.

In addition to charging the for-profit companies a subscription fee, some companies also charge a success fee for making a successful match that results in a deal between the parties (i.e., licensor and licensee). The success fee is generally some percentage of the overall license fee.

One company, Pharma-Transfer, actively solicits faculty to publish current research summaries (of 250 words) on the Pharma-Transfer Web site that are then distributed to corporate subscribers. Users of the Pharma-Transfer service should note that although the site warns users about posting confidential information (that could jeopardize future patent rights), many faculty can easily miss or overlook this warning.

One way inventors can help to market technology is by writing a Scientific American-type article in a trade journal. Each major industry has dedicated trade journals, for example, *In Vitro Diagnostics*, *Advance Laboratory*, and *LabMedica International* are journals, for the vitro diagnostic industry; *Medical Device & Diagnostic Industry* is a publication for the medical device industry; *Pharmaceutical Technology*, *BioPharma*, and *Modern Drug Discovery* for the pharmaceutical industry; *Genetic Engineering News* and *Biotech Lab International* cover the biotechnology indus-

try; and, for general industry coverage, there is *R&D*. One of the advantages of publishing in a trade journal is to reach a wider audience than through technical journals because trade journals are read by business personnel as well as scientists. A well-written article in a trade journal can capture the attention of a business manager.

If the invention or discovery is of major importance, a press release, developed with the help of the institution's public relations office, may be warranted. Press releases are distributed to the mass media, often published in newspapers and weekly news magazines, and often reported on the evening TV news. Once a release is issued, it is important to become available to answer questions from news reporters. Obviously press releases have the best potential to generate general public and, therefore, market interest in a new technology.

Displaying technology at regional and national conferences is another excellent way to market your technology because it encourages one-on-one interaction. Some organizations, like Association of University of Technology Managers (AUTM) and Licensing Executives Society, have created networking fairs at their annual meetings to give universities and other service providers (e.g., law firms) the opportunity to exhibit their technology and/or products to conference attendees. Recently, *Scientific American* has begun to offer licensors the opportunity to advertise technology in the journal. Some magazines, like Cahner's *R&D*, have sections dedicated exclusively to new and interesting emerging technologies from academia.

It is a good practice to keep track of the mailings (or e-mailings) made and the responses that they generate. This is particularly important as it can provide an opportunity to reassess your marketing plan if it appears a marketing campaign is striking out (not leading to any inquires). This information is also useful for institutions that send out annual reports to inventors reporting the results of marketing.

Future

In the future, the importance of the Internet will enhance an institution's efforts to market its technologies. However, the Internet will never replace the human element. E-mail is already replacing regular mail, and we envision a day where technology transfer offices' Web sites will be supplemented with multimedia presentations, including the advent of video conferencing to host technology transfer networking fairs.

The best way to achieve successful technology marketing is through a two-step process: one must first conduct market research to identify target companies, then complete the actual marketing of the technology. Recently, Techqusition, Inc.[24] has launched a brokering Web site that combines the market research and marketing functions. The services also allow sellers and buyers of technology to communicate and negotiate their needs and available technologies to one another.

Marketing an institution's technology is not easy. With the increasing amount of resources and information about potential licensees that are available to a technology transfer office, it takes a significant amount of effort to do an effective job. However, the completion of a license deal makes all the effort worthwhile.

Acknowledgment

The author wishes to gratefully acknowledge the helpful suggestions and comments provided by Dan O'Neill, Associate Director at the University of Cincinnati.

• • • References

1. Jansen, C., and Dillon, H. "Where Do the Leads for Licenses Come From? Source Data from Six Institutions." *Journal University Technology Managers XI* (1999): 51–66.

2. Strategic Research Institute Web site, http://www.srinstitute.com (accessed June 10, 2005).

3. International Business Forum Conferences Web site, http://www.ibfconferences.com (accessed June 10, 2005).

4. Greene, J., Carey, J., Arndt M., and Port O. "Reinventing Corporate R&D." *Businessweek*, June 10, 2005, 74–76.

5. Foraker, S. "Plenary Session, Leaders of Corporate Licensing Panel Discussion." Presentation at the Licensing Executives Society 39th annual meeting, San Diego, CA, September 21–25, 2003.

6. AstraZeneca International, "Licensing," http://www.astrazeneca.com/Article/11223.aspx (accessed June 10, 2005).

7. BioWorld Online Web site, http://www.bioworld.com (accessed June 10, 2005).

8. BioCentury Web site, http://www.biocentury.com (accessed June 10, 2005).

9. Biotechnology Industry Organization Web site, http://www.bio.org (accessed June 10, 2005).

10. Genetic Engineering News, "Biotechnology Database," http://www.gendirectonline.com (accessed June 10, 2005).

11. Available from Peak Publishing, Inc., PO Box 54051, Cincinnati, OH 45254.

12. Wisdomain Web site, http://www.wisdomain.com (accessed June 10, 2005).

13. Metrics Group Web site, http://www.metricsgroup.com (accessed June 10, 2005).

14. Association of University Technology Managers Web site, http://www.autm.net (accessed June 10, 2005).

15. Licensing Executives Society Web site, http://www.les.org (accessed June 10, 2005).

16. Abbott Laboratories Global Licensing and Business Development Web site, http://licensing.abbott.com (accessed June 10, 2005).

17. University of Cincinnati Intellectual Property Office, http://www.ipo.uc.edu (accessed June 10, 2005).

18. Harvard Biomedical Community Technology Gateway Web site, http://techgate.med.harvard.edu/tech.html (accessed June 10, 2005).

19. TechEx Web site, http://www.techex.com (accessed June 10, 2005).

20. UVentures.com Web site, http://www.uventures.com (accessed June 10, 2005).

21. Pharma-Transfer Web site, http://www.pharma-transfer.com (accessed June 10, 2005).

22. Yet2.com Web site, http://www.yet2.com/app/about/home (accessed August 30, 2005).

23. Pharmalicensing Web site, http://www.pharmalicensing.com (accessed June 10, 2005).

24. Techquisition Web site, http://www.techquisition.com (accessed June 10, 2005).

67

Licensing Technologies

Robert MacWright, PhD

Skydiving

I have never jumped out of a flying airplane and, though I am sure I could find a good book about parachute jumping, I am also quite sure that actually doing it is a lot different than reading a book about it. Packing your own parachute is a serious business, and it must be scary to jump from an airplane and to experience free-fall. However, it must be both very dramatic and comforting to feel the parachute open; and then so very satisfying to stand on the ground again and to look up to see where you have been. It must be incredibly tempting to try it again.

I have said that I have never gone skydiving—but maybe I have spoken too soon: my experience with technology licensing has actually been a lot like sky-diving. Preparing for the deal (defining your needs list, your wish list, your starting positions, and your fall-back positions) is like packing a parachute. If not perfectly prepared, the results can be excruciating, to put it mildly! Walking into that first negotiating session, focusing on the big issues of license scope, royalty rate, upfront and milestone fees, is probably exactly what it feels like to jump from a perfectly safe airplane into nothing but air: you just can't be sure at that point how things will turn out. And all the time that you are in the free-fall of batting numbers back and forth across the table, you know you will have to eventually pull the rip cord and say "yes" to a set of basic terms that you hope reduces the tension in the

room enough to more easily work through the relatively tedious process of resolving the myriad of smaller issues. As you work toward resolution of the smaller and smaller issues (increasingly legalistic in nature), you can feel the deal get closer and closer to closing, much like a landing. But as the closing comes into focus, you know that the agreement will yet need final management approval on both sides. Landing the agreement can be hard or soft; but by the time it happens, there is little you can do to affect the outcome. When the approval finally comes and the deal is signed, sealed, and delivered, you smile a big smile because when you look back to the beginning, it is damn amazing that you have safely arrived to where you are now. The experience has been so amazing and so rewarding, that you can not wait to do it again. Best of all, it feels the same way every time you jump, which is why many who become involved in technology licensing never want to stop.

Unfortunately, though, just like with parachute jumping, you can not really tell what licensing is like until you actually do it. And you can not become a licensing expert unless you personally do it many times, because every deal is different, and no matter how many times you negotiate a deal, you always learn something new. Fortunately, this chapter and other materials offer you the basic structure, processes, and challenges of technology licensing. But remember, once you have the basics down, there is only one way to really find out what it is like. Jump!

An Amalgam of Knowledge and Skills

Like many university licensing professionals, I came to licensing through a combination of choice and chance, starting in a career as a scientist. At the outset, I knew that my background in science would be enormously valuable in dealing with complex university inventions. But I am not sure I appreciated at the outset what an amalgam of knowledge and skills I would need to develop in order to excel in this new and sometimes baffling field. In licensing, the areas of law, business, psychology, and logic are every bit as important as science.

People sometimes ask me if a background in science is essential for success in academic technology transfer. Simply put, the answer is no. This has been proven by the many outstanding licensing professionals who first came to this business in the early days of technology transfer, with little or no formal training in science. It is also proven by the fact that many technology transfer professionals regularly handle inventions that are far removed from the field of their formal scientific training. However, I do believe that it is easier for a scientist to learn the necessary nonscience skills than it is for a person with a background in a nonscience field to learn about the field of science. Learning science is harder, but science is the primary language of faculty inventors. If a person has no scientific training, there is much to learn in order to become a credible representative of science to a very discerning audience of faculty scientists. This credibility is extremely important. Faculty inventors are usually poor judges of legal or business expertise, but are keen judges of scientific expertise and are more likely to assume a person's credibility in those other key process areas regarding technology transfer if they respect a person's scientific knowledge. Conversely, if you lack credibility in science, faculty are more likely to doubt your credibility in law and business, which may lead to harsh criticism, even before you start. So, indeed, a strong background in science is a very valuable asset in academic technology transfer, and if you do not have it, you will need to study every technology quite carefully before having any discussions with inventors.

Besides science, technology transfer requires the field of law. Legal knowledge is needed, not a law degree; and if you have a good mentor, or if you are dedicated to self-study, it is possible to learn what you need to know. First, you need to understand the basics of patent law in order to understand technology rights, and the legal conditions for the transfer of technology. You need to know the basics of contract law to know what can and cannot lawfully be accomplished within a contract, and how contracts are properly interpreted. In addition, you need to know the basic principles of licensing law (e.g., that patent royalties can not be collected after a patent has expired, but that trade secret royalties can be collected indefinitely); and also what license terms can cross the line of legality (e.g., patent misuse or if a license fails to fall within the European Block Exemptions). Do not worry. None of these issues are as daunting as they may seem.

To take advantage of this legal knowledge, however, you must develop special legal skills. The most fundamental is to be able to use words with the same precision with which a mathematician speaks of numbers. This skill is the essence of contract drafting, because imprecision leads to ambiguity, which can lead to a licensee or a court interpretation of the contract in a completely unintended way. Another fundamental skill is what lawyers call "issue spotting": finding potential problems or glitches that might arise downstream, that can be headed off in the contract. You may appreciate that this sometimes leads to lawyers being accused of focusing too much on doom and gloom prediction, but some of this kind of thinking is important. A third skill is to be able to stretch beyond what may be very typical terms and to find creative solutions to apparent impasses. Some of this comes with experience; the more twists and turns found in agreements, the easier they are to create.

Now, you may be thinking that you can not do licensing, because you don't have this knowledge or experience. But if you have an experienced mentor, whether an outside attorney, colleague, or consultant, you can begin to learn what you need to know to develop the necessary legal skills. The best way to learn how to apply these skills is by doing.

Business knowledge and skills are important, too. In order to understand the viewpoint of the company negotiator, you need to know something about what effort is involved to turn a raw inventive concept into a new product or service. The better you are able to get into that person's head, the easier it is to work out a deal. You also need to know how to investigate the marketplace for inventions in a variety of fields, so that you can understand what the relative value of an invention is, and to whom you might market the invention. Perhaps most importantly, you need to learn what are considered reasonable terms and conditions in different technology markets. Although some of this business knowledge and skill may be taught in business schools, much is not. These are things to learn from experience. Again, an experienced mentor can help you get up to speed and start off on the right foot.

The one critically important field largely overlooked regarding technology licensing is psychology. License negotiation is an inherently human process. I realize that today emotions have a very strong effect on the licensing process; yet, I did not see this nearly as well when I was new to this business. But the kind of psychology I am talking about here is not really something you can learn from a psychology textbook. It is something that executive education institutions call "psychological mindedness," which is the ability to look beyond what someone says or does to understand from a human experience point of view why they did so. For example, if someone yells at you over the phone, is it because that person is under a lot of pressure from his or her boss to get you to agree to what they want? Is it because that person is frustrated that you do not see his or her side of the argument? Is it because that person thinks he or she can intimidate you into submission? If you can figure out the motivation, perhaps by asking a few revealing questions, it can very much change how you handle that outburst.

You also need to know how to distinguish between logic and illogic. There are some arguments that are based entirely on logic: those you more or less have to accept. For example, if the company can show that profit margins are low on products like the proposed licensed product, you really can not easily discount that factor. But there are also many illogical arguments that people make when trying to persuade others, e.g., appeals to emotion ("If I can not get these terms, I will lose everything"); false analogies (saying the royalty rate should be the same as in another license for a less valuable technology); ad hominem attacks (attacking your background or skill, rather than the issue at hand); appeals to fear (threatening to go to the dean, your boss, etc.); appeals to tradition ("we always got these terms before"); appeals to flattery ("I am very impressed with your program, and you are the most experienced person I have ever dealt with at a university...I'm sure you can understand why we need to keep the royalty down to 1%.").

Fortunately, logic is something that you can learn quite a bit about from books. But you do not want a book on logic, as they are often mathematics books; you want a book about logic and language. You can also find much good information about logic and language from the Internet, if you do a search on "fallacies."

Lastly, and perhaps the hardest thing to learn, is to pay attention to your gut and to your creative abilities. Licensing is a complex art; no two technologies, no two companies, and no two deals are the same. Nevertheless, as you gain experience with licensing, you develop an intuitive sense about many things (e.g., how a deal is going; when there is likely to be an impasse; and when the company negotiator might try to go over your head, etc.). You also develop a heightened sense of when a creative term or a clever matrix of trade-offs might resolve the seemingly unresolvable. Along with this, you develop a greater ability to craft unique contract language that gives flight to those creative ideas. However, none of this helps you if you do not learn to trust this growing gut-level intuition and your new creative abilities.

It is a tall order to learn these things and to become skilled in applying them in the licensing context. When I came to the licensing industry as a scientist, I suddenly had to widen my perspective from the molecular level to a vastly broader horizon. From my own experience and from the experience of others that I have mentored, it takes about a year on the job to grasp the scope of the licensing manager's role. It takes at least another year to become comfortable in that newfound skin. But you can get there if you just jump in and start doing.

Stages of Progress

The technology licensing process can be dissected into several reasonably well-defined stages. These do not necessarily align with any discrete set of actions: they are general points along the way to completing the deal. Like any other complex job, it is easier to succeed if you break the licensing process down into smaller, more manageable pieces: you feel some sense of accomplishment as each one is completed, and you know what is likely to happen next. The stages that I define here may not mesh with what some other licensing experts may describe, as others may take a more formalistic view. I tend to view these stages from a pragmatic, human experience of view. So, the stages I define here correlate with the need to change perspectives on the deal, and how you may feel along the way.

In the *preparation* stage, you gather information about the company, the technology, the marketplace for such technologies, and the company's negotiator. In the *evaluation* stage, you decide what you need to ask for initially, what your fall-back position will be, and what your bottom line is, i.e., the least you are willing to accept. In the *exploration* stage, you make your first offer and hear the first offer (not necessarily in that order): these set the stage by bracketing the range of the final terms. In the *horse-trading* stage, you try to make trade-offs between issues, to preserve value for your side while at the same time accommodating the apparent needs of the other side. In the *crunch* stage, you have to find ways to resolve apparent impasse issues that may have crystallized. In the *legal* stage, you haggle over definitions of terms, a large amount of dense legal prose, and deal with those issues that only a lawyer can love, which may not have been discussed before. Finally, in the *closing* stage, you clean up the final language and get signatures from both sides.

Preparation

Preparing to negotiate involves collecting information and is usually the weak link in the licensing process. Everyone prepares to some degree, but those who spend more time on preparation are always at an advantage over those who do not. For a company, licensing a new product technology is not an everyday thing like it is to university tech transfer offices; and when a company takes a license, it comes with serious commitments of money and other resources. So, you can usually be sure that the company negotiator will invest considerable effort at this stage, both personally and in consultation with company experts in marketing, product development, and accounting. As a result, if you shortcut the preparation stage, you will probably be at a significant disadvantage at the negotiating table.

Getting started is often the hard part. At the outset, you may feel somewhat overwhelmed, as if looking for a needle in a haystack. That is perfectly normal. But you probably already have a head start. When you were evaluating the invention and looking for a licensee, you probably collected a good bit of information, and this is a great place to start. To begin with, dig into the technical details about the invention you are licensing. You want to dig deeper than before, to look for features and benefits that may bolster your negotiations. When you hit a rough spot in getting what you want out of the license, you can soften the company's resistance by pointing to the unique and advantageous features of the invention they are licensing. This technical review also yields dividends later, when you write and negotiate the license. You may discover that the particular technology at issue raises

special licensing concerns, for example, the storage and retrieval of biological materials, charging royalties on diagnostic testing services as well as on testing kits, etc.

You also want to review the marketing information collected earlier, at the time you were still looking for a licensee. You now want to look at that information with a somewhat different focus. You are looking for the comparative value of the technology. Take a look at the companies that you identified as possible licensing candidates, and see what comparable products they may be making (those products that led you to consider them as licensing prospects in the first place). Search around on the Internet for information about those products to see if you can get a sense of which ones dominate the market; how competitive your new technology might make the licensee; and, if you can find it, what relative market share the existing products have. One avenue to this kind of information that is often overlooked is patent searching. If you have already filed a patent application, and your application has been classified by the US Patent and Trademark Office (PTO), you can go to the PTO Web site and simply browse through the other patents and published applications that are in the same class and subclass. Look for technologies that are similar or close to yours, and then speculate about what market share the new technology might attract. If you extrapolate and estimate some projected sales figures, you can calculate the dollar impact of different royalty rates on your income, and determine how much the licensee will likely be willing to pay for milestone payments, up-fronts, etc.

You also want to look at the information you have about the company you are planning to license to, and then probe the Internet for more information. If it is a publicly traded company, the Edgar database of SEC filings can be a treasure trove of information. Also, see if you can get a copy of the company's annual report from its Web site; you may be able to decipher what relative portion of its business is related to the technology you plan to license them. Is it right in the middle of its business, is it a modest offshoot, or is it a new venture? If the intended licensee is a small company, there will be fewer sources of information; but almost all companies today have Web sites that tell about their business, and some have product brochures and the like that can be downloaded. In addition, there are often reports that can be purchased (e.g., from Dun & Bradstreet) that are available even for relatively small companies. Collect every tidbit of information you can find, evaluate carefully, and read between the lines. As you progress, you should find yourself with a growing sense of the company's philosophy, market focus, and its corporate environment. All of this information will help you understand why the company is interested in a license, and how important it might be to the company.

If you are clever, you can get the company's negotiator to give you all the information you want about the company without revealing its potential value to you as you prepare to negotiate. But you have to plan ahead. Well before any negotiations begin, perhaps about the time you are going to sign a confidentiality agreement and to send the company confidential information about your invention, you can simply ask for whatever information you would like, for example, a copy of the company's annual report, information about the company's finances, etc. You can also ask lots of questions about the size of the company, its product lines, its future plans, how it is organized, etc. After all, you do need to know who you are licensing to—licenses are often 20-year commitments—and you need to know that the company has the financial ability to develop and market the licensed product. You also need to know what level of resource commitment is likely to be made. To also get the information you need while preparing to negotiate, you have to resist the urge to take a superficial view if the company looks strong on the surface or if they are your only "live one." Even Fortune 500 companies will be glad to provide you with detailed information if you ask; after all, they want you to like them, and they want you to want to license to them.

Perhaps the most important information—and the most often overlooked—is information about the person with whom you will be negotiating. This is important because licensing is an inherently human process; it only makes sense that the more you know about the only other human involved, the better you are able to manage the process. Every person has his or her own perspective on the world, which is founded on educational background, relative position at the workplace, past work experience, level of experience in the current job, etc. The more you can learn about these things, the more you will be able to tell bluff from threat, experience from puffery, and bottom-line from wishful thinking.

If you are lucky, the company Web site will provide a biography of the negotiator and biographies of the other employees as well. If the company negotiator is a lawyer, the Martindale-Hubble database usually provides a very detailed biography (if you do not

have access to that database, have one of your patent lawyers look it up for you). You might learn from this kind of information about one or more of his or her previous jobs, and then you can size up those companies to get a sense of his or her experience base.

You also want to know about the company negotiator's role in the company. For a big company, you might find an organizational chart if you probe the Internet carefully. At the very least, you should be able to learn the person's job title from e-mail or letters he or she may have sent you. But don't take the person's title at face value: titles can often be quite inflated, especially when the company knows its negotiators need to look authoritative. That's why learning something about the company's organizational structure can be very helpful.

In addition, do some Web searching on the negotiator's name, and see what comes up. You might, for example, find a home address. Then, if you peek into a real estate database, you may be able to tell if he or she lives in a mansion or in a modest ranch, which will tell you something about how well he or she is paid, which, in turn, will tell you something about how important he or she really is at the company. You also might find that he or she coaches a Little League baseball team or that he or she belongs to an astronomical society. Anything that helps you to know that person better helps you understand where that person is coming from in the negotiations.

Perhaps the best source of information about the company's negotiator comes from that person directly. But again, you have to plan ahead. When you first start talking with the company negotiator, whether the dialogue begins with a marketing call, or in the early stages of negotiation, just be cordial and relaxed.

As you may know, the traditional American business style is to begin a business meeting with a bit of small talk. Don't discount the importance of that phase! Foreigners and extremely driven people sometimes shortcut or eliminate that opening, but they often miss out on useful information about the other side's negotiator, and they also may lose the relaxed atmosphere that is conducive to reaching compromise later on. Starting such small talk is easy—bad weather, good weather, better weather there than here—all are common openers. Or, by looking in the AUTM or LES membership directory ahead of time, you may find that you are both members, and may have attended the same conferences.

Now, you might say that such relaxed dialogue helps the person learn more about you, which may have strategic benefit to him or her in preparing to negotiate. But there is little risk here. Whatever he or she learns about you will probably help smooth the negotiations, too. The person probably has greater independent resources to find out about you than you have to find out about him or her anyway.

Once you have collected all of the information you can find, you will probably have many printouts to look at. You probably skimmed them as you retrieved them, and already have much more developed perspectives than before. But you will have a far more concrete sense if you prepare a summary, perhaps only a page or two long, listing key findings in each category: the company, the negotiator, the technology, and the relevant marketplace. This will be a handy resource to have while you are negotiating.

Evaluation

Having completed the exploration phase, you now have the information you need to evaluate what your starting, fall-back, and bottom-line positions are for this deal. But before addressing this, we need to first look at an important way to dissect the license into manageable pieces.

Term Sheets In virtually every negotiation, the price terms are the first things on the minds of the negotiators. What will the licensee have to pay for the license? Of course, there are many factors that affect the price terms, including the number and breadth of the patent rights; whether know-how and/or software rights are included; whether future rights to improvements and other related inventions are included; the field limitation, if any (e.g., for human therapeutic use, with veterinary uses reserved for another possible licensee); the geographic scope of the license (e.g., Europe only vs. worldwide); and other factors as well. The price terms themselves include the royalty rate, the up-front payment, milestone payments and patent cost reimbursement, and perhaps other payments. Other threshold issues in licensing include warranties (or more typically, the lack thereof), product liability insurance requirements and diligence requirements.

Of course, a license agreement covers many more topics and generally has 20 to 40 pages of fairly dense legal prose. I have to admit, as a younger man, I used to just jump right in with a proposed license and negotiate the key issues along with everything else. But I would never do that today. Today, I always start with a term sheet (see the example in Appendix A at the end of this chapter).

There are several reasons why starting with a term sheet is much, much better. First, it makes negotiating the big issues more manageable. A term sheet separates the key business issues from the nitty-gritty legal terms. This makes agreement on the key business terms far easier, because you are less distracted by side issues, and at a glance you can easily appreciate the overall balance of benefits and burdens for both sides. It becomes easy to say, "Let's increase the royalty to 6%, and decrease the up-front fee to $50,000," and both parties can easily pencil in those changes. A second reason using a term sheet is much better is that it is less foreboding, formal, and rigid. A detailed license is an imposing document, and digging into it takes a considerable amount of patience, which may be hard to have when you do not yet know if the basic terms are reasonable. A detailed license agreement also has a very formal tone, with many terms that become important only if and when one or the other party behaves badly. A license agreement also has a rather fixed structure, and changing one thing in the text may unintentionally also affect many other terms. A third reason that term sheets work best is that many companies have woven such an approach into their negotiating process; the business people negotiate the basic terms and then the company's lawyers negotiate the remaining terms.

The example term sheet shown at the end of this chapter is a fairly detailed one. In many cases, the term sheet will be much simpler at the outset, but will become more complex and detailed as the negotiations proceed. You will also note that some terms do seem to have a bit of a legalistic flavor. This is because you want to make sure the language is unambiguous and specific. Lastly, and quite importantly, you will note a paragraph at the beginning of the term sheet that points out that the term sheet is not a binding contract. I began using this some time ago, after learning about a case where the parties could not agree on the language of the final license, and the prospective licensee sued the patent owner to enforce the terms of the term sheet claiming that it actually was a license!

The "Ask" Even though you may have collected tons of information in the preparation phase, you will almost certainly feel uneasy about deciding what to ask for. Everyone does. Ask for too little, and you have needlessly given away value. Ask for too much, and they will reject your offer out of hand. Fortunately, there are some simple rules to guide you.

You Can Not Have What You Do Not Ask For. This seems like a silly and obvious rule, but it is one often disobeyed. When you consider what to ask for, do not forget to explore all of the things you could possibly want, and also less important things that you feel they will probably not mind giving! It is surprising to me that so many times, people could have received more, had they just asked. For example, many companies will gladly pay an issue fee of a few thousand dollars or more when the key patent issues, but few people ask for it.

Ask for More Than You Want, because You Will Not Get Everything You Ask For. This seems obvious too, but in many cases, people are reluctant to pile too much onto the deal, fearing they will push it too far; but later on, they do not have much to give away in bargaining, because they did not build in enough room to maneuver.

Aim for the top of the Range of Reasonableness. There is a simple visual approach that makes it easier to decide what your opening ask should be. For illustration purposes, I will focus on the royalty rate, but you can do the same thing for each value term, such as the up-front fee and milestone payments.

Grab a piece of graph paper, and make a vertical value line. Now, put a mark at the bottom of that line to represent the lowest royalty rate that you would ever accept from this deal. Most of us find it easy to decide what that is! Some refer to this as your bottom line, others speak of it as the best alternative to a negotiated agreement (BATNA), still others call it your walk away. Using the graph paper as a scale, put another mark at the very highest royalty rate you can ever imagine the other side paying. That is not as hard as you might think; for example, few companies would pay a 20% royalty for a largely untested drug compound! Now, think about other licenses you have negotiated, and the information you have collected, and try to make your lower end as realistic as possible. Then, look at that high end, and ask yourself, "Would I be shocked if they agreed to that?" If your answer is yes, you are probably too high. Continue to think back and forth, until you have settled on the upper and lower rates. What is in between is the range of reasonableness.

If you think back to how you decided on the lowest end of that range, you will see that if the licensee offers a royalty rate that falls even slightly below your lower limit, it would be outside the range of reasonableness, and you would reject it out of hand. This does not mean that you would walk away from the table, but you would probably insist it was not even in the ballpark, and expect them to make a better offer without a counteroffer from you. But what if it were just half a point over your lower limit? Would you reject it as unreasonable, or would you have to respond with a counter-offer? You would not reject it out of hand; you would see it as too low, but not unreasonable, and you would

give a counteroffer with a higher rate. So, when you think about what royalty rate you want to ask for, you want to make it a number just below their upper limit of reasonableness, but not above it.

If you were to draw these scales for all of the primary value elements in the proposed license, and lay them side-by-side, you would find that they all vary in true dollar value, and also in the risk that you might never get paid. An up-front fee is a sure thing, but whether you ever get running royalties depends on a myriad of unknowable variables. Nevertheless, they are all fungible: if you get a half-point less in royalties, but get an extra $1 million in milestone fees, would that be a reasonable trade? The MBAs would reduce each item to net present value, and calculate an exact answer. But this is in my view unnecessary, and quite frankly, undoable, given that the future variables and risks are impossible to accurately predict. So, you ultimately need to make trade-offs, and you will likely do so based on your intuition, gut sense, and generalized view of the deal as a whole, and, often, you will do it on the fly, while in the heat of negotiations. That is just the nature of the beast. But you can do some planning, and have some intermediate thresholds in mind.

The Fall-Back Position. Looking back at your royalty value line, you can see what is the least you would accept—your bottom line, and the most you could reasonably hope for—the dream deal. But what would make you comfortable? What would be a fair, but neither exciting nor disappointing, result? This is often considered your fall-back position. By now, you can probably just pencil it into your value line. If you feel uncertain, go back and look at other deals for technologies in the same field, to get a feeling for it. If you do not have any such deals, call a few friends at other universities and ask them what they feel would be a fair deal, and they may be able to give examples.

The fall-back position is important, because you really want to negotiate for something between your dream deal and the fallback. You do not want to take the range between the fallback and your bottom line into consideration when you decide what your various counteroffers might be, because you really do not want to wind up there. Taking that part of the range into consideration will make your counteroffers too low. If try as you might, you just can not get out of the basement, there will be time enough to consider that part of the range.

The Working Term Sheet. Once you have decided on opening, fall-back, and bottom-line positions for each value term, prepare a term sheet for your own use and pencil all three numbers in for each value term. Needless to say, you *never* want the licensee to see this piece of paper! Guard it closely and do not make copies. If you are negotiating in person, do not lay it on the table, because reading upside down could be a skill enjoyed by the company negotiator! The best bet is to put it in your pocket or purse, where you can easily refer to it during a caucus break (discussed below).

Exploration

This is where all of your hard work first goes into action. You know what you want to ask for: it represents the best you could hope for, and it will most likely prompt a counteroffer from the other side. That counteroffer will be at the low end of what you are willing to accept. If it is too low, reject it out of hand, and be prepared to offer some explanation as to why the technology is worth far more (do not tell them it is below your bottom line, or they will start probing to find where that bottom line is). Once each side has made an offer, you will have bracketed a range within which the final rate will fall. If you use your scale, or visualize it, it can also help you evaluate what to counteroffer, and how fair any counteroffers they make might be. For example, if you moved down by 5% and they moved up only 0.5%, you can see that the natural progression will wind up with a fairly low rate. So, you may want to make your next counteroffer move by a far smaller amount than before, to signal that you have gone about as far as you want to. The give-and-take of negotiation is covered in more detail in a later chapter of this book.

One question that always comes up is, who will make the first offer? Whoever makes the first offer gives away information about where they think the range of reasonableness lies, and a skilled negotiator on the other side can take that into account in making his or her counteroffer. For example, if you ask for 5%, and the company negotiator was expecting to pay 4%, he or she now knows that your range is lower than the company's! He or she might also reasonably assume that your bottom line is lower than he or she might have thought, so, the counteroffer may be considerably lower than originally planned.

This is not something to fear: both sides have to make offers sooner or later. But people do tap-dance to try to get the other side to make the first offer! It is sometimes comical, and laughing at it is often the best way to encourage the other side to jump in first.

Keep in mind that first offers are often quite narrow, i.e., they often only address the royalty term and the up-front fee, with something mumbled about also having minimum annual royalties and milestone payments. The scope of the patents and other rights to be licensed are often implied rather than stated.

If you make the first offer, and later feel you came in too low, do not worry about it. You can always recover by asking for more than you planned for the milestones and minimums, and any other value terms that are on your working term sheet.

A strong caution is in order here. Whatever you do, do not agree to anything! Even if your proposed terms are close, and even if you are willing to accept the offer, do not say so. You need to probe their value sense, not make any commitments. If you agree to anything here, you give up any leverage you may have to get what you want in the horse-trading stage to follow, where you will address the other value items on the working term sheet that is in your pocket or purse. Although in the abstract, avoiding agreement may seem awkward, in practice it is easy. Just say, "Well, we are still fairly far apart, but let us see where we are on the other issues," or just simply move on to another value term. They will know that it is the total package, not just the one term, that you are focusing on.

You also do not want to unintentionally let on your satisfaction by the tone of your voice, or, if you are negotiating in person, by the expression on your face. Experience in playing poker can come in handy here! Any hint that you like what they offered on one term may encourage them to come in lower on other terms.

When this stage has been completed—there are now starting offers on the table from both sides—it will be invigorating. Your earlier uncertainties will fade, and you will have a concrete sense that there is a deal to be had. But there is still much work left to do.

Horse Trading

It is now time to bargain. There will not be any clear transition from the exploration phase to this horse trading phase, except that you will see many more issues on the table. Either side can start it, by injecting other ask terms besides the royalty rate and up-fronts (as described earlier, all matters should at this point remain unresolved). Once the horse trading has begun, you want to make sure all of the value items in your working term sheet get on the table. Naturally, you will make opening asks or counteroffers on each term using the starting terms on your working term sheet, unless of course, you decide that you just might go higher, given what you have observed of the other side.

The other side may put issues on the table that you do not expect. Do not worry, you will just have to wing it here. Do not come too close to their proposals; 100 percent to 300 percent higher for your side may still be quite reasonable. Remember, so long as you leave the issue open, you can balance out value between these new issues and those you expected to have on the table.

After all the issues are on the table, the real give-and-take begins. It is worthwhile, at this point, to envision the carnival game "whack-a-mole," where every time you whack one mole with the rubber hammer, another mole pops up somewhere else. You should treat the various value terms that are on the table the same way. If the other side says they want to keep the running royalty low, and insist on a particular royalty rate, then you can insists on something more on another term or terms, for example, perhaps a higher up-front payment, and/or higher minimum annual royalties. Your goal is to retain good value for the deal as a whole.

As you horse-trade, try to keep as many items open as you can; do not lock anything in, so that you can still increase it if you need to in exchange for something else. The best way to keep things open is to haggle until you feel you are fairly close, and then bring in something else. Here is an example: suppose your last offer was a 6% royalty, and their last offer was a 4% royalty. They had previously offered an up-front fee of $25,000 and you asked for $150,000. Your brain will want to focus on the royalty issue, which seems kind of close; the urge will be to say, "How about we split the difference, at 5%?" But you want to hold back a bit, and think. Would you not be better off to link the royalty and up-front issues together, and offer a $5^1/_2$% royalty, provided that you get your $150,000 up-front? In most cases, you would. Only going down to $5^1/_2$% illustrates another general principle, too: do not make big concessions when little ones may suffice. You can always concede further after they make another offer, which may help you sense how much value you will be able to retain.

The actual discussion will be far more complex than the hypothetical one I have described; you will have many other items open, and your counter-offers may be rather complex. At some point, you naturally start to view all of the issues from the perspective of your working term sheet.

As the horse trading proceeds, do not neglect opportunities for creative solutions. For example, if the company says the royalty is too high because its profits will not be very good until reaching some level of market penetration, then consider a ramping-up royalty. This is quite common in pharmaceutical licenses, and is generally keyed to reaching a fixed goal of lifetime royalties. Or, if the company says it can not afford much up-front money, consider taking some equity as part of the up-front fee. There are endless variations; none are good or bad, right or wrong. It really depends on the circumstances, needs, and limitations of the two sides.

In addition, you will have to work hard to remember that *nothing is cast in stone*. Just because you uttered, "3.5%" does not mean you are stuck with that. Remember, you have many other issues in play: you can always trade off some value elsewhere to bump the royalty higher. You can also caucus for a few minutes, talk with your negotiating partner or call the office, and then come back and say, "Well, I am very sorry, but I went too far. I am afraid we just can't live with a 3.5% royalty." Will they like it? No. But what can they do, walk away because they are not going to get something they only just started thinking they would get? It is very doubtful. And sometimes, you really have gone too far, for example, you call the boss and he says he will not accept it. The usual result is some serious grumbling, and, usually, some complaints about your lack of honor or authority. Do not take the bait and reverse yourself; it will pass.

Back to the term sheet. Here is where a term sheet really helps. Once you have a variety of issues in play, you can begin to mold them into a term sheet. There are two ways to do this. One is to simply offer the other side a draft you prepared ahead of time, with all of your ask positions written in. Another approach is to bring a blank one with you, and pencil in your figures and pass it over the table. But my own approach is to draft a term sheet onto a blank piece of paper, right there at the bargaining table. That way, you can add items as you go along, maybe even ones you had not initially thought of, and they will not seem like second thoughts; they will have the same weight as those things you expected to be there. If you take this approach, you will not need to worry about formalities, because you would never sign such a handwritten document.

Feel Free to Caucus. If you have someone else from your office at the bargaining table, keep in mind that only one of you can do the horse trading, because everything is tied to everything else. The person who is largely observing is very important, too, because he or she will often have different and often better perspectives than the one who is doing the talking, because talking limits the lead person's thinking time. In addition, if you have been at it for more than 30 to 45 minutes, you are probably wearing down and will be less effective than you were at the beginning. These are the reasons that good bargainers will take time out to caucus privately. It is easy to do, just say, "Well, we have covered a lot of ground here, so I think we would like to talk privately for a few minutes." Or, "Well, it looks like we may have a logjam here; let me go talk with Jane for a few minutes, and see if we can come up with any new ideas." Then go to another room, where you are sure you will not be overheard. You may be surprised by how helpful this is; you can get good feedback, good ideas, and clear your head. If the meeting is very long, you should plan to caucus several times. If there is a sticking point in the discussions, you just may find a solution or come away feeling more certain that you want to hold your ground.

If you are alone at the table, you should still take some time out along the way. A restroom break is an easy way to get a few minutes; and if you make a cell phone call to someone back in the office, you can bounce a few ideas around before returning to the bargaining table.

Consider a Fixed Execution Date. If there is an indeterminate time period in which to negotiate the final license, completing the deal will always take longer. The reason is that when the big issues have been resolved, then medium-sized issues become the big issues, and when the medium ones are resolved, the small-sized issues become the big issues. You lose all sense of relative importance when time is no object. To avoid this problem, consider setting a firm execution date in the term sheet, for example, 30 days out. Companies usually like this, because they are far more time-sensitive than universities. You will learn to like it too; you will suffer less frustration, and as a bonus, you will find that you get more deals done each year, because they can not drag on and on.

Executing the Term Sheet. I generally try to get all terms of the term sheet agreed to by both parties in a single session. If people go back to the office and think for a few days, they usually come back with a lower value perception than they had at the meeting. Besides, if the basic terms have been agreed upon at the end of the meeting, everyone is usually very satisfied and upbeat, which sets a good tone for negotiating the contract details.

But even if there is agreement, you are not quite there yet. One of you will need to draft a formal version of the term sheet, so that both parties can sign. Although it says on its face that the term sheet is not a binding contract, as a matter of honor, both sides will generally accept those terms as negotiation of the license contract proceeds. I might point out that I always volunteer to draft the term sheet, to make sure it properly reflects my view of the deal. The other side may wish to edit it somewhat before it is signed, which should be treated as additional horse trading.

The Crunch

Unfortunately, working out the business terms of a license is not usually the smooth, collegial affair that it may at first seem to be. This is especially true if the person on the other side is an experienced negotiator. Such a person will have a very keen sense of when to compromise and when to stand firm, and how to handle the strain of taking a hard line. So, you often wind up in the situation where there are one or two issues that you just can not reach agreement, and the royalty term is often one of them. Or, you may have come to your bottom line on certain issues, and you may draw the line yourself. By this point, you have usually traded away everything you are willing to give, as the other person probably has, too. What do you do?

First, recognize it as a "crunch," and remember that emotion is the greatest hazard. One or both of you can easily become angry and frustrated, and once that emotion comes out, it makes further compromise more difficult. Second, take heed that those feeling the crunch sometimes resort to indirect ways around the issue, such as complaining to your boss or the university (which is why they need to know that complaints are sometimes negotiating tactics). And third, recognize that the vast majority of crunches are resolved. That is why I do not refer to them as "impasses." Remind yourself that neither of you would be at the table if you did not both want to reach an agreement.

Given these realities, it is usually best if you can work to resolve a crunch before it gets too adversarial. Unfortunately, there is no one-size-fits-all way to resolve a crunch. However, there are a few avenues that are always worth exploring.

One thing to consider is whether there might be a *combination* of other concessions that would allow one party to concede on the crunch issue. For example, if the company managers say they just will not go over a 2% royalty and your bottom line is 3%, maybe if they increase the up-front fee *and* the milestone fees *and* the sublicensing share *and* the minimum annual royalty, you could justify conceding the additional 1% in royalty rate. It might seem very expensive to you when you propose it, but you never know why the other side digs in its heels. Maybe senior management said, "Don't pay more than 2% for it," without limiting other financial terms.

Another thing to explore is whether the crunch issue can be resolved by varying a value term over time. Here, you have to listen carefully about why they feel what you ask is too high. If they say the royalties will be too expensive because of start-up costs, consider a ramp-up royalty that starts lower and increases in several stages with increasing sales levels. Or, if the company managers feel they will add a great deal of value over time, you might consider a ramp-down royalty rate, which decreases as sales volume goes up and the company's contributions to the product's success increase. I have seen both. Yet another possible crunch-breaker is to spread out payments. Disagreements about upfront fees can often be resolved by providing an installment plan.

Overall, creativity is the most important factor in resolving crunch situations. You need to look beyond what is in dispute, and beyond what is in your working term sheet. Some people are naturally creative, and they tend to resolve these situations more easily than others. For those who are less creative, experience is a perfectly acceptable substitute! Once you have seen a few hundred crunches, you will surely find it much easier to resolve them, because you will have a large palette to choose from and you will know what works. Fortunately, you do not have to wait years and years to get this experience: ours is a very open profession, and most seasoned licensing people at other universities are more than willing to help you come up with some ideas. So, keep the AUTM membership directory handy, and do not be bashful about calling for some impromptu advice.

Even after years of licensing experience, you will still get the feelings of shock and discouragement when a crunch situation arises. Fortunately, you can also enjoy the tremendous sense of accomplishment that comes when you work through it. Resolving such seemingly unsolvable problems is what makes licensing so rewarding.

Legal Language Negotiation

Once a term sheet has been signed, attention moves on to the often foreboding task of negotiating the legal language of the license agreement itself. For many, this stage seems tedious and focused on minutiae. But if you approach it with the degree of care it needs, it is a very cerebral undertaking.

Before you can negotiate the legal terms, however, someone needs to write them. It will almost always be best if you volunteer to do this work. University licenses have to address a considerable number of issues that are of special importance because the university mission is decidedly noncommercial. For example, the faculty's ability to freely publish research findings is paramount. State universities often can not agree to follow the laws of other states. Universities will not warrant anything about the technology, and require indemnification by the company. And universities almost always require patent cost reimbursement. There are a number of other issues, as well. If the company writes the first draft and you address these issues in a revised draft, your revisions may seem too severe, and may even require restructuring the text.

There is a later chapter in this book that addresses contract negotiation in considerable detail. But generally, there are only four things you need to keep in mind:

License Agreements Are Often 20-Year Relationships. Given that there is usually a lag of 7 to 10 years between signing a license and making a good royalty return, there is a good chance that the license you negotiate will be interpreted by your successor. In addition, although a licensee may initially see the license as a source of opportunity, as time goes on, he or she is likely to think of it as a tax bill to pay.

Ambiguity Is Your Enemy. Most people understand that a contract seeks to precisely explain what the parties are giving up in exchange for what they want to get. Only with some experience will you fully appreciate the exquisite degree of precision needed. If there is more than one way to interpret any given provision or set of provisions, you can expect that the company will someday interpret it in the way least favorable to you. This is why ambiguity is the ever present enemy of the license negotiator.

Avoid "Wobble Words." The biggest ambiguity trap for those new to licensing is the use of words like "relating" and "pertaining." Although they can properly be used in contract language, many reach for these words for convenience and with a single interpretation in mind, which may not be the only interpretation. For example, if you were to include in a license all of Professor Jones' future inventions that "relate to neurosurgery," would that include a new anesthetic he later invents? Anesthesia is surely important when having brain surgery! How about a new scalpel blade design? Using "specifically relating to neurosurgery" would not really have been much better, since "specifically" is subject to interpretation, too. Instead, you have to spell out exactly what you mean. For example, there is little chance for misinterpretation if you include in the license all "mechanical device and apparatus inventions that are specially adapted for use in brain surgical procedures, and are not suitable for use in other, nonbrain surgical procedures."

Contracts Are Word Puzzles. Remember that ambiguity can arise from structure as well as from language. I have seen some perfectly lovely looking licenses that had the most horrifying structural ambiguities. There are many ways ambiguities can creep into a license, but you should at least watch out for these:

- *Circularity:* Virtually every license contains a set of defined terms, which are then used as shorthand throughout the text. It is quite common for these definitions to refer to one another; for example, "licensed products" are defined as products covered by one or more "licensed patents." But such a chain of definitions must start with a definition that is independent! If licensed patents are defined as the patents in Schedule A that cover licensed products, can you concretely figure out what the licensed products are? It is implied that they are the patents in Schedule A; but from the language, you can not know what the licensed products are unless you know what the licensed patents are, which you can not determine without knowing what the licensed products are. Keep in mind you can create such awkwardness in other parts of the contract too, if you are not careful.

- *Disconnects.* Another common problem is failing to use the correct defined terms. I have seen quite a few licenses where one "Witnesseth" in the preamble said the "technology" invented by the university was being licensed without defining it in any detail. The grant clause gave the company the right to make, use, and sell products covered by the licensed patents. But the royalty provision charged a royalty on products covered by the technology. You can infer what was meant here, but you can not say for certain.

The most troubling disconnect of all is where the grant clause and the obligation to pay royalties do not match exactly. For example, suppose you license a patented diagnostic technology, and the company agrees to pay royalties on sales of licensed products, i.e., products covered by the licensed patents. The grant clause gives the company the right to make, use, sell, offer for sale, and import products covered by the licensed patents. What if the company decides not to sell diagnostic kits, but instead to provide diagnostic testing services? Are they really selling licensed products? Or are they using them, for which there does not seem to be a royalty obligation? Although it is clearly the intention of the parties that the company should pay a royalty in exchange for enjoying the benefits of the license, such disconnects can lead to very fundamental disputes.

- *String Definitions.* You can wind up with difficult ambiguities if you repeatedly use a long string of words or definitions to define something. For example, if in one clause you refer to "running royalties, up-front fees, milestone payments, and minimum annual royalties," and in another clause you refer to "royalties, licensing fees, milestone fees, and minimum royalties," are these the same things? If you later refer to "running royalties, milestone fees and minimum annual royalties," did you leave out "up-front fees" on purpose, or was it an oversight? All of these problems can be avoided by adding a definition such as "payments" for this list of payments due, and using that term throughout the agreement.

Make it Sing. As any lawyer will tell you, the trick in drafting and negotiating contracts, as in most other legal matters is issue spotting—seeing that something that might come up is not addressed, that there is an ambiguity, or that the clause does not do what you want it to. To spot all of the issues, you will need to read the entire contract many times, especially if you are new at it. Once you have combed out all of the issues, you will be able to read the entire license from start to finish, without finding a single issue; if the document is smoothly written, it will sing like a fine melody in your mind.

How to Read a Contract. You may think that those with experience can read a contract like a novel, even if contract reading puts you to sleep. But your self-criticism is unwarranted. Very few people can read an entire contract with a uniform degree of attention. Indeed, a great many contracts have the first five pages very well-honed, and the quality deteriorates thereafter because those on both sides consistently lost their focus.

Because of our human failings, to become a top contract negotiator, you need to give up on the typical brute force approach and adopt a systematic method for reading and editing contracts. You will have to learn to work on them in manageable bites. This is really quite simple. Most people can manage to concentrate through five pages of contract language at a time, so just do not try to cover more than five pages in one sitting. Most importantly, put a sticky note with an arrow to where you left off, to help you resist the urge to start from the beginning again. Between sessions, go do something else besides reading and editing. Once you have gone through the entire document, read it again, in five-page bites, starting from the end, and working your way forward. You will be surprised to see how many new issues you will see this way.

Haggling with Lawyers. After your term sheet is signed, you may find that the company asks its lawyer to take over from there, and work out the contract terms with you. This is very often the case with large companies. If you are not a lawyer yourself, you may feel a bit out-gunned, but you should not have a real handicap. If they raise esoteric concerns or insist on impenetrable language, you can always have your lawyer call them back to discuss and haggle out those few provisions. You will, however, have to pay special attention to the change in tone. Company lawyers sometimes are considerably more aggressive than the business people were. As long as you are aware of the change, you should be able to rise to the challenge, and give as good as you get.

"Don't Let the Perfect Be the Enemy of the Good Enough." These sage words from Congressman Henry Hyde (6th District, Illinois) are important to keep in mind. Every contract is a complex set of compromises and the language used usually winds up being a mixture of writing styles and formats. You could spend an eternity trying to get every word just right! You will never get the person on the other side to agree with you about what just right looks like. When you get down to the little issues, ask yourself, "What is the worst that could happen if we just signed this deal, and moved on to the next one?" If the worst you can imagine is a tolerable risk, get on to the next deal. Your time is best spent there.

Closing the Deal

Occasionally, a licensee will want to have a formal signing ceremony where those on both sides of the transaction have their pictures taken as they sign the license. In some other cases, a licensee will be in a great rush to close the license at a certain date and time, with both sides leaning over a fax machine to exchange signatures. This usually happens because the company needs the license as a condition to closing a stock purchase agreement with investors. But more typically, closing is a bit of an anticlimax. One party prints off two copies of the agreed-on language and signs them, then sends them off to the other side for signature. Each party gets a signed copy, and the deal is done, with very little fanfare.

But never, ever take it on faith that contracts printed and signed by the other side are what you agreed to! You would be surprised how often people slip up and send you a previous draft (more favorable to them, of course), or add things that you never discussed. You have to read through the signature copies line-by-line before you sign.

Although signing a license (or having it signed by the boss) may happen with little fanfare, you will find that you can not help smiling. It has been a long and sometimes craggy road, but finally, the deal is done. It will put a spring in your step, as you move on to work on the dozen other deals you have going on!

Conclusion

Here, we have tried to look at technology licensing as a step-by-step process. But it is really an art, not a science. There are no hard-and-fast rules, only guiding principles gained through your own experience and what you have been able to learn from the experiences of others. Sometimes, doing something you have never seen or heard of before can make all the difference. And just like parachute jumping, the only way to learn what it is really like, and the only way to get better at it, is to *jump*. You will find that with experience, the fear will fade away, but the exhilaration will always be there. That's why so many licensing professionals love what they do.

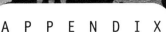

APPENDIX

67-A

Term Sheet

Hypothetical Therapeutics, Inc./UVAPF License for Compounds for Treating Ovarian Cancer

This term sheet is not meant to be a binding contract, but rather is intended to set forth the primary licensing terms as agreed upon by the undersigned parties, to be codified in a License Agreement to be negotiated between the parties.

Licensing Terms

Parties to the Agreement:	Hypothetical Therapeutics, Inc. ("HP") University of Virginia Patent Foundation ("UVAPF")
Effective Date:	August 1, 2004 (anticipated)
Licensed Rights:	US application 09/562,821; Australian application 1102639948; European application 017057.9; and Canadian and Japanese equivalents of same (application numbers not known), all of which claim priority from PCT/US01/09650 (now expired); all continuations and divisionals of the foregoing, and all patents issuing therefrom; and all know-how rights regarding these technologies.
Scope of Rights:	Exclusive, worldwide license in the Field, with right to sublicense, subject to the Reservations of Rights below
Reservations of Rights:	The License Agreement shall be subject to the following reservations of rights: 1. To UVA for internal research and educational purposes, and for compliance with the NIH Guidelines on the Dissemination of Research Tools. 2. To the Federal Government, as required by 35 U.S.C. §§200-206. 3. To Northwest Reagent Co. for sales of certain of the Licensed Products as research tools for nonclinical research purposes. 4. UVA may publish its research findings in academic journals, without any liability to HP, even though such publication may limit or destroy certain know-how rights licensed hereunder.
Field of Use:	Human therapeutic treatment of disease
Licensing Fee:	$100,000 due on or before the Effective Date
Patenting Costs:	All past patenting costs will be reimbursed by HP within 30 days after the Effective Date. Future patenting costs will be covered by HP as incurred, either by reimbursement to UVAPF or by direct payment to UVAPF's counsel, as UVAPF may elect.

Royalty Rate:

According to the following table:

Royalty	Limitation
4%	Until cumulative Net Sales exceeds $250M
5%	Thereafter, until cumulative Net Sales exceeds $500M
6%	Thereafter, for term of License Agreement

Royalties payable on sales in nonpatent countries will be at one-half (1/2) of the rates shown above.

Diligence Provisions:

1. By January 1, 2005, submit a reasonably complete written development plan for a Licensed Product for a first indication, including estimated money and personnel needed to execute such plan;
2. Complete toxicology and pharmacokinetics work and initiate an IND application for a Licensed Product by July 1, 2006;
3. Completion of a first Phase II clinical trial for a Licensed Product by July 1, 2008;
4. Completion of a first Phase III clinical trial for a Licensed Product by July 1 2010;
5. Submit an NDA for a Licensed Product by January 1, 2011; and
6. Achieve 1st commercial sale of a 1st Licensed Product by January 1, 2012.

Minimum Annual Royalty:

Due at the end of the relevant calendar year, as follows:

Year	MAR
2007 through and including the year in which a first NDA is filed for a 1st Licensed Product with the FDA or foreign equivalent	US $50,000
All subsequent years	US $250,000

Milestone Payments:

The following payments will be due for each distinct compound comprising a Licensed Product, for a 1st indication.
1. $25,000 upon filing of an IND;
2. $100,000 upon initiation of a 1st Phase I clinical trial;
3. $200,000 upon initiation of a 1st Phase II clinical trial;
4. $300,000 upon initiation of a 1st Phase III clinical trial;
5. $200,000 upon filing of an NDA;
6. $1,000,000 upon marketing approval in a 1st major country; and
7. $300,000 upon marketing approval in a 2nd major country.

Nonroyalty
Sublicensing Fees:

Shared equally between the parties

Maintenance Fees:

$10,000 annually at the end of each calendar year, starting in 2005—fully creditable against Minimum Annual Royalties

Insurance/Indemnification:

Required as a condition of the license (such insurance policy to name UVA and UVAPF as insured parties).

Agreed by:

HP _____   Date _____

UVAPF _____   Date _____

68

Elements of a License Agreement

Katherine Chou, MS, MBA

Academic institutions rely on the resources of industry to move inventions from their raw origins as data in a laboratory notebook into practical use. From the university perspective, the license agreement enables the commercial development of a technology, such as medical diagnostic or therapeutic, for widespread public benefit. Licensing revenue, in turn, flows back to the university to fund continued research. From a company standpoint, a license agreement ensures the ability to practice and develop a valued technology. A license agreement is a written contract that details the agreed-upon intent of the participating parties. The participating parties consist of the licensor (owner of the technologies) and the licensee(s) (parties who license the technologies from the licensor). Every agreement, although based on a standard template, has unique elements that can be modified to address each party's concerns and, in general, each element is negotiable.

There are many ways to reach the execution stage of a license agreement. The process commonly starts with discussions between party representatives, who exchange and modify a term sheet, complete an agreed-upon term sheet and, ultimately, translate the term sheet into a license agreement. The negotiation process can be lengthy, depending on the flexibility or steadfastness of each party regarding the individual licensing terms.

License Structure

In general, the licensee decides the type of agreement into which it will enter. In the event that the technology is a research tool (e.g., a cell line or an antibody) or provides a broad range of application, a licensor may predetermine the licensing terms. A sample license agreement is in Appendix A. Inventions arising from federal government funding may have such licensing restrictions in order to make the technology more widely available for research and commercial use. Some standard formats in which a license agreement can be structured include an option agreement, exclusive license, co-exclusive license, or nonexclusive license arrangements. Types of agreements are briefly described include:

- Option Agreement: provides a company a set period (option period) of time for exclusive evaluation of a technology. An option arrangement is favored in a situation in which a company requires additional time to assess the technology, or to research the market size, or to raise more funding before making its licensing decision. The company may exercise its option and enter into license agreement negotiations any time during the option period. However, should the company not exercise its option, the licensor has no further obligation to the company and may consider other commercial interest in the technology.
- Exclusive License: allows only one company to commercialize the technology. In the event that

761

the technology is developed using federal funding then the federal government shall have the free ("march-in") right to use the technology in addition to the company/licensee. This type of license structure is most frequently applied to therapeutic drug application technologies because a licensee must invest vast amounts of time and resources in order to commercialize such technologies. The Food and Drug Administration (FDA) requires extensive preclinical and clinical testing of potential therapeutic drugs. In addition to these obstacles to commercialization, there is the possibility that a licensee may neglect or defer development of an exclusively licensed technology or attempt to conceal that technology as a means of thwarting competitors. The licensor has a duty to ensure that commercialization of an exclusively licensed technology is not unduly delayed by the licensee. Therefore, in exchange for exclusivity, this type of license agreement usually demands high financial compensation from the licensee.

- Co-exclusive License: allows a minimum of two companies to commercialize the technology. There is no maximum number of companies in a co-exclusive arrangement, but typically up to three participating companies are involved in this type of license arrangement. The licensor may select such a deal structure when more than one potential licensee is interested in licensing a technology. In some cases, the co-exclusive licensees may partner to develop the technology (described in the next section on Field of Use and Territory). In the example, two companies interested in practicing the technology in particular parts of the world may enter into a co-exclusive license agreement that lists the territories (countries) in which they may practice the technology. Each company may have an established presence in its respective licensed territory, and the partnership enables both companies to work together to bring the technology into the world market. The co-exclusive license outlines both the individual and collective rights and obligations of the licensees.

- Nonexclusive License: provides many companies with opportunities to commercialize the technology. This type of deal structure is common for research tool or reagent technologies. Nonexclusive licensees have restricted rights to practice the technology for particular purposes. However, they generally also have fewer responsibilities; for instance, they may be exempt from reimbursing patent-related expenses for the technology.

Field of Use and Territory

Certain defined terms in a license agreement specify the areas in which a licensee may practice a licensed technology. These terms can be tailored to meet the business focus of the licensee and may enable the licensor to license the technology more broadly to different companies.

The phrase "field of use" refers to how the licensee may apply the technology. Different fields of use can be licensed separately depending on the licensee's business interest. Field of use definitions such as "all field of use," "therapeutic applications," "diagnostic applications," and "internal research use only" are commonly used in a license agreement with a pharmaceutical or biotechnology licensee. The type of technology licensed determines how the field of use is defined; for example, a chemical compound may have both diagnostic and therapeutic applications and, in such a case, the licensor may split the therapeutic applications and diagnostic applications into two distinct fields of use and license each field of use separately. Such arrangement is possible if the licensor identifies two companies interested in licensing an individual field of use.

Rights to practice in specific geographic areas can also be licensed separately depending on a company's business focus and needs. For example, for the same technology, Company A may have a license to practice only in China and Company B may have a license in the rest of the world. In this case, a co-exclusive license would be appropriate and some of the considering factors should include alliance strategy in marketing partners and a technology's application in certain designated area.

Monetary Compensation

In consideration of the owner of a technology granting a licensee the right to use a technology, a licensee provides financial compensation to the licensor. There are no guidelines or standard rules regarding the range of the financial compensation the licensor can demand or regarding what the licensee is willing to pay. The development stage of the technology plays a big role in determining the amount. The more a licensee has to invest to commercialize the technology, the less financial compensation a licensor can demand. The utility, originality, competition, advantages, status as intellectual property, and potential market of a technology are also important factors in determining its value. The scope of applications for which the technology will be licensed is another critical factor. All other factors being equal, therapeutic applications usually demand higher compensation.

Listed below are terms commonly used in a license agreement:

- Upfront License/Option Fee

  The upfront license/option fee is usually a one-time fee that is nonrefundable. This fee indicates the commitment of the licensee to enter into the license agreement. The fee can be in the form of cash and/or stock (equity) of a company. Each university has its own policy regarding acceptance of stock as full or partial licensing compensation as well as the amount of stock that can be accepted due to conflict of interest considerations.

- Royalty

  A licensee pays a licensor royalty based on net sales (including sublicensing revenues) of a licensed product. Various approaches can be applied to royalty rates in a license agreement. Two examples are: (1) a single royalty rate based on a licensed product; or (2) a tier system in which a different royalty rate is applied based on the aggregated sales volume

- Monetary Performance Milestone

  Universities often require licensees to share financial rewards when the licensed technologies achieve certain milestones during the commercialization process. For example, it is commonly accepted that licensees pay a prenegotiated financial compensation when a licensee completes a satisfactory phase II clinical trial or obtains FDA approval on a licensed product. Completion of these objectives indicates that a company has made substantial strides in bringing the product to the marketplace.

- Maintenance Fee

  A licensee pays an annual fee to maintain the license with the licensor. This fee usually is credited against the running royalty. This is a desirable tool for a licensor to provide incentive to its licensee in continuing to develop/commercialize the licensed technology.

Nonmonetary Performance Milestone

In order to ensure that a licensee diligently develops licensed technologies, universities sometimes set up nonmonetary performance milestones to monitor

the time line for commercial development of a licensed technology. For example, a university/licensor may require its licensee to complete certain preclinical animal model studies and to initiate a human clinical trial within two years after a company obtains a license. For early stage technologies in particular, licensee-sponsored research in the inventor's laboratory may also provide additional data for further development of the technology.

Legal Expenses and Patent Prosecution

Universities provide their potential commercial partners a competitive edge in commercializing their technologies through patent protection for intellectual property. Therefore, universities usually require an exclusive licensee to reimburse past legal expenses and to take responsibility for all future legal expenses. In a co-exclusive arrangement, the incurred past legal expenses would be shared by all licensees. The co-exclusive licensees are also responsible for all future legal expenses. Universities seldom require nonexclusive licensees to be responsible for legal expenses. In the case of an option arrangement, the optionee usually is required to pay for the legal expenses incurred during the option period.

Once an exclusive license agreement is established, both licensor and licensee(s) usually cooperate in guiding patent prosecution, with universities (licensor) taking the lead. In a co-exclusive arrangement, universities take input from co-exclusive licensees and maintain a leading role in the patent prosecution process. In a nonexclusive arrangement, universities take a leading role in the patent prosecution process.

Infringement

In the event that a third party is infringing a licensed technology, university licensors may or may not take a leading role in pursuing the infringer depending on the type of license arrangement. An exclusive licensee usually has the responsibility for taking a leading role in going after the infringer. For a co-exclusive arrangement, there is often a preagreed condition indicating which co-exclusive licensee will take the leading role. Alternatively, the licensor may take the lead. Universities usually take a leading role in going after infringers of nonexclusively licensed technologies, if the universities decide to pursue the infringer.

Publication

Publication freedom is essential for universities and the license agreements for university licensors are structured to preserve their research freedom and rights to freely publish their research results. However, when a university licenses its technology and adopts an external partner to commercialize its technology, the university as licensor would have to consider its commercial partner's welfare in allowing a set period of time for the company/licensee to request filing for patent protection before publishing its scientific findings.

Each university has specific guidelines for such requests. Both universities and companies often accept a review period of thirty days prior to submission of a manuscript for publication review, followed by a maximum of sixty additional days to allow for the filing of a patent application.

Name Use

Universities and their commercial partners usually have different missions. Therefore, use of the other party's name becomes a challenge once a license business relationship is established. In general, universities require an opportunity to review and approve public announcements (both verbal and print) to ensure that no misleading statements are presented in such announcements. Each university has its own policy providing guidelines for name use.

Successful negotiations, although often prolonged and intense, culminate in a license agreement between the licensor and the licensee. During their "courtship," each party worked to accommodate the reasonable interests and concerns of the other party while simultaneously remaining faithful to its own policies, guidelines, and interests. Once their partnership has been established, it is equally important that the licensor and licensee keep their mutual passion for the technology alive. In order for their relationship to prosper, each party must demonstrate its commitment, either through providing technical input or meeting payment deadlines and milestone obligations. Both parties will benefit from their collective dedication to developing the licensed technology. A future chapter considers how the licensor and licensee can build and improve a long-term relationship following the "honeymoon period" when the licensing vows have been exchanged.

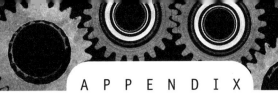

68-A

Sample License Agreement

Exclusive License Agreement
Between
Angel University
And
Wincell, Inc.
Effective as of January 1, 2004
Re: CLA_JOH.001, entitled "The use of Aba the anti-cancer compound"

For and in consideration of the mutual promises and covenants set forth below, intending to be legally bound, the parties hereto agree as follows:

ARTICLE I

DEFINITIONS

As used in this Agreement, the following terms shall have the following meanings:

1.1 ACADEMIC RESEARCH PURPOSES: use of PATENT RIGHTS for academic research or other not-for-profit scholarly purposes which are undertaken at a nonprofit or governmental institution that does not use the PATENT RIGHTS in the production or manufacture of products for commercial sale or the performance of services for a fee.

1.2 AFFILIATE: shall mean any entity which controls, is controlled by, or is under common control with LICENSEE. For the purposes of this definition, "control" shall mean beneficial ownership (direct or indirect) of more than fifty percent (50%) of the shares of the subject entity entitled to vote in the election of directors (or, in the case of an entity that is not a corporation, for the election of the corresponding managing authority). Unless otherwise specified, the term LICENSEE includes AFFILIATES.

1.3 CONSIDERATION: shall mean and include without limitation, money, services, property and any other thing of value such as payment of costs, cancellation or forgiveness of indebtedness, discounts, rebates, barter and the like. If any such CONSIDERATION is in a form other than cash (such as in kind, equity interests, indebtedness earn-outs, or other deferred payments, consulting fees, etc.) then the value of such CONSIDERATION shall be determined in good faith by the Parties.

1.4 FIELD: All fields of use.

1.5   AU: Angel University, a nonprofit Pennsylvania educational corporation having offices at 1000 Market Street, Philadelphia, PA 19100.

1.6   LICENSED PROCESSES: the processes covered by at least one VALID CLAIM included within the PATENT RIGHTS.

1.7   LICENSED PRODUCTS: product(s) covered by at least one VALID CLAIM included within the PATENT RIGHTS or products made or services provided in accordance with or by means of LICENSED PROCESSES.

1.8   LICENSEE: Wincell, Inc., a corporation organized under the laws of Delaware having its principal offices at 1000 Pine Street, Rochester, New York 14500.

1.9   NET RESEARCH AND DEVELOPMENT INCOME: RESEARCH AND DEVELOPMENT INCOME less LICENSEE's actual direct cost for research, development and/or research development services provided.

1.10 NET SALES: the amount collected or received (whichever occurs first) from non-affiliated third parties for sales, leases, or other transfers (other than sublicenses) of LICENSED PRODUCTS, less:

   (a) customary trade, quantity, wholesaler, distributor, prompt payment or cash discounts and non-affiliated brokers', agents' or other resellers' commissions actually allowed and taken;

   (b) amounts repaid or credited by reason of rejection, return or retroactive price reduction;

   (c) taxes levied on and/or other governmental charges made as to production, sale, transportation, storage, delivery or use and paid by or on behalf of LICENSEE or SUBLICENSEES; and

   (d) reasonable charges for delivery, transportation, storage, packing and insurance provided by third parties, if separately stated.

   NET SALES also includes the fair market value of any CONSIDERATION whatsoever received by LICENSEE or SUBLICENSEES for the sale, lease, or transfer of LICENSED PRODUCTS, other than NON-ROYALTY SUBLICENSE INCOME; provided, however that any transfers among LICENSEE, its AFFILIATE, SUBLICENSEES or third party resellers shall not be considered a sale and shall be excluded from NET SALES, and only the subsequent sales of LICENSED PRODUCTS to unrelated third parties shall be deemed NET SALES hereunder.

1.11 RESEARCH AND DEVELOPMENT INCOME: the total financial CONSIDERATION of any kind (excluding amounts taken into account for purposes of calculating NET SALES) received as a result of the utilization of LICENSED PRODUCTS or LICENSED PROCESSES by LICENSEE as a result of a contract with a third party.

1.12 SUBLICENSE INCOME: the amount paid to LICENSEE by a third party (other than an AFFILIATE of LICENSEE) for the granting of a sublicense under Section 3.1 hereinafter, including but not limited to (i) license fees, (ii) milestone payments, (iii) the fair market value in cash of any non-cash CONSIDERATION of any kind for such sublicense, (iv) in the event that LICENSEE receives any payment for equity in connection with such sublicense that included a premium over the fair market value of such equity, the amount of such premium, and (v) NET RESEARCH AND DEVELOPMENT INCOME.

1.13 PATENT RIGHTS: The applications and patents as listed in Appendix A of this Agreement, the VALID CLAIMS of such applications and patents, the inventions described and claimed therein, and any divisions, or continuations, or continuations-in-part of the applications and patents as listed in Appendix A, and specific claims of any continuations-in-part of such applications to the extent the specific claims are directed to subject matter described in the applications and patents listed in Appendix A in a manner sufficient to support such specific claims under 35 U.S.C., patents issuing thereon or reissues thereof, and any and all foreign patents and patent applications corresponding thereto, all to the extent owned or controlled by AU.

1.14 SUBLICENSEE: as used in this Agreement shall mean any third party to whom LICENSEE has granted a license to make, have made, use and/or sell the LICENSED PRODUCT or LICENSED PROCESS under PATENT RIGHTS, provided said third party has agreed in writing with LICENSEE to accept the conditions and restrictions agreed to by LICENSEE in this Agreement.

1.15 TERRITORY: Worldwide.

1.16 VALID CLAIM: either (a) a claim of an issued patent that has not been held unenforceable or invalid by an agency or a court of competent jurisdiction in any unappealable or unappealed decision or (b) a claim of a pending patent application that has not been abandoned or finally rejected without the possibility of appeal or refiling and that has been pending for less than five (5) years from its priority date.

1.17 The terms "Public Law 96-517" and "Public Law 98-620" include all amendments to those statutes.

1.18 The terms "sold" and "sell" include leases and other legal transfers and similar transactions involving CONSIDERATION.

ARTICLE II

REPRESENTATIONS

2.1 AU is owner by assignment from inventors of their entire right, title and interest in the PATENT RIGHTS, and in the inventions described and claimed therein as listed in the Appendix.

2.2 AU has the authority to issue licenses under PATENT RIGHTS.

2.3 AU is committed to the policy that ideas or creative works produced at AU should be used for the greatest possible public benefit, and believes that every reasonable incentive should be provided for the prompt introduction of such ideas into public use, all in a manner consistent with the public interest.

2.4 LICENSEE is prepared and intends to diligently develop the invention and to bring products to market which are subject to this Agreement.

2.5 LICENSEE is desirous of obtaining an exclusive license in the TERRITORY in order to practice the above-referenced invention covered by PATENT RIGHTS in the United States and in certain foreign countries, and to manufacture, use and sell in the commercial market the products made in accordance therewith, and AU is desirous of granting such a license to LICENSEE in accordance with the terms of this Agreement.

ARTICLE III

GRANT OF RIGHTS

3.1 AU hereby grants to LICENSEE and LICENSEE accepts, subject to the terms and conditions hereof, in the TERRITORY and in the FIELD an exclusive license under PATENT RIGHTS to research and develop, to make and have made, to use and have used, to sell and have sold the LICENSED PRODUCTS, and to practice the LICENSED PROCESSES, for the life of the PATENT RIGHTS.

3.2 AU also grants to LICENSEE the right to issue sublicenses to third parties to make, have made, use, and sell LICENSED PRODUCTS and to practice LICENSED PROCESSES, providing LICENSEE has current exclusive rights thereto under this Agreement. LICENSEE shall within thirty (30) days of executing any such sublicense provide AU a copy of such sublicense agreement. To the extent applicable, such sublicenses shall include all of the rights of and obligations due to AU (and, if applicable, the United States Government) that are contained in this Agreement. LICENSEE shall collect and guarantee payment of all royalties due AU from SUBLICENSEES, and summarize and deliver all reports due AU from SUBLICENSEES.

3.3 The granting and exercise of this license is subject to the following conditions:

(a) AU's "Patent Policy," Public Law 96-517 and Public Law 98-620. Any right granted in this Agreement greater than that permitted under Public Law 96-517, or Public Law 98-620, shall be subject to modification as may be required to conform to the provisions of those statutes.

(b) AU reserves the right to make and use, and grant to others nonexclusive licenses to make and use for ACADEMIC RESEARCH PURPOSES the subject matter described and claimed in PATENT RIGHTS.

(c) LICENSEE shall use commercially reasonable diligent efforts to effect introduction of the LICENSED PRODUCTS into the commercial market as soon as practicable, consistent with sound and reasonable business practice and judgment; thereafter, until the expiration of this Agreement, LICENSEE shall endeavor to keep LICENSED PRODUCTS reasonably available to the public.

(d) Pursuant to Section 9.2(c), at any time after five (5) years from the effective date of this Agreement, AU may terminate or render this license nonexclusive if, in AU's reasonable judgment, the Progress Reports furnished by LICENSEE substantially demonstrate that LICENSEE:

(i) has not put the licensed subject matter into commercial use in a country or countries in the TERRITORY, directly or through a sublicense (provided, however, that any such termination or rendering of this license nonexclusive shall only terminate or render it nonexclusive with respect to such country or countries), and is not keeping the licensed subject matter reasonably available to the public; and

(ii) is not engaged in research, development, manufacturing, marketing or sublicensing activity reasonably appropriate to achieving (i) above.

(e) AU understands and acknowledges that LICENSEE will be spending considerable resources, both human and financial, on the development of the LICENSED PRODUCTS in an effort to obtain the necessary approvals of LICENSED PRODUCTS in the Territory. LICENSEE further acknowledges that it is AU's mission to make the LICENSED PRODUCTS available to the public.

(f) In all sublicenses granted by LICENSEE hereunder, LICENSEE shall include a requirement that the SUBLICENSEE(S) use commercially reasonable efforts to bring the subject matter of the sublicense into commercial use as quickly as is reasonably possible. LICENSEE shall further provide in such sublicenses that such sublicenses are subject and subordinate to the terms and conditions of this Agreement, except: (i) the SUBLICENSEE may not further sublicense; and (ii) the rate of royalty on NET SALES paid by the SUBLICENSEE to the LICENSEE. AU agrees to maintain any information contained in such provisions in confidence, except as otherwise required by law, however, AU may include in its usual reports annual amounts of royalties paid.

(g) A license in any other field of use in addition to the FIELD shall be the subject of a separate agreement and shall require LICENSEE's submission of evidence, satisfactory to AU, demonstrating LICENSEE's willingness and ability to develop and commercialize in such other field of use the kinds of products or processes likely to be encompassed in such other fields. Prior to entering into negotiations with any third party for an exclusive license in any territory or field of use in addition to the TERRITORY and/or FIELD, AU agrees to notify LICENSEE, and provides opportunity for LICENSEE to make license proposals.

(h) To the extent that federal funds are used to support research leading to a patent or patent application in the PATENT RIGHTS, LICENSEE shall cause any LICENSED PRODUCT produced for sale by LICENSEE or SUBLICENSEES in the United States to be manufactured substantially in the United States during the period of exclusivity of this license in the United States.

3.4 All rights reserved to the United States Government and others under Public Law 96-517, and Public Law 98-620, shall remain and shall in no way be affected by this Agreement.

ARTICLE IV

ROYALTIES

4.1 (a) LICENSEE shall pay to AU a nonrefundable license royalty fee in the sum of fifty thousand dollars ($50,000). Twenty thousand dollars ($20,000) is due to AU upon execution of the Agreement and the remaining balance is due to AU three months (3) months after the execution date of this Agreement.

(b) As further consideration for the rights granted hereunder, LICENSEE shall pay to AU during the term of this Agreement a royalty in the form of stock of LICENSEE. LICENSEE shall issue to AU restricted shares of common stock ("Shares") equivalent to five percent (5%) of LICENSEE's outstanding shares of common stock on the date hereof pursuant to the terms of a mutually acceptable Stock Subscription Agreement, provided, however, that AU shall be, now and in the future, subject to and enter into such agreements and related documents as are required of other stockholders of LICENSEE. Additional shares shall be issued to AU to maintain such percentage until LICENSEE raises aggregated paid-in capital in the amount of one and one half (1.5) million dollars.

AU's ownership rights to Shares shall not be affected should the license pursuant to this Agreement be converted to a nonexclusive one.

4.2 (a) In accordance with Section 5.4, LICENSEE shall pay to AU during the term of this Agreement a royalty of three percent (3%) of NET SALES by LICENSEE.

(b) For each LICENSED PRODUCT or LICENSED PROCESS sold by LICENSEE, LICENSEE may credit up to one half (1/2) of royalties that LICENSEE is paying to third parties on LICENSEE's NET SALES of that LICENSED PRODUCT or LICENSED PROCESS against royalty payments due AU pursuant to (a) above, provided that the royalty paid to AU pursuant to (a) above shall not be reduced below one and one-half percent (1.5%) of the NET SALES of that LICENSED PRODUCT for which such third party royalties are being paid.

(c) In the case of sublicenses, in accordance with Section 5.4 LICENSEE shall pay to AU a royalty of twenty-two and one-half percent (22.5%) of all SUBLICENSE INCOME.

4.3 As further consideration for the rights granted hereunder, LICENSEE shall pay to AU during the term of this Agreement the following cash milestone payments within thirty (30) days of their occurrence (time of payment is of the essence):

For the first two licensed human therapeutic products:

(i) One hundred thousand dollars ($100,000) upon the filing of a LICENSEE sponsored Phase III clinical trial, and

(ii) Two hundred thousand dollars ($200,000) upon the filing of a New Drug Application ("NDA")

4.4 Anything herein to the contrary, if the license pursuant to this Agreement is converted to a nonexclusive one and if other nonexclusive licenses in the same field and territory are granted, the above royalties in Sections 4.1 and 4.2 shall not exceed the royalty rate to be paid by other licensees in the same field and territory during the term of the nonexclusive license and the milestone payments provided in Section 4.3 shall not be payable.

4.5 No later than January 1st of each calendar year after the effective date of this Agreement, LICENSEE shall pay to AU the following nonrefundable advance on those royalties due AU pursuant to Sections 4.1 and 4.2 above. Such payments may only be credited against running royalties due for that calendar year and Royalty Reports shall reflect such a credit. Such payments shall not be credited against milestone payments in Section 4.3 (if any) nor against royalties due for any subsequent calendar year nor for any other payments made pursuant to this license.

January 1, 2005	$ 10,000
January 1, 2006	$ 15,000
January 1, 2007	$ 15,000
each year thereafter	$ 15,000

ARTICLE V

REPORTING

5.1 Six (6) months after signing this Agreement, LICENSEE shall provide to AU a written research and development plan under which LICENSEE intends to bring the subject matter of the licenses granted hereunder into commercial use. Such plan includes projections of sales and proposed marketing efforts.

5.2 No later than sixty (60) days after June 30 of each calendar year, LICENSEE shall provide to AU a detailed written annual Progress Report describing progress on research and development, regulatory approvals, manufacturing, sublicensing, marketing and sales during the most recent twelve (12) month period ending June 30 and plans for the forthcoming year. If multiple technologies are covered by the license granted hereunder, the Progress Report shall provide the information set forth above for each technology. If progress differs from that anticipated in the plan required under Section 5.1, LICENSEE shall explain the reasons for the difference and propose a modified research and development plan for AU's review. LICENSEE shall also provide any reasonable additional data AU reasonably requires to evaluate LICENSEE's performance.

5.3 LICENSEE shall report to AU the date of first sale of LICENSED PRODUCTS (or results of LICENSED PROCESSES) in each country within thirty (30) days of occurrence.

5.4 (a) LICENSEE shall submit to AU within sixty (60) days after each calendar half year ending June 30 and December 31, a Royalty Report setting forth for such half year at least the following information:

(i) the number of LICENSED PRODUCTS sold by LICENSEE and SUBLICENSEE in each country;

(ii) total billings and amounts actually received by LICENSEE for such LICENSED PRODUCTS;

(iii) an accounting for all LICENSED PROCESSES used or sold;

(iv) deductions applicable to determine the NET SALES thereof;

(v) the amount of SUBLICENSE INCOME received by LICENSEE; and

(vi) the amount of royalty due thereon, pursuant to Sections 4.1 and 4.2 less any credits pursuant to Section 4.5, or, if no royalties are due to AU for any reporting period, the statement that no royalties are due.

Such report shall be certified as correct by an officer of LICENSEE and shall include a detailed listing of all deductions from royalties.

(b) LICENSEE shall pay to AU with each such Royalty Report the amount of royalty due with respect to such half (1/2) year.

(c) All payments due hereunder shall be deemed received when funds are credited to AU's bank account and shall be payable by check or wire transfer in United States dollars. Conversion of foreign currency to U.S. dollars shall be made in accordance with LICENSEE's standard accounting practices relating to recognition of revenue from foreign sales. No transfer, exchange, collection or other charges shall be deducted from such payments.

(d) Late payments shall be subject to a charge of one and one-half percent (1.5%) per month, or $250, whichever is greater.

5.5 In the event of acquisition, merger, change of corporate name, or reorganization, LICENSEE shall notify AU in writing within thirty (30) days of such event and provide AU with reasonable assurance that such changes shall not effect payment to AU or the commercialization of the LICENSED PRODUCT and or LICENSED PROCESS.

5.6 If LICENSEE or any AFFILIATE or SUBLICENSEE does not qualify as a "small entity" as provided by the United States Patent and Trademark Office, LICENSEE must notify AU immediately.

ARTICLE VI

RECORD KEEPING

6.1 LICENSEE shall keep, and shall require its AFFILIATES and SUBLICENSEES to keep, accurate records (together with supporting documentation) of LICENSED PRODUCTS made, used or sold under this Agreement, appropriate to determine the amount of royalties due to AU hereunder. Such records shall be retained for at least three (3) years following the end of the reporting period to which they relate. They shall be available during normal business hours for examination by an accountant selected by AU, for the sole purpose of verifying reports and payments hereunder. In conducting examinations pursuant to this Section, AU's accountant shall have access to all records which AU reasonably believes to be relevant to the calculation of royalties under Article IV.

6.2 AU's accountant shall not disclose to AU any information other than information relating to the accuracy of reports and payments made hereunder.

6.3 Such examination by AU's accountant shall be at AU's expense, except that if such examination shows an underreporting or underpayment in excess of five percent (5%) for any twelve (12) month period, then LICENSEE shall pay the cost of such examination as well as any additional sum that would have been payable to AU had the LICENSEE reported correctly, plus interest on said sum at the rate of one and one-half percent (1.5%) per month.

ARTICLE VII

DOMESTIC AND FOREIGN PATENT FILING AND MAINTENANCE

7.1 Upon execution of this Agreement, LICENSEE shall pay AU $_____ as a partial reimbursement of the expenses AU has incurred for the preparation, filing, prosecution and maintenance of PATENT RIGHTS prior to the execution date of this Agreement. Six (6) months after execution of this Agreement, LICENSEE shall pay AU $_____ as reimbursement for the remaining expenses AU has incurred for the preparation, filing, prosecution and maintenance of PATENT RIGHTS prior to the execution date of this Agreement.

Subject to Section 7.4, after the execution date of this agreement, LICENSEE shall reimburse AU for all such future reasonable expenses for preparation, filing, prosecution and maintenance of PATENT RIGHTS as described in Section 7.2 upon receipt of invoices from AU. Late payment (thirty (30) days from first invoice) of these invoices shall be subject to interest charges of one and one-half percent (1.5%) per month.

7.2 AU shall be responsible for the preparation, filing, prosecution and maintenance of any and all patent applications and patents included in PATENT RIGHTS. AU will instruct counsel to directly notify AU and LICENSEE and provide them copies of any official communications from the United States and foreign patent offices relating to said prosecution, and to provide LICENSEE and AU with advance copies of all relevant communications to the various patent offices, so that LICENSEE may be informed and apprised of the continuing prosecution of patent applications in PATENT RIGHTS. LICENSEE shall have reasonable opportunities to participate in decision making on all key decisions affecting filing, prosecution and maintenance of patents and patent applications in PATENT RIGHTS. AU will use reasonable efforts to incorporate LICENSEE's reasonable suggestions regarding said prosecution. AU shall use all reasonable efforts to amend any patent application to include claims reasonably requested by LICENSEE to protect LICENSED PRODUCTS.

7.3 AU and LICENSEE shall cooperate fully in the preparation, filing, prosecution and maintenance of PATENT RIGHTS and of all patents and patent applications licensed to LICENSEE hereunder, executing all papers and instruments or requiring members of AU to execute such papers and instruments so as to enable AU to apply for, to prosecute and to maintain patent applications and patents in AU's name in any country. Each party shall provide to the other prompt notice as to all matters which come to its attention and which may affect the preparation, filing, prosecution or maintenance of any such patent applications or patents. In particular, LICENSEE must immediately notify AU if LICENSEE or any AFFILIATE or SUBLICENSEE does not qualify as a "small entity" as provided by the United States Patent and Trademark Office.

ARTICLE VIII

INFRINGEMENT

8.1 LICENSEE may elect to surrender its PATENT RIGHTS in any country upon sixty (60) days written notice to AU and upon expiration of such 60 day period LICENSEE shall have no further obligation under Section 7.1 above to reimburse AU for fees associated with such country. Such notice shall not relieve LICENSEE from responsibility to reimburse AU for patent-related expenses incurred prior to the expiration of the (60) day notice period (or such longer period specified in LICENSEE's notice).

8.2 With respect to any PATENT RIGHTS that are exclusively licensed to LICENSEE pursuant to this Agreement, LICENSEE shall have the right to prosecute in its own name and at its own expense any infringement of such patent, so long as such license is exclusive at the time of the commencement of such action. (For purposes of clarification, although AU has reserved certain rights pursuant to Section 3.3(b), the parties still deem the license hereunder to be "exclusive.") AU agrees to notify LICENSEE promptly of each infringement of such patents of which AU is or becomes aware. Before LICENSEE commences an action with respect to any infringement of such patents, LICENSEE shall give careful consideration to the views of AU and to potential effects on the public interest in making its decision whether or not to prosecute.

(a) If LICENSEE elects to commence an action as described above, AU may, to the extent permitted by law, and at its own expense, join as a party in that action and AU shall cooperate fully with LICENSEE in connection with any such action.

(b) Other than as set forth in Section 8.2(a), LICENSEE shall reimburse AU for any costs AU incurs, including reasonable attorneys' fees, as part of an action brought by LICENSEE.

8.3 If LICENSEE elects to commence an action as described above, LICENSEE may deduct from its royalty payments to AU with respect to the patent(s) subject to suit an amount not exceeding fifty percent (50%) of LICENSEE's expenses and costs of such action, including reasonable attorneys' fees; provided, however, that such reduction shall not exceed fifty percent (50%) of the total royalty due to AU with respect to the patent(s) subject to suit for each calendar year. If such fifty percent (50%) of LICENSEE's expenses and costs exceeds the amount of royalties deducted by LICENSEE for any calendar year, LICENSEE may to that extent reduce the royalties due to AU from LICENSEE in succeeding calendar years, but never by more than fifty percent (50%) of the total royalty due in any one year with respect to the patent(s) subject to suit.

8.4 No settlement, consent judgment or other voluntary final disposition of any suit that materially adversely affects a party's rights may be entered into without the prior written consent of the other party, which consent shall not be unreasonably withheld.

8.5 Recoveries or reimbursements from actions commenced pursuant to this Article shall first be applied to reimburse LICENSEE and AU for litigation costs not paid from royalties and then to reimburse AU for royalties deducted by LICENSEE pursuant to Section 8.3. Any additional recoveries shall shared by LICENSEE and AU, fifty percent (50%) to LICENSEE and fifty percent (50%) to AU.

8.6 If LICENSEE elects not to exercise its right to prosecute an infringement of the PATENT RIGHTS pursuant to this Article, AU may do so at its own expense, controlling such action and retaining all recoveries therefrom. LICENSEE shall cooperate fully with AU in connection with any such action.

AU shall reimburse LICENSEE for any costs LICENSEE incurs, including reasonable attorneys' fees, as part of an action brought by AU.

8.7 Without limiting the generality of Section 8.6, AU may, at its election and by notice to LICENSEE, establish a time limit of ninety (90) days for LICENSEE to decide whether to prosecute any infringement of which AU is or becomes aware. If, by the end of such ninety (90) day period, LICENSEE has not commenced such an action, AU may prosecute such an infringement at its own expense, controlling such action and retaining all recoveries therefrom. With respect to any such infringement action prosecuted by AU in good faith, LICENSEE shall pay over to AU any payments (whether or not designated as "royalties") made by the alleged infringer to LICENSEE under any existing or future sublicense authorizing LICENSED PRODUCTS, up to the amount of AU's unreimbursed litigation expenses (including, but not limited to, reasonable attorneys' fees).

8.8 If a declaratory judgment action is brought naming LICENSEE as a defendant and alleging invalidity of any of the PATENT RIGHTS, AU may elect to take over the sole defense of the action at its own expense. LICENSEE shall cooperate fully with AU in connection with any such action.

ARTICLE IX

TERMINATION OF AGREEMENT

9.1 This Agreement, unless terminated as provided herein, shall remain in effect until the last patent or patent application containing a VALID CLAIM in PATENT RIGHTS has expired or been abandoned.

9.2 AU may terminate this Agreement as follows:

(a) If LICENSEE does not make a payment due hereunder and fails to cure such nonpayment (including the payment of interest in accordance with Section 5.4(e)) within thirty (30) days after the date of notice in writing of such nonpayment by AU.

(b) As described in Section 10.3(d) if LICENSEE defaults in its obligations under Section 10.3(c) to procure and maintain insurance.

(c) If, at any time after five years from the date of this Agreement, AU determines that the Agreement should be terminated pursuant to Section 3.2(d).

(d) If LICENSEE shall make an assignment for the benefit of creditors, shall have been declared bankrupt by a court of competent jurisdiction, makes use of any law or regulation for relief from creditors, or reorganizes or restructures in order to avoid creditors. Such termination shall be effective immediately upon AU giving written notice to LICENSEE.

(e) If an examination by AU's accountant pursuant to Article VI shows an underreporting or underpayment by LICENSEE of amounts owned under Sections 4.1 and 4.2 in excess of twenty percent (20%) for any twelve (12) month period and in excess of fifty thousand dollars ($50,000) and LICENSEE fails to cure such underpayment within thirty (30) days after the date of notice in writing from AU of such underpayment.

(f) If LICENSEE is convicted of, or pleads nolo-contendere to, a felony relating to the manufacture, use, or sale of LICENSED PRODUCTS.

(g) Except as provided in Subsections (a), (b), (c), (d), (e) and (f) above, if LICENSEE defaults in a material respect in the performance of any obligations under this Agreement and the default has not been remedied within sixty (60) days after the date of notice in writing of such default by AU.

9.3 LICENSEE shall provide, in all sublicenses granted by it under this Agreement, that such sublicenses shall survive the termination of this Agreement and that LICENSEE's interest in such sublicenses shall be assigned to AU upon termination of this Agreement; provided, however, that AU shall not be subject to LICENSEE's obligations to its SUBLICENSEEs under such assigned sublicenses.

9.4 LICENSEE may terminate this Agreement by giving ninety (90) days advance written notice of termination to AU. Upon termination, LICENSEE shall submit a final Royalty Report to AU and any royalty payments and unreimbursed patent expenses due to AU shall become immediately payable. Upon termination by LICENSEE, all obligations and duties under this LICENSEE shall cease and terminate and LICENSEE agrees to execute all reasonable documentations requested evidencing such termination.

9.5 Sections 6.1, 6.2, 6.3, 8.5, 9.5, 10.2, 10.4, 10.5 and 10.8 of this Agreement shall survive termination.

ARTICLE X

GENERAL

10.1 AU does not warrant the validity of the PATENT RIGHTS licensed hereunder and makes no representations whatsoever with regard to the scope of the licensed PATENT RIGHTS or that such PATENT RIGHTS may be exploited by LICENSEE, an AFFILIATE, or SUBLICENSEE without infringing other patents.

10.2 AU EXPRESSLY DISCLAIMS ANY AND ALL IMPLIED OR EXPRESS WARRANTIES AND MAKES NO EXPRESS OR IMPLIED WARRANTIES OF MERCHANTABILITY OR FITNESS FOR ANY PARTICULAR PURPOSE OF THE PATENT RIGHTS OR INFORMATION SUPPLIED BY AU, LICENSED PROCESSES OR LICENSED PRODUCTS CONTEMPLATED BY THIS AGREEMENT. IN NO EVENT WILL AU BE LIABLE FOR ANY INCIDENTIAL, SPECIAL OR CONSEQUENTIAL DAMAGES RESULTING FROM EXERCISE OF THIS LICENSE OR THE USE OF THE INVENTIONS OR LICENSED PRODUCTS.

10.3 (a) LICENSEE shall indemnify, defend and hold harmless AU and its current or former directors, governing board members, trustees, officers, faculty, medical and professional staff, employees, students, and agents and their respective successors, heirs and assigns (collectively, the "INDEMNITEES"), from and against any claim, liability, cost, expense, damage, deficiency, loss or obligation of any kind or nature (including, without limitation, reasonable attorney's fees and other costs and expenses of litigation) (collectively, "Claims"), based upon, arising out of, or otherwise relating to any cause of action relating to product liability concerning any product, process, or service made, used or sold pursuant to any right or license granted under this Agreement.

(b) LICENSEE shall, at its own expense, provide attorneys reasonably acceptable to AU to defend against any actions brought or filed against any Indemnitee hereunder with respect to the subject of indemnity contained herein, whether or not such actions are rightfully brought.

(c) Beginning at the time any such product, process or service is being commercially distributed or sold (other than for the purpose of obtaining regulatory approvals) by LICENSEE or by a SUBLICENSEE, AFFILIATE or agent of LICENSEE, LICENSEE shall, at its sole cost and expense, procure and maintain commercial general liability insurance in amounts not less than $2,000,000 per incident and $2,000,000 annual aggregate and naming the Indemnitees as additional insureds. During clinical trials of any such product, process or service, LICENSEE shall, at its sole cost and expense, procure and maintain commercial general liability insurance in such equal or lesser amount as AU shall reasonably require, naming the AU as additional insureds. Such commercial general liability insurance shall provide: (i) product liability coverage; and (ii) broad form contractual liability coverage for LICENSEE's indemnification under this Agreement. If LICENSEE elects to self-insure all or part of the limits described above (including deductibles or retentions which are in excess of $250,000 annual aggregate) such self-insurance program must be reasonably acceptable to AU. The minimum amounts of insurance coverage required shall not be construed to create a limit of LICENSEE's liability with respect to its indemnification under this Agreement.

(d) LICENSEE shall provide AU with written evidence of such insurance upon request of AU. LICENSEE shall provide AU with written notice at least fifteen (15) days prior to the cancellation, nonrenewal or material change in such insurance; if LICENSEE does not obtain replacement insurance providing comparable coverage within such fifteen (15) day period, AU shall have the right to terminate this Agreement effective at the end of such fifteen (15) day period without notice or any additional waiting periods.

(e) LICENSEE shall maintain such commercial general liability insurance beyond the expiration or termination of this Agreement during: (i) the period that any product, process, or service, relating to, or developed pursuant to, this Agreement is being commercially distributed or sold by LICENSEE or by a SUBLICENSEE, AFFILIATE or agent of LICENSEE; and (ii) a reasonable period after the period referred to in Subsection (e)(i) above which in no event shall be less than fifteen (15) years.

10.4 LICENSEE shall not use AU's name or insignia, or any adaptation of them, or the name of any of AU's inventors in any advertising, publicity, promotional activities or sales literature without the prior written approval of AU except in announcing to the public the existence of this agreement, consistent with LICENSEE's legal responsibility as a public company. Nothing contained in this Agreement shall be construed as conferring any right to use in advertising, publicity, or other promotional activities any name, trade name, trademark, or other designation of either party hereto (including contraction, abbreviation or simulation of any of the foregoing). Unless required by law, the use by Licensee of the name, "Angel University" or the name of any campus of Angel University is expressly prohibited.

10.5 This License Agreement and the rights and duties hereunder may not be assigned by either party without first obtaining the written consent of the other, which consent will not be unreasonably withheld. Any such purported assignment, without the written consent of the other party, will be null and of no effect. Notwithstanding the foregoing, LICENSEE may assign this License Agreement to a purchaser, or successor in-interest or acquirer of substantially all of the LICENSEE's assets or business and/or pursuant to any reorganization qualifying under section 368 of the Internal Revenue Code of 1986 as amended, as may be in effect at such time.

10.6 The interpretation and application of the provisions of this Agreement shall be governed by the laws of the Commonwealth of Pennsylvania.

10.7 LICENSEE shall comply with all applicable laws and regulations. In particular, it is understood and acknowledged that the transfer of certain commodities and technical data is subject to United States laws and regulations controlling the export of such commodities and technical data, including all Export Administration Regulations of the United States Department of Commerce. These laws and regulations among other things, prohibit or require a license for the export of certain types of technical data to certain specified countries. LICENSEE hereby agrees and gives written assurance that it will comply with all United States laws and regulations controlling the export of commodities and technical data, that it will be solely responsible for any violation of such by LICENSEE or its AFFILIATES or SUBLICENSEEs, and that it will defend and hold AU harmless in the event of any legal action of any nature occasioned by such violation.

10.8 LICENSEE agrees: (i) to obtain all regulatory approvals required for the manufacture and sale of LICENSED PRODUCTS and LICENSED PROCESSES; and (ii) to utilize appropriate patent marking on such LICENSED PRODUCTS. LICENSEE also agrees to register or record this Agreement as is required by law or regulation in any country where the license is in effect.

10.9 Any notices to be given hereunder shall be sufficient if signed by the party (or party's attorney) giving same and either: (i) delivered in person; (ii) mailed certified mail return receipt requested; or (iii) faxed to other party if the sender has evidence of successful transmission and if the sender promptly sends the original by ordinary mail, in any event to the following addresses.

   Any notice or payment required to be given to either party shall be deemed to have been properly given and to be effective (a) on the date of delivery if delivered in person or (b) five (5) days after mailing if mailed by first-class certified mail, postage paid, to the respective addresses given below, or to such other address as it shall designate by written notice given to the other party.

If to LICENSEE:
Wincell, Inc.
1000 Pine Street
Rochester, New York 14500
Attention: President
Fax:
With copy to:
BB, LLP
500 Pine Street
Rochester, New York 14505
Attention: Bob Brown
Fax:
If to AU:
Office for Technology Transfer
Angel University
1000 Market Street
Philadelphia, PA 19100
Attention: Director, Office of Technology Transfer
Fax:
With copy to University Counsel at:
University Counsel
1000 Walnut Street
Philadelphia, PA 19100

By such notice either party may change their address for future notices.

10.10 Should a court of competent jurisdiction later hold any provision of this Agreement to be invalid, illegal, or unenforceable, and such holding is not reversed on appeal, it shall be considered severed from this Agreement. All other provisions, rights and obligations shall continue without regard to the severed provision, provided that the remaining provisions of this Agreement are in accordance with the intention of the parties.

10.11 In the event of any controversy or claim arising out of or relating to any provision of this Agreement or the breach thereof, the parties shall try to settle such conflict amicably between themselves. Subject to the limitation stated in the final sentence of this section, any such conflict which the parties are unable to resolve promptly shall be settled through arbitration conducted in accordance with the rules of the American Arbitration Association. The demand for arbitration shall be filed within a reasonable time after the controversy or claim has arisen, and in no event after the date upon which institution of legal proceedings based on such controversy or claim would be barred by the applicable statute of limitation. Such arbitration shall be held in Philadelphia, Pennsylvania. The award through arbitration shall be final and binding. Either party may enter any such award in a court having jurisdiction or may make application to such court for judicial acceptance of the award and an order of enforcement, as the case may be. Notwithstanding the foregoing, either party may, without recourse to arbitration, assert against the other party a third-party claim or cross-claim in any action brought by a third party, to which the subject matter of this Agreement may be relevant. The prevailing party in any arbitration shall be afforded reasonable costs and attorney fees.

10.12 This Agreement constitutes the entire understanding between the parties and neither party shall be obligated by any condition or representation other than those expressly stated herein or as may be subsequently agreed to by the parties hereto in writing.

IN WITNESS WHEREOF, the parties hereto have caused this Exclusive License Agreement to be executed by their duly authorized representatives.

_____   _____

Angel University   Wincell, Inc.

_____   _____

President for Science Policy and Technology Transfer   President

_____   _____

Date   Date

Appendix

The following comprise PATENT RIGHTS:

CLA_JOH.001

Inventors

Last Name	First Name	Institution
Claude	John	AU

Country	Patent Relation	Patent Status	Application Number	Filing Date	Patent #	Issue Date
EPO	NATIONAL PHASE	Abandoned	97285466.1	4/2/1995		
PCT	FOREIGN	Abandoned	PCT/US96/04522	1/8/1996		
USA	PROVISIONAL	Expired	60/095,178	5/3/1995		
USA	REGULAR	Issued	08/347,854	5/6/1997	5,108,251	8/4/1998

69

Negotiating a License Agreement

Christopher McKinney, MBA, DA

Introduction

The successful license negotiator uses a variety of skills and capabilities in developing and nurturing commercially viable agreements. Key ideas and tips are presented to help improve negotiation skills by discussing negotiation, its application to licensing, a series of points for improvement, and finally a set of tips for strengthening the overall skill set.

Negotiation is a basic element of the human condition and, when done effectively, often makes the difference between success and failure in the business world. Well developed negotiation skills and capabilities are particularly valuable in the licensing of intellectual property rights either into or out of an organization and represent a topic of special interest to those involved in the research enterprise.

This chapter has three areas of focus: 1) the art of negotiation; 2) negotiation in the context of intellectual property licensing; and 3) tips for becoming a more effective negotiator.

Negotiation: The Art of Working with People

While there are many definitions of negotiation, the author would define negotiation most broadly as *the process of seeking mutual understanding, developing creative methods for maximizing the perceived benefits to all parties, and acting on the resulting agreement*. In addition, negotiation often includes the subsequent nurturing and refinement of a relationship that requires amending an understanding. In short, negotiation is about the art of working with (as opposed to against) other people. It is definitely most effective when applied in a long-term context, i.e., the parties think of their relationship as having a life *after* the initial arrangements are negotiated.

Whether in a business partnership, a marriage, in the workplace, through community activities, or elsewhere, we find ourselves needing to understand, work through and resolve, and act upon areas of differing interests and opportunities. Sometimes, of course, negotiation per se does not result in an outcome that is satisfactory for all parties involved. In such cases, in fact, doing *nothing* is possibly better than doing a bad deal.

Consider this long-term, relationship-oriented focus in structuring business agreements as compared to buying a car. When you structure a long-term deal, you have an incentive, as well as a good opportunity, to develop that deal for the mutual benefit of all parties over time. By contrast, buying a car is generally more focused on the *transaction* than on the *relationship*. The image of the plaid-jacketed used car salesman comes to mind when one thinks about the look and feel of buying a car. In fact, many people find the car buying experience to be among the most unpleasant that they experience. Why? Perhaps it is the very fact that the car purchase is virtually always treated as a one-off transaction. It is rare to have a long-term affiliation with a given car salesman, isn't it? In the context of licensing, as is discussed shortly, we focus broadly on not just today and tomorrow, but on three, five, ten, or more years in the future. Think of negotiating a license as something akin to a marriage, one where the parties hear about each other, perhaps meet, maybe even date, and so forth.

Another construct the author likes to use in discussing negotiation is the proverbial "pizza pie metaphor." The question here is, "Can I develop a larger pizza pie, e.g., market share, market penetration, even if I have a smaller slice?" In many cases, the smaller slice of the larger pie is a better deal, especially when dealing with key financial terms and conditions. The alternative case, where you hold your breath until you turn blue in order to obtain a larger share of a smaller pie, often strangles the deal, as seen in the case of the "inventor's deadly embrace." The reason the pizza pie illustration works is that it forces you to think about the overall good that can be created in a relationship, rather than just your own share of the deal. Remember, too, that a smaller slice of a bigger pie may create the desire by your partner to "make pizza" again with you in the future. Another way to look at this principle is to think of "leaving some goodwill on the table," i.e., don't beat the last concession or dollar out of your partner. Simply, sometimes less is more when doing negotiation.

In thinking about negotiation as a skill that can be developed and honed, it is important to characterize negotiation in relation to other forms of problem solving or, in less pleasant circumstances, dispute resolution. Negotiation, in order to be placed in context, can be compared to mediation, arbitration, and litigation.

- *Mediation* can be thought of as negotiation where the principals are assisted in the negotiating process by a third party.
- *Arbitration* is where a third party, unlike the mediator, may recommend or even decide the outcome of a matter brought by the parties.
- *Litigation* is, of course, where parties turn to the legal system with judges and juries to help resolve differences.

Taken as a continuum, negotiation is the most direct method for the parties, mediation is a bit less direct given the third party helper, arbitration tends toward the litigation end of the continuum by involving a third party who—as opposed to the situations in negotiation or mediation—actually recommends or, in some cases, even imposes an answer on the parties. Litigation is the most detached from the standpoint of the principals and is, for all practical purposes, an adversarial form of conflict resolution.

The student of negotiation must bear in mind that negotiation is at least as much based on character and motive as on technique and hot tips. Modern business literature, really a creature of the twentieth century now continuing into the twenty-first century, tends toward the "quick fix," the "magic bullet," and the "killer app" business tool. If only it were so easy! It turns out that tips and techniques for negotiation really function as the icing on an already well-baked cake, where your effectiveness as a negotiator is directly related not just to the specific approaches you use, but also to the underlying character you display. Trustworthy people tend to be better long-term relationship negotiators. People who care about the feelings of others tend, also, to perform better. Good listeners who can really appreciate the views, concerns, and perspectives of others fare better in the world of license negotiation, as do those who display solid communication and organization skills.

Another theme that is useful in the art of negotiation is the notion of *congruence*, the degree of alignment of what you believe and feel (who you are inside) with what you say and do (who you are outside). Congruent people tend to come across as more genuine, honest, and displaying higher integrity than those who are less so. What does this mean to you as a negotiator? Two things: 1) it is important for *you* to be as congruent as possible given social norms and propriety; and 2) being aware of the congruence level of others can help you more clearly identify problem areas. Does this mean that you should always say what you think when you think it? No, but it does mean that you should make sure your overall behavior aligns with your overall thinking about a given deal lest you send mixed messages to your partners.

Congruence is particularly important in a world where communication can often be garbled, mishandled, and misunderstood, especially in the case of e-mail and other noninteractive media. If you are not congruent *and* not well understood, your relationship is in for problems. To be congruent, however, does *not* mean that you are not adaptive to new situations, i.e., using different approaches in negotiation as circumstances warrant. Thus, the congruent negotiator can be soft, hard, firm, fair, assertive, passive, pleasant, strong-willed, stubborn, etc. while remaining true to the inner self.

Before turning to some key tips that build upon your basic personality in negotiating, we will explore the more specific context of negotiation in the licensing business.

The Licensing Context: The Importance of Negotiation Skills

To bring negotiation directly into the licensing context, we must start by defining the key players in the normal intellectual property licensing discussion. We refer here to the technical, business, and legal professionals. Without an alignment of those key players both within and across the principal organizations, negotiations are likely to be ineffective or at least suboptimal.

How does one become effective at rallying the key functional players both within and between principal organizations? The first, and most critical, point is to recognize and act upon the reality that *all negotiation is about developing, enhancing, sustaining, improving, and nurturing relationships*. Technology licensing is, as is oft-quoted in the press, a "contact sport" where we focus at least as much on people and people issues as on technology and the technical details. In fact, the author would characterize successful negotiation as an 80/20 proposition where 80% of the success comes from working effectively in negotiating and 20% arises from the great technology itself. Does this mean one should advocate licensing a poor technology? Hardly. It does mean that the psychological aspects matter most.

Also, it can be helpful to consider for the practice of licensing a metaphor: How is intellectual property licensing like golf? Students of golf spend a fair amount of time developing their follow-through *after* the ball has left the tee. Why? It turns out that how one follows through with the club affects how the golfer hits the ball. In licensing, the parallel is that we must focus on the long-term implications of a deal in order to make sure it works in the near-term. Counterintuitive to some, this is an essential aspect of excellent negotiation skills in the intellectual property licensing context.

Before turning to specific tips for improving the enterprise of license negotiation, let us note several assumptions:

You Know This Stuff

Much of what we discuss is considered to be somewhat common sense in nature. However, what seems to be common sense is not always what we actually do. Therefore, taking a careful look at how we negotiate licenses is a productive use of time and energy, as well as a way to generally acquire new ideas and methods.

You Focus on the Deal, Not the "Four Corners" of the License Document

A mistake often made is to believe (and act upon the belief) that the license agreement *is* the relationship. This could not be further from the truth. The license agreement should *reflect* the relationship and, as with all relationships, be flexible enough to adapt to changing circumstances. Negotiators who hide behind the document often have difficulty with more complex and interpersonally challenging negotiation projects.

You Want a Long-Term Relationship

Given that technology commercialization is often an extended effort over a period of many years, and includes the expenditure of thousands or millions of dollars, the desired outcome of the parties is a strong and sustaining relationship. Anything less makes our work more akin to the famed used car salesperson.

You Recognize That a Good Relationship Can Overcome a Bad Deal

It turns out that strong relationships can withstand mistakes, errors, and other things that happen in life. The same is true in licensing. The converse, though, is also true: A *bad* relationship can overcome a *good* deal (otherwise known as "snatching defeat from the jaws of victory").

The "Mirror Test" Matters

When negotiating business relationships, negotiators do care about being successful. Being successful includes many things, in particular the "mirror test." Do you feel good about *how* you do your work when you look in the mirror?

Having discussed negotiation and its context, we turn now to a more specific look at how we can improve our negotiation efforts.

Key Methods for Negotiating Improved License Agreements

We now turn to challenges in negotiating license agreements, brief suggestions for generally improving how we do our business, and spend the balance of our time in reviewing a dozen tips that have been time proven and effective in becoming a better negotiator.

A few primary challenges exist in negotiating license agreements:

- Time
- Issues—real and perceived
- Personalities
- Agendas
- Honesty and trust

Time is a nonrenewable resource that both limits our ability to dither endlessly in working a deal yet also provides a source of healing when relations might be strained. In some cases, we are negotiating in what the pro wrestling world might call a "cage match," where we *must* conclude some deal in a given timeframe due to external circumstances. These situations can be very stressful indeed, yet can also result in a level of focus that helps the parties work rapidly toward closure. To explore this concept, consider the following. If you were in your house and it was on fire, and you only had five minutes to remove from the house whatever you could, what would you take? Doing this exercise mentally provides an important, and possibly surprising, view of what you value most in your home. The same approach can happen in a pressure-cooker license negotiation, particularly if the parties all work from the premise that they must cut to the chase in order to finish the deal not only in a timely fashion, but also considering the mutual best interests of all concerned.

In other situations, we have time to do the deal but have hit a rough spot which may be related to interpersonal tension (*within* or *between* parties) that threatens the deal's further development. In some of those cases, actually deliberately and openly delaying work (and communicating to the entire team that you are doing this) can be a healthy way to sooth hurt feelings and allow for a bit of a fresh start in developing the deal.

The handling of issues—real and perceived, can be critical to the success of a deal—both in its execution and future. The focus here is on the principle that real issues and perceived issues are *essentially the same thing*. As human beings act from their senses, both physical and mental, we do not necessarily differentiate between what is real and what we perceive to be real. As our colleagues in the behavioral sciences like to say, "Perception *is* reality." Does this mean that we cannot overcome what we might believe to be incorrect perceptions of ourselves or others? No! What it does mean is that we must work very diligently to communicate effectively (with others) and reflect thoroughly (within ourselves) in order to clear up misconceptions, errors, and other sources of misperception.

We as human beings are inherently individual—we have our own personalities. Without a doubt,

licensing technologies is an endeavor that places very different people in a variety of situations in close proximity (at least from a business standpoint) and requires them to listen, learn, and interact effectively enough to overcome personal style issues and the like. Yet, there are some people who we might find to be difficult in the licensing business. What do we do to overcome this? Perhaps one of the best pieces of advice for such circumstances is to focus on the issues and opportunities, rather than on the likeability of the other players. In fact, people probably can work together effectively without a great deal of personal affinity provided the levels of trust and mutual respect are sufficiently high.

A common expression over the last several decades has been to characterize someone's underlying motives as their agenda for a relationship. The presence (real or perceived) of agendas by any parties to a relationship may stall the development of the relationship. How do we overcome this? Again, thorough communication that starts with careful listening can help people discover those underlying purposes and act accordingly. Does this mean we will not have difficulties due to the motives that people do not share, i.e., their agendas? Not at all. It means that we have the opportunity explore more deeply—and react appropriately—to those underlying drivers.

Honesty is something people demonstrate, while *trust* is something they give to others. Both involve action by you. You can make a direct contribution to a positive outcome. Dishonest and untrustworthy people may succeed in isolated circumstances, but the ethical and personal binds in which they find themselves may be far more painful than the rewards for treachery are pleasurable. Being honest is its own reward in negotiation. Placing trust in others also tends to strengthen relationships and facilitate business dealings.

Having explored a few challenges in negotiation, we now turn to some ideas for improving our efforts.

How Can We Improve?

One of the most important things a negotiator can do is be self-aware, a practice the author likes to call "looking inside." The goal, here, is to understand yourself. What motivates you? What are your hot buttons? What tends to frustrate you? What makes you happy? Having some answers to these questions will allow you to proactively accommodate not only the realities of the world (and people) around you, but also will foster a better sense of how to operate in the negotiating environment. It is quite simple—if you know yourself well and can incorporate that knowledge into your business life, you will be more successful. One of the best pieces of advice is to know yourself as you are, not as you would like to be. Accept who you are, and capitalize on the strengths you possess. Bing Crosby said it best: "Accentuate the positive."

Profit from mistakes in order to both synthesize from your experiences and also know where the mine fields are for future negotiation endeavors. Consider the definitions of "expertise" and "ignorance." Expertise is the accumulation of mistakes from which you *have* learned; ignorance is the accumulation of mistakes from which you have *not* learned. In learning from mistakes—and we all make them—we can become more expert in our work.

In addition to being self-aware and learning from errors, developing the ability to *learn from others* is essential to our task. Here, the emphasis is on adopting best practices, to use the contemporary phrase, not so much from organizations as from individuals. Of course, we can learn from both good and bad examples of individual behavior. Watching others and observing how they use effective approaches to negotiating can help you become more skilled. Consider that bad examples are also educational. Just do not emulate the later cases.

"*Risk failure to achieve success*" is a personal favorite in the licensing business. The focus here is on considering that eliminating the risk of failure, whether through the deal itself or even from trying new and creative ways to do business, is a sure path to mediocre performance at best. We in the licensing business are not in the risk-taking business, but we are in the risk management business. We have to balance downside risk with upside potential in order to make our license agreements as viable, flexible, and workable as possible.

Know when to take "yes" for an answer when doing licensing. All too often, people become so target fixated in their negotiations that they lose sight of the fact that the parties may be in agreement, but the negotiator is still trying to sell or pitch an argument. Once the parties agree on a given point, move on! The risk of overselling is a big one. Take the good feelings of agreement on point A and apply them to solving problem B.

Know when you need face-to-face communications to make good things happen. In a world of e-mail, fax, telephones, video conferencing, personal digital assistants, and the like, why would this be suggested? Can we not just work it out over the phone line, so to speak? Perhaps. However, licensing is inherently a people-centered business, and sometimes there is no good substitute for being together in working through challenging issues and opportunities. Consider the impact of body language. It has been often suggested that over 70% of what we communicate, we do so through body language. That may be why, though, some folks prefer to not get together! Despite those who think the body language element is not important, meeting face-to-face can build more of a sense of "team," of "us working together," and of mutual respect and affinity—all good things in developing long-term relationships.

With these initial suggestions in mind, let us turn now to the author's favorite "dozen tips" for enhancing the negotiation of license agreements.

A Dozen Tips

Be Outcome-Oriented

Many negotiations often fall prey to the "he said, she said" mindset, where process overcomes product. This is a poison pill to doing business! Focusing on the question of where we are headed and what we want is essential to both crafting and breathing life into license agreements. Focus on the end point, and then check everything you do against that end state. If others get bogged down in process management, help them refocus on managing to a desired outcome.

A particularly memorable case where the author did not do this well involved a lengthy negotiation with a company for an agricultural biotechnology with a company famous for other, more mundane, household products. The author became so fixated with the manipulations of the business executive, the internal legal counsel, and the external legal counsel that sight of the larger goal—doing a good deal for all parties—was lost. We worked this deal during late December and finally decided it was not a good thing for the parties. Might we have arrived at a different conclusion had the author been less process-focused and more outcome-focused? With time comes enhanced perspective, and a very positive "Yes!" in response to the question.

Help Your Partner, and You Will Help Yourself

In the world of "me first," it might sound counter-intuitive to suggest that helping the other guy is a personal and professional strategy for negotiation success. However, that is precisely what it is. Helping other parties succeed, both by your methods of working with them and by offering substantive assistance, can bear much fruit in making a license agreement more successful. While you may not see direct and immediate benefits to this approach, be assured that long-term relations are definitely positively impacted by this style.

The author ran into this one a few years ago where a partner's key player was having personal problems. In a face-to-face visit, the author realized that negotiation was not the right topic for the moment. Rather, there was a need to attend to the individual's other concern—and at least recognize it as valid and important. While not much headway was made that day on the terms and conditions of the deal, a relationship was certainly further cemented. The ultimate deal was probably better for all concerned due to the deeper relationship and rapport.

Also, you can help your partner by letting him or her make a mistake and not charging for fixing it (e.g., when an error is discovered in a final draft agreement). First, helping another identify the problem, and, second, helping to resolve that issue without having to have a quid pro quo sends a powerful message about the partnership.

Focus on Intent, Then Content

All too often, we exchange large, bulky, and frightening documents with substantial quantities of complex language too early in the negotiation. Use a term sheet (a brief document of one to two pages that highlights key details of the agreement) as a means of working the major 80% to 90% of issues in a deal before turning to the full-blown agreement process. Focusing first on *intent*—what we are trying to do together—is more important in the early steps than focusing on *content*, the precise instrument of how we do it. This is not to say that we do not want to flesh out key issues early (such as with the term sheet), but that we do want to focus on the intent of the parties before slogging too deeply into the documents and language. "Cocktail napkin analysis" is not just an expression but a viable way to start the licensing process.

This message has never been as clear as when the author was involved in a large deal where time was short and enthusiasm was high to conclude a complex, yet workable, arrangement. Although the parties knew we had to conclude the full, formal agreements in very short order due to the funding for the project being subject to recall after a near-term date, we decided together to flesh out the key points in a term sheet just so we could focus a bunch of busy people on the essentials without getting bogged down in the full contracts. By doing so, we both forged a great partnership and closed our deals on time.

Know When to Do "No-deal"

Sometimes, the best answer to resolving seemingly impossible problems in a negotiation is to ... walk away. Is this pessimistic? No, it is a strategy of being realistic. Sometimes, the deal just will not make sense. It is better to agree to disagree, shake hands, and live to do business another day; of course, you might want to first consider the viability of your options should you do "no-deal."

Sadly, the author has been known for being too much of an optimist when it comes to closing deals. However, that is who the author is. In one particular arrangement a few years ago, several of us working the terms and conditions just could not find a rhythm for the deal. We tried, tried, and tried some more. No luck. Finally, in the spirit of disagreeing agreeably and leaving the door open for another day, we walked away from the mutual opportunity. The happy upshot to that example is that the personal affinity and mutual respect helped bring us back together for another deal sometime down the road—a deal that is now very profitable for all concerned.

Be Creative

Often times, we find ourselves in what military pilots refer to as "target fixation," the state where we are so intent on some specific objective within an agreement that we lose sight of the larger deal, and crash into the ground. Avoid target fixation by being creative, focusing not just inside the box of possibilities, but also outside the box of present ideas. Even if the creative solutions do not work for the parties, sharing them tends to both lighten the mood a bit (a nontrivial thing when times are tough) and also turn the discussion in a more positive direction.

One approach to encourage creativity (besides buying beer) is to switch sides for a while to try to articulate the other person's position on the deal. This can have the wonderful effect of both promoting communication and understanding and also helping everyone understand the bigger picture. In addition, you may come up with some pretty good ideas for your partner to suggest to you!

Use Time Effectively (Both Acting and Waiting)

Timing can be everything. There are times to allow people to cool down (professional version of time out), and there are times to move quickly (strike while the iron is hot). If the parties clearly communicate that they are pushing for a fast resolution or allowing time to pass, their relationships can be enhanced and the likelihood of a viable deal will increase.

This can be a tough tip, because you have to explain to all of your constituents that you may hold at some points and hurry up at others based on your intuitive sense of the best timing. As actors say, "Timing is everything."

Practice "Servant Leadership"

In the "me generation" orientation of doing what is best for number one first, the notion of demonstrating leadership by serving others may sound pretty strange. However, this is an excellent approach for building friendships, professional ties, and helping to make good things happen. Also, you will find that others react very favorably to someone who focuses on helping people achieve great things. The results are contagious and exciting!

Some of the greatest figures in world history have effectively served others and, by doing so, demonstrated extraordinary leadership. I am always impressed, for example, by the "service above self" orientation of Rotary International, a worldwide organization of professionals who want to give something back to their communities. Interestingly, many Rotarians are actually more well-known for their service through Rotary than through their day job occupation and other accomplishments.

Make Partners for Life

Since we are in the long-term relationship business, focusing on the idea of working not just with a particular partner, but also with particular people, can create the environment where mutual respect, creative problem solving, and general good working relations blossom. Thinking as you do licenses that you will work with those folks again and that can really enhance the quality of your business relationships.

This brings us back to the golf analogy, i.e., where the follow-through affects how you hit the ball. Imagine what you would like your partners to say about you five to ten years from now, and manage to that expectation!

Dispute-proof the Deal

A problem in far too many license agreements is that they are too complex and hard to interpret. Besides the virtue of simplicity (noted in the

"K.I.S.S." section), there is also the value of trying to iron out dispute potential before signing the deal. If this means simplifying language, clarifying difficult provisions, and the like, do it!

Another virtue of dispute-proofing is that you clearly demonstrate your desire to foster a long-term relationship that is valuable to all. In addition, in today's increasingly litigious business world in the United States, you are helping to save your employer and your partners money over the years by attending to the little things right now.

K.I.S.S. ("Keep It Simple Strategy")

As a general rule in licensing, simpler is better. When fewer layers of definitions, for example, will work as well as more layers, do it. The simpler deal is easier for others to read and understand. Besides, one must consider the "beer truck analogy"—if all the principals to a deal were hit by a beer truck tomorrow, how would the remaining folks pick up on the spirit—the intent—of the deal?

As a personal commentary on this tip, people who *do not want* to simplify give cause for concern. Please do not be one of those people!

Coalition-build

Consider licensing to be an exercise in team- (or coalition-) building. Our goal is to align people (simultaneously!) both within and outside of our respective organizations. Not a trivial task. By focusing on licensing as more than a one-on-one exercise, we can keep all the key parties involved and help streamline not only the license agreement's execution, but also its implementation and, as is often the case, later amendment.

Working on the internal and external team relationships also enhances communications, mutual exchange, and, frankly, is more interesting. Keeping the deal interesting is a very functional investment of your time and attention.

Know the Decision Makers to Make It Go

Nothing is more frustrating in working a license agreement than to do it and then find out that the people with whom you have been working are not principals, i.e., empowered to execute the agreement, but rather have to ask for other approvals, etc. Does this mean that you do not negotiate with nonprincipal players? This would not be an effective approach, because many license negotiators do, in fact, have to seek the approval of others. What it does mean is that you will want to determine up front who can sign, whose sign-off is required, etc. This suggestion cuts both ways, too, so be sure to tell others about your approval path early in the negotiation process. The good faith demonstrated will help.

As an example of what not to do, the author was engaged in a deal many years ago where he worked diligently with a point person from a large industrial firm—pushing hard to hammer out a fair deal in just a few weeks. When both gave the most valiant efforts to arrive at closure, the author was thrilled to send off signature copies of the final agreement. Nothing was heard in the first week. Nothing in the second week, either. By the third week, the author called his contact only to learn that the agreement had been forwarded to a stand-

ing management committee in the top of the organization. That deal fell apart quickly thereafter and prompted us to turn to other more credible partners.

Conclusion

Taken as a whole, licensing is very much the art of the possible, rather than the art of the easy-to-do. Thus, people working closely with people is an essential and core ingredient of success. Our efforts in this chapter are directed at providing ideas and tips for the new, as well as the seasoned, license negotiator.

70

Role of Technology Transfer Office after the Deal

Katherine Chou, MS, MBA

A partnership is sealed upon the execution of a license agreement. Just like a marriage, this relationship requires continuous nurturing, monitoring, and strengthening. A technology transfer office (TTO) serves as its university's representative to maintain good relationships with licensees. There are two primary areas in which a TTO interacts with its commercial partners:

1. Monitoring the execution of the license agreement and sponsored research program, if any; and,
2. Maintaining an ongoing relationship.

Monitoring the Execution of the License Agreement and Sponsored Research Program

A TTO usually accepts responsibility for monitoring licensee compliance regarding the execution of terms stipulated in a license agreement. These responsibilities include collecting fees that a licensee promises to pay in the agreement; billing the licensee for ongoing legal expenses; and monitoring the licensee's due diligence obligations. If a sponsored research program is structured together with a license agreement, the TTO may facilitate the interaction between the scientists and the commercial partner. At times, the TTO also participates in fee collection for an existing license relationship with the commercial partner.

Fee Collection

TTOs usually bill a licensee for the fees stipulated in a license agreement: these fees include an upfront license fee, past incurred legal expenses, and an annual maintenance fee. The TTO also monitors and collects the licensee's royalty payments. The TTO also initiates auditing action and takes proper measures in the event that a dispute arises about royalty distribution due to the licensor. If the licensee fails to pay fees, the TTO may initiate termination action. However, in a license agreement, there is usually a prenegotiated period of time during which a licensee can cure its breach and remain in good standing with the licensor.

Legal Reimbursement

When a law firm bills the university/licensor for patent prosecution expenses, the TTO is responsible for collecting such reimbursement from its licensees and the TTO can also arrange for the licensee to be billed directly by the law firm. A TTO also is responsible for coordinating patent prosecution and for mediating any disputes between its licensee and the law firm. The licensor may permit the licensee to communicate directly with the law firm. However, the university licensor may have intellectual property reporting obligations to agency sponsors of the research. Universities, therefore, usually take the lead in coordinating patent prosecution so that the individual applications in a patent family can be closely monitored.

Even when a law firm bills directly to a licensee, the TTO remains responsible for coordinating patent prosecution and intervening in any disputes between the licensee and the law firm.

Due Diligence Monitoring

Universities as licensors often require demonstration of annual progress in developing a licensed technology from licensees. The TTO is required to monitor such progress and to maintain a constant dialogue with its licensees to ensure the actual development of the licensed technologies.

Maintaining an Ongoing Relationship

Constant and open communication between universities/licensor and their commercial partners/licensees is essential to maintaining successful and fruitful relationships. Repeat customers are the best customers; when each party is familiar with the other party's working style, future transactions become more efficient.

It is always good practice for a TTO to communicate openly with its commercial partners about its university policies and politics. Such communication provides guiding principles, but also can create practical impediments to any ongoing relationship. In most cases, such obstacles may be more easily overcome when the licensor and licensee have established a strong rapport and understanding of the internal conflicts that might otherwise hamper a business arrangement.

Another potential challenge faced by university technology transfer when dealing with companies is the preservation of the mission of its nonprofit academic organizations. For instance, the policies of a nonprofit research university or hospital may clash with industry regarding confidentiality and publication. Companies often keep innovations under wraps in order to prevent theft of their ideas and products by competition. Universities, however, have mandates and obligations to publish research results. Nonprofit institutions and corporations alike must be mindful of the restrictions under which the other works and be willing to compromise to resolve differences. Certain issues may remain nonnegotiable, but the parties may find other areas on which they can agree, as long as each keeps an open mind.

Making the effort to establish a strong relationship with a licensee offers lasting benefits that cannot be overstated. Every licensing office dreams of return customers and future licensing opportunities that are more quickly negotiated. This is especially important as university TTOs must attempt to match the fast-paced business tempo of corporate licensees. Having a receptive ear when offering a promising new technology can minimize the marketing, evaluation, and licensing timelines.

As the overall business pace quickens in relationships between institutions and for-profit entities, TTOs must be adept at packaging their technologies, showcasing their technologies to attract company interest, and be able to take advantage of the new multidisciplinary approaches in science to appeal to companies with diverse business interests. Having a roster of satisfied licensees ready to undertake new technologies is an equally valuable asset.

The TTO and its licensee are part of a commercialization team. Appreciation, respect, and communication are tools to achieve consensus building among such a commercialization team.

71

Spin-Off Companies from University Technologies

Jayne Carney, MS, PhD, MBA

Introduction

As noted by many sources and as detailed more thoroughly in this chapter, "Entrepreneurs are the engine of growth and innovation in the competitive market economy."[1] There are various definitions of spin-offs, spinouts, or start-ups companies, as noted by the Association of University Technology Managers (AUTM) and other technology transfer organizations. AUTM defines start-ups as those companies initiated solely on the basis of university technology. The AUTM's 2001 survey summary reports that 17% of US university technology agreements were with start-up companies, 51% with small companies, and 32% occurred with larger companies.[2] As discussed later in this chapter, start-ups are an increasingly important licensing vehicle for universities, as well as an important source of growth for the US economy.

This chapter reviews the most recent data on start-ups from academic institutions and explores what start-ups need for success. There is also discussion about what universities gain from start-up collaboration and about the conditions when a university or research foundation accepts equity. Also included in the chapter are models illustrating the successful practices being used today to foster entrepreneurship. This chapter, however, only introduces and briefly explains these concepts to provide general understanding of critical topics of technology transfer. The chapter in no way provides enough information for action, unless the action is to start on an MBA degree or to work for a start-up!

The types of skills and experience needed for competency in technology transfer have grown enormously in the past few years. The opportunity to use a wide variety of skills makes technology transfer positions much more interesting and challenging. Some academics are increasingly focused on industrial funding and the opportunity to be an agent for new product development may attract increasing numbers of experienced people who have industrial backgrounds. Salaries appear to be increasing (anecdotal evidence), and these changes should reduce turnover in technology transfer offices or technology commercialization offices as they are increasingly called. Of course, both of these factors lead to more stability in offices, which in a positive feedback loop, result in better service to the faculty, the disclosure of more inventions from truly creative faculty, and the in-house skills to manage more complex licensing processes.

A Look at Start-Up Activity at Academic Institutions

According to AUTM, between 1980 and 2002 there were a total of 4,320 start-ups that resulted from licenses issued by academic institutions; and 2,741 or 63.4 percent of these start-ups were still in operation by the end of 2002. AUTM's survey included US and Canadian universities, hospitals, and nonprofit research institutes.[3] Figure 71-1, a graphical compilation of data from the 1994 to 2002 fiscal

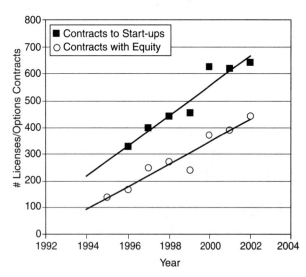

FIGURE 71-1 Contracts to Start-Up Companies and Those in Which the Institution Took Equity.

year AUTM licensing surveys, shows that there has been an increase in the number of licenses to start-up businesses and in the number of licenses in which equity was taken in the start-up by the licensing institution.[4,5,6] However, upon closer examination, the FY 2002 data show a decrease in company formation over the previous two years of almost 9%; this decrease is probably a reflection of the period of overall economic downturn and decrease in investment capital.

Analysis of the AUTM data shows that the average number of start-ups per reporting institution was slightly more than 1.5 in FY 1994 and slightly fewer than 2.5 per institution in FY 2000. However, this average is misleading in two regards: first, it masks the very high variance among universities. For example, while MIT and the University of California system granted licenses to 23 start-ups in FY 2002, 46 universities reported none at all.[7] Second, the average masks the increase in the overall number of universities which have licensed to start-ups and taken equity. For example, in FY 1996, 66 of 129 US university respondents reported start-up licensing deals, while 101 of 147 did so in FY 2002.[8,9] That more than two-thirds of universities reporting in 2002 were involved in start-ups shows the importance of this topic.

What Start-Ups Need for Success

To be successful, companies need some basic ingredients: a good idea, great people, and capital. Start-ups, with early-stage technologies, also require a degree of nurturing, which must start early on. It is not enough to work with a technology transfer office (TTO) which knows how to market to companies and/or how to efficiently complete licenses (although these are important skills); it is also necessary for the TTO to search out those highly entrepreneurial scientists who not only have creative, useful ideas and can also find funding for the applied work not covered by the federal research institutes and foundations, but still support those scientists who regard patenting and applications as a distraction from their true interest, science.

Many universities now have funds of $30,000 to $50,000 per project (or more) targeted to develop prototypes or performance data to demonstrate functionality of concepts. Some technology transfer offices have partnerships with their business schools to provide market assessments; others even prepare business plans. This type of support for university start-ups is much needed for situations where there is an inexperienced entrepreneur. To help facilitate start-up efforts, enterprising universities sometimes allow the university-related start-up to rent lab benches within in the university. Others provide support services both before and after the license is complete. One of the most critical support components includes finding the person to lead the enterprise, or the "investable entrepreneur."[10]

In the early years of university-start-up licensing, inventors themselves most often held the dual responsibilities of university-affiliated scientist and start-up CEO. As noted in *Utah Business*, "The entrepreneur is probably the single most important factor in a strong economy—individuals willing to step forward and take the risk to start new businesses."[11]

What Universities Gain from Start-Ups

Most universities (especially state universities) receive a benefit, though usually intangible, from licensing to a start-up company, since more than 80% of start-ups are in the same state as the institution from which they licensed the technology.[12] With the increased pressure on local and state governments for increased tax revenues, most governments strongly emphasize programs that will create new jobs. Whether there is a formal report to the state legislature or merely requests from the university public relations office for company start-up numbers and job creation numbers, successful local start-ups can be an important measure of success for a TTO. Some universities recognize that entrepreneurial faculty will highly value faculty positions at those universities whose policies are faculty-startup and equity friendly. These same universities may recognize the benefits that a TTO may provide in terms of faculty attraction and retention.

Universities benefit in a number of ways if they take equity. If no existing companies are willing to take on a traditional license, an equity-based license may be the only way for the TTO to complete its mission of facilitating the development of products and services for the public good.

Should a start-up be successful, there are at least two ways the university may receive income in excess of revenue from a typical license issue fee: for example, the TTO takes equity and the company eventually goes public and the stock price rises, buoyed by a successful Phase III clinical trial. The TTO may also greatly benefit when the start-up is acquired by a public company, and, in turn, the TTO (the university) receives stock from the larger company for their equity. However, it should be understood that there have been only a few cases where universities have profited in such manner.

Equity

Institutional Considerations

It is important for the TTO to carefully consider whether to accept equity in lieu of a cash up-front fee in a licensing agreement. As a general policy, if the university wants to encourage this special group of companies, start-ups, the university has to have or develop a policy that allows the TTO to take equity, whether directly or through a research foundation. To do so, some state universities may even need to modify the state law or the state constitution.

Although people may think that taking equity means giving up cash, in most cases where equity is the consideration, the company would not be able to start if a cash payment were required. This leads to the recognition that taking equity is an exchange of one high-risk good, the equity, for another high-risk good, an early-stage technology. Whether this has been clearly articulated in policies or not, the fact that most universities will accept equity in lieu of cash as the license issue fee, but not as payment for patent costs (an example of a situation where the university has already paid out cash), suggests an inherent understanding of this key point.

The normal risks involved in licensing any technology exist, of course, compounded by the special challenges in working with start-ups, plus the lost opportunity costs for the increased amount of time spent by people in the TTO in these situations. But there are also special risks involved in equity situations. Some of these are at the institutional level and include potential impact on taxable income and tax-exempt status, as well as institutional conflicts of interest/commitment. Other situations have an impact on both the TTO and the institution: income loss though equity dilution; and individual conflicts of interest/commitment not only for faculty, as earlier discussed, by also for TTO personnel in terms of stock they may own as individuals, their influence on the sale of stock by their institution, and other related issues.[13] Many of these risks can be reduced if the institution permits only a passive investment role with neither board nor voting memberships in these start-ups, and if the TTO insulates licensing people from certain negotiations. The risk of equity dilution from future investment rounds can be reduced to a degree by a standard term sheet, which requires protection from dilution to some specific investment level, for example, $2 million dollars.

This raises the question of how an institution deals with equity. Some empower the TTO to put their equity with an outside firm that holds it until the equity has become publicly negotiable and any restriction period has passed, and then sells the stock at intervals. Other institutions or their research foundations comingle the equity with the university's investments and the decision is made in the same manner as for the general funds by the university's investment committee. In either case, the stock may not be sold at its highest point, hence the full potential value may not be realized by the institution. There are many approaches to managing equity, but the key commonality is that the university is shielded from institutional conflicts and the TTO personnel and any university inventors are shielded from individual real or apparent conflict of interest (COI) issues resulting from insider information. Of course the TTO loses any control over whether or when proceeds from cashed-in equity are added to the TTO's bottom line, but that is less important than the COI issues.

TTO Considerations

While the decision of whether or not to accept equity may be a major issue for the university regents or the state legislators, the TTO may have its own issue with accepting equity. In the long run, all TTOs want and need their licensees to successfully develop their technology into products and/or services and manufacture and market them as quickly as possible. But the situation is considerably different with start-ups. Interestingly, but not surprisingly, while slightly fewer than half (or 46.5 percent) of all FY 02 licenses were exclusive; 91 percent of the licenses to start-ups were exclusive. This is understandable, as companies whose entire technology portfolio is based on licensed technology usually need to be protected from competition, at least from the same technology. The TTO also must consider that the additional effort involved in an exclusive license to a start-up cannot be amortized over a series of nonexclusive licenses. It is important to recognize this as licenses to start-ups, particularly those involving equity, truly take additional effort.

However, less effort on the part of the TTO would be needed, and certainly the likelihood of success would be enhanced when licensing to a start-up, if there were an experienced businessperson, other than the inventor, involved. Besides the benefits of experience, access to investment capital may increase and potential COI issues are reduced. It is uncomfortable for TTO professionals to negotiate with their own university professors; moreover, such situations can place professors at risk for potential COI. Should the technology have been developed with federal funds, it is also necessary for any potential COI to be disclosed by the professor to the COI committee, whereby the conflict, if it cannot be eliminated, must be reduced or managed, through a written management plan.

When a TTO licenses to an existing company, a formal written development and/or business plan, depending on the stage of development of the technology, is typically requested and delivered. However, this is more difficult to accomplish when licensing to a start-up and, in such cases, a TTO alliance with the university business school can be very helpful in the development of business plans and market assessments. In addition, an understanding of the potential applications, time to market, size of potential markets and competitive technologies can provide valuable information to both the start-up and the TTO, particularly for the development of a term sheet agreeable to both parties.

So now you have an early-stage technology, an experienced businessperson, and a "fit" between their plans and your TTO's comfort level. Do you take equity? If so, how and how much? First, you must check that your university or foundation allows equity-based licenses, and you must know

whether your office has a policy or practice requiring at least some up-front cash.

The situation is actually a little more complex since some universities are free to take an equity interest for any portion of the financial components of a license, while others are prohibited from taking equity where the organization has already paid cash. Many institutions are not permitted to invest financially in a company. It is very important to understand the boundaries of your institution; for example, whether the university can accept warrants (options to purchase stock at a later date for a predetermined price); whether you can accept equity as reimbursement for your institution's investment in the patent application; and whether the university can, at a later date, accept additional equity in lieu of cash for a milestone payment. It is important to understand what your institution's charter, laws, and policies permit, but even if permitted a sound understanding of the risks incurred in taking equity needs to underpin the decision of whether or not it is good practice. The circumstances under which an exchange of cash for equity may occur need to be carefully thought through.

Perhaps the biggest surprise for TTOs in recent economic times has been the dilution of their equity in "cram-downs." This developed in the first few years of this millennium as venture capital dried up and companies were unable to proceed with expensive developments (e.g., clinical trials). Investors were then able to exact new requirements on early equity participants; for example, new investors might require early investors to pay-in thousands of dollars per share or risk dilution. An interesting discussion of issues and conflicts of interest may be found in Jaffe's article.[14] Sometimes, these investments result in highly successful companies; other times they do not. But most TTOs do not have the expertise to evaluate whether such investment is warranted, and many, if not most, are not permitted to invest cash. Hence, their shares may be severely diluted. A well articulated set of conditions to reduce these potential negative situations may be found in the "Structuring Equity Transactions" section on the University of British Columbia's Web site.[15]

A final consideration is unconscious bias for those TTOs that are not self-supporting. If a TTO does not bring in sufficient royalty and issue fees to pay its costs, and has to be subsidized by the university, then there may be a subtle or unconscious pressure not to spend time on equity-based licenses. All of the factors need to be weighed and dealt with when deciding whether and how to license technologies to start-ups, particularly when equity is a factor.

Comparative Approaches

This section contrasts the most passive start-up strategy (where the university receives equity as a consideration for the license) with a middle role (where the university acquires a larger percent of the equity in consideration of their efforts). This section also discusses the most complex choice, to take founder's equity as compensation for the additional role the university plays in the formation of the company.

If the startup lacks an experienced entrepreneur, universities may take a percentage of the initial formative equity and may choose to license only a limited field. An early or underdeveloped commercial platform provides an opportunity to seek Small Business Innovation Research (SBIR) development funds. But whether there is a license grant to a limited field of use or to all fields, each TTO needs to decide the percentage of equity that is appropriate based on the technology, the level of development by university personnel, the breadth of the field granted, and other licensing considerations.

A more midrange approach is that of Isis, the technology transfer company of the University of Oxford:

> The University expects to be a significant shareholder in the spin-out company because of the resources and permissions it makes available to the spin-out. Isis will provide advice about the division of the equity spilt [sic] between the University, the researchers and the investors. The university expects that its shareholding [will] be the same as the founder researchers. There are a number of factors to be taken into account: for example, the roles of the individual researchers, the value of the intellectual property, the amount

of capital required, the involvement of the University in reaching the stage where a spin-out is possible, and the importance of the association with the University.[16]

An example of this approach is shown in Stage 1 of Table 71-1, where Stages 2 and 3 show the impact of dilution with increased levels of investment.

A more complex situation occurs where a university participates in both founder's equity and receives equity for the license. In the briefest explanation, founder's equity may be divided among in various proportions among those critical to company development. The par value may vary from a nominal $0.001/share for the founders to $0.01/share when the license is negotiated. By tracking through Table 71-2, the valuation of two sample technologies, originally valued at a total of $300,000 can be compared to founders' shares and their subsequent dilution through various investment rounds can be seen.

The previous discussion is more illustrative of concepts that need to be understood than it is explanatory in a textbook sense. For a more thorough discussion of start-up equity, consult Buz Brown and Jon Soderstrom's excellent chapter in the AUTM's training manual.[17]

Models for Universities to Support Start-Ups

Increasingly, universities understand that it is to their advantage to provide seed funding for early-stage development of a concept or for applications testing either directly or through their foundations.[18,19] Some create protected mini-incubators

TABLE 71-1	Initial Share Dilution.*					
Illustration of Share Dilution						
	Stage 1 shares	%	**Stage 2** shares	%	**Stage 3** shares	%
Founders	50	50.0	50	33.3	50	29.4
University	50	50.0	50	33.3	50	29.4
Investors	0	0	50	33.3	50	29.4
Management	0	0	0	0	20	11.8
Total Shares	100		150		170	
Total %		100		100		100

*From " Starting a Spin-out Company," page 12.[21]

TABLE 71-2	Sample Deal Structure.									
(M = Millions of Dollars)										
Shareholder	**Founders Equity**	**% Class**	**Option Pool**	**% Class**	**Common Stock**	**% Class**	**Series A Preferred**	**% Class**	**Total Issued & Outstanding**	**% Total**
Yale University	2.0 M	25		0	2.0 M	19		0	2.0 M	7.8
Yale Inventor	2.0 M	25		0	2.0 M	19		0	2.0 M	7.8
Yale Scientist	2.0 M	25		0	2.0 M	19		0	2.0 M	7.8
CEO	2.0 M	25		0	2.0 M	19		0	2.0 M	7.8
Option Pool		0	2.25 M	100	2.25 M	21		0	2.25 M	8.8
Technology A		0		0	0.2 M	2		0	0.2 M	0.8
Technology B		0		0	0.1 M	1		0	0.1 M	0.4
Lead Investor		0		0		0	7.0 M	47	7.0 M	27.4
Investor 2		0		0		0	4.0 M	27	4.0 M	15.7
Investor 3		0		0		0	4.0 M	27	4.0 M	15.7
Totals	8.0 M	100	2.25 M	100	10.55 M	100	15.0 M	100	25.55	100

Used with permission from Brown and Soderstrom's chapter in AUTM's Technology Transfer Practice Manual.[22] Modified to fit page.

on-campus,[20] while the most advanced institutions themselves find seasoned entrepreneurs and venture capital.[23] Additionally, many universities partner with state, federal, and commercial groups to speed up this important economic development process. For example, some states fund university researchers to develop platform technologies with the potential to spin-out a number of local companies;[24] some universities partner in regional incubator organizations;[25] others partner directly with venture capitalists.[26] Overall, there are a number of reasons for technology transfer or commercialization offices to become directly and actively involved in the development of technology, not the least of which is to avoid the "valley of death" situation that can occur between the time when R&D funding may run out and when a commercial interest can be identified, as characterized by Betten.[27]

Following are examples of cases that only begin to illustrate the many ways in which universities, local economic groups, and states can enhance growth and development processes. If these examples do not seem appropriate for your institution or situation, it is recommended that you read through Tornatzky, Waugaman, and Gray's review[28] of programs at twelve different universities, which provides an additional array of ideas for consideration.

Many universities have development program funds. For example, a review of the results of the Technology Commercialization Program at the University of Utah[29] shows how even small amounts of funding, if carefully distributed and monitored, can have large economic returns. At the University of Utah, individual programs are funded for $35,000 per year and are renewable for a second year and results from an unpublished report (J.F. Carney, University of Utah) show that from the $1.98 million invested over the five-year period from 1999 to 2003, more than $6.75 million in return was realized (this includes license income and grant monies received, excluding value of job creation or potential sales of equity).

A new approach to a mini-incubator has been also been developed at Utah State University. Their Office of Technology Management and Commercialization (OTMC) established what they refer to as a "bridge fund." "This fund, coupled with business and marketing support from OTMC, is directed at providing marketing and sales efforts for developed products/services. The concept is to create a business incubator for 'inside' spinout companies that will allow them to move rapidly from a cash-consuming development phase to a cash-producing business with revenues. Once profitable, these business can be transferred to 'external' spinout companies or moved to an independent unit of the USU Research Foundation."[30] These funds have subsequently allowed the office to hire a market development manager with direct commercial experience to develop a business strategy for a new software system.[31]

In a state and university partnership effort, the Utah State Legislature funded a university-based Centers of Excellence Program to support, "Highly targeted, market-driven projects that perform the applied research, prototype development and business planning necessary to successfully commercialize promising technical innovations..." In 2001, $1.6 million in state program funding at four Utah universities resulted in matching funds of $20.5 million, an 11:1 ratio. As a result of the multiyear centers program, at least 150 Utah-based companies have been started and by 2001, those companies directly employed over 1,300 people at an average salary of $68,000.[32]

The University of Central Florida's incubator has received a number of awards in the brief time since it was formed:

> Since its founding in 1999, the UCF Technology Incubator (UCFTI) has helped more than 70 emerging technology companies create over $100 million in revenue and more than 400 new jobs with an average salary of $68,000. As a result of this success, the UCFTI has been lauded as one of the top 10 performing technology incubators in the country by the National Business Incubation Association. Headquartered in Research Park adjacent to the University, the Incubator is a collaboration in economic development between UCF, Orange County, the City of Orlando and the Florida High Tech Corridor Council.[33]

The programs referenced heretofore have each resulted in technologies that have been directly licensed to start-ups. While any individual TTO may not be equipped to support the extent of these efforts, these examples show the success that can be realized from even one program. Perhaps the most important thing for any TTO to consider is that any development program starts with an invention, and so the starting place is the inventiveness of the University's faculty.

While working and investing in a start-up can be time-consuming and undoubtedly risky, there can be enormous rewards. The author writes these words in a TTO office in a university research park, surrounded by several dozen companies that were started with university technologies licensed years ago by technology transfer people in this very office. Now, thousands of people are gainfully employed, lives around the world have been improved by prod-

ucts from these start-ups, and royalties from these products support today's tech transfer people and further provide funding to inventors for exciting new research inventions that will become inspiration for tomorrow's start-up companies.

References

1. Haynes, G. W., and C. Ou. "A Profile of Owners and Investors of Privately Held Businesses in the United States, 1989–1998," *Annual Conference of the Academy of Entrepreneurial and Financial Research*, New York, 2003, available at http://www.sba.gov/advo/stats/wkp02co.pdf (accessed July 11, 2005).
2. The Association of University Technology Managers, Inc. "AUTM Licensing Survey: FY 2001," http://www.autm.net/surveys/dsp.surveyDetail.cfm?pid=18 (accessed July 11, 2005).
3. The Association of University Technology Managers, Inc. "AUTM Licensing Survey: FY 2002," http://www.autm.net/events/File/Surveys/02_Member_Survey_Summary.pdf (accessed October 25, 2005).
4. The Association of University Technology Managers, Inc., 2001.
5. The Association of University Technology Managers, Inc., 2002.
6. The Association of University Technology Managers, Inc. "AUTM Licensing Survey: FY 1996 Survey Summary," http://www.autm.net/events/File/Surveys/96_AUTUM_Lic_Survey_public.pdf (accessed October 25, 2005).
7. The Association of University Technology Managers, 2001.
8. The Association of University Technology Managers, 2001.
9. The Association of University Technology Managers, 1997.
10. Brown, A., and J. Soderman. "Yale Do [sic] it Differently," *TransPharma*, December 2002/January 2003, p. 45.
11. "Industry Outlook," *Utah Business 2003* 17, no. 12 (2003): 56.
12. The Association of University Technology Managers, 2002.
13. Council on Governmental Relations. "Recognizing and Managing Personal Financial Conflicts of Interest," Washington, DC, 2002.
14. Jaffe, D. "Conflicts of Interest in Venture Capital 'Cram Down' Transactions." *The Metropolitan Corporate Counsel*, April 2002, p. 15.
15. University of British Columbia. "Acceptance, Management and Sale of Technology Licensing

Equity." *Policies, Policy* 105, p. 3, 4. http://www.universitycounsel.ubc.ca/policies/policy105.pdf (accessed July 11, 2005).

16. Cook, T. "Starting a Spin-out Company." *Isis Innovation Limited*, http://www.isis-innovation.com/researchers/spinout-9.html (accessed July 8, 2005).

17. Brown, A., and J. Soderstom. "Start-Up and Equity Primer." In *Technology Transfer Practice Manual*, 1–24. Washington, DC: The Association of University Technology Managers, Inc., 2002.

18. Tornatzky, L. G., P. G. Waugaman, and D. O. Gray. *Innovation U.: New University Roles in a Knowledge Economy*. Research Triangle Park, NC: Southern Technology Council, 2002.

19. University of Utah. "Funding Opportunities, Technology Commercialization Project," http://www.research.utah.edu/funding/tcp.html (accessed July 11, 2005).

20. Utah State University, Office Technology Management and Commercialization, "Business of Technology Briefs," http://www.usu.edu/techcomm/fy04qtr1.pdf (accessed July 11, 2005).

21. Cook.

22. Brown and Soderstom, 2002.

23. Brown and Soderstom, 2002.

24. Utah State, Centers of Excellence. *Annual Report, Fiscal Year July 2001–June 2002*, http://goed.utah.gov/COE/documents/01-02Centers report.pdf (accessed October 25, 2005).

25. University of Central Florida. "UCF Technology Incubator to Share Secrets of Success with Other Universities and Incubators," January 28, 2004, http://www.incubator.ucf.edu/newscenter/2004_PressReleases/01-28_AUTMNBIA. html (accessed October 25, 2005).

26. Thayer, A. "Universities Back Venture Funds." *Chem. and Eng. News*, May 19, 2003, p. 12.

27. Betten, P. "Pharmaceutical Up-Front Licensing Fees." *Les Nouvelles* 38 (2003): 201–205.

28. Tornatzky, Waugaman, and Gray, 2002.

29. University of Utah.

30. Utah State University, p. 3.

31. Utah State University.

32. Utah State, Centers of Excellence.

33. University of Central Florida, 2004.

Establishing a Spin-Off Company

Janet E. Scholz

What Is a Spin-Off Company?

For the purpose of this discussion, a "spin-off company" is a small, newly founded company formed around one or more innovations arising from the results of academic-based research, and there is involvement of the inventor and cooperation/participation of the institution, usually through the technology transfer office (TTO) and/or through an institutional organization established to facilitate technology transfer and spin-off company development. There exists considerable debate about definitions of the terms "spin-off company" and "start-up company." In many of the referenced materials supporting this discussion, the term "start-up company" is used, thus it is important for the reader to keep the foregoing definition in mind.

Why Engage in Spin-Off Company Development?

Academic-based research institutions encourage and participate in new venture creation encompassing technologies developed within their research facilities. They do so for many reasons, including to:

- Increase perception of and contribution to public benefit.
- Support of the academic mission.
- Enhance the reputations of the institution and its researchers.
- Increase opportunities for relevant industrial development experiences for faculty, staff, and students.
- Maximize the opportunity for success of a particular technology.
- Provide a positive impact on economic development.
- Aid in faculty recruitment and retention.
- Extend service and supply opportunities to local and regional business.
- Expand employment opportunities for graduates.
- Provide financial incentives.
- Attract investment to the community.

Most spin-off companies are located and remain within the region in which they were created. Since it first began to collect data on spin-off company creation, the Association of University Technology Manager's (AUTM) annual licensing survey has determined that companies tend to locate and stay near the institution from which their technology was sourced or created.[1] This provides the local and regional businesses with new opportunities and also serves to attract new investment into the community.

Institutions in the United States, Canada, and in many other countries are increasingly challenged to contribute to public benefit, not only through the graduation of highly qualified personnel and the expansion of knowledge, but by providing public access to information on government-funded (and some industry-funded) research that is conducted at their institutions. In fact, in some countries, such as in the United Kingdom, regional economic development is a stated part of the new academic mission. In Canada and the United States, economic development is often a less obvious part of missions that more broadly capture the concept. Nonetheless, the concept of institutions as contributors to and catalysts for economic development is cited in mission statements. For example:

- Georgia Tech is a leading center for research and technological development that continually seeks opportunities to advance society and the global economic competitiveness of Georgia and the nation. *From the "Vision and Mission" section of the Georgia Institute of Technology Strategic Plan, in which the term "economic development" is frequently cited.*

- Our mission is to educate young men and women to be industry and academic leaders, and to create new technologies that will fuel economic prosperity. Partnerships with industry are essential to both our education and research missions. *From the Mission Statement of the Jacobs School of Engineering at the University of California, San Diego.*

The publication *The New Idea Factory*[2] suggests that large corporate entities, multinationals, and the like have large research and development operations of their own. It is known that these companies spend billions of dollars each year inventing and nurturing hundreds of their own research and development projects, and therefore it seems obvious that they will be unlikely to consider early stage technologies from academic-based research institutions. Increasingly, it appears that large companies would rather wait until a technology is proven to be marketable before it considers whether or not the technology is of any interest. Of course by then, a new technology may have been lost due to lack of investment in the continuing research or in the development of the opportunity by way of licensing, codevelopment or otherwise.

For this reason, as well as many others similarly expressed, creating a new spin-off company around an appropriate technology opportunity may be the best commercialization strategy for that technology ensuring it a place in the market, or perhaps a place in the mergers and acquisitions market. Either way, a return on investment is realizable.

As stated by Angus Livingstone in the 1998 University of British Columbia's spin-off company report:

> A growing number of large national and multi-national organizations have realized they are not well suited, by internal means, to generate new products and new lines of business to respond to changing market opportunities. For them it is too difficult and time-consuming to create a new successful division when their existing policies and organization structures are resistant. Instead, they are turning to mergers and acquisitions to meet these objectives. Many are now willing to pay a significant amount for a smaller operating company which has potential and is synergistic with their business mission. Herein lies the opportunity for investors in a successful spin-off or start-up venture to recoup their capital and earn significant returns.[3] Contributions to economic development take many forms. The creation of new spin-off companies established to provide a vehicle for investment in, and the commercialization of, new technologies actively promotes and contributes to the development of the local economy. Among the benefits of spin-off companies are employment opportunities, attraction of investment to the community, enhanced public visibility of the institution and its scientists, and the purchasing power of these new companies not to mention the tax base, all contributing to the local and regional economies.[3]

In relation to faculty recruitment and retention, new faculty being recruited to an institution will often inquire about the opportunities related to intellectual property that they may bring to or create at the institution. They are directly concerned about the opportunities for participation in spin-off company development. Experienced technology transfer professionals have expressed the view that to the extent spin-off companies remain in the local region and the faculty inventors have the opportunity to remain active consultants and/or advisors to the company, the spin-off can be a powerful force in keeping faculty inventors at the institution.

Sourcing Technologies Suitable for Spin-Off Companies

To many, the creation of a new company is one of the more exciting options for commercialization of technologies or innovations arising from academic-based research institutions. To be a candidate for new company creation, the technology or innovation must be unique, have diverse application, and have the potential for multiple products or other commercial opportunities.

Some issues to consider in determining if spin-off company development is the most effective method of transferring or translating the technology or innovation are:

- If the invention is sufficient for creating a new venture, including a strong intellectual property position and the potential for a wide range of products in multiple markets.
- The effort required, including staff time during the preparation period for creating the new venture and the management of the conflicts of interest issues.
- The likelihood of creating a viable business opportunity through identification of a champion and knowledgeable management.
- The most effective and efficient path to market for the technology—either licensing to an existing company or creating a new business venture.
- The impact on economic development in the local economy—employment, taxes, access to and use of complementary local businesses.

Institutions are creating programs within their TTOs to identify and support technologies suitable for spin-off company creation. For example, programs such as the VentureLab at Georgia Tech,[4] the University of British Columbia Prototype Development Program,[5] and VentureBox at the University of Manitoba[6] (all described in more detail in the following paragraphs) serve to accelerate the commercial opportunity for suitable innovations that are identified through diligent intellectual property assessments, market assessments, and technology positioning exercises.

VentureLab. VentureLab is a relatively new initiative of the Georgia Institute of Technology's Office of Economic Development and Technology Ventures (EDTV). VentureLab's mission is to be a one stop shop for faculty members interested in commercializing new technologies or innovations arising from their laboratories. The program provides educational outreach workshops for faculty, staff, and students on the principles and practices involved in technology commercialization. Venture-Lab can also facilitate access to preseed funding for the development of prototypes, demonstration of proof-of-concept or other activities to make the spin-off more attractive to other potential investors. VentureLab conducts technology assessments, which include recommendations for commercial applications, in order to evaluate the commercial potential of technology. Unique to the program are the VentureLab Fellows, experienced technology entrepreneurs who serve as advisors to program-affiliated spin-off company creation.

UBC Prototype Development Program. The University of British Columbia has one of the most productive prototype development programs in Canada.[7] The primary goal of the Prototype Development Program is to develop the commercial potential of a given technology by:

- Demonstrating proof-of-concept;
- Demonstrating technology scale-up;
- Conducting detailed market and technical evaluations; and,
- Broadening the coverage of the intellectual property position.

As stated in the "UBC Spin-Off Company Report":

> Without spin-off companies the opportunity to maximize regional economic and social benefits would be lost, or at best, greatly diminished. Many new technologies might be abandoned, have their development delayed or be exploited outside of British Columbia. By transferring UBC technologies to custom companies with high growth potential, the university is helping to foster entrepreneurship, create jobs, and build a stronger high technology industrial base in the province.[8]

VentureBox Program of the University of Manitoba.[9] VentureBox is a comprehensive program designed to successfully create, mentor, and grow high-tech and biotech start-up companies. It is an institution-to-business interface committed to fostering start-up business opportunities from academic based research activities of the University of Manitoba and its affiliated research partners. Once an invention disclosure is received, the disclosure is reviewed for potential intellectual property position and market potential. Each qualifying disclosure is reviewed by a committee consisting of representatives of the financial community, the business community, senior university administration, and entrepreneurs. Upon review of the technology and the recommended commercialization strategy, an invention may be identified for the VentureBox program. The researcher must be interested in proceeding under the VentureBox program and the research supporting an intellectual property position will be monitored and assessed regularly. Once research outcomes, intellectual property, and business indicators meet standards necessary for considering spin-off company creation, a company will be incorporated and investment sought. For spin-offs, VentureBox offers:

- Incorporation for an eligible technology;
- Provision of workshops and materials for VentureBox researchers on start-up operations, term sheets, and venture capital fund expectations;

- Development of business and research plans as well as identifying interim management for each VentureBox company;
- Introduction to alliance partners related to the incubator facility in the research park; and
- Access to the Springboard Fund, a small pre-seed fund dedicated to start-up business opportunities in the VentureBox program.

Described previously are only three of the numerous venture programs at research intensive institutions throughout the world. These programs have and continue to contribute significantly to the success of new venture spin-off companies.

Mechanisms for Access to IP by a Spin-Off Company

At the outset, usually at the point of trying to determine whether or not to proceed through spin-off company creation, frequently used vehicles allowing access to the spin-off for the purpose or raising initial funding include:

- Option to obtain/license
- Memorandum of understanding
- Letter of intent

Once there is a commitment to establish the spin-off evidenced through the commitment or presence of preseed or seed funding, the legal and practical issues must be managed. These will include incorporating and structuring the company, developing shareholder and employee agreements, assembling interim management for the company, and identifying additional preseed, seed, and/or venture capital funding. Activities in these areas may also include identifying regulatory and taxation issues including recommendations on addressing these.

At this point, the institution may transfer or license the technology into the company in exchange for equity and other financial considerations. Equity is sometimes used in lieu of license fees or license initiation fees and is very often seen positively by the investment community as a vote of confidence for the technology being positioned in the spin-off company. Equity in the spin-off is only one of several financial considerations in the license or transfer agreement: others include royalty and milestone payments, share of income from sublicensing, and sublicensing fees. These other fees come into play as the technology is further developed, regulatory requirements met, sales and mar-

keting activities well underway. This is often referred to as "back-loading" the license in order to provide for the most optimum opportunity for the spin-off company. This allows the spin-off to concentrate on the success of the innovation and is seen as sharing the risk by the financial community.

It should be noted that in most institutions, technologies are not transferred into the spin-off company but rather licensed to the company in exchange for equity, royalties, and/or other consideration with the institution retaining ownership of the technology. In some circumstances (for example, where a spin-off company would be sufficiently capitalized to move the technology to the marketplace and the continued investment in and development of the technology appears relatively certain), the institution may be in a position to transfer the entire right to the technology to the company over a period of time. This is traditionally done by using a staged approach, where ownership of the technology may be transferred based on the successful completion of certain milestones, the culmination of which is the complete ownership of the technology being transferred to the company. In the United States, this may be quite difficult given the obligations imposed on the institutions through the Bayh-Dole Act. However, where federal funds subject to the Bayh-Dole Act have not been used in the development of the technology, a scenario, such as that posed above, may be possible. This also is dependent upon the institution's policies on ownership and transfer of intellectual property.

There are many beneficial ways in which a spin-off company can access the intellectual assets including the employment of the students or graduate students who may have been involved in the development of the innovation and the continued involvement of the faculty inventor(s). The company obtains not only the intellectual property (for example, the patent through the license or transfer), but also significant intellectual assets of the hands-on, know-how resident with the students and faculty.

Downsides to Keep in Mind and Strive to Overcome

While the promise of positive return on investment is the cornerstone of the decision to create a new spin-off company, there are several downsides that may need to be considered and carefully overcome, including:

- Very high risk in nascent technologies or innovations.
- Difficulty in finding financing for early stage ventures.
- Complexity and difficulty in negotiations.

- Difficulty in attracting an experienced management team.

In their presentation at the Fall 2002 AUTM Start-up Business Development, Berneman and Denis discussed the following deal-breaking issues:[10]

- Open-ended patent rights (investors may seek rights to all future related inventions created by faculty founders).
- Patent costs and control of prosecution.
- Indemnification (institutions accept no liability and require insurance).
- Warranty (the lack thereof).

Basic Elements Required for Establishing Spin-Off Companies

Besides having all the important technical, scientific, and intellectual property and market indicators suitable for spin-off company development, there are a few other elements that are critical for establishing spin-off companies, as further discussed next.

Funding

There are many traditional sources of funding, but for new spin-off company creation, gaining access to early stage (angel, preseed, and seed) investment funding is incredibly difficult. Absence of experienced investors is regularly cited as the barrier to spin-off company creation. Investors need to be aware that new and innovative technologies require a longer time to develop into marketable products, while also requiring a greater investment of time and money before being ready for market. Some institutions are trying to overcome this very early hurdle in the initiation of new spin-off companies through the creation of internal or at-arms-length, preseed venture funds. Some examples of these funds are:

- University of Manitoba's Springboard Fund
- Purdue University/Purdue Research Foundation's Trask Technology Innovation and Pre-Seed Awards
- Boston University, Office of Technology Development's VC Limited Partnership Funds

Business Partners and Mentors

Suitable business partners and mentors can often be found through the local or regional community and can be identified through the academic business school, the board of governors or trustees of the institution, the financial and venture community, alumni of the institution, and local business entrepreneurs. The role of these partners is quite varied depending on the circumstances at hand, but it is clear that the kinds of expertise such partners would bring to a spin-off is of paramount importance to the success of the venture.

Facilities and Location

In order to establish a spin-off company based on the outcome of academic-based research, it is advantageous to locate as near as possible to the licensing institution. In recognition of this, many institutions and organizations are establishing research parks and other facilities to better foster and promote spin-off company development.

Role of the Technology Transfer Office

Depending on the depth and breadth of the institution's commitment to the development of spin-off company development, the role of the TTO can be either a passive or active one. The most passive activity occurs when a TTO facilitates spin-off company discussions and aids in the development of the business concept, technology assessment, intellectual property due diligence, or in the proposal of venture financing. Traditionally, TTOs have taken more passive roles, but recent data from the AUTM Licensing Survey indicates the level of TTOs' effort and participation is changing by becoming far more aggressive in the creation of start-up ventures. TTOs' active roles include participation in:

- Development of the business concept or preliminary business plan.
- Intellectual property due diligence (including ownership, freedom to operate).
- Intellectual property assessment.
- Market assessment and technology positioning.
- Introduction to financial community (angels, venture capital, etc.).
- Identification of the initial management team (mentors).

Creative development and use of partnerships to support and develop entrepreneurial infrastructure are some ways in which the TTO can add value to the spin-off company venture. In addition to the foregoing list of possible TTO services, other mechanisms can support and add value to new business creation and can include the identification and access to assistance programs from various government agencies. Some examples of these include the Small Business Innovation Research (SBIR) program in the United States and the National Research Council's Industrial Research Assistance Program (NRC-IRAP) in Canada. There may also be opportunities for funding of the research supporting patent or other intellectual property activities of the scientist laboratories such as local, state, or regional assistance programs; university-industry programs of federal research sponsors; economic development agencies and so on. The institutional partner in a spin-off is often best positioned to provide advice, guidance, and access to these programs.

Some institutions prefer to use contracted or partnered services (e.g., as offered through Research Corporation Technologies, Inc.). These organizations and others like them provide many of the same services that are offered by the TTO, but are focused solely on the commercial opportunity of the technology. Under some circumstances, this type of service may be the most optimum for a technology, even where the TTO is an active partner. One of the keys for success is to maximize the opportunity for any given technology through effective use of available resources.

Working with Faculty Interested in Spin-Off Companies

Role of Researcher

To form a successful spin-off company, a solid invention or technology is needed, preferably already issued patent or other intellectual property protection. Desire, commitment, and cooperation of the inventor/creator is also critical to the success of a spin-off. Working with faculty who are interested in seeing the commercial fruits of their research is one of the more unique and rewarding aspects of working in an institutional technology transfer capacity. Researchers often have difficulty understanding that to develop the commercial strategy, focus shifts to market-related issues, business financing, scale-up of technology, regulatory issues and barriers, and ultimately on return on investment—none of these activities that appear to the scientist as having much to do with the science behind the innovation or even the innovation itself. To address this paradox, the TTO must work closely with faculty researchers to facilitate their understanding of the commercialization process as it relates to their science. This includes increasing faculty understanding of time scale development and of the legal and financial aspects of the business to be addressed early on in the venture.

The ultimate role of the faculty researcher or inventor can depend upon the acuity of the individual related to the business opportunity or can be related to the desire of the inventor to be intimately involved or to take a more passive role. These are all possible roles, but ones often dictated, at least in part, by the financing partner(s). A most appropriate role for academic inventors might be that of chief scientific officer. Rarely should an academic inventor take on the role of president and chief executive officer. The TTO should provide guidance on these various roles accordingly.

Conflict of Interest, Conflict of Commitment

There has been significant discussion in a variety of sources of the inherent conflicts of interest in research conducted for or with private sector/industry partners. Even more so, the perception and reality of conflict is paramount in spin-off company creation from academic-based research. Recalling that the definition at the beginning of this discussion included the element of active participation of the inventor in the company, it is easily seen where conflict can and does occur.

Conflict of commitment can occur where a faculty member who is actively involved in a spin-off company experiences or demonstrates difficulty in prioritizing their obligations to their students, employer, and to the spin-off.

Although there is more discussion of these concepts elsewhere in this publication, a few comments are worthy of consideration here.

The University of Wisconsin, Madison. There is a very positive and effective approach to identifying and managing conflicts of interest at the University of Wisconsin, Madison. For example, it is permissible for faculty-owned companies to support research on campus in the faculty member's own laboratory. These arrangements are complex and therefore involve considerable oversight and review, but are nonetheless allowed within existing policy.[11]

The University of Utah. Faculty at the University of Utah can simultaneously hold equity in a company and be full-fledged members of their academic units, although conflict of interest disclosures and management are expected/required. Companies owned by faculty can contract with the university for research projects, including the participation of a faculty member and his/her laboratory. Oversight and management of these relationships is required.[12]

Purdue University. Purdue has a well-written document, "Policy, Guidelines and Procedures Document on Faculty-Owned and Operated Businesses," which offers clear, concise guidance on issues involving conflict of interest and conflict of commitment.[13]

Statistical Evidence of Spin-Off Company Development

The Association of University Technology Managers, through its annual licensing surveys, has been collecting information and statistics on spin-off company development since 1994 when the survey requested respondents to include the number of spin-off companies formed since 1980 through FY 1993. Starting in 1995, the survey asked how many start-ups had been formed in the year of reporting. The AUTM definition of start-ups (called spin-offs for the purpose of this discussion) is deliberately narrow in that it is restricted to companies that were dependent on the license of the reporting institution's technology for initiation. The question of equity as consideration or partial consideration for the license to the spin-off was not asked until 2000 when respondents reported holding equity in 252 or the 454 start-ups reported for FY 2000 or 55%. Based on the data for years subsequent, this number appears fairly consistent. Based on data for the previous years reporting, this number has remained consistent.[14]

The AUTM Licensing Survey: FY 2002 survey reported a decline in the number of spin-off companies from 2001,[15] and a further decline was reported in the FY 2003 survey[16] noting the difficult conditions for raising early stage funding for such ventures in both 2002 and 2003. Given the activities of the investment community in 2004, it is possible that this downward trend will continue. The number of companies in which the licensing institutions took equity however appears to be at a significantly increased level since 2000. The proportion of licenses with equity executed with existing small companies almost tripled from FY 2001 to FY 2002, although it declined in FY 2003. One interpretation of this dataset may be that given the difficult financial climate for new spin-off company formation, an increased number of licenses were executed with equity as part of the consideration for the license rather than cash payments of up-front license fees. This is possibly also due to the more sophisticated licensing activities at institutions, the increased willingness to be creative in

order to support early stage technologies, and establishing the mechanisms through which institutions can actually hold equity in a spin-off.

Spin-Off Company Activity

In the AUTM Licensing Survey: FY 2003, 432 new spin-off companies based on academic discovery were reported, down almost 10% from the previous year. Of the new companies created, 84.3% were located in the state or province of the academic institution where the technology was created. Since 1980, 4,748 new companies have been formed based on a license or transfer of technology from an academic-based research institution. Of those start-ups, 2,769 or 58.3% were still operational as of the end of FY 2003.[17]

> This start-up survival rate is quite high, approaching the rate experienced by the venture capital industry overall. This observation isn't necessarily unexpected, considering the large proportion of university start up companies that received funds from venture capitalists.[18]

The AUTM Licensing Survey and resources available through the AUTM Web site (www.autm.org) include many references to the activities of companies created around technologies licensed from institutions and the new products these companies are marketing. These vignettes are a very worthwhile read and are evidence of the enhanced contribution to public benefit that can be made by considering spin-off company formation as an important tool in the technology transfer tool box and an important contribution to economic and social benefit.

Licenses and Options

For the 4,964 licenses and options executed in FY 2003 for which data on both exclusivity type and the size and nature of the licensee was reported (98.3% of the total reported licenses and options):

- 63.1% of new licenses and options executed were with newly formed or existing small companies (fewer than 500 employees), while 36.8% were with large companies;
- 95.5% of licenses and options to start-ups were exclusive;
- 44.2% of licenses to existing small companies were exclusive.

Keeping Perspective

Of the measured technology transfer activities including licensing options and spin-off company development, spin-off company development represents only about 10% of activities directed to commercialization. While it is thought that the measurable returns on investment may be increased through spin-off company development, the statistics have yet to certify this as fact. It is also imperative to consider the mission of the institution, the investment in the technology transfer activities of that institution, and the expertise available to support a spin-off company development program.

Dr. Howard Bremer, in his keynote address to the International Patent Licensing Seminar 2002, in Tokyo, Japan, stated: "In today's globally competitive economy we must remember and understand that no matter how much money is spent on research and development, the results of those efforts are not going to benefit society unless there is suitable incentives to invest in commercialization."[19]

• • • References

1. The Association of University Technology Managers, Inc. *AUTM Licensing Survey, FY 2002: A Survey Summary of Technology Licensing (and Related) Performance for U.S. and Canadian Academic and Nonprofit Institutions, and Patent Management Firms.* Chicago: AUTM, 2002: 14.

2. Gross, C. M., Reischl, U., and Abercrombie, P. *The New Idea Factory: Expanding Technology Companies with University Intellectual Capital.* Columbus, Ohio: Battelle Press, 2000.

3. Livingstone, A. *Report on UBC Spin-off Company Formation and Growth.* Vancouver, Canada: University-Industry Liaison Office, University of British Columbia, 1997.

4. Georgia Tech VentureLab Web site, http://venturelab.gatech.edu (accessed September 29, 2005).

5. The University of British Columbia, University-Industry Liaison Office Web site, http://www.uilo.ubc.ca (accessed September 29, 2005).

6. The University of Manitoba Web site, http://www.umanitoba.ca/research (accessed September 29, 2005).

7. The University of British Columbia, University-Industry Liaison Office, UILO Prototype Development Program, http://www.uilo.ubc.ca/researcher_Prototype.asp?sID=05C08570B06941BEA66DD144AFEBC8C2 (accessed October 17, 2005).

8. Livingstone, 1997.

9. The University of Manitoba Web site.

10. Berneman, L., and Denis, K. Course material presented at the Association of University Technology Managers, Inc., Start-up Business Development course, AUTM, Hollywood, CA. October 6–8, 2002.

11. University of Wisconsin Alumni Research Foundation Web site, www.warf.ws/inventors (accessed September 29, 2005).

12. University of Utah. "University Faculty Profit-Making Corporations," http://www.admin.utah.edu/ppmanual/6/6-3.html (accessed October 17, 2005).

13. Purdue University. "Faculty-owned and Operated Businesses: Policy, Guidelines, and Procedures." http://www.purdue.edu/Research/IRTPOffice/faculty-owned.pdf (accessed October 17, 2005).

14. The Association of University Technology Managers, Inc. *AUTM Licensing Survey, FY 2000: A Survey Summary of Technology Licensing (and Related) Performance for U.S. and Canadian Academic and Nonprofit Institutions, and Patent Management Firms.* Chicago: AUTM, 2000.

15. The Association of University Technology Managers, Inc., 2002.

16. The Association of University Technology Managers, Inc. *AUTM Licensing Survey, FY 2003: A Survey Summary of Technology Licensing (and Related) Performance for U.S. and Canadian Academic and Nonprofit Institutions, and Patent Management Firms.* Chicago: AUTM, 2003.

17. Association of University Technology Managers, 2003.

18. Association of University Technology Managers, 2003.

19. Bremer, H. "Technology Transfer: The American Way." Keynote address, international patent licensing seminar, Tokyo, Japan, June 2002.

• • • Other Reference Materials and Recommended Reading

Jonash, R. S., and Sommerlatte, T. *The Innovation Premium: How Next-Generation Companies Are Achieving Peak Performance and Profitability.* Arthur D. Little, Inc., 1999.

Rice, M. P., and Matthews, J. B. *Growing New Ventures, Creating New Jobs: Principles and Practices of Successful Incubation.* United Kingdom: Quorum Books, 1995.

Tornatzky, L. G., Waugaman, P. G., and Gray, D. O. *Innovation U.: New University Roles in a Knowledge Economy,* Southern Growth Policies Board, 2002.

73

The Role of Universities and Research Institutions in Economic Development

Elliott C. Kulakowski, PhD, FAHA

Introduction

A comprehensive definition of economic development is

a community's collective efforts to:

- Create expanded employment and business opportunities for local residents
- Provide support for existing employees and businesses
- Improve local productivity
- Promote the development of quality jobs and qualified workers
- Increase wages and local business profitability
- Help diversify employment sources and the local economy
- Stimulate growth and private investment in the community
- Maintain and enhance local property tax values and the property tax base
- Retain and attract young people for the community
- Enhance the community's quality of life.[1]

The community can exist at the local or state levels, and, in terms of the world economies, at the federal level. Federal, state, and local governments, therefore, are all concerned about economic development efforts within their spheres of influence, and undertake efforts in a number of ways to stimulate and support such development. As new technologies are great factors in driving modern economic development, governments increasingly recognize the importance of and provide support to research institutions as engines for economic development.

Research institutions (academic institutions, research hospitals, and nonprofit research organizations) are becoming hubs around which major economic development takes place. Universities educate the workforces that add value to communities and their research programs engage in basic, applied, and developmental research that yields new products and processes that can generate new businesses. As research institutions increase their activities, they also contribute to the local economy by expanding their facilities and by hiring additional researchers, technical staff, and other workers. Overall, the success of research universities benefits local, state, regional, and national economies.

Support for Economic Development to Research Institutions

Federal Government

The federal government has undertaken several major programs to stimulate economic development within the last twenty-five years. Four of the programs are summarized in this chapter.

Bayh-Dole Act In 1980, during a time of slow economic growth and high unemployment, the federal government looked at many opportunities to stimulate economic growth. This included recognition that federal financial support served to nurture the growth of research at research institutions that led to technological advances. However, the technological fruits from federally funded research were not picked because access to the intellectual property was freely available. There were virtually no incentives for either research institutions to harvest the fruits or for industry to develop them.

It was the Bayh-Dole Act that in 1980 allowed research institutions to retain title to inventions developed with federal funds. The institutions were allowed to seek patent protection and to share any royalty income with the research faculty inventors from any licenses with industry. The program was intended to stimulate economic development by allowing the outcome of the research to be transferred to industry for development of new products and processes, contributing to the overall development of technical industry. (Note: For a complete description of the Bayh-Dole Act, refer to Chapter 59 authored Howard Bremer in this book.)[2]

Small Business Innovation Research (SBIR) Program

The 1982 establishment of the Small Business Innovation Research (SBIR) program was another effort by the federal government to stimulate economic growth through technology innovation and to meet the R&D needs of federal agencies. The purpose of the SBIR program supports further development and commercialization of inventions developed at small companies or research institutions that are licensed to small companies. In fact, many small companies supported by this program are spin-off companies of the research institutions. Many of these companies retain close ties with the research institutions that helped to found them.

The SBIR program originally required that federal research agencies, providing over $100 million in extramural research support, set aside 2.5% of their extramural research budget for the SBIR program. The SBIR program was so successful that it was reauthorized in December 2000 through Federal Fiscal Year 2008. In 2004 over $1.5 billion was appropriated by the federal agencies participating in the program.[3,4]

Small Business Technology Transfer (STTR) Program

The STTR program is another federally established program that, unlike SBIR, requires participation from a nonprofit research institution (the principal investigator can, however, be from either the research institution or the small company). This program is supported by the five federal agencies (Department of Defense, Department of Education, National Aeronautics and Space Administration, National Institutes of Health, and National Science Foundation) that provide over $1 billion in research support. As of Fiscal Year 2004, the sponsoring federal agencies were required to set aside 0.3% of their extramural budget for this program. Public Law 107-50, enacted in October 2001, authorizes STTR through Fiscal Year 2009.[3,4]

Partnership Intermediary

A partnership intermediary is another federal mechanism to stimulate economic development and enhance technology. As of January 6, 2003, US Code Title 15, Commerce and Trade (Chapter 63, Technology Innovation, Section 3715) defines a partnership intermediary as when "an agency of a State or local government ... assists, counsels, advises, evaluates, or otherwise cooperates with small business firms, institutions of higher education that need or can make demonstrably productive use of technology-related assistance from a Federal laboratory."[5]

The mechanism for support of a partnership intermediary is through a memorandum of understanding or a contract. An example of a intermediary memorandum of understanding has been published by the federal government.[6]

Several programs are supported through a partnership intermediary. Three of these are summarized below.

Maryland Technology Development Corporation (TEDCO) and the US Navy established a partnership to more effectively develop an outreach program to small businesses, state agencies, and academic institutions to increase technology transfer and the collaborative use of the Navy's Indian Head facilities.[7]

TechLink, established in 1996 at Montana State University, is supported by the Department of Defense and NASA. TechLink was established to license technologies from the two federal agencies and to commercialize the technology and to partner on joint technology research and development.[8]

In 2004 the University of Utah entered into an agreement with the US Army at Dugway Proving Ground through a partnership intermediary to identify and develop technologies that would benefit Dugway and to partner with them to develop technologies related to chemical and biological defense.

State Governments

In support of economic development, states undertake a number of different efforts to support technology development, maturization, productization, and commercialization through the establishment of quasi-government organizations for economic development or through support of technology centers. Depending on the state, such support can be managed through the state's commerce department or through an office of economic development. In certain instances, states can provide direct appropriations to research institutions to support economic development activities.

For example, the Commonwealth of Pennsylvania established greenhouse centers located throughout the Commonwealth to stimulate technology development and spur job creation. The basic premise of the centers is to leverage and expand the Commonwealth's technology clusters. Both state and local governments finance the initiative and the greenhouse centers are established in collaboration with the regional research institutions, which also provide support. The greenhouses provide start-up companies with seed funding; incubation and business services; technology transfer management; shared laboratory facilities and equipment; and gap funding.

Greenhouses have been created for the areas of life science, biotechnology, and chip technologies. The centers are located across the Commonwealth, in the Southeastern region, in Central Pennsylvania, and in the Pittsburgh area. The Life Sciences Greenhouse is located in Central Pennsylvania.[9] BioAdvance is the biotechnology greenhouse to stimulate economic development in Southeastern Pennsylvania, the hub of the pharmaceutical industry in the United States.[10] In Pittsburgh, there are the Life Sciences Greenhouse and the Digital Greenhouse. The Pittsburgh Digital Greenhouse merged with the Robotics Foundry in 2005 to form The Technology Collaborative to support economic development by leveraging the industries related to agile robotics and digital technologies.[11]

The Commonwealth of Pennsylvania also supports The Ben Franklin Technology Partners, another state economic development program supported through the Commonwealth's Office of Economic Development. Since its establishment in 1982, the Technology Partners program has evolved from supporting research institutions and their technology development efforts to fostering collaborative efforts between young entrepreneurial companies and the Commonwealth's research institutions. The program can boast that for every dollar invested since the program's inception there has been $23 of additional income to the state; the creation of 93,105 new jobs; an increase in tax revenues by $400 million; and an overall $8 billion boost to the Commonwealth's economy.[12]

Technology Centers State governments often support state economic developments through a Centers of Excellence program. These programs vary widely, however, in their design, management, levels of support, and mechanism of economic stimulation.

The state of Utah is a leader in supporting a Centers of Excellence program. As in other states, the purpose of Utah's program is to stimulate economic growth in high technology fields that yield new products or processes and the expansion of employment in the state. The program supports centers located at the three research universities, University of Utah, Utah State University, and Brigham Young University, in areas such as biotechnology, information technology, and material sciences. The Utah legislature provides $2 million a year to the State Office of Business and Economic Development to support the centers. The program requires that $2 in matching funds be obtained by the company for every dollar provided by the state. The state has invested $36 million in the program since its inception in 1986. The program's efforts have resulted in approximately $400 million (more than ten times the state's investment) through the creation of about 150 spin-off companies and the creation of thousands of technology-related jobs.[13]

The state of New York's Centers of Excellence program is funded through the state's Office of Science Technology and Academic Research Centers of Excellence. During Fiscal Year 2002 to 2003 the program provided $250 million in support for the upgrade of "research facilities and other high technology and biotechnology capital projects, allowing colleges, universities and research institutions to secure research funding that will lead to job creation."[14] New York anticipates another $1 billion to be leveraged by industry and other contributions to support Centers of Excellence at academic institutions in technology areas such as in bioinformatics, environmental systems, and nanoelectronics.[14]

Research Institutions

Federal and state governments support research institutions through a variety of programs that are designed to increase technology development, stimulate new business ventures in technology areas, and support the creation of new high technology jobs. Academic institutions contribute significantly to economic development locally and nationally. This is accomplished through education of the future workforce, research activities, the transfer of the results of the research to industry, and creation of an entrepreneurial atmosphere through research parks and support of start-up companies, and support of local economy. Other types of research institutions also contribute in many of the same ways as academic institutions by providing an atmosphere to stimulate research and the technology that derives from it.

Educating Students

The primary objective of academic institutions is to educate individuals. It was once said that the economy of a nation is tied to the education of its workforce. These individuals, upon graduation, make up the local, regional, and national workforce.

The number of students attending colleges and universities has grown from about 7 million in 1967 to 15.6 million in 2000. In addition the number of post-secondary students graduating also has increased steadily: in 1980, 22 per 100 twenty-four-year-olds held bachelor degrees; 34 per 100 in 2000.[15]

The growth in the number of undergraduate students pursuing degrees in science and engineering increased respectively by 21% and 24%.[15] In the United States, there are 127 designated research universities that enroll about 19% of all students in academia. It is notable that these research-intensive institutions award over 42% of all baccalaureate degrees in science and engineering.[16]

Graduate enrollment in science and engineering, after faltering in the mid- to late 1990s, is recovering. The 127 US research universities awarded 52% of all science and engineering master's degrees in 2003[16] and in 2001 there were 27,100 doctoral degrees awarded in the science and engineering areas.[15]

Universities conduct about 50% of all basic research in the United States, where about 90% of all postdoctoral training occurs.[15] There were roughly 47,000 postdoctoral trainees at US academic institutions in 2003. However, only about 42% of postdoctoral trainees remain in academia after their training experience.[15] The majority, who are not in academia, pursue employment in industry.

With the recent technology boom over the last twenty years, it is not surprising that the science and engineering workforce has grown from 2.6% to 3.8%.[15] The economic impact of university graduates is that they tend to remain in the workforce, have higher paying jobs, and stimulate other sectors of the economy through the purchase of homes, goods, and services.

Research   Second to providing an educated work force, universities participate in research activities. University expenditures for research and development activities have grown almost sevenfold since 1979, the year before Bayh-Dole was enacted. In 1979, total academic research and development (R&D) expenditures were $5.4 billion, compared to $36.3 billion in 2002. Industry's share of total university R&D expenditures increased from $200 million (3.7% of the total) in 1979 to $2.2 billion (6.0% of the total) in 2002. This is a 62% increase in industry's share of the total.[17]

The growth in industry support of research and development is in part due to the increasing competition and the desire to develop new products or processes. Universities can provide expert faculty or access to instrumentation that small business may not have the continual need or the capital to acquire. This has significantly increased the numbers of joint ventures between industry and academia.

Industry also gained a greater appreciation of the importance of collaborations with universities, even at the early stages of basic science research. Between 1991 and 1997, US industry investment in basic research increased by 20% in constant dollars. In 1997, industry supported 6.5% of all basic research or $1.05 billion and 9.1% of all applied and developmental research, which amounted to $545 million.[18]

The increase in the relationship between industry and academia, independent research institutes, government research laboratories, and research hospitals also can be seen in the growing number of joint publications. Between 1981 and 1995 the number of industry publications increased from 2,905 to 7,479. During this same time period the number of articles coauthored between industry and academia increased from 21.6% to 40.8%.[18]

The increase in research support to institutions also had other effects on local and national economies. As research efforts expanded, so did the need for new research facilities. The increase stimulated the construction industry and provided employment in the construction trades. The facilities had to be furnished and new equipment and supplies purchased. The new research facilities also attracted new faculty and researchers who brought their research funding with them. It also provided employment opportunities for skilled technical staff and other support staff.

Intellectual Property

In an effort to increase technology competitiveness and improve the economy, the federal government sought new ways to stimulate innovation through the programs aimed at research institutions, such as those earlier described. It was hoped that the development of new technologies with federal research dollars would translate into new patents and inventions. The patents would be licensed to companies that would hire more workers to produce the products. The products would be available for industry, government and/or the general public, and, thus, the economy of the US would be improved.

Prior to passage of the Bayh-Dole Act, the main products of research endeavors were in the form of publications. The act added a new dimension to measure the success of researchers; these were inventions. To manage the entire technology transfer process, research institutions had to either create or expand Technology Transfer Offices (TTOs) or hire external companies or individuals to manage their programs. After Bayh-Dole, the field of technology transfer expanded greatly. This resulted in new highly technical positions being created for individuals with business and marketing degrees; for technologists with specialized training in fields (e.g., engineering, biotechnology, and computer sciences) to understand the inventions; and lawyers with specialization in intellectual property.

While research institutions had to make new investment in technology transfer programs, they were also forced to think about measures of success in these efforts. Success can be measured on different levels. First, research institutes measure the numbers of invention disclosures, patent applications, and license agreements executed. They also look at the revenues generated, products that make it to market, and economic impact. Success can also be measured by the increase in the reputation of the investigators and the institution and the institution's ability to expand its research activities by attracting high quality researchers and trainees.

Industry Trends in Research Support and Links to Public Research reports that in high tech research areas such as biotechnology, US patents are increasingly linked to research from public institutions such as academia, nonprofit research institutes, research hospitals and government research facilities.[18] Statistics from the Association of University Technology Managers' (AUTM) *Licensing Survey—2002* support the concept that research institutions are an important source of high technology innovation.[19]

The successes are even more pronounced when AUTM reported that in Fiscal Year 1999, research institutions and patent management firms through licensing activities added more than $40 billion to the US economy and supported 270,000 jobs.[20]

Not only is the impact felt at the national level, it impacts state economies. A Texas State report, "Economic Development Activities at Public Universities and Health Sciences Centers in Texas," shows that the institutions in Texas generated about $27 million in license income in fiscal year 2000.[21] This compares to other public institutions cited in the Texas report, such as the University of California System, $252 million; Florida State University, $67 million; and the University of Washington, $30 million.

AUTM also looks at the technology revenues as a proportion of research dollars received. The national average is that technology revenues are about 2% of the research dollars. In 2004, the Office of Technology Transfer at the University of Utah reported revenues of $15 million and research revenues of $275 million. The license revenues are about 5% of the amount of research that the institution receives. This is a tremendous accomplishment for the University of Utah.

Whether you look at the national, state, or individual school figures, it is difficult not to see measures of success sparked by the Bayh-Dole Act. This is especially true considering that prior to 1980 there were fewer than 250 patents annually awarded to academic institutions, while 3,673 were issued in 2002.[19]

Many researchers also took advantage of the SBIR program, which allowed them entrepreneurial opportunities to establish their own small business; license their own inventions back from their institution; establish consortium arrangements with the university; and apply to the federal government research agencies to support their devel-

TABLE 73-1	Intellectual Property Activity of Research Institutions		
Invention Disclosures	**New Patent Applications**	**Patents Issued**	**New Licenses or Options**
15,573	7,224	3,673	4,673

Source: AUTM Licensing Survey—2002

opment activities through the SBIR or STTR programs. These programs also provided research funds for universities and companies for job creation of highly trained technical positions required to further develop and commercialize the technology.

The success of the small business program can be seen by the numbers of patents and licenses to new or small companies. These small or new companies are usually located in relatively close proximity to the institutions that hold the patent and with which the inventor is associated. Of the new license or options agreements reported to AUTM in 2002, about 68% were given to new or small businesses.[19]

Research Parks   The establishment of research parks is another mechanism whereby economic development can be stimulated. Over 80% of research parks in the United States are owned by or closely affiliated with academic institutions. A research park's mission "is to encourage research, development, and commercialization of the University's intellectual assets, and to foster economic growth."[22]

Research parks that are owned by universities work in collaboration with governments and industry. The Virginia Biotechnology Research Park was created as a partnership among the University of Virginia, the City of Richmond, the Commonwealth of Virginia, other academic institutions, industry and nonprofit organizations.[23] The concept and general missions of a research park are not unique to the United States. Other countries also support research parks. The University of Waterloo's Research and Technology Park is supported in collaboration with government of Canada, the Province of Ontario, local government, Canada's Technology Triangle, and industry collaborators.[24]

Other research parks may be privately owned or are the outgrowth of government activities. The Australian government has established cooperative research centers that are collaborations between universities, public research agencies, and businesses.[25]

It is not surprising that the focus of research parks would mimic the research strengths of the university to which they are affiliated and the local technology clusters, which are not mutually exclusive. The focus of the Virginia BioTechnology Research Park, with its close relationship to the Virginia Commonwealth University Medical Center, is in the biological and biomedicine area with about 50 related companies located at the park.[23]

The success of a research park is what it contributes to the university and local economy.

Research parks support the orderly transition of inventions from universities and into the industrial arena.[26] Many start-up companies that are built around university inventions take up residence at the university-affiliated research parks. The research parks serve as incubators for the university technologies. The university envisions their technologies being developed and commercialized in companies at the research park. University faculty are often able to participate in the development of the product through research agreements or a consulting relationship, or the faculty member may become an owner of the start-up company. Research parks also support the growth of the university because the research parks, "contribute to the success of faculty recruitment and retention by creating opportunities for faculty to participate in the commercialization of their intellectual property."[22]

Often research parks add value by providing services to the high technology occupants. They may provide legal, technology transfer, business planning, and financial assistance programs. The university and its faculty may provide some of the services. For example, the university's technology transfer office may be used, associations may be formed with the business school to provide training and internships for students in return for business plan development, and legal support may be provided by professors or students at the law school.

One of the biggest benefits to the local and state economy is the creation of jobs as a result of the creation of new businesses or their expansion at the research park. The opportunities can be in the high technology areas and in the support services sector. There can be local hiring and/or an influx of new highly skilled people to the area. There also is the opportunity to provide training for students. Since the opening of its research park in January 2001, the University of Illinois has reported the creation of over 700 high technology jobs (over 180 of these are student internships and other similar positions).[22]

Spin-Off Companies

Research institutions are becoming more involved in the establishment of start-up companies. Start-up companies are centered around the institution's intellectual property with hope that the relationship will bring economic benefit to the institution and to the region if a successful product reaches market.[27,28]

Research institutions are becoming more entrepreneurial. In the past institutions had a hands-off approach, whereby they would license only to established companies. As successes at other institutions became public and a role of universities began to assume a more prominent role in economic development, institutional philosophies began to change. Despite the allure of start-up companies, not every technology is important enough to engender a start-up company.

With an appropriate technology, institutions increasingly are participating in start-up companies. However, the degree of an institution's participation can vary greatly depending on the technology and the institution's philosophy to risk tolerance. Examples of an institution's participation include:

- Allowing a start-up company to license a technology.
- Allowing faculty participation in start-up companies.
- Encouraging start-up companies.
- Taking an active role in establishment and management of the start-up.
- Having an equity position in the start-up company.

The degree of participation depends on the entrepreneurial culture of the institution. As the risks grow with each increasing level of involvement, so too does the level of reward should the venture prove successful.

Institutions must work with and within the local economic and social framework to make such ventures possible. Before a product is developed, start-ups from research institutions already play a role in economic development. There must also be local business talent hired to provide the corporate framework; there must be available financial resources such as angel investors or venture capital available; and the presence of an entrepreneurial local or state government support for such ventures. It is easier to coordinate resources when the start-up company is centered within a research park.

University of Utah serves as an excellent model to demonstrate the impact of start-up companies on economic development. In September 2004, Brent Brown, the university's Acting Director of the Technology Transfer Office, reported that the university had established 86 spin-off companies. Of these companies, in 2004 sixty-four remained in existence (56% in the state of Utah), a 75% success rate.

The University of Utah's research park is home to many of the university's spin-off companies, including Myriad Genetics, a company based on research conducted by Mark Skolnick and other researchers at the Center for Cancer Genetic Epidemiology. Established in 1991, the company is based on the concept that certain individuals have a genetic predisposition to specific cancers. Today, with a market capitalization of over $500 million, they are seeking to identify genetic predisposition to

other diseases (e.g., Alzheimer's, hypertension, and cardiovascular diseases).[29,30]

The impact of the three research universities' entrepreneurial efforts on the economy in Utah has been substantial. There has been about $150 million in direct investments in these companies, and the companies have added to the employment in Utah by the direct creation of over 1,000 jobs.[13] In addition there has been indirect job creation in the services needed by the new hires. Benefits also accrue to the local Salt Lake City area and to the state of Utah through an increased tax base.

Conclusion

Our research universities and other research institutions are expanding their spheres of influence into the area of economic development. Governments (federal, state, and local) are recognizing the importance of research in economic development and are supporting the efforts of their research institutions.

Research institutions are being considered as central in the perpetual cycle of economic development. Research universities attract highly skilled and entrepreneurial faculty, who train successive generations of high tech workers at all levels (undergraduate, graduate, and postgraduate) in science. Faculty are responsible for conducting cutting-edge research in science and engineering fields. The outcome of their basic, applied, and developmental research is new knowledge, which is disseminated to the public through publications and intellectual property. In the high technology areas, companies are created or expanded to license research technology and are utilizing the talent and facilities available at the research institutions. In turn, the research institutions are becoming more involved in establishing start-up companies that are often located in university research parks, which are increasing in number. The cycle comes full circle, as companies need a more highly trained workforce and again look to the universities to supply technology and business graduates to meet staffing needs. The royalties that the research institutions receive are used to reward inventors and are also used, in part, to build and to expand the research facilities, to purchase high tech equipment, and to support institutional infrastructure. The reputations of the research institutions increase as they are viewed as having entrepreneurial cultures. Such reputations, in turn, attract additional highly trained science and engineering researchers, as well as students—the next generations of technology trainees.

Research institutions cannot accomplish these goals by themselves; however, they rely on support from government agencies and the local business community. The partnership among research institutions, government, industry, and the community is the new paradigm for economic development.

• • • References

1. Clark, Cal. "How Do You Define Economic Development?" *The Developer* 34, no. 3, http://www.edam.org/06_01_news_define.cfm (accessed September 26, 2004).

2. Bremer, Howard. "University Technology Transfer Evolution or Revolution." In *Research Administration and Management*, edited by Elliott C. Kulakowski and Lynne U. Chronister, 627–639. Sudbury, MA: Jones and Bartlett Publishers, 2006.

3. Nixon, R A., Shindell, R., and Goodnight, J. "SBIR/STTR Programs." In *Research Administration and Management*, edited by Elliott C. Kulakowski and Lynne U. Chronister, 865–872. Sudbury, MA: Jones and Bartlett Publishers, 2006.

4. United States Small Business Administration. "SBIR and STTR Programs and Awards," http://www.sba.gov/SBIR/indexsbir-sttr.html#sbir (accessed September 16, 2005).

5. *U.S. Code* 15 Commerce and Trade Chapter 63 Technology Innovation § 3715, http://caselaw.lp.findlaw.com/casecode/uscodes/15/chapters/63/sections/section_3715.html (accessed September 16, 2005).

6. Air Force Research Laboratory, "VI. Partnership Intermediary Memorandum of Understanding," Air Force Technology Transfer Handbook. Updated September 1, 2005, http://64.233.161.104/search?q=cache:iD38xxx6eTQJ:www.afrl.af.mil/techtran/handbk/transferdocs/pia_model.doc+paternership+intermediary+memorandum+of+understanding&hl=en&client=firefox-a (accessed September 16, 2005).

7. Maryland Technology Development Corporation. "U.S. Navy Signs First Ever Partnership Intermediary Agreement Between Indian Head Division and TEDCO," http://www.marylandtedco.org/news/pdfs/PIA_IndianHead.pdf (accessed September 16, 2005).

8. TechLink Web site, http://techlink.msu.montana.edu/services/services.html (accessed September 16, 2005).

9. Life Sciences Greenhouse of Central Pennsylvania Web site, http://www.lsgpa.com/html/ (accessed September 16, 2005).

10. BioAdvance Web site, http://bioadvance.com/home/ (accessed September 16, 2005).

11. The Technology Collaborative Web site, http://www.techcollaborative.org/ (accessed September 12, 2005).

12. Ben Franklin Technology Partners. "BFTP: Returning Dividends for Pennsylvania," http://www.benfranklin.org/our_impact/index.asp (accessed September 16, 2005).

13. Utah Governor's Office of Economic Development. "Centers of Excellence," http://goed.utah.gov/COE/index.html (accessed September 12, 2005).

14. New York State, Office of Science Technology and Academic Research Centers of Excellence Web site, http://www.nystar.state.ny.us/coes.htm (accessed September 16, 2005).

15. National Science Foundation. "Science and Engineering Indicators 2004," http://www.nsf.gov/sbe/srs/seind04/start.htm (accessed September 26, 2004).

16. National Science Foundation. "Science and Engineering Indicators 2002." http://www.nsf.gov/sbe/srs/seind02/start.htm (accessed September 26, 2004).

17. National Science Foundation. "Academic Research and Development Expenditures—Fiscal Year 2002," http://www.nsf.gov/sbe/srs/nsf04330/pdfstart.htm (accessed September 26, 2004).

18. National Science Foundation. "Industry Trends in Research Support and Links to Public Research," http://www.nsf.gov/pubs/1998/nsb9899/nsb9899.htm (accessed September 26, 2004).

19. Association of University Technology Managers. "AUTM Licensing Survey: 2002 Survey Summary," http://www.autm.net/events/File/Surveys/02_Abridged_Survey.pdf (accessed September 15, 2005).

20. "Common Questions & Answers About Technology Transfer," *AUTM Surveys*, http://www.autm.net/pubs/survey/qa.html (accessed September 30, 2004).

21. Strayhorn, C.K. "Economic Development Activities at Public Universities and Health Sciences Centers in Texas," *Special Report*, http://www.window.state.tx.us/specialrpt/ecodev03/07ch4.html (accessed September 30, 2004).

22. University of Illinois Research Park, http://www.tech.com/researchpark/index.asp (accessed September 16, 2005).

23. Virginia BioTechnology Research Park Web site, http://www.vabiotech.com/ (accessed September 16, 2005).

24. The University of Waterloo Research and Technology Park Web site, http://www.uwrtpark.uwaterloo.ca/ (accessed September 16, 2005).

25. Australian Government, Austrade. "Cooperative Research Centres," http://www.austrade.gov.au/IT/layout/0,,0_S4-1_wqcrz29-2_3_

PWB110362883-4_23j258z1-5_-6_-7_,00.html (accessed September 16, 2005).

26. Association of University Research Parks. "What Is a Research Park?" http://www.aurp. net/about/whatis.cfm (accessed September 16, 2005).

27. Carney, J. "Spin-Off Companies from University Technologies." In *Research Administration and Management,* edited by Elliott C. Kulakowski and Lynne U. Chronister, 787–794. Sudbury, MA: Jones and Bartlett Publishers, 2006.

28. Scholz, J. "Establishing a Spin-Off Company." In *Research Administration and Management,* edited by Elliott C. Kulakowski and Lynne U. Chronister, 795–802. Sudbury, MA: Jones and Bartlett Publishers, 2006.

29. University of Utah Technology Commercialization Office, "Creativity Collaboration Commercialization" http://www.tto.utah.edu/about/ TCO_brochure.pdf (accessed September 16, 2005).

30. Myriad Genetics, Inc., http://www.myriad.com/ index.php (accessed September 16, 2005).

74

Material Transfer Agreements

Fred Reinhart, MBA

Introduction

Most research administrators know that MTA is short for "Material Transfer Agreement." However, the more experienced administrators suspect that the acronym really stands for Masochistic Torture Assignment! MTAs are often complicated. They take too much of your precious time to handle and the work you do to process MTAs is rarely acknowledged and is likely not compensated. Often, MTAs seem to multiply like bunnies, and each comes with a little sign around its neck that reads, "Help me," or "Can you guess what's wrong with me?" My personal favorite is the sign that reads, "My advisor has had me for a month, but he just dropped me off and I need to be looked at yesterday because I am very, very sick." MTAs can bring up many issues, especially for administrators, who aren't familiar with them or who process only a few agreements each month.

So why bother doing MTAs? Why is it worth spending the time to negotiate them, track their compliance, etc.? The key reason is: they are important to your researchers, and to the agreement itself, just to obtain the materials. Somewhere in another academic or corporate lab—in Kansas, New York, Maryland, or Stockholm—some other researcher has a cell line, an antibody or a compound that your researcher wants. And he or she wants it now, if not yesterday! You and the spiteful MTA are all that stand in the way of scientific progress for your scientist.

If you suspect that your researchers don't think too deeply about adhering to the terms of an MTA covering incoming materials, you are probably right. If you believe your researchers are not especially concerned about the rights of your institution under MTAs covering outgoing materials, you are probably right again.

The bottom line and the most important take-away message: MTAs make it possible for your talented researchers to get valuable and proprietary material needed to make speedy research progress, to make your investigators more competitive in grants and in publications, and to facilitate collaboration with top scientists around the world. The MTA is a critical fact of professional life for your researchers and are your responsibility. Reminding yourself of their importance may take some of the drudgery out of doing them.

This chapter is intended to assist research administrators who review MTAs and covers only the key aspects of handling this unique agreement. Further, the chapter focuses on the most challenging kind of MTA, the one that covers the transfer of material from industry to academia.

What Is an MTA?

"Material Transfer Agreement" pretty much sums up the MTA's definition and purpose. An MTA is an agreement by which two independent organizations state the ground rules for a transfer of proprietary materials owned by one of them (i.e., the "material").

Often, proprietary information accompanies the materials and is also covered by the MTA.

What Kinds of Materials Are Transferred Using an MTA?

Just when you thought you had seen every kind of material needing an MTA, something new comes along! The list is as long as your arm and can include any material one party deems proprietary, valuable, or even hazardous. Specific examples include biological materials (cell lines, antibodies, DNA or RNA, viral vectors, proteins, peptides, enzymes, growth factors) or whole biological systems (disease-causing pathogens, bacteria, yeast, roundworms, zebra fish, transgenic mice, or knock-out animal models). Another category includes chemical compositions or structures ("small molecule" pharmaceutical agents, research reagents, industrial chemicals and formulations; samples of metal alloys, advanced ceramics; coatings, nano-materials or even components of sensors chips or medical devices).

What Is the Purpose of an MTA?

MTAs serve several purposes. First, they protect the provider of the material from mistreatment by the recipient. Often the materials (or "inventions") to be transferred represent a significant investment in time and money by the providing institution and by scientist(s) who have developed them. Given the value of the materials, the provider, therefore, would like assurance that the recipient will not sell the materials; will not attempt to claim ownership of them; will not distribute them to others; and will not use them inappropriately. The provider also wants to be acknowledged as the source of the materials; to have access to any related future inventions; to be informed about any scientific results obtained using the materials; to be assured that the recipient's scientists are capable of using the materials; and to be sheltered from any liability or loss arising from the recipient's use of the materials. Also, the provider wants assurance that the materials will only be used for the purpose as described by the recipient when the request was made and that, if any subsequent inventions are made by the recipient, the provider will be notified and, if appropriate under patent law, be cited as a coinventor. With most MTAs that involve industrial materials, the provider requires license rights covering recipient inventions or can even attempt to assert ownership over such inventions.

Second, MTAs outline the rights of the recipient by confirming that he/she has permission to use the materials, by specifying how long such rights last and by clarifying ownership of inventions made by the recipient while using the materials.

Finally, MTAs supply certain legal, logistical and housekeeping information:

- The name and signatures of those officials who have authority to sign the agreement and bind their institutions.
- The names of the provider and recipient scientists, including addresses and contact information.
- Technical description and quantity of the material.
- Fees to be charged, if any.
- Term of the agreement.

What Is at Stake with an MTA?

In principle, there is potentially much at stake. A properly executed MTA is a legal document that gives one party recourse, if the other party breaches the agreement. Some materials are really quite valuable and their misappropriation could be a serious matter. Some materials are hazardous and their misuse or improper disposal might cause harm to people or the environment or violate applicable laws. Failure on the part of the recipient to adhere to the terms of an MTA can jeopardize intellectual property rights of the provider or even the recipient. Likewise, the failure of the provider to utilize an MTA in the first place could have the same effect.

How Serious Are the Problems That Arise with MTAs?

In spite of the foregoing, on a purely statistical basis, you might conclude that it is a case of much ado about nothing. Considering the thousands of MTAs signed each year, very, very few provoke a dispute between parties, and it is extremely rare that litigation results from a material transfer. This goes to the essence of MTA frustration for research administrators. MTAs take a lot of time, they are absolutely necessary for moving your research mission forward, and they are complex and contentious to negotiate. But, at the end of the day, the provisions of the agreement are almost never invoked and the document itself, though properly archived and accessible, is rarely, if ever, read again. Like many a legal document, it protects signers from unlikely events that may result from either intentional or inadvertent actions by a tiny fraction of those involved. The good news is that so few MTAs cause strife or legal action. The bad news, for you, is that someone still has to negotiate and process them.

What Kinds of Problems Do Come up with MTAs?

During the MTA Special Interest Group meetings at the 2002 and 2003 annual meeting of the Association of University Technology Managers (AUTM), surveys were conducted by Fred Reinhart (Wayne State University), Terry Donaghue (Mount Sinai Hospital, Toronto), and Wendy Streitz (University of California) to identify the problems of greatest concern to academic technology transfer professionals. The top twelve problems were as follows starting with those most significant:

1. Definition of materials is too broad.
2. Provider wants nonexclusive, royalty-free license, with unlimited right to sublicense.
3. Tracking/honoring obligations to provider.
4. Ownership by provider (either sole or joint) of solely-made recipient inventions.
5. Definition of invention or joint invention.
6. Differing points of view on control of patent prosecution.
7. Publication restrictions on recipient.
8. Penalty clause for inventions resulting from unauthorized use of material.
9. Choice of law.
10. Confidentiality obligations.
11. Principal investigator signs for university.
12. Indemnification/product liability concerns.

Who is Typically Involved When an MTA Is in Place?

Stakeholders include the providing and receiving scientists, their organizations (academic or corporate), and the sponsors whose funds supported the research that created the materials or will support future research utilizing such materials. Internally, and depending on the organizational chart, the relevant organizational units may include the academic department, the sponsored programs office, your provost, technology transfer office, legal counsel, business development office and heads of research units or teams.

Who Handles or Should Handle MTAs Covering Incoming Material?

Who handles MTAs covering incoming material depends entirely on the research institution. There are many unique administrative and authority models for the drafting, negotiation, execution and compliance monitoring of MTAs. In my opinion, the best arrangements for handling incoming materials possess several common features such as:

1. A recognized entry point and consistent approach for review of incoming MTAs.

2. Review of the most problematic language by highly experienced contracts professionals regardless of their title or department.
3. An efficient process for negotiating changes in the MTA.
4. Use of a standard affirmation memo or check list by the recipient scientist.
5. Diligent filing of MTAs and appropriate compliance monitoring.
6. Reasonable timelines for negotiation and execution.

With respect to the last point, there is no reason that a simple letter agreement or uniform biological MTA implementing letter (each later described in more detail) cannot be completed in a day or two, even sooner if fax signatures are accepted. Other routine MTAs that do not require negotiating can be completed within about a week. For difficult MTAs covering unique or valuable materials or with problematic terms that will require back and forth negotiation, the process may go on for several months.

Who Should Handle MTAs Covering Outgoing Material?

Who handles MTAs covering outgoing material depends on how important or how valuable (commercially) the material is. Handling of routine material is discussed below. For material with significant value, the technology transfer office is more likely to know about such material because of a prior invention disclosure and is probably best qualified to manage this kind of transaction in a way that protects the provider institution.

When Is an MTA Ordinarily Used and When Should It Be Used?

The decision to use an MTA is usually made by the provider because it is usually their call. Historically, we seem to have come full circle. During the 1980s, few MTAs were used. Scientists exchanged materials freely with a simple cover letter memorializing the transfer. As the biotechnology industry developed and certain materials proved to be commercially valuable, MTA use increased dramatically. In the mid-1990s, MTA use was so prevalent (and possibly excessive) that groups of scientists complained that progress in science was being impeded by MTA disputes and the associated administrative burden. Several steps were taken to alleviate the situation. The uniform biological MTA (UBMTA) and simple letter agreement were developed in cooperation with the National Institutes of Health (NIH).

NIH carried things one step further and several years later released, "Principles and Guidelines For Recipients of NIH Research Grants and Contracts on Obtaining and Disseminating Biomedical Research Resources,"[1] and asked all recipients of NIH funding to adhere to these guidelines when providing or receiving proprietary materials. At the same time, NIH encouraged institutions to use the simple letter agreement for transfers or to forgo MTAs altogether unless there was a strong rationale to use one.

If your institution is providing material to another party, it is fine to ask yourself (and your providing scientist) if an MTA is even necessary. Factors that point to the need for an MTA:

1. The material was developed at significant cost to your institution.
2. The material has significant commercial value.
3. You wish to maintain the proprietary status of the material.
4. The material is toxic, dangerous, or risky to handle or dispose.
5. You will be exporting the material to another country.
6. Your legal counsel prefers that an agreement cover the transfer.
7. Your institution will receive financial or other consideration from the transfer.
8. Your providing scientist wishes to be acknowledged as the source of the material.
9. The material has been licensed to one or more companies.
10. Your providing scientist does not know or trust the recipient scientist.
11. You must pass along to the Recipient institution an existing obligation you have to another party such as a federal or industry sponsor or a provider of material which has been incorporated into your material.
12. The material has been licensed commercially or is covered by patents which have been licensed commercially.

On the other hand, if the material to be transferred is not particularly valuable, can be easily duplicated by the recipient or obtained from other sources, is a benign substance, is not proprietary, and assuming your general counsel or risk management office has no objection, it can be transferred without use of a formal agreement.

Types of MTAs

The Uniform Biological Material Transfer Agreement (UBMTA)

My favorite. The UBMTA was developed as a result of cooperative discussions between several universities (e.g., Harvard University) and NIH. It is used primarily for transfers between academic institutions or between academia and government labs. It consists of two parts: the master agreement, which has been signed previously by both the providing and receiving organizations, and a situation-specific implementing letter.[2] (See Appendix 74-A at the close of this chapter for a sample implementing letter.) The letter is short and needs three signatures: those of the providing scientist, the recipient scientist, and a recipient official, who can attest that his/her organization has signed the UBMTA master agreement. It also specifies the material (and amounts) to be transferred along with the necessary addresses.

If your institution has not signed the UBMTA master agreement,[3] you should try to find out why. As of this writing, over 250 organizations have signed it. Use of the UBMTA dramatically reduces the time and administrative burden of transfers.

The Simple Letter Agreement

Another favorite, developed by the same group as the UBMTA, the simple letter agreement is a much shorter, much simpler cousin of the UBMTA and is also extremely useful, for example, with less important materials and when an exchange is to occur between two organizations and one has not signed the UBMTA master agreement. It can also be used for academia-to-industry transfers, although is

---

[1] National Institutes of Health, Principles and Guidelines for Recipients of NIH Research Grants and Contracts on Obtaining and Disseminating Biomedical Research Resources: Final Notices, December 23, 1999, http://ott.od.nih.gov/RTguide_final.html (accessed September 25, 2005).

[2] Sample Copy of a UBMTA Implementing Letter, www.autm.net/aboutTT/implementingLetter.doc (accessed September 25, 2005).

[3] Sample Copy of the UBMTA Master Agreement, http://www.net/aboutTT/aboutTT_ubmta.cfm (accessed September 25, 2005).

rarely used for the reverse because of the inherent value of many commercial materials.[4] (For a sample copy, see Appendix 74-B at the close of this chapter.)

In cases where a non-profit provider such as a university or research hospital chooses not to use an unmodified version of the UBMTA or simple letter agreement, it is not uncommon to see a variation of one of those two agreements. Though not as ideal a situation, this is progress, nevertheless, and shows that these agreements serve as useful benchmarks if nothing else. The problem is that you now have to wade through the document and figure out where changes were made. Surprisingly, you will often see agencies within the federal government, NIH included, not using the UBMTA or simple letter agreement. Their MTAs tend to be fairly benign, however, so this does not present a serious problem.

Organization-Specific and Customized Form Agreements

Remember the bunny with the sign that said, "Can you guess what's wrong with me?" There are hundreds of variations in these customized MTAs, many with hidden flaws (at best) or time bombs (at worst). These types of agreements are the high maintenance time-wasters because you have to review them carefully and try to spot the unique approaches people dream up.

It is an annoyance to see a customized MTA coming from another university because both parties miss out on the efficiencies and benefits that come from using the UBMTA implementing letter or the simple letter agreement. Nevertheless, most academic-academic MTAs contain few problem areas. Look to see if the inventions and publication clauses are acceptable, check on governing law, and whether there are any unusual strings attached, e.g., option rights for the provider resulting from an obligation the provider has to an existing licensee. (See Appendix 74-C for a sample of an academic MTA.)

For industry to academia transfers, you can be certain that you will be looking at a customized MTA that might have any number of surprising or difficult clauses. You can always tell when a colleague is reviewing an industry MTA because within one minute you will hear the famous phrase, "Ohhh Nooo" usually accompanied by a deep, drawn-out sigh. There are a few enlightened companies which, either because of progressive atti-

tudes or because some weary mid-level agreements administrator has tired of hearing the same complaints from university recipients, have created user-friendly MTA boilerplates. These marvelous rarities walk a fine line of reasonableness and protection for both parties and, shock and awe, offer a pleasant first read needing no modifications prior to signing. These agreements should not come as a complete surprise. Remember that at the other end of many transactions is a company researcher who believes there will be a benefit in getting the material into the hands of your ingenious researcher.

There is also one type of industry-provided MTA that tends to be a no-brainer. It covers the exchange of some well-characterized, well-tested material, perhaps even a drug already on the market, and is very short. Often these MTAs require only the signature of your investigator. Typical provisions stipulate that the recipient scientist knows how to use the material properly, will report results, will dispose of it in accordance with applicable regulations, agrees not to put the material into people or food animals, and is, in general, not a lunatic. (See Appendices 74-D and 74-E for samples of industry MTAs.)

Special note: Be especially careful with agreements from institutions or companies in other countries. They sometimes have clauses which, although common in regions such as Europe or Asia, are rarely seen in the United States. You may see demands relating to publication or invention ownership that are unacceptable. Governing law in these situations can also be a problem.

Components of an MTA

The key parts of an MTA are sections that deal with definitions, ownership of the material, the grant of rights, reports to provider, publication and confidentiality provisions, invention ownership and rights, and liability. Other sections are found in an MTA but these are familiar and routine, (e.g., preamble, representations and warranties, notices, integration clauses, assignment, validity, etc.).

Definitions. A straightforward listing of provider, recipient, principal investigator (or recipient dcientist), material and so on. The important question here is how broadly the provider defines "material." If defined so broadly as to cover all derivatives or Inventions made by the recipient, this is a potential problem.

Ownership of material. The not-so-surprising reiteration that the provider is claiming ownership of the material, however that term is

---

[4]Sample Copy of Simple Letter Agreement for the Transfer of Materials, http://autm.net.aboutTT/simpleLtrWord.doc (accessed September 25, 2005).

defined, and reserves the right to do any number of things with it besides lending it to your scientist.

Grant of rights. This assures the recipient and recipient scientist that they have the limited right to use the material for a specified purpose that the provider is comfortable with, for example, to carry out the proposed study, but not for any other purpose.

Reports to provider. The provider wants recipient and recipient scientist to promptly report results of the study in which the material was used. In addition, providers usually want notification of inventions and copies of both manuscripts and publications citing the material and study results.

Publication provisions. These specify procedures the recipient must follow in publishing study results. Typical terms obligate the recipient to: (i) delete any confidential information that was previously developed by the provider and given to recipient; and (ii) delay publication for a specified period of time (ideally no more than 60 to 90 days) to allow the parties to seek patent protection.

Confidentiality provisions. Confidential information previously developed by the provider may often accompany material and must be kept secret. Some providers try to include the recipient's study results within the definition of confidential information. Such attempts conflict with federal regulations and most university policies and should be firmly rejected by the recipient.

Invention ownership and rights. These provisions clarify which party owns inventions made by the recipient using the material and should address scenarios such as sole and joint inventorship. The logical next question after ownership is licensing, including the procedure for electing rights, negotiating a license agreement and the specific terms of the license agreement.

Liability. This is an allocation of risk between the parties in the event of loss or damages occurring as a result of recipient's use or disposal of material or provider's use of study results or inventions.

Negotiating MTAs

Providers usually have more leverage than recipients. There is a limit to how much the recipient can demand before the provider says, "thanks, but we don't really want (or need) to do this." After all, there is little or no financial compensation paid to

the provider, so if you are asking him to waive all access to inventions made using the materials, use the recipient's state for governing law, or to forgo any liability obligation by your institution, you may experience resistance or long delays.

Of the twelve problems listed earlier under "What Kinds of Problems Come up with MTAs?" all but two (numbers 3 and 11) can be handled by negotiation. Those that are amenable to negotiation fall into four general categories: invention ownership; licensing rights; publication provisions and confidentiality obligations; and legal issues.

Invention Ownership

Unfortunately, many for-profit providers still attempt either to claim ownership of inventions made by the recipient using the material or to obtain a royalty-free exclusive license for such inventions. Some providers even insert a punitive clause which says that if the recipient scientist goes outside the agreed-upon limits for using the material and makes an invention, the provider will own that invention outright. In most cases, recipients can get favorable modifications to this language by citing their internal policies, impracticality, precedent, or, where the research to be done will be funded by the federal government, federal law and NIH or NSF policies. In any event, the provider will want at the very least a royalty-free nonexclusive research license, often with an option or right of first refusal to obtain a royalty-bearing exclusive license. In the latter case, a time-limited option period is preferable with the company covering patent expenses while the option is in effect. Issues can arise around control of patent prosecution, which, though not an issue of invention ownership per se, is related. Of the small number of providers that seek such control, most will bend on this if you give them the right to review patent correspondence and comment on substantive patent decisions.

Licensing Rights

For-profit providers will usually accept a royalty-free nonexclusive license as an alternative to an exclusive license but in many cases will still want the right to sublicense their nonexclusive rights. Such rights will undermine your ability to find other licensees because the provider's sublicense rights represent an unknown risk for licensees. In some cases, you can simply get the sublicensing right taken out of the MTA. In many others, the provider will hang firm and the best you can do then is to have the sublicensing right narrowed or carefully defined. Almost all MTAs will feature a clause giving the provider an option or right of first refusal to negotiate a royalty-bearing exclusive license, and there is great variety concerning the process to accomplish this. Given that so few MTAs actually result in an exercise of rights by the provider, having minimal details about the process is not a great concern. On the whole, there is a fair amount of hairsplitting that goes on when negotiating licensing rights clauses.

Publication Provisions and Confidentiality Obligations

Most for-profit providers now understand that academic recipients cannot agree to give them control over publications or their content and do not put such provisions in their standard MTAs. However, you may still see such onerous terms in MTAs involving smaller, unsophisticated biotechnology companies, non-U.S. life science companies, and companies that are developing potentially valuable human therapies and are concerned that publications containing negative data about their drug will sharply decrease its value or that of the company itself. There have been some bitter disputes or threats of lawsuits as a result of attempts by a provider to block potentially damaging publications on the grounds that the publication contained incorrect data or was a violation of confidentiality provisions in an MTA or nondisclosure agreement signed by the recipient. In addition, we continue to see "innovative" clauses or creative wordsmithing that purport to give recipients control over content and publication but do the opposite. Recipients would do well to adhere strictly to a freedom-to-publish position and to cite internal policies, federal regulations and concerns about maintaining the organization's nonprofit status. This is also important in relation to export controls so universities can regard their research as "fundamental research" and thus exempt from requiring export licenses.

Legal Issues Such As Risk Allocation and Governing Law

Legal issues are less common and rarely a deal breaker for providers. A provider's desire not to incur liability as a result of the recipient's use of material, material which is usually given for free, is reasonable. Subject to state law limitations, recipient institutions are usually willing to accept liability for risks that result from their use of material. On the other hand, if a provider exercises its right to a

license covering inventions made using material, it should accept liability for losses resulting from commercialization of those inventions. With regard to governing law, even though there is precedent for the provider to choose the venue, this presents a problem for both public and private universities so many providers will bend on this issue and allow the MTA to remain silent on governing law or even accept the recipient's state law.

In general, when reasonable and experienced people are negotiating an MTA, there are few issues that should stand in the way of finalizing the agreement. Unless the provider is insisting on approval of publications (or their content); ownership of or a royalty-free exclusive license covering recipient inventions or some other similar demand, you should be able to work things out. Someone at the recipient organization needs to have experience and skill in dealing with the more challenging clauses and be comfortable getting on the phone to speak with the provider's negotiator or sending an intelligently-worded email response which outlines why the agreement as written cannot be signed.

In terms of the time required to negotiate an MTA, however, one significant problem is the delay caused by simple communication logistics, miscommunication, and procedural snafus. Let's assume the both provider and recipient have their acts together and have assigned one individual to handle negotiating the MTA and that person has the requisite expertise and authority to get the job done. Sounds great, but if they spend the next two weeks playing phone tag, you can bet the agreement they are trying to execute starts getting buried by the two dozen new ones that come in after they start. These agreement handlers need to be trained on effective strategies for efficient and timely communication with the other side so that agreements are wrapped up quickly.

In addition to interorganizational problems, you have the process snafus that are strictly internal. Here are three common ones: your researcher doesn't know where to send the MTA for review and signing; no one knows where the agreement is physically (shocking but true); and the agreement is signed but the involved parties aren't informed about what needs to happen next! These kinds of problems often add weeks or even months to the time needed to receive valuable materials and can increase dramatically the level of faculty frustration. The irony, of course, is that these problems are easily solved.

One trick to watch for: company providers sometimes have multiple versions of MTAs. Let's call them the Sucker version (alternative name: "The Nubie Research Administrator-Who-Doesn't-Know-Any-Better" version); the Most Egregious Terms-Deleted version; and the Savvy-Sophisticate version that has been refined over the years to be acceptable to most academic organizations that execute a lot of MTAs. Be sure to ask for the last one!

Whole books have been written on how to negotiate agreements, and this chapter has not attempted a comprehensive discussion. Suffice it to say that clear, timely and straightforward communication with the appropriate, hopefully accessible, person on the other side, and an open discussion of concerns and needs will go a long way to reducing negotiation time. Sometimes, however, you will find that the other side is not going to bend on unacceptable language and you will have to abandon that particular MTA. Just tell your researcher as soon as possible and explain the reasons.

Record-Keeping

Once an MTA has been fully executed, make sure that all relevant parties receive a copy for their files. Ordinarily, the principal investigator, departmental administrator, technology transfer office and/or sponsored programs office should receive a copy. If you know for a fact that the MTA relates to an existing invention file, you should also put a copy there.

If you have a small research operation, the original agreement will probably go to an appropriate hard copy file under the investigator's name, but cross-referenced, at the very least, with the name of the provider (e.g., the company or university) and other identifiers. If you are with a big university, you might be using digitized or scanned images of the MTA stored on CD with the original document archived off site. Regardless of your filing method, the MTA should be accessible by the recipient scientist and individuals in sponsored programs, technology transfer and your legal department to assure compliance with its terms, especially when an Invention has been made utilizing the material.

Educating Researchers

Experienced research administrators will say that you can never overeducate your researchers about matters such as MTAs. New faculty come in, and existing faculty forget. It is a good idea to schedule MTA training sessions on a regular basis and to prepare instructional materials or brochures for distribution to the relevant faculty and graduate students.

One very effective way to simultaneously educate faculty, uncover or head off potential problems relating to material transfers is through the use of affirmation memos. There are several other names applied to these documents, but they are essentially a check box form that a recipient scientist is required to sign before an MTA covering incoming material is reviewed. An affirmation memo typically asks several questions including:

1. The source of funding which will support the study in which the material will be used and disclosure of any obligations which will accompany such funding. If federal funds will be used, there will be certain obligations relating to proper handling of results and inventions. If funding from a for-profit organization (other than the provider) will be used, this could very well create a conflict of obligations and a breach of the MTAs provisions on invention rights.

2. Whether a patentable invention is likely to result from the study in which the material will be used. This alerts the research administrator to a potential problem and helps determine your negotiating stance vis-à-vis invention ownership and licensing rights.

3. Whether the material will be combined with material previously licensed to a company or proprietary material from a third party or if the study is a collaboration with scientists at another organization or company.

4. Whether the material poses special risks in handling or disposal.

Tracking Compliance

Tracking compliance is really important so it is a wonder so few offices do it! Once you set up a data storage system, either in database or paper file form, the idea is to use it! When do you use it? The most common triggers are when:

- Your researcher is preparing a publication based on work done using the materials.
- An invention is disclosed.
- Technology is going to be licensed which relates to use of material received by your institution.
- Faculty leave your institution.
- Tracking obligations to the provider of the material.
- You send in an affirmative final invention statement to a federal agency or the federal sponsor.

You do not have to track compliance, but if you fail to, you may have to endure the consequences which can be severe, for example, breach of a license agreement, potential litigation, or an unhappy federal, foundation, or corporate sponsor.

Recommendations and Conclusion

Remember those cute little bunnies from the beginning of the chapter and our new definition for the MTA acronym (Masochistic Torture Assignment)? I hope the information presented helps you to retain the true meaning of MTA and to get those bunny critters under control. With a little background and experience, you can work with MTAs more gracefully to the benefit of your faculty and researchers; area departments; your institution overall; and of the collaborators, sponsors, and the various government agencies that support your research program.

Additional Web Site Resources

1. Council on Government Relations. www.cogr. edu.
2. Association of University Technology Managers. Material Transfer Agreements, www. autm.net.

74-A

Sample UBMTA Implementing Letter

Once your organization has signed the UBMTA master agreement, this is all that needs to be signed!

The purpose of this letter is to provide a record of the biological Material transfer, to memorialize the agreement between the PROVIDER SCIENTIST (identified below) and the RECIPIENT SCIENTIST (identified below) to abide by all terms and conditions of the Uniform Biological Material Transfer [[Page 12775]] Agreement ("UBMTA") March 8, 1995, and to certify that the RECIPIENT's (identified below) organization has accepted and signed an unmodified copy of the UBMTA. The RECIPIENT organization's Authorized Official also will sign this letter if the RECIPIENT SCIENTIST is not authorized to certify on behalf of the RECIPIENT organization. The RECIPIENT SCIENTIST (and the Authorized Official of RECIPIENT, if necessary) should sign both copies of this letter and return one signed copy to the PROVIDER. The PROVIDER SCIENTIST will forward the Material to the RECIPIENT SCIENTIST upon receipt of the signed copy from the RECIPIENT organization.

Please fill in all of the blank lines below:

1. PROVIDER: Organization providing the ORIGINAL MATERIAL:
   Organizat _____
   Address: _____
2. RECIPIENT: Organization receiving the ORIGINAL MATERIAL:
   Organizat _____
   Address: _____

3. ORIGINAL MATERIAL (Enter description):
4. Termination date for this letter (optional):
5. Transmittal Fee to reimburse the PROVIDER for preparation and distribution costs (optional). Amount:_____.

This Implementing Letter is effective when signed by all parties. The parties executing this Implementing Letter certify that their respective organizations have accepted and signed an unmodified copy of the UBMTA, and further agree to be bound by its terms, for the transfer specified above.

PROVIDER SCIENTIST

Name: _____

Title: _____

Address: _____

_____

Signature: _____

Date: _____

RECIPIENT SCIENTIST

Name: _____

Title: _____

Address: _____

_____

Signature: _____

Date: _____

RECIPIENT ORGANIZATION CERTIFICATION

    Certification: I hereby certify that the RECIPI-ENT organization has accepted and signed an unmodified copy of the UBMTA (May be the RECIPIENT SCIENTIST if authorized by the RECIPIENT organization):

Authorized

Official: _____

Title: _____

Address: _____

Signature: _____

Date: _____

74-B

Sample Simple Letter Agreement

In response to the RECIPIENT's request for the MATERIAL [insert description] the PROVIDER asks that the RECIPIENT and the RECIPIENT SCIENTIST agree to the following before the RECIPIENT receives the MATERIAL:

1. The above MATERIAL is the property of the PROVIDER and is made available as a service to the research community.

2. THIS MATERIAL IS NOT FOR USE IN HUMAN SUBJECTS.

3. The MATERIAL will be used for teaching or not-for-profit research purposes only.

4. The MATERIAL will not be further distributed to others without the PROVIDER's written consent. The RECIPIENT shall refer any request for the MATERIAL to the PROVIDER. To the extent supplies are available, the PROVIDER or the PROVIDER SCIENTIST agree to make the MATERIAL available, under a separate Simple Letter Agreement to other scientists for teaching or not-for-profit research purposes only.

5. The RECIPIENT agrees to acknowledge the source of the MATERIAL in any publications reporting use of it.

6. Any MATERIAL delivered pursuant to this Agreement is understood to be experimental in nature and may have hazardous properties. THE PROVIDER MAKES NO REPRESENTATIONS AND EXTENDS NO WARRANTIES OF ANY KIND, EITHER EXPRESSED OR IMPLIED. THERE ARE NO EXPRESS OR IMPLIED WARRANTIES OF MERCHANTABILITY OR FITNESS FOR A PARTICULAR PURPOSE, OR THAT THE USE OF THE MATERIAL WILL NOT INFRINGE ANY PATENT, COPYRIGHT, TRADEMARK, OR OTHER PROPRIETARY RIGHTS. Unless prohibited by law, Recipient assumes all liability for claims for damages against it by third parties which may arise from the use, storage or disposal of the Material except that, to the extent permitted by law, the Provider shall be liable to the Recipient when the damage is caused by the gross negligence or willful misconduct of the Provider.

7. The RECIPIENT agrees to use the MATERIAL in compliance with all applicable statutes and regulations.

8. The MATERIAL is provided at no cost, or with an optional transmittal fee solely to reimburse the PROVIDER for its preparation and distribution costs. If a fee is requested, the amount will be indicated here: [insert fee]_____.

The PROVIDER, RECIPIENT and RECIPIENT SCIENTIST must sign both copies of this letter and return one signed copy to the PROVIDER. The PROVIDER will then send the MATERIAL.

PROVIDER INFORMATION and AUTHORIZED SIGNATURE

Provider
Scientist: _____

Provider
Organization:_____

Address: _____

825

Name of Authorized
Official: _____

Title of Authorized
Official: _____

   Certification of Authorized Official: This Simple Letter Agreement __has / __has not [check one] been modified. If modified, the modifications are attached.

_____

Signature of Authorized Official   Date

RECIPIENT INFORMATION and AUTHORIZED SIGNATURE

Recipient
Scientist: _____

Recipient
Organization:
Address: _____

Name of Authorized
Official: _____

Title of Authorized
Official: _____

Signature of Authorized
Official/Date Signed:_____

   Certification of Recipient Scientist: I have read and understood the conditions outlined in this Agreement and I agree to abide by them in the receipt and use of the MATERIAL.

_____   _____

Recipient Scientist   Date

Sample Academic MTA

(Used with permission of Wayne State University)

Materials Transfer Agreement

This Agreement is made as of _____ by and between Wayne State University, having its principal place of business at 656 West Kirby, Detroit, MI 48202 ("Provider") and _____, having its principal place of business at _____ ("Recipient"). Provider is the owner of the Materials ("Materials") identified below and all rights, title and interest therein. Provider and Recipient hereby agree as follows with respect to access to and use of the Materials:

Agreement

1. **Materials.** "Materials" shall mean (a) the following cells or molecules and any related biological Material which will be received by Recipient from Provider: _____; and (b) any cells or molecules that are replicated or derived by Recipient from the cells and molecules identified in (a).

2. **Transfer of Materials.** Subject to the provisions of this Agreement, Provider shall transfer to Recipient such amount of the Materials as is mutually agreed upon and hereby grants Recipient a non-exclusive, royalty-free license to use the intellectual property rights embodied in the Materials for the sole purpose of enabling Recipient to perform the research or investigation described in the request letter attached as Exhibit A. [Optional: Recipient will not attempt to create any analog, homolog, modification or modified derivative of Materials or to in any way reverse engineer Materials.] Recipient acknowledges that this Agreement conveys no other rights of any sort with respect to the Materials or the intellectual property rights embodied therein.

3. **Inventions.** Recipient agrees to inform the Provider of any inventions made during the research using the Material. If Recipient seeks patent coverage on such inventions, Recipient agrees to inform the Provider to determine ownership interests, if any, to which Provider may be entitled. [Optional: Provider shall be entitled to a non-exclusive royalty free license to use for non-commercial research and teaching purposes any inventions, methods and/or discoveries that arise from Recipient's use of the Material.]

4. **Reporting; Publication.** Recipient agrees to inform Provider of the data and research results from Recipient's use of the Materials. Recipient agrees to acknowledge Provider as the source of the Materials in any publication reporting on Recipient's use thereof.

5. **Confidentiality.** Recipient acknowledges that the Materials (and the intellectual property rights embodied therein) are considered proprietary to Provider and hereby covenants that it and each of its employees shall receive and hold the Materials in trust and confidence. Recipient shall use all reasonable efforts to protect the confidentiality of the Materials, including efforts fully commensurate with those employed by Recipient for the protection of its own proprietary information. Recipient shall restrict disclosure of the Materials to those of its employees who in Recipient's judgment have a need to use the Materials for the purposes

authorized under Section 2. Recipient has and will maintain an appropriate arrangement with each of its employees provided access to the Materials, sufficient to enable Recipient to comply with the provisions of this Agreement. Recipient shall not transmit or otherwise provide access to the Materials by any third party without the prior written consent of Provider.

6. **Disclaimer.**   Recipient accepts the Materials with the knowledge that they are experimental in nature and hereby covenants to comply with all applicable laws and regulations relating to the handling, use, storage and disposal of such Materials. PROVIDER MAKES NO WARRANTIES, EXPRESS OR IMPLIED, INCLUDING BUT NOT LIMITED TO THE WARRANTIES OF MERCHANTABILITY AND FITNESS FOR A PARTICULAR PURPOSE AND HEREBY DISCLAIMS SAME. PROVIDER MAKES NO EXPRESS OR IMPLIED WARRANTY THAT THE MATERIALS DO NOT INFRINGE PATENTS OR OTHER PROPRIETARY RIGHTS OF THIRD PARTIES AND HEREBY DISCLAIMS THE SAME.

7. **Waiver.**   Recipient hereby waives any claims that might arise against Provider relating to the Materials and hereby covenants and agrees that it shall indemnify and hold Provider and its affiliates, trustees, officers, medical staff, employees and agents (and their respective successors, heirs and assigns) harmless against any cost, damage, liability, loss or expense (including reasonable attorney's fees and litigation expenses) incurred by or imposed upon them in connection with any actions, claims, demands, suits or judgments arising out of or relating to Recipient's handling, use, storage or disposal of the Materials.

8. **Termination.**   Provider may terminate this Agreement with five days written notice to Recipient at the address set forth below if Recipient breaches any of its obligations set forth herein, unless Recipient cures such breach within said five-day period. Upon termination, Recipient shall return all Materials to Provider if requested to do so by Provider or destroy all Materials and any other Materials embodying the intellectual property rights embodied in the Materials and shall provide Provider with a written certification of same within five business days of termination. Sections 3, 4, 5, 6 and 7 shall survive any termination of this Agreement.

9. **Miscellaneous.** (a) Any notice to be given hereunder shall be in writing and shall be deemed given when delivered personally or one busi-ness day after it is mailed by Express Mail, postage prepaid to the addresses set forth below or to such other place as any party may designate by written notice to the other parties; (b) this Agreement shall be governed by and construed in accordance with the law (other than the choice of law provisions) of the State of Michigan; (c) this Agreement represents the entire understanding between the parties with respect to the subject matter described, supersedes all prior or contemporaneous understandings and agreements, oral or written, between the parties with respect to the subject matter and cannot be modified except by a written instrument signed by the authorized representative of each party; (d) this Agreement shall inure to the benefit of and be binding upon the parties, and their successors and permitted assigns; this Agreement is not intended to confer on any other person any rights, remedies, obligations or liabilities under or by reason of this Agreement. Recipient may not assign its rights or delegate its obligations under this Agreement.

IN WITNESS WHEREOF, the parties have caused this agreement to be executed by their duly authorized representatives effective as of the date set forth above.

WAYNE STATE UNIVERSITY _____
                                                                 (Recipient)

By: _____   By: _____

Name   Name

Director   Title: _____

Technology Transfer   _____
Office   (Institutional Representative)

Wayne State University   _____

4032 FAB, 656 West Kirby   _____

Detroit, MI 48202   _____

(fax: 313-577-3626)   _____

[Please return this form   Agreed and Accepted:
to the above address.]

_____
Investigator/Requestor
[address: c/o RECIPIENT]

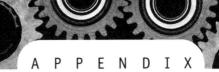

74-D

Sample Long Form Industry MTA

Courtesy of: Faber Daeufer & Rosenberg PC, Waltham, Massachusetts

Material Transfer Agreement

THIS MATERIAL TRANSFER AGREEMENT (together with its Appendix, the "Agreement") is made as this _____ day of _____, 2005 ("Effective Date") between XXXX, having a principal office at XXXXXXX ("Supplier") and XXXXX, having a principal address at XXXXXXXX ("Recipient").

1. **Background.** Recipient desires to obtain the Material and/or information described in **Appendix A** (together, in the case of chemical Material, with all analogs, formulations, mixtures or compositions thereof, and in the case of biological Material, with all progeny, fragments and unmodified derivatives, and, the "Material") from Supplier for use by Recipient investigator ("Recipient Investigator") solely in the non-commercial research described in **Appendix A** (the "Research") under the terms and conditions of this Agreement. Certain obligations of Recipient herein described (e.g. use and transfer of Material) will apply to any biological Material that incorporates the Material or any recombinant version thereof (e.g., Supplier's gene into a vector or combination of Supplier's gene with other polynucleotides) ("Modified Material").

2. **The Material and the Research.** Recipient acknowledges that Supplier owns, or has exclusive rights to, the Material. Supplier will use commercially reasonable efforts to provide Recipient with the quantity of the Material described in **Appendix A.** Recipient will use the Material and Modified Material solely in its Research and for no other purpose. The Research will be conducted solely by or under the direction of the Recipient Investigator in his/her laboratory at Recipient's research facilities. None of the Material or Modified Material will be transferred or sold to third parties. If the Research is funded either in whole or in part by the U.S. Government, Recipient agrees to take title to any Subject Inventions as defined in 37 CFR 401 ("Subject Inventions") made in the performance of the Research.

3. **Use of Material.** The Material is intended exclusively for investigational use in laboratory animals or for in vitro studies, and is not for use in humans. Recipient Investigator will exercise due care to ensure that all Material is handled by trained laboratory personnel only. Recipient and Recipient Investigator will use the Material in compliance with all applicable laws and regulations, including, in the case of animal studies, any applicable animal welfare laws and regulations. Any Material remaining upon completion of the Research either will be returned to Supplier or discarded, consistent with Supplier's instructions.

4. **Inventions.**
   4.1. **Disclosure Notice.** Recipient will promptly and fully disclose in writing to Supplier any and all inventions, know-how and other rights (whether or not protectible under state, federal, or foreign intellectual property laws) related to the Material or its use, or developed using the Material, which are conceived and/or reduced to practice by Recipient, alone or jointly with others, in the course of its Research ("Inventions").

4.2. Option for Exclusive License. Subject to any non-exclusive license retained by the U.S. Government, Recipient hereby grants to Supplier an option to obtain an exclusive, royalty-bearing license, including the right to grant sublicenses, to Recipient's interest in all Inventions. For each Invention, Supplier's option must be exercised within ninety (90) days of receipt by Supplier of the Disclosure Notice describing that Invention. The terms and conditions of any exclusive license will be negotiated in good faith by the parties and will include license terms standard for agreements between academic institutions and industry, including, but not limited to, appropriate provisions for reimbursement of patent expenses incurred by Recipient under Section 4.4 below.

4.3. Licenses. Recipient grants to Supplier the following irrevocable rights which Supplier may sublicense to its development and/or marketing collaborators:

a. **Improvements.** A non-exclusive, royalty-free license to Recipient's interest in Inventions which are "improvements" to or modified derivatives of the Material;

b. **New Uses.** A non-exclusive, royalty-free license to Recipient's interest in Inventions which are "new uses" of the Material; and

c. **New Substances.** A non-exclusive, royalty-free license, limited to research purposes only, to Recipient's interest in Inventions which are "new substances" developed using the Material.

4.4. Patent Applications.

a. **Joint Inventions.** Any patent applications necessary to protect the proprietary positions of the parties in any Inventions made jointly by Supplier and Recipient will be prepared, filed and prosecuted by Supplier, jointly in its and Recipient's names, with expenses shared equally by the parties. If Supplier elects not to prepare, file, prosecute or maintain an application or patent arising from any joint Invention, Supplier will promptly notify Recipient, and Recipient will have the right to prepare, file, prosecute and maintain those applications or patents, in Recipient's and Supplier's names, and at Recipient's expense. Subject only to Recipient's grant of an option to Supplier under Section 4.2, each of Supplier and Recipient will have the right to license, transfer and/or sell its respective rights in

each joint Inventions without the consent of the other.

b. **Recipient's Sole Inventions.** Any patent applications necessary to protect the proprietary positions of the parties in any Inventions made solely by Recipient will be prepared, filed and prosecuted by Recipient, solely in Recipient's name, with the expenses paid by Recipient. If Recipient elects not to prepare, file, prosecute or maintain an application or patent arising from any sole Inventions, Recipient will promptly notify Supplier, and Supplier will have the right to prepare, file, prosecute and maintain those applications or patents, in Recipient's name and at Supplier's expense. In the event an Invention made solely by Recipient is a Subject Invention and Supplier elects not to exercise its right to prepare and prosecute patent applications or patents covering that Invention, then Recipient will be relieved of its obligation under Section 2 above to take title from the U.S. Government to that Subject Invention.

c. **Inventorship.** Inventorship will be determined according to U.S. patent law or other national patent law that may apply.

d. **Patent Cooperation.** Each party will provide the other party with copies of all substantive communications from all patent offices regarding applications or patents on any joint Inventions and Recipient's sole Inventions promptly after the receipt thereof. Each party will provide the other party with copies of all proposed substantive communications to such patent offices regarding applications or patents on any such Inventions in sufficient time before the due date in order to enable the other party an opportunity to comment on the content thereof. Each party will make available to the other party or its authorized attorneys, agents, or representatives, such of its employees whom the other party in its reasonable judgment deems necessary in order to assist it in obtaining patent protection for such Inventions. Each party will sign or use its best efforts to have signed all legal documents necessary to file and prosecute patent applications or to obtain or maintain patents at no cost to the other party.

5. Reports. Recipient Investigator will submit to Supplier, within thirty (30) days following the end of each six-month calendar period, a written report summarizing the status of the

Research and any Inventions developed during the preceding six-month period. Recipient Investigator will also submit to Supplier a comprehensive final report within ninety (90) days after completion of the Research.

6. **Confidentiality.** Except as provided in Section 7, Recipient and Recipient Investigator will not publish or disclose to third parties any of the Supplier's non-public proprietary information ("Confidential Information"). Recipient and Recipient Investigator will use Confidential Information solely in connection with the Research. Confidential Information will include information which is (a) disclosed in writing or other tangible form and is labeled or identified as "CONFIDENTIAL" at the time of disclosure or, by written notice to Recipient or Recipient Investigator, within thirty (30) days following disclosure; (b) disclosed verbally and reduced to writing or other tangible form and similarly labeled, within thirty (30) days of verbal disclosure; or (c) commonly regarded as confidential and/or proprietary in the life sciences industry.

This confidentiality obligation does not apply to information which is lawfully and in good faith made available to Recipient or Recipient Investigator from an independent source, is already published through no breach of this Agreement, or is/was known by Recipient or Recipient Investigator independent of the Supplier's disclosure as evidenced by written records at the time of disclosure.

7. **Publication.** Recipient will have the right to publish and disclose the results of the Research. In order to balance this right with the Supplier's proprietary interests, Recipient will submit the proposed disclosure to Supplier for its review at least thirty (30) days prior to the earlier of the date of submission to any journal for review or the date of publication or disclosure. Supplier will complete its review within thirty (30) days of receipt of the submitted documents. Supplier may require that Recipient delete from its documents any reference to the Supplier's Confidential Information. If, during the thirty (30) day review period, Supplier notifies Recipient that it desires to file a patent application on any Inventions disclosed in the documents, Recipient will defer publication/disclosure for up to sixty (60) additional days from the date of submission of the document to Supplier to permit Supplier to prepare and file a patent application.

8. **No Warranty.** THE MATERIAL IS PROVIDED TO RECIPIENT "AS-IS" AND WITHOUT ANY WARRANTY, EXPRESS OR IMPLIED, INCLUDING ANY WARRANTY OF MERCHANTABILITY, TITLE, FITNESS FOR A PARTICULAR PURPOSE OR NON-INFRINGEMENT.

9. **No Conflict.** Neither Recipient nor Recipient Investigator has entered into any agreements with any third party commercial entity providing Material for the Research which could result in a claim by such third party that it has commercial rights to any Inventions made by Recipient under this Agreement. Recipient will not involve any third party commercial entity in the Research nor use Material provided by a third party commercial entity in the Research, without first (a) providing to Supplier a copy of the agreement governing Recipient's obligations to such third party regarding the Research and (b) obtaining Supplier's written consent to such third party's involvement in the Research.

10. **Indemnification.** To the extent not prohibited under law, Recipient will indemnify and hold Supplier harmless from any claims or liability resulting from Recipient's use of the Material, except insofar as such claims or liability result from Supplier's gross negligence or willful misconduct.

11. **Completion of Research/Termination.** Either party may terminate this Agreement upon thirty (30) days' prior written notice to the other party. Upon completion of the Research or any termination, Recipient will immediately return to Supplier its Confidential Information, and any unused samples of the Material, and all of Recipient's rights to use the Material will end. Following completion of the Research or termination, neither party will have any further obligations under this Agreement, except that Sections 4 through 7 and 10 through 12 will survive.

12. **Miscellaneous.** This Agreement (a) may not be assigned or transferred by Recipient without Supplier's prior written consent, and (b) will be governed by and construed in accordance with the law of the Commonwealth of Massachusetts, U.S.A., without regard to any choice of law principle that would dictate the application of the law of another jurisdiction and (c) may only be modified by written agreement of the parties.

XXXXXXXX.

By _____
duly authorized

Print Name_____
Title_____

[INSERT RECIPIENT NAME]

_____
By _____
duly authorized

Print Name_____

Title_____

Address _____

_____

Telephone _____

Facsimile_____

I have read this Agreement and agree to its provisions.

_____

Recipient Investigator, [Name]

* *

Appendix A

Material: TEXT

Research: TEXT

74-E

Industry Short Form MTA

Used with permission of Pfizer, Inc.

October 6, 2005

Researchers Name

Dear <<Salutation>> <<Last_Name>>:

We have received your (the "Investigator") request for a sample of a Pfizer Compound, , , (the "Material"), to be used in your laboratory under your supervision. Please complete the attached Statement of Investigation Form, which will inform Pfizer of your intended use of our compound. Before the Material can be sent to you, we will require that you confirm your agreement to the conditions of delivery by signing the Compound Transfer Agreement ("Agreement") below and having the Agreement signed by an authorized individual at (Institution). The execution of this Agreement places no obligation on Pfizer to supply the Material to you. Any decision to supply the Material will be made at Pfizer's sole discretion upon review of the completed Statement of Investigation Form.

1. PARTIES OF THE AGREEMENT:

The parties to this Agreement are Pfizer and its Affiliates ("Pfizer") and [insert institution], (the "Institution"), effective as of [insert date].

2. SCOPE OF WORK:

The research ("Research") is described in the Statement of Investigation Form, which is attached to and made part of this Agreement as Exhibit A. The use of the Material is limited to the Research under the Investigator's direction

3. MATERIAL:

(a) The Investigator and the Institution acknowledge that the Material is for laboratory use only and is not for consumption by, or treatment of, humans or non-laboratory animals.

(b) The Investigator and the Institution will use the Material in compliance with all applicable federal, state and local laws, regulations and ordinances.

(c) The Investigator and the Institution will not make the Material available to any third party or to any person who is not subject to the Investigator's direct supervision.

(d) At the conclusion of the Research, the Investigator will return any unused portion of the Material to Pfizer at the following address: Manager, Sample Bank, Pfizer Inc, Eastern Point Road, Groton, Connecticut 06340-5146.

4. REPORT:

The Investigator will inform Pfizer of the results of the Investigator's work with the Material in the Research ("Results"). The Investigator will inform Pfizer in writing of the Results at the conclusion of the Research or within one (1) year of receiving the Material, whichever is sooner. The Results will be provided as a written report, one copy being supplied to [insert name] and a second copy being supplied to: Manager, Compound Transfer, Research and Development Operations, Pfizer Inc, Eastern Point Road, Groton, Connecticut 06340-5146.

5. **PUBLIC DISCLOSURE:**

(a) Pfizer shall not publish any of the Investigator's data without the Investigator's written permission.

(b) Pfizer encourages the exercise of academic freedom and shall have no right to prevent the Investigator and the Institution from publishing or presenting any findings from the Research. Notwithstanding the foregoing, the Investigator and the Institution acknowledge Pfizer's role as discoverer of the Material and, before they publish or present any findings from the Research relating to the Material, they will provide Pfizer with an opportunity to respond to such findings. In the case of any publications planned by the Investigator or the Institution, they will provide Pfizer with a copy of the proposed submission for publication at least thirty (30) days before its submission. In the case of any oral presentation to a third party, they will provide Pfizer with copies of any audiovisual Materials, including slides, at least twenty-one (21) days before the presentation.

6. **INTELLECTUAL PROPERTY:**

Neither the Investigator nor the Institution shall have any property rights in the Material or in any information that Pfizer discloses to either of them relating to the Material. Except and only to the extent necessary for the Investigator to use the Material in the Research, neither the Investigator nor the Institution is granted any license, express or implied, under any Pfizer patent or patent application, or under any patent or patent application under which Pfizer is licensed.

7. **INVENTION:**

(a) "Invention" means any invention or discovery, patentable or not, relating to the manufacture, use or sale of the Material which is first conceived or first reduced to practice by the Investigator, by any person under the Investigator's direct supervision, or by the Institution in performance of the Research.

(b) The Institution will inform Pfizer in writing of any Invention promptly upon its occurrence.

(c) The Institution hereby grants Pfizer a worldwide, perpetual license in and to all Inventions. Such license shall be royalty-free and nonexclusive, to make, use, import, offer for sale and sell the subject matter of such Inventions.

Sincerely,

_____

Pfizer Inc.   Date

INSTITUTION I represent to have authority to execute this Agreement on behalf of Institution:

By:_____
Institution Signature   do/<<Request_Number>>

_____
Printed Name

_____
Title

_____
Date

INVESTIGATOR while not a party to this agreement, acknowledges that they have read this agreement and understands their obligations as an Institution employee:

_____
Investigator's Signature

_____
Printed Name

_____
Date

STATEMENT OF INVESTIGATION FORM

Courtesy of Pfizer

Date: Request Number: <<Request_Number>>	Sponsor: <<Sponsor>>
Compound Requested: <<Compound>> <<Compound_2>> <<Compound_3>>	Amount: <<Compound_Amount>> <<Compound_2_Amount>> <<Compound_3_Amount>>
Investigator: <<Salutation>> <<First_Name>> <<Last_Name>> <<Initials>>	Institution: <<Institution>>
Title: <<Title>>	Department: <<Department>>
Phone: <<Phone_Number>> Fax: <<Fax>> e-mail: <<email>>	Address: <<Address 1>> <<Address 2>> <<Address 3>> <<City>>, <<State>> <<Zip>> <<Country>>

Please type a detailed explanation of the proposed studies using Pfizer compound(s) in the space provided below

Study Title:

Key Words:

Please type a brief justification for the amount of compound(s) requested.

PFIZER USE ONLY		
Is active ingredient available locally for supply?		
Medical Director:		Date:
Team Leader:		Date:
Director, Medical Operations:		Date:
VP, Quality Control:		

75

Drafting and Enforcing Nondisclosure Agreements

Kathleen D. Rigaut, PhD, JD

Ideas and innovations are often the most valuable assets companies, universities and individual inventors possess. Accordingly, effective protection of such assets can be obtained via execution of nondisclosure agreements (NDAs) or secrecy agreements prior to disclosing confidential proprietary information. NDAs enable parties who wish to exchange information to maintain the confidentiality or secrecy of the disclosed materials. Employers often require potential employees to agree to confidentiality. Small businesses in the process of negotiation with competitors frequently enter into NDAs. In the university technology transfer arena, such agreements are often drafted prior to disclosing a technology to a commercial partner.

Effective NDAs contain several key pieces of information, including the names of the parties exchanging information; the effective date of the agreement; the purpose of the disclosure; the type of information being exchanged; a mechanism for termination of the agreement; a provision regarding breach of the agreement; and list of exceptions to confidentiality. NDAs may also include standard choice-of-law provisions, as well as modification, integration and assignment provisions. A typical NDA is provided at the end of this chapter.

Frequently, the importance of an NDA is downplayed or overlooked altogether. Many businesses and universities rely on standard one- or two-page forms, which simply fail to address aspects of the agreement with the appropriate level of specificity. Accordingly, it is prudent to tailor each agreement to the particular technology and material to be disclosed. Additionally, it is advisable that all written

or tangible confidential materials exchanged be marked as "Confidential" to clearly identify those materials that should not be disclosed to third parties. If oral information is disclosed, it should be memorialized in writing and then also marked as confidential. The NDA should also clearly delineate the purpose of the disclosure, i.e., for the parties to consider entering into a further relationship. Finally, if there is any uncertainty on the part of the disclosing party regarding the integrity or ability of the recipient party to maintain the disclosed materials in confidence, it may be wise to file a provisional patent application or a copyright application to protect the invention or idea prior to disclosing the information. Alternatively, the parties may wish to enlist the aid of an objective third party to render an opinion. Using this approach minimizes concerns on the part of the disclosing parties that their ideas will be usurped by the recipient parties and also diminishes the chance of contamination of the recipient parties, particularly in cases where the recipient parties are engaged in a similar and/or competitive business.

In circumstances of disclosure of intellectual property or trade secrets having significant commercial value, the disclosing party should avoid setting a predetermined time period for maintaining conditions of confidentiality. It is typical in an NDA to specify a three- to five-year period under the assumption that information having high commercial value will reach the public domain within that period. However, in cases where trade secrets are disclosed, maintenance of conditions of confidentiality should continue indefinitely or until the trade secret is disclosed to the public. The NDA should clearly differentiate between that information considered confidential and that viewed as a trade secret.

Upon termination of the agreement, the NDA should provide for the immediate return of all confidential materials to the disclosing parties. The agreement may permit the receiving parties to maintain an archival copy for their records but restrictions should be placed upon access and use of any such materials.

Often NDAs are executed between parties having unequal bargaining power, i.e., the small start-up business vs the large commercial partner. It is important that the parties agree to include a provision addressing breach of the NDA. Breach of an NDA can cause irreparable harm to the disclosing party, thus, an effective agreement should contemplate a remedy for such damage as a review of the following case will demonstrate.[1]

In 1993, Celeritas Technologies was assigned the rights in US Patent 5,386,590 that claimed an apparatus for increasing the rate of data transmission over analog cellular telephone networks. This deemphasis technology improved the integrity of cell phone transmissions. In September 1993, officials of Celeritas met with representatives of Rockwell International to demonstrate the proprietary deemphasis technology as Rockwell was the leading manufacturer of modem "chip sets," containing the core functions of commercial modems including the modulation function where deemphasis is performed. The parties entered into a nondisclosure agreement wherein Rockwell agreed, "not to disclose or use any proprietary information except for the purpose of evaluating the prospective business arrangements between Celeritas and Rockwell."[2] Notably, the NDA also provided for injunctive relief or any other damages which may be appropriate should either party breach the agreement.

In March 1994, AT&T Paradyne began to sell a modem that incorporated deemphasis technology. In that same month, Rockwell informed Celeritas that it would not license the use of Celeritas proprietary technology, and concurrently began a development project to incorporate deemphasis technology into its modem chip sets. Significantly, Rockwell did not independently develop its own deemphasis technology, but instead assigned the same engineers who had learned of Celeritas technology under the NDA to work on the deemphasis development project. In January 1995, Rockwell began shipping its first prototype chip sets that contained deemphasis technology.[3]

Following commencement of these sales, Celeritas sued Rockwell, alleging breach of contract, misappropriation of trade secrets, and patent infringement. The jury returned a verdict for over $57 million on the breach of contract claim and awarded $900,000 in attorney's fees for the patent infringement claim. Rockwell appealed. The patent was held invalid as anticipated by prior art, thus the award for attorney's fees was dismissed. The court did not consider the misappropriation of trade secrets claim as Celeritas had stipulated that it would accept the liability theory with the highest damage award. The court upheld the breach of contract claim and also found that the $57 million award for damages for breach of the NDA was proper. The court reasoned that following the disclosure of the confidential information, Rockwell had two choices—to enter into a license agreement with Celeritas or refrain from using the information. Rockwell chose to use the information illegally. The jury award was likened to a license fee Rockwell would have paid Celeritas had it not breached the NDA. Accordingly, Rockwell's motion for a new trial on damages was denied.

As mentioned above, most NDAs contain provisions excluding certain information from confidentiality. Commonly, "information that is already in the public domain is excluded."[4] The patent at issue in Celeritas was ultimately held invalid as anticipated by the prior art. Accordingly, Rockwell asserted that its liability ended once the information was readily available to the public. Rockwell also argued that "any competent engineer could reverse engineer the AT&T modem." The Court of Appeals was not persuaded by these arguments and concurred with Celeritas' position that "for a trade secret to enter the public domain in California, it must be ascertained by proper means and not merely ascertainable."[5] In upholding the jury verdict for damages for breach of contract, the court also found that Celeritas had "disclosed implementation details and techniques that went beyond the public domain information available to Rockwell."[6]

NDAs serve as important legal documents, which can provide the only legal protection for the disclosing party should negotiations with the potential commercial partner fall through. Accordingly, while the standard one- or two-page forms serve as a good starting point, NDAs should be reviewed by a competent attorney who is well versed in the technology area and has an appreciation for the client's ultimate business goals. It is also prudent to have an attorney review the materials that are to be disclosed to ascertain whether the confidentiality of the concept has been properly documented by the disclosing party. In litigation, courts favor the parties who have clearly maintained confidential information in secrecy and has taken the necessary steps to protect themselves. Such practices should be standard operating procedure. Indeed as mentioned above, protection of the idea, via the filing of a patent application or copyright application, may be warranted prior to making the disclosure.

In summary, the simple NDA is really not so simple after all. The disclosure of confidential and proprietary information should never be undertaken without careful consideration and forethought. By addressing the points raised above, NDAs that can pique the commercial party's interest without placing the disclosing party at great risk of losing a valuable company asset can be drafted.

••• Endnotes

1. See *Celeritas Technologies, Ltd. v. Rockwell International Corporation*, 150 F.3d 1354 (Fed. Cir. 1998), *cert. denied*, 525 U.S. 1106 (1999).
2. *Celeritas Technologies, Ltd. v. Rockwell International Corporation*, at 1357.
3. *Celeritas Technologies, Ltd. v. Rockwell International Corporation*, at 1357.
4. *Celeritas Technologies, Ltd. v. Rockwell International Corporation*, at 1357.
5. *Celeritas Technologies, Ltd. v. Rockwell International Corporation*, at 1358.
6. *Celeritas Technologies, Ltd. v. Rockwell International Corporation*, at 1358.

75-A

Sample Disclosure Agreement

CONFIDENTIAL DISCLOSURE AGREEMENT

This Agreement, entered into this _____ day of _____, by and between DISCLOSING PARTY (hereinafter "_____") and RECIPIENT (hereinafter "_____").

WHEREAS, DISCLOSING PARTY has developed and is the owner of certain proprietary information relating to _____, which information DISCLOSING PARTY now maintains and wishes to continue to maintain in confidence, such information being referred to hereinafter as "Confidential Information";

WHEREAS, RECIPIENT desires to evaluate the Confidential Information to determine its potential interest therein and RECIPIENT desires DISCLOSING PARTY to disclose said Confidential Information to RECIPIENT for such purpose; and

WHEREAS, DISCLOSING PARTY is agreeable to disclose the Confidential Information to RECIPIENT for the purpose and under the conditions set forth herein.

NOW, THEREFORE, in consideration of the foregoing premises and of the mutual promises set forth herein, the parties intending to be legally bound, agree as follows:

1. DISCLOSING PARTY agrees to disclose in confidence to RECIPIENT as much of the Confidential Information as RECIPIENT may reasonably require for the limited purpose of evaluating the Confidential Information.
2. RECIPIENT acknowledges that the Confidential Information received by it pursuant to paragraph 1 is proprietary to DISCLOSING PARTY and is to be used by RECIPIENT solely for the above-stated purpose and for no other purpose, in the absence of a separate agreement entered into between the parties hereto.
3. RECIPIENT agrees that the Confidential Information will be accepted and held by it in confidence and that it shall make no disclosure of the Confidential Information except to RECIPIENT employees and consultants who have a need to know by reason of their participation in RECIPIENT's evaluation of the Confidential Information. RECIPIENT further agrees that all reasonable diligence will be used to prevent disclosure to others by its employees.
4. The obligation of nondisclosure and nonuse assumed by RECIPIENT hereunder shall apply to all Confidential Information disclosed to RECIPIENT in a writing marked "confidential" or if disclosed orally is reduced to a writing marked "confidential" and transmitted to RECIPIENT within thirty (30) days of the original disclosure. The obligations of nondisclosure and nonuse shall not apply to any Confidential Information that RECIPIENT can prove:

   (a) is in the public domain at the time of disclosure to

   RECIPIENT by DISCLOSING PARTY or thereafter becomes a part of the public domain other than through unauthorized disclosure by RECIPIENT; or

(b) was in the possession of RECIPIENT in recorded, or other verifiable form prior to DISCLOSING PARTY's disclosure to RECIPIENT; or

(c) was disclosed to RECIPIENT by a third party not under any obligation of confidence to DISCLOSING PARTY with respect to the Confidential Information; or

(d) was expressly authorized by DISCLOSING PARTY in writing to be released from confidential status.

For the purpose of this paragraph 4, no specific portion of the Confidential Information shall be deemed to be a part of the public domain, or within the knowledge or possession of RECIPIENT merely because it is embraced by more general information, which is part of the public domain or within the knowledge or possession of RECIPIENT.

5. The obligation of nondisclosure and nonuse assumed by RECIPIENT hereunder shall remain in effect until no restrictions exist and full disclosure of the Confidential Information has occurred.

6. It is understood and agreed that any Confidential Information disclosed by DISCLOSING PARTY to RECIPIENT pursuant to this Agreement shall remain the sole and exclusive property of DISCLOSING PARTY. Subject to the next sentence hereof, all of said Confidential Information, including any duplications that RECIPIENT may have made shall, upon request of DISCLOSING PARTY, be immediately returned to DISCLOSING PARTY, and RECIPIENT shall forthwith cause any reports, memoranda, notes, drawings, source code or other documents and all copies thereof not so supplied by DISCLOSING PARTY to RECIPIENT, but relating to any of said Confidential Information disclosed to RECIPIENT by DISCLOSING PARTY to be destroyed. Notwithstanding the foregoing, counsel for RECIPIENT may retain one (1) copy of all such documents incorporating or relating to the Confidential Information for record purposes only.

7. It is understood that no right or license of any kind is hereby granted to either party of this Agreement and that the disclosure of Confidential Information pursuant hereto shall not result in any obligation to grant either party any rights in or to property of the other party.

8. DISCLOSING PARTY and RECIPIENT acknowledge that the extent of damages in the event of the breach of any provision of this Agreement would be difficult or impossible to ascertain, and that there will be available no adequate remedy at law in the event of any such breach. Further such breach will cause irreparable harm to the DISCLOSING PARTY. Each party therefore agrees that in the event it breaches any provision of this Agreement, the other party will be entitled to injunctive or other equitable relief, in addition to any other relief to which it may be entitled. The parties hereby waive any requirement for the posting of a bond or other security in connection with the granting of injunctive relief.

9. This Agreement constitutes the entire agreement between the parties relating to _____.
There are no understandings or representations of any kind except those expressly set forth herein. No amendment of this Agreement shall be valid unless in writing and signed by the parties hereto.

10. This Agreement may not be assigned by either party without the prior written consent of the other party, and this Agreement shall inure to the benefit of the successors and assigns of the respective parties.

IN WITNESS WHEREOF, the parties hereto, have executed this Agreement as of the day and year first written above.

BY

_____
        DISCLOSING PARTY

Title _____

BY   _____
        RECIPIENT

Title

76

Copyrights, Trademarks, and Trade Secrets

David Huizenga, JD, PhD, and Hope Slonim, JD

Introduction

The US government provides or allows varying levels of protection for four areas of intellectual property: patents, copyrights, trademarks, and trade secrets. This chapter specifically discusses copyrights, trademarks, and trade secrets. Before outlining these rights, the chapter provides an important perspective and understanding about these rights: where these rights come from; and why arguably the most capitalistic market in the world would not only allow these various limited monopolies, but in fact, promote them. A basic understanding of the policy behind each right makes a nonexpert in these areas functional in discourse and able to issue spot for each right, which arguably are the most important goals for the technology director or research director.

Two of the rights, patent and copyright, arise directly from the US Constitution. Article I, § 8 of the US Constitution states that:

> Congress shall have the power . . . To promote the progress of science and useful arts, by securing for limited times to authors and inventors the exclusive right to their respective writings and discoveries.

Thus, for patents and copyrights, the rationale for society granting the monopoly flows from the goal of promoting "the progress of science and useful arts." Our founding fathers created a quid pro quo. Inventors and authors who give to society their ideas and work receive, in return, a period of exclusive rights to the results of their ideas and work because this, it was believed in the eighteenth century, promoted the production of more art and more science, the benefits of which resided in and raised up society as a whole. As will be discussed in the copyright section in this chapter, and in the chapters dealing with patents in this book, all fundamental laws and rules regarding patents and copyrights, such as laws governing what they are, how they are obtained, and for how long, can be traced back to this fundamental quid pro quo.

Noticeably absent from Article I, § 8, however, is any mention of protection for a trademark or trade secret. This absence itself instructs because it implies that neither trademarks nor trade secrets promote a general benefit for society, there is no quid pro quo. A trade secret actually contradicts the quid pro quo underlying the justification for patents and copyrights. By its very definition, a person holding a trade secret is keeping his or her idea secret, thus hindering the promotion of the related science or art. Why then should a trade secret be allowed? Although, not entirely satisfactory, one argument is that by allowing people to derive value from their business secrets, they are rewarded for expending the effort for obtaining the secret.[1] Again, approaching any trade secret question, such as what is a trade secret, from this basic view point can lead one to the likely answer under the law.

Lastly, while trademarks are not directly mentioned in Article I, § 8, it has been said that the constitutional basis for trademarks can be found as well in Article I, § 3, which states:

Congress shall have the power to . . . regulate Commerce with foreign Nations, and among the several States, and with the Indian Tribes.

This section has become known as the Commerce Clause and has been used to find a Constitutional granting of power to the federal government to regulate everything from racial integration to interstate pricing constraints. This connection of trademarks with the Commerce Clause, however, reveals the rationale for allowing trademarks: they are associated with commerce and consumers. There is no promotion of the arts or science, but they do something arguably even more important—they protect the consumer. Trademarks exist so that consumers not only can expect the quality and characteristics they have come to associate with a given trademark, but to provide a direct link between the consumer and the holder of the mark should the consumer desire recourse for some reason.

Thus, four intellectual property rights exist, but they exist for varying reasons. As discussed below, the policy by which the federal government justifies its involvement within these spheres can be used to come to an off-the-cuff or rule-of-thumb assessment of many of the issues that arise within each of these areas of IP that a technology director or research administrator may confront.

Copyright

Copyright is likely the oldest form of statutory intellectual property, tracing its origins all the way back to the British Statute of Anne from 1709-1710, and the basis for the Statute of Anne formed the underpinning of Article 1, § 8 of the US Constitution providing a copyright in the United States.[2] Like patents, copyright arises exclusively under federal law.[3] The US government provides a very helpful Web site related to the copyright office at http://www.copyright.gov/.

Copyright vests in authors of original works, and prevents people from copying or manipulating the work created by the author. 17 USC 102 states:

Copyright protection subsists, in accordance with this title, in original works of authorship fixed in any tangible medium of expression, now known or later developed, from which they can be perceived, reproduced, or otherwise communicated, either directly or with the aid of a machine or device. Works of authorship include the following categories:

(1) literary works;

(2) musical works, including any accompanying words;

(3) dramatic works, including any accompanying music;

(4) pantomimes and choreographic works;

(5) pictorial, graphic, and sculptural works;

(6) motion pictures and other audiovisual works;

(7) sound recordings; and

(8) architectural works.

(b) In no case does copyright protection for an original work of authorship extend to any idea, procedure, process, system, method of operation, concept, principle, or discovery, regardless of the form in which it is described, explained, illustrated, or embodied in such work.[4]

Thus, copyright can arise in a number of different areas including written works, art works, such as sculptures and pictures, and motion pictures and audio works. Songs, paintings, sculptures, books, speeches that are recorded, labels, jingles, movies, TV shows, and computer programs are just a few of the different types of creations copyrights can vest in.

Title 35 § 102 of the US Code also makes clear that only original and creative works of authorship create a copyright. "Original" means that the work arose independently from the author, not that it is absolutely new. Thus, if, for example, two different people, independently and without any influence from the other's work, wrote the song, "Blowin' in the Wind," both Bob Dylan and the second person would receive copyright in the song. In addition, the work must also be creative; however, almost any work will be seen as creative, if there is any modicum of creativity that can be found.

To be copyrighted, a work must be in a fixed tangible form of expression, such as a written or recorded medium.[5] Copyright cannot protect ideas, only the expression of an idea.[6] This contrasts with patents and trade secrets, which can protect ideas. Thus, for example, computers utilizing algorithms can be patented, but the algorithms themselves cannot be copyrighted. However, the software implementing the algorithm on the computer can be copyrighted.

The owner of the copyright has the exclusive right to reproduce the copyrighted work; to prepare new versions (or derivative works) based upon the copyrighted work; to publicly distribute copies of the copyrighted work; to perform the copyrighted work publicly in the case of literary, musical, dramatic and choreographic pantomimes, motion pictures and other audio visual works; and to display the work publicly.[7] Should anyone other than the owner of the copyright perform any of these actions without permission, the owner of the copyright can bring an infringement suit in which injunctive relief, monetary damages, and attorney's fees can be sought.[8]

A copyright occurs the moment an author creates a work in a fixed and tangible medium.[9] Since 1989 it has not been necessary to place a notice of copyright on a work and its copies. However, it is still good practice to include the notice on all published and unpublished copies of the work.[10] The notice should include the owner's name, the date of publication, and the copyright symbol or word copyright. Additionally, the phrase "All Rights Reserved" can be added to the notice for protection in Latin American countries.[11]

The duration of a copyright is the life of the author plus seventy years. In the case of a work for hire, the copyright endures for a term of ninety-five years from its first publication, or one hundred years from its creation.[12]

Copyright vests in the author of the work or in those who have acquired the rights of the copyright from the author.[13] Coauthors are automatically joint owners unless there is an agreement to the contrary.[14] One particular type of ownership transfer is a work for hire arrangement,[15] under which the person creating the work has an arrangement with another entity, such as a company or a person who commissioned the work, such that when the work is created it is the entity or person who commissioned the work that is actually considered the author. The copyright statute defines "work made for hire" as a work prepared by an employee within the scope of his or her employment; or a work specially ordered or commissioned for use as a contribution to a collective work, as a part of a motion picture or other audiovisual work, as a translation, as a supplementary work, as a compilation, as an instructional text, as a text, as answer material for a test, or as an atlas, if the parties expressly agree in a written instrument signed by them that the work shall be considered a work made for hire.[16] It is important to note that not every work made at the request of someone else is considered a work for hire.

Copyright vests automatically in the creation of the work and its fixation in a tangible medium, however this does not mean that the copyright has been registered.[17] However, registration of the copyright is important because registration (before or within five years after the first publication of the work) is prima facie evidence of the validity of the

copyright and of the facts stated on the registration certificate; the registration is required to file suit for copyright infringement; attorneys' fees, and statutory damages, even in the absence of lost profits, are not available where a work was unregistered at the time of the infringement unless the work was registered within three months after the first publication; registration establishes a public record of the copyright claim; and the registration may be recorded with the US Customs Service, which will impound (and possibly destroy) imported infringing copies of the copyrighted work.[18]

Typically to prove copyright infringement one has to show that the alleged infringer had access to the work and that the accused work is substantially similar in appearance to the copyrighted work. Should infringement be proven, injunctions and impounding of the work are available,[19] as are lost profits and actual damages, and statutory damages as high as $100,000 can be provided if the infringement was found to be willful.[20]

The advantages of copyright flow from the ease of obtaining the registration and the long time the right lasts, relative to patents. The disadvantages of copyright, however, arise from the narrow breadth that is afforded the scope of the work when infringement is alleged and in the fact that the copyright can cover only the expression of the idea, not the idea itself. This makes designing around a copyright relatively easy.

Trademark

Introduction

A trademark is not a patent and it is not a copyright. It does not protect the underlying invention itself nor does it protect an original work of authorship or artistic expression. Instead, trademarks are the words, slogans, designs, and other symbols that identify different products and services in the marketplace. They are the brands that consumers encounter every day and they frequently are the basis for making purchasing decisions.

The federal trademark law provides a working definition for "trademark." It explains that a trademark includes any word, name, symbol, or device (or any combination thereof) used to identify and distinguish goods or services and to indicate their source.[21] Key terms are "any," "identify and distinguish goods and services," and "indicate their source." The word "any" demonstrates that the trademark field is flexible. That is, trademarks can be words and designs, but they can be more creative than that. They also can be shapes (e.g., the shape of Hershey's Kisses® candy[22]), colors (e.g., the color of brown used by United Parcel Service® on trucks and uniforms for its delivery services[23]), and sounds (e.g., the sound of the lion's roar used by MGM® to identify its motion picture services[24]). "Any" keeps the law open to new possibilities for trademark protection. The wording "identify and distinguish goods and services" is critical because that is what trademarks do. Trademarks are not symbols that exist in a vacuum. Instead, they are applied to products or services, and they distinguish one product or service from another. For example, Campbell's® used on a soup can label identifies a particular type of soup and serves to distinguish that soup from another, such as Progresso®.[25] Finally, the wording "and indicate their source" specifies the main purpose of trademarks. Trademarks are "source identifiers"; they identify the source of a particular product or service and consumers use this information along with their experience in the marketplace to determine the quality of a product or service and to make a purchasing decision.

Technically, the terms "trademark" and "service mark" identify whether a designation is used on a product or in connection with a service. Coca-Cola® used on beverages and beverage syrups is a "trademark."[26] McDonalds® used on signs to identify restaurant services is a "service mark."[27] The same term can be both a trademark and a service mark. For example, when applied to packaging for hamburgers, McDonalds® is being used as a trademark.[28] However, the umbrella term is "trademarks," and the same laws and policies cover both. The federal trademark law and all of its provisions apply to trademarks as well as service marks.

Common Law, State Registration, and Federal Registration

There are three sources of trademark protection: common law, state registration, and federal registration through the United States Patent and Trademark Office (the USPTO), an agency within the US Department of Commerce. Rights in a trademark arise as soon as the trademark is used in the marketplace on a product or with a service. Those are common law rights, and although they mark the beginnings of trademark rights, they are limited to the geographic area(s) in which the trademark actually is used. That geographic limitation is due to the fact that others outside the immediate area of use typically would not encounter the trademark or

have knowledge of its existence. Therefore, to provide greater notice to others, trademark owners may take the additional step of registering their trademarks at the state level.

Almost all states in the United States have laws that provide some form of protection for trademarks.[29] Under those laws, trademarks may be registered in the state or states where they are used. Typically, a government office such as a secretary of state maintains a public registry of trademarks.[30] In this way, state registration is a means for a trademark owner to put the public on notice about its claim of ownership in that state. In other words, because the trademark now is a matter of public record, others can learn of its existence and hopefully will avoid using a similar trademark for related goods or services. Trademark owners who rely on their common law rights or a state registration may use the symbols "TM" (for trademark) or "SM" (for service mark). It should be noted that TM and SM do not procure substantive rights in a trademark. Instead, they are merely a means for providing informal notice to others of a claim of ownership. The symbol ® is reserved for those trademarks that have been registered at the federal level with the USPTO.

Trademarks become eligible for federal protection once the owner uses, or intends to use, its trademark in a type of commerce that Congress can regulate, such as interstate commerce or commerce between the United States and a foreign country.[31] At that time, a trademark owner may file an application for federal registration with the USPTO. Notably, the federal law permits a trademark owner to file an application for registration even before use in commerce has begun, based on its bona fide intent to use the trademark in commerce.[32] These are called "intent-to-use applications." However, the USPTO will not register the trademark until the owner establishes actual use of its mark in commerce within prescribed time frames.[33]

The federal trademark law is the Trademark Act of 1946, as amended, also known as the Lanham Act. Under this law and the Trademark Rules of Practice, the USPTO examines each trademark application for compliance with substantive law and procedural requirements.[34] A trademark owner may use the federal registration symbol, ®, only after its application has been reviewed, approved, and registered by the USPTO.[35]

Federal trademark registration with the USPTO is not mandatory. Trademark owners maintain their common law rights and, if applicable, state law protections even without a registration from the USPTO. However, federal registration gives the trademark owner certain legal presumptions and benefits which the owner otherwise could not claim. For example, it creates a legal presumption, in the registrant's favor, that the registered mark is valid, that the registrant is the owner of the trademark, and that the registrant has the exclusive right to use the trademark nationwide.[36] In addition, it permits the trademark owner to bring legal actions in federal court.[37] Federal registration provides nationwide constructive notice of the federal registrant's claim of ownership.[38] That is, while others may not have actual knowledge of use of a particular trademark, they are deemed to know about it by nature of its existence on the federal register. In this manner, constructive notice essentially eliminates a good faith defense that a party innocently and unknowingly adopted another's registered trademark.[39] Another benefit of federal registration is that it gives its owner the right to request US Customs officials to bar the importation of goods bearing infringing trademarks.[40] Additionally, subject to certain limitations, the owner's exclusive right to use its federally registered trademark may become incontestable if the mark has been in continuous use in commerce for five years after the date of registration.[41]

Issues Concerning Use in Commerce

The concept of "use" is central to trademarks. As previously stated, common law rights arise only when a trademark is actually used. A trademark owner generally cannot obtain a federal registration unless it establishes use of its mark in commerce, meaning a type of commerce that Congress can regulate.[42] From the purchaser's point of view, that makes sense. A trademark has no significance to the purchaser unless he or she actually encounters it in the marketplace.

The federal law defines "use in commerce" as the "bona fide use of a mark in the ordinary course of trade, and not made merely to reserve a right in a mark."[43] It also explains that, with respect to goods, a trademark is used in commerce when it is placed on the goods themselves, on containers, associated displays, tags or labels, and when "the goods are sold or transported in commerce"; with respect to services, the trademark must be used in connection with sales or advertising.[44] This definition contains two important ideas. First, that use must be bona fide and not merely to reserve trademark rights, sometimes referred to as "token

use."[45] Second, the federal law does not necessarily require a commercial sale or transaction, but rather that goods bearing the trademark be sold or transported in commerce.

While actual use is needed to obtain rights under common law as well as a federal registration, the federal trademark law also recognizes the concept of "constructive use."

The date that a trademark owner files its application for federal registration constitutes "constructive use" of its mark. Once the trademark is in fact registered, the constructive use date establishes the trademark owner's priority rights over subsequent users throughout the United States. The federal trademark law states:

> Contingent on the registration of a mark on the principal register provided by this Act, the filing of the application to register such mark shall constitute constructive use of the mark, conferring a right of priority, nationwide in effect, on or in connection with the goods or services specified in the registration . . . .[46]

Constructive use is particularly beneficial to a trademark owner who files an intent-to-use application in the USPTO. When it eventually provides evidence of actual use, the owner must provide the date it first used its trademark in commerce that is regulated by Congress. Typically the date of use in commerce is later than the date the application was filed. However, based on the concept of constructive use, the trademark owner's national priority rights are based on the earlier application filing date (i.e., the constructive use date) rather than the date of first use in commerce.[47]

The law also recognizes limitations on a federal registrant's constructive use rights, such as parties who used the trademark before the registrant's application filing date and owners of previously registered federal trademarks or earlier-filed pending applications for registration.[48]

Generally, the owner of a trademark is the party that directly uses it by placing the trademark on products or using it with services, and distributing those products or services to consumers in the marketplace. However, the federal law recognizes circumstances where the owner himself does not use the trademark, but rather authorizes its use by other parties, or related companies.[49] Typical related company situations involve licensors and licensees, franchisers and franchisees, and parent and wholly-owned subsidiary corporations.[50] In each case, the owner of the trademark is the party that maintains control over the nature and quality of the goods or services on which the mark is used. In these instances, use of the trademark by the related company inures to the benefit of the owner, so long as the owner continues to exercise the requisite control.[51]

Putting together many of the use concepts described previously may lead to the following scenario. A party develops a trademark for its product and, rather than use the trademark itself, the party intends to use it through a related company—a licensee. That party may file an application for federal registration based on its bona fide intention to use the trademark in interstate commerce through a licensee. Once the licensee begins to use the trademark in interstate commerce, the licensor (who controls the quality of the goods on which the trademark is used) must provide evidence of such use to the USPTO in order to obtain a federal registration. Once the registration issues, the licensor's national priority rights date back to the original application filing date (i.e., the constructive use date) rather than the date its licensee first began using the trademark in interstate commerce.

Like other forms of property, trademarks can be sold or otherwise transferred from one party to another. A trademark owner can legally assign its ownership interest with the associated good will of the business in which the trademark is used. In this regard, a trademark cannot be assigned unless it actually is being used. With respect to pending applications for federal registration, a trademark owner generally cannot assign an intent-to-use application before use in commerce is established.[52] The federal law permits assignment of intent-to-use applications in one instance: when the assignment is made to a successor to the applicant's business or portion of the business to which the mark pertains, if that business is ongoing and existing.[53] The primary purpose of this limitation is to ensure that trademarks are assigned only with the underlying business or goodwill to which the trademark pertains, and to prevent trafficking in trademarks.[54]

A final note on use. Just as trademark protection begins with use, it ends with nonuse. A trademark owner abandons its trademark when it ceases to use the trademark and when it has no intention to resume such use.[55]

Federal Registration Terms and Maintenance

Federal trademark registrations issued on or after November 16, 1989 remain in force for ten years and may be renewed for subsequent ten-year periods.[56] Unlike patents and copyrights, a federal trademark may be renewed as many times as the owner wishes. There is no set time after which the federal registration must end and the trademark enters the public domain. Instead, the registration may last indefinitely so long as the trademark owner continues to use its mark in commerce and properly maintains it by filing the required documents in the USPTO at the appropriate times.

To maintain its federal registration, the trademark owner first must file an affidavit of continued use or excusable nonuse between the fifth and sixth year after the date of registration.[57] The purpose of this document is to remove dead wood from the federal register, i.e., those trademarks that no longer are being used in commerce.[58] If the owner fails to file its affidavit during the prescribed time period, the USPTO will cancel the registration.

Every ten years from the date of registration, the trademark owner must file both a request for renewal and an affidavit of continued use or excusable nonuse.[59] The trademark registration will expire if the owner fails to request renewal within the proper time period.

Grounds for Refusal of Federal Trademark Registration

As noted above, the USPTO examines each trademark application for compliance with substantive and procedural law set forth in the Trademark Act of 1946, as amended, and the Rules of Practice. Registration may be refused if the trademark fails to satisfy legal requirements. Two of the most common grounds for refusing federal registration are likelihood of confusion with a previously registered trademark, and lack of distinctiveness. While those issues are discussed here with respect to federal registration, they also are relevant in trademark litigation.

Likelihood of Confusion   A trademark owner cannot obtain a federal registration if its trademark is likely to cause confusion with a previously registered trademark.[60] Similarly, trademark infringement occurs when one party uses a trademark that is likely to cause confusion with another party's trademark.[61] The test is likelihood of confusion, rather than actual confusion, meaning that the courts and the USPTO must decide whether the respective trademarks used in the marketplace are *likely* to cause consumers confusion as to the source of the goods and services, not whether actual confusion exists. The purpose behind the likelihood of confusion concept is, in large part, to protect consumers in the marketplace, to enable them to properly identify the source of a particular product or service, to help them determine quality and ultimately make an informed purchasing decision.

There are several factors used to determine whether a likelihood of confusion exists between different parties' trademarks. The principal ones are the similarity between the trademarks with respect to sound, appearance, meaning, and overall commercial impression; whether the goods or services on which the trademarks are used are closely related; and the channels of trade through which the respective goods and services travel to reach consumers.[62]

The following case demonstrates how the USPTO applies the likelihood-of-confusion analysis. The agency refused to register "Strategyn," used on computer software for developing business strategies, based on a previous registration for "Strategen," used on computer software that performs statistical data analysis for marketing and sales management.[63] The USPTO determined that even though the trademarks are spelled differently, they sound the same and they create the identical commercial impression in that both suggest the idea of a strategy.[64] As to the goods, it was noted that the respective software products are different, but they are closely related because they overlap in significant ways. Both may be used to study various financial aspects of a business. As such, they travel through the same channels of trade to the same type of consumer.[65]

In litigation, the parties may furnish survey evidence to show consumer perceptions of the respective trademarks in the marketplace. Such evidence may aid courts in reaching final determinations as to whether confusion is likely, but the parties first must consider the time, cost, and anticipated benefit associated with it as survey evidence generally involves considerable expense.[66]

Nondistinctiveness: Descriptive, Generic and Geographic Terms and Surnames

Trademarks must be distinctive. That is, a trademark must contain a certain level of uniqueness, imagination, and thought in order to distinguish one party's goods or services from others. Otherwise, the USPTO may refuse registration. The underlying rationale is that competitors need to use descriptive terminology to identify their products and services in the marketplace and that, as a matter of public policy, it would be unfair for one person or entity to own such a term and have exclusive rights to use it as a trademark.

Trademarks travel on a continuum between distinctiveness and descriptiveness, between strong and weak. Generally, the more distinctive or unique a trademark is, the stronger it is and the wider its scope of protection. The more descriptive the trademark is in relation to the product or service on which it is used, the weaker it is and the narrower its scope of protection.[67] In descending order from strongest to weakest, the continuum comprises terms that are coined or fanciful, arbitrary, suggestive, merely descriptive, and finally generic.

The most distinctive type of trademark is a coined or fanciful term, such as "Kodak," "Kleenex," "Xerox," "Pepsi," and "Clorox."[68] These terms have no meaning in the English language other than their trademark significance and they are considered to be very strong trademarks. Arbitrary terms are words that have English significance but, as applied to a particular product or service, they have no actual meaning. Examples of arbitrary terms used as trademarks are "Apple" for computers, "Camel" for cigarettes and "Old Crow" for whiskey.[69] Suggestive terms are words that imply some aspect or quality about the products or services. For example, "Coppertone" used on suntan lotion suggests that the product will give skin a "copper tone."[70]

Coined, arbitrary, and suggestive terms are inherently distinctive and, as such, may become federally registered trademarks through the USPTO. However, a line is crossed and registration may be refused when a trademark is merely descriptive of a product or service.[71] The determination of whether or not a trademark is merely descriptive is made in relation to the goods or services on which it is used, not in the abstract.[72] This requires consideration of how consumers encounter the trademark in the marketplace, and whether they would attribute any descriptive significance to it.[73] Examples of merely descriptive terms used as trademarks are "Apple Pie" for potpourri, "Bed & Breakfast Registry" for lodging reservations services and "Food & Beverage On-Line" for a news and information service for the food processing industry.[74]

Terms that are merely descriptive are not absolutely barred from federal registration. The USPTO maintains two registers: the Principal Register and the Supplemental Register. The Principal Register carries all the legal presumptions and benefits that come with federal registration, listed previously.[75] However, to be on the Principal Register, the trademark must be "distinctive"; it must identify the source of the product or service on which it is used. If it is not distinctive, but capable of becoming distinctive, the trademark may be registered on the Supplemental Register.[76] Since coined, arbitrary, and suggestive terms are inherently distinctive, they are immediately eligible for registration on the Principal Register. Merely descriptive terms are not distinctive, but they are capable of acquiring distinctiveness through the owner's continued use in the marketplace, advertising, and marketing efforts to associate the descriptive term with the product or service. Thus, descriptive terms may be registered as trademarks on the Supplemental Register. A registration on the Supplemental Register does not carry all the legal benefits as one on the Principal Register, but it does carry some, such as the right to use the federal registration symbol® and the right to file suit in federal court. It also may be the basis for a likelihood of confusion refusal by the USPTO if another party seeks to register a confusingly similar trademark used on related goods or services.[77]

Eventually, the owner of a trademark on the Supplemental Register may reapply for federal registration on the Principal Register claiming that its trademark has acquired distinctiveness. In that instance, the USPTO may permit registration on the Principal Register under Section 2(f) of the Trademark Act, a designation that indicates the trademark is not inherently distinctive, but has acquired distinctiveness through the owner's continued use and/or advertising.[78] Once a trademark has acquired distinctiveness, it is said to have "secondary meaning." That is, the trademark not only has its original descriptive significance but, through use and marketing, it has developed a second meaning in the minds of the purchasing public—its trademark significance.

Surnames and geographic terms are treated the same as terms that are merely descriptive. A trademark that is primarily, merely a surname, such as "Johnson" or "Jones," is not inherently distinctive. It may be registered on the Supplemental Register or on the Principal Register after a showing of acquired distinctiveness.[79] Similarly, the USPTO may refuse registration to a trademark that uses a geographic term depicting the origin of the goods or services. For example, the USPTO refused federal registration to "The Nashville Network" used in connection with television program production and distribution services emanating from Nashville, Tennessee.[80] Like merely descriptive terms and surnames, trademarks that are primarily geographically descriptive of the goods or services that they identify may be registered on the Supplemental Register or on the Principal Register after a showing of acquired distinctiveness.[81]

Generic terms are common names for categories of products and services.[82] "Kleenex" and "Clorox" are, of course, trademarks; "tissue" and "bleach" are the generic terms for the products that these trademarks identify.[83] Generic terms by themselves, like "tissue" and "bleach" used on tissue and bleach products, are incapable of ever becoming distinctive. In other words, generic terms are incapable of identifying a single source for the products or services on which they are used. Therefore, they cannot be registered as trademarks in the USPTO on either the Principal or the Supplemental registers.[84] To illustrate, the USPTO has refused as generic "Web communications" for Web site consulting services and "e-Ticket" for computerized reservation and ticketing of transportation services.[85]

Some terms that began as distinctive trademarks became generic over time. For example, "Aspirin," "Escalator," and "Linoleum" once were trademarks. However, consumers began to use those terms as the generic names for the products themselves and they eventually lost their trademark significance. When that occurs, the trademark is said to have become abandoned, and is subject to cancellation at any time by the USPTO.[86] For that reason, legal advisors often warn trademark owners to use trademarks as adjectives and not as nouns or verbs. For example, rather than the expression "use a Kleenex" in advertising, a trademark owner often is advised to use wording such as "use a Kleenex® tissue."

Conclusion: A Brief Note about Protecting One's Trademark

The role of the USPTO is to register eligible trademarks that comply with federal law, not to enforce trademark rights. Although federal registration confers certain legal advantages, it still is the owner's job to protect its trademark and to assert its rights against possible infringers. Some trademark owners employ businesses or law firms to police their trademarks in the marketplace.

Similarly, a trademark owner protects its trademark by continuing to use it in commerce and by using it properly so that it does not become the generic name for the goods or services that it identifies. A trademark owner may abandon its rights if it ceases to use the trademark in commerce or if its mark loses all trademark significance by turning into a generic term.

Finally, the owner of a federal registration must keep its registration active by filing the required documents in the USPTO at the proper times. Protecting and maintaining a registered trademark requires continuous effort, but the reward is great because, unlike copyrights and patents, federal trademark protection can last forever.

Trade Secrets

Trade secret law protects confidential and proprietary information from being disclosed to third parties by people who have a duty to the owner of the information to keep the information confidential. State law governs most trade secret law, and most states now have adopted some form of the Uniform Trade Secrets Act (UTSA).[87] However, the federal government has recently enacted the Economic Espionage Act (EEA) of 1996,[88] which provides both federal civil penalties as well as federal criminal penalties for theft of a trade secret.

Prior to statutory law surrounding trade secrets, common law legal theories for trade secrets were based in contract or property rights. The contract theory flowed from situations in which there were specific agreements between individuals about the status of information. As relationships between employees and employers matured and the law around these relationships grew, the contract theory evolved into situations where there might not have been an explicit contract, but in which there was an implied contractual relationship to maintain the status of a company's or individual's information. Trade secret law can also find a basis in property law in which the information itself is seen as a property to which ownership rights can attach. Modern statutory constructions and theories follow more of a property theory than a contractual theory, although contracts regarding trade secret information are employed routinely in the form of, for example, noncompete and confidentiality agreements.

The UTSA defines a trade secret as information, including a formula, pattern, compilation, program, device, method, techniques, or process, that: (i) derives independent economic value, actual or potential, from not being generally known to, and not being readily ascertainable by proper means by, other persons who can obtain economic value from its disclosure or use, and (ii) is the subject of efforts that are reasonable under the circumstances to maintain its secrecy.[89]

Today a trade secret can be almost anything. For example, specific chemical formulas or specific steps in a manufacturing process can be trade secrets. Lists of customers or lists of inventory or purchasers or suppliers can all be trade secrets.

Designs for building machines as well as the very know-how contained in an employee's brain as to how to perform a certain aspect of a business, such as manufacturing a particular product, can also be trade secrets. Possibly the most famous trade secret is the formula of Coca-Cola® or Coke Classic® as it is known today. To this day, the Coca-Cola Company maintains that the formula for making its nearly 100-year-old flagship product has been, is, and always will be a trade secret. Whether the exact composition of Coke Classic®, with all of the technological capabilities of the twenty-first century available to Coca-Cola's competitors, remains a mystery is anybody's guess. However, what is clear is that the Coca-Cola Company still gets mileage from its secret formula.[90]

A trade secret must be more than just a secret. There must be economic value derived from the secret and the efforts to keep it a secret must be reasonable.[91] Thus, to qualify as a trade secret, information must relate to a trade or business; it must be a secret (i.e., not known publicly or known generally within the trade or business concerned); and it must be used, or if not used, intended for use in a trade or business.

A trade secret only provides protection as long as it remains a secret, however, it arises without the creation of any written document. A trade secret does not protect the owner from reverse engineering or unintentional loss of the secret. Typically, the test for whether the owner of a secret has acted in such a way as to maintain a trade secret as a secret is a test of reasonableness. Things such as computer security, requirements for confidentiality agreements with outside parties, restricted access to business premises, control of employees through nondisclosure documents, not providing source code on the user end, and marking documents and other items "confidential" are characteristics courts will examine in determining the reasonableness of the efforts to keep the information secret.

Typically, trade secret law prevents those who are under a legal duty from disclosing trade secrets and other confidential and proprietary information to any third party who does not have a right to know the information. Under the UTSA, the trade secret cannot be misappropriated.[92] Under the UTSA, misappropriation means:

(i) acquisition of a trade secret of another by a person who knows or has reason to know that the trade secret was acquired by improper means; or (ii) disclosure or use of a trade secret of another without express or implied consent by a person who (A) used improper means to acquire knowledge of the trade secret; or (B) at the time of disclosure or use knew or had reason to know that his knowledge of the trade secret was (I) derived from or through a person who has utilized improper means to acquire it; (II) acquired under circumstances giving rise to a duty to maintain its secrecy or limit its use; or (III) derived from or through a person who owed a duty to the person seeking relief to maintain its secrecy or limit its use; or (C) before a material change of his position, knew or had reason to know that it was a trade secret and that knowledge of it had been acquired by accident or mistake.[93]

This definition of misappropriation requires an understanding of the meaning of "improper means." The UTSA defines improper means as including "theft, bribery, misrepresentation, breach or inducement of a breach of duty to maintain secrecy, or espionage through electronic or other means."[94]

As discussed above, in 1996 the federal government enacted laws drawn to the protection of trade secrets.[95] The main reason according to the legislative history of the EEA for creating the EEA arose from foreign espionage and theft of American technological secrets.[96] However, the EEA makes it clear that not only foreigners can be prosecuted. It defines a theft of a trade secret as:

Whoever, with intent to convert a trade secret, that is related to or included in a product that is produced for or placed in interstate or foreign commerce, to the economic benefit of anyone other than the owner thereof, and intending or knowing that the offense will, injure any owner of that trade secret, knowingly . . . [97]

The definition of a trade secret and the requirements that must be met to obtain trade secret protection are similar to those of the UTSA.[98] However, the EEA provides for criminal prosecution of theft of trade secrets, where as the UTSA provides only for civil remedies.[99]

There are several advantages of a trade secret relative to other types of intellectual property protection. First, a trade secret can cover things that cannot be covered by a copyright or a patent, such as an idea or information contained in a list or something not otherwise qualified for patent or copyright protection. A second advantage is that no outside action, such as filing a patent application or copyright registration, must be taken to create or extend the right. Lastly, trade secrets can be very valuable where the competitive advantage actually arises, not just from exclusion of action based on the knowledge, but rather from the information itself. In other words, a trade secret is appropriate when the owner or creator of the knowledge receives little or no incentive for disclosing the information. The disadvantage of a trade secret is that it only exists as long as it remains a secret, and in today's business environment where collaborations are increasingly important to successful business models and employees are increasingly mobile, this can be difficult or nearly impossible.

Author's Note

The opinins expressed herein are those of the authors and do not necessarily reflect the views of the US Patent and Trademark Office or any other federal agency.

• • • Endnotes

1. See, for example, *Kewanee Oil Company v. Bicron Corp.*, 416 U.S. 470 (1990).
2. Patterson, L. Ray, and Stanley W. Lindberg. *The Nature of Copyright*. Athens: University of Georgia Press, 1991.
3. 17 USC §§ 100–1332.
4. 17 USC § 102.
5. 17 USC § 102.
6. 17 USC § 102.
7. 17 USC § 106.
8. 17 USC §§ 501–505.
9. 17 USC § 102.
10. 17 USC §§ 401–406.
11. 17 USC § 401(b).
12. 17 USC § 302.
13. 17 USC § 201(a).
14. 17 USC § 201(a).
15. 17 USC § 201(b).
16. 17 USC § 101.
17. 17 USC § 408.
18. 17 USC § 411.
19. 17 USC §§ 502–503.
20. 17 USC § 504.
21. *Trademark Act of 1946*, as amended, 15 USC § 1127.
22. See U.S. trademark registration numbers 0165248 (registered March 6, 1923) (for the

words *Hershey's Kisses*) and 0186828 (registered July 22, 1924) (for the shape of the candy).

23. See U.S. trademark registration number 0815191 (registered September 13, 1966) (for the acronym UPS); see also U.S. trademark registration numbers 2131693 (registered January 27, 1998) (for the color brown used on delivery trucks) and 2159865 (registered May 26, 1998) (for the color brown used on uniforms).

24. See U.S. trademark registration numbers 1060489 (registered March 1, 1977) (for the acronym MGM) and 1395550 (registered June 3, 1986) (for the sound of the lion's roar).

25. See U.S. trademark registration number 0048461 (registered January 2, 1906) and 2052959 (registered April 15, 1997) (Campbell's); see U.S. trademark registration number 0708478, (registered December 13, 1960) (Progresso).

26. See U.S. trademark registration number 0238145 (registered January 31, 1928).

27. See U.S. trademark registration number 0743572 (registered January 8, 1963).

28. See U.S. trademark registration number 1426681 (registered January 27, 1987).

29. See McCarthy, J. Thomas. *McCarthy on Trademarks and Unfair Competition*. Deerfield, IL: Clark Broadman Callaghan § 22:10 (2004).

30. McCarthy, 2004. In Utah, for example, the state trademark law is the *Registration and Protection of Trademarks and Service Marks Act*, § 70-3a-101 et seq, administered by the state Department of Commerce, Division of Corporations and Corporate Code.

31. See United States Patent and Trademark Office, *Trademark Manual of Examining Procedure*, § 901.03, "Commerce That May Be Lawfully Regulated by Congress," www.uspto.gov/web/offices/tac/tmep/0900.htm (accessed October 20, 2005).

32. 15 USC § 1051(b).

33. 15 USC §§ 1051(c) and (d). See also *Trademark Manual of Examining Procedure*, § 1103.

34. The trademark rules of practice are located in the *Code of Federal Regulations* at 37 CFR § 2.1 et seq.

35. The owner of a federally registered trademark must use the federal symbol, ®, in order to collect statutory damages in an infringement action, unless it can show that the defendant had actual notice of the registration. 15 USC § 1111. See 15 USC § 1117 regarding statutory damages.

36. 15 USC § 1057(b).

37. 15 USC § 1121. This statutory section states that federal court jurisdiction is "without

regard to the amount in controversy or to diversity or lack of diversity of the citizenship of the parties."

38. 15 USC § 1072.

39. See McCarthy, 2004, § 26:32.

40. 15 USC § 1124.

41. 15 USC § 1065; *Trademark Manual of Examining Procedure*, § 1605. Incontestable trademark registrations may be challenged only on certain grounds, such as the trademark becoming the generic name for the good or services, or abandonment. See 15 USC §§ 1064 and 1115. See also *Park 'N Fly, Inc. v. Dollar Park & Fly*, 469 U.S. 189, 196, 83 L. Ed. 2d 582, 105 S. Ct. 658, 224 USPQ 327, 331 (1985).

42. Foreign trademark owners who seek U.S. registration based on registrations from their countries of origin are not required to establish use in commerce to obtain a U.S. registration. 15 USC § 1126(e). However, in order to maintain their registrations, they eventually are required to show use in commerce or excusable nonuse. 15 USC § 1058.

43. 15 USC § 1127.

44. 15 USC § 1127.

45. *Trademark Manual of Examining Procedure*, § 901.02.

46. 15 USC § 1057(c).

47. For further information regarding constructive use and priority issues, See *generally*, McCarthy, § 26 (2004).

48. 15 USC § 1057(c); *Trademark Manual of Examining Procedure*, § 201.02.

49. The federal trademark law defines *related company* as: "any person whose use of a mark is controlled by the owner of the mark with respect to the nature and quality of the goods or services on or in connection with which the mark is used." 15 USC § 1127.

50. See *Trademark Manual of Examining Procedure*, §§ 1201.03(c) and 1201.03(f). Ownership rights in a trademark or service mark may be acquired and maintained through the use of the mark by a controlled licensee even when the only use of the mark has been made, and is being made, by the licensee. *Turner v. HMH Publishing Co., Inc.*, 380 F.2d 224, 154 USPQ 330, 334 (5th Cir. 1967), cert. denied, 389 U.S. 1006, 156 USPQ 720 (1967); *Central Fidelity Banks, Inc. v. First Banker's Corp. of Florida*, 225 USPQ 438, 440 (Trademark Trial and Appeal Board [TTAB] 1984). *Trademark Manual of Examining Procedure*, § 1201.03(f).

51. See 15 USC § 1055; See also *Smith International, Inc. v. Olin Corp.*, 209 USPQ 1033, 1044 (Trademark Trial and Appeal Board

1981); *Trademark Manual of Examining Procedure*, § 1201.03.

52. 15 USC § 1060; 37 CFR § 3.16.

53. 15 USC § 1060; 37 CFR 3.16.

54. *Trademark Manual of Examining Procedure*, § 501.01(a).

55. 15 USC § 1127. Nonuse for three consecutive years is prima facie evidence of abandonment. *Trademark Manual of Examining Procedure*, § 501.01(a).

56. 15 USC §§ 1058 and § 1059. Registrations issued before November 16, 1989 remain in force for twenty years and may be renewed for subsequent ten-year periods.

57. 15 USC § 1058. The law provides a six-month grace period after the sixth year for filing the affidavit. 15 USC § 1058(c).

58. See Morehouse Manufacturing Corp. v. J. Strickland & Co., 407 F.2d 881, 160 U.S.P.Q. 715, 750 (CCPA 1969).

59. 15 USC 15 USC §§ 1058 and 1059. The law provides a six-month grace period at the end of each successive ten-year period. §§ 1058(c) and 1059(a).

60. 15 USC § 1052(d).

61. 15 USC § 1125.

62. Additional factors are listed in *In re E. I. du Pont de Nemours & Co.*, 476 F.2d 1357, 177 USPQ 563 (C.C.P.A. 1973). This case lists thirteen factors which, in addition to the ones stated earlier, include the degree of care that consumers use when purchasing the goods or services at issue (i.e., impulse vs. careful, sophisticated purchasing), the fame of the prior trademark, whether similar trademarks already are in use on similar goods or services, the amount of time that both trademarks have been used without actual confusion in the marketplace, whether the parties have entered into a consent agreement, etc. See also *Trademark Manual of Examining Procedure*, § 1207.01.

63. *In re The Total Quality Group, Inc.*, 51 USPQ2d 1474 (Trademark Trial and Appeal Board 1999).

64. *Total Quality Group*. 51 USPQ2d at 1476.

65. *Total Quality Group, Inc.* 51 USPQ2d at 1477.

66. See McCarthy, 2004, § 32:163.

67. *Trademark Manual of Examining Procedure*, § 1209.01.

68. See U.S. trademark registration number 0195218 (registered February 17, 1925) ("Kodak"); U.S. trademark registration number 0191941 (registered November 25, 1924) ("Kleenex"); U.S. trademark registration number 0525717 (registered May 30, 1950) ("Xerox"); U.S. trade-mark registration number 0824150 (registered February 14, 1967) ("Pepsi"); U.S. trademark registration number 0251292 (registered January 1, 1929) ("Clorox"); *Trademark Manual of Examining Procedure* § 1209.01(a).

69. See U.S. trademark registration number 1078312 (registered November 29, 1977) ("Apple"); U.S. trademark registration number 0126760 (registered September 30, 1919) ("Camel"); U.S. trademark registration number 0042919 (registered June 28, 1904) ("Old Crow"); *Trademark Manual of Examining Procedure*, § 1209.01(a).

70. See U.S. registration number 0917825 (registered August 3, 1971) ("Coppertone").

71. 15 USC § 1052(e)(1).

72. *Trademark Manual of Examining Procedure*, § 1209.01(b).

73. *Trademark Manual of Examining Procedure*, § 1209.01(b).

74. *In re Gyulay*, 820 F.2d 1216, 3 USPQ2d 1009 (Fed. Cir. 1987) ("Apple Pie" held merely descriptive of potpourri); *In re Bed & Breakfast Registry*, 791 F.2d 157, 229 USPQ 818 (Fed. Cir. 1986) ("Bed & Breakfast Registry" held merely descriptive of lodging reservations services); *In re Putnam Publishing Co.*, 39 USPQ2d 2021 (Trademark Trial and Appeal Board 1996) "Food & Beverage Online" held merely descriptive for a news and information service updated daily for the food processing industry, contained in a database). See also *Trademark Manual of Examining Procedure*, § 1209.01(b).

75. See, e.g., 15 USC § 1057(b) regarding prima facie evidence of the validity of the registered mark, the registrant's ownership of the mark, and the registrant's exclusive right to use the registered mark; see also 15 USC § 1057(c) regarding constructive use, 15 USC § 1072 regarding constructive notice, 15 USC § 1124 regarding the right to request U.S. Customs to bar importation of goods with infringing trademarks and 15 USC § 1065 regarding incontestability.

76. 15 USC § 1091.

77. See McCarthy, 2004, §§ 19:36 and 19:37.

78. 15 USC § 1052(f). This statutory section states that five years of substantially exclusive and continuous use of the trademark in commerce may, in some instances, establish acquired distinctiveness.

79. 15 USC § 1052(e)(4); *Trademark Manual of Examining Procedure*, § 1211 et seq.

80. *In re Opryland USA Inc.*, 1 USPQ2d 1409, 1413 (Trademark Trial and Appeal Board 1986).

81. 15 USC § 1052(e)(2); § 1210 et seq. Note, however, that trademarks are absolutely barred from registration on the principal and the supplemental registers if they identify a place other than the place where the goods or services originate and the public would be deceived and mistakenly believe that the goods or services come from there. 15 USC § 1052(e)(3); 15 USC § 1052(a); *Trademark Manual of Examining Procedure* §§ 1203.02, 1210.01(b) and (c). See e.g., *In re Boyd Gaming Corporation,* 57 USPQ2d 1944 (TTAB 2000) (holding that Havana Resort & Casino used on clothing that does not come from Cuba is geographically deceptively misdescriptive).

82. See *Trademark Manual of Examining Procedure,* § 1209.01(c).

83. See endnote 68.

84. Many registered trademarks combine generic terms with other distinctive matter. See, e.g., U.S. trademark registration number 0176970 (registered December 11, 1923) for Buster Brown Shoes with a design for shoes. The wording *shoes* is generic. In these instances, the trademark owner must disclaim the exclusive right to use the generic term apart from the trademark. 15 USC § 1056; *Trademark Manual of Examining Procedure,* § 1213.08(a)(i).

85. *In re Web Communications,* 49 USPQ2d 1478 (TTAB 1998) (concerning Web Communications); *Continental Airlines, Inc. v. United Air Lines, Inc.,* 53 USPQ2d 1385 (TTAB 1999) (concerning e-Ticket).

86. 15 USC § 1056 and 15 USC § 1064.

87. UTSA, § 1–4.

88. 18 USC §§ 1831–9.

89. UTSA, § 1(4).

90. See for example, The Coca-Cola Company, "Coke Lore," http://www2.coca-cola.com/heritage/cokelore_newcoke.html and Tucker, R. "How Has Coke's Formula Stayed a Secret?" *Fortune,* http://www.fortune.com/fortune/print/0%2C15935%2C368701%2C00.html.

91. UTSA, § 1(4).

92. UTSA, §§ 2 and 3.

93. UTSA, § 1(2).

94. UTSA, § 1(1).

95. 18 USC §§ 1831–9.

96. Legislative history of 18 USC §§ 1831–9.

97. 18 USC §§ 1832.

98. 18 USC §§ 1839(3).

99. 18 USC §§ 1834.

77

Export Control

James Taylor, JD

Introduction

Following the events of September 11, 2001, compliance with export control regulations has become a priority with the US Government. However, export control regulations are a unique challenge to universities. These laws require universities to balance concerns about national security with the traditional concept of academic freedom. For instance, universities often employ foreign nationals to conduct research, which in many cases means training foreign nationals on equipment that is controlled by US export regulations. If the piece of equipment is controlled by export regulations, then the university has to either receive a license from the government or ban foreign nationals from working on the research project. In order to understand the balance, research administrators and researchers need to understand how export regulations apply to their respective research projects. Therefore it is important to understand two basic concepts related to export regulations. First, one must know when the research of the university is controlled by US export regulations. Second, one must determine whether the fundamental research exclusion applies if the research is controlled by export regulations.

Export control laws (EAR, trade protection and ITAR, national security) restrict and regulate the exports of goods and services to foreign entities and foreign nationals for reasons of national security and foreign policy. An export law applies whenever a foreign national, whether on US soil or abroad, has access to an export-controlled item. Exports covered by EAR (Export Administration Regulations) and ITAR (International Traffic In Arms Regulations) can include the shipment of certain physical goods (i.e., equipment) and services, as well as disclosure of information and data, including verbal disclosures, and visual inspections of any technology, software, or data to any foreign national or entity. Therefore, research and activities of universities at times are subject to US export regulations. In some instances, export regulations will require that the university obtain a special license from the Commerce, State, or Treasury Department.

The potential impact export laws can have on universities can be dramatic. These laws can restrict the university's ability to conduct research in several ways. First, they can restrict the ability to allow foreign students to participate in research involving a controlled technology. Second, the university may be precluded from providing services or training on the use of controlled equipment to foreign nationals. Third, the university may not be able to send items to foreign countries.

If the university is required to receive a license, one of two things may happen. First, the research can be delayed: applying for and receiving a license from the appropriate government agency is time-intensive. A research project can be delayed by months or even years. Second, the appropriate government agency can deny the license. In many cases the denial of a license can lead to the termination of the research project. The consequences of violating these regulations can be quite severe, ranging from loss of research awards to monetary penalties and/or jail time.

Fortunately, export laws do not control the vast majority of exports. Only exports that are controlled under EAR and ITAR require licenses. Even if export regulations control a certain item, ITAR and EAR provide that no license is needed to disclose technical information to foreign nationals if the information is in the public domain. Information in the public domain is information that is published and is generally accessible to the public through unlimited and unrestricted distribution. This is typically referred to as the "fundamental research" exemption.

In many cases, the university is not required to receive a license because the research falls under a research exemption. However, vigilance is required to ensure that the availability of the fundamental research and other exemptions are not lost due inadvertent acceptance of contractually imposed restrictions on research.

The purpose of this chapter is to provide basic information to help university administrators identify export control issues. This chapter is designed to help administrators ensure that fundamental research exemptions are not lost to inadvertent acceptance of restrictive contractual clauses. This chapter provides an overview of the EAR and ITAR regulations, a list of key terms, and compares significant differences between the two sets of regulations. This chapter concludes with some suggested best practices with regard to export control compliance for research institutions.

Definitions

It is important to have a general familiarity with the key words that are often used in regard to export regulations. Below is a general summary of the words often found within export regulations. However, it should be noted that the official regulatory definition should always be consulted for specific applications.

Deemed Export

This is generally defined as: actual shipment of any covered goods or items outside the United States, and release or disclosure, including verbal disclosures or visual inspections of any covered technology, software, or technical data to any foreign national whether in the United States or abroad.[1] It should be noted that ITAR also includes the performance of a defense service on behalf of or for the benefit of a foreign national, whether in the United States or abroad.[2] If an item is controlled by an

export regulation, it means that the item cannot be exported without first securing a license from the appropriate federal agency or qualifying for an exemption. Any item that is sent from the United States to a foreign destination is an export. How an item is transported outside of the United States does not matter in determining export license requirements. An item is also considered an export even if it is leaving the United States temporarily or if it is going to a wholly owned US subsidiary in a foreign country. Even a foreign-origin item exported from the United States, transmitted, or transshipped through the United States, or being returned from the United States to its foreign country of origin is considered an export.

Fundamental Research

This refers to basic or applied research in science and/or engineering at an accredited institution of higher learning in the United States, where the resulting information is ordinarily published and shared broadly in the scientific community and in other cases, where the resultant information has been or is about to be published.[3] Fundamental research is distinguished from research that results in information that is restricted for proprietary reasons or pursuant to specific US government access and dissemination controls. The Fundamental Research Exclusion is destroyed if an individual or institution accepts contract clauses that forbid the participation of foreign nationals or gives the sponsor a right to approve publications resulting from the research.[4] However, it should be noted that the fundamental research applies only to disclosure to foreigners in the United States and to technical data. It does not apply to actual shipments of things (physical items including, for example, specified scientific equipment) or services (e.g. training foreign nationals inside or outside the United States) outside our borders.

Fundamental research also encompasses the following exclusions that can be found in EAR and ITAR:

Educational Exclusion. No License is required to share with foreign nationals if the information under consideration is commonly taught in universities or the information is in the public domain. Students using controlled equipment to conduct research should be registered for a research credit class.[5]

Employment Exclusion. No license is required to share covered technical data with a foreign national if the foreign national is a full-time, bona fide university employee.[6] This means that the employee has a permanent address in the United States while employed. Many researchers, particularly postdoctoral candidates and students, cannot qualify for the exclusion because they are not full-time employees of the university.

Public Domain. Information that is published and that is generally accessible or available to the public through sales at newsstands and bookstands; through subscriptions that are available without restriction to any individual who desires to obtain or purchase the published information; through second class mailing privileges granted by the US government; at libraries open to the public or from public documents; through patents available at any patent office; through unlimited distribution at a conference, meeting, seminar, trade show, or exhibition; through public release in any form after approval by the cognizant US government department or agency; and through fundamental research in science and engineering at accredited institutions of higher learning in the United States where the resultant information is ordinarily published and shared broadly in the scientific community.[7]

Defense Article. This is any designated item in the International Traffic In Arms Regulations that include chemical agents, cameras designated for military purposes, specified lasers, and GPS equipment. It also means any technical data recorded or stored in any physical form, models, mock-ups, or other items that reveal technical data directly relating to the particular item.[8]

Defense Service. This is the furnishing of assistance anywhere (inside the United States or abroad) to foreign nationals in connections with the design, development, engineering, manufacture, production, assembly, testing, repair, maintenance, notification, manufacture, demilitarization, destruction, processing, or use of defense articles, and the furnishing of any controlled technical data to foreign nationals anywhere.[9]

Technical Data. This includes information required for the design, development, production, manufacture, assembly, operations, repair, testing, maintenance, and modification of controlled articles. This includes information in the form of blueprints, drawings, plans, instructions, diagrams, photographs, etc.[10]

Overview

Export control laws cover virtually all fields of science. Fortunately, universities do not need to obtain a license to transfer scientific, technical, or engineering information to their foreign national students and faculty members if the information qualifies for the fundamental research exemption.

The fundamental research exemption applies to the majority of university research controlled by export regulations. Therefore, when the research exemption applies, research may be conducted with the participation of foreign nationals, and research information may be disclosed without the need to obtain a license from the US government. However both ITAR and EAR state that the fundamental research exemption will be lost for any research project where a university or its researchers accept restrictions on the publications of research findings. It is important that all research agreements are reviewed to make sure that the "public domain" aspect of the work is unimpaired. University research will not be deemed to qualify as fundamental research if the university accepts a restriction on the publication of the information resulting from the research. Limited prepublication reviews by research sponsors to prevent inadvertent divulging of proprietary information provided to the researcher (by the sponsor or to ensure the publication will not compromise patent rights of the sponsor) is acceptable.[11] If the research is not considered fundamental research and is controlled by the export regulations, the university will need to apply for an export license.

EAR versus ITAR

There are some key differences between EAR and ITAR. EAR covers dual-use items or items that are designed for a commercial use, but those which can have military applications (e.g., computers, pathogens, civilian aircraft). ITAR strictly covers military items (e.g., munitions, missiles, tanks, bombers). EAR licensing regime balances competing interests, including foreign availability, commercial and research objectives with national security. ITAR is a strict regulatory regime, with the sole purpose of ensuring US security; ITAR does not balance commercial or research objectives.

EAR

EAR regulates the export of most commercial items. EAR often refers to the items as dual-use items having both commercial and military or proliferation applications. However, purely commercial items without an obvious military use are also subject to the EAR.[12]

The Bureau of Industry (BIS) in the Department of Commerce is responsible for EAR licensing. The Commerce Control List (CCL) categorizes the goods and related technology it covers into ten topical categories and one catch-all category:

0. Nuclear materials, facilities and equipment, and miscellaneous
1. Materials, chemicals, microorganisms, and toxins
2. Materials processing
3. Electronics
4. Computers
5. Telecommunication and information security
6. Lasers and sensors
7. Navigation and avionics
8. Marine
9. Propulsion systems, space vehicles and related equipment[13]

Each of these categories is subdivided into lists of specific items. Within each category items are arranged into five groups that are then further divided. In the EAR regulations, there is a catch-all category of coverage known as "EAR 99." Any item subject to EAR that does not fall under one of the ten specific CCL categories falls into EAR 99.[14] Licenses are not required for goods or technologies in this category except in limited circumstances, such as a country that is on the US embargo list.[15]

Under EAR, university research conducted by scientists, engineers, or students normally is considered fundamental research and is therefore exempt from licensing requirements.[16] However without careful management of export issues, a university can lose the exemption under EAR. University-based research is not considered fundamental if the university or its researchers have accepted restrictions on the publication of scientific and technical information. The university can accept prepublication review to ensure that publication would not inadvertently divulge proprietary information furnished by the sponsor or comprise patent rights.[17] The EAR exemption for fundamental university research is broader than under the ITAR.

Violations of the EAR can have both criminal and civil consequences. Criminal violations can include a $50,000 to $1 million fine or five times the value of the export, whichever is greater per violation, and up to ten years in prison. Civil penalties can include fines from $10,000 to $120,000 per violation and can ultimately end with the loss of export privileges.[18]

If an export license is required, the university must prepare a "Multipurpose Application Form" (Form BIS-748P) and submit it for review and approval. The best and fastest way to submit an export application form is through the agency's online system.*

ITAR

ITAR deals with items that the state department has deemed to be inherently military in character. ITAR controls the export of articles, services, and related technical data. These items are organized into twenty-one categories, which include equipment, software algorithms, and, under each category, technical data and services related to the items specified. These defense articles and related technical data are listed on the US munitions list (USML). Some items listed include articles and technologies that are not readily identifiable as inherently military in nature (e.g., research satellites). The categories vary in breadth of coverage, although some are fairly specific:

1. Firearms, close assault weapons and combat shotguns
2. Guns and armament
3. Ammunition/ordnance
4. Launch vehicles, guided missiles, ballistic missiles, rockets, torpedoes, bombs and mines
5. Explosives and energetic materials, propellants, incendiary agents and their constituents
6. Vessels of war and special naval equipment
7. Tanks and military vehicles
8. Aircraft and associated equipment
9. Military training equipment
10. Protective personnel equipment
11. Military electronics
12. Fire control, range finder, optical and guidance and control equipment
13. Auxiliary military equipment
14. Toxicological agents, including chemical agents, biological agents, and associated equipment

---

*See http://www.bis.doc.gov/SNAP/index.htm. The university can also request a Form BIS-748P by fax at (202) 482-3617; by phone at (202) 482-3617; in writing, to the U.S. Department of Commerce Office of Exporter Services, P.O. Box 273, Washington, DC 20044; or by e-mail (through the agency's Web site).

15. Spacecraft systems and associated equipment
16. Nuclear weapons, design and testing related items
17. Classified articles, technical data and defense services not otherwise enumerated
18. Directed energy weapons
19. Reserved
20. Submersible vessels, oceanographic and associated equipment
21. Miscellaneous[19]

ITAR, like EAR, allows the fundamental research exemption. The fundamental research exemption is more limited under ITAR, however. For instance, there is no reference in ITAR that allows a limited prepublication review by a sponsor, while most universities presume that such a review is permitted. ITAR also provides that university research is not considered fundamental research if the university or its researchers accept other restrictions on the publication of scientific and technical information resulting from the project. Also, the ITAR contains language that implies that the provision to a foreign national of even public domain information may be considered a defense service that requires a license under ITAR.[20]

In response to concerns expressed by universities about university-based research involving satellites and the relationship to the ITAR, the US State Department attempted to clarify the research exemption in March 2002.[21] In so doing, the State Department reiterated that it does not control or regulate fundamental research; and it also indicated that the 1999 transfer of commercial communications satellites from the CCL to the USML did not change this policy and did not affect the longstanding ITAR jurisdiction over research, experimental, and scientific satellites. The amendment clarified that the fundamental research exemption allows accredited US institutions to export articles under ITAR without a license as long as it is to certain universities and research centers in countries that are members of NATO, the European Union, the European Space Agency, or to major non-NATO allies such as Japan and Israel.

ITAR also exempts disclosures of unclassified technical data in the United States by US institutions of higher learning to foreign nationals who are *bona fide* full-time regular employees (these do not include students or graduate students).[22]

ITAR, like EAR, states that a university is not considered for fundamental research exclusion if the university accepts restrictions on the publication of scientific and technical information.

Violations of ITAR are quite severe. Criminal violation can result in fines up to $1 million per violation and up to ten years imprisonment. Civil penalties include seizure and forfeiture of the articles.[23]

If an export license is required, it can be obtained from the State Department Web site.* The State Department also has an online submission Web site called the Electronic Licensing Entry System (ELLIE). In addition to electronic submissions, official forms may be submitted, and are available from an online ordering system.†

The Treasury Department's Office of Foreign Assets Control (OFAC) prohibits transactions with countries subject to boycotts, trade sanctions, and embargoes without a license. OFAC sanctions focus on the end-user or country, rather than on the technology. This government agency has the authority to impose controls on transactions and exports from the United States to specific foreign nationals, countries, and entities. OFAC also has the power to freeze foreign assets that are under the jurisdiction of the United States (embargoed countries frequently are referred to as the "T-& 7s").

Universities do not frequently encounter OFAC issues. However, occasionally OFAC sanctions may impact university activities. For example, in October 2003 the Treasury Department issued an advisory opinion indicating that publication activities (including Web sites that provided even the most minimal assistance to their users) may be forced to exclude users from OFAC-embargoed countries. [The issue arose in the context of a US engineering journal providing editing services on articles submitted by authors from embargoed countries.] A US university was also recently sanctioned by OFAC for providing funding to a nonprofit foundation in an embargoed country. As a final check before exporting research articles, universities should check the OFAC's list of embargoed entities. Currently under embargo are Cuba, Iran, Iraq, Libya, Liberia, Sudan, Syria, and North Korea. For a full up-to-date listing visit the OFAC Web site.‡

Violations of OFAC have similar consequences to those of ITAR and EAR. Criminal violations

---

*See http://www.pmdtc.org/licenses.htm. Forms may also be ordered by calling the DUTCH receptionist at (202) 663-2980. You must identify which form(s) and the quantity to be sent to you. For any other assistance, you may also call the Response Team at (202) 663-1282.

†See http://www.pmdtc.org.

‡See http://www.treas.gov/offices/eotffc/ofac/sanctions/index.html.

include fines of up to $1 million per violation and up to ten years in prison; civil penalties include fines between $12,000 to $55,000 per violation.

Best Practices

Here are some suggested practices and procedures currently in place at various institutions. These practices are primarily meant to raise awareness of export control issues and how to manage those issues.

A. Researchers can include a standard statement in the executive summary or abstract of their proposals, such as following:

> This is a fundamental research project and, as such, the University shall be free to publish or disseminate the results of this research or otherwise treat such results as in the public domain, and it will conduct the research in accord with National Security Decision Directive 189 and the applicable export control implementing regulations.

Including such a statement should make sponsors aware of the institution's position on publication and should further support the exercise of the fundamental research exemption by the institution. This statement should be added to the proposal itself, not just within a cover letter.[24]

B. During the proposal submission process, it is important to add questions to internal proposal routing forms inquiring of the researcher. For example, questions regarding:

1. Any restrictions placed on publication in the Requests for Proposals or program announcements.
2. Whether the export of controlled technology or items is expected.[25]
3. On the part of the research administrator staff, when reviewing a proposal submitted by a researcher, the administrator should review the proposal and RFP to see whether they contain any language or terms that:
   - Reference US export regulations;
   - Restrict non-US entity participation based on country of origin;
   - Prohibit the hiring of non-US persons;
   - Address security concerns;
   - Grant the sponsor preapproval right on publications;
   - Grant the sponsor a right to prepublication review for matters other than the inclusion of patent and/or proprietary sponsor information; or

- Allow the sponsor to claim resulting research information as proprietary or trade secret.

As research administrators you should look for these kinds of provisions. In particular, it is advantageous to address these issues at the proposal stage so as to minimize any delay in securing the funding.[26]

In negotiating modifications to a government contract, you should point out whether the clause does not comply with National Security Decision Directive (NSDD) 189 or the Federal Acquisition Regulations (FAR) data rights clause for universities. NSDD states, as a matter of federal policy, that papers or other publications resulting from unclassified basic research are exempt from prepublication controls. NSDD further states that when national security requires controls on publication, the mechanism that must be used to restrict the dissemination of information generated during federally-funded fundamental research is through classification. In other words, NSDD 189 stands for the proposition that no restrictions may be placed upon the conduct or reporting of federally funded fundamental research that has not received national security classification.

In negotiating the change, you should also note that NSDD 189 has been codified in the FAR 27.404 Basic Rights in Data clause. The first sentence of 27.404 (g) (2) states:

> In contracts for basic or applied research with university or colleges, no restrictions may be placed upon the conduct of or reporting on the results of unclassified basic or applied research, except as provided in applicable U.S. statutes.[27]

C. Each university administration should select an individual in research administration or the legal office to serve as the official contact person for both the governmental agency and the researchers, regarding export control issues. This official should also be closely supported by the outside counsel engaged for export control matters.

The university should also form a relationship with an outside counsel skilled at dealing with export control issues. When export control questions do arise, they are generally complex and it is unrealistic to assume that any institution's legal staff is trained to handle the issues.

Each university should establish an export policy and training program to help make researchers and research administrators aware of export issues. The training program should pay special attention to those departments or laboratories that are most likely to have projects that will be covered by export laws (e.g. engineering, computer sciences, and space science.) At the minimum, a Web site providing information both on the export control laws in general and specific institutional policies and procedures should be developed and made available institution-wide.[28]

Inspector General's Reports

The Office of the Inspector General (OIG) in its most recent audit is suggesting the fundamental research exemption be reevaluated. In the audit, the OIG stated concerns that the fundamental research exemption is allowing foreign nationals and foreign entities access to items and information that should receive a license under EAR and ITAR. It is possible in the near future that the fundamental research exemption could either be eliminated or at the least be narrowed.

The OIG reports recommended changes that would have serious impacts on universities. If the reports' changes are implemented, they will have a dramatic effect on how research is performed at universities. For instance, if the OIG's interagency report is implemented and the fundamental research exemption is eliminated, universities would need to receive export licenses for the vast majority of their research. If the Department of Defense report is implemented and a university concludes that it is not feasible to receive a license because of time constraints or when a license was denied by the government, then the university would need to have facilities that denied access to foreign nationals. This would likely require a badge system and facilities separate from the normal university in order to exclude access of foreign nationals.

Below is a summary of the individual interagency reports.

1. *The Department of Defense (DOD)* The OIG report recommends that the Defense Acquisition Regulations (DFARS) be amended to incorporate an export control compliance clause. This clause would require that in all DOD contracts involving export controlled technology, contractors implement access control plans including badging of foreign nationals, export compliance training, periodic self-assessments, and obtaining licenses for any foreign national who requires access to export

controlled technology or information. The university fundamental research exemption from export requirements is mentioned only in passing and its status, should DOD implement such a clause, is unclear.

2. *The Department of Commerce.* The OIG report recommends that this department make clear that technology for the use of export controlled equipment is subject to licensing requirements, even if the research being conducted with that equipment is fundamental, since its use is likely to be accompanied by transmittal of information about the technology. Thus, many universities would need to seek export licenses for foreign nationals working with the equipment, or otherwise restrict their access. This approach is quite different from the current approach taken by most universities for research conducted under the auspices of the fundamental research exemption.

3. *The Department of Energy.* The OIG report is much along the lines of the Department of Commerce report.

4. *Interagency.* The OIG report directly questions university fundamental research and educational exemptions. It calls for reexamination of these exemptions, on the grounds they might allow transfer of sensitive US technology to entities of concern and affect national security. Apparently similar recommendations were made in a previous 2000 interagency OIG report, and the new report says it is again necessary to raise awareness. It recommends that both Congress and the National Security Council reexamine the export license exemptions accordingly.

The individual OIG reports are available via Web sites:

DOD OIG Report, http://www.dodig.osd.mil/audit/reports/FY04/04-061.pdf.

Interagency OIG Report, http://www.dodig.osd.mil/audit/reports/fy04/04-062.pdf.

Commerce OIG Report, http://www.oig.doc.gov/oig/reports/2004/BIS-IPE-16176-03-2004.pdf.

Energy OIG Report, http://www.ig.doe.gov/pdf/ig-0645.pdf.

Since the release of the Inspector General reports, the Department of Commerce issued an Advance Notice of Proposed Rulemaking (ANPR) published in the *Federal Register* on March 28, 2005 asking for comments on the recent recommendations of the Department of Commerce Inspector General (IG) with regard to deemed exports in the context of university fundamental research. In response to the ANPR, the Council of Governmental Relations (COGR) issued a memo in response. In the memo, COGR has asked for the Department of Commerce to reconsider the following points:

1. reconsider and not accept the IG's interpretation of the scope of the fundamental research exclusion from export controls;
2. clarify the Export Administration Regulations;
3. increase the communication between the federal government and the regulated communities.[29]

Summary

Export control regulations are federal law. Do not rely on contract grants or other agreement terms to tell you whether the export regulations apply or challenge the assertion that the research being proposed is subject to export controls, if you believe it is not. Fundamental research is clearly defined as basic and applied research in science and technology, performed by the US institutions of higher education, the results of which will be shared widely and within the interested community. Additional information and technology generated by fundamental research information or technology to foreign persons in the United States is permissible.

In order to ensure that the university does not lose its fundamental research exemption, university administrators need to be vigilant as to the following:

1. Make sure that are no restrictions on the university's ability to publish.
2. Make sure there are no restrictions on the personnel who may be used on the project or restrictions on those who may have access to the research.

Watch out for flow-down clauses from other organizations that incorporate publication clauses and personnel restrictions. Some of these may be obvious, others less so. Remember, you will always need a license to ship an actual device, piece of equipment, or other embodiment of a controlled technology outside the shores of the United States.

• • • References

1. Title 15 *Code of Federal Regulations* § 734.2.
2. Title 22 *Code of Federal Regulations* § 120.17(5).
3. Title 15 *Export Administration Regulations* § 734.8(b).
4. Title 15 *Export Administration Regulations* § 120.11(8).
5. Title 15 *Export Administration Regulations* § 734.9.
6. Title 15 *Export Administration Regulations* § 734.9.
7. Title 22 *Code of Federal Regulations* § 120.11.
8. Title 22 *Code of Federal Regulations* § 120.6.
9. Title 22 *Code of Federal Regulations* § 120.9.
10. Title 22 *Code of Federal Regulations* § 120.10(5).
11. Title 15 *Export Administration Regulations* § 734.8(b).
12. Title 15 *Export Administration Regulations* § 730.3.
13. Title 15 *Export Administration Regulations* § 738.2.
14. Title 15 *Export Administration Regulations* § 738.2(b).
15. Title 15 *Export Administration Regulations* § 730.2.2.
16. Title 15 *Export Administration Regulations* § 734.8(b).
17. Title 15 *Export Administration Regulations* § 734.8(b).
18. Title 15 *Export Administration Regulations* §§ 734.8(b), 764.2 and 764.3.
19. Title 22 *Code of Federal Regulations* § 121.1.
20. Title 22 *Code of Federal Regulations* § 120.11.
21. *Federal Register* 67, no. 61 (March 29, 2002): 15099–15101.
22. Title 22 *Code of Federal Regulations* § 120.11(8).
23. Title 22 *Code of Federal Regulations* § 127.1-12.
24. Council on Governmental Relations, *Export Controls and Universities: Information and Case Studies*. Washington, DC: Council on Governmental Relations, 2004, 39.
25. *Export Controls and Universities*, 2004, 39.
26. *Export Controls and Universities*, 2004, 39.
27. *Export Controls and Universities*, 20.
28. *Export Controls and Universities*, 40.
29. Council on Governmental Relations. *Council on Governmental Relations*, Letter to Alexander Lopes, Director, Deemed Exports and Electronics Division, US Department of Commence, June 24, 2005, 2.

CHAPTER

78

SBIR/STTR Programs

Roberta A. Nixon, Jo Anne Goodnight, and Rick Shindell

Small Business Innovation Research (SBIR) Program

The Small Business Innovation Research (SBIR) program is a competitive program currently administered by eleven federal agencies. The Small Business Administration plays an important role as the coordinating agency for the SBIR program and in providing policy oversight to the agencies that administer an SBIR program. The SBIR program is designed to support small businesses in the conduct of innovative research or research and development (R/R&D) that has potential for commercialization and public benefit and that addresses priority areas of the sponsoring federal agency. In addition, SBIR-supported technologies are expected to lead to commercial products and processes that engender economic growth.

The statutory purposes of the SBIR program are:

1. to stimulate technological innovation;
2. to use small business to meet federally funded research or research and development (federal R/R&D) needs;
3. to foster and encourage participation in technological innovation by socially and economically disadvantaged small businesses, as well as small businesses that are 51% owned and controlled by women; and
4. to increase private sector commercialization of innovations derived from federal R/R&D, thereby increasing competition, productivity, and economic growth.

Since its inception in 1982, the SBIR program has supported more than 14,000 small businesses throughout the United States in the development of new technologies and in taking these concepts as products to the marketplace. One example of such a technology development is provided by Noesis, Inc., a small company in Arlington, Virginia. Noesis is currently engaged in "the development of enhanced metal fiber electrical brushes that significantly improve the operating efficiencies of electrical systems and drastically reduce the requirement for costly periodic maintenance" on US Navy submarines.[1]

Under the 1982 Small Business Innovation Development Act, agencies with extramural R&D budgets of $100 million or greater are required to conduct an SBIR program. A set percentage of a federal agency's total extramural R&D budget is set aside as a line item in the agency's budget for the fiscal year. The initial percentage was 1.25% in 1987 and currently is 2.5% of an agency's external R&D budget, which translates into a total of almost $2 billion, reserved for eligible small, R&D firms each year. This is a significant infusion of funds, which has proven to be a worthy investment. The news release by the SBA Office of Advocacy on January 27, 2004, stated "Small highly innovative firms have a big impact on many high tech industries, according to a report issued today by the Office of Advocacy. The report shows that large firms in the biotechnology, medical electronics, semiconductor, and telecommunications industries are citing patents by small firms in higher than expected numbers."[2]

In this chapter, we describe the components of the SBIR program; list the agencies involved; describe how a companion program, the Small Business Technology Transfer (STTR) program came into being; explain how the SBIR and STTR programs are used as mechanisms to link colleges and universities to small businesses; and describe possible changes in the eligibility requirements for the programs.

History of SBIR

The concept for the SBIR program goes back to the mid-1970s. At that time, researchers at small businesses were concerned about being shut out of funding for their research ideas by the National Science Foundation (NSF). If they worked at a university, grants would be available to them. But since they worked in small businesses, no mechanism existed to fund their research. Several companies went to Senator Ted Kennedy, who was then Chairman of the Senate subcommittee that had jurisdiction over the annual NSF budget authorization. To address this small business concern about R&D funding, Senator Kennedy included in the NSF budget a "floor" or minimum percentage of the applied research budget to go to small businesses. This budget requirement was placed on a program called Research Applied to National Needs (RANN). The set-aside for small businesses was ratcheted up to 12.5% over a period of three years, during which time the NSF inaugurated the SBIR program to meet the interests and capabilities of this new constituency.

The NSF tapped Roland Tibbetts, who worked in the Applied Research Directorate, to design a research program for the high-tech small business community. A Harvard MBA who had worked in the venture capital industry as well as in two high-tech companies in the Washington metropolitan area, Mr. Tibbetts consulted widely with government and business managers to develop the original three-phase program design of SBIR. The first NSF SBIR solicitation appeared in Fiscal Year 1977 and contained topics drawn from the RANN Program. In FY 1978 NSF funded follow-on Phase II grants, omitting a solicitation for new Phase I proposals. FY 1979 saw a new SBIR solicitation, and NSF has since conducted SBIR solicitations and funded projects in every following year. In FY 1979 the Department of Defense (DOD) began a program similar to the SBIR Program and called it DESAT. Roland Tibbetts worked closely with the DOD's program manager to make DESAT a fitting precursor to the eventual government-wide SBIR program.

As the earliest program manager of the SBIR program, Mr. Tibbetts is widely acknowledged today in the SBIR community as the "Father of SBIR." In honor of this distinction, the SBA has annually given the national Tibbetts Award to exemplary small businesses and organizations in recognition of superior SBIR technological innovation, economic impact, and business achievements. Approximately sixty companies and individuals receive this prestigious award annually.[3]

The Small Business Innovation Development Act of 1982 (P.L. 97-219) established a federal SBIR program to assist small businesses in the areas of high-tech research and development. The 1982 act had a sunset clause and needed to be legislatively renewed. Thus, it was extended and revised by amendments in 1988, 1992, and 2001.

The 1992 Reauthorization Act was developed for the following purposes: "1) to expand and improve the SBIR Program; 2) to emphasize the goal of increasing private sector commercialization; 3) to increase small business participation in federal R&D; and 4) to improve dissemination of information on SBIR Program."[4]

Key provisions of the most recent reauthorization (Small Business Reauthorization Act of 2000, P.L.106-554) included the following:[5]

- Extension of the SBIR program through September 30, 2008.
- A new mentoring program for companies in areas underserved by the program.
- An annual reporting requirement on the SBIR program.
- Improved SBA reporting and database requirements.
- A comprehensive study of the SBIR program by the National Research Council.
- Policy directive modifications requiring commercialization plans for Phase II proposals.
- Agency reports for Phase III follow-on funding agreements.
- A federal and state technology partnership (FAST) program.

In the early days of SBIR, large corporations and universities were interested in learning more about this new program. In April 1984, the School of Engineering and Applied Science at the University of Virginia presented one of the first SBIR conferences entitled, "How High Tech Corps Acquire R&D, Capital and Federal Grants." This was a one-day seminar modeled after a similar event held at the University of Texas, Dallas by John A. Rodman in 1983. Bobbe Nixon worked with both academic and state entities to organize the conference. Sponsors included the governor's office, the School of

Engineering and Applied Science, the University of Virginia, and Center for Innovative Technology. Of particular note is the conference sponsorship provided by Arthur Andersen & Co., Packard Press, and the Commonwealth of Virginia. Speakers were drawn from SBA, DOD, NASA, and NSF to talk about their SBIR programs. In addition to describing the SBIR program, the seminar presented:

1. How the university could be a catalyst by working with small businesses to perform research;
2. How to find alternative financing sources;
3. How to promote the growth of high technology businesses in Virginia.

When this early seminar took place, the federal agencies participating in SBIR were awarding 780 grants to small businesses for a total value of $44 million nationwide. At the time, they were expecting SBIR funding to triple within the next few years. In fact, the SBIR program has grown from $44 million in 1983 to $2 billion in 2004. This is a growth of fifty times the 1983 funding.[6]

The makeup of the 1984 Charlottesville conference is not so different from what we find today at state-sponsored SBIR conferences, agency conferences, FAST meetings, and national conferences. It is the magnitude of the program and the small business involvement that has grown tremendously. Industry–university partnership is still strongly encouraged, agencies are still detailing the SBIR program and providing information about how to win awards, and small businesses are working to identify alternative financing techniques for later-stage projects. These are the necessary components for success in the SBIR program.

Description of the SBIR Program

For the purpose of the SBIR and STTR programs, the SBA defines a small business concern as one that, at the time of award for both Phase I and Phase II funding agreements, meets all of the following criteria:

1. It is organized for profit, with a place of business located in the United States, which operates primarily within the United States or which makes a significant contribution to the United States economy through payment of taxes or use of American products, materials, or labor;
2. It is in the legal form of an individual proprietorship, partnership, limited liability company, corporation, joint venture, association, trust or cooperative, except that where the form is a

joint venture, there can be no more than 49% participation by foreign business entities in the joint venture;
3. It is at least 51% owned and controlled by one or more individuals who are citizens of, or permanent resident aliens in, the United States, except in the case of a joint venture, where each entity to the venture must be 51% owned and controlled by one or more individuals who are citizens of, or permanent resident aliens in, the United States; and
4. It has, including its affiliates, not more than 500 employees, and meets the other regulatory requirements found in 13 CFR, Part 121.

In addition, under the SBIR program, the principal researcher must be primarily employed by the small business concern. Each year federal agencies participating in the SBIR program are required by law to apportion a set percentage (currently 2.5%) of their extramural R&D funds to award to small businesses through announced agency solicitations. Once a solicitation is issued, small businesses review the topics in the solicitation and submit a proposal.

The SBIR program consists of three phases:

- *Phase I.* The objective of Phase I is to establish the technical merit and feasibility of the proposed R/R&D efforts and to determine the quality of performance of the small business awardee's organization prior to providing further federal support in Phase II. Support under Phase I is normally provided for six months/$100,000 for SBIR and one year/$100,000 for STTR.
- *Phase II.* The objective of Phase II is to continue the R/R&D efforts initiated in Phase I. Only Phase I awardees are eligible for a Phase II award. SBIR and STTR Phase II awards normally may not exceed $750,000 total.
- *Phase III.* The objective of Phase III, where appropriate, is for the small business concern to pursue with non-SBIR/STTR funds the commercialization objectives resulting from the Phase I/II R/R&D activities. In some federal agencies, Phase III may involve follow-on non-SBIR/STTR funded R&D or production contracts for products, processes, or services intended for use by the US Government. In some agencies where a project will directly benefit an agency's mission, e.g., the building of a component on a Navy submarine, Phase III may be funded by non-SBIR sources within the agency. Generally, Phase III funds come from the private sector and are employed in product and market development.[7,8]

Eligibility Requirements

To receive SBIR funds, each recipient of an SBIR Phase I or Phase II award must qualify as a small business. Other requirements apply in all of the SBIR funding agencies, as follows:

Phase I A minimum of two-thirds of the research or analytical effort must be performed by the awardee. Occasionally, deviations from this requirement may occur, and must be approved in writing by the funding agreement officer after consultation with the agency SBIR program manager/coordinator.

Phase II A minimum of one-half of the research or analytical effort must be performed by the awardee. Occasionally, deviations from this requirement may occur and these must be approved in writing by the funding agreement officer after consultation with the agency SBIR program manager/coordinator.

Phases I and II For both Phase I and Phase II, the primary employment of the principal investigator must be with the small business at the time of award and during the conduct of the proposed project. Primary employment means that more than one-half of the principal investigator's time is spent in the employ of the small business. This precludes full-time employment with another organization. Occasionally, deviations from this requirement may occur and must be approved in writing by the funding agreement officer after consultation with the agency SBIR program manager/coordinator. A small business may replace the principal investigator on an SBIR Phase I or Phase II award, subject to approval in writing by the funding agreement officer. For purposes of the SBIR Program, personnel obtained through a Professional Employer Organization or other similar personnel leasing company may be considered employees of the awardee. This is consistent with SBA's size regulation (13 CFR 121.106, Small Business Size Regulations).

For both Phase I and Phase II, the R/R&D work must be performed in the United States. However, in rare and unique circumstances, agencies may approve a particular portion of the R/R&D work to be performed or obtained in a country outside of the United States, for example, when a supply or material or other item or project requirement is not available in the United States. The funding agreement officer must approve each such specific condition in writing, according to the 2002 SBIR policy directive:

> In the SBIR program, a research institution may partner with a small business through a subcon-

tracting arrangement. This is encouraged but not required. In Phase I, 33% of the award may be outsourced to a university and/or consultants. In Phase II, the allowed figure for such outsourcing is 50%.

Statistics Regarding the Size of the Program

The following statistics for Fiscal Year 2002 give an idea of the size of the program: 4,138 Phase I grants awarded to small businesses in all fifty states; 1,595 Phase II grants awarded; and a combined total of $1.5 billion appropriated for both Phase II awards. This is a large investment into small companies to develop new, high-tech products for the marketplace. California received the largest number of SBIR dollars, a total of $299,262,647 for 1,197 Phase I and Phase II awards. Massachusetts was second with $215,459,825 in 799 awards. Virginia was a distant third with $89,717,760 in 333 awards. Of the nearly $300 million California received, $89,952,185 was in the form of 892 Phase I awards and $209,310,462 for 305 Phase II awards. The significance of these statistics is that California is submitting and receiving considerable start-up technologies with their Phase I projects. The 305 Phase II awards show that California is also developing these technologies toward products in the Phase II R&D process.

Participating Federal Agencies

Federal agencies with R&D budgets over $100 million dollars participate in the SBIR Program. Currently these agencies are:[9]

- Department of Agriculture (USDA)
- Department of Commerce (DOC)
- National Institute of Standards & Technology (NIST)
- National Oceanic & Atmospheric Administration (NOAA)
- Department of Defense (DOD)
- Army
- Air Force
- Missile Defense Agency (MDA)
- Chemical and Biological Defense (CBD)
- Defense Advanced Research Projects Agency (DARPA)
- Defense Threat Reduction Agency (DTRA)
- Office of the Secretary of Defense (OSD)
- National Geospatial-Intelligence Agency (NGA)
- Navy
- Special Operations Command (SOCOM)
- Department of Education (DoEd)
- Department of Energy (DOE)
- Department of Health & Human Services (HHS)

- National Institutes of Health (NIH)
- Centers for Disease Control (CDC)
- Federal Drug Administration (FDA)
- Agency for Healthcare Research and Quality (AHRQ)
- Department of Transportation (DOT)
- Environmental Protection Agency (EPA)
- National Aeronautics & Space Administration (NASA)
- National Science Foundation (NSF)
- Department of Homeland Security (DHS)
- Homeland Security Advanced Research Projects Agency (HSARPA)

Together, these agencies currently provide over $2 billion to the SBIR program annually.

At least annually, each participating agency must issue a program solicitation that sets forth a substantial number of R/R&D topic and subtopic areas consistent with stated agency needs or missions. Both the list of topics and the description of the topics and subtopics must be sufficiently comprehensive to provide a wide range of opportunities for small businesses to participate in the agency R&D programs. Topics and subtopics must emphasize the need for proposals with advanced concepts to meet specific agency R/R&D needs. Each topic and subtopic must describe the needs in sufficient detail to assist in providing on-target responses, but cannot involve detailed specifications of prescribed solutions of the problems.

Many agencies release only one solicitation per year, while others may vary from year to year. Historically, the DOD has released two separate SBIR solicitations per year. However, for FY 2002, the DOD released four SBIR solicitations, the most ever. In additional to its annual omnibus solicitation of the NIH, CDC, and FDA for SBIR/STTR grant solicitations,[10] NIH releases funding opportunities to small business concerns through the NIH guide for grants and contracts as program announcements and requests for applications.[11]

SBIR Proposal and Award Process

The SBIR process begins with an agency announcing a solicitation with the R&D topics it plans to fund during a given competition. All agencies now release their solicitations in electronic format only. Small businesses prepare proposals in response to the solicitation according to specific guidelines. The guidelines vary somewhat according to agency, and/or the agency component (i.e., Army, Navy, and Air Force). Submissions are due on a specified date with no allowance for late submissions. More and more agencies are moving to electronic submission-only systems, so applicants/offerors need to be somewhat fluent with the World Wide Web and with using PDF format files.

Agencies base their award selections on technical merit, the firm's qualifications, and the potential for commercialization of the technology. Normally, SBIR agencies establish a proposal review cycle wherein successful and unsuccessful applicants are notified of final award decisions within six months of the awarding agency's Phase I solicitation closing date. However, agencies may extend that notification period up to 12 months based on individual agency needs.

Each agency has its own set of review criteria. In general, a quality proposal addresses the following areas:

Significance. What problem is going to be solved? What is the significance of the problem or business opportunity? What difference will the solution make?

Innovation. Does the project challenge existing paradigms or employ novel technologies, approaches, or methodologies? Are the aims original and innovative?

Approach. How is the identified issue going to be resolved? What are the technical objectives? What is the research plan for accomplishing the objectives?

Investigators. Why is this the right firm to perform the work? What credentials, experience in related R&D, and qualifications of key personnel make this firm the best choice?

Environment. Is there sufficient access to resources (e.g., equipment, facilities)? Does the scientific and technological environment in which the work will be done contribute to the probability of success? Do the experiments take advantage of unique features of the scientific environment or employ useful collaborative arrangements?

It is important to understand that each agency prescribes in its solicitation its own proposal format that must be adhered to closely.[12]

Small Business Technology Transfer Program (STTR)

In 1992, Congress enacted the Small Business Technology Transfer Act of 1992 (P.L. 102-564). The STTR Act established the Small Business Technology Transfer Program as a pilot program that requires Federal agencies with extramural budgets for research or research and development in excess of $1 billion per fiscal year to enter into funding agreements with small business concerns that engage in a collaborative relationship with a research institution. The purpose of the STTR

Program is to stimulate a partnership of ideas and technologies between innovative small business concerns and research institutions.[13]

The STTR program was developed to "stimulate and foster scientific and technological innovation through cooperative research and development carried out BETWEEN small business concerns AND research institutions."[14] In the STTR program, primary employment is not stipulated. This means that the principal investigator can be employed by the research institution and/or a small business, although the award must go to the small business with a subcontract to the research institution.[15]

Reauthorization of the STTR program runs through Fiscal Year 2009. The mandated set-aside increased from 0.15% to 0.30% of participating agencies' external R&D budget in Fiscal Year 2004.[16]

There are some differences between the SBIR and the STTR programs, including the dollar amounts of the awards and the length of the award periods of performance.

- *Phase I.* Awards normally do not exceed $100,000 for a period of 12 months.
- *Phase II.* Awards increased from $500,000 to $750,000 for a period of 24 months in Fiscal Year 2004.[17]
- *Phase III.* Non-STTR funds are used for commercialization.

In the SBIR program, research institution partnerships are optional. With the STTR program, however, the program requires research institution participation. Of the award, 40% to 70% may be allotted to small business. A total of 30% to 60% may be allotted to the academic partner.[18]

Universities may participate in the SBIR/STTR program in many different ways. The STTR program was created to attract more academics who own an interest in a small business to become involved in developing their technologies. With the National Science Foundation's (NSF) SBIR/STTR Programs, faculty can own small businesses. They also may be senior personnel in a budget. Faculty members may even be principal investigators with official leave from their university. Faculty may be subcontractors to an award. University laboratories may be used for analytical and other service support for an STTR project.[19]

The NSF also provides additional assistance through supplemental grants to Phase II SBIR/STTR awardees. A Research Experience for Undergraduates (REU) supplement may be used to add an additional $6,000 to the SBIR/STTR award for an undergraduate student to work on the grant. One or two students per year may be awarded this supplement. The Research Experience for Teachers (RET) supplement can provide up to $10,000 per K-12 teacher to participate on these grants.[20]

STTR Solicitations

The number of STTR solicitations varies somewhat from year to year. Some agencies such as the DOD report their schedules far in advance, while others merely place an announcement on Fedbizopps (http://fedbizopps.gov) if contracts format or on (http://www.grants.gov) if grants format. Some agencies issue presolicitation notices while others do not. Occasionally, the Federal Register is used for presolicitations. For Fiscal Year 2004, the number of solicitations per agency for both SBIR and STTR are listed below:

- Department of Agriculture: 1 SBIR
- Department of Commerce
- National Institutes of Standards & Technology: 1 SBIR
- National Oceanic & Atmospheric Administration: 1 SBIR
- Department of Defense: 4 SBIR, 1 STTR
- Department of Education: 2 SBIR
- Department of Energy: 1 SBIR, 1 STTR
- National Institutes of Health: 1 SBIR, 1 STTR (NIH omnibus solicitation runs all calendar year but has three submission dates during the year and its STTR shares the same topics as its SBIR omnibus topics. NIH also releases several special program announcements [PAs] and requests for applications [RFAs] for extended Phase II opportunities.)
- Department of Homeland Security: 2 SBIR
- Department of Transportation: 1 SBIR
- Environmental Protection Agency: 1 SBIR (may have additional special solicitations, but all areas are released and due at the same time, usually in the spring)
- National Aeronautics & Space Administration: 1 SBIR, 1 STTR
- National Science Foundation: 2 SBIR, 2 STTR (SBIR and STTR share the same topics)

Where the SBIR and STTR Programs Are Today

According a 2004 report prepared by CHI Research, Inc., "Small Firms and Technology: Acquisitions, Inventor Movement and Technology Transfer," the overall findings show positive results:

> Small firms are a vital element of new technology in many industries. Their importance is not immediately apparent when all industries are considered, because small firms tend to be excluded from such key capital intensive industries as automotive, aerospace, and oil research. In newer high technology industries, such as biotechnology, medical electronics, medical equipment, and telecommunications, large firms frequently rely on small firms' discoveries and inventions.[21]

Highlights from the "Small Firms and Technology" report include:

- The influence of small firms in technology is increasing. Small firms represented 40 percent of the highly innovative firms in 2002, as opposed to 33 percent in the 2000.
- Between the mid-1990s and the early 2000s, large firms' share of elite inventors (those with at least 10 patents in a two-year period) fell from 72 percent to 69 percent. The share of elite inventors employed by small firms rose from 12 percent to 16 percent during the same period. . . .
- Small firms have a greater technological impact in industries that tend to consist of many young, small innovative firms. Industries that fit these characteristics include biotechnology, computers and peripherals, medical electronics, medical equipment, semiconductors and electronics, and telecommunications. More than half of the small firms in these industries only obtained their first patents after 1990.[22]

At the time of writing, lobbyists of influential and well-funded organizations such as the Biotechnology Industry Organization (BIO) and the National Venture Capital Association (NVCA) are working to influence legislation to change the SBIR eligibility rules. They seek changes that would allow large-scale venture capital organizations to own and control small businesses competing for SBIR funding. Many seasoned SBIR veterans believe that this change would result in greatly diminished opportunities for the small businesses. Rural and smaller states would be put at a major disadvantage because of the lack of venture capital funding in those states. The overall result would be a "widening gap between the richest SBIR states (California and Massachusetts) and the smaller rural states such as Wyoming, New Mexico, Montana and Maine."[23]

Acknowledgment

The authors would like to acknowledge and thank Mr. Ritchie Coryell, SBIR program manager at the National Science Foundation, for his review of this chapter. His excellent suggestions, corrections, and additions were invaluable in its preparation.

The authors would like to acknowledge and recognize Mrs. Liesl Amos for her invaluable editing skills and suggestions for improvement on very short notice.

Authors' Note

The opinions expressed herein are those of the authors and do not necessarily represent the views of the National Institutes of Health, Department of Health and Human Services, or any other federal agency.

• • • Endnotes

1. See The Department of Defense, "A DoD SMIR Success Story," http://www.dodsbir.com/Materials/SuccessStories/Noesis.htm (accessed October 1, 2005).
2. SBA Office of Advocacy News release, SBA # 04-04ADVO, January 27, 2004.
3. Ritchie Coryell (SBIR Program Manager, NSF), in discussion with the author, September 29, 2004.
4. Lee Eiden and Jo Anne Goodnight (presentation at the national SBIR conference, Anaheim, California, March 22, 2002).
5. Eiden and Goodnight, 2002.
6. Small Business Administration Technology–SBIR/STTR, "What We Do," http://www.sba.gov.sbir/indexwhatwedo/html (accessed October 16, 2005).
7. SBA Technology—SBIR/STTR, "SBIR and STTR Programs and Awards," http://www.sba.gov/sbir/indexsbir-sttr.html#sbir (accessed on July 2, 2005).
8. Eiden and Goodnight, "General Session" (presentation at the national SBIR spring conference, Arlington, VA, April 22–24, 2003).
9. See SBA, "SBIR Representatives of Participating Federal Agencies," http://www.sbaonline.sba.gov/sbir/indexcontacts-reps.html (accessed October 1, 2005).
10. See National Institutes of Health, Office of Extramural Research, "Small Business Funding Opportunities," http://grants1.nih.gov/grants/funding/sbir.htm#sol (accessed October 1, 2005).

11. See National Institutes of Health, Office of Extramural Research, "Special Announcements for Small Business Research Opportunities," http://grants1.nih.gov/grants/funding/sbir_announcements.htm (accessed October 1, 2005).

12. See the *SBIR/STTR Proposal Preparation Handbook* from the SBIR conference in Charlottesville, NC, September 12, 2001.

13. SBA, Document 03-14635, "Small Business Technology Transfer Program Policy Directive," *Federal Register* (June 16, 2003): 1.

14. Eiden and Goodnight, 2003.

15. Eiden and Goodnight, 2003.

16. Eiden and Goodnight, 2003.

17. Extramural Programs Reserved for Small Businesses, http://www.sba.gov/sbir/SBIRSTTR_3 CourseFullOverview.ppt (accessed on October 16, 2005).

18. Kesh Narayanan (presentation at the national SBIR spring conference, April 22–24, 2003, Arlington, VA).

19. Narayanan, 2003.

20. Narayanan, 2003.

21. CHI Research, Inc., under contract SBA-HQ-02-M-0491, "Small Firms and Technology: Acquisitions, Inventor Movement and Technology Transfer," Haddon Heights, NJ, January, 2004, p. 1.

22. CHI Research, 2004.

23. SBIR Gateway, "VCs & Biotech Lobbyists Push for Last-Minute SBIR Legislation Change: Attempt to Avoid Public Hearings," updated September 19, 2004, http://www.zyn.com/sbir/articles/bnews-vc2-s.htm (accessed September 19, 2004).

79

Cooperative Research and Development Agreements

Kathleen Sybert, PhD, JD, and Concetta Bartosh, JD

General Introduction

What a CRADA Is and Is Not

A cooperative research and development agreement (CRADA) is an agreement, "between one or more Federal laboratories and one or more non-Federal parties . . . toward the conduct of specified research or development efforts which are consistent with the missions of the laboratory."[1] CRADAs are usually multiyear agreements involving significant research projects.

A CRADA is the only agreement under which the government, "may grant, or agree to grant in advance, to a collaborating party patent licenses or assignments, or options thereto, in any invention made in whole or in part by a laboratory employee."[2] Prospective CRADA collaborators often see the grant of CRADA inventions rights as a prerequisite to their making the significant corporate investment required by most CRADA research projects.

In addition to the promise of intellectual property rights in advance, a CRADA can offer other significant advantages to a CRADA collaborator. Companies are able to leverage their existing personnel, facilities, and equipment, and to complement the skill sets of their employees with the scientific and engineering expertise of government professionals. Under a CRADA the federal laboratory may provide, "personnel, services, facilities, equipment . . . or other resources."[3]

Under a CRADA, the collaborator may provide, "funds, personnel, services, facilities, equip-

ment . . . or other resources."[4] CRADAs are one of the few mechanisms that the federal government has to receive nonappropriated funds from the private sector.[5]

CRADAs are not funding agreements. That is, the nonfederal party to a CRADA may not receive funds from the federal party under the agreement. In fact, under a CRADA, quite the opposite is true. As discussed above, the nonfederal party *may provide* funds to the federal party under the CRADA.

CRADAs are also not acquisition contracts for the procurement of the research and development services of a federal laboratory. CRADAs should not divert the research and development activities of the federal laboratory to serve only the purposes of the collaborating party. The CRADA research project must be consistent with the missions of the federal laboratory involved.[6]

CRADAs also are not an alternative route to the licensing of already existing federal laboratory patents. If such patents comprise background intellectual property rights necessary to practice a CRADA invention, the collaborator must separately license such patents according to the terms and conditions of the relevant federal regulations.[7]

Legislation Related to CRADAs

The Stevenson-Wydler Technology Innovation Act of 1980 made federal agencies responsible for transferring federal technology to state and local governments and to the private sector.[8] The Federal Technology Transfer Act (FTTA) of 1986, the first amendment to the Stevenson-Wydler Technology

Innovation Act, made technology transfer a specific responsibility of each and every federal science or engineering laboratory professional.[9] The Federal Technology Transfer Act of 1986 also gave federal agencies and their scientific and engineering professional staff the authority to enter into CRADAs.[10] Several public laws have amended the Stevenson-Wydler Technology Innovation Act since 1986, with only minor modifications to the basic CRADA authority.[11]

The purpose of the Federal Technology Transfer Act of 1986 was "to improve the transfer of commercially useful technologies from the Federal laboratories and into the private sector."[12] The FTTA addressed the concern that agencies, "need[ed] clear authority to do cooperative research and that they need[ed] to be able to exercise that authority at the laboratory level."[13] The CRADA authority would improve the ability of federal laboratories to interact with state, local and private sector institutions. A major goal of the legislation was to realize the full potential of federal research to the benefit of the national defense, the public health, and the national economy.[14] Among the economic considerations of the legislation was the welfare of small businesses, as well as those businesses agreeing to manufacture CRADA subject inventions in the United States. The FTTA provided that in deciding whom to collaborate with, each federal laboratory director, "shall . . . give special consideration to small business firms and consortia involving small business firms;[15] and . . . give preference to business units located in the United States which agree that products made under the [CRADA] . . . will be manufactured substantially in the United States."[16]

Case Law Related to CRADAs

There are only a few significant cases related to CRADAs to date. They have involved deciding between a procurement contract and a CRADA; defining a federal "laboratory"; and exempting CRADA data from disclosure under the Freedom of Information Act (FOIA).

In *Chem. Service, Inc. v. Environmental Protection Agency*,[17] the court dealt with an issue that many technology transfer professionals have faced. That is, deciding whether a particular proposed relationship is more appropriately a procurement contract or a CRADA. The Third Circuit's decision drew the distinction between the two mechanisms based on the amount of research and development that still needed to be done. That is, if the govern-

ment can simply contract for services or products that require no further R&D, then it should.

In *Edmonds Institute v. Babbitt*,[18] the court determined that a National Park (in this case, Yellowstone) qualified as a "laboratory" that could enter into a CRADA because it had facilities and staff engaged in the conduct of research.

In *DeLorme Publishing Co., Inc. v. Nat'l Oceanic & Atmospheric Admin.*,[19] government records generated in anticipation of entering into a CRADA were exempted from disclosure under the FOIA pursuant to 15 USC § 3710a(c)(7), which provides protection from disclosure through 5 USC § 552(b)(3) ("FOIA Exemption 3").[20]

Patent Rights under CRADAs

Definition of a Subject Invention

The intellectual property terms of CRADAs relate to subject inventions. Subject inventions are inventions "conceived or first actually reduced to practice" under the CRADA.[21] Therefore, it is possible for an invention that is conceived (or conceived and constructively reduced to practice by filing a patent application) to become a subject invention if it is first actually reduced to practice under the CRADA.

The CRADA's Core Promise

There is one major reason why a nonfederal party would both want and need to use a CRADA to formalize its research collaboration with the government—during the research project, government laboratory staff may invent. If a license to the resulting government patent is not promised in advance to the collaborator under a CRADA, the government patent may be licensed to the collaborator's competitors or other interested parties under federal licensing regulations. Since companies are usually very interested in maintaining as much control as possible over inventions related to their existing portfolios, a CRADA is often the mechanism of choice for collaborating with federal government scientists. As discussed above, a CRADA is the only mechanism under which the government can grant intellectual property rights in advance to a collaborator.

Patent Rights the Government Conveys and Retains under CRADAs

Under a CRADA, "[t]he laboratory shall ensure . . . that the collaborating party has the option to choose an exclusive license for a pre-negotiated field of use for any such invention under the agreement."[22] In consideration for this option, the collaborator grants the government the right to a nonexclusive license to CRADA subject inventions made solely by the collaborator.[23] The collaborator must also agree that for those CRADA subject inventions made by the government and licensed exclusively to the collaborator, the government shall retain a nonexclusive license[24] and the right to require the grant of a license to a third party.[25]

The government use license to sole collaborator inventions is a "nonexclusive, nontransferable, irrevocable, paid-up license to practice the invention or have the invention practiced throughout the world by or on behalf of the Government for research or other Government purposes."[26] Under the law, this government use license is to be "normally" granted.[27] That is, the government has some discretion in this regard. It is the policy and practice of the National Institutes of Health (NIH) to always require the grant of this government use license.[28]

The government also retains a nonexclusive license to government CRADA inventions that are licensed exclusively to the collaborator.[29] This license is not intended to complicate a CRADA collaborator's commercialization efforts. Exclusive licensing can be a reasonable and necessary incentive to acquire the investment and make the expenditure to bring a CRADA invention to practical application or to otherwise promote the invention's utilization by the public. Therefore, in the exercise of this retained nonexclusive license, the government cannot "publicly disclose trade secrets or commercial or financial information that is privileged or confidential."[30]

If a government CRADA invention is exclusively licensed to the collaborator, the government also retains the right to "require the collaborating party to grant to a responsible applicant a nonexclusive, partially exclusive, or exclusive license to use the invention . . . or . . . to grant the license itself."[31] The government can only require such a third party license under "exceptional circumstances and only if the Government determines that . . . the action is necessary to meet health or safety needs . . . not reasonably satisfied by the collaborating party; . . . to meet requirements of public use . . . not reasonably satisfied by the collaborating party; or . . . the collaborating party has failed to comply with an agreement [relating to U.S. manufacture]."[32] Collaborators disagreeing with a determination can pursue an administrative appeal and/or seek judicial review.[33]

Nonpatent Issues Related to CRADAs

Data, Publications, FOIA

Depending upon the missions of the laboratory involved, the duration of the government's confidentiality obligation will be limited to varying degrees. For example, the NIH, which has among its missions the maintenance of research freedom for its scientists and the dissemination of research results,[34] normally agrees to maintain confidential information for only three years after termination of a CRADA.[35]

Similarly, the NIH will normally delay publication only for as long as it takes to file any necessary patent application.[36]

Regardless of which federal agency is involved, certain CRADA-related information is subject to public disclosure under the Freedom of Information Act (FOIA).[37] However, there are statutory bases for withholding from disclosure the commercial or financial confidential information of a collaborator. These include 5 USC § 552(b)(4) (FOIA Exemption 4) and 15 USC § 3710a(c)(7)(A), which is applicable through 5 USC § 552(b)(3) (FOIA Exemption 3). *The Freedom of Information Act Guide and Privacy Act Overview* describes FOIA Exemption 4 as "intended to protect the interests of both the Government and submitters of information," including "safeguarding [submitters of information] from the competitive disadvantages that could result from disclosure." It goes on to state that "[e]xamples of items regarded as commercial or financial information include: . . . research data . . . and operating costs."[38]

Chapter 15 USC §3710a(c)(7)(A) specifically prohibits the disclosure of the commercial or financial confidential information of a CRADA collaborator, and is applicable through 5 USC § 552(b)(3) (FOIA Exemption 3), which states that FOIA "does not apply to matters that are . . . specifically exempted from disclosure by statute."

In addition, 35 USC § 122 and 35 USC § 205 provide protection from disclosure for materials specifically related to patent applications. Chapter 35 USC § 122 exempts unpublished patent applications from disclosure under FOIA,[39] and 35 USC § 205 exempts, for a reasonable time, records relating to inventions not yet filed as patent applications.

Human Subjects Data, Human Subjects Regulations, and the Privacy Rule Under HIPAA

The NIH often conducts human clinical trials under CRADAs with pharmaceutical companies. Human subjects research data is shared with pharmaceutical companies collaborating with the NIH under the following four conditions: (1) the data "cannot be linked to individual subjects, either directly or through codes;" (2) the data is coded and there is "a written agreement that unequivocally prohibits release of identifiers to the company;" (3) the company has access and review of the data "solely for purposes of on-site quality auditing, where (i) a written agreement unequivocally prohibits use or release of such information for other purposes, and (ii) the IRB-approved protocol and informed consent document clearly describe this practice;" (4) "[the c]ompan[y] . . . receive[s] identifiable private information solely for purposes of satisfying FDA reporting requirements, where (i) a written agreement unequivocally prohibits use or release of such information for other purposes, and (ii) the IRB-approved protocol and informed consent document clearly describe this practice." [40]

Parties to clinical trial CRADAs should ensure that they are in compliance with any relevant Department of Health and Human Services (DHHS) and Food and Drug Administration (FDA) Protection of Human Subjects Regulations.[41,42] Parties to clinical trial CRADAS should also ensure that they are in any necessary compliance with the "Privacy Rule" (Standards for Privacy of Individually Identifiable Health Information)[43,44] recently issued by the DHHS under the Health Insurance Portability and Accountability Act (HIPAA) of 1996.[45,46]

Copyrights, Trademarks, and Service Marks

The Federal Technology Transfer Act does not address intellectual property rights in copyrights, trademarks, or service marks. Yet, these types of intellectual property can certainly be important to a CRADA research project. For example, CRADAs for the development of software or software-related products can result in copyrightable material. While federal employees cannot copyright the work product of their official duties,[47] the federal government can accept assignment of copyrights from nongovernment owners of such rights. It is often important to the federal laboratory to be able to reproduce and disseminate copyrightable materials generated by the CRADA collaborator, so this issue should be addressed up front.

Trademarks and service marks may also be issues that should be addressed. They become important when, for example, the CRADA project will improve a product or service that the collaborator already has on the market or an information product that the government already maintains for the public.

The Naval Research Laboratory (NRL) CRADA boilerplate deals with copyrights and both trademarks and service marks in the following way. The collaborator can take copyright, and then grants a nonexclusive, irrevocable, paid-up license to the government.[48] Both collaborator and the government may establish and file applications to register trademarks and service marks, and each grants to the other a paid-up, irrevocable, nonexclusive license.[49,50]

Indemnification

There are general Constitutional and statutory prohibitions against federal employees committing government funds in advance of their appropriation by Congress, absent specific statutory authority.[51,52] Inasmuch as federal budgets are appropriated by Congress on a fiscal year cycle, indemnification against future years' claims would therefore be prohibited absent specific statutory authorization. The government receives no authority from the CRADA statutes to indemnify CRADA collaborators. If a federal agency has no other statutory authority under which to indemnify its CRADA collaborator, this may be of special concern to the collaborator when the research project could give rise to liability to third parties, such as in human clinical trials. With respect to those CRADAs involving state government-based institutions, and in particular academic research institutions that are state and/or land-grant institutions, indemnification by the state institutions also may specifically be prohibited by state statute and/or constitution. In the case of the clinical trials CRADA, these prohibitions may pose unique challenges to the acquisition of good and sufficient data to satisfy the objectives of the collaboration.

Governing Law

Because the federal government is a party to the CRADA, the law governing the CRADA is federal law, as applied by the federal courts in the District of Columbia. Because state universities are subject to the laws and constitutions of their own individual states, when a state university is a party to a CRADA, the language concerning governing law can be changed to be both federal law and the laws of the state, with federal law prevailing in the event of a conflict.

Absence of Endorsement

The government's participation in a CRADA, and in the development of products thereunder, must not be used by the collaborator as an endorsement of its commercial activities. This is usually expressly stated in the CRADA document and reflected in language providing for government review and comment on proposed press releases.

Model CRADA Agreements, Examples of Agency-Specific Policies and Terms

This section examines the distinctions between two federal laboratories' implementation of the CRADA authority to grant licenses or options to licenses in advance.[53] The distinctions demonstrate how different federal agencies have adopted different policies for the conveyance of intellectual property under their CRADA programs. The distinctions emphasize why, in addition to becoming familiar with the relevant statutes, a company considering entering into a CRADA with a laboratory should also become familiar with the CRADA policy of that laboratory.

NIH

The National Institutes of Health (NIH) is an agency of the Public Health Service in the Department of Health and Human Services. It conducts and supports research to advance the public health.[54] The standard NIH CRADA grants the collaborator an exclusive option to elect an exclusive or nonexclusive commercialization license. The NIH CRADA boilerplate does not address rights in copyrights or trademarks—rights that are not addressed by the CRADA statute. These rights are negotiated on a case-by-case basis, depending upon the nature of the research project.

The PHS model CRADA used by the NIH consists of a boilerplate agreement and related appendices.[55] The appendices include a research plan, a description of the financial and staffing contributions of the parties, and a list of exceptions or modifications to the standard agreement. In addition, the NIH has developed specialized appendices for use in CRADAs involving human clinical trials.

NRL

The NRL describes itself as the Navy's "corporate research laboratory," engaged in scientific research and technology development related to the Navy's environment.[56] It is the policy and practice of the NRL to grant CRADA collaborators a paid-up royalty-free, nonexclusive license to CRADA subject inventions made by NRL investigators.[57] This is in addition to the option for an exclusive license to

subject inventions made by NRL investigators. The NRL CRADA also includes cross-licenses between the parties for rights in copyrights and trademark—rights that are not addressed by the CRADA statute.

The standard Navy CRADA used by the NRL also consists of a boilerplate agreement and related appendices.[58] The appendices to the NRL CRADA include a statement of work and a confirmatory license agreement.

Parties to a CRADA

Government and Corporation

The CRADA between the government (either a federal agency or a national lab) and a commercial enterprise is perhaps the most common CRADA relationship. This relationship is designed to promote and enhance the development of US industry and the US manufacture of goods. The federal government has gone further to specifically promote the development of small business interests by providing that federal agencies give "special consideration" to small businesses when deciding on a CRADA collaborator.[59] In addition, federal agencies are to give "preference" to those "business units located in the United States which agree that products embodying inventions made under the [CRADA] . . . will be manufactured substantially in the United States . . . ."[60] It should be noted, however, that the United States has prohibitions against doing business with certain foreign entities, and that if there is a question with regard to a particular proposed collaborator, that advice of counsel should be sought in order to avoid potentially severe penalties.

Government and Nonprofit/University

A CRADA between an academic research institution and a federal agency or national laboratory takes on a unique flavor, by virtue of the nonprofit status of the academic institution (where such nonprofit status is established pursuant to Internal Revenue Service regulations). It is important to keep in mind that the CRADA instrument establishes the terms of the research relationship, including the option granted for license of technology that may be developed by the federal participant(s), but the CRADA instrument stops short of defining the details of the economic and legal relationship of the parties postinvention. When an invention is born from the research relationship, the parties must enter into a new, inter-institutional agreement (IIA). The IIA defines the roles and responsibilities of each party for patent and commercialization purposes. Further, the IIA establishes guidelines for patent enforcement, as well as a mutually acceptable royalty sharing and distribution framework.

Pre- and postinvention terms are necessarily separate, since a CRADA is unable to establish terms related to the commercialization of intellectual property that has yet to be created. This is further bolstered by the limitations imposed on academic research institutions and other nonprofit entities by the Internal Revenue Service, through the Private Activity Bond Act, as set out in Revenue Procedure 97-14.

Government and More Than One Collaborator

The CRADA relationship may incorporate more than two collaborating parties. The most frequent example of a multiple party CRADA is the case of the clinical trial CRADA that contemplates a multi-center clinical trial. The CRADA statute provides that "if there is more than one collaborating party, that the collaborating parties are offered the option to hold licensing rights that collectively encompass the rights that would be held . . . by one party." [61]

How a Company or a University May Be a Participant in a CRADA, but Not a Party to the CRADA

Quite often, a portion of what either the federal laboratory or the collaborator has agreed to do under the CRADA will be done on their behalf by others (for example, by grantees or contractors). This has the potential to result in third parties holding rights to inventions that would otherwise have been CRADA-subject inventions. Therefore, corresponding provisions must be made in the CRADA document and in the separate third party agreements, to maintain the integrity of the parties' mutual CRADA promises with regard to intellectual property.

Conducting Clinical Trials as a Grantee under a Federally Funded Cooperative Agreement

The National Cancer Institute (NCI), a component institute of the NIH, can conduct human clinical trials under CRADAs through its extramural cooperative group grantees. Under the Bayh-Dole Act, these grantees would normally retain rights to their own inventions. However, in order to assure

CRADA collaborators of the intellectual property exclusivity that they desire, NCI asks its grantees to voluntarily agree to "grant to collaborator: (i) a paid-up nonexclusive, nontransferable, royalty-free, world-wide license to all [grantee] Institution Inventions for research purposes only; and (ii) a time-limited first option to negotiate an exclusive, world-wide royalty-bearing license for all commercial purposes." [62] This promise is sufficient to make these extramural inventions as if they had been government inventions under the CRADA.

Contracting to the Government or Its CRADA Collaborator

Collaborators often conduct a portion of their obligations under CRADAs through contracts. In negotiating these contracts, a collaborator should ensure that all contractor inventions are assigned to the collaborator. The inventions then are as if they had been collaborator inventions under the CRADA.

CRADA Case Studies

A CRADA for the Development of a New Pharmaceutical

In this example, a government contractor has identified a natural product extract that arrests the growth of cancer cells *in vitro*. The active ingredient is purified, and enough compound is finally generated to do preclinical and early clinical studies. These studies show great promise against a type of cancer for which there is currently no effective treatment. Expanded clinical trials are warranted. But if the government works alone, extraction of sufficient quantities of the naturally occurring compound will consume the agency's human and financial resources at the expense of many other projects. In addition, harvesting the natural product will negatively impact protected old growth forestland and the habitat of endangered animal species, unless carefully coordinated with other federal agencies responsible for these natural resources. A synthetic or semisynthetic version of the compound that would avoid these complications is years away—and lives are at stake. The government decides to establish a CRADA with a pharmaceutical company with the expertise and the resources to assume responsibility for the rapid, large-scale procurement of the needed raw material and its purification into clinical grade material. In addition, the collaborator will be expected to collaborate in the conduct of clinical trials and to seek regulatory approval from the FDA for the new compound. There is no patent on the compound, and so a license cannot be used to give a company the promise of exclusivity to provide the necessary incentive to engage in these activities. And there is no promise that the compound will ultimately obtain FDA approval for marketing (in fact, most new compounds never make it to final approval). A CRADA is used to provide the necessary incentive, by providing the collaborator with exclusive access to the clinical data, as well as an option in advance to license any CRADA subject inventions made by the government. At the same time, and separate from the CRADA, both the federal agency and the pharmaceutical company fund research grants directed at identifying a synthetic or semisynthetic method of production of the compound. A semisynthetic method is successfully developed under a grant from the pharmaceutical company, and is ultimately used to produce the FDA-approved version of the drug developed under the CRADA.

A CRADA for the Development of a New Genomics/Proteomics Research and Clinical Laboratory Device

In this example, government scientists have developed a manual procedure to dissect out single cancer cells from diseased tissue. This procedure will greatly facilitate the genomic and proteomic study of cancer cells in different stages of the disease's progression. Hundreds of research labs around the world will want to be able to practice this invention quickly, easily and reproducibly. An automated device would also have utility for the clinical diagnosis and treatment of cancer. The government enters into a CRADA with a company that has licensed the government invention. Under the CRADA, an automated clinical workstation and related products are developed. These are successfully marketed and placed in labs throughout the world.

CRADA "Legends"

There are several commonly held beliefs, or CRADA "legends," that have caused some organizations to avoid collaborating with the government.

Potential CRADA collaborators of the NIH are often concerned that because they collaborate with the government for the development of new drugs, the government will set the market price for that drug. The reality is that, while the government certainly has a concern that the public benefit from the

results of its participation, there is no pricing clause in the NIH CRADA boilerplate. What was previously referred to as the "pricing clause" was removed by NIH after public discussion.

Potential CRADA collaborators are often concerned that the government will require modification of their CRADA license and force a sublicense to a third party. The reality is that the CRADA provides for a third party license only in exceptional circumstances and only if the action is necessary to meet health or safety needs that are not reasonably satisfied by the collaborator. Any such determination is subject to administrative appeal and judicial review.

Potential CRADA collaborators are often concerned that the nonexclusive license that the government retains when it exclusively licenses its CRADA subject inventions to the collaborator will complicate the collaborator's commercialization efforts. As discussed earlier, the government recognizes that exclusivity can be a necessary incentive to invest in new product development, and in the practice of its use license, the government cannot "publicly disclose trade secrets or commercial or financial information that is privileged or confidential." [63]

Potential CRADA collaborators are often concerned that their confidential information will become publicly available if they work with the government. The reality is that the Freedom of Information Act provides exemption from disclosure for "trade secrets and commercial or financial information . . . [that is] privileged or confidential." [64]

Potential CRADA collaborators are often concerned that a CRADA will take forever to negotiate because of the government bureaucracy. The reality is that the complexity of the project and the bureaucracies on both sides determine the duration of the negotiation. In addition, a letter of intent can be used to let the research begin, while negotiations are concluded.

Past, Present, and Future of the CRADA Program

When the CRADA legislation was passed, several federal agencies entered into CRADAs in numbers sufficient to be characterized as a CRADA "bubble" once the activity decreased. In the case of some of these agencies, CRADA activity decreased because more flexible, alternative mechanisms were available. Not all agencies experienced the CRADA bubble, however. For example, within the DHS, the

NIH has had a moderate number of CRADAs executed on a more consistent basis. And for those organizations without more flexible alternative public private partnership mechanisms, CRADAs will likely take on even more importance in the future as organizations face ever-increasing demands on their limited resources.

Authors' Note

This chapter provides educational information only, and does not constitute legal advice on the subject matter of CRADAs. This chapter is a derivative work based substantially on a portion of an earlier paper co-authored by K. Sybert, entitled "Government Funding and Research & Development Collaborations with Biotech Companies," which appeared in the Practicing Law Institute course handbook, "Biotechnology 2003: Biotechnology Patents and Business Strategies" (R. Berholtz and S.P. Ludwig, co-chairs). K. Sybert co-authored this chapter as part of her official duties while an employee of the US Government. In accordance with 17 USC § 105, no copyright protection is available for either work under US law.

• • • Endnotes

1. *15 U.S. Code* § 3710a(d)(1) (2000).
2. *15 U.S. Code* § 3710a(b)(1) (2000).
3. *15 U.S. Code* § 3710a(d)(1) (2000).
4. *15 U.S. Code* § 3710a(d)(1) (2000).
5. Other ways in which the federal government can receive nonappropriated funds from the private sector include gifts and license royalties.
6. *15 U.S. Code* § 3710a(d)(1) (2000).
7. *37 Code of Federal Regulations*, part 404 (2002).
8. *Stevenson-Wydler Technology Innovation Act of 1980*, Pub. L. 96-480, § 11, 94 Stat. 2311 (1980).
9. *Federal Technology Transfer Act of 1986*, Pub. L. 99-502, § 4, 100 Stat. 1785 (1986), codified at 15 U.S. Code 3710(a)(2) (2000).
10. *Federal Technology Transfer Act*, § 2, codified at 15 U.S. Code § 3710a(a)(1) (2000).
11. Pub. L. 100-418, 102 Stat. 1107 (1988); Pub. L. 100-519, 102 Stat. 2589 (1988); Pub. L. 101-189, 103 Stat. 1352 (1989) (enabling government-owned contractor-operated federal laboratories to enter into CRADAs); Pub. L. 102-25, 105 Stat. 75 (1991); Pub. L. 102-245,

106 Stat. 7 (1992); Pub. L. 102-484, 106 Stat. 2640 (1992); Pub. L. 104-113, 110 Stat. 775 (1996) (further defining the option to an exclusive license to CRADA subject inventions); Pub. L. 106-404, 114 Stat. 1742 (2000).
12. S. Rep. 99-283, at 1 (1986).
13. H.R. Conf. Rep. 99-953, at 15 (1986).
14. S. Rep. 99-283, at 2 (1986).
15. *15 U.S. Code* § 3710a(c)(4)(A) (2000).
16. *15 U.S. Code* § 3710a(c)(4)(B) (2000).
17. 12 F. 3d 1256 (3d Cir. 1993).
18. 42 F. Supp. 2d 1 (D.D.C. 1999), *sum. j. granted*, 93 F. Supp. 2d 63 (2000).
19. 917 F. Supp. 867 (D. Me. 1996).
20. See a more detailed discussion of these grounds for exemption from disclosure infra under "Data, Publications, FOIA."
21. *35 U.S. Code* § 201(e) (2000).
22. *15 U.S. Code* § 3710a(b)(1) (2000).
23. *15 U.S. Code* § 3710a(b)(2) (2000).
24. *15 U.S. Code* § 3710a(b)(1)(A) (2000).
25. *15 U.S. Code* § 3710a(b)(1)(B) (2000).
26. *15 U.S. Code* § 3710a(b)(2) (2000).
27. *15 U.S. Code* § 3710a(b)(2) (2000).
28. PHS CRADA Model Agreements, http://ott.nih.gov/docs/CRADAModel/2005.doc (accessed October 16, 2005). Includes the grant of a government use license to sole collaborator inventions at article 7.4.
29. *15 U.S. Code* § 3710a(b)(1)(A) (2000).
30. *15 U.S. Code* § 3710a(b)(1)(A) (2000).
31. *15 U.S. Code* § 3710a(b)(1)(B) (2000).
32. *15 U.S. Code* § 3710a(b)(1)(C) (2000).
33. *15 U.S. Code* § 3710a(b)(1)(C) (2000).
34. PHS CRADA Policy, last updated March 6, 2000, http://ott.od.nih.gov/crada_policy.html (accessed October 16, 2005).
35. The NIH model CRADA at article 8.6 provides that "[t]he Collaborator may request an extension to this term when necessary to protect Proprietary Information relating to products not yet commercialized." PHS CRADA Model Agreements http://ott.nih.gov/docs/CRADAModel/2005.doc (accessed October 16, 2005).
36. PHS CRADA Model Agreement at article 8.7.
37. *5 U.S. Code* § 552 (2000).
38. U.S. Department of Justice, Office of Information and Privacy, *The Freedom of Information Act Guide* (2004). http://www.usdoj.gov/oip/foi_act.htm (accessed October 16, 2005).
39. See Irons & Sears v. Dann, 577 F. 2d 610 (9th Cir. 1978), cert. denied, 439 U.S. 1073 (1978).
40. Memorandum from Director, Division of Human Subject Protection, OPRR, to Director

Division of Human Subject Protections, OPRR, December 23, 1999, http://www.hhs.gov/ohrp/humansubjects/guidance/guid1223.pdf (accessed October 16, 2005). Note that the Office for Protection from Research Risks (OPRR) is now the Office of Human Research Protections (OHRP) within the OPHS, DHHS.

41. HHS Protection of Human Subjects Regulations, 45 *Code of Federal Regulations*, part 46 (2002).

42. FDA Protection of Human Subjects Regulations, 21 *Code of Federal Regulations*, part 50, 56 (2003).

43. Standards for Privacy of Individually Identifiable Health Information, 45 *Code of Federal Regulations*, part 160, 164 A, E (2002).

44. DHHS Office for Civil Rights—HIPAA. "National Standards to Protect the Privacy of Medical Health Information," http://www.hhs.gov/ocr/hipaa (accessed June 16, 2003) (linking to the text of the HIPAA privacy rule).

45. *Health Insurance Portability and Accountability Act of 1996*, Pub. L. 104-191, 110 Stat. 1936 (1996) (codified as amended in scattered sections of 18, 26, 29, and 42 U.S. Code).

46. DHHS Office for Civil Rights—HIPAA.

47. 17 *U.S. Code* § 105 (2000).

48. "Standard Navy Cooperative Research and Development Agreement between the Naval Research Laboratory and XYZ Corporation," at article 7.2 (5th ed., rev. May 3, 2001), http://techtransfer.nrl.navy.mil/pdfs/standard_crada.pdf (accessed June 16, 2003).

49. "Standard Navy Cooperative Research and Development Agreement between the Naval Research Laboratory and XYZ Corporation," at article 7.3, 2001.

50. For a more thorough discussion of the treatment of nonpatent intellectual property under CRADAs, see Bruce D. Goldstein et al., "Cooperative Research and Development Agreements," at § 10.4 in *Association of University Technology Managers (AUTM) Manual* (2002) (manuscript on file with author).

51. U.S. Const. art. I, § 9.

52. 31 *U.S. Code* § 1341(a)(1)(B)(2004).

53. For a broader overview of the CRADA programs of several federal agencies, including how to find out about CRADA opportunities with them, see Bruce D. Goldstein et al., at § 10.5. For example, NASA will not enter into a CRADA unless the proposed collaboration cannot be established using a *Space Act* agreement.

54. USDHHS. "National Institutes of Health: The Nation's Medical Research Agency," last updated May 17, 2004, http://www.nih.gov/about/NIHoverview.html (accessed October 3, 2005).

55. See discussion of key provisions of this and other CRADA boilerplates *infra* Section II J.

56. US Naval Research Laboratory Web site, http://www.nrl.navy.mil (accessed June 16, 2003).

57. "Standard Navy Cooperative Research and Development Agreement between the Naval Research Laboratory and XYZ Corporation," 2001.

58. "Standard Navy Cooperative Research and Development Agreement between the Naval Research Laboratory and XYZ Corporation," 2001.

59. 15 *U.S. Code* § 3710a(c)(4)(A)(2000).

60. 15 *U.S. Code* § 3710a(c)(4)(B)(2000).

61. 15 *U.S. Code* § 3710a(b)(1)(2000); referring specifically to the option to choose an exclusive license for a prenegotiated field of use for CRADA subject inventions.

62. National Cancer Institute. "Intellectual Property Option to Collaborator," revised September 12, 2003, http://ctep.cancer.gov/industry/ipo.html (accessed October 3, 2005).

63. 15 *U.S. Code* § 3710a(b)(1)(A) (2000).

64. 5 *U.S. Code* § 552(b)(4) (2000).

A

Selected Glossary of Common Terms

This glossary contains short, concise definitions of common terms in research administration. The definitions provided here may not be complete or all-encompassing.

A

A-21 Cost Principles for Educational Institutions Outlines the principles for determining costs applicable to federal grants, contracts, and other federal agreements (also known as "sponsored projects") with educational institutions.

A-87 Cost Principles for State and Local Governments and Recognized Indian Tribal Governments Uniform administrative requirements for grants, contracts and other agreements for state and local governments and Recognized Indian Tribal Governments.

A-110 Grants and Agreements with Institutions of Higher Education Defines uniform administrative requirements for federal grants and agreements with institutions of higher education, hospitals, and other nonprofit organizations.

A-122 Cost Principles for Nonprofit Organizations Uniform administrative requirements for grants, contracts and other agreements; does not cover educational institutions, state and local governments or recognized Indian Tribal Governments *Also see A-87.*

A-133 Audits of States, Local Governments, and Nonprofit Organizations Federal agency standards for the audit of states, local governments, and non-profit agencies who are recipients of federal awards.

Allocable Costs Allowable costs that benefit the grant or contract to which they are charged.

Allowable Costs Appropriate costs that can be charged to a grant (e.g., salaries and equipment, but not alcoholic beverages).

Application Request for financial support of a project and/or activity that is submitted to a sponsoring agency.

Appropriation Funds authorized by Congress and provided to federal agencies to support grant awards.

Assistance Agreement *See* Grant.

Assurance Statement attesting to institution's or organization's compliance with federal regulations (e.g., Civil Rights, Title IX, Human Subjects) that is necessary in order to qualify for federal funding.

Audit Formal examination of an organization's or individual's financial account management. An audit may also include examination of compliance with applicable terms, laws, and regulations.

Authorization Congressional legislation establishing a specific program.

Authorized Signature Signature of person legally responsible for making agreements on behalf of an organization; signature must appear on an application before it can be officially considered; implies that if an award is accepted, the responsibility for its proper administration is assured.

Authorizing Official The individual or individuals authorized to act on behalf of the organization.

Award   Provision of funds, based on an approved application or proposal and budget, to an organizational entity or an individual to carry out an activity or project.

B

Billing, Third Party   The party (typically an insurance company or Medicare or Medicaid) responsible for covering the cost of medical care or procedure. Especially relevant to clinical trials.

Block Grant   Lump sum funding given to a state or local governing agency based on a formula to be spent in generally eligible areas. Purposes are broadly defined and few restrictions are mandated from the funding source. Restrictions can be imposed by the agency to subrecipients.

Broad Agency Announcement (BAA)   Announcement (typically from the Department of Defense and/or defense-related agencies) regarding targeted research areas within a time period, and which reflects approved budget authorities for particular research areas.

Budget   Estimated cost of conducting the proposed project, consisting of direct/indirect costs, matching contribution (cost-sharing), and justification.

Budget Justification (Budget Explanation)   Clarification of the budget, noting determination of dollar amounts; the rationale for the requested budget amounts.

Budget Negotiation   Discussion between submitting organization and funding source prior to an award; initiated by the funding source; often involves modification of budget request, and results in budget reduction.

Budget Period   The interval of time—typically one year—into which the project period is divided for budgetary and funding purposes.

C

Carry-over or Carry-forward   Unexpended award funds that are allowed by the sponsor agency to be moved into the next funding period (typically one year).

CASB (Cost Accounting Standards Board)   A legislatively established board that oversees uniformity and consistency in cost accounting practices governing measurement, assignment, and allocation of contract funding by the US federal government.

Categorical Grants   Typically awarded to state or local governments for broad expenditures; somewhat more restricted than block grants.

Clinical Investigations   A scientific treatment plan or study outline for experimental procedures or treatments on human subjects; also known as Clinical Study or Clinical Trial.

Close Out   The final act or completion of all internal procedures and sponsor requirements needed to terminate or complete a research project.

Competing-Continuation   The extension of an actively funded project based on an application made in the same manner as a new application; the application is competitively reviewed.

Compliance Officer   Individual who is responsible for the oversight and day-to-day management of the integrity and/or regulatory compliance program of an institution.

Confidentiality Agreement   Agreement (may also be labeled secrecy agreement or nondisclosure or mutual nondisclosure agreement) signed by two or more parties that agree to maintain specified confidential information as confidential for a specified period of time. Agreement is typically subject to governing laws of the state or federal government. Depending on organizational policy, agreement may be signed by the institutional official or other individual(s) officially designated by the parties to the agreement.

Conflict of Commitment   When a party assumes responsibility outside of a primary employment and/or contract agreement, negatively affecting responsibility and duty to a primary employer and/or contractor.

Conflict of Interest   When a party receives compensation or holds an external position and the party can influence the conduct of a project that results in that party's personal gain.

Consultant   A participant, typically external to the institution, whose work on a project does not require a sub-award or subcontract, and who is compensated via a personal service agreement.

Contract   Legal document specifying type, scope, budget, and time period of work; typically resulting in a tangible product (deliverables).

Contracting Officers' Technical Representatives (COTRs)   Individuals appointed by sponsors' contracting officers to act as authorized representatives in the monitoring and administration of a contract. *Also see Program/Project Officer.*

Cooperative Agreement   An award similar to a grant, but in which the sponsor's staff may be actively involved in proposal preparation and have substantial involvement in research activities once the award has been made.

Copyright A form of protection provided by the laws of the United States (title 17, US Code) to the authors of "original works of authorship," including literary, dramatic, musical, artistic, and certain other intellectual works.

Cost Accounting Standards (CAS) Federally mandated accounting standards intended to ensure uniformity in budgeting and spending.

Cost Reimbursement Type Contract/Grant A contract/grant for which the sponsor funds all costs incurred (up to an agreed-upon amount) over the course of the project.

Cost Sharing Financial contribution by the grantee or a third party to project; typically less than one-third of the total cost; more common in research grants; a form of matching.

Cost Transfer Accounting term for the transfer of cost from one source to another. In federal funding, extensive or delayed cost transfers from one account or fund source can trigger concern regarding the appropriate expenditure of funds.

D

Data *See Research Data.*

Data Rights The maintenance of ownership and stewardship of scientific data and records for research projects. In the case of federal contracts/grants, FAR Clause Subpart 27.4-Rights in Data and Copyrights prescribes policies, procedures, and contract clauses pertaining to patents, and assists agencies in development of appropriate data and copyright coverage.

Debarment Action taken by a debarring official in accordance with regulations to exclude a person from participating in covered transactions. A person so excluded is debarred.

Demonstration Grant An award that allows a grantee to create a working model, typically meant to be reproduced by others.

Departmental Research Research, development, and other scholarly activities that are not organized research and are not separately budgeted and accounted. Defined in OMB A-21. *Also see Organized Research.*

Direct Costs Costs directly associated in the conduct of the sponsored project, including but not limited to salaries, fringe benefits, consultants, travel, equipment, supplies, patient care costs, and other project-specific costs.

Disallowance or Disallowed Costs Charges to a grant or contract that the federal agency determines to be unallowable in accordance with the applicable federal cost principles or other terms and conditions contained in the award. Typically, the sponsor does not pay for these expenditures, and the disallowed expenditure becomes the responsibility of the PI and must be transferred to another budget (non-federal) or receive after-the-fact approval from the sponsor.

Discretionary Grant An award made in accordance with legislation allowing the funding source to exercise reasonable freedom in selecting the project and the grantee and determining the amount of the award.

E

Effective Date Start date of an award; project costs generally may not be charged to a project until this date.

Effort Reporting Time reporting of effort on a sponsored project. For universities, effort on externally sponsored projects is reported based on a percent of time expended in overall effort (up to 100%) compared to other activities (e.g., teaching, service, research on other grants or contracts, patient care, consulting for the institution, etc.). Effort is not reported based on a forty-hour week or hours per week.

Electronic Data Interchange (EDI) Computer-application-to-computer-application exchange of business information in a standard electronic format. Translation software can aid in the exchange through the conversion of data from the application database into standard EDI format for transmission to one or more trading partners.

Electronic Funds Transfer (EFT) The electronic transfer of funds from one account to another; typically through an EFT software program.

Electronic Research Administration (ERA) The conduct of research administration utilizing electronic resources (e.g., the Internet, the World Wide Web, form templates, databases, and other electronic tools).

Encumbrances Obligations in the form of purchase orders, contracts or salary commitments chargeable to an award and for which a portion of the awarded amount is reserved. When paid, these cease to be encumbrances.

Environmental Health and Safety Frequently used to describe the collection of offices responsible for organizational compliance broadly relating to environment, health, and safety, also including radiological safety, laboratory safety, chemical safety, bio-safety, hazardous waste oversight and removal, and other areas as designated by an institution. Generally overseen by individuals and committees governed by federal regulations.

Equipment   Tangible assets over $5,000 with a life expectancy of more than one year, which are acquired through donation, gift, purchase, capital lease, or self-construction (federal definition).

Equity Investment into a program or company. The amount of equity is generally based upon a percent of gross or net profit accrued by a company and paid to the investing organization. For example, an institution may take equity interest in a company started by licensing the institution's intellectual property with a low royalty rate or waiver of fees.

Expanded Authorities   Operating authorities provided to grantees under certain research grant mechanisms that waive the requirement for agency approval for specified actions.

Expiration Date (Termination Date)   Last date of a project; no charges may be made to a project after this date. *Also see Duration Dates and Grant Period.*

Export Administration Regulation (EAR)   Designated in the Export Administration Act of 1979 (as amended), 50 USC app 2401-24220, controls the export, reexport, and other activities regarding the export of sensitive materials, person, or activities.

Export Control   *See Export Administration Regulation (EAR).*

F

Facility and Administration (F&A) Costs   Also known as Indirect Costs, overhead expenses indirectly associated with the sponsored project. Included are administrative expenses, utilities, physical plant maintenance, library facilities, etc.

False Claims Act   Covers fraud involving any federally funded contract or program with the exception of tax fraud. (US Code Title 31, Subtitle III, Financial Management, Chapter 3)

False Statement Act   Covers any false, fictitious or fraudulent statements or representations in any matter within the jurisdiction of any department or agency of the United States. (US Code, Title 18, Part I, Chapter 44, SC 1001)

FASB (Financial Accounting Standards Board)   Established to improve the financial standards, accounting, and reporting to the public. Many private institutions of higher education use FASB principles for accounting for gifts and endowments.

Federal Demonstration Program (FDP)   Program responsible for simplification of the federal rules governing all activities relating to submission and acceptance of grants and contracts between institutions of higher education and the federal government.

Federal Flow-through Funds   Funds received by the institution from nonfederal sponsor when the initial funding source is directly attributable to the federal government through a grant or contract to a nonfederal sponsor. Federal flow-through funds become federal funds upon receipt of an award to the institution, whereupon federal rules apply to the receipt, spending, and accounting of the funds, unless expressly exempted by the federal agency initially making the award.

Federal Sentencing Guidelines   Sentencing policies and practices for the federal criminal justice system. 2005 guidelines were published that define implementation of compliance programs for institutions, including sentencing guidelines for noncompliance. (US Sentencing Commission, US Code Title 28, Section 9941 (a)).

Fellowship   Award made directly to an individual in support of specific educational pursuits; recipients may be subject to service and/or payback requirements after the fellowship terminates.

Fiscal Compliance   Written or unwritten assurance that funds are appropriately spent and that the work is completed and at the highest standards.

Fixed-Price (FP) Type Contract/Grant   Contract/grant for which one party pays the other a predetermined price, regardless of actual costs, for services rendered; often a fee-for-service agreement.

Fraud   May be defined as a deliberate misrepresentation or misinterpretation which causes another individual or organization to suffer damages; includes lying to government agencies.

Freedom of Information Act (FOIA)   Federal statute that allows any person the right to obtain federal agency records unless the records (or part of the records) are protected from disclosure by any of the nine exemptions contained in the law. (US Code Section 552 (1), www.usdoj.gov)

Fringe Benefits   Employee benefits paid by the employer (e.g., FICA, Worker's Compensation, Withholding Tax, Insurance, etc.).

Full-Time Equivalent (FTE)   Percentage of full-time employment. For hourly paid personnel, FTE is used in the generation of time reports to calculate the number of hours to assign on the report. For salaried personnel, it is not used for calculation of hours, but to show general distribution of time and effort that equates to the distribution of cost. *Also see Percent of Effort.*

G

GASB (Government Accounting Standards Board)   Standards set by the GAS board to govern financial accounting and reporting for state and local governments, including public institutions. The Board consists of seven members from constituency groups that form the Financial Accounting Foundation, a 501 (c) 3 organization.

Gifts and Bequests   Awards given with few or no specified conditions. Gifts may establish an endowment or provide direct support for existing programs. Frequently, gifts are used to support developing programs for which other funding is not available. Lack of restrictions make gifts attractive sources of support.

Goals   General statements about anticipated project outcomes, more global in scope than objectives, and not typically measurable. Goals should be supported by well-stated objectives.

Grant   Award of financial or other assistance that does not hold the grantee to a rigid work plan; more flexible than a contract; grantee or the public are typical beneficiaries.

Grant Period   Period between "effective date" and "expiration date" when items may be charged against the grant or contract.

Grant/Contract Officer/Administrator   The sponsor's designated official responsible for the business management of a grant, cooperative agreement or contract. Typically serving as the counterpart to the business officer of the grantee/contractor organization, the grant/contract officer oversees the comprehensive review, negotiation, award, and administration of a grant or contract, and associated policies, regulations, and provisions. *Also see Program/Project Officer.*

Grantee Institution   Organization that receives a grant from a sponsor or cooperative agreement.

H

Health Insurance Portability and Accountability Act (HIPAA)   Provides standards for the electronic transmission of health information, regulates legal access of health information and areas related to human subjects research.

Human Tissue   Includes any tissue or fluid from the human body (e.g., tears, nails, blood, skin, etc.). Depending on the purpose and/or use by an organization, may not include identifiable organs or anatomical specimens or entire bodies.

I

Indirect Costs   Overhead expenses indirectly associated with the sponsored project. Included are administrative expenses, utilities, physical plant maintenance, library facilities, etc. *Also see Facility and Administration Costs.*

In-Kind Contribution   Service or item donated in lieu of dollars to the operation of a funded project; usually given by the grantee or a third party (e.g., donated equipment, speaker's time); if required should be referenced in budget as direct project cost, but as in-kind; must be auditable with letter of agreement as minimum of paper trail.

Institution   For purposes of research administration, refers to colleges, universities, independent research institutes, hospitals, other nonprofit organizations, and industry that conduct externally sponsored projects.

Institutional Animal Care and Use Committee (IACUC)   Reviews and approves all use of vertebrate animals in teaching and research; monitors care and use of animals in laboratory and research programs to ensure humane treatment of animals in accordance with applicable laws and regulations.

Institutional Review Board (IRB) for Research with Human Subjects   Reviews and approves all proposed research projects that involve human subjects to ensure that the rights of subjects are protected, that adequate and informed consent for their participation is obtained, and that any possible benefits of the research are commensurate with the risks involved.

Intellectual Property   As defined by the USPTO, it is a creative work or idea embodied in a form that can be shared or can enable others to recreate, emulate, or manufacture; protected by trademark, trade secret, or copyright.

Interdisciplinary Research   Generally defines research that crosses the boundaries of more than one scientific or scholarly discipline, and may focus on specific issues (also termed Cross-Disciplinary Research or Research at the Interface of Disciplines).

Intergovernmental Personnel Act (IPA)   Temporary assignments of personnel between governmental agencies and other qualified institutions for projects of mutual concern and benefit; under the Intergovernmental Personnel Act (IPA) Mobility Program. ((5 US Code, Section 3371 through 3375) (5CFR, Part 334)).

Invention   The USPTO defines an invention as any art or process, machine, manufacture, design or composition of matter, or any new and useful improvement thereof, or any variety of plant, which is or may be patentable under the patent laws of the United States.

Invention Disclosure   Formal disclosure of information regarding potentially legally protected invention.

ITAR (International Traffic in Arms Regulation)   Section 38 of the Arms Export Control Act (22 USC 2778) authorizes the President of the United States to control the export and import of defense articles and services.

J

Just in Time   In the research arena, generally refers to the process of providing assurances and other information at the point that it is needed. For example, NIH requires various approvals and assurances prior to an award being made, but not at the proposal stage.

L

License   Agreement between parties that allows intellectual property owned by one party to be transferred to another party for its use, manufacture, distribution, sales, and/or sublicensing. Terms and conditions are defined within the license agreement.

Licensing Fee   Fee charged by licensor to licensee when a license is issued for use of a protected intellectual property.

Limited Submission   The limitations placed by a sponsor on the submission of proposals. Generally these refer to the number of proposals that will be accepted from any given institution.

M

Matching Funds   Financial contribution by the grantee; common to capital and/or equipment grants when grantee and/or grantee's clients are the primary beneficiary; typically one-third or greater; a form of cost sharing.

Material Transfer Agreement (MTA)   Agreement between parties regarding the use and disposition of materials or information shared from one party to another. For example, if an industry shares a drug with a research institution, the MTA defines the terms for the use, ownership, and disposition of the drug.

Misconduct Integrity (Scientific Misconduct)   Fabrication, plagiarism, fraud, or other practices that seriously deviate from those that are commonly accepted within the scientific community for proposing, conducting, or reporting research. Does not include honest error or honest differences in interpretations or judgments of data.

Mission Agency   An agency of the federal government that has a specific or special mission (e.g., NIH, ONR, DOD, etc.)

MOA (Memoranda of Agreement)/MOU (Memoranda of Understanding)   Used by two or more parties to agree to specific activities, collaborations, and partnerships. The memoranda set the terms of the parties' relationship, but generally do not include the provision of funding to be handled by a grant or contract arrangement or other procurement.

Modified Total Direct Costs (MTDC)   Basic indirect costs calculated on a subset of direct costs, normally excluding equipment, patient care, space rental, alterations and renovations, and subcontract costs in excess of the first $25,000 of an award.

Modular Grants   Under the NIH Modular Grant Application and Award Initiative, applicants prepare simplified proposals that provide limited budget information in a narrative format; applicants do not have to submit other research support information until just prior to award. Applications are to request direct costs in $25,000 modules, up to a total direct costs request of $250,000 per year for all unsolicited new, revised, and competing continuation R01, R03, R15, R21, R41, and R43 grants and competing supplements. These include applications responding to RFAs for these mechanisms.

N

No Cost Extension   An extension of the period of performance beyond the expiration data that allows the principal investigator to complete a project; typically, no additional costs are provided.

Notice of Grant Award   The legally binding document that notifies the grantee and others that an award has been made, contains or references all terms and conditions of the award, and documents the obligations of federal funds. May be issued in letter or electronic format.

O

OAS–C3–Cost Principles for Hospitals   A guide for hospitals to establish cost principles and procedures for establishing indirect cost and patient care rates for grants and contracts.

Office of Management and Budget   US government office overseeing federal budgeting and expending; part of the Executive Branch.

Option Agreement   Agreement whereby the owner of intellectual property grants another party the right to review the intellectual property for a finite period of time before offering its use to other parties.

Organized Research   Research and development that is separately budgeted and accounted, as defined in OMB Circular A-21, including sponsored activities that are supported by external funds, university research that is supported by funds allocated internally, and other sponsored activity that is not considered instruction or organized research (e.g., public service).

Other Institutional Activities   Activities that may include health service projects, community service projects, testing services, clinical services, or consulting through the institution where the institution receives compensation for these activities conducted by an institution without sponsor support.

Other Sponsored Activities   Activities as defined in *Other Institutional Activities*, but those conducted by an institution with sponsor support.

Other Transaction Agreements (OTA)   Variation of a contractual agreement with fewer bid restrictions; the Bayh-Dole Act does not apply, therefore the sponsoring agency may retain all rights to intellectual property. *Also see Technology Investment Agreement.*

Overhead   *See Facility and Administration (F&A) Costs.*

P

Partnership Intermediary   Defined by the federal government as a program whereby an agency of a state or local government assists, counsels, advises, evaluates or otherwise cooperates with small business firms and institutions of higher education that can make demonstrably productive use of technology-related assistance from a federal laboratory.

Patent   A new, novel, and nonobvious invention qualified to receive protection under the US Patent law; may take many forms.

Patriot Act (USA Patriot Act of 2001)   The Uniting and Strengthening America by Providing Appropriate Tools Required to Intercept and Obstruct Terrorism Act gives broad powers to US government entities to carry out activities to ensure safety and protection of the United States. Includes numerous clauses pertaining to the conduct of academic institutions in education and research.

Personnel Action Notification (PAN)   Communication to human resources about information or data regarding an individual's employment at the institution; provides both job-related and personal information. A relatively new term, some institutions may use other terms or acronyms to define this activity.

Personnel Activity Report (PAR)   A system in accordance with government regulation, which consists of after-the-fact effort reports for all exempt employees who expend effort on sponsored projects for which reimbursement is claimed from the grantor and, in addition, exempt employees in a department associated with grants and contracts. A relatively new term, some institutions may use other terms or acronyms to define this activity.

Principal Investigator   Individual responsible for the conduct of research or other activity as designated in a proposal, usually for a single project.

Prior Approval   Written documentation of permission to alter any aspect of a funded project; includes programmatic and financial changes; may be obtained within grantee organization or from grantor depending upon the case in point and grantor policy.

Procurement   Agreement to purchase a specified good or service from a particular entity. Document can be used in place of a grant or contract document and may contain specific terms and conditions for the procurement.

Program Announcement   Announcement or solicitation by a sponsor of a program of funding; often used to stimulate research or interest in a particular area, but might have set aside funding amounts.

Program Income   Gross income earned by a grantee that is directly generated by the grant-supported project or activity or earned as a result of the award.

Program/Project Officer   Sponsor's designated individual officially responsible for the technical, scientific or programmatic aspects of a particular grant, cooperative agreement, or contract. Serving as the counterpart to the principal investigator/project director of the grantee/contractor organization, the program/project officer deals with the grantee/contractor organization staff to ensure program progress. *For definition of business officer, see Grant/Contract Officer.*

Project Period   The total time for which support of a project has been approved. The total project period is comprised of the initial competitive segment and subsequent competitive segment(s) resulting from a competing continuation award(s) and noncompeting extensions.

Project/Program Director Individual responsible for supervising the sponsored program for the funded agency. Usually applies to a large, multiproject part, cooperative agreement, or contract.

Proposal Application for funding that contains all information necessary to describe project plans, staff capabilities, and funds requested. Formal proposals are officially approved and submitted by an organization in the name of a principal investigator.

Publication Rights Terms in an agreement that define any limitations on publication of results or products of research or other sponsored activity.

R

Real Property Land, including land improvements, structures, and appurtenances, but not movable machinery and equipment.

Recharge Centers Operating centers that provide specialized services to the institution's community; services may be provided on an incidental basis to external users.

Regulatory Compliance Requirements and assurances with which an organization must comply if in receipt of federal funds. Noncompliance can result in debarment, fines, and legal recourse through the federal court system.

Representations and Certifications (Reps and Certs) Statements of compliance completed by the institution that must accompany federal contracts and proposals.

Request for Applications (RFA) Announcement by a funding source and distributed to potential grantees, which defines a targeted area of interest; used to stimulate research in a specific area; funding mechanism is by grant.

Request for a Proposal (RFP) Announcement by a funding source and distributed to potential grantees which defines a specific project and scope of work, and deliverable work product; funding mechanism is a contract.

Request for a Quotation (RFQ) Announcement by a funding source and distributed to potential respondents which generally defines the type of services/items in accordance with specifications within the price or price limitation, if any, set forth for each service/item.

Research Data Laboratory notebooks and/or any form or media format that records the necessary data to reconstruct and evaluate reported results, and the events and processes leading to research results.

Research, Training, and Other Sponsored Activity The three primary categories of activities covered by a federally negotiated cognizant agency that determines the facility and administrative rate for an organization.

Royalty Payments made by an entity that licenses intellectual property from a licensor. Terms and conditions of the payments vary according to license agreement.

S

Select Agent The US Departments of Health and Human Services and Agriculture regulations that govern the use of select agents that pose severe threat to public health and safety. The list of toxins and biologic agents are listed under 42 CFR, 7 CFR, and 9 CFR.

Small Business Innovation Research (SBIR) Program Federal program supporting private sector commercialization and R&D of federally sponsored technology projects; the program is especially supportive of small business participation.

Small Business Technology Transfer (STTR) Program Federal program that requires that a percentage of federal agency extramural research or R&D budget be reserved for small business awards to develop cooperative R&D with nonprofit research institutions.

Sponsored Research Research funded by an outside agency, either through grant, contract, or other transaction.

Stipend Payment made to an individual under a fellowship or training grant in accordance with pre-established support for the individual's living expenses during the period of training.

Subcontract/Award/Grant/Recipient Agreement or secondary contract in which a third party agrees to perform some of the activities defined in a primary proposal; terms are agreed to at the time of submission, but are not consummated until after the award has been made to the submitting organization.

Suspension Action taken by an official that immediately excludes a person from participating in covered transactions pending the completion of investigation and any subsequent legal, debarment, or Program Fraud Civil Remedies Act proceedings.

T

Technology Investment Agreement (TIA)   Used to carry out basic, applied, or advanced research projects when it is appropriate to use assistance agreements. The research will be performed in part by for-profit firms, especially if they are members of consortia. TIAs allow Department of Defense agencies to leverage financial investments made by for-profit firms in research related to commercial products and processes.

Technology Transfer   The process of moving laboratory based research into the marketplace. An institution's technology transfer office oversees the legal and administrative requirements of the transfer.

Technology Transfer Office (TTO)   Also known as Technology Commercialization Office (TCO), office within an institution responsible for the protections of the institution's intellectual property and the commercialization of it, including the legal and administrative requirements of the transfer.

Total Cost   The total cost of a project, including direct and indirect costs and voluntary and involuntary cost sharing or matching.

Total Direct Cost (TDC)   The total of all direct costs of a project.

Trade Secret   All forms and types of financial, business, scientific, technical, economic, or engineering information, whether tangible or intangible. Trade secret covers information whether or how stored, compiled, or memorialized physically, electronically, graphically, photographically or in writing, if (A) the owner thereof has taken reasonable measures to keep such information secret; and (B) the information derives independent economic value, actual or potential, from not being generally known and not being readily ascertainable through proper means by the public.

U

Unallowable Costs   Costs determined to be unallowable in accordance with the applicable cost principles or other terms and conditions contained in a grant award.

Unsolicited Proposal   Proposal initiated by the applicant that defines the project concept.

W

Warfighter   Used by the Department of Defense and other agencies and organizations to define the soldiers engaged in some aspect of war.

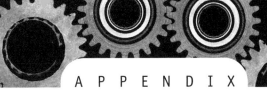

B

Acronyms

Index of Commonly Used Research Abbreviations and Acronyms

Agencies/Offices/Government

AFOSR	Air Force Office of Scientific Research
AFRRI	Armed Forces Radiobiology Research Institute
APHIS	Animal and Plant Health Inspection Service
ARO	Army Research Office
ARPA	Advanced Research Projects Agency
BLM	Bureau of Land Management (DOI)
CDC	Centers for Disease Control
DARPA	Defense Advanced Research Projects Agency
DED	Department of Education
DHHS or HHS	Department of Health and Human Services
DHS	Department of Homeland Security
DOC	Department of Commerce
DOD	Department of Defense
DOE	Department of Energy
DOI	Department of Interior
DOJ	Department of Justice
DOT	Department of Transportation
EPA	Environmental Protection Agency
FDA	Food and Drug Administration
FICE	Federal Interagency Committee on Education
FIPSE	Fund for the Improvement of Postsecondary Education
GAO	Government Accountability Office
HSARPA	Homeland Security Advanced Research Projects Agency
NAS	National Academy of Sciences
NASA	National Aeronautics and Space Administration
NATO	North Atlantic Treaty Organization
NEA	National Endowment for the Arts
NEH	National Endowment for the Humanities
NIH	National Institutes of Health
NIST	National Institute of Standards and Technology
NSF	National Science Foundation
OJJDP	Office of Juvenile Justice and Delinquency Prevention
ONR	Office of Naval Research
OSTP	Office of Science and Technology Policy
PHS	Public Health Service
PTO (USPTO)	Patent and Trademark Office
SAMHSA	Substance Abuse and Mental Health Services Administration
SBA	Small Business Administration

USAMRIID	United States Army Medical Research Institute of Infectious Diseases
USDA	United States Department of Agriculture
USGS	United States Geological Survey (DOI)
USUHS	Uniformed Services University of the Health Sciences
WHO	World Health Organization

National Institutes of Health (NIH) Institutes and Offices

CC	Clinical Center (Warren Grant Magnuson Clinical Center)
CIT	Center for Information Technology
CSR	Center for Scientific Review
FIC	John E. Fogarty International Center
NCCAM	National Center for Complementary and Alternative Medicine
NCI	National Cancer Institute
NCMHD	National Center on Minority Health and Health Disparities
NCRR	National Center for Research Resources
NEI	National Eye Institute
NHGRI	National Human Genome Research Institute
NHLBI	National Heart, Lung, and Blood Institute
NIA	National Institute on Aging
NIAAA	National Institute on Alcohol Abuse and Alcoholism
NIAID	National Institute of Allergy and Infectious Diseases
NIAMS	National Institute of Arthritis and Musculoskeletal and Skin Disease
NIBIB	National Institute of Biomedical Imaging and Bioengineering
NICHHD	National Institute of Child Health and Human Development
NIDA	National Institute on Drug Abuse
NIDCD	National Institute on Deafness and Other Communication Disorders
NIDCR	National Institute of Dental and Craniofacial Research
NIDDK	National Institute of Diabetes and Digestive and Kidney Diseases
NIEHS	National Institute of Environmental Health Sciences

NIGMS	National Institute of General Medical Sciences
NIMH	National Institute of Mental Health
NINDS	National Institute of Neurological Disorders and Stroke
NINR	National Institute of Nursing Research
NLM	National Library of Medicine
OD	Office of the Director

Regulatory, Policy, Accreditation, and Oversight Offices or Organizations

AAALAC	American Association for Accreditation of Laboratory Animal Care International
AAHRPP	Association for the Accreditation of Human Research Participant Protection
AALAS	American Association for Laboratory Animal Science
ACRP	Association of Clinical Research Professionals
CAS	Cost Accounting Standards
CASB	Cost Accounting Standards Board
CBO	Congressional Budget Office
DCAA	Defense Contract Audit Agency
EHS	Environmental Health and Safety
FASB	Financial Accounting Standards Board
FDP	Federal Demonstration Project
GASB	Government Accounting Standards Board
GSA	General Services Administration
IACUC	Institutional Animal Care and Use Committee
IBC	Institutional Biosafety Committee
IRB	Institutional Review Board (*human subjects protections*)
NRA	Nuclear Regulatory Agency
OHRP	Office of Human Research Protection
OMB	Office of Management and Budget
ORI	Office of Research Integrity
OSHA	Occupational Safety and Health Administration
PHRP	Partnership for Human Research Protection

Associations, Professional Organizations, and Interest Groups

AAAS	American Association for the Advancement of Science
ALF	Animal Liberation Foundation
ARMA	Association of Research Managers and Administrators (UK) (formerly RAGnet)
ARMS	Australian Research Management Society
AUTM	Association of University Technology Managers
CASE	Council for Advancement and Support of Education
CAURA	Canadian Association of University Research Administrators
COGR	Council on Governmental Relations
EARMA	European Association of Research Managers and Administrators
ELF	Environmental Liberation Foundation
LES	Licensing Executive Society
NACUA	National Association of College and University Attorneys
NACUBO	National Association of College and University Business Offices
NAS	National Academy of Science
NASULGC	National Association of State Universities and Land Grant Colleges
NCURA	National Council of University Research Administrators
NRC	National Research Council
PETA	People for the Ethical Treatment of Animals
RAGnet	Research Administrators Group Network (now ARMA)
SARIMA	South African Research and Innovation Management Association
SRA	Society of Research Administrators International

Regulatory Documents

AGAR	Agriculture Acquisition Regulation
CFDA	Catalog of Federal Domestic Assistance
CFR	Code of Federal Regulations
DEAR	Department of Energy Acquisition Regulations
DFAR	Defense Federal Acquisition Regulations
EAR	Export Administration Requirements
EDGAR	Education Department General Administrative Regulations
FAR	Federal Acquisition Regulations
FMC	Federal Management Circular
FOIA	Freedom of Information Act
HIPAA	Health Insurance Portability and Accountability Act
ISO (9000)	International Organization for Standardization
ITAR	International Treaty for Arms Regulations
NIHGPS	National Institutes of Health Grants Policy Statement
OMB	Office of Management and Budget

Publications and Information Sources

CBD	Commerce Business Daily
CFDA	Catalog of Federal Domestic Assistance
COS	Community of Science
DIALOG	An extensive information retrieval system
FEDBIZOPPS	Federal Business Opportunities
FEDIX	Federal Information Exchange
FR	Federal Register
GPG	Grant Proposal Guide
GRC	Grant Resource Center
IRIS	Illinois Research Information System
SPIN	Sponsored Programs Information Network

Other Terms and Concepts

ACO	Administrative Contracting Officer
AREA	Academic Research Enhancement Award
BAA	Broad Agency Announcement
BAFO	Best and Final Offer (now referred to as Final Proposal Revision)
BMTA	Biological Material Transfer Agreement
BRDPI	Biomedical Research and Development Price Index
BSL	Bio-Safety Level
CDA	Confidential Disclosure Agreement

CICA	Competition in Contracting Act	**MIPR**	Military Interdepartmental Purchase Request
CO	Contracting Officer	**MOA**	Memorandum of Agreement
COA	Contracting Officer Approval	**MOU**	Memorandum of Understanding
COTR	Contracting Officer Technical Representative	**MSDS**	Material Safety Data Sheet
CPSR	Contractor Procurement/Property System Review	**MTA**	Material Transfer Agreement
		MTDC	Modified Total Direct Costs
CR	Cost Reimbursable (Contract/Grant)	**MTDC+S**	Modified Total Direct Costs + Stipend
CRADA	Cooperative Research and Development Agreement	**NDA**	Nondisclosure Agreement
CRF	Case Report Form	**NPRM**	Notice of Proposed Rulemaking
CY	Calendar Year	**OSP or SPO or RO**	Office of Sponsored Projects or Sponsored Projeccts Office or Research Office
CYTD	Calendar Year-to-Date		
DA	Department Administration	**OTA**	Other Transactional Agreement
DC	Direct Costs	**PA**	Program Announcement
DSMB	Data Safety and Monitoring Board	**PAN**	Personnel Action Notification
DUNS	Data Universal Numbering System for businesses	**PAR**	Personnel Activity Report
		PI	Principal Investigator
EA	Expanded Authorities	**PO**	Program/Project Officer
EDI	Electronic Data Interchange	**QA**	Quality Assurance
EFT	Electronic Fund Transfer	**R&D**	Research and Development
ERA	Electronic Research Administration	**RDNA**	Recombinant DNA
F&A	Facilities and Administration	**RFA**	Request for Application
FAR	Federal Acquisition Regulations	**RFP**	Request for Proposal
FASR	Financial Status Report	**RFQ**	Request for Quotation
FDP	Federal Demonstration Partnership	**SBIR**	Small Business Innovation Research Program
FP	Fixed-Price (Contract/Grant)		
FPR	Final Proposal Revision (formerly Best and Final Offer)	**SNAP**	Streamlined Noncompeting Award Process
		SOP	Standard Operating Procedures
FSR	Financial Status Report	**SPA**	Sponsored Programs Administration
FTE	Full-Time Equivalent	**STTR**	Small Business Technology Transfer Program
FY	Fiscal Year		
FYTD	Fiscal Year-to-Date	**S&W**	Salaries and Wages
GA	General Administration	**SW&EB**	Salaries, Wages, and Employee Benefits
GCP	Good Clinical Practices		
GLP	Good Laboratory Practices	**TADC**	Total Allocable Direct Costs
GMO	Grants Management Officer	**TBSR**	Total Business Systems Review
GMP	Good Manufacturing Practices	**TC**	Total Cost
GTP	Good Tissue Practices	**T&Cs**	Terms and Conditions
IDC	Indirect Costs (see F&A)	**TDC**	Total Direct Costs
IFB	Invitation For Bid	**TIA**	Technology Investment Agreement
IND	Investigational New Drug	**T&M**	Time and Materials
IPA	Intergovernmental Personnel Act	**TTO**	Technology Transfer Office
IR&D	Independent Research and Development	**UBIT**	Unrelated Business Income Tax
JIT	Just in Time	**YTD**	Year To Date

Index